KU-016-880

LEEDS BECKETT UNIVERSITY
LIBRARY
DISCARDED

Leeds Metropolitan University
17 0221698 4

Principles and Practice of

Disinfection, Preservation and Sterilization

Principles and Practice of

Disinfection, Preservation and Sterilization

EDITED BY

A.D. RUSSELL

BPharm, DSc, PhD, FRPharmS, FRCPath
Professor of Pharmaceutical Microbiology,
Cardiff University, Cardiff

W.B. HUGO

BPharm, PhD, FRPharmS
Formerly Reader in
Pharmaceutical Microbiology,
University of Nottingham

G.A.J. AYLIFFE

BSc, MD, FRCPath
Emeritus Professor of Medical Microbiology,
University of Birmingham;
Formerly Director,
Hospital Infection Research Laboratory,
City Hospital NHS Trust
Birmingham

THIRD EDITION

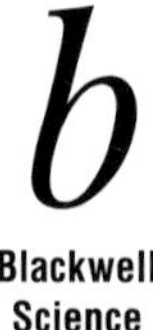

Blackwell
Science

Editorial Offices:
Osney Mead, Oxford OX2 0EL
25 John Street, London WC1N 2BL
23 Ainslie Place, Edinburgh EH3 6AJ
350 Main Street, Malden
MA 02148 5018, USA
54 University Street, Carlton
Victoria 3053, Australia
10, rue Casimir Delavigne
75006 Paris, France

Other Editorial Offices:
Blackwell Wissenschafts-Verlag GmbH
Kurfürstendamm 57
10707 Berlin, Germany

Blackwell Science KK
MG Kodenmacho Building
7-10 Kodenmacho Nihombashi
Chuo-ku, Tokyo 104, Japan

First published 1982
Second Edition 1992
Reprinted 1994 (twice)
Third Edition 1999

Set by Setrite Typesetters, Hong Kong
Printed and bound in
Great Britain at the
University Press, Cambridge

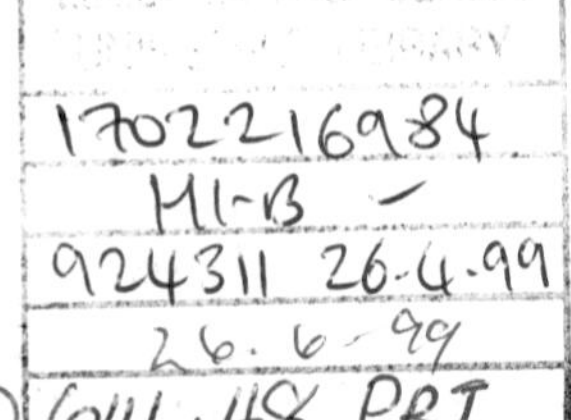

DISTRIBUTORS

Marston Book Services Ltd
PO Box 269
Abingdon, Oxon OX14 4YN
(*Orders*: Tel: 01235 465500
Fax: 01235 465555)

USA
Blackwell Science, Inc.
Commerce Place
350 Main Street
Malden, MA 02148 5018
(*Orders*: Tel: 800 759 6102
781 388 8250
Fax: 781 388 8255)

Canada
Login Brothers Book Company
324 Saulteaux Crescent
Winnipeg, Manitoba R3J 3T2
(*Orders*: Tel: 204 837-2987)

Australia
Blackwell Science Pty Ltd
54 University Street
Carlton, Victoria 3053
(*Orders*: Tel: 3 9347 0300
Fax: 3 9347 5001)

A catalogue record for this title is available from the British Library

ISBN 0-632-04194-3

Library of Congress
Cataloging-in-publication Data

Principles and practice of disinfection, preservation, and sterilization/edited by A.D. Russell, W.B. Hugo, G.A.J. Ayliffe.—
—3rd ed.
p. cm.
Includes bibliographical references and index.
ISBN 0-632-04194-3
1. Disinfection and disinfectants.
2. Antiseptics
3. Sterilization.
I. Russell, A.D. (Allan Denver)
II. Hugo, W.B. (William Barry) III. Ayliffe, G.A.J. IV. Title:
Principles and practice of disinfection, preservation, and sterilization
RA761.P84 1998
614.4'8—dc21 98-14781
CIP

For further information on Blackwell Science, visit our website: www.blackwell-science.com

Contents

List of Contributors

M.C. ALLWOOD *School of Health and Community Studies, University of Derby, Mickleover, Derby DE3 5GX*

G.A.J. AYLIFFE *Hospital Infection Research Laboratory, City Hospital NHS Trust, Dudley Road, Birmingham B18 7QH*

J.R. BABB *Hospital Infection Research Laboratory, City Hospital NHS Trust, Dudley Road, Birmingham B18 7QH*

R.M. BAIRD *Lyes House, Hummer, Trent, Sherbourne, Dorset, D19 4SH*

E.G. BEVERIDGE *School of Health Sciences, Fleming Building, University of Sunderland, Sunderland SR2 7EE*

S.F. BLOOMFIELD *Unilever Research, Port Sunlight Laboratory, Quarry Road East, Bebington, Wirral L63 3JW*

C.R. BRADLEY *Hospital Infection Research Laboratory, City Hospital NHS Trust, Dudley Road, Birmingham B18 7QH*

A.F. BRAVERY *Building Research Establishment, Garston, Watford WD2 7JR*

F.F. BUSTA *Department of Food Science and Nutrition, University of Minnesota, 1334 Eckles Avenue, St Paul, Minnesota 55108-6099, USA*

M.E. CARTER *Department of Veterinary Microbiology & Parasitology, Faculty of Veterinary Medicine, University College Dublin, Ballsbridge, Dublin 4, Ireland*

R.E. CHILD *National Museums and Galleries of Wales, Cathays Park, Cardiff CF1 3NP*

J.V. DADSWELL *Pinewoods, Soke Road, Silchester, Reading RG7 2PD*

M.J. DAY *School of Pure and Applied Biology, Cardiff University, Cardiff CF1 3XF*

S.P. DENYER *Department of Pharmacy, University of Brighton, Moulsecoomb, Brighton BN2 4GJ*

R. ELSMORE *Robert McBride Ltd, Middleton Way, Middleton, Manchester M24 4DP*

J.R. FURR *Welsh School of Pharmacy, Cardiff University, Cardiff CF1 3XF*

G.W. GOULD *17 Dove Road, Bedford MK41 7AA*

G.W. HANLON *Department of Pharmacy, University of Brighton, Moulsecoomb, Brighton BN2 4GJ*

E.A. HILDITCH *12 Manor Lane, Clanfield, Bampton, Oxon OX18 2TR*

E.C. HILL *ECHA Microbiology Ltd, Unit M210, Cardiff Workshops, Lewis Road, Cardiff CF 5EJ*

G.C. HILL *ECHA Microbiology Ltd, Unit M210, Cardiff Workshops, Lewis Road, Cardiff CF 5EJ*

N.A. HODGES *Department of Pharmacy, University of Brighton, Moulsecoomb, Brighton BN2 4GJ*

E.V. HOXEY *Medical Devices Agency, Hannibal House, Elephant and Castle, London SE1 6TQ*

W.B. HUGO *618 Wollaton Road, Nottingham NG8 2AA*

E.L. JARROLL *Department of Biology, Northeastern University, 414 Mulgar Building, Boston, MA 02115, USA*

J.B. KING *Safety Services Section, Cardiff University, Cardiff CF1 3XF*

L. LAWRENCE *Food Microbiology, Agriculture and Food Science Centre, Queen's University of Belfast, Newforge Lane, Belfast BT9 5PX*

J.-Y. MAILLARD *Welsh School of Pharmacy, Cardiff University, Cardiff CF1 3XF*

B.K. MARKEY *Department of Veterinary Microbiology & Parasitology, Faculty of Veterinary Medicine, University College Dublin, Ballsbridge, Dublin 4, Ireland*

B.J. McCARTHY *Shirley Technology Centre, BTTG, Shirley House, Wilmslow Road, Didsbury, Manchester M20 2RB*

A. MEGAN *Food Microbiology, Agriculture and Food Science Centre, Queen's University of Belfast, Newforge Lane, Belfast BT9 5PX*

S.W.B. NEWSOM *Papworth Hospital, Papworth St Agnes, Cambridge*

P.J. QUINN *Department of Veterinary Microbiology & Parasitology, Faculty of Veterinary Medicine, University College Dublin, Ballsbridge, Dublin 4, Ireland*

G. REYBROUCK *Public Health Laboratory, School of Public Health, Katholicke Universiteit Leuven, B-3000 Leuven, Belgium*

A.D. RUSSELL *Welsh School of Pharmacy, Cardiff University, Cardiff CF1 3XF*

A.S. SATTAR *Faculty of Medicine, Microbiology and Immunology, University of Ottowa, Ontario K1H 8MS, Canada*

J.N. SOFOS *Department Of Animal Sciences, Colorado State University, Fort Collins, Colorado 80523-1171, USA*

W.R. SPRINGLE *Paint Research Association, 8 Waldegrave Road, Teddington, Middlesex TW11 8LD*

S. SPRINGTHORPE *Faculty of Medicine, Microbiology and Immunology, University of Ottowa, Ontario K1H 8MS, Canada*

D.J. STICKLER *School of Pure and Applied Biology, Cardiff CF1 3XF*

D.M. TAYLOR *Neuropathenogenesis Unit, Institute for Animal Health, Ogston Building, West Mains Road, Edinburgh EH9 3JF*

N. THOMAS *Medical Devices Agency, Hannibal House, Elephant and Castle, London SE1 6TQ*

E. UNDERWOOD *Wyeth Laboratories Ltd, Huntercombe Lane South, Taplow, Maidenhead, Berks SL6 0PH*

Preface to the Third Edition

All chapters in the new edition have been updated to meet the rapidly expanding fields of antisepsis, disinfection, preservation and sterilization. The chapter on viricidal agents has been remodelled, and new chapters introduced on *Listeria* (a topic we felt was underemphasized in the previous edition), *Acanthamoeba* and contact-lens solutions, hospital wastes and laundry, reuse of disposable equipment, resistant enterococci and new emerging technologies for food preservation. The problems of biofilms have been mentioned in several chapters as the special difficulties encountered in inactivating sessile bacteria become more and more apparent.

The new edition will continue to be of value to microbiologists, physicians and pharmacists involved in all aspects of health care, as well as to all others who have an interest in the underlying mechanisms of microbial inactivation and resistance.

We thank our contributors for their sterling efforts and the publishers for their help and expertise.

A.D.R., W.B.H.
G.A.J.A.

Preface to the First Edition

Sterilization, disinfection and preservation, all designed to eliminate, prevent or frustrate the growth of microorganisms in a wide variety of products, were incepted empirically from the time of man's emergence and remain a problem today. The fact that this is so is due to the incredible ability of the first inhabitants of the biosphere to survive and adapt to almost any challenge. This ability must in turn have been laid down in their genomes during their long and successful sojourn on this planet.

It is true to say that, of these three processes, sterilization is a surer process than disinfection, which in turn is a surer process than preservation. It is in the latter field that we find the greatest interactive play between challenger and challenged. The microbial spoilage of wood, paper, textiles, paints, stonework, stored foodstuffs, to mention only a few categories at constant risk, costs the world many billions of pounds each year and if it were not for considerable success in the preservative field this figure would rapidly become astronomical. Disinfection processes do not suffer quite the same failure rate and one is left with the view that failure here is due more to uninformed use and naïve interpretation of biocidal data. Sterilization is an infinitely more secure process and, provided that the procedural protocol is followed, controlled and monitored, it remains the most successful of the three processes.

In the field of communicable bacterial diseases and some virus infections, there is no doubt that these have been considerably reduced, especially in the wealthier industrial societies, by improved hygiene, more extensive immunization and possibly by availability of antibiotics. However, hospital-acquired infection remains an important problem and is often associated with surgical operations or instrumentation of the patient. Although heat sterilization processes at high temperatures are preferred whenever possible, medical equipment is often difficult to clean adequately, and components are sometimes heat-labile. Disposable equipment is useful and is widely used if relatively cheap, but is obviously not practicable for the more expensive items. Ethylene oxide is often used in industry for sterilizing heat-labile products, but has a limited use for reprocessing medical equipment. Low-temperature steam with or without formaldehyde has been developed as a possible alternative to ethylene oxide in the hospital.

Although aseptic methods are used for surgical techniques, skin disinfection is still necessary and a wider range of non-toxic antiseptic agents suitable for application to tissues is required. Older antibacterial agents have been reintroduced, e.g. silver nitrate for burns, alcohol for hand disinfection in the general wards and less corrosive hypochlorites for disinfection of medical equipment.

Nevertheless, excessive use of disinfectants in the environment is undesirable and may change the hospital flora, selecting naturally antibiotic-resistant organisms, such as *Pseudomonas aeruginosa*, which are potentially dangerous to highly susceptible patients. Chemical disinfection of the hospital environment is therefore reduced to a minimum and is replaced where applicable by good cleaning methods or by physical methods of disinfection or sterilization.

A.D.R.
W.B.H.
G.A.J.A

PART I

Disinfection and Antisepsis

The inactivation of microorganisms by chemical agents forms the basis of antisepsis, disinfection (both described in Part I) and preservation (Part II). It is always useful to look back in time and examine the historical aspects (Chapter 1) of a topic. A large number of chemical compounds can be used for medical, industrial and other purposes (Chapter 2) and it is essential to maximize their effects by considering the factors that influence their activity (Chapter 3). Methods for evaluating their antibacterial, antifungal and antiviral activity need to be critically assessed (Chapters 4A, B and 6C).

The responses to biocides of individual groups of microorganisms are discussed for bacteria (Chapters 2, 3 and 10), fungi (Chapter 5), human (Chapter 6A) and veterinary (Chapter 6B) viruses, prions (Chapter 7) and *Acanthamoeba* and other protozoa (Chapters 8A and 8B, respectively). It is always important to evaluate the mechanisms of action of antimicrobial agents and useful information is provided in Chapters 5 (antifungal), 6D (antiviral) and 9 (antibacterial). Reasons for the reduced sensitivity to biocides of some important groups are comprehensively reviewed in Chapter 10 (A-G).

The applications of many of these principles are put into practice in Chapters 11 (good manufacturing practice), 12 and 13 (hospital disinfection and antisepsis, respectively), 14 (hospital wastes and laundry) and 15 (recreational waters and hydrotherapy pools), as well as in the preservation of many types of industrial products (Part II).

CHAPTER 1

Historical Introduction

1 Early concepts

In any account dealing with the history of microbiology, it is necessary to keep in mind the watershed between the empirical and the theoretical. This historical divide is marked by a period concerning both the discovery of bacteria and their later implication in disease, putrefaction and spoilage.

Throughout the empiric era it is quite amazing the extent to which hygienic precepts were being applied. These may be read in, for example, the literature of the Near and Middle East when written records became available and readable and no doubt these records were preceded by an oral code. An interesting example of early written codes of hygiene may be found in the Bible, especially in the Book of Leviticus, chapters 11–15. This in turn reflects the accumulating wisdom of western Asiatic medicine.

The process of flaming, used every day in bacteriological laboratories, was recorded in the Book of Numbers, where the passing of metal objects, especially cooking vessels, through fire was declared to cleanse them. Again it may be inferred that there was an awareness that something more than mechanical cleanness was required, and this represents an early empirical example of heat sterilization.

Chemical disinfection of a sort could be seen in the practice recorded at the time of Persian imperial expansion, *c.* 450 BC, of storing water in vessels of copper or silver to keep it potable. Water stored in pottery vessels soon acquired a foul odour and taste. Aristotle recommended to Alexander the Great the practice of boiling the water to be drunk by his armies.

Wine, vinegar and honey were used on dressings and as cleansing agents for wounds and it is interesting to note that diluted acetic acid has been recommended comparatively recently for the topical treatment of wounds and surgical lesions infected by *Pseudomonas aeruginosa*.

The art of mummification, which so obsessed the Egyptian civilization (although it owed its success largely to desiccation in the dry atmosphere of the country), also employed a variety of balsams which contained natural preservatives. Natron, a crude native sodium carbonate, was also used to preserve the bodies of human and animal alike.

Not only in hygiene but in the field of food preservation were practical procedures discovered. Thus tribes which had not progressed beyond the status of hunter-gatherers discovered that meat and fish could be preserved by drying, salting or mixing with natural spices. As the great civilizations of the Mediterranean and Near and Middle East receded, so arose the European high cultures and, whether through reading or independent discovery, precepts of empirical hygiene were also developed. There was, of course a continuum of contact between Europe and the Middle and Near East through the Arab and Ottoman incursions into Europe, but it is difficult to find early European writers acknowledging the heritage of these empires.

An early account of procedures to try and combat the episodic scourge of the plague may be found in the writings of the fourteenth century, where one Joseph of Burgundy recommended the burning of juniper branches in rooms where the plague sufferers had lain. Sulphur, too, was burned in the hope of removing the cause of this terrible disease.

The association of malodour with disease and the belief that matter floating in the air might be responsible for diseases, a Greek concept, led to these procedures. If success was achieved it may be due to the elimination of rats, later to be shown as the bearers of the causal organism. In Renaissance Italy at the turn of the fifteenth century a poet, philosopher and physician, Girolamo Fracastoro, who was professor of logic at the University of Padua, recognized possible causes of disease, mentioning contagion and airborne infection; he thought there must exist 'seeds of disease', as indeed there did! Robert Boyle, the sceptical chemist, writing in the mid-seventeenth century, wrote of a possible relationship between fermentation and the disease process. In this he foreshadowed the views of Louis Pasteur. There is no evidence in the literature that Pasteur even read the opinions of Robert Boyle or Fracastoro.

The next landmark in this history was the discovery by Antonie van Leeuwenhoek of small living creatures in a variety of habitats, such as tooth scrapings, pond water and vegetable infusions. His drawings, seen under his simple microscopes (×300), were published in the *Philosophical Transactions of the Royal Society* in 1677 and also in a series of letters to the Society before and after this date. Some of his illustrations are thought to represent bacteria, although the greatest magnification he is said to have achieved was 300 times. When considering Leeuwenhoek's great technical achievement in microscopy and his painstaking application of it to original investigation, it should be borne in mind that bacteria in colony form must have been seen from the beginning of human existence. A very early report of this was given by the Greek historian Siculus, who, writing of the siege of Tyre in 332 BC, states how bread, distributed to the Macedonians, had a bloody look. This was probably attributable to infestation by *Serratia marcescens*; this phenomenon must have been seen, if not recorded, from time immemorial.

Turning back to Europe, it is also possible to find other examples of workers who believed, but could not prove scientifically, that some diseases were caused by invisible living agents, *contagium animatum*. Among these workers were Kircher (1658), Lange (1659), Lancisi (1718) and Marten (1720).

By observation and intuition, therefore, we see that the practice of heat and chemical disinfection, the inhibitory effect of desiccation and the implication of invisible objects with the cause of some diseases were known or inferred from early times.

Before passing to a more rationally supported history it is necessary to report on a remarkable quantification of chemical preservation published in 1775 by Joseph Pringle. Pringle was seeking to evaluate preservation by salting and he added pieces of lean meat to glass jars containing solutions of different salts; these he incubated, and judged his end-point by the presence or absence of smell. He regarded his standard 'salt' as sea salt and expressed the results in terms of the relative efficiency as compared with sea salt; nitre, for example, had a value of 4 by this method. One hundred and fifty-three years later, Rideal and Walker were to use a similar method with phenolic disinfectants and *Salmonella typhi*; their standard was phenol.

2 Chemical disinfection

Now, newer and purer chemical disinfectants began to be used. Mercuric chloride, corrosive sublimate, found use as a wound dressing; it had been used since the Middle Ages and was introduced by Arab physicians. In 1798 bleaching powder was first made and a preparation of it was employed by Alcock in 1827 as a deodorant and disinfectant. Lefevre introduced chlorine water in 1843. In 1839 Davies had suggested iodine as a wound dressing. Semmelweis was to use chlorine water in his work on childbed fever occurring in the obstetrics division of the Vienna General Hospital. He achieved a sensational reduction in the incidence of the infection by insisting that all attending the birth washed their hands in chlorine water; later (in 1847) he substituted chlorinated lime.

Wood and coal tar were used as wound dressings in the early nineteenth century and in a letter to the *Lancet* Smith (1836–7) describes the use of creosote (Gr. *kreas* flesh, *soter* saviour) as a wound dressing. In 1850 Le Beuf, a French pharmacist, prepared an extract of coal tar by using the natural saponin of quillaia bark as a dispersing agent. Le Beuf asked a well-known surgeon, Jules Lemair, to evaluate his product. It proved to be highly efficacious. Küchenmeister was to use pure phenol in solution as a wound dressing in 1860 and Joseph Lister also used phenol in his great studies on antiseptic surgery during the 1860s. It is also of interest to record that a number of chemicals were being used as wood preservatives. Wood tar had been used in the 1700s to preserve the timbers of ships, and mercuric chloride was used for the same purpose in 1705. Copper sulphate was introduced in 1767 and zinc chloride in 1815. Many of these products are still in use today.

Turning back to evaluation, Bucholtz (1875) determined what is called today the minimum inhibitory concentration of phenol, creosote and benzoic and salicylic acids to inhibit the growth of bacteria. Robert Koch made measurements of the inhibitory power of mercuric chloride against anthrax spores but overvalued the products as he failed to neutralize the substance carried over in his tests. This was pointed out by Geppert, who, in 1889, used ammonium sulphide as a neutralizing agent for mercuric chloride and obtained much more realistic values for the antimicrobial powers of mercuric chloride.

It will be apparent that, parallel with these early studies, an important watershed already alluded to in the opening paragraphs of this brief history had been passed. That is the scientific identification of a microbial species with a specific disease. Credit for this should go to an Italian, Agostino Bassi, a lawyer from Lodi (a small town near Milan). Although not a scientist or medical man, he performed exacting scientific experiments to equate a disease of silkworms with a fungus. Bassi identified plague and cholera as being of microbial origin and also experimented with heat and chemicals as antimicrobial agents. His work anticipated the great names of Pasteur and Koch in the implication of microbes with certain diseases, but because it was published locally in Lodi and in Italian it has not found the place it deserves in many textbooks.

Two other chemical disinfectants still in use today were early introductions. Hydrogen peroxide was first examined by Traugott in 1893, and Dakin reported on chlorine-releasing compounds in 1915. Quaternary ammonium compounds were introduced by Jacobs in 1916.

In 1897, Kronig and Paul, with the acknowledged help of the Japanese physical chemist Ikeda, introduced the science of disinfection dynamics; their pioneering publication was to give rise to innumerable studies on the subject lasting through to the present day.

3 Sterilization

As has been stated above, heat sterilization has been known since early historical times as a cleansing and purifying agent. In 1832 William Henry, a Manchester physician, studied the effect of heat on contagion by placing contaminated material, i.e. clothes worn by sufferers from typhus and scarlet fever, in air heated by water sealed in a pressure vessel. He realized that he could achieve temperatures higher than 100°C by using a closed vessel fitted with a proper safety valve. He found that garments so treated could be worn with impunity by others, who did not then contract the diseases. Louis Pasteur also used a pressure vessel with safety valve for sterilization.

Sterilization by filtration has been observed from early times. Foul-tasting waters draining from ponds and percolating through soil or gravel were sometimes observed on emerging, spring-like, at a lower part of the terrain to be clear and potable (drinkable), and artificial filters of pebbles were constructed. Later, deliberately constructed tubes of unglazed porcelain or compressed kieselguhr, the so-called Chamberland or Berkefeld filters, made their appearance in 1884 and 1891, respectively.

Although it was known that sunlight helped wound healing and in checking the spread of disease, it was Downes and Blunt in 1887 who first set up experiments to study the effect of light on bacteria and other organisms. Using *Bacillus subtilis* as test organism, Ward in 1892 attempted to investigate the connection between the wavelength of light and its toxicity; he found that blue light was more toxic than red.

In 1903, using a continuous arc current, Barnard and Morgan demonstrated that the maximum bactericidal effect resided in the range 226–328 nm, i.e. in the ultraviolet–light is now a well-established agent for water and air sterilization (see Chapter 20B).

At the end of the nineteenth century, a wealth of pioneering work was being carried out in subatomic physics. In 1895, the German physicist, Rontgen, discovered X-rays, and 3 years later Rieder found these rays to be toxic to common pathogens. X-rays of a wavelength between 10^{-10} and 10^{-11} are one of the radiations emitted by ^{60}Co, now used extensively in sterilization processes (Chapter 20A).

Another major field of research in the concluding years of the nineteenth century was that of natural radioactivity. In 1879, Becquerel found that, if left near a photographic plate, uranium compounds would cause it to fog. He suggested that rays, later named Becquerel rays, were being emitted. Rutherford, in 1899, showed that when the emission was exposed to a magnetic field three types of radiation (α, β and γ) were given off. The γ-rays were shown to have the same order of wavelength as X-rays. Beta rays were found to be high-speed electrons, and α-rays were helium nuclei. These emissions were demonstrated to be antimicrobial by Mink in 1896 and by Pancinotti and Porchelli two years later. High-speed electrons generated by electron accelerators are now used in sterilization processes (Chapter 20A).

Thus, within 3 years of the discovery of X-rays and natural radiation, their effect on the growth of microorganisms had been investigated and published. Both were found to be lethal. Ultraviolet light was shown in 1993 to be the lethal component of sunlight.

These and other aspects have been discussed by Hugo (1996).

After this time the science of sterilization and disinfection followed a more ordered pattern of evolution, culminating in the new technology of radiation sterilization. However, mistakes—often fatal—still occur and the discipline must at all times be accompanied by vigilance and critical monitoring and evaluation.

4 References

GENERAL REFERENCES

Brock, T.D. (ed.) (1961) *Milestones in Microbiology*. London: Prentice Hall.

Bullock, W. (1938) *The History of Bacteriology*. Oxford: Oxford University Press.

Collard, P. (1976) *The Development of Microbiology*. Cambridge: Cambridge University Press.

Hugo, W.B. (1991) A brief history of heat and chemical preservation and disinfection. *Journal of Applied Bacteriology* **71**, 9–18.

Hugo, W.B. (1996) A brief history of heat, chemical and radiation preservation and disinfection. *International Biodeterioration and Biodegradation*, **36**, 197–221.

Reid, R. (1974) *Microbes and Men*. London: British Broadcasting Corporation.

SPECIFIC REFERENCES

Crellin, J.K. (1966) The problem of heat resistance of microorganisms in the British spontaneous generation controversies of 1860–1880. *Medical History*, **10**, 50–59.

Gaughran, E.R. & Goudie, A.J. (1975). Heat sterilisation methods. *Acta Pharmaceutica Suecica*, **12** Suppl., 15–25.

Hugo, W.B. (1978) Early studies in the evaluation of disinfectants. *Journal of Antimicrobial Chemotherapy*, **4**, 489–494.

Hugo, W.B. (1978) Phenols: a review of their history and development as antimicrobial agents. *Microbios*, **23**, 83–85.

Selwyn, S. (1979) Early experimental models of disinfection and sterilization. *Journal of Antimicrobial Chemotherapy*, **5**, 229–238.

Smith, Sir F. (1836–7) External employment of creosote. *Lancet*, **ii**, 221–222.

CHAPTER 2

Types of Antimicrobial Agents

1 Introduction

Many different types of antimicrobial agents are now available and serve a variety of purposes in the medical, veterinary, dental and other fields (Russell *et al.*, 1984; Gorman & Scott, 1985; Gardner & Peel, 1986, 1991; Russell & Hugo, 1987; Russell, 1990a,b, 1991a,b; Russell & Gould, 1991a,b; Fleurette *et al.*, 1995; Marianos, 1995; Rossmore, 1995; Russell & Russell, 1995; Rutala, 1995a,b; Ascenzi, 1996a; Russell & Chopra, 1996). Subsequent chapters will discuss the factors influencing their activity and their role as disinfectants and antiseptics and as preservatives in a wide range of products or materials (Akers, 1984; Fels *et al.*, 1987; Eklund, 1989; Gould & Jones, 1989; Wilkins & Board, 1989; Russell & Gould, 1991a,b; Kabara & Eklund, 1991; Seiler & Russell, 1991). Lists of preservatives are provided by Denyer & Wallhäusser (1990) and by Hill (1995). Additional information is provided on their mechanism of action and on the ways in which microorganisms show resistance. Recent British Standards (1997a,b,c) describe tests for basic bactericidal and fungicidal activity and for hygienic handwashes.

The present chapter will concentrate on the antimicrobial properties and uses of the various types of antimicrobial agents. Cross-references to other chapters are made where appropriate. A comprehensive summary of inhibitory concentrations, toxicity and uses is provided by Wallhäusser (1984).

2 Phenols

The historical introduction (Chapter 1) and the papers by Hugo (1979, 1991) and Marouchoc (1979) showed that phenol and natural-product distillates containing phenols shared, with chlorine and iodine, an early place in the armoury of antiseptics. Today they enjoy a wide use as general disinfectants and as preservatives for a variety of manufactured products (Freney, 1995). The main general restriction is that they should not be used where they can contaminate foods.

As a result of their long history, a vast literature has accumulated dealing with phenol and its analogues, with bactericidal and bacteriostatic indices and phenol coefficient values measured against a large array of microorganisms. Unfortunately, many different parameters have been used to express their biocidal and biostatic power but the phenol coefficient (Chapter 4A) has probably been the most widely employed and serves as a reasonable cross-referencing cipher for the many hundreds of papers and reports written.

A feature of the work in the 1930s is the frequent exclusion of *Pseudomonas* species from the list of test organisms. At that time the pseudomonads were not regarded with the same degree of apprehension as they are today. The purpose of this section is not to repeat the mass of data but to take advantage of the passage of time and the present position to consider those phenolic derivatives which are likely to be found in common usage. The same accumulation of biological data has, however, enabled a reasonable assessment of the relationship between structure and activity in the phenol series to be compiled (Suter, 1941). The main conclusions from this survey were:

1 *para*-Substitutions of an alkyl chain up to six carbon atoms in length increases the antibacterial action of phenols, presumably by increasing the surface activity and ability to orientate at an interface. Activity falls off after this due to decreased water-solubility. Again, due to the conferment of polar properties, straight chain *para*-substituents confer greater activity than branched-chain substituents containing the same number of carbon atoms.

2 Halogenation increases the antibacterial activity of phenol. The combination of alkyl and halogen substitution which confers the greatest antibacterial activity is that where the alkyl group is *ortho* to the phenolic group and the halogen *para* to the phenolic group. Russell *et al.* (1987) compared the activity of phenol, cresol and chlorocresol on wild-type and envelope mutant strains of *Escherichia coli* and found that chlorocresol was the most active against all strains and especially against deep rough mutants.

3 Nitration, while increasing the toxicity of phenol towards bacteria, also increases the systemic toxicity and confers specific biological properties on the molecule, enabling it to interfere with oxidative phosphorylation. This has now been shown to be due to the ability of nitrophenols to act as uncoupling agents. Studies (Hugo & Bowen, 1973) have shown that the nitro group is not a prerequisite for uncoupling, as ethylphenol is an uncoupler. Nitrophenols have now been largely superseded as plant protection chemicals, where at one time they enjoyed a large vogue, although 4-nitrophenol is still used as a preservative in the leather industry.

4 In the bis-phenol series, activity is found with a direct bond between the two C_6H_5–groups or if they are separated by $-CH_2-$, –S– or –O–. If a –CO–, –SO– or –CH(OH)– group separates the phenyl groups, activity is low. In addition, maximum activity is found with the hydroxyl group at the 2,2′- position of the bis-phenol. Halogenation of the bis-phenols confers additional biocidal activity.

2.1 Sources of phenols—the coal-tar industry

Most of the phenols that are used to manufacture disinfectants are obtained from the tar obtained as a by-product in the destructive distillation of coal. This process was carried out primarily, until the advent of North Sea gas, to produce coal gas, and is still used to produce coke and other smokeless fuels. Coal is heated in the absence of air and the volatile products, one of which is tar, condensed. The tar is fractionated to yield a group of products, which include phenols (called tar acids), organic bases and neutral products, such as alkyl naphthalenes, which are known in the industry as neutral oils. Phenols may be separated by extraction with alkali, from which they are regenerated by reaction with acid, e.g. carbon dioxide (CO_2) from flue gas.

The yield of tar acids from tar depends on the type of oven or retort used, the type of coal and the temperature of carbonization. Coal heated in a coke oven yields a tar with about 2% tar acid content; in the low-temperature process used to produce smokeless fuels, some 25% of the weight of tar consists of tar acids.

A typical but abridged analysis of the 50 or more phenolic substances produced is shown in Table 2.1. These figures are based on a low-temperature carbonization process.

The cresols consist of a mixture of 2-, 3- and 4-cresol. The 'xylenols' consist of the six isomeric dimethylphenols plus ethylphenols. The combined fraction, cresols and xylenols, is also available as a commercial product, which is known as cresylic acid. High-boiling tar acids consist of higher alkyl homologues of phenol, e.g. the diethylphenols, tetramethylphenols, methylethylphenols, together with methylindanols, naphthols and methylresorcinols, the latter being known as dihydrics. There may be traces of 2-phenylphenol. The chemical constituents of some of the phenolic components are shown in Fig. 2.1. Extended information on coal tars and their constituents is given in the *Coal Tar Data Book* (1965).

As tar distillation is a commercial process, it should be realized that there will be some overlap between fractions. Phenol is obtained at 99% purity. Cresol of the *British Pharmacopoeia* (1998) (2-, 3- and 4-cresols) must contain less than 2% of

Table 2.1 Typical analysis of a coal tar produced by the low-temperature carbonization process.

Phenol	Boiling range (°C)	Percentage
Phenol	182	7
Cresols	189–205	15
Xylenols	210–230	22
High-boiling tar acids	230–310	16

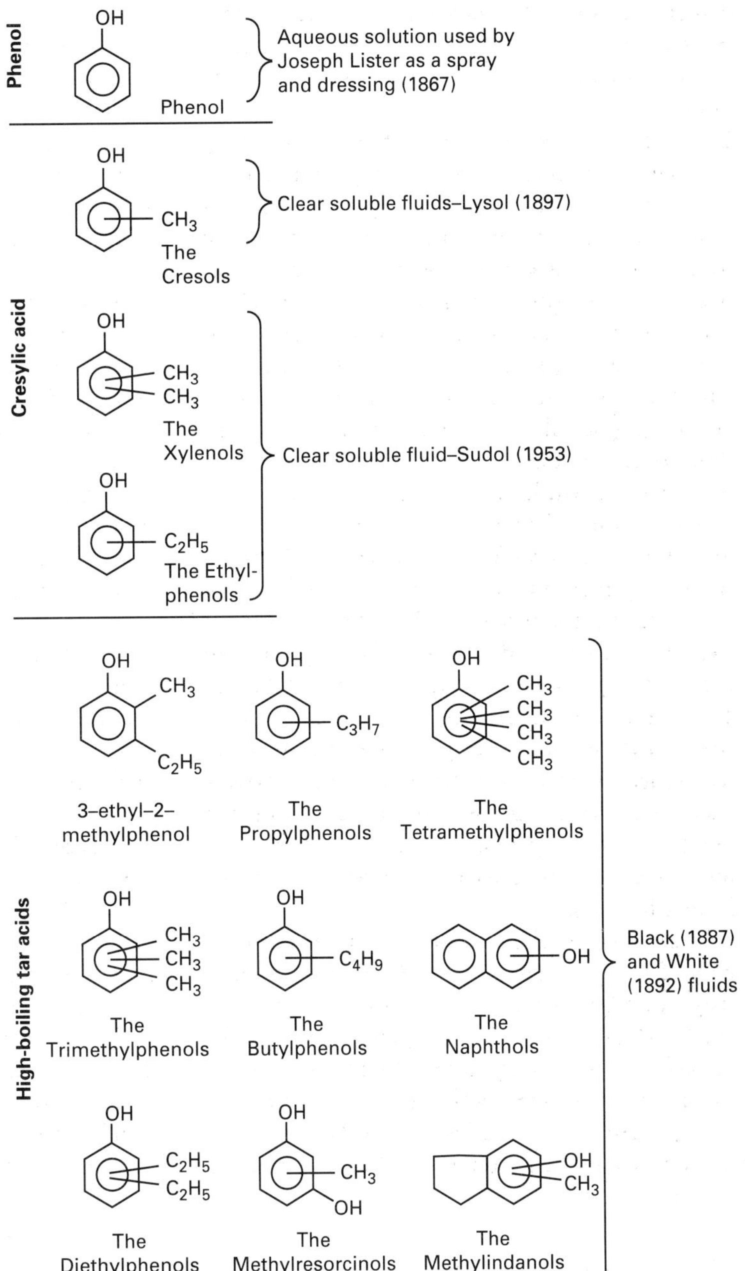

Fig. 2.1 Phenol, cresols, xylenols, ethylphenols and high-boiling tar acids.

phenol . A commercially mixed xylenol fraction contains no phenols or cresols but may contain 22 of the higher-boiling phenols. High-boiling tar acids may contain some of the higher-boiling xylenols, e.g. 3,4-xylenol (boiling-point (b.p.) 227°C).

Mention must be made of the neutral oil fraction, which has an adjuvant action in some of the formulated disinfectants to be considered below. It is devoid of biocidal activity and consists mainly of hydrocarbons, such as methyl- and dimethylnaphthalenes, *n*-dodecane, naphthalene, tetramethylbenzene, dimethylindenes and tetrahydronaphthalene. Some tar distillers offer a neutral oil, boiling range 205–296°C, for blending with phenolics destined for disinfectant manufacture (see also Section 2.4.3).

2.2 Properties of phenolic fractions

The passage from phenol (b.p. 182°C) to the higher-boiling phenols (b.p. up to 310°C) is accompanied by a well-defined gradation in properties, as follows: water-solubility decreases, tissue trauma decreases, bactericidal activity increases, inactivation by organic matter increases. The ratio of activity against Gram-negative to activity against Gram-positive organisms, however, remains fairly constant, although in the case of pseudomonads, activity tends to decrease with decreasing water-solubility; see also Table 2.2.

2.3 Formulation of coal-tar disinfectants

It will be seen from the above data that the progressive increase in desirable biological properties of the coal-tar phenols with increasing boiling-point is accompanied by a decrease in water solubility. This presents formulation problems and part of the story of the evolution of the present-day products is found in the evolution of formulation devices.

The antiseptic and disinfectant properties of coal tar had been noted as early as 1815, and in 1844 a Frenchman called Bayard made an antiseptic powder of coal tar, plaster, ferrous sulphate and clay, an early carbolic powder. Other variations on this theme appeared during the first half of the nineteenth century.

In 1850, a French pharmacist, Ferdinand Le Beuf, living in Bayonne, prepared an emulsion of coal tar using the bark of a South American tree, the quillaia. This bark contained a triterpenoid glycoside with soap-like properties belonging to the class of natural products called saponins. By emulsifying coal tar, Le Beuf made a usable liquid disinfectant, which in the hands of the French surgeon, Lemaire, proved a very valuable aid to surgery. A 'solution' of coal tar prepared with quillaia bar was described in the *Pharmaceutical Codex* (1979); it would be interesting to know how many people attribute this formula to Le Beuf, who developed it 130 years ago. Quillaia is replaced by polysorbate 80 in formulae for coal-tar 'solutions' in the *British Pharmacopoeia* (1998).

In 1887 the use of soap and coal tar was first promulgated, and in 1889 a German experimenter, T. Damman, patented a product which was prepared from coal tar, creosote and soap and which involved the principle of solubilization. Thus, between 1850 and 1887, the basis for the formulation of coal-tar disinfectants had been laid and

Table 2.2 Phenol coefficients of coal-tar products against *Salmonella typhi* and *Staphylococcus aureus*.

Product and m.p., m. range (°C)	Phenol coefficient		Water-solubility (g/100 ml)
	S. typhi	*S. aureus*	
Phenol 182	1	1	6.6
Cresols 190–203	2.5	2.0	2.0
4-Ethylphenol 195	6	6	Slightly
Xylenols 210–230	5	4.5	Slightly
High-boiling tar acids 230–270	40	25	Insoluble
High-boiling tar acids 250–275	60	40	Insoluble

subsequent discoveries were either rediscoveries or modifications of these two basic themes of emulsification and solubilization. Better-quality tar acid fractions and products with clearer-cut properties aided the production of improved products.

In 1887 John Jeyes of Northampton patented a coal-tar product, the well-known Jeyes fluid, by solubilizing coal-tar acids with a soap made from the resin of pine trees and alkali. It is difficult, from the written history of the Jeyes Company (Palfreyman, 1977), to learn how John acquired the background knowledge for his product, but his brother, Philadelphus, was apprenticed to a pharmacist and might have supplied information on formulation.

In 1897, Engler and Pieckhoff in Germany prepared the first Lysol by solubilizing cresol with soap.

2.4 The modern range of solubilized and emulsified phenolic disinfectants

Black fluids are essential coal-tar fractions solubilized with soaps; white fluids are prepared by emulsifying tar fractions. Their composition as regards phenol content is shown in Fig. 2.1. The term 'clear soluble fluid' is also used to describe the solubilized products Lysol and Sudol.

2.4.1 *Cresol and soap solution British Pharmacopoeia (BP) 1963 (Lysol)*

This consists of cresol (a mixture of 2-, 3- and 4-cresols) solubilized with a soap prepared from linseed oil and potassium hydroxide; it forms a clear solution on dilution. Most vegetative pathogens, including mycobacteria, are killed in 15min by dilutions of Lysol ranging from 0.3 to 0.6%. Bacterial spores are much more resistant, and there are reports of the spores of *Bacillus subtilis* surviving in 2% Lysol for nearly 3 days. Even greater resistance has been encountered among clostridial spores. Lysol still retains the corrosive nature associated with the phenols and should be used with care. Both the method of manufacture and the nature of the soap used have been found to affect the biocidal properties of the product (Tilley & Schaffer, 1925; Berry & Stenlake, 1942). Rideal–Walker (RW) coefficients (British Standard (BS) 541: 1985; see Chapter 4A) are of the order of 2.

2.4.2 *Xylenol-rich cresylic acid and soap solution (Sudol: Tenneco Organics Ltd, Avonmouth, Bristol)*

By using a coal-tar fraction devoid of cresols but rich in xylenols and ethylphenols, a much more active but less corrosive product (Sudol) is obtained. Rideal–Walker coefficients as high as 7 gave been reported for this product. Sudol has a Chick–Martin coefficient (BS 808: 1986; see Chapter 4A) of 3.9 and is thus seen to be quite potent in the presence of organic matter; in fact, this phenol fraction seems to be the best of those normally used for disinfectant manufacture in retaining activity in the presence of organic debris. Other solubilized phenolic products in this category include Printol and Clearsol (also produced by Tenneco).

Sudol is active against *Mycobacterium tuberculosis* (phenol coefficient 6.3) and *Staphylococcus aureus* (phenol coefficient 6). The phenol coefficient against *Pseudomonas aeruginosa* is 4. It also possesses sporicidal activity: a 2% solution killed a suspension of *Clostridum perfringens* spores in 4 h; however, a suspension of *B. subtilis* spores needed 6 h in a 66% solution for inactivation. A full bacteriological protocol of activity against non-sporing organisms is given by Finch (1953).

Printol and Clearsol are similar to Sudol in general properties (all from Tenneco Organics, Avonmouth, BS11 0YT, UK). Another is Stericol (Sterling Health, Sheffield, S30 4YP, UK).

2.4.3 *Black fluids*

These are defined in a British Standard (BS 2462: 1986). They consist of a solubilized crude phenol fraction prepared from tar acids, of the boiling range 250–310°C (Fig. 2.1, Table 2.1).

The solubilizing agents used to prepare the black fluids of commerce include soaps prepared from the interaction of sodium hydroxide with resins (which contain resin acids) and with the sulphate and sulphonate mixture prepared by heating castor oil with sulphuric acid (called sulphonated castor oil or Turkey red oil).

Additional stability is conferred by the presence of coal-tar hydrocarbon neutral oils. These have already been referred to in Section 2.1 and comprise such products as the methylnaphthalenes, indenes and naphthalenes. The actual mechanism whereby they stabilize the black fluids has not been adequately explained; however, they do prevent crystallization of naphthalene present in the tar acid fraction. Klarmann & Shternov (1936) made a systematic study of the effect of the neutral oil fraction and also purified methyl- and dimethylnaphthalenes on the bactericidal efficiency of a coal-tar disinfectant. They prepared mixtures of cresol and soap solution (Lysol type) of the *United States Pharmacopoeia* with varying concentrations of neutral oil. They found, using a phenol coefficient-type test and *Salmonella typhi* as test organism, that a product containing 30% cresols and 20% neutral oil was twice as active as a similar product containing 50% cresols alone. However, the replacement of cresol by neutral oil caused a progressive decrease in phenol coefficient when a haemolytic streptococcus and *M. tuberculosis* were used as test organisms. The results were further checked using a pure 2-methylnaphthalene in place of neutral oil and similar findings were obtained. It is worth noting in parenthesis that, because of these divergent organism-dependent results, the authors argued against the use of *S. typhi* as the sole test organism in disinfectant testing.

Depending on the phenol fraction used and its proportion of cresylic acids to high-boiling tar acid, black fluids of varying RW coefficients reaching as high as 30 can be produced; however, as shown in Section 2.2, increasing biocidal activity is accompanied by an increasing sensitivity to inactivation by organic debris.

To obtain satisfactory products, the method of manufacture is critical and a considerable expertise is required to produce active and reproducible batches.

Black fluids give either clear solutions or emulsions on dilution with water, those containing greater proportions of higher phenol homologues giving emulsions. They are partially inactivated by the presence of electrolytes.

2.4.4 *White fluids*

These are also defined in BS 2462: 1986. They differ from the foregoing formulations in being emulsified, as distinct from solubilized, phenolic compounds. The emulsifying agents used include animal glue, casein and the carbohydrate extractable from the seaweed called Irish moss. Products with a range of RW coefficients may be manufactured by the use of varying tar-acid constituents.

As they are already in the form of an oil-in-water emulsion, they are less liable to have their activity reduced on further dilution, as might happen with black fluids if dilution is carried out carelessly. They are much more stable in the presence of electrolytes. As might be expected from a metastable system — the emulsion — they are less stable on storage than the black fluids, which are solubilized systems. As with the black fluids, products of varying RW coefficients may be obtained by varying the composition of the phenol. Neutral oils from coal tar may be included in the formulation.

An interesting account of the methods and pitfalls of manufacture of black and white fluids is given by Finch (1958).

2.5 Non-coal-tar phenols

As has been seen, the coal-tar (and to a lesser extent the petrochemical) industry yields a large array of phenolic products; phenol itself, however, is now made in large quantities by a synthetic process, as are some of its derivatives. Three such phenols, which are used in a variety of roles, are 4-tertiary octylphenol, 2-phenylphenol and 4-hexylresorcinol (Fig. 2.2).

2.5.1 *4-Tertiary octylphenol*

This phenol (often referred to as octylphenol) is a white crystalline substance, melting-point (m.p.) 83°C. The cardinal property in considering its application as a preservative is its insolubility in water, 1 in 60 000 (1.6×10^{-3}%). The sodium and potassium derivatives are more soluble. It is soluble in 1 in 1 of 95% ethanol and proportionally less soluble in ethanol containing varying proportions of water. It has been shown by animal-

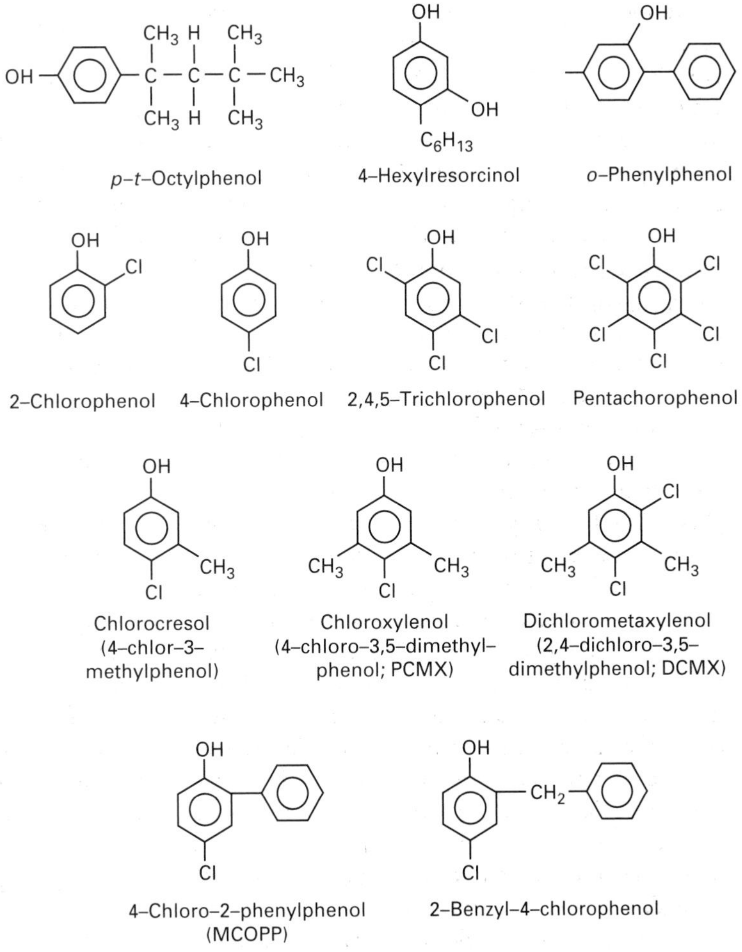

p-t-Octylphenol 4-Hexylresorcinol *o*-Phenylphenol

2-Chlorophenol 4-Chlorophenol 2,4,5-Trichlorophenol Pentachorophenol

Chlorocresol (4-chlor-3-methylphenol) Chloroxylenol (4-chloro-3,5-dimethyl-phenol; PCMX) Dichlorometaxylenol (2,4-dichloro-3,5-dimethylphenol; DCMX)

4-Chloro-2-phenylphenol (MCOPP) 2-Benzyl-4-chlorophenol

Fig. 2.2 Examples of phenolic compounds.

feeding experiments to be less toxic than phenol or cresol.

Alcoholic solutions of the phenol are 400–500 times as effective as phenol against Gram-positive organisms but against Gram-negative bacteria the factor is only one-fiftieth. Octylphenol is also fungistatic, and has been used as a preservative for proteinaceous products, such as glues and non-food gelatins. Its activity is reduced in the presence of some emulgents, a property that might render it unsuitable for the preservation of soaps and cutting oils.

2.5.2 2-Phenylphenol (2-phenylphenoxide)

This occurs as a white crystalline powder, melting at 57°C. It is much more soluble than octylphenol, 1 part dissolving in 1000 parts of water, while the sodium salt is readily soluble in water. It is both antibacterial and antifungal and is used as a preservative, especially against fungi, in a wide variety of applications. Typical minimal inhibitory concentrations (MICs, μg/ml) for the sodium salt are *E. coli*, 32; *S. aureus*, 32; *B. subtilis*, 16; *Pseudomonas fluorescens*, 16; *Aspergillus niger*, 4; *Epidermophyton* spp., 4; *Myrothecium verrucaria*, 2; *Trichophyton interdigitale*, 8. Many strains of *P. aeruginosa* are more resistant, requiring higher concentrations than those listed above for their inhibition.

Its main applications have been as ingredients in disinfectants of the pine type, as preservatives for cutting oils and as a general agricultural disinfectant. It has been particularly useful as a slimicide and fungicide in the paper and cardboard industry, and as an addition to paraffin wax in the preparation of waxed paper and liners for bottle and jar caps.

2.5.3 *4-Hexylresorcinol*

This occurs as white crystalline needles (m.p. 67°C). It is soluble 0.5% in water but freely soluble in organic solvents, glycerol and glycerides (fixed oils). It is of low oral toxicity, having been used for the treatment of round- and whipworm infections in humans. It is used as a 0.1% solution in 30% glycerol as a skin disinfectant and in lozenges and medicated sweets for the treatment of throat infections.

2.6 Halo and nitrophenols

The general effect of halogenation (Fig. 2.2) upon the antimicrobial activity of phenols is to increase their activity but reduce their water solubility (Section 2.1). There is also a tendency for them to be inactivated by organic matter. The work on substituted phenols dates from the early twentieth century and was pioneered by Ehrlich and studied extensively by Klarmann *et al.* (1929, 1932, 1933).

To illustrate the effect of chlorination on the biocidal activity of phenols, RW coefficients are as follows: 2-chlorophenol, 3.6; 4-chlorophenol, 4; 3-chlorophenol, 7.4; 2,4-dichlorophenol, 13; 2,4,6-trichlorophenol, 22; 4-chloro-3-methylphenol, 13; 4-chloro-3,5-dimethylphenol, 30.

Chlorophenols are made by the direct chlorination of the corresponding phenol or phenol mixture, using either chlorine or sulphuryl chloride.

2.6.1 *2,4,6-Trichlorophenol*

This is a white or off-white powder, which melts at 69.5°C and boils at 246°C. It is a stronger acid than phenol with a pK_a (negative logarithm of acidic ionization constant; see Section 3.2) of 8.5 at 25°C. It is almost insoluble in water but soluble in alkali and organic solvents. This phenol has been used as a bactericidal, fungicidal and insecticidal agent. It has found application in textile and wood preservation, as a preservative for cutting oils and as an ingredient in some antiseptic formulations. Its phenol coefficient against *S. typhi* is 22 and against *S. aureus* 25.

2.6.2 *Pentachlorophenol (2-phenylphenoxide)*

A white to cream-coloured powder, m.p. 174°C, it can crystallize with a proportion of water, and is almost insoluble in water but soluble in organic solvents. Pentachlorophenol or its sodium derivative is used as a preservative for adhesives, textiles, wood, leather, paper and cardboard. It has been used for the in-can preservation of paints but it tends to discolour in sunlight. As with other phenols, the presence of iron in the products which it is meant to preserve can also cause discoloration.

2.6.3 *4-Chloro-3-methylphenol (chlorocresol)*

Chlorocresol is a colourless crystalline compound, which melts at 65°C and is volatile in steam. It is soluble 0.38% in water and readily soluble in ethanol, ether and terpenes. It is also soluble in alkaline solutions. Its pK_a at 25°C is 9.5. Chlorocresol is used as a preservative in pharmaceutical products and an adjunct in a former UK pharmacopoeial sterilization process called 'heating with a bactericide', in which a combination of heat (98–100°C) and a chemical biocide enabled a sterilization process to be conducted at a lower temperature than the more usual 121°C (see Chapter 3). Its RW coefficient in aqueous solution is 13 and nearly double this value when solubilized with castor oil soap. It has been used as a preservative for industrial products, such as glues, paints, sizes, cutting oils and drilling muds.

2.6.4 *4-Chloro-3,5-dimethylphenol (chloroxylenol; PCMX)*

Chloroxylenol is a white crystalline substance, melting at 155°C. It is soluble in water at 0.03% and readily soluble in ethanol, ether, terpenes and alkaline solutions. Its pK_a at 25°C is 9.7. It is used chiefly as a topical antiseptic, solubilized in a suitable soap solution and often in conjunction with terpineol or pine oil. Phenol coefficients for the pure compound were: *S. typhi*, 30; *S. aureus*, 26; *Streptococcus pyogenes*, 28; *Trichophyton rosaceum*, 25; *P. aeruginosa*, 11. It is not sporicidal and has little activity against the tubercle bacillus (in other words, it is a narrow-spectrum bactericide). It is also inactivated in the presence of organic matter. Its formulation into a solubilized, clear, liquid disinfectant will be considered below (Section 2.8). Its properties have been re-evaluated (Bruch, 1996).

2.6.5 *2,4-Dichloro-3,5-dimethylphenol (dichloroxylenol; DCMX)*

This is a white powder, melting at 94°C. It is volatile in steam and soluble in water at 0.02%. Although it is slightly less soluble than PCMX, it has similar properties and antimicrobial spectrum. It is used as an ingredient in pine-type disinfectants and in medicated soaps and hand scrubs.

2.6.6 *Monochloro-2-phenylphenol*

This is obtained by the chlorination of 2-phenylphenol and the commercial product contains 80% of 4-chloro-2-phenylphenol and 20% of 6-chloro-2-phenylphenol. The mixture is a pale straw-coloured liquid, which boils over the range 250–300°C. It is almost insoluble in water but may be used in the formulation of pine disinfectants, where solubilization is effected by means of a suitable soap.

2.6.7 *2-Benzyl-4-chlorophenol*

This occurs as a white to pink powder, which melts at 49°C. It has a slight phenolic odour and is almost insoluble in water. Suitably formulated by solubilization with vegetable-oil soaps, it has a wide biocidal spectrum, being active against Gram-positive and Gram-negative bacteria, viruses, protozoa and fungi.

2.6.8 *Mixed chlorinated xylenols*

A mixed chlorinated xylenol preparation can be obtained for the manufacture of household disinfectants by chlorinating a mixed xylenol fraction from coal tar.

2.6.9 *Other halophenols*

Brominated and fluorinated monophenols have been made and tested but they have not found extensive application.

2.6.10 *Nitrophenols*

Nitrophenols in general are more toxic than the halophenols. 3,5-Dinitro-*o*-cresol was used as an ovicide in horticulture, but the nitrophenol most widely used today is 4-nitrophenol, which is amongst a group of preservatives used in the leather manufacturing industry at concentrations of 0.1–0.5%. For a general review on the use and mode of action of the nitrophenols, see Simon (1953).

2.6.11 *Formulated disinfectants containing chlorophenols*

It will be seen from the solubility data recounted above that some formulation device, such as solubilization, already applied successfully to the more insoluble phenols, might be used to prepare liquid antiseptics and disinfectants based on the good activity and the low level of systemic toxicity and of the likelihood of tissue damage shown by chlorinated cresols and xylenols. Indeed, such a formula was patented in Germany in 1927, although the use of chlorinated phenols as adjuncts to the already existent coal-tar products had been mooted in England in the early 1920s.

In 1933, Rapps compared the RW coefficients of an aqueous solution and a castor-oil soap-solubilized system of chlorocresol and chloroxylenol and found the solubilized system to be superior by a factor of almost two. This particular disinfectant recipe received a major advance (also in 1933) when two gynaecologists, seeking a safe and effective product for midwifery and having felt that Lysol, one of the few disinfectants available to medicine at the time, was too caustic, made an extensive evaluation of the chloroxylenol–castor-oil product; their recipe also contained terpineol (Colebrook & Maxted, 1933). It was fortunate that this preparation was active against β-haemolytic streptococci, which are a hazard in childbirth, giving rise to puerperal fever. A chloroxylenol–terpineol–soap preparation is the subject of a monograph in the *British Pharmacopoeia (1998)*.

The bacteriology of this formulation has turned out to be controversial; the original appraisal indicated good activity against β-haemolytic streptococci and *E. coli*, with retained activity in the presence of pus, but subsequent bacteriological examinations by experienced workers gave divergent results. Thus Colebrook in 1941 cast doubt upon the ability of solubilized chloroxylenol–terpineol to destroy staphylococci on the skin, a finding which was refuted by Beath (1943). Ayliffe *et al.* (1966) indicated that the product was more active against *P. aeruginosa* than *S. aureus*. As so often happens, however, *P. aeruginosa* was subsequently shown to be resistant and Lowbury (1951) found that this organism would actually multiply in dilutions of chloroxylenol–soap.

Although still an opportunistic organism, *P. aeruginosa* was becoming a dangerous pathogen, especially as more and more patients received radiotherapy or radiomimetic drugs, and attempts were made to potentiate the disinfectant and to widen its spectrum so as to embrace the pseudomonads. It had been well known that ethylenediamine tetraacetic acid (EDTA) affected the permeability of pseudomonads and some enterobacteria to drugs to which they were normally resistant (Russell, 1971a; Russell & Chopra, 1996) and both Dankert & Schut (1976) and Russell & Furr (1977) were able to demonstrate that chloroxylenol solutions with EDTA were most active against pseudomonads. Hatch & Cooper (1948) had shown a similar potentiating effect with sodium hexametaphosphate. This phenomenon may be worth bearing in mind when formulating hospital disinfectants.

2.6.12 *Phenol*

The parent compound C_6H_5OH (Fig. 2.1) is a white crystalline solid, m.p. 39–40°C, which becomes pink and finally black on long standing. It is soluble in water 1:13 and is a weak acid, pK_a 10. Its biological activity resides in the undissociated molecule. Phenol is effective against both Gram-positive and Gram-negative vegetative bacteria but is only slowly effective towards bacterial spores and acid-fast bacteria.

It is the reference standard for the RW and Chick–Martin tests for disinfectant evaluation (Chapter 4A). As has been mentioned (Chapter 1), it was used by Lister and others in pioneering work on antiseptic surgery. It finds limited application in medicine today, but is used as a preservative in such products as animal glues.

Although first obtained from coal tar, it is now largely obtained by synthetic processes, which include the hydrolysis of chlorobenzene of the high-temperature interaction of benzene sulphonic acid and alkali.

2.7 Pine disinfectants

As long ago as 1876, Kingzett took out a patent in Germany for a disinfectant deodorant made from oil of turpentine and camphor and which had been allowed to undergo oxidation in the atmosphere. This was marketed under the trade name Sanitas. Later, Stevenson (1915) described a fluid made from pine oil solubilized by a soap solution. This had a pine oil content of over 60°C.

The chief constituent of turpentine is the cyclic hydrocarbon pinene (Fig. 2.3). The odour of pinene, whether in turpentine or from pine oils made by distilling wood chips or leaves (needles) from various coniferous trees, has long held an association in the public's mind with freshness, cleanliness and a safe, disinfected environment, but the terpene hydrocarbons, of which pinene is but one example, have little or no biocidal activity.

The terpene alcohol terpineol (Fig. 2.3), which may be produced synthetically from pinene or turpentine via terpin hydrate, or in 80% purity by steam-distilling pine-wood fragments, is another ingredient of pine disinfectants and has already been exploited as an ingredient of the Colebrook

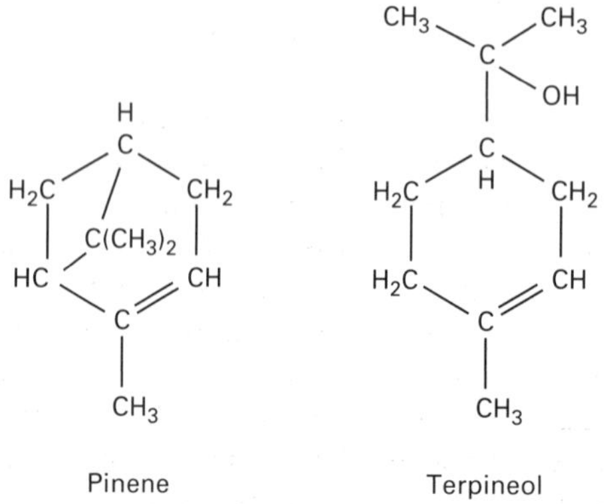

H
C
H_2C
CH_2
$C(CH_3)_2$
HC
CH
C
CH_3
Pinene

CH_3
CH_3
C
OH
C
H
H_2C
CH_2
H_2C
CH
C
CH_3
Terpineol

Fig. 2.3 Pinene and terpineol.

& Maxted (1933) chloroxylenol formulation. Unlike pinene, it possesses antimicrobial activity in its own right and it shares with pinene the property of modifying the action of phenols in solubilized disinfectant formulations, although not in the same way for all microbial species. An interesting experiment by Moore & Walker (1939) showed how the inclusion of varying amounts of pine oil in a PCMX/soap formulation modified the phenol coefficient of the preparation, depending on the test organism used.

Pine oil concentrations of from 0% to 10% caused a steady increase in the phenol coefficient from 2.0 to 3.6 when the test organism was *S. typhi*. With *S. aureus* the value was 0% pine oil, 0.6; 2.5% pine oil, 0.75; thereafter the value fell, having a value of only 0.03 with 10% oil, a pine-oil concentration which gave the maximum *S. typhi* coefficient. In this respect, pinene and terpineol may be compared with the neutral oils used in the coal-tar phenol products (Section 2.4.3), but it should be remembered that terpineol possesses intrinsic biocidal activity.

Terpineol is a colourless oil, which tends to darken on storing. It has a pleasant hyacinth odour and is used in perfumery, especially for soap products, as well as in disinfectant manufacture. A series of solubilized products has been marketed, with 'active' ingredients ranging from pine oil, pinene through terpineol to a mixture of pine oil and/or terpineol and a suitable phenol or chlorinated phenol. This gave rise to a range of products, extending from those which are really no more than deodorants to effective disinfectants.

Unfortunately there has been a tendency to ignore or be unaware of the above biocidal trends when labelling these varied products, and preparations containing a small amount of pine oil or pinene have been described as disinfectants. Attempts to remedy this situation have been made through the publication of a British Standard entitled *Aromatic Disinfectant Fluids* (BS 5197: 1976). The standard makes it clear that it specifies the requirements for a general-use disinfectant and does not imply use in hospitals or in other situations where there is a risk of infectious disease. The active ingredients, as stated in the standard, are substituted phenols together with pine oil or related terpenes and aromatic oils. A typical recipe for such a product would contain 4-chloro-3,5-xylenol, monochloro-2-phenylphenol, 2-phenylphenol, pine oil, terpineol and lime oil solubilized in water by means of potassium ricinoleate. Products with RW coefficients ranging from 3 to 10 may be produced, depending on the phenol content.

A further important requirement set out in the standard is that none of the products should be used at a use dilution more than 20 times the RW value, i.e. a product of RW 5 should never be used at dilutions greater than 1:100. Unrealistic use dilutions have contributed as much as uninformed formulation to the unreliability of some of these products.

It is very important that the labelling of this group of products should be carefully scrutinized before use and the mere possession of pine odour not used as the sole and final assessment for disinfectant potential.

2.8 Theory of solubilized systems

It will be apparent from the foregoing account that the art of obtaining aqueous solutions of relatively water-insoluble substances with the aid of soaps has been known since the late nineteenth century, when this technique was certainly applied to antiseptic systems.

Solubilization is achieved when anionic or cationic soaps aggregate in solution to form multiple particles of micelles, which may contain up to 300 molecules of the constituent species. These micelles are so arranged in an aqueous solution that the charged group is on the outside of the particle and the rest of the molecule is within the particle. It is in this part, often a hydrocarbon chain, that the phenols are dissolved, and hence solubilized, in an aqueous milieu.

The nature and antibacterial action of solubilized systems have intrigued many workers, notably Berry and his school, and Alexander and Tomlinson. The relationship between solubilization and antimicrobial activity was explored in detail by Bean & Berry (1950, 1951, 1953), who used a system consisting of 2-benzyl-4-chlorophenol (Section 2.6.7) and potassium laurate, and of 2,4-dichloro-3,5-dimethylphenol (Section 2.6.5) and potassium laurate. The advantage to a fundamental understanding of the system is that potassium laurate can be prepared in a pure state and its physical properties have been well documented. 2-Benzyl-4-chlorophenol is almost insoluble in water and the antimicrobial activity of a solubilized system containing it will be uncomplicated by a residual water-solubility. The concepts were then extended to chlorocresol.

A plot of weight of solubilized substance per unit weight of solubilizer against the concentration of solubilizer at a given ratio of solubilized substance to solubilizer usually shows the type of curve illustrated in Fig. 2.4, curve OXYZ. Above the line OXYZ a two-phase system is found; below the curve a one-phase system consequent upon solubilization is obtained. Upon this curve has been superimposed a curve (O′ABC) which illustrates the change in bactericidal activity of such a system which is found if the solubilized substance possesses antibacterial activity. Such data give some indication of the complex properties of solubilized systems, such as Lysol and Roxenol. Bactericidal activity at O′ is no more than that of the aqueous solution of the bactericide. The increase (O′–A) is due to potentiation of the action of the bactericide by unassociated soap molecules. At A, micelle formation and solubilization begin and thereafter (A–B) activity declines because, it has been suggested, the size of the micelle increases; the amount of drug per micelle decreases, and this is accompanied by a corresponding decrease in the toxicity of the system. However, at B an increase in activity is again found, reaching a maximum at C. This has been explained by the fact that at B, although increase in micellar size no longer occurs, increase in micellar number does, hence the gradual increase in activity.

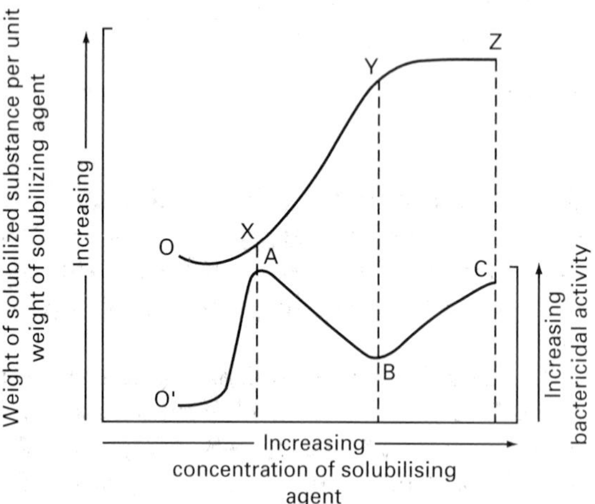

Fig. 2.4 The relationship between solubilization and antibacterial activity in a system containing a constant ratio of solubilized substance to solubilizer and where the solubilized substance possesses low water-solubility. *Curve OXYZ*, weight of solubilized substance per unit weight of solubilizing agent plotted against the concentration of solubilizing agent. *Curve O′ABC*, bactericidal activity of the system.

The lethal event at cell level has been ascribed to an adsorption of the micelles by the bacterial cell and a passage of the bactericide from the micelle on to and into the bacterial cell. In short, this theory postulates that the bactericidal activity is a function of the concentration of the drug in the micelle and not its total concentration in solution. This was held to be the case for both the highly insoluble benzylchlorophenol and the more water-soluble chlorocresol (Bean & Berry, 1951, 1953). Alexander & Tomlinson (1949), albeit working with a different system, suggest a possible alternative interpretation. They agree that the increase, culminating at A, is due to the potentiation of the action of phenol by the solubilizing agent, which because it possesses detergent properties acts by disrupting the bacterial membrane, thereby permitting more easy access of the drug into the cell. The decline (A–B), however, was thought to be due to the removal of drug from the aqueous milieu into the micelles, thereby decreasing the amount available for reacting with the cell. They reject the notion that a drug-bearing micelle is lethal and capable itself of adsorption on the cell and passing its drug load to the cell, and declare that the activity of this system is a function of the concentration of bactericide in the aqueous phase. It must also be pointed out that high concentrations of soaps may themselves be bactericidal (reviewed by Kabara, 1978) and that this property could explain the increase in activity noted between B and C.

The above is only an outline of one experimental system in a very complex family. For a very complete appraisal together with further patterns of interpretation of experimental data of the problem, the papers of Berry *et al.* (1956) and

Berry & Briggs (1956) should be consulted. Opinion, however, seems to be settling in favour of the view that activity is a function of the concentration of the bactericide in the aqueous phase. Indeed, Mitchell (1964), studying the bactericidal activity of chloroxylenol in aqueous solutions of cetomacrogol, has shown that the bactericidal activity here is related to the amount of chloroxylenol in the aqueous phase of the system. Thus a solution which contained, as a result of adding cetomacrogol, 100 times as much of the bactericide as a saturated aqueous solution was no more bactericidal than the saturated aqueous solution. Here again, this picture is complicated by the fact that non-ionic surface-active agents, of which cetomacrogol is an example, are known to inactivate phenols (Beckett & Robinson, 1958).

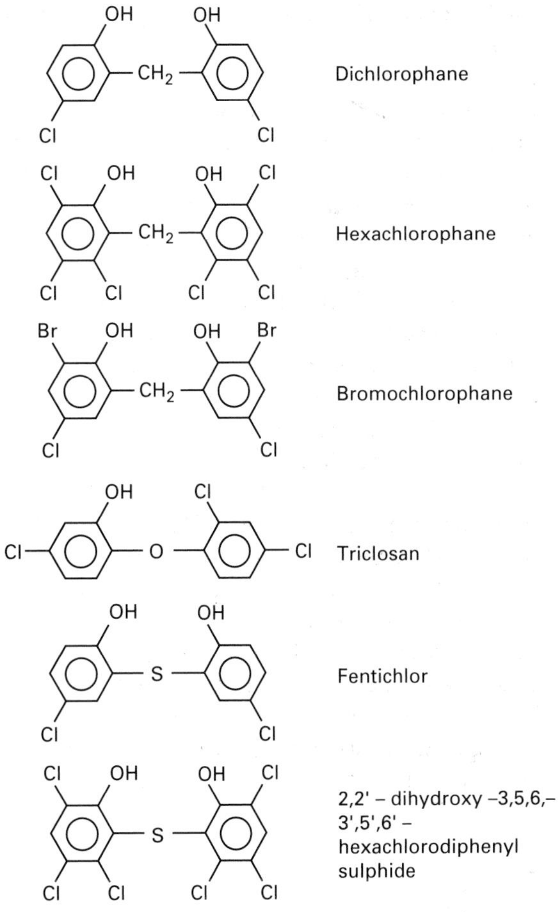

Dichlorophane

Hexachlorophane

Bromochlorophane

Triclosan

Fentichlor

2,2' – dihydroxy –3,5,6,– 3',5',6' – hexachlorodiphenyl sulphide

Fig. 2.5 Bis-phenols.

2.9 The bis-phenols

Hydroxy halogenated derivatives (Fig. 2.5) of diphenyl methane, diphenyl ether and diphenyl sulphide have provided a number of useful biocides active against bacteria, fungi and algae. They all seem to have low activity against *P. aeruginosa*, however, i.e. they show the '*Pseudomonas* gap'; they also have low water solubility and share the property of the monophenols in that they are inactivated by non-ionic surfactants.

Ehrlich and co-workers were the first to investigate the microbiological activity of the bis-phenols and published their work in 1906. Klarmann and Dunning and colleagues described the preparation and properties of a number of these compounds (Klarmann & von Wowern, 1929; Dunning *et al.*, 1931). A useful summary of this early work has been made by Suter (1941). Later, Gump & Walter (1960, 1963, 1964) and Walter & Gump (1962) made an exhaustive study of the biocidal properties of many of these compounds, especially with a view to their use in cosmetic formulations.

2.9.1 *Derivatives of dihydroxydiphenylmethane*

1 Dichlorophane, G-4,5,5′-dichloro-2,2′-dihydroxydiphenylmethane (Panacide, registered BDH, Poole, UK). This compound is active to varying degrees against bacteria, fungi and algae. It is soluble in water at 30 µg/ml but more soluble (45–80 g/100 ml) in organic solvents. The pK_a values at 25°C for the two hydroxyl groups are 7.6 and 11.6.

Typical killing concentrations in µg/ml in broth for bacteria at 25°C after 24 h incubation were: *S. aureus*, 2.5; *Streptococcus faecalis*, 7.5; *B. subtilis*, 7.5; *E. coli*, 10; *S. typhi*, 7.5; *P. aeruginosa* , 80; *Proteus mirabilis*, 50. The toxicity of the compound is low and it has been used for the treatment of tapeworm in humans and domestic animals at dose levels of 6 g on two successive days. It has also been used in the treatment of athlete's foot, indicating low skin-irritancy.

It has found application as a preservative for toiletries, textiles and cutting oils and to prevent the growth of bacteria in water-cooling systems and humidifying plants. It is used as a slimicide in paper manufacture. It may be added to papers and other packing materials to prevent microbial growth and has been used to prevent algal growth in greenhouses.

2 Hexachlorophane, 2,2′-dihydroxy-3,5,6,3′,5′,6′-hexachlorodiphenylmethane, G11. This compound is almost insoluble in water but soluble in ethanol, ether and acetone and in alkaline solutions. The pK_a values are 5.4 and 10.9. Its mode of action has been studied in detail by Gerhardt, Corner and colleagues (Corner *et al.*, 1971; Joswick *et al.*, 1971; Silvernale *et al.*, 1971; Frederick *et al.*, 1974; Lee & Corner, 1975).

It is used mainly for its antibacterial activity but it is much more active against Gram-positive than Gram-negative organisms. Typical MICs (bacteriostatic) in μg/ml are: *S. aureus*, 0.9; *B. subtilis*, 0.2; *Proteus vulgaris*, 4; *E. coli*, 28; *P. aeruginosa*, 25.

It has found chief application as an active ingredient in surgical scrubs and medicated soaps and has also been used to a limited extent as a preservative for cosmetics. Its use is limited by its insolubility in water, its somewhat narrow antibacterial spectrum and by the fact that in the UK it is restricted by a control order made in 1973. In general, this order restricted the use of this product to 0.1% in human medicines and 0.75% in animal medicines. Its toxicity has restricted its use in cosmetic products, and the maximum concentration allowed is 0.1%, with the stipulation that it is not to be used in products for children or personal hygiene products.

3 Bromochlorophane, 3,3′-dibromo-5,5′-dichlor-2,2′-dihydroxydiphenylmethane. This product is soluble in water at 100 μg/ml and is markedly more active against Gram-positive organisms than bacteria. Strains of *S. aureus* are inhibited at from 8 to 11μg/ml, whereas 100 times these concentrations are required for *E. coli* and *P. aeruginosa*. It has been used as the active ingredient in deodorant preparations and toothpastes.

2.9.2 *Derivatives of hydroxydiphenylether*

1 Triclosan, 2,4,4′-trichlor-2′-hydroxydiphenylether (Irgasan, registered Ciga-Geigy Ltd, Basle, Switzerland). This derivative is only sparingly soluble in water but soluble in solutions of dilute alkalis and organic solvents. It inhibits staphylococci at concentrations ranging from 0.1 to 0.3 μg/ml. Paradoxically, a number of *E. coli* strains are inhibited over a similar concentration range. Most strains of *P. aeruginosa* require concentrations varying from 100 to 1000 μg/ml for inhibition. It inhibits the growth of several species of mould at from 1 to 30 μg/ml. It has a similar use potential to other bis-phenols and was the most widely used phenolic preservative reported in the survey by Richardson (1981), appearing in 52 formulations. It is used in some medicated soaps and hand-cleansing gels.

2.9.3 *Derivatives of diphenylsulphide*

1 Fenticlor, 2,2′-dihydroxy-5,5′-dichlorodiphenylsulphide. This chemical is a white powder, soluble in water at 30 μg/ml, but is much more soluble in organic solvents and oils. In common with its bisphenol cogeners, it shows more activity against Gram-positive organisms and a '*Pseudomonas* gap'. Typical inhibitory concentrations (μg/ml) are *S. aureus*, 2; *E. coli*, 100; *P. aeruginosa*, 1000. Typical inhibitory concentrations (μg/ml) for some fungi are: *Candida* spp., 12; *Epidermophyton interdigitale*, 0.4; *Trichophyton granulosum*, 0.4.

Fenticlor has found chief application in the treatment of dermatophytic conditions. It can cause photosensitization and this might limit its use as a cosmetic preservative. Its low water-solubility and narrow spectrum are further disadvantages, but it has potential as a fungicide. Its mode of action was described by Hugo & Bloomfield (1971a,b,c) and Bloomfield (1974).

2 Chlorinated analogue of fenticlor, 2,2′-dihydroxy-3,4,6,3′4′,6′-hexachlorodiphenylsulphide; 2,2′-thiobis(3,4,6-trichlorophenol). This is a more highly chlorinated analogue of fenticlor. It is almost insoluble in water. In a field test, it proved to be an effective inhibitor of microbial growth in cutting-oil emulsions.

An exhaustive study of the antifungal properties of hydroxydiphenylsulphides was made by Pfleger *et al.* (1949).

3 Organic and inorganic acids: esters and salts

3.1 Introduction

A large family of organic acids (Fig. 2.6), both aromatic and aliphatic, and one or two inorganic acids have found application as preservatives, more especially in the food industry. Some, for example benzoic acid, are also used in the preservation of pharmaceutical products; others (salicylic, undecylenic and again benzoic) have been used, suitably formulated, for the topical treatment of fungal infections of the skin.

Vinegar, containing acetic acid (ethanoic acid), has been known as long as alcohol, from which it would be formed by natural oxidation, and early on it had been found to act as a preservative. It was also used as a wound dressing. This application has been revived in the use of dilute solutions of acetic acid as a wound dressing where pseudomonal infections have occurred.

Hydrochloric and sulphuric acids are two mineral acids sometimes employed in veterinary disinfection. Hydrochloric acid at high concentrations is sporicidal and has been used for disinfecting hides and skin contaminated with anthrax spores. Sulphuric acid, even at high concentrations, is not sporicidal, but in some countries it is used, usually in combination with phenol, for the decontamination of floors, feed boxes and troughs (Russell & Hugo, 1987).

Citric acid is an approved disinfectant against foot-and-mouth virus. It also appears, by virtue of its chelating properties, to increase the permeability of the outer membrane of Gram-negative bacteria (Shibasaki & Kato, 1978; Ayres *et al.*, 1993) when employed at alkaline pH. Malic acid and gluconic acid, but not tartaric acid, can also act as permeabilizers at alkaline pH (Ayres *et al.*, 1993); see also Section 14.4.

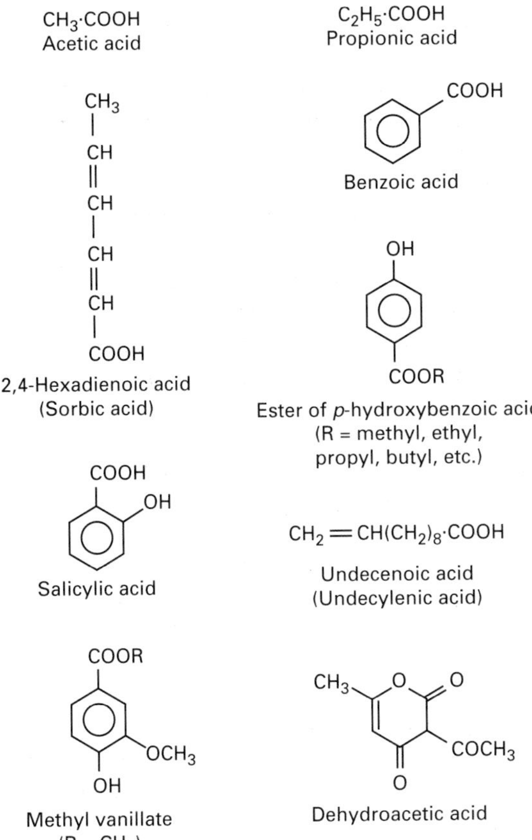

Fig. 2.6 Organic acids and esters.

3.2 Physical factors governing the antimicrobial activity of acids

At first sight, it might be thought that the special ability of acids to generate protons (hydrogen ions) when dissolved in water underlies their general toxicity; it is well known that acid conditions are inimical to the growth of many microorganisms. However, many successful antimicrobial acids are weak acids, i.e. they have dissociation constants between 10^{-3} and 10^{-5}; see below.

If an acid is represented by the symbol AH, then its ionization will be represented by A^-H^+. Complete ionization, as seen in aqueous solutions of mineral acids, such as hydrogen chloride (where AH = ClH), is not found in the weaker organic acids and their solutions will contain three components: A^-, H^+ and AH. The ratio of the concentration of these three components is called the ionization constant of that acid, K_a, and $K_a = A^- \times H^+/AH$. By analogy with the mathematical device used to define the pH scale, if the negative logarithm of K_a is taken, a number is obtained, running from about 0 to about 14, called pK_a. Some typical pK_a values are shown in Table 2.3.

An inspection of the equation defining K_a shows

Table 2.3 pK_a values of acids and esters used as antimicrobial agents.

Acid or esters	pK_a
Acetic (ethanoic) acid	4.7
Propionic (propanoic acid)	4.8
Sorbic acid (2,4-hexadienoic acid)	4.8
Lactic acid	3.8
Benzoic acid	4.2
Salicylic acid	3.0
Dehydroacetic acid	5.4
Sulphurous acid	1.8, 6.9
Methyl-*p*-hydroxybenzoic acid	8.5
Propyl-*p*-hydroxybenzoic acid	8.1

that the ratio A^-/AH must depend on the pH of the solution in which it is dissolved, and Henderson and Hasselbalch derived a relationship between this ratio and pH as follows:

$$\log \frac{A^-}{AH} = pH - pK_a$$

The application of this equation to the relative proportions of C_6H_5OOH and $C_6H_5COO^-$ in solutions of benzoic acid dissolved in buffers of varying pH is shown in Table 2.4. An inspection of the formula will also show that at the pH value equal to the pK_a value the product is 50% ionized. These data enable an evaluation of the effect of pH on the toxicity of organic acids to be made.

Typically it has been found that a marked toxic effect is seen only when the conditions of pH ensure the presence of the un-ionized molecular species AH. As the pH increases or, to put it in another way, the equilibrium $HA = HA^- + A^+$ moves to the right, the concentration of HA falls and the toxicity of the system falls; this may be indicated by a higher MIC, longer death time or higher mean single-survivor time, depending on the criterion of toxicity (i.e. antimicrobial activity) chosen.

Table 2.4 Effect of pH on ionization of benzoic acid, pK_a 4.19.

pH	Molecular form (C_6H_5COOH) (%)	Ionic form ($C_6H_5COO^-$) (%)
3.24	90	10
3.59	80	20
3.82	70	30
4.01	60	40
4.19	50	50
4.36	40	60
4.55	30	70
4.79	20	80
5.14	10	90

An inspection of Fig. 2.7 would suggest that HA is more toxic than A^-. However, an altering pH can alter the intrinsic toxicity of the environment. This is due to H^+ alone, the ionization of the cell surface, the activity of transport and metabolizing enzymes and the degree of ionization of the cell surface and hence sorption of the ionic species on the cell. Too simplistic a view, therefore, of the undoubted pH effect on the activity of weak acids must not be assumed. The ideal test organism would be one which is insensitive to changes in pH over a wide range.

Some few pages have been devoted to the above but in the authors' experience predictions for preservative ability of acids validated at one pH are rendered meaningless when such a preservative is added without further consideration to a formulation at a higher pH. The pK_a of the acid preservative should always be ascertained and any pH shift of 1.5 units or more on the alkaline side of this can be expected to cause progressive loss of activity quite sufficient to invalidate the originally determined performance. That pH modifies the antimicrobial effect of benzoic acid has been known for a long time (Cruess & Richert, 1929). For more detailed accounts of the effect of pH on the intensity of action of a large number of ionizable biocides, the papers of Simon & Blackman (1949) and Simon & Beeves (1952a,b) should be consulted.

3.3 Mode of action

The mode of action of acids used as food preservatives has been studied by Freese *et al.* (1973), Sheu *et al.* (1975), Krebs *et al.* (1983), Salmond *et al.* (1984), Eklund (1980, 1985, 1989), Sofos *et al.* (1986), Booth & Kroll (1989) Cherrington *et al.* (1990, 1991) and Russell (1992). Convincing evidence has been produced that many acid preservatives act by preventing the uptake of substrates which depend on a proton-motive force for their entry into the cell, in other words they act as uncoupling agents (Chapter 9).

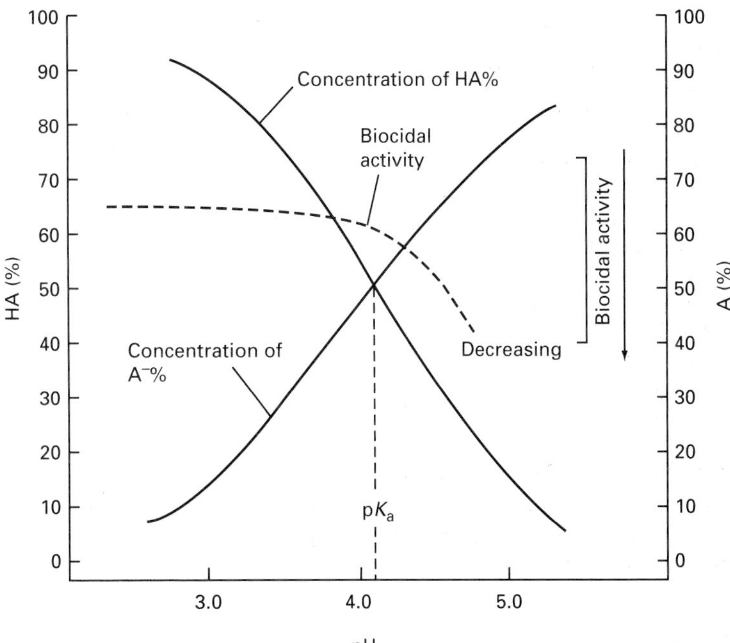

Fig. 2.7 A generalized diagram of the effect of pH on the ionization and biocidal activity of an acid (HA) of pK_a 4.1.

In addition to acids such as benzoic, acetic and propionic, the esters of *p*-hydroxybenzoic acid (the parabens) were also included in some of the above studies; they too acted as uncoupling agents but also inhibited electron transport.

Equally interesting were experiments on the pH dependence of the substrate uptake effect. The intensity of uptake inhibition by propionate, sorbate and benzoate declined between pH 5 and 7, while that induced by propyl-*p*-hydroxybenzoic acid (pK_a 8.5) remained constant over the same pH range. As has been stated, the growth-inhibitory effect of ionizable biocides shows pH dependence and this, as might be expected, is applicable to a biochemical effect upon which growth in turn depends. The total complement of compounds investigated by Freese *et al.* (1973) and Freese & Levin (1978) were acetic, benzoic, propionic, sorbic, caprylic and sulphurous acids and the methyl, propyl and heptyl esters of *p*(4)-hydroxybenzoic acid.

Organic acids, such as benzoic and sorbic, are deliberately used as preservatives. Acids such as acetic, citric and lactic are often employed as acidulants, i.e. to lower artificially the pH of foods. A low pK_a value is not the only significant feature of acidulants, however, since: (i) sorbate and acetate have similar pK_a values but the latter is a less potent preservative; (ii) organic acids used as preservatives are more potent inhibitors than other weak acids of similar pH; and (iii) weak organic acid preservatives are more effective inhibitors of pH homoeostasis than other acids of similar structure.

3.4 Individual compounds

3.4.1 Acetic acid (ethanoic acid)

This acid, as a diluted petrochemically produced compound or as the natural product vinegar, is used primarily as a preservative for vegetables, of which the onion (pickled onions) is the most familiar example. It is an ingredient of many sauces, pickles and salad cream, although the latter may need additional preservation. As it is a weak acid (pK_a 4.7), it is not likely to destroy the intracellular pectin of plant tissue, thus causing unsightly fragmentation.

Vinegars vary in strength but a wine vinegar may contain 8% of acetic acid. Vinegars made from acetic acid contain not less than 4% of acid, may be artificially coloured brown with caramel and must be clearly labelled as artificial. The toxicity of vinegars and diluted acetic acid must rely to an extent on the inhibitory activity of the molecule itself, as solutions of comparable pH made from mineral acid do not exhibit the same preservative activity. A 5% solution of acetic acid contains 4.997% CH_3COOH and 0.003% H^+. As might be expected from the pK_a value, 4.7, the activity is rapidly lost at pH values above this value. This suggests that the acetate ion is less toxic than the undissociated molecule, although, as has been said, the concomitant reduction in hydrogen ion concentration must play some part in the reduction of toxicity. As has been stated, diluted 1–5% acetic acid has been used as a wound dressing where infection with *Pseudomonas* has occurred (Phillips *et al.*, 1968).

3.4.2 *Propionic acid*

This acid is employed almost exclusively as the sodium, and to a lesser extent the calcium, salt in the baking industry, where it is used to inhibit mould and bacterial growth in breads and cakes. It is particularly useful in inhibiting the growth of the spore-forming aerobe *Bacillus macerans*, which gives rise to an infestational phenomenon called ropy bread.

Manufacturers give explicit directions as to the amount to be used in different products, but in general 0.15–0.4% is added to the flour before processing. Other products that have been successfully preserved with propionates include cheeses and malt extract. In addition to foods, wrapping materials for foods have also been protected from microbial damage with the propionates.

3.4.3 *Undecanoic acid (undecylenic acid)*

This has been used either as such or as the calcium or zinc salt in the treatment of superficial dermatophytoses. It is usually applied in ointment form at concentrations of 2–15%.

3.4.4 *2,4-Hexadienoic acid (sorbic acid)*

This unsaturated carboxylic acid, which is also available as its potassium salt, is assimilated by mammals as food. It is effective against a wide range of microorganisms (Bell *et al.*, 1959) and has been used as the acid itself, or its potassium salt, at concentrations of 0.01–0.1% to preserve bakery products, soft drinks, alcoholic beverages, cheeses, dried fruits, fish, pickles, wrapping materials and pharmaceutical products. As with all acids, there is a critical pH, in this case 6.5, above which activity begins to decline. Again it is the undissociated acid which is the active antimicrobial species (Beneke & Fabian, 1955; Gooding *et al.*, 1955). Sorbic acid was believed to act by interfering with the functioning of the citric acid cycle (York & Vaughan, 1955; Palleroni & de Prinz, 1960).

Sorbic acid is known to interfere with the uptake of amino and oxo acids in *E. coli* and *B. subtilis*; it affects the proton-motive force in *E. coli* and accelerates the movement of H^+ ions from low media pH into the cytoplasm. It probably acts overall by dissipating ΔpH across the membrane and inhibiting solute transport. The membrane potential ($\Delta\psi$) is reduced but to a much smaller extent than ΔpH (Eklund, 1989; Cherrington *et al.*, 1991; Kabara & Eklund, 1991; Russell & Chopra, 1996). A combination of sorbic acid with monolaurin has been shown to be often more active than parabens or sorbic acid alone (Kabara, 1980).

3.4.5 *Lactic acid*

Lactic acid shares with some other hydroxyacids the interesting property of being able to destroy airborne microorganisms (Lovelock *et al.*, 1944; see also Section 19). A careful study of hydroxyacids, including lactic acid, as, air disinfectant was made by Lovelock (1948). Lactic acid was found to be a cheap, efficient aerial bactericide when sprayed into the area to be sterilized. It has, however, a slight irritant action on the nasal mucosa, which tends to limit its use. It could be used in emergencies for sterilizing glove boxes or hoods if other means of sterilization are not provided (see also Section 19).

Lactic acid in liquid form is less active than several other organic acids (Eklund, 1989) but nevertheless is used as an acidulant for low-pH foods and fruit juices (Russell & Gould, 1991a,b).

3.4.6 *Benzoic acid*

This organic acid occurs naturally in many natural

balsams and gums and these were used as preservatives early in human history. Benzoic acid, first shown to be antifungal in 1875, is a white crystalline powder, which is soluble 1:350 in water. It is used as a preservative for foods and pharmaceutical products, but is rapidly inactivated at pH values above 5.0 (Eklund, 1989; Kabara & Eklund, 1991; Russell & Gould, 1991b).

As with other preservatives, its activity may also be modified by the milieu in which it acts (Anderson & Chow, 1967; Beveridge & Hope, 1967. Resistance may develop (Ingram, 1959) and the acid may be metabolized by a contaminant it is meant to inhibit (Stanier *et al.*, 1950; Hugo & Beveridge, 1964; Stanier & Orston, 1973). In addition to its use as a preservative, benzoic acid has been combined with other agents for the topical treatment of fungal infections.

Benzoic acid, like many other compounds, inhibits swarming of *Bacillus* spp. (Thampuran & Surendran, 1996). Studies with benzoic acid derivatives have demonstrated that lipophilicity and pK_a are the two most important parameters influencing activity (Ramos-Nino *et al.*, 1996). The mode of action of benzoic acid is discussed in Chapter 9.

3.4.7 *Salicylic acid*

This is often used, in combination with benzoic acid and other antifungal agents, for the topical treatment of fungal infections. Salicylic acid has keratinolytic activity and in addition affects metabolic processes. For an account of the action of benzoic and salicylic acids on the metabolism of microorganisms, see Bosund (1962) and Freese *et al.* (1973).

3.4.8 *Dehydroacetic acid (DHA)*

Wolf (1950), looking at a general relationship between the structures of organic molecules possessing antimicrobial properties, noticed activity in a group of compounds containing an α,β unsaturated ketone residue. Wolf selected for study a series of 1,2 and 1,4 pyrones (Wolf & Westveer, 1950). Of these, 3-acetyl-6-methyl-1,2-*H*-pyran-2,4(3*H*)-dione (3-acetyl-4-hydroxy-6-methyl-2-acetyl-5-hydroxy-3-oxo-4-hexanoic acid-γ-lactone) or dehydroacetic acid showed especial promise.

Dehydroacetic acid is a white or light yellow, odourless, crystalline compound, which is soluble at less than 0.1% in water; the sodium salt is soluble to the extent of 33%. Typical inhibitory concentrations (%) of the latter for selected microorganisms are: *Aerobacter aerogenes*, 0.3; *Bacillus cereus*, 0.3; *Lactobacillus plantarum*, 0.1; *S. aureus*, 0.3; *P. aeruginosa*, 0.4; *A. niger*, 0.05; *Penicillium expansum*, 0.01; *Rhizopus nigricans*, 0.05; *T. interdigitale*, 0.005; *Saccharomyces cerevisiae*, 0.1. Extensive toxicological studies have indicated that the product is acceptable as a preservative for foods, cosmetics and medicines. The pK_a value of DHA is 5.4 but an inspection of pH/activity data suggests that activity loss above the pK_a value is not as great as with other preservative acids (propionic, benzoic) and indeed, in Wolf's 1950 paper, the MIC against *S. aureus* remained at 0.3% from pH 5 to 9. Loss of activity at alkaline pH values was, however, noted by Bandelin (1950) in his detailed study of the effect of pH on the activity of antifungal compounds, as would be predicted by the pK_a value.

Little was known about its mode of action, although Seevers *et al.* (1950) produced evidence that DHA inhibited succinoxidase activity in mammalian tissue, while Wolf & Westveer (1950) showed that it did not react with microbial –SH enzymes.

Dehydroacetic acid has found application in the preservation of foods, food wrappings, pharmaceuticals and toiletries. In the survey made by Richardson (1981) of the preservatives used in 18 500 cosmetic formulae, sodium dehydroacetate was used in 73 and dehydroacetic acid in 145.

3.4.9 *Sulphur dioxide, sulphites, bisulphites*

The fumes of burning sulphur, generating sulphur dioxide, have been used by the Greeks and Egyptians as fumigants for premises and food vessels to purify and deodorize. Lime sulphur, an aqueous suspension of elementary sulphur and calcium hydroxide, was introduced as a horticultural fungicide in 1803. Later, the salts, chiefly sodium, potassium and calcium, of sulphurous acid were used in wine and food preservation.

In addition to their antimicrobial properties, members of this group also act as antioxidants helping to preserve the colour of food products, as enzyme inhibitors, as Maillard reaction inhibitors and as reducing agents (Gould & Russell, 1991).

A pH-dependent relationship exists in solution between the species SO_2, HSO_3^- and SO_3^{2-}. As the pH moves from acid to alkaline, the species predominance moves from SO_2, the toxic species, through HSO_3^- to SO_3^{2-}. Above pH 3.6, the concentration of SO_2 begins to fall, and with it the microbicidal power of the solution. It is postulated that SO_2 can penetrate cells much more readily than can the other two chemical species (Rose & Pilkington, 1989).

Yeasts and moulds can grow at low pH values, and hence the value of sulphites as inhibitors of fungal growth in acid environments, such as fruit juices. For reviews on the antimicrobial activity of sulphur dioxide, see Hammond & Carr (1976), Wedzicha (1984), Rose & Pilkington (1989) and Gould & Russell (1991).

3.4.10 Esters of p-*hydroxybenzoic acid (parabens)*

The marked pH-dependence of acids for their activity and the fact that the biocidal activity lay in the undissociated form led to the notion that esterification of an aromatic hydroxy carboxylic acid might give rise to compounds in which the phenolic group was less easily ionized.

Sabalitschka (1924) prepared a series of alkyl esters of *p*-hydroxybenzoic acid and tested their antimicrobial activity (Sabalitschka & Dietrich, 1926; Sabalitschka *et al.* 1926). This family of biocides, which may be regarded as either phenols or esters of aromatic hydroxy carboxylic acids, has stood the test of time and is today among the most widely used group of preservatives (Richardson, 1981).

As might be imagined for compounds which have been in use for over 60 years, there is an extensive literature. The esters usually used are the methyl, ethyl, propyl, butyl and benzyl compounds and are active over a wider pH range (4–8) than acid preservatives (Sokol, 1952), as has also been shown in biochemical experiments. Their pK_a values (8–8.5) compare with around 4 for preservative acids (Table 2.3). They have low water-solubility, which decreases in the order methyl–benzyl (Table 2.5). A paper which gives extensive biocidal data is that of Aalto *et al.* (1953). Table 2.5 shows typical data from the literature. Again it can be seen that activity increases from the methyl to the benzyl ester. The compounds show low systemic toxicity (Mathews *et al.*, 1956). Russell & Furr (1986a,b, 1987) and Russell *et al.* (1985, 1987) studied the effects of parabens against wild-type and envelope mutants of *E. coli* and *Salmonella typhimurium*, and found that, as the homologous series was ascended, solubility decreased but activity became more pronounced, especially against the deep rough strains.

In summary, it can be said that the parabens are generally more active against Gram-positive bacteria and fungi, including yeasts, than against Gram-negative bacteria, and in the latter *P. aeruginosa* is, as is so often seen, more resistant, especially to the higher homologues.

Hugo & Foster (1964) showed that a strain of *P. aeruginosa* isolated from a human eye lesion could metabolize the esters in dilute solution, 0.0343%, a solution strength originally proposed as a preservative vehicle for medicinal eye-drops. Beveridge & Hart (1970) verified that the esters could serve as a carbon source for a number of Gram-negative bacterial species. Rosen *et al.* (1977) studied the preservative action of a mixture of methyl (0.2%) and propyl (0.1%) *p*-hydroxybenzoic acid in a cosmetic lotion. Using a challenge test, they found that this concentration of esters failed to kill *P. aeruginosa*. It was part of their work indicating that these esters + imidazolindyl urea (Section 17.2.2) were ideal to provide a broad-spectrum preservative system, pseudomonads being successfully eliminated

It has been traditional to use these esters in mixtures, as for example in Rosen's experiments recounted above. The rationale for this might be seen in the preservation of water-in-oil emulsion systems, where the more water-soluble methyl ester protected the aqueous phase while the propyl or butyl esters might preserve the oil phase. This point is discussed by O'Neill *et al.* (1979).

Another factor which must be borne in mind when using parabens is that they share the property found with other preservatives containing a phenolic group of being inactivated by non-ionic

Table 2.5 Chemical and microbiological properties of esters of *p*-hydroxybenzoic acid.

	Ester			
Property*	Methyl	Ethyl	Propyl	Butyl
Molecular weight	152	166	180	194
Solubility in water (g/100 g) at 15°C)	0.16	0.08	0.023	0.005
K_w^o (arachis oil)	2.4	13.4	38.1	239.6
Log *P* (octanol:water)	1.96	2.47	3.04	3.57
MIC values (molar basis)†				
E. coli (wild type)	3.95×10^{-3}	2.7×10^{-3}	1.58×10^{-3}	1.03×10^{-3}
E. coli (deep rough)	2.63×10^{-3}	1.2×10^{-3}	2.78×10^{-4}	1.03×10^{-4}
MIC values (μg/ml)‡				
E. coli	800	560	350	160
P. aeruginosa	1000	700	350	150
Concentration (mmol/l) giving 50% inhibition of growth and uptake process in§				
E. coli	5.5	2.2	1.1	0.4
P. aeruginosa	3.6	2.8	> 1.0	> 1.0
B. subtilis	4.3	1.3	0.9	0.46

*K_w^o, partition coefficient, oil:water; *P*, partition coefficient, octanol:water.
†Russell *et al.* (1985).
‡El-Falaha *et al.* (1983).
§Eklund (1980).

surface agents. Hydrogen bonding between the phenolic hydrogen atom and oxygen residues in polyoxyethylated non-ionic surfactants is believed to be responsible for the phenomenon. Experiments to support this inactivation are described by Patel & Kostenbauder (1958), Pisano & Kostenbauder (1959) and Blaug & Ahsan (1961). Various ways of quenching paraben activity, including the use of polysorbates, are considered by Sutton (1996).

As has been stated, methyl and propyl parabens topped the league table of cosmetic preservatives (Richardson, 1981) and, provided their limitations are borne in mind, they form a very useful set of preservatives.

The mode of action of the parabens has been studied by Furr & Russell (1972a,b,c), Freese *et al.* (1973), Freese & Levin (1978), Eklund (1980, 1985, 1989) and Kabara & Eklund (1991). Haag & Loncrini (1984) have produced a comprehensive report of their antimicrobial properties.

3.4.11 *Vanillic acid esters*

The methyl, ethyl, propyl and butyl esters of vanillic acid (4-hydroxy-3-methoxy benzoic acid) possess antifungal properties when used at concentrations of 0.1–0.2%. These esters are not very soluble in water and are inactivated above pH 8.0. The ethyl ester has been shown to be less toxic than sodium benzoate and it has been used in the preservation of foods and food-packing materials against fungal infestation.

3.5 Regulations for the use of preservatives in foods

Certain of the foregoing substances described are used as food preservatives. The use of food preservatives is controlled by law in this and many other countries. Lloyd & Drake (1975) discuss problems associated with the addition of preservatives to foodstuffs. Legislative aspects have been comprehensively reviewed by Pollard (1991).

The special problems of food preservation are dealt with in Chapter 17 and of pharmaceutical products in Chapter 16, Lueck (1980) has published a detailed monograph on food preservatives, which includes a consideration of their history, uses, health aspects and regulatory status, while Tilbury (1980) discusses developments in food preservatives.

4 Aromatic diamidines

Diamidines are a group of organic compounds of which a typical structure is shown in Fig. 2.8. They were first introduced into medicine in the 1920s as possible insulin substitutes, as they lowered blood-sugar levels in humans. Because of these lowered levels, the notion was sustained that they might possess antitrypanosomal activity because of the exogenous requirement for glucose of this parasite. Later, they were found to possess an intrinsic trypanocidal activity not related to their action on blood sugar, and from this arose an investigation into their antimicrobial activity (Thrower & Valentine, 1943; Wien *et al.*, 1948). From these studies two compounds, propamidine and dibromopropamidine, emerged as useful antimicrobial compounds, being active against both bacteria and fungi.

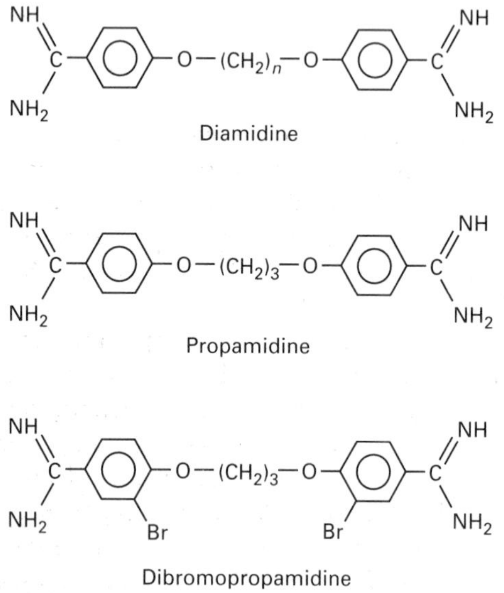

NH, NH₂ — C — O—$(CH_2)_n$—O — C — NH, NH₂

Diamidine

O—$(CH_2)_3$—O

Propamidine

O—$(CH_2)_3$—O, Br, Br

Dibromopropamidine

Fig. 2.8 Typical structure of a diamidine; propamidine; dibromopropamidine.

4.1 Propamidine

Propamidine is 4,4′-diamidinophenoxypropane; in order to confer solubility on this molecule, it is usually supplied as the di(2-hydroxyethane-sulphate), the isethionate. This product is a white hygroscopic powder, which is soluble in water, 1 in 5. Antimicrobial activity and clinical applications are described by Thrower & Valentine (1943). A summary of its antibacterial and antifungal activity is given in Table 2.6. Its activity is reduced by serum, by blood and by low pH values. Microorganisms exposed to propamidine quickly acquire a resistance to it by serial subculture in the presence of increasing doses. Methicillin-resistant *S. aureus* (MRSA) strains may show appreciable resistance to propamidine (see Chapter 10F). It is chiefly used in the form of a cream containing 0.15% as a topical application for wounds.

4.2 Dibromopropamidine

Dibromopropamidine is 2,2′-dibromo-4,4′-diamidinodiphenoxypropane, which is again usually supplied as the isethionate. It occurs as white crystals, which are readily soluble in water. Dibromopropamidine is active against Gram-positive, non-spore-forming organisms; it is less active against Gram-negative organisms and spore formers, but is active against fungi (Table 2.6). Resistance is acquired by serial subculture, and resistant organisms so induced also show a resistance to propamidine. Russell & Furr (1986b, 1987) found that Gram-negative bacteria present a permeability barrier to dibromopropamidine isethionate, and MRSA strains may be resistant to the diamidine (Chapter 10F). Its activity is reduced in acid environments and in the presence of blood and serum. It is usually administered as an oil-in-water cream emulsion containing 0.15% of the isethionate.

More detailed reviews on this group of compounds will be found in Hugo (1971) and Fleurette (1995).

5 Biguanides

Various biguanides show antimicrobial activity,

Table 2.6 Antimicrobial properties of propamidine and dibromopropamidine isethionates.

Microorganism	MIC (μg/ml) of Propamidine isethionate*	Dibromopropamidine isethionate†
Staphylococcus aureus	1–16	1
Staphylococcus albus	6	
MRSA‡	800/100	
MRSE§	250–800	
Streptococcus pyogenes	0.24–4	1
Streptococcus viridans	1–4	2
Streptococcus faecalis	25	
Pseudomonas aeruginosa	250–400	32 (64)
Proteus vulgaris	125–400	128 (256)
Escherichia coli	64–100	4 (32)
Clostridium perfringens	3–32	512
Clostridium histolyticum	256	256
Shigella flexneri	32	8
Salmonella enteriditis	256	65
Salmonella typhimurium	256	64
Actinomyces kimberi	100	10
Actinomyces madurae	100	50
Actinomyces hominis	1000	1000
Trichophyton tonsurans	100	25
Epidermophyton floccosum	250	
Achorion schoenleinii	3.5	
Blastomyces dermatitidis	3.5	
Geotrichum dermatitidis	3.5	200
Hormodendron langevonii		500

*Data from various sources, including Wien *et al.* (1948).
†Data from Wien *et al.* (1948).
‡MRSA, methicillin-resistant *Staph. aureus* carrying *qacA*/*qacB* gene (data of Littlejohn *et al.*, 1992).
§MRSE, methicillin-resistant *Staph. epidermidis* (data of Leelaporn *et al.*, 1994).
Figures in parentheses denote bactericidal concentrations.

including chlorhexidine, alexidine and polymeric forms.

5.1 Chlorhexidine

Chlorhexidine (Fig. 2.9a) is one of a family of N^1, N^5-substituted biguanides which has emerged from extensive synthetic and screening studies, primarily by research workers at Imperial Chemical Industries (ICI) (Curd & Rose, 1946; Davies *et al.*, 1954; Rose & Swain, 1956). It is available as a dihydrochloride, diacetate and gluconate. At 20°C the solubilities of the dihydrochloride and diacetate are 0.06 and 1.9% w/v, respectively; the digluconate is freely soluble.

Chlorhexidine and its salts occur as white or faintly cream-coloured powders and are available in a number of pharmaceutical formulations. It is widely used combined with cetyltrimethylammonium bromide as a topical antiseptic (Savlon, Zeneca Ltd., Alderley Park, Macclesfield, Cheshire, UK).

Chlorhexidine has a wide spectrum of antibacterial activity against both Gram-positive and Gram-negative bacteria. Some bacteria, notably strains of *Proteus* and *Providencia* spp., may be highly resistant to the biguanide (Stickler *et al.*, 1983; Ismaeel *et al.*, 1986a,b; Russell, 1986; Baillie, 1987; see also Chapter 10A). It is not sporicidal (Shaker *et al.*, 1986, 1988a,b; Russell, 1990a,b, 1991b; Russell & Day, 1993; Ranganathan, 1996; Russell & Chopra, 1996). Chlorhexidine is not

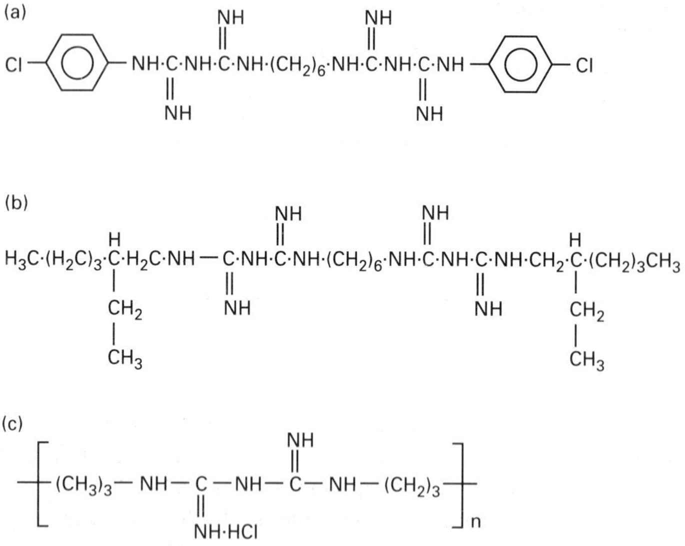

(a)

$$Cl-C_6H_4-NH\cdot C(=NH)\cdot NH\cdot C(=NH)\cdot NH\cdot (CH_2)_6\cdot NH\cdot C(=NH)\cdot NH\cdot C(=NH)\cdot NH-C_6H_4-Cl$$

(b)

$$H_3C\cdot (H_2C)_3\cdot CH(CH_2CH_3)\cdot H_2C\cdot NH-C(=NH)\cdot NH\cdot C(=NH)\cdot NH\cdot (CH_2)_6\cdot NH\cdot C(=NH)\cdot NH\cdot C(=NH)\cdot NH\cdot CH_2\cdot CH(CH_2CH_3)\cdot (CH_2)_3CH_3$$

(c)

$$\left[(CH_3)_3-NH-C(=NH\cdot HCl)-NH-C(=NH)-NH-(CH_2)_3 \right]_n$$

Fig. 2.9 Chlorhexidine (a), alexidine (b) and Vantocil 1B, a polymeric biguanide (c), in which mean n is 5.5.

lethal to acid-fast organisms, although it shows a high degree of bacteriostasis (Russell, 1995, 1996; Russell & Russell, 1995; Table 2.7). It is, however, tuberculocidal in ethanolic solutions and sporicidal at 98–100°C. A range of bacteriostatic and bactericidal values against a variety of bacterial species is shown in Tables 2.7 and 2.8, respectively.

Activity is reduced in the presence of serum, blood, pus and other organic matter. Because of its cationic nature, its activity is also reduced in the presence of soaps and other anionic compounds. Another cause of activity loss is due to the low solubility of the phosphate, borate, citrate, bicarbonate, carbonate or chloride salts. Any system which contains these anions will precipitate chlorhexidine.

Its main use is in medical and veterinary antisepsis (Holloway *et al.*, 1986). An alcoholic solution is a very effective skin disinfectant (Lowbury & Lilley, 1960). It is used in catheterization procedures, in bladder irrigation and in obstetrics and gynaecology. It is one of the recommended bactericides for inclusion in eyedrops and is widely used in contact-lens solutions (Gavin *et al.*, 1996). In the veterinary context (Russell & Hugo, 1987), chlorhexidine fulfils the major function of the application of a disinfectant of cows' teats after milking and can also be used as an antiseptic wound application. Chlorhexidine is

Table 2.7 Bacteriostatic activity of chlorhexidine against various bacterial species.

Organism	Concentration of chlorhexidine (μg/ml) necessary for inhibition of growth
Streptococcus lactis	0.5
Streptococcus pyogenes	0.5
Streptococcus pneumoniae	1.0
Streptococcus faecalis	1.0
Staphylococcus aureus	1.0
Corynebacterium diphtheriae	1.0
Salmonella typhi	1.67
Salmonella pullorum	3.3
Salmonella dublin	3.3
Salmonella typhimurium	5.0
Proteus vulgaris	5.0
Pseudomonas aeruginosa (1)	5.0
Pseudomonas aeruginosa (2)	5.0
Pseudomonas aeruginosa (3)	12.5
Enterobacter aerogenes	10
Escherichia coli	10⁺
Vibrio cholerae	3.3
Bacillus subtilis	0.5
Clostridium welchii	10
Mycobacterium tuberculosis	0.5
*Candida albicans**	5.0

Inoculum: one loopful of 24-h broth culture per 10 ml Difco heart–brain infusion medium.
Incubation: 24 h at 37°C.
* Yeast.
⁺ Much higher than normally recorded.

Table 2.8 Bactericidal activity of chlorhexidine against various bacterial species.

	Concentration of chlorhexidine (μg/ml)		
Organism	To effect 99% kill	To effect 99.9% kill	To effect 99.99% kill
Staphylococcus aureus	8	14	25
Streptococcus pyogenes	–	–	50
Escherichia coli	6.25	10	20
Pseudomonas aeruginosa	25	33	60
Salmonella typhi	5	–	8

Inoculum: 10^5 in distilled water. Contact time: 10 min at room temperature. Neutralizer: egg-yolk medium.

also widely employed in the dental field (Gorman & Scott, 1985; Molinari, 1995; Cottone & Molinari, 1996).

Its mode of action has been studied by various authors (Hugo & Longworth, 1964a,b, 1965, 1966; Longworth, 1971, Hugo, 1978; Fitzgerald *et al.*, 1989, 1992a,b; Kuyyakanond & Quesnel, 1992; Barrett-Bee *et al.*, 1994; Russell & Day, 1996). ^{14}C-chlorhexidine gluconate is taken up very rapidly by bacterial (Fitzgerald *et al.*, 1989) and fungal (Hiom *et al.*, 1995a,b) cells. At lower concentrations, up to 200 μg/ml, it inhibits membrane enzymes and promotes leakage of cellular constituents; this is probably associated with bacteriostasis. As the concentration increases above this value, cytoplasmic constituents are coagulated and a bactericidal effect is seen (Chapter 9). Chlorhexidine has low oral toxicity and it may be administered for throat medication in the form of lozenges.

Extensive details on uses and application, together with relevant biocidal data, will be found in the booklet *Hibitane* (Imperial Chemical Industries, n.d.). Comprehensive surveys of its activity and uses have been published (Russell & Day, 1993; Reverdy, 1995a; Ranganathan, 1996).

5.2 Alexidine

Alexidine (Fig. 2.9b) is a bisbiguanide that possesses ethylhexyl end-groups as distinct from the chlorophenol end-groups found in chlorhexidine. Alexidine is considerably more active than chlorhexidine in inducing cell leakage from *E. coli*, and concentrations of alexidine (but not of chlorhexidine) above the MIC induce cell lysis (Chawner & Gilbert, 1989a,b). Alexidine has been recommended for use as an oral antiseptic and antiplaque compound (Gjermo *et al.*, 1973).

Unlike chlorhexidine, both alexidine and polyhexamethylene biguanide (PHMB) (Section 5.3) induce membrane lipid-phase separation and domain formation.

5.3 Polymeric biguanides

A novel compound, a polymer of hexamethylene biguanide (Fig. 2.9c), with a molecular weight of approximately 3000 (weight average), has found particular use as a cleansing agent in the food industry. Its properties have been described by Davies *et al.* (1968) under the trade name Vantocil 1B.

Polyhexamethylene biguanide is soluble in water and is usually supplied as a 20% aqueous solution. It is also soluble in glycols and alcohols but is insoluble in non-polar solvents, such as petroleum ethers or toluene. It inhibits the growth of most bacteria at between 5 and 25 μg/ml but 100 μg/ml is required to inhibit *P. aeruginosa* while *P. vulgaris* requires 250 μg/ml. It is less active against fungi; for example, *Cladosporium resinae*, which has been implicated as a spoilage organism in pharmaceutical products, requires 1250 μg/ml to prevent growth.

Polyhexamethylene biguanide is believed to gain access to Gram-negative bacteria by a mechanism of self-promotion through cation displacement from, predominantly, core lipopolysaccharide in the outer membrane (Gilbert *et al.*, 1990a). Antimicrobial activity of PHMB increases with increasing polymer length (Gilbert *et al.*, 1990b). It is a membrane-active agent (Broxton *et al.*, 1983, 1984a,b; Woodcock, 1988), inducing phospholipid phase separation (Ikeda *et al.*, 1984). A complete loss of membrane function ensues, with precipitation of intracellular constituents leading to a bactericidal effect.

Because of the residual positive charges on the polymer, PHMB is precipitated from aqueous solutions by anionic compounds, which include soaps and detergents based on alkyl sulphates. It is also precipitated by detergent constituents, such as sodium hexametaphosphate, and in a strongly alkaline environment.

It finds use as a general sterilizing agent in the food industry, provided the surfaces to which it is applied are free from occlusive debris, a stricture that applies in all disinfection procedures. Because it is not a surface-active agent, it can be used in the brewing industry, as it does not affect head retention on ales and beers. Contact should be avoided with one commonly used material in food manufacture, anionic caramel, as this will, like other anionic compounds, inactivate the polymer. It has also been used very successfully for the disinfection of swimming pools. Apart from copper, which it tarnishes, this polymeric biguanide has no deleterious effect on most materials it might encounter in use.

Polyhexamethylene biguanide has activity against both the trophozite and the cyst forms of *Acanthamoeba castellanii* (Khunkitti *et al.*, 1996, 1997, 1998; see also Chapter 8A).

6 Surface-active agents

Surface-active agents (surfactants) have two regions in their molecular structure, one being a hydrocarbon water-repellent (hydrophobic) group and the other a water-attracting (hydrophilic or polar) group. Depending on the basis of the charge or absence of ionization of the hydrophilic group, surface-active agents are classified into anionic, cationic, non-ionic and ampholytic (amphoteric) compounds.

6.1 Cationic agents

Cationic surfactants possess strong bactericidal, but weak detergent, properties. The term 'cationic detergent' usually signifies a quaternary ammonium compound (QAC, onium compound), but this is not strictly accurate, as the smallest concentration at which a QAC is microbicidal is so low that its detergent activity is negligible (Davis, 1960).

Lawrence (1950), D'Aray & Taylor (1962a,b), Merianos (1991), Joly (1995) and Reverdy (1995b) have reviewed the surface-active quaternary ammonium germicides, and useful data about their properties and activity are provided by Wallhäusser (1984) and about their uses by Gardner & Peel (1986,1991) and Denyer & Wallhäusser (1990). Early references to their use are found in Jacobs (1916), Jacobs *et al.* (1916a,b) and Domagk (1935).

6.1.1 *Chemical aspects*

The QACs may be considered as being organically substituted ammonium compounds, in which the nitrogen atom has a valency of five, and four of the substituent radicals (R^1–R^4) are alkyl or heterocyclic radicals and the fifth (X^-) is a small anion (Fig. 2.10: general structure). The sum of the carbon atoms in the four R groups is more than 10. For a QAC to have a high antimicrobial activity, at least one of the R groups must have a chain length in the range C_8 to C_{18} (Domagk, 1935). Three of the four covalent links may be satisfied by nitrogen in a pyridine ring, as in the pyridinium compounds, such as cetylpyridinium chloride. This and the other important QACs are listed in Fig. 2.10. The cationic onium group may be a simple aliphatic ammonium, a pyridinium or piperidinium or other heterocyclic group (D'Arcy & Taylor, 1962b).

Apart from the monoquaternary compounds, monoquaternary derivatives of 4-aminoquinaldine (e.g. laurolinium) are potent antimicrobial agents, as are the bisquaternary compounds, such as hedaquinium chloride and dequalinium. These are considered in more detail in Section 10 (see also Fig. 2.22).

In addition to the compounds mentioned above, polymeric QACs are used as industrial biocides. One such compound is poly(oxyethylene(dimethylimino)ethylene)dichloride.

Organosilicon-substituted (silicon-bonded) qua-

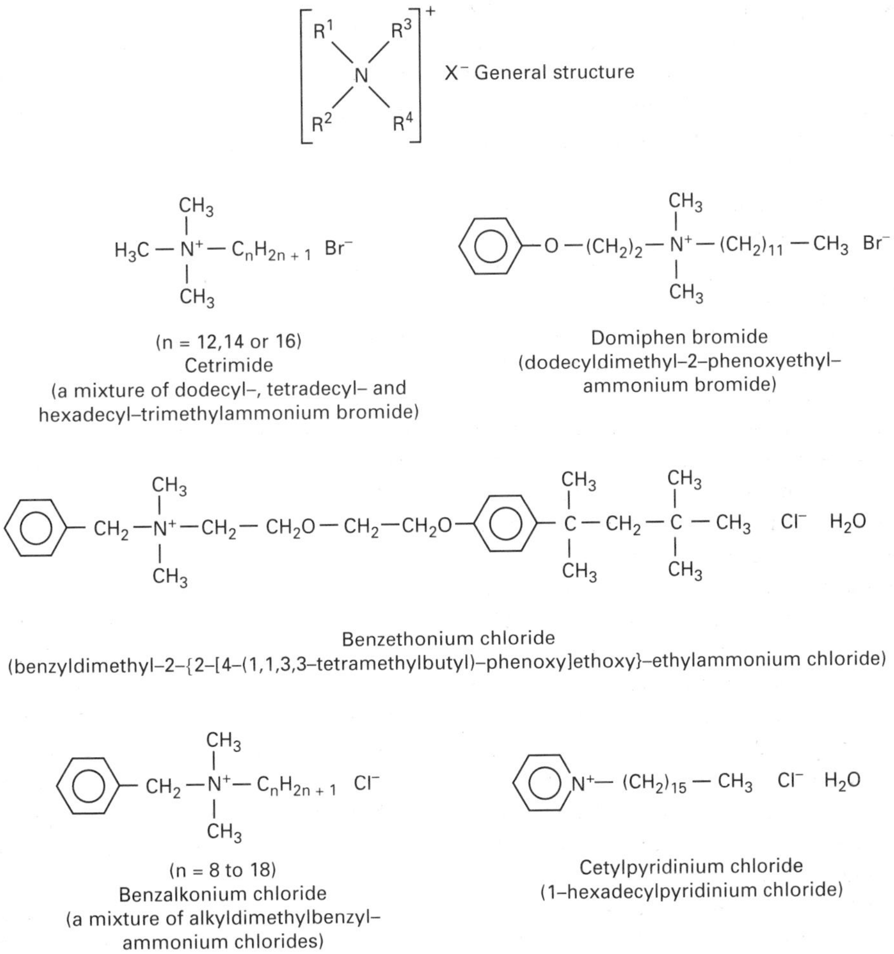

$$\left[R^1R^2N R^3R^4 \right]^+ X^- \quad \text{General structure}$$

$$H_3C-N^+(CH_3)_2-C_nH_{2n+1}\ Br^-$$

(n = 12,14 or 16)
Cetrimide
(a mixture of dodecyl–, tetradecyl– and hexadecyl–trimethylammonium bromide)

$$C_6H_5-O-(CH_2)_2-N^+(CH_3)_2-(CH_2)_{11}-CH_3\ Br^-$$

Domiphen bromide
(dodecyldimethyl–2–phenoxyethyl–ammonium bromide)

$$C_6H_5-CH_2-N^+(CH_3)_2-CH_2-CH_2O-CH_2-CH_2O-C_6H_4-C(CH_3)_2-CH_2-C(CH_3)_2-CH_3\ Cl^-\ H_2O$$

Benzethonium chloride
(benzyldimethyl–2–{2–[4–(1,1,3,3–tetramethylbutyl)–phenoxy]ethoxy}–ethylammonium chloride)

$$C_6H_5-CH_2-N^+(CH_3)_2-C_nH_{2n+1}\ Cl^-$$

(n = 8 to 18)
Benzalkonium chloride
(a mixture of alkyldimethylbenzyl–ammonium chlorides)

$$C_5H_5N^+-(CH_2)_{15}-CH_3\ Cl^-\ H_2O$$

Cetylpyridinium chloride
(1–hexadecylpyridinium chloride)

Fig. 2.10 General structure and examples of quaternary ammonium compounds (QACs).

ternary ammonium salts, organic amines or amine salts have been introduced recently. Compounds with antimicrobial activity in solution are also highly effective on surfaces. One such compound, 3-(trimethoxysily)propyloctadecyldimethyl ammonium chloride, demonstrates powerful antimicrobial activity while chemically bonded to a variety of surfaces (Malek & Speier, 1982; Speier & Malek, 1982). Schaeufele (1986) has pointed out that fatty alcohols and/or fatty acids, from both natural and synthetic sources, form the basis of the production of modern QACs, which have improved organic soil and increased hard-water tolerance.

6.1.2 *Antimicrobial activity*

As stated above, the antimicrobial properties of the QACs were first recognized in 1916, but they did not attain prominence until the work of Domagk in 1935. Early workers claimed that the QACs were markedly sporicidal, but the fallacy of this hypothesis has been demonstrated by improved testing methods. In particular, the experimental procedures devised by Davies (1949) are of considerable importance. He found that suspensions of *B. subtilis* spores were apparently sterilized after 1 h by various QACs when no precautions were made to prevent bacteriostasis in the recovery medium; however, the inclusion in the recovery medium of Lubrol W (Bergan & Lystad, 1972; Mackinnon, 1974) showed the lack of sporicidal activity (Russell, 1971b). Weber & Black (1948) had earlier recommended the use of lecithin as a neutralizer for QACs. Lawrence (1948) showed that soaps and anionic detergents failed to inactivate QACs, and suggested suramin sodium for this purpose. British Standard 647 (1984) recommends lecithin (2%) solubilized with Lubrol W (3%), although Lubrol W itself may be toxic to streptococci, a point discussed more fully by Russell *et al.* (1979) and Russell (1981). Sutton (1996) describes appropriate neutralizing systems for QACs and other biocides; cyclodextrin (Simpson, 1992) may prove to be useful.

The QACs are primarily active against Gram-positive bacteria, with concentrations as low as 1 in 200 000 (0.0005%) being lethal; higher concentrations (*c.* 1 in 30 000 or 0.0033%) are lethal to Gram-negative bacteria (Hamilton, 1971), although *P. aeruginosa* tends to be highly resistant (Davis, 1962). Nevertheless, cells of this organism which are highly resistant to benzalkonium chloride (1 mg/ml, 0.1%) may still show ultrastructural changes when grown in its presence (Hoffman *et al.*, 1973). The QACs have a trypanocidal activity (reviewed by D'Arcy & Taylor, 1962b) but are not mycobactericidal (Sykes, 1965; Smith, 1968), presumably because of the lipid, waxy coat of these organisms. Gram-negative bacteria, such as *E. coli*, *P. aeruginosa* and *S. typhimurium*, exclude QACs, but deep rough mutants are sensitive (El-Falaha *et al.*, 1983; Russell & Furr, 1986a,b, Russell *et al.*, 1986; (Russell & Chopra, 1996). Contamination of solutions of QACs with Gram-negative bacteria has often been reported (Frank & Schaffner, 1976; Kaskow *et al.*, 1976).

Viruses are more resistant than bacteria or fungi to the QACs. This is clearly shown in the excellent review of Grossgebauer (1970), who points out that the QACs have a high protein defect, and that, whereas they are active against lipophilic viruses (such as herpes simplex, vaccinia, influenza and adenoviruses), they have only a poor effect against viruses (enteroviruses, e.g. polio, Coxsackie and Echo) that show hydrophilic properties. The QACs have, however, been demonstrated in laboratory tests to exhibit anti-human immunodeficiency virus (HIV) activity (Bond, 1995).

Activity of QACs against hepatitis B virus (HBV) has been shown by Prince *et al.* (1993). These findings led Bond (1995) to conclude that HIV and HBV are readily killed *in vitro* by a variety of biocidal agents, including QACs, but he emphasized the importance of the absence of organic matter.

The antiviral properties of QACs and other biocides are considered in detail in Chapter 6A.

The QACs possess antifungal properties, although they are fungistatic rather than fungicidal (for a review, see D'Arcy, 1971). This applies not only to the monoquaternary compounds, but also to the bisonium compounds, such as hedaquinium and dequalinium (Section 10; see also Chapter 9).

The Ferguson principle stipulates that compounds with the same thermodynamic activity will exert equal effects on bacteria. Weiner *et al.* (1965) studied the activity of three QACs (dodecyltrimethylammonium chloride, dodecyldimethylammonium chloride and dodecylpyridinium chloride) against *E. coli*, *S. aureus* and *Candida albicans*, and correlated these results with the surface properties of these agents. A clear relationship was found between the thermodynamic activity (expressed as a ratio of the surface concentration produced by a solution and the surface concentration at the critical micelle concentration (CMC)) and antibacterial activity.

Because most QACs are mixtures of homologues, Laycock & Mulley (1970) studied the antibacterial activity of mono- and multicomponent solutions, using the homologous series *n*-dodecyl, *n*-tetradecyl and *n*-hexadecyl trimethylammonium bromides individually, binary systems containing C_{12}/C_{14} or C_{14}/C_{16} mixtures, and a ternary mixture (centrimide) of the $C_{12}/C_{14}/C_{16}$ compounds. Antibacterial activity was measured as the concentrations needed to produce survivor levels of 1.0 and 0.01%; CMC was measured by the surface-tension method. In almost every instance, the thermodynamic activity (CMC/concentration to produce a particular survivor level) producing an equivalent biological response was reasonably constant, thereby supporting the Ferguson principle for these micelle-forming QACs.

The QACs are incompatible with a wide range

of chemical agents, including anionic surfactants (Richardson & Woodford, 1964), non-ionic surfactants, such as lubrols and tweens, and phospholipids, such as lecithin and other fat-containing substances. Benzalkonium chloride has been found to be incompatible with the ingredients of some commercial rubber mixes, but not with silicone rubber; this is important when benzalkonium chloride is employed as a preservative in multiple-dose eye-drop formulations (*Pharmaceutical Codex* 1994, *British Pharmacopoeia*, 1998).

Although non-ionic surfactants are stated above to inactivate QACs, presumably as a consequence of micellar formation (see Elworthy, 1976, for a useful description of micelles), nevertheless potentiation of the antibacterial activity of the QACs by means of low concentrations of non-ionic agents has been reported (Schmolka, 1973), possibly as a result of increased cellular permeability induced by the non-ionic surfactant (see Chapter 3 for a more detailed discussion).

The antimicrobial activity of the QACs is affected greatly by organic matter, including milk, serum and faeces, which may limit their usefulness in practice. The uses of the QACs are considered below (Section 6.1.3) and also in more general terms in Section 20. They are more effective at alkaline and neutral pH than under acid conditions. The action of benzalkonium chloride on *P. aeruginosa* is potentiated by aromatic alcohols, especially 3-phenylpropanol (Richards & McBride, 1973).

6.1.3 Uses

The QACs have many and varied uses. They have been recommended for use in food hygiene in hospitals (Kelsey & Maurer, 1972). Benzalkonium chloride has been employed for the preoperative disinfection of unbroken skin (0.1–0.2%), for application to mucous membranes (up to 0.1%) and for bladder and urethra irrigation (0.005%); creams are used in treating nappy (diaper) rash caused by ammonia-producing organisms, and lozenges for the treatment of superficial mouth and throat infections. In the UK, benzalkonium chloride (0.01% is one of four antimicrobial agents officially recognized as being suitable preservatives for inclusion in eye-drop preparations (*Pharmaceutical Codex* 1994, *British Pharmacopoeia*, 1993). Benzalkonium chloride is also widely used (at a concentration of 0.001–0.01%) in hard contact lens soaking (disinfecting) solutions; EDTA (see Section 13) at a concentration of 0.1% may be included to enhance its action (Kay, 1980). The QAC is too irritant to be used with hydrophilic soft (hydrogel) contact lenses because it can bind to the lens surface, be held within the water present in hydrogels and then be released into the eye (Davies, 1980).

Benzethonium chloride is applied to wounds as an aqueous solution (0.1%) and as a solution (0.2%) in alcohol and acetone for preoperative skin disinfection and for controlling algal growth in swimming pools.

Cetrimide is used for cleaning and disinfecting burns and wounds and for preoperative cleansing of the skin. For general disinfecting purposes, a mixture (Savlon) of cetrimide with chlorhexidine is often employed. At pH 6, but not at pH 7.2, this product may be liable to contamination with *P. aeruginosa* (Bassett, 1971). Solutions containing 1–3% of cetrimide are employed as hair shampoos (e.g. Cetavlon P.C., a concentrate to be diluted with water before use) for seborrhoea capitis and seborrhoeic dermatitis.

Cetylpyridinium chloride is employed pharmaceutically, for skin disinfection and for antiseptic treatment of small wound surfaces (0.1–0.5% solutions), as an oral and pharyngeal antiseptic (e.g. lozenges containing 1–2 mg of the QAC) and as a preservative in emulsions. Cosmetically (see also Quack, 1976), it is used at a concentration of between 0.1 and 0.5% in hair preparations and in deodorants; lower concentrations (0.05–0.1%) are incorporated into face and shaving lotions.

Several investigations have been made of the use of QACs in the disinfection of bedding and blankets (Schwabacher *et al.*, 1958; Gillespie & Robinson, 1959; Thomas *et al.*, 1959; Crewther & McQuade, 1964). Blankets and bedding comprise an important source of cross-infection in hospital wards. The bacteria associated with this cross-infection are usually non-sporing, and *S. aureus* is a particularly troublesome organism. Contamination of the air in a ward is very marked when beds are being made. The QACs were one of the first methods of disinfecting hospital woollen blankets, which, however, are now rarely used.

In the veterinary context, the QACs have been used for the disinfection of automatic calf feeders and have been incorporated into sheep dips for controlling microbial growth in fleece and wool. They are not, however, widely used on farm sites because of the large amount of organic debris they are likely to encounter.

In general, then, the QACs are very useful disinfectants and pharmaceutical and cosmetic preservatives. Further information on their uses and antimicrobial properties is considered in Section 20 and in Chapters 3 and 16; see also BS 6471: 1984, BS 6424: 1950 and Reverdy (1995b).

6.2 Anionic agents

Anionic surface-active agents are compounds which, in aqueous solution, dissociate into a large complex anion, responsible for the surface activity, and a smaller cation. Examples of anionic surfactants are the alkali-metal and metallic soaps, amine soaps, lauryl ether sulphates (e.g. sodium lauryl sulphate) and sulphated fatty alcohols.

They usually have strong detergent but weak antimicrobial properties, except in high concentrations, when they induce lysis of Gram-negative bacteria (Salton, 1968). Fatty acids are active against Gram-positive but not Gram-negative bacteria (Galbraith *et al.*, 1971). More recent information will be found by consulting Kabara (1984).

6.3 Non-ionic agents

These consist of a hydrocarbon chain attached to a non-polar water-attracting group, which is usually a chain of ethylene oxide units, e.g. cetomacrogols. The properties of non-ionic surfactants depend mainly on the proportions of hydrophilic and hydrophobic groups in the molecule. Other examples include the sorbitan derivatives, such as the polysorbates (tweens).

The non-ïonic surfactants are considered to have no antimicrobial properties. However, low concentrations of polysorbates are believed to affect the permeability of the outer envelopes of Gram-negative cells (Brown, 1975), which are thus rendered more sensitive to various antimicrobial agents. High concentrations of tweens overcome the activity of QACs, biguanides, parabens and phenolics. This is made use of in designing appropriate neutralizing agents (Russell *et al.*, 1979; Sutton, 1996) and is considered in more detail in Chapter 3.

6.4 Amphoteric (ampholytic) agents

Amphoteric agents are compounds of mixed anionic–cationic character. They combine the detergent properties of anionic compounds with the bactericidal properties of the cationic. Their bactericidal activity remains virtually constant over a wide pH range (Barrett, 1969) and they are less readily inactivated than QACs by proteins (Clegg, 1970). Examples of amphoteric agents are dodecyl-β-alanine, dodecyl-β-aminobutyric acid and dodecyl-di(aminoethyl)-glycine (Davis, 1960). The last-named belongs to the Tego series of compounds, the name Tego being a trade name (Goldschmidt, Essen).

The Tego compounds are bactericidal to Gram-positive and Gram-negative bacteria, and, unlike the QACs and anionic and non-ionic agents, this includes the mycobacteria (James, 1965; Croshaw, 1971), although the rate of kill of these organisms is less than that of the others (Block, 1983). Compounds based on dodecyl-di(aminoethyl)-glycine find use as disinfectants in the food industry (Kornfeld, 1966).

6.5 Betaines

Betaine itself is trimethylglycine. It is a natural constituent of beetroot and sugar beet and is obtained as a by-product of the sugar-beet industry.

Analogues, in which one of the methyl groups is replaced by a long-chain alkyl residue (Fig. 2.11), find application as detergents and as a basis for

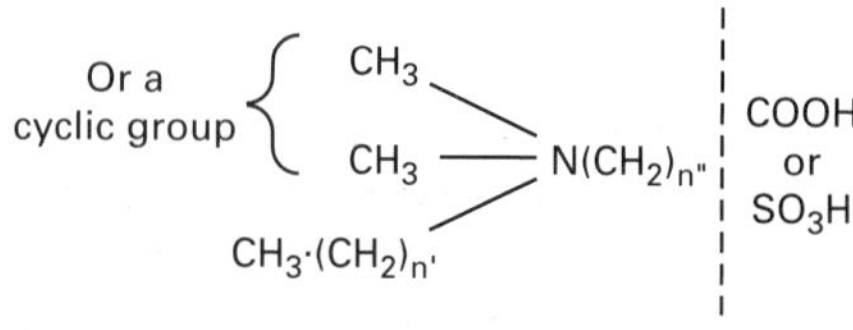

Fig. 2.11 General structure of betaines ($n' = 14-16$, $n'' = 1$ or 2).

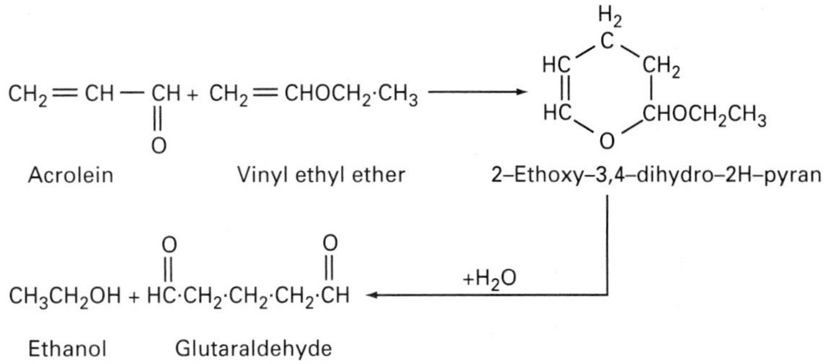

$$CH_2{=}CH{-}\underset{\underset{O}{\|}}{CH} + CH_2{=}CHOCH_2{\cdot}CH_3 \longrightarrow \text{2-Ethoxy-3,4-dihydro-2H-pyran}$$

Acrolein   Vinyl ethyl ether   2–Ethoxy–3,4–dihydro–2H–pyran

$$\xrightarrow{+H_2O} CH_3CH_2OH + \overset{\overset{O}{\|}}{HC}{\cdot}CH_2{\cdot}CH_2{\cdot}CH_2{\cdot}\overset{\overset{O}{\|}}{CH}$$

Ethanol   Glutaraldehyde

Fig. 2.12 Industrial production of glutaraldehyde.

solubilizing or emulsifying phenolic biocides. They have also been used in quaternary ammonium biocides (More & Hardwick, 1958) but are not considered as biocides *per se*.

Other chemical variants include the replacement of the –COOH group by $-SO_3H$ (Fig. 2.11) and of the two methyl groups by a ring system.

7 Aldehydes

Two aldehydes are currently of considerable importance as disinfectants, namely glutaraldehyde and formaldehyde, although others have been studied and shown to possess antimicrobial activity. Glyoxal (ethanedial), malonaldehyde (propanedial), succinaldehyde (butanedial) and adipaldehyde (hexanedial) all possess some sporicidal action, with aldehydes beyond adipaldehyde having virtually no sporicidal effects (Pepper & Chandler, 1963). Succinaldehyde is sometimes used as an antimicrobial agent, and this aspect is considered later (Section 7.3), in the form of Gigasept.

This section on aldehydes will deal mainly with glutaraldehyde and formaldehyde, although a 'new' aldehyde, *o*-phthalaldehyde, will also be considered briefly.

7.1 Glutaraldehyde (pentanedial)

7.1.1 Chemical aspects

Glutaraldehyde is a saturated 5-carbon dialdehyde with an empirical formula of $C_5H_8O_2$ and a molecular weight of 100.12. Its industrial production (Fig. 2.12) involves a two-step synthesis via an ethoxydihydropyran. Glutaraldehyde is usually obtained commercially as a 2, 25 or 50% solution of acidic pH, although for disinfecting purposes a 2% solution is normally supplied, which must be 'activated' (made alkaline) before use.

The two aldehyde groups may react singly or together to form bisulphite complexes, oximes, cyanohydrins, acetals and hydrazones. Polymerization of the glutaraldehyde molecule occurs by means of the following possible mechanisms.

1 The dialdehyde exists as a monomer, with an equilibrium between the open-chain molecule and the hydrated ring structure (Fig. 2.13a,b).

2 Ring formation occurs by an intramolecular mechanism, so that aqueous solutions of the aldehyde consist of free glutaraldehyde, the cyclic hemiacetal of its hydrate and oligomers of this is equlibrium (Fig. 2.13c).

3 Different types of polymers may be formed at different pH values, and it is considered that polymers in the alkaline range are unable to revert to the monomer, whereas those in the neutral and acid range revert easily (Boucher, 1974; Fig. 2.14).

Polymerization increases with a rise in pH, and above pH 9 there is an extensive loss of aldehyde groups. Glutaraldehyde is more stable at acid than alkaline pH; solutions at pH 8 and above generally lose activity within 4 weeks. Novel formulations have been produced, and continue to be designed, to overcome the problems of loss of stability (Babb *et al.*, 1980; Gorman *et al.*, 1980; Power, 1997).

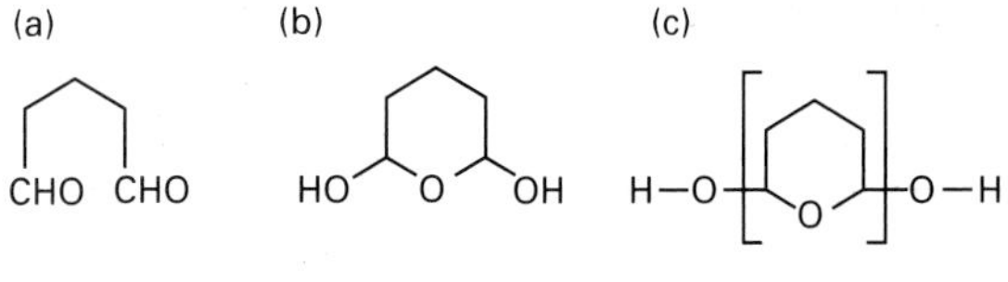

(a) CHO CHO   (b) HO O OH   (c) H–O–[O]–O–H

Fig. 2.13 (a) Free glutaraldehyde; (b) hydrated ring structure (cyclic hemiacetal of its hydrate); (c) oligomer.

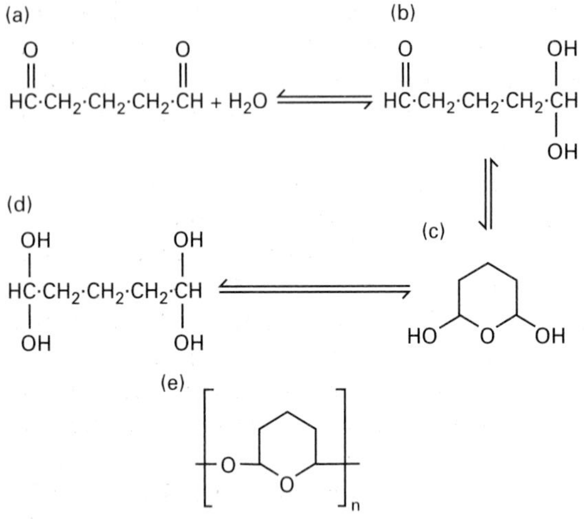

(a) $HC\cdot CH_2\cdot CH_2\cdot CH_2\cdot CH(=O)$ with O on both terminal carbons + H_2O ⇌ (b) $HC(=O)\cdot CH_2\cdot CH_2\cdot CH_2\cdot CH(OH)_2$ ⇌ (c) cyclic hemiacetal (HO, O, OH) ⇌ (d) $(HO)_2HC\cdot CH_2\cdot CH_2\cdot CH_2\cdot CH(OH)_2$; (e) polymer $[-O-(\text{ring O})-]_n$

Fig. 2.14 (a) Open-chain molecule of glutaraldehyde; (b), (c) and (d) formation of several more stable 'polymers' (hydrated) in aqueous alkaline solution; (e) polymer with an acetal-like structure, in neutral and acid ranges (after Boucher, 1974).

7.1.2 *Interactions of glutaraldehyde*

Glutaraldehyde is a highly reactive molecule. It reacts with various enzymes (but does not sterically alter them to loss all activity) and with proteins; the rate of reaction is pH-dependent, increasing considerably over the pH range 4–9, and the reaction product is highly stable (Hopwood *et al.*, 1970). Glutarldehyde prevents dissociation of free ribosomes (Russell & Hopwood, 1976), but under the normal conditions of fixation (Hopwood, 1975) little reaction appears to occur between nucleic acids and glutaraldehyde. There is little published information on the possible reactions of glutaraldehyde and lipids (Russell & Hopwood, 1976).

7.1.3 *Microbicidal activity*

Glutaraldehyde possesses high microbicidal activity against bacteria and their spores, mycelial and spore forms of fungi and various types of viruses (Borick, 1968; Borick & Pepper, 1970). Although there was some doubt about its mycobactericidal potency, glutaraldehyde is now considered to be an effective antimycobacterial agent (Collins, 1986; Broadley *et al.*, 1991; Russell, 1994, 1996; Ascenzi, 1996c). Additional information is provided in Chapter 10D; see also Power (1997).

A summary of the antimicrobial efficacy of glutaraldehyde is presented in Table 2.9, which demonstrates the effect of pH on its activity. However, acid-based products are also available commercially which are claimed to be of equal activity to potentiated alkaline glutaraldehyde. Acid glutaraldehyde is itself an effective microbicide provided that long contact periods are used. The exact mechanism of action of the dialdehyde is unknown, but the fact that its rate of interaction with proteins and enzymes increases with increasing pH (Hopwood *et al.*, 1970; Russell & Munton, 1974) is undoubtedly of importance. The cross-linking mechanism is also influenced by time, concentration and temperature (Eager *et al.*, 1986; Bruch, 1991; Russell, 1994, 1996). Acid glutaraldehyde is a markedly inferior disinfectant to alkaline glutaraldehyde, but this discrepancy disappears with increasing temperature. Resistance development to glutaraldehyde is a late event in sporulation (Power *et al.*, 1988; Russell, 1990a,b, 1994, 1995; Knott *et al.*, 1995) and sodium hydroxide-induced revival of spores of *Bacillus* spp. has been demonstrated (Dancer *et al.*, 1989;

Table 2.9 Microbicidal activity of glutaraldehyde*.

Form of glutaraldehyde	Approximate pH value	Fungicidal activity†	Viricidal activity	Bactericidal activity‡	Sporicidal activity
Acid	4–5	Low	Low to high	Low	Low to very high
Alkaline	8	High	High	High	Reasonable to very high

*See also Gorman *et al.* (1980), Russell (1994) and Favero (1995).

†Use of low dialdehyde concentrations (0.01–0.02%); 2% solutions of acid and alkaline glutaraldehyde are both highly active against bacteria and probably viruses. A high-concentration (3.2%) glutaraldehyde solution is also available (Akamatsu *et al.*, 1997).

‡Activity of acid glutaraldehyde increases markedly with temperature and at *c.* 37°C its activity approaches that of alkaline glutaraldehyde. Acid glutaraldehyde may also be sporicidal at ambient temperatures, provided that long periods of time (*c.* 10 h) are used (Rutala *et al.*, 1993a,b).

Power *et al.*, 1989, 1990; Williams & Russell, 1992a,b).

Organic matter is considered to have no effect on the antimicrobial activity of the aldehyde. In view of the interaction of glutaraldehyde with the amino groups in proteins, this would appear to be a rather unusual finding. It is, however, true to state that it retains a considerable degree of activity in the presence of high levels of organic matter, such as 20% serum (A.D. Russell, unpublished data).

Dried spores are considerably more resistant to chemical disinfectants than are spores in suspension, and it would appear that glutaraldehyde is no exception. The use of the Association of Official Analytical Chemists (AOAC) test with dried spores of *B. subtilis* has shown that 2% alkaline glutaradehyde may require up to 10 h to achieve sterilization at 20°C (Rubbo *et al.*, 1967).

The antimicrobial activity of glutaraldehyde has been reviewed by Gorman *et al.* (1980), Bruch (1991), Russell (1994), Ascenzi (1996c) and Power (1997).

7.1.4 Uses of glutaraldehyde

The uses of glutaraldehyde as a fixative in electron microscopy, in leather tanning and biochemically have been discussed by Russell & Hopwood (1976). In a microbiological context, glutaraldehyde has been recommended for the disinfection/sterilization of certain types of medical equipment, notably cystoscopes and anaesthetic equipment.

Favero and Bond (1991) have rightly drawn attention to the differences between physical methods of sterilization and liquid chemical germicides and point out that 2% alkaline glutaraldehyde is capable of acting as a sterilizing agent but only after prolonged periods of contact. Bearing this comment in mind, glutaraldehyde has long been used for the high-level disinfection of endoscopes, although problems have arisen because of its toxicity. Glutaraldehyde has also been employed for the disinfection of arthroscopes and laparoscopes (Loffer, 1990).

As pointed out, alkaline glutaraldehyde is more active, but less stable, than the acid form. However, 2% activated alkaline glutaraldehyde should not be used continuously to disinfect endoscopes for 14 days after activation, although it is effective over this period if not repeatedly reused (Babb, 1993; Babb & Bradley, 1995). These authors recommend reuse for endoscopes provided that the concentration does not fall appreciably below 1.5%.

Problems in reusing glutaraldehyde are associated with accumulation of organic matter, dilution of disinfectant, change in product pH and difficulties in accurately assaying residual concentrations (Mbithi *et al.*, 1993; Rutala & Weber, 1995; Springthorpe *et al.*, 1995). Colour indicators are not always satisfactory (Power & Russell, 1988). Glutaraldehyde has been employed in the veterinary field for the disinfection of utensils and of premises (Russell & Hugo, 1987), but its potential mutagenic and carcinogenic effects (Quinn, 1987) make these uses hazardous to personnel. The main advantages claimed for glutaraldehyde are as follows: it has a broad spectrum of activity with a rapid microbicidal action, and it is non-corrosive to metals, rubber and lenses. Its toxicity (*vide supra*) remains a problem.

7.2 Formaldehyde (methanal)

Formaldehyde is used as a disinfectant as a liquid or vapour. Gaseous formaldehyde is referred to briefly in Section 18 and in more detail in Chapter 21. The liquid form will be considered mainly in this section.

The Health and Safety Executive of the UK has indicated that the inhalation of formaldehyde vapour may be presumed to pose a carcinogenic risk to humans. This indication must have considerable impact on the consideration of the role and use of formaldehyde and formaldehyde releasers in sterilization and disinfection processes.

7.2.1. Chemical aspects

Formaldehyde occurs as formaldehyde solution (formalin), an aqueous solution containing *c.* 34–38% w/w CH_2O. Methyl alcohol is present to delay polymerization. Formaldehyde displays many typical chemical reactions, combining with amines to give methylolamines, carboxylic acids to give esters of methylene glycol, phenols to give methylphenols and sulphides to produce thiomethylene glycols.

7.2.2 Interactions of formaldehyde

Formaldehyde interacts with protein molecules by attaching itself to the primary amide and amino groups, whereas phenolic moieties bind little of the aldehyde (Fraenkel-Conrat *et al.*, 1945). Subsequently, it was shown that formaldehyde gave an intermolecular cross-linkage of protein or amino groups with phenolic or indole residues.

In addition to interacting with many terminal groups in viral proteins, formaldehyde can also react extensively with the amino groups of nucleic acid bases, although it is much less reactive with deoxyribonucleic acid (DNA) than with ribonucleic acid (RNA) (Staehelin, 1958).

7.2.3 Microbicidal activity

Formaldehyde is a microbicidal agent, with lethal activity against bacteria and their spores, fungi and many viruses. Its first reported use as a disinfectant was in 1892. Its sporicidal action is, however, slower than that of glutaraldehyde (Rubbo *et al.*, 1967). Formaldehyde combines readily with proteins (Section 7.2.2) and is less effective in the presence of protein organic matter. Plasmid-mediated resistance to formaldehyde has been described, presumably due to aldehyde degradation (Heinzel, 1988). Formaldehyde vapour may be released by evaporating formalin solutions, by adding potassium permanganate to formalin or alternatively by heating, under controlled conditions, the polymer paraformaldehyde ($HO(CH_2O)_nH$), urea formaldehyde or melamine formaldehyde (Tulis, 1973). The activity of the vapour depends on aldehyde concentration, temperature and relative humidity (r.h.) (Section 18.2).

7.2.4 Formaldehyde-releasing agents

Noxythiolin (oxymethylenethiourea; Fig. 2.15a) is a bactericidal agent (Kingston, 1965; Wright & McAllister, 1967; Browne & Stoller, 1970) that apparently owes its antibacterial activity to the release of formaldehyde (Kingston, 1965; Pickard, 1972; cf. Gucklhorn, 1970):

$$CH_3{\cdot}NH{\cdot}CS{\cdot}NH{\cdot}CH_2OH \rightarrow CH_3{\cdot}NH{\cdot}CS{\cdot}NH_2H + CHO$$

Noxythiolin has been found to protect animals

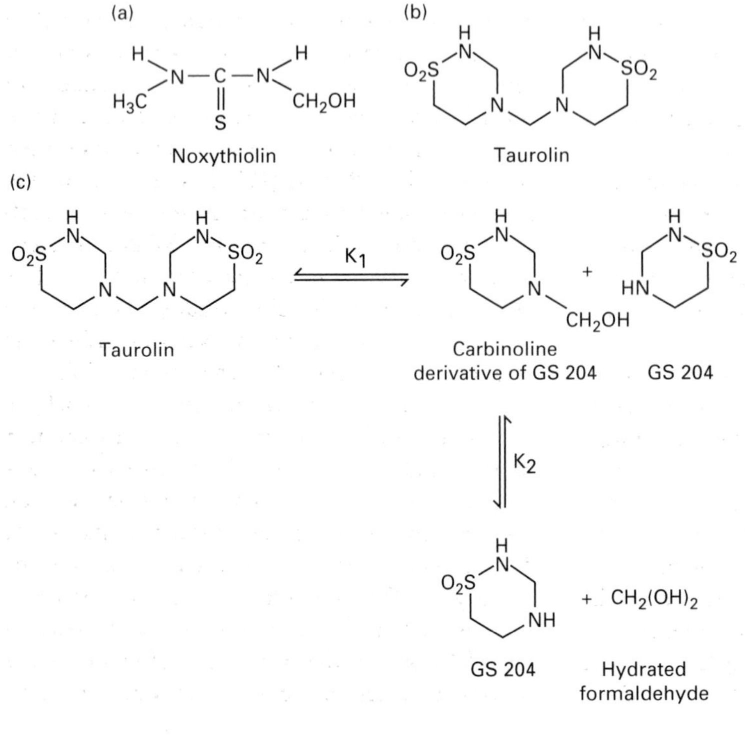

(a) Noxythiolin (b) Taurolin

(c) Taurolin $\underset{K_1}{\rightleftharpoons}$ Carbinoline derivative of GS 204 + GS 204 $\underset{K_2}{\rightleftharpoons}$ GS 204 + $CH_2(OH)_2$ Hydrated formaldehyde

Fig. 2.15 (a) Noxythiolin; (b) taurolin; (c) postulated equilibrium of taurolin in aqueous solution (after Myers *et al.*, 1980).

from lethal doses of endotoxin (Wright & McAllister, 1967; Haler, 1974) and is claimed to be active against all bacteria, including those resistant to other types of antibacterial agents (Browne & Stoller, 1970).

Noxythiolin has been widely used both topically and in accessible body cavities, notably as an irrigation solution in the treatment of peritonitis (Pickard, 1972). Unfortunately, solutions are rather unstable (after preparation they should be stored at 10°C and used within 7 days). Commercially, noxythiolin is available as Noxyflex S and Noxyflex (Geistlich Ltd., Chester, UK), the latter containing amethocaine hydrochloride as well as noxythiolin. Solutions of Noxyflex (containing 1 or 2.5% noxythiolin) are employed where local discomfort is experienced.

More recently, the amino acid taurine has been selected as the starting-point in the design of a new antibacterial agent, taurolin (Fig. 2.15b), which is a condensate of two molecules of taurine and three molecules of formaldehyde. Taurolin (bis-(1,1-dioxoperhydro-1,2,4-thiazinyl-4)methane) is water-soluble and is stable in aqueous solution. It has a wide spectrum of antimicrobial activity *in vitro* and *in vivo* (Reeves & Schweitzer, 1973; Browne *et al.*, 1976, 1977, 1978).

Taurine is considered to act as a non-toxic formaldehyde carrier, donating methylol groups to bacterial protein and endotoxin (Browne *et al.*, 1976). According to these authors, taurine has a lower affinity for formaldehyde than bacterial protein, but a greater affinity than animal protein, the consequence of which is a selective lethal effect. Taurolin has been shown to protect experimental animals from the lethal effects of *E. coli* and *Bacteroides fragilis* endotoxin (Pfirrman & Leslie, 1979).

This viewpoint that the activity of taurolin results from a release of formaldehyde which is adsorbed by bacterial cells is, however, no longer tenable. When taurolin is dissolved in water (Myers *et al.*, 1980), an equilibrium is established (Fig. 2.15c) to release two molecules of the monomer (1,1-dioxoperhydro-1,2,4-thiadizine (GS 204)) and its carbinolamine derivative. The antibacterial activity of taurolin is considerably greater than that of free formaldehyde (Myers *et al.*, 1980; Allwood & Myers, 1981) and these authors thus concluded that the activity of taurolin was not due entirely to bacterial adsorption of free formaldehyde but also to a reaction with a masked (or latent) formaldehyde. Since GS 204 has only a low antibacterial effect, then the carbinolamine must obviously play an important role.

Clinically, the intraperitoneal administration of taurolin has been shown to bring about a significant reduction of morbidity in peritonitis (Browne *et al.*, 1978).

A third formaldehyde-releasing agent is hexamine (methenamine); hexamine itself is inactive but it breaks down by acid hydrolysis to release formaldehyde. It has been reviewed by Allwood & Myers (1981). Derivatives of hexamine are considered in Section 17.4 and other formaldehyde-releasing agents in Sections 17.2 (imidazole derivatives), 17.5 (triazines) and 17.6 (oxazolo-oxazoles). Table 2.18 should also be consulted, as well as Section 18.2 (which deals with release of gaseous formaldehyde) and Paulus (1976).

7.2.5 Uses of formaldehyde

Formaldehyde is employed as a disinfectant in both the liquid and gaseous states. Vapour-phase formaldehyde is used in the disinfection of sealed rooms; the vapour can be produced as described above, or alternatively an equal volume of industrial methylated spirits (IMS) can be added to formaldehyde and the mixture used as a spray. Other uses of formaldehyde vapour have been summarized by Russell (1976). These include the following: low-temperature steam plus formaldehyde vapour (LTSF) for the disinfection/sterilization of heat-sensitive medical materials (see also Chapter 19A); hospital bedding and blankets; and fumigation of poultry houses, of considerable importance in hatchery hygiene (Anon., 1970).

Aerobic spores exposed to liquid formaldehyde can be revived by a sublethal post-heat treatment (Spicher and Peters, 1976, 1981). Revival of LTSF-treated *Bacillus stearothermophilus* spores can also be accomplished by such means (Wright *et al.*, 1996), which casts considerable doubt on the efficacy of LTSF as a potential sterilizing process.

Formaldehyde in liquid form has been used as a viricidal agent in the production of certain types of viral vaccines, e.g. polio (inactivated) vaccine.

Formaldehyde solution has also been employed for the treatment of warts, as an antiseptic mouthwash, for the disinfection of membranes in dialysis equipment and as a preservative in hair shampoos. Formaldehyde-releasing agents were considered in Section 7.2.4. Formaldehyde and formaldehyde condensates have been reviewed in depth by Rossmore & Sondossi (1988).

7.3 Other aldehydes

Other aldehydes have been studied but results have sometimes been conflicting and they have thus been reinvestigated (Power & Russell, 1990). Sporidicin, used undiluted and containing 2% glutaraldehyde plus 7% phenol and 1.2% phenate, is slightly more active against spores than is 2% activated, alkaline glutaraldehyde. Gigasept, containing butan-1,4-dial, dimethoxytetrahydrofuran and formaldehyde, and used at 5% and 10% v/v dilutions, is considerably less active (Power & Russell, 1990).

o-Phthalaldehyde (Fig. 2.16) is a 'new' aldehyde. It is claimed to have potent bactericidal and viricidal activity (Alfa & Sitter, 1994) but information about its antimicrobial properties is currently based on limited experimentation. Further data about its activity and mechanisms of action are needed.

Glyoxal (2%) is weakly sporicidal, and butyraldehyde has no activity. It is essential that adequate procedures are employed to remove residual glutaraldehyde (and phenol/phenate, if present) or other aldehyde in determining survivor levels. This has not always been appreciated (Pepper, 1980; Leach, 1981; Isenberg, 1985).

The properties and uses of various aldehydes have been reviewed by Bartoli and Dusseau (1995).

8 Antimicrobial dyes

There are three groups of dyes which find application as antimicrobial agents: the acridines, the triphenylmethane group and the quinones.

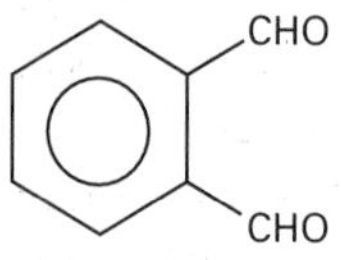

CHO

CHO

Fig. 2.16 *o*-Phthalaldehyde (OPA).

8.1 Acridines

8.1.1 Chemistry

The acridines (Fig. 2.17) are heterocyclic compounds that have proved to be of some value as antimicrobial agents. Acridine itself is feebly basic, but two of the five possible monoaminoacridines are strong bases, and these (3-aminoacridine and 9-aminoacridine) exist as the resonance hybrid of two canonical formulae. Both these monoacridines are well ionized as the cation at pH 7.3, and this has an important bearing on their antimicrobial activity (see below and Table 2.10). Further information on the chemistry of the acridines can be found in Albert's excellent book (Albert, 1966).

8.1.2 Antimicrobial activity

The acridines are of considerable interest because they illustrate how small changes in the chemical structure of the molecule cause significant changes in antibacterial activity. The most important limiting factor governing this activity is the degree of ionization, although this must be cationic in nature (Table 2.10). Acridine derivatives that form anions or zwitterions are only poorly antibacterial in comparison with those that form cations. In general terms, if the degree of ionization is less than 33% there is only feeble antibacterial activity, whereas above about 50% there is little further increase in activity (Albert, 1966).

In contrast to the triphenylmethane dyes (Section 8.2), the acridines do not display a selective action against Gram-positive organisms, nor are they inactivated by serum. Acridines compete with H^+ ions for anionic sites on the bacterial cell and are more effective at alkaline than acid pH (Browning *et al.*, 1919–20). They are relatively slow in their action and are not sporicidal (Foster & Russell, 1971). Resistance to the acridines develops as a result of mutation and indirect selection (Thornley & Yudkin, 1959a,b). Interestingly, acridines can eliminate ('cure') resistance in R^+ strains (see Watanabe, 1963, for an

Table 2.10 Dependence of antibacterial activity of acridines on cationic ionization (based on the work of Albert and his colleagues (see Albert, 1966)).

Substance	Predominant type (and percentage) of ionization at pH 3 and 37°C	Inhibitory activity
9-Aminoacridine	Cation (99%)	High
9-Aminoacridine-2-carboxylic acid	Zwitterion (99.8%)	Low
Acridine	Neutral molecule (99.7%)	Low
Acridine-9-carboxylic acid	Anion (99.3%)	Low

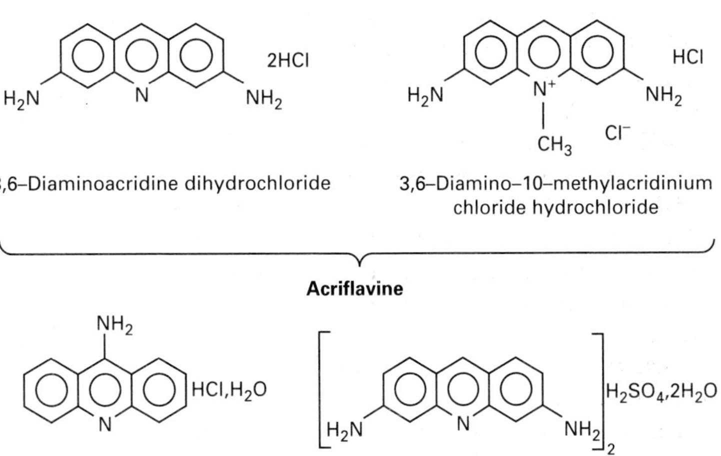

Fig. 2.17 Acridine compounds.

early review). Viljanen & Boratynski (1991) provide more recent information about plasmid curing.

The MRSA and methicillin-resistant *Staphylococcus epidermidis* (MRSE) strains are more resistance to acridines than are antibiotic-sensitive strains, although this resistance depends on the presence of *qac* genes, especially *qac*A or *qac*B Littlejohn *et al.*, 1992; Leelaporn *et al.*, 1994).

8.1.3 Uses

For many years, the acridines held a valuable place in medicine. However, with the advent of antibiotics and other chemotherapeutic agents, they are now used infrequently. Their major use has been the treatment of infected wounds. The first compound to be used medically was acriflavine (a mixture of 3,6-diaminoacridine hydrochloride and 3,6-diamino-10-methylacridinium hydrochloride, the former component being better known as proflavine). Proflavine hemisulphate and 9-aminoacridine (aminacrine) have found use in treating wounds; aminacrine is particularly useful as it is non-staining.

8.2 Triphenylmethane dyes

The most important members of this group are cyrstal violet, brilliant green and malachite green (Fig. 2.18). These were used as local antiseptics for application to wounds and burns, but were limited in being effective against Gram-positive bacteria (inhibitory concentrations 1 in 750 000 to 1 in 5 000 000) but much less so against Gram-negative organisms, and in suffering a serious decrease in activity in the presence of serum. Their selective activity against Gram-positive bacteria has a practical application in the formulation of selective media for diagnostic purposes, e.g. crystal violet lactose broth in water filtration-control work.

The activity of the triphenylmethane dyes is a property of the pseudobase, the formation which is established by equilibrium between the cation and the base; thus, both the ionization and the equilibrium constants will affect the activity (Albert, 1966). Antimicrobial potency depends on external pH, being more pronounced at alkaline values (Moats & Maddox, 1978).

For an extensive account of the antibacterial dyestuffs, see Browning (1964).

The MRSA and MRSE strains containing *qac* genes are more resistant to crystal violet than are plasmidless strains of *Staph. aureus* and *Staph. epidermidis*, respectively (Littlejohn *et al.*, 1992; Leelaporn *et al.*, 1994). This is believed to be the result of an efficient efflux system in the resistant strains (Paulsen *et al.*, 1996a,b). However, crystal violet finds little, if any, use nowadays as an antibacterial agent, and the clinical relevance of this finding thus remains uncertain (Russell & Chopra, 1996; Russell, 1997).

8.3 Quinones

Some members of this group of dyes are important agricultural fungicides. The quinones are natural dyes, which give colour to many forms of plant and animal life. Chemically (Fig. 2.19), they are diketocyclohexadienes; the simplest member is 1,4-benzoquinone. In terms of toxicity to bacteria, moulds and yeast, naphthaquinones are the most toxic, followed (in this order) by phenanthrenequinones, benzoquinones and anthraquinones.

Antimicrobial activity is increased by halogenation and two powerful agricultural fungicides are chloranil (tetrachloro-1,4-benzoquinone) and dichlone (2,3-dichloro-1,4-naphthaquinone); see D'Arcy (1971) and Owens (1969).

9 Halogens

The most important microbicidal halogens are iodine compounds, chlorine compounds and

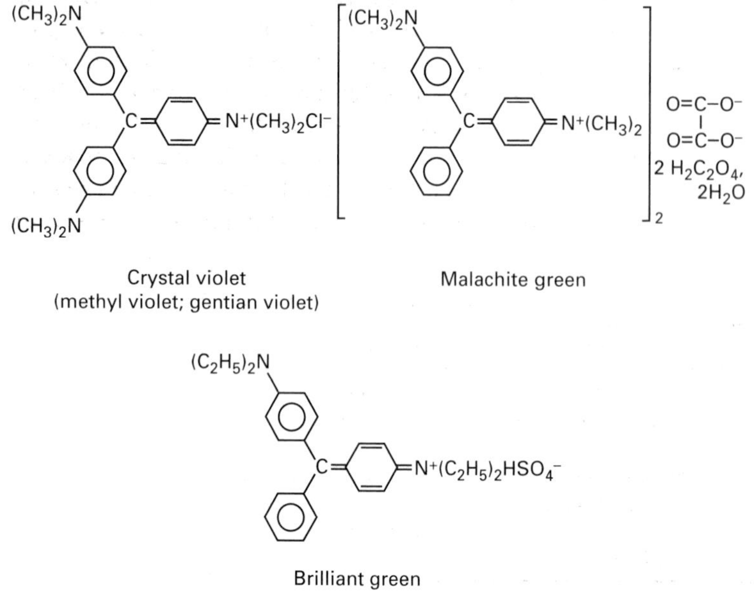

$(CH_3)_2N$, $(CH_3)_2N$, $=N^+(CH_3)_2Cl^-$

Crystal violet
(methyl violet; gentian violet)

$[(CH_3)_2N \ldots =N^+(CH_3)_2]_2$ $O=C-O^-$ / $O=C-O^-$, $2\ H_2C_2O_4$, $2H_2O$

Malachite green

$(C_2H_5)_2N \ldots =N^+(C_2H_5)_2HSO_4^-$

Brilliant green

Fig. 2.18 Triphenylmethane dyes.

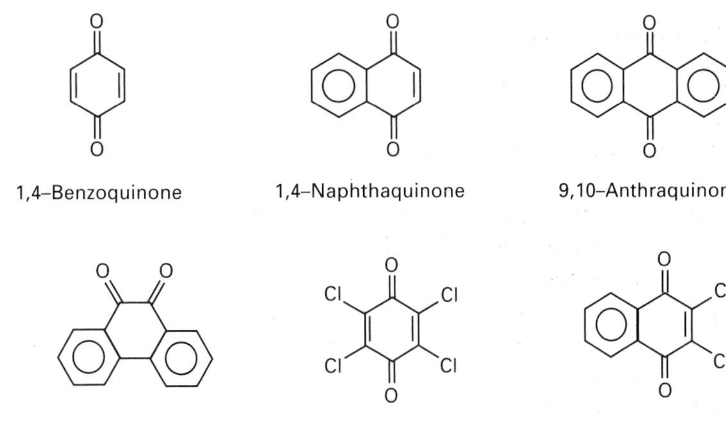

Fig. 2.19 Quinones.

bromine. Fluorine is far too toxic, irritant and corrosive for use as a disinfectant (Trueman, 1971), although, interestingly, fluoride ions have been shown to induce bacterial lysis (Lesher *et al.*, 1977). This section will deal predominantly with iodine, iodophors and chlorine-releasing compounds (those which are bactericidal by virtue of 'available chlorine'), but bromine, iodoform and (considered here for convenience) chloroform will be considered briefly.

9.1 Iodine compounds

9.1.1 Free iodine

Iodine was first employed in the treatment of wounds some 140 years ago and has been shown to be an efficient microbicidal agent with rapid lethal effects against bacteria and their spores, moulds, yeasts and viruses (Gershenfeld, 1956; Anon., 1965; Sykes, 1965; Russell, 1971b; Kelsey & Maurer, 1972). It is normally used in aqueous or alcoholic solution; it is only sparingly soluble in cold water but solutions can be made with potassium iodide. Iodine is less reactive chemically than chlorine, and is less affected by the presence of organic matter than is the latter; however, it must be added that, whereas the activity of high concentrations of iodine is little affected by organic matter, that of low concentrations is significantly lowered. The activity of iodine is greater at acid than at alkaline pH; see Table 2.11. Unfortunately, iodine solutions stain fabric and tend to be toxic.

9.1.2 Iodophors

Certain surface-active agents can solubilize iodine to form compounds (the iodophors) that retain the germicidal action but not the undesirable properties of iodine. The uses of the iodophors as detergent-sterilizers have been described by Blatt & Maloney (1961) and Davis (1962). The term iodophor itself means, literally, iodine-carrier. It must be noted that different concentrations of iodophors are used for antiseptic and disinfectant

Table 2.11 Effect of pH on the antimicrobial activity of iodine compounds (based on Trueman, 1971).

pH	Active form	Comment
Acid and neutral	I_2(diatomic iodine) Hypo-iodous acid	Highly bactericidal Less bactericidal
Alkaline	Hypo-iodite ion Iodate (IO_3^-), iodide (I^-) and tri-iodide (I_3^-) ions	Even less bactericidal All inactive

purposes, and that the lower concentrations employed in antisepsis are not claimed to be sporicidal (Favero, 1985, 1995).

Gershenfeld (1962) has shown that povidone-iodine is sporicidal, and Lowbury *et al.* (1964) found that povidone-iodine compressess reduced the numbers viable spores of *Bacillus globigii* on the skin by >99% in 1 h, suggesting that this iodophor had a part to play in removing transient sporing organisms from operation sites. The importance of povidone-iodine in preventing wound infection was re-emphasized as a result of the studies of Galland *et al.* (1977) and Lacey (1979).

The concentration of free iodine in aqueous or alcoholic iodine solutions is responsible for microbicidal activity. Likewise, the concentration of free iodine in an iodophor is responsible for its activity: this was proved by Allawala & Riegelman (1953), who made a log–log plot of the killing time against the amount of free iodine, and who showed that the 99% killing time against *B. cereus* spores was a function of the concentration of free iodine in the presence or absence of added surface-active agents.

In most iodophor preparations, the carrier is usually a non-ionic surfactant, in which the iodine is present as micellar aggregates. When an iodophor is diluted with water, dispersion of the micelles occurs and most (80–90%) of the iodine is slowly liberated. Dilution below the CMC of the non-ionic surface-active agent results in iodine being in simple aqueous solution. A paradoxical effect of dilution on the activity of povidone-iodine has been observed (Gottardi, 1985; Rackur, 1985). As the degree of dilution increases, then beyond a certain point bactericidal activity also increases. An explanation of this arises from consideration of physicochemical studies, which demonstrate that, starting from a 10% commercially available povidone-iodine solution, the concentration of non-complexed iodine (I_2) initially increases as dilution increases. This reaches a maximum value at about 0.1% and then falls. In contrast, the content of other iodine species, e.g. I^- and I_3^- decreases continuously. These properties affect the sporicidal activity of iodine solutions (Williams & Russell, 1991).

The iodophors, as stated above, are microbicidal, with activity over a wide pH range. The presence of a surface-active agent as carrier improves the wetting capacity. Iodophors may be used in the dairy industry (when employed in the cleansing of dairy plant it is important to keep the pH on the acid side to ensure adequate removal of milkstone) and for skin and wound disinfection. Iodophors, such as Betadine, in the form of alcoholic solutions are widely used in the USA for disinfection of hands for operation sites (see also Chapter 13). Pseudobacteraemia (false-positive blood cultures) has been found to result from the use of contaminated antiseptics. Craven *et al.* (1981) have described such an outbreak of pseudobacteraemia caused by a 10% povidone-iodine solution contaminated with Burkholderia (*Pseudomonas*) *cepacia*.

The properties, antimicrobial activity, mechanisms of action and uses of iodine and its compounds have been described by Rutala (1990), Favero & Bond (1991), Banner (1995), Favero (1995) and Bloomfield (1996). Information about the revival of iodine-treated spores of *B. subtilis* is provided by Williams & Russell (1992, 1993a, b,c).

9.1.3 Iodoform

When applied to tissues, iodoform (CHI_3) slowly releases elemental iodine. It thus has some weak antimicrobial activity. It is not often used in practice, and thus will not be considered further.

9.2 Chlorine compounds

9.2.1 Chlorine-releasing compounds

Until the development of chlorinated soda solution, surgical (Dakin's solution), in 1916, the commercial chlorine-releasing disinfectants then in use were not of constant composition and contained free alkali and sometimes free chlorine. The stability of free available chlorine in solution is dependent on a number of factors, especially the following (Dychdala, 1983):

1 Chlorine concentration.
2 pH of organic matter.
3 Presence the solution.
4 Light.

These factors are considered below.

The types of chlorine compounds that are most frequently used are the hypochlorites and *N*-chloro compounds (Trueman, 1971; Dychdala, 1983; Gardner & Peel, 1986, 1991; Favero & Bond, 1991; Bloomfield & Arthur, 1994; Banner, 1995; Favero, 1995; Bloomfield, 1996).

Hypochlorites. These have a wide antibacterial spectrum, although they are less active against spores than against non-sporulating bacteria and have been stated to be of low activity against mycobacteria (Anon., 1965; Croshaw, 1971). Recent studies have suggested that chlorine compounds are among the most potent sporicidal agents (Kelsey *et al.*, 1974; Coates & Death, 1978; Death & Coates, 1979; Coates & Hutchinson, 1994). The hypochlorites show activity against lipid and non-lipid viruses (Morris & Darlow, 1971; Favero, 1995; Bloomfield, 1996).

Two factors that can affect quite markedly their antimicrobial action are organic matter, since chlorine is a highly reactive chemical, and pH, the hypochlorites being more active at acid than at alkaline pH (Table 2.12). The former problem can, to some extent, be overcome by increasing the hypochlorite concentration, and it has been shown that the sporicidal activity of sodium hypochlorite (200 parts/10^6 available chlorine) can be potentiated by 1.5–4% sodium hydroxide, notwithstanding the above comment about pH (Russell, 1971b, 1982). The sporicidal activity can also be potentiated by low concentrations of ammonia (Weber & Levine, 1944) and in the presence of bromine (Farkas-Himsley, 1964); chlorine-resistant bacteria have been found to be unaffected by bromine but to be readily killed by chlorine–bromine solutions (Farkas-Himsley, 1964). Such mixtures could be of value in the disinfection of natural waters.

Organic chlorine compounds. N-chloro compounds, which contain the =N–Cl group, show microbicidal activity. Examples of such compounds, the chemical structures of which are shown in Fig. 2.20, are chloramine-T, dichloramine-T, halazone, halane, dichloroisocyanuric acid, sodium and potassium dichloroisocyanurates and trichloroisocyanuric acid. All appear to hydrolyse in water to produce an imino (=NH) group. Their action is claimed to be slower than that of the hypochlorites, although this can be increased under acidic conditions (Cousins & Allan, 1967). A series of imidazolidinone *N′,N′*-dihalamine disinfectants has been described (Williams *et al.*, 1987, 1988; Worley *et al.*, 1987). The dibromo compound (Fig. 2.20) was the most rapidly acting bactericide, particularly under halogen demand-free conditions, with the mixed bromo-chloro compound (Fig. 2.20) occupying an intermediate position. However, when stability of the compounds in the series was also taken into account, it was concluded that the mixed product was the most useful as an aqueous disinfectant solution.

Coates (1985) found that solutions of sodium hypochlorite (NaOCl) and sodium dichloroisocyanurate (NaDCC) containing the same levels of available chlorine had similar bactericidal activity despite significant differences in their pH. Solutions of NaDCC are less susceptible than NaOCl

Table 2.12 Factors influencing activity of hypochlorites.

Factor	Result
pH	Activity decreased by increasing pH (see text and use of NaOH also)
Concentration of hypochlorite (pH constant)	Activity depends on concentration of available chlorine
Organic matter	Antimicrobial activity reduced considerably
Other agents	Potentiation may be achieved by **1** addition of ammonia **2** 1.5–4% sodium hydroxide* **3** addition of small amounts of bromide†

*Cousins & Allan (1967).

†In the presence of bromide, hypochlorite also has an enhanced effect in bleaching cellulosic fibres.

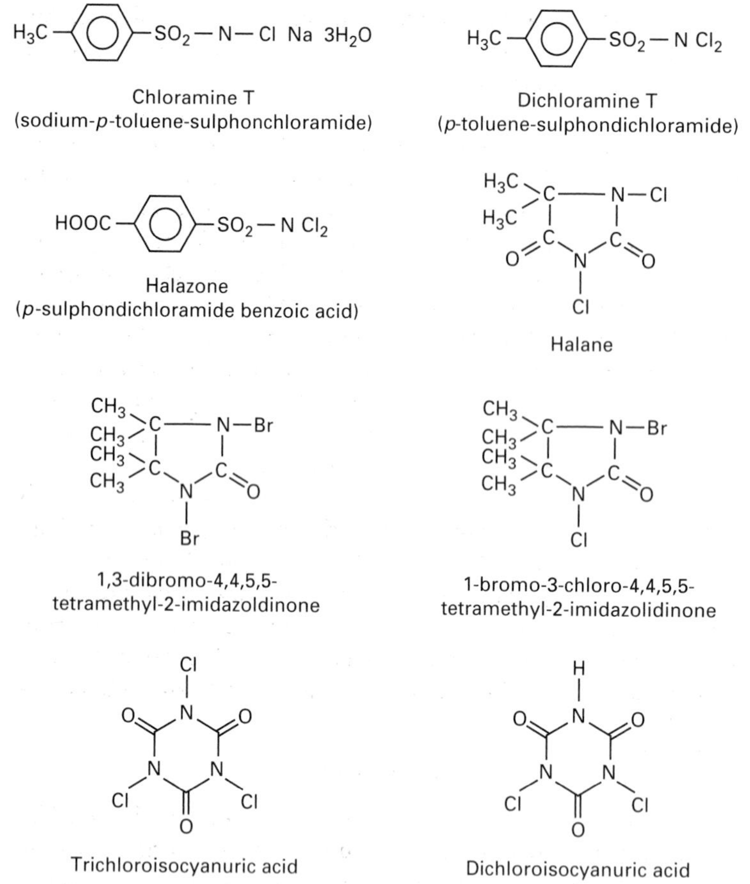

Chloramine T
(sodium-*p*-toluene-sulphonchloramide)

Dichloramine T
(*p*-toluene-sulphondichloramide)

Halazone
(*p*-sulphondichloramide benzoic acid)

Halane

1,3-dibromo-4,4,5,5-tetramethyl-2-imidazoldinone

1-bromo-3-chloro-4,4,5,5-tetramethyl-2-imidazolidinone

Trichloroisocyanuric acid

Dichloroisocyanuric acid

Fig. 2.20 Organic chlorine compounds.

to inactivation by organic matter (Bloomfield & Miles, 1979a,b; Bloomfield & Uso, 1985; Coates, 1985, 1988).

Uses of chlorine-releasing compounds. Chlorinated soda solution (Dakin's solution), which contains 0.5–0.55% (5000–5500 parts/10^6) available chlorine, and chlorinated lime and boric acid solution (Eusol), which contains 0.25% (2500 parts/10^6) available chlorine, are chlorine disinfectants that contain chlorinated lime and boric acid. Dakin's solution is used as a wound disinfectant or, when appropriately diluted, as an irrigation solution for bladder and vaginal infections. Eusol is used as a wound disinfectant, but Morgan (1989) has suggested that chlorinated solutions delay wound healing.

Chlorine gas has been employed to disinfect public water-supplies. Sodium hypochlorite is normally used for the disinfection of swimming-pools.

Blood spillages containing HIV or HBV can be disinfected with NaOCl solutions containing 10 000 parts/10^6 available chlorine (Working Party, 1985). Added directly to the spillage as powder or granules, NaDCC is also effective, may give a larger margin of safety because a higher concentration of available chlorine is achieved and is also less susceptible to inactivation by organic matter, as pointed out above (Coates, 1988). Furthermore, only a very short contact time (2–3 min) is necessary before the spill can be removed safely (Coates & Wilson, 1989). Chlorine-releasing powder formulations with high available chlorine concentrations are particularly useful for this purpose (Bloomfield & Miller, 1989; Bloomfield *et al.*, 1990).

Chlorine dioxide, an alternative to sodium

hypochlorite, is more active at alkaline pH and in the presence of organic matter and more environmentally satisfactory (BS 7152, 1991).

Additional information. Chlorine-releasing agents continue to be widely studied. Their sporicidal activity has been described by Te Giffel *et al.* (1996) and Coates (1996), their antiviral efficacy by Bellamy (1995), van Bueren (1995), Bond (1995) and Hernandez *et al.* (1996, 1997) and their usefulness in dental practice by Molinari (1995), Cottone & Molinari (1996) and Gurevich *et al.* (1996).

9.2.2 *Chloroform*

Chloroform ($CHCl_3$) has been used as a preservative in many pharmaceutical products intended for internal use, for more than a century. In recent years, with the object of minimizing microbial contamination, this use has been extended. Various authors, notably Westwood & Pin-Lim (1972) and Lynch *et al.* (1977), have shown chloroform to be a bactericidal agent, although it is not sporicidal and its high volatility means that a fall in concentration could result in microbial growth. For details of its antibacterial activity in aqueous solutions and in mixtures containing insoluble powders and the losses, through volatilization, under 'in-use' conditions, the paper by Lynch *et al.* (1977) should certainly be consulted.

The present position is that chloroform may be used in oral pharmaceutical products at concentrations of no greater than 0.5%; in cosmetic products its use (at a maximum concentration of 4%) will be restricted to toothpaste. It is totally banned in the USA. It is noteworthy that, in an article on the preservation of cosmetics and toiletries, Hill (1995) describes those cosmetic preservatives allowed in the European Union (EU): chloroform is not included in this list.

9.3 Bromine

The antimicrobial activity of bromine was first observed in the 1930s, but it was not until the 1960s that it was used commercially in water disinfection. The most commonly used oxidizing biocide in recirculating waters is chlorine, but bromine has been put forward as an alternative (Elsmore, 1993).

Elemental bromine is not itself employed commercially. The two available methods (Elsmore, 1995) are: (i) activated bromide produced by reacting sodium bromide with a strong oxidizing agent, such as sodium hypochlorite or gaseous chlorine; and (ii) organic bromine-releasing agents, such as *N*-bromo-*N*-chlorodimethylhydantoin (BCDMH; Fig. 2.21a). When BCDMH hydrolyses in water, it liberates the biocidal agents hypobromous acid (HOBr) and hypochlorous acid (HOCl), together with the carrier, dimethylhydantoin (DMH; Fig. 2.21b).

Both HOBr and HOCl would appear to contribute towards the overall germicidal activity of BCDMH. However, Elsmore (1993, 1995) has pointed out that the primary agent present in water is HOBr. Hypochlorous acid is used up in regenerating 'spent bromine' produced when HOBr reacts with organic materials and microorganisms:

$$HOCl + Br^- \rightarrow HOBr + Cl^-$$

Bromine is claimed to have a greater bactericidal activity than chlorine. It is effective against *Legionella pneumophila* in the laboratory and in field studies (McCoy & Wireman, 1989). The pK_a for HOBr (8.69) is higher than that for HOCl (7.48) and thus, at the normal alkaline pH values found in cooling towers, there is a significantly higher amount of active biocide present with HOBr than with HOCl.

10 Quinoline and isoquinoline derivatives

There are three main groups of derivatives:

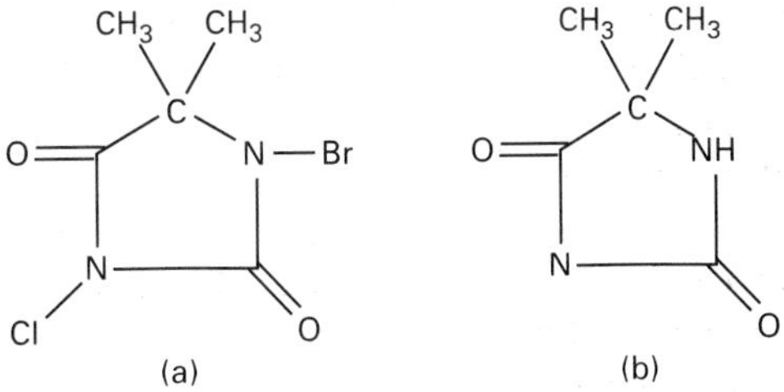

Fig. 2.21 (a) Bromochlorodimethylhydantoin (BCDMH); (b) dimethylhydantoin (DMH).

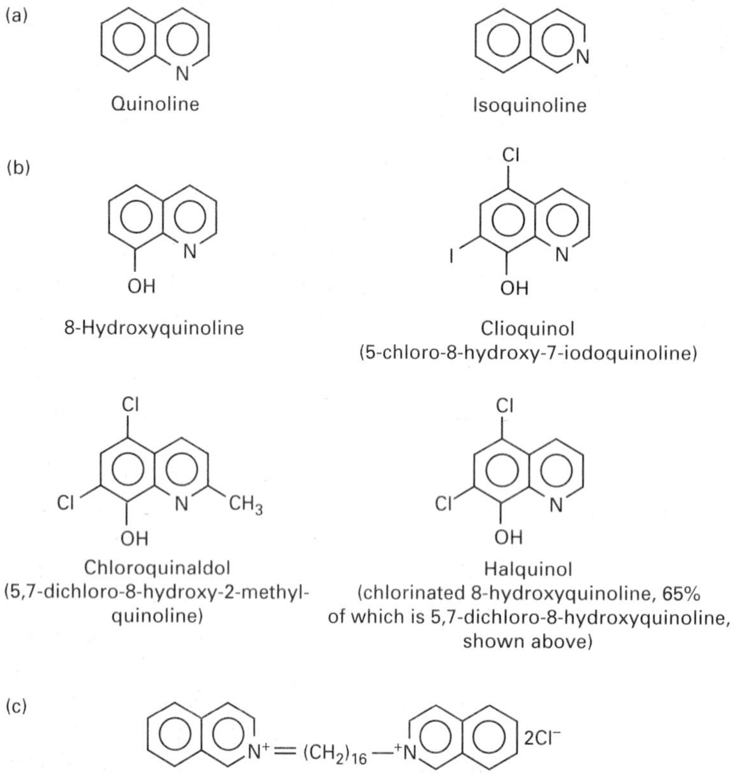

(a)

Quinoline

Isoquinoline

(b)

8-Hydroxyquinoline

Clioquinol (5-chloro-8-hydroxy-7-iodoquinoline)

Chloroquinaldol (5,7-dichloro-8-hydroxy-2-methyl-quinoline)

Halquinol (chlorinated 8-hydroxyquinoline, 65% of which is 5,7-dichloro-8-hydroxyquinoline, shown above)

(c)

$N^+ = (CH_2)_{16} — {}^+N$ $2Cl^-$

Fig. 2.22 (a) Structures of quinoline and isoquinoline; (b) 8-hydroxyquinoline derivatives with antimicrobial properties; (c) hedaquinium chloride.

8-hydroxyquinoline derivatives, 4-aminoquinaldinium derivatives and isoquinoline derivatives. They are described in Figs. 2.22 and 2.23.

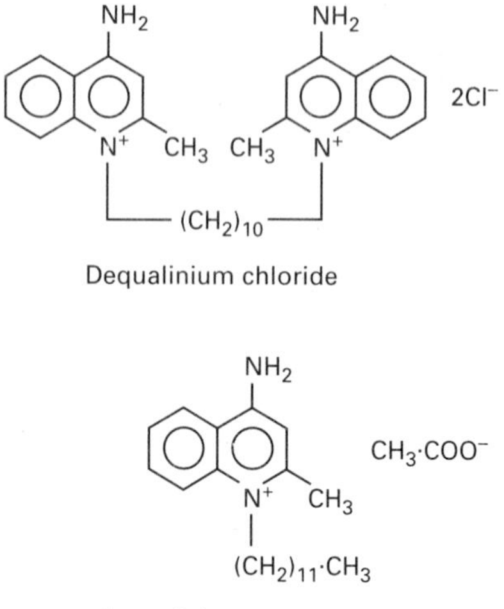

10.1 8-Hydroxyquinoline derivatives

8-Hydroxyquinoline (oxine) possesses antibacterial activity against Gram-positive bacteria, but much less against Gram-negative organisms. It also has antifungal activity, although this occurs at a slower rate. Other useful compounds are depicted in Fig. 2.22a). Like oxine, clioquinol, chlorquinandol and halquinol have very low water solubilities, and are generally employed as applications to the skin. An interesting feature of their activity (discussed in more detail in Chapter 9) is the fact that they are chelating agents, which are active only in the presence of certain metal ions.

Dequalinium chloride

Laurolinium acetate

Fig. 2.23 4-Aminoquinaldinium derivatives with antimicrobial properties.

10.2 4-Aminoquinaldinium derivatives

These are QACs (see Fig. 2.23), which also fall into this grouping. The most important members are laurolinium acetate and dequalinium chloride (a bis-QAC). Both compounds possess antibacterial activity, especially against Gram-positive bacteria (Collier *et al.*, 1959; Cox & D'Arcy, 1962), as well as significant activity against many species of yeasts and fungi (Frier, 1971; D'Arcy, 1971). Their activity is decreased in the presence of lecithin; serum decreases the effectiveness of laurolinium but not of dequalinium. Dequalinium chloride is used as lozenges or paint in the treatment of infections of the mouth and throat. Laurolinium has been used as a preoperative skin disinfectant, although this was never widely adopted.

10.3 Isoquinoline derivatives

The most important isoquinoline derivative is hedaquinium chloride (Fig. 2.22c), another bisquaternary salt. This possesses antibacterial and antifungal activity (Collier *et al.*, 1959; D'Arcy, 1971), and is regarded as one of the most active antifungal QAC agents (D'Arcy, 1971).

11 Alcohols

Several alcohols have been shown to possess antimicrobial properties. Generally, the alcohols have rapid bactericidal activity (Morton, 1950), including acid-fast bacilli, but are not sporicidal; they have low activity against some viruses, but are viricidal towards others. Their chemical structures are shown in Fig. 2.24.

11.1 Ethyl alcohol (ethanol)

Ethanol is rapidly lethal to non-sporulating bacteria and destroys mycobacteria (Croshaw, 1971) but is ineffective at all concentrations against bacterial spores (Russell, 1971b). The presence of water is essential for its activity, but concentrations below 30% have little action. Activity, in fact, drops sharply below 50% (Rutala, 1990).

The most effective concentration is about 60–70% (Price, 1950; see also Croshaw, 1977; Morton, 1977; Scott & Gorman, 1987). Solutions of iodine or chlorhexidine in 70% alcohol may be employed for the preoperative disinfection of the skin. Ethanol is the alcohol of choice in cosmetic products because of its relative lack of odour and irritation (Bandelin, 1977).

Some variable results have been reported about the effects of ethanol on HIV. Tjøtta *et al.* (1991) showed that 70% ethanol in the presence of 2.5% serum produced a 3-log/ml reduction in virus titre after a 10-min contact period, as determined by plaque assay or immunofluorescence. In contrast, using a $TCID_{50}$ assay, Resnick *et al.* (1986) found that 70% alcohol after 1min and in the presence of 50% plasma yielded a 7-log reduction in $TCID_{50}$/ml, again in a suspension test. Van Bueren *et al.* (1994) also described a rapid inactivation of HIV-1 in suspension, irrespective of the protein load. The rate of inactivation decreased when high protein levels were present when a carrier test was employed. A notable feature of the experiments carried out by van Buesen *et al.* (1994) was the care taken to ensure that residual alcohol was neutralized to prevent toxicity to the cell line employed in detecting uninactivated virus.

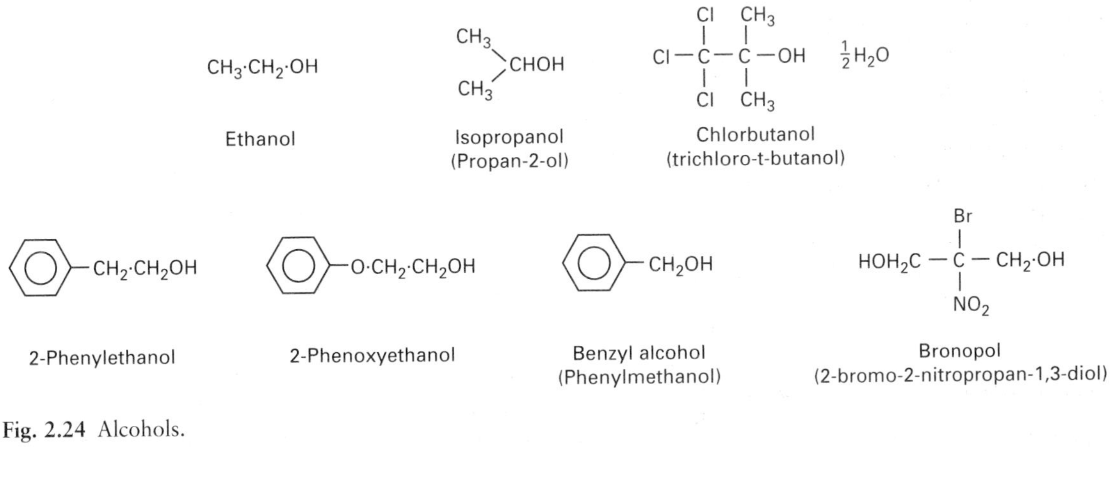

$CH_3{\cdot}CH_2{\cdot}OH$ — Ethanol

$(CH_3)_2CHOH$ — Isopropanol (Propan-2-ol)

$Cl_3C{-}C(CH_3)_2{-}OH \cdot \frac{1}{2}H_2O$ — Chlorbutanol (trichloro-t-butanol)

$C_6H_5{-}CH_2{\cdot}CH_2OH$ — 2-Phenylethanol

$C_6H_5{-}O{\cdot}CH_2{\cdot}CH_2OH$ — 2-Phenoxyethanol

$C_6H_5{-}CH_2OH$ — Benzyl alcohol (Phenylmethanol)

$HOH_2C{-}C(Br)(NO_2){-}CH_2{\cdot}OH$ — Bronopol (2-bromo-2-nitropropan-1,3-diol)

Fig. 2.24 Alcohols.

The non-enveloped poliovirus is more resistant to biocides in general than the herpesvirus, and ethanol caused no inactivation of poliovirus in a suspension test (Tyles *et al.*, 1990).

11.2 Methyl alcohol (methanol)

Methyl alcohol has poor antibacterial activity and is not sporicidal (Russell, 1971b; Bandelin, 1977; Coates & Death, 1978; Death & Coates, 1979). Furthermore, it is potentially toxic, and is thus little used. However, freshly prepared mixtures of alcohols (especially methanol) and sodium hypochlorite are highly sporicidal (Coates & Death, 1978). Although it was then considered that methanol was potentiating the activity of hypochlorites, it is, in fact, more likely that hypochlorites, by virtue of their effects on the outer spore layers (Bloomfield and Arthur, 1994), are aiding the penetration of methanol into the spore.

11.3 Isopropyl alcohol (isopropanol)

Isopropyl and *n*-propyl alcohols are more effective bactericides than ethanol (Anon., 1965; Kelsey & Maurer, 1972), but are not sporicidal. They are miscible with water in all proportions, but isopropanol has a less objectionable odour than *n*-propanol and is considered as a suitable alternative to ethanol in various cosmetic products, either as a solvent or as a preservative (Bandelin, 1977; Hill, 1995).

Isopropanol has viricidal activity, but not towards 'hydrophilic' (non-lipid-enveloped) viruses (Rutala, 1990). Van Bueren *et al.* (1994) have demonstrated inactivation of HIV type 1 by isopropanol. For further information, the papers by Tyler *et al.* (1990) and Sattar & Springthorpe (1991) should be consulted.

11.4 Benzyl alcohol

In addition to having antimicrobial properties, benzyl alcohol is a weak local anaesthetic. It has activity against Gram-positive and Gram-negative bacteria and against moulds (D'Arcy, 1971).

Benzyl alcohol is incompatable with oxidizing agents and is inactivated by non-ionic surfactants; it is stable to autoclaving and is normally used at a concentration of 1% v/v (Denyer & Wallhäusser, 1990).

11.5 Phenylethanol (phenylethyl alcohol)

Phenylethyl alcohol is an antimicrobial agent with selective activity against various bacteria (especially Gram-negative (Lilley & Brewer, 1953) and which has been recommended for use as a preservative in ophthalmic solutions, often in conjunction with another microbicide. Because of its higher activity against Gram-negative bacteria, phenylethyl alcohol may be incorporated into culture media for isolating Gram-positive bacteria from mixed flora, e.g. phenylethyl alcohol agar.

Phenylethanol is commonly used at a concentration of 0.3–0.5% v/v; it shows poor stability with oxidants and is partially inactivated by non-ionic surfactants (Denyer & Wallhäusser, 1990).

11.6 Bronopol

Bronopol, 2-bromo-2-nitropropan-1,3-diol, is an aliphatic halogenonitro compound with antibacterial and antifungal activity, although bacterial spores are unaffected. It is effective against *P. aeruginosa*. Its activity is reduced somewhat by 10% serum and to a greater extent by sulphydryl compounds, but is unaffected by 1% polysorbate or 0.1% lecithin. It has a half-life of about 96 days at pH and 25°C (Toler, 1985).

Bronopol is most stable under acid conditions; the initial decomposition appears to involve the liberation of formaldehyde and the formulation of bromonitroethanol (Fig. 2.25a). A second-order

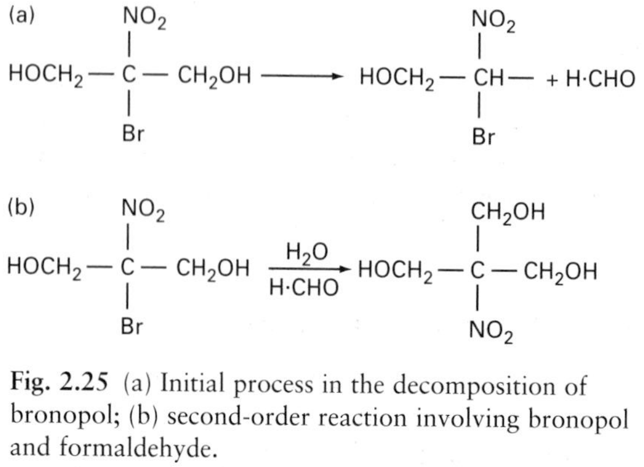

(a)

$$HOCH_2-C(NO_2)(Br)-CH_2OH \longrightarrow HOCH_2-CH(NO_2)(Br)- + H{\cdot}CHO$$

(b)

$$HOCH_2-C(NO_2)(Br)-CH_2OH \xrightarrow[H{\cdot}CHO]{H_2O} HOCH_2-C(CH_2OH)(NO_2)-CH_2OH$$

Fig. 2.25 (a) Initial process in the decomposition of bronopol; (b) second-order reaction involving bronopol and formaldehyde.

reaction involving bronopol and formaldehyde occurs simultaneously to produce 2-hydroxymethyl-2-nitro-1,3-propanediol (Fig. 2.25b), which itself decomposes with the loss of formaldehyde.

Details of the microbiological activity, chemical stability, toxicology and uses of bronopol are documented by Bryce *et al.* (1978), Croshaw & Holland (1984), Toler (1985) and Rossmore & Sondossi (1988). Denyer & Wallhäusser (1990) have provided useful information about bronopol, the typical in-use concentration of which is 0.01–0.1% w/v. Sulphydryl compounds act as appropriate neutralizers in preservative efficacy tests.

11.7 Phenoxyethanol (phenoxetol)

The antimicrobial activity of phenoxyethanol and other preservatives has been reviewed by Gucklhorn (1970, 1971). Phenoxyethanol was shown by Berry (1944) to possess significant activity against *P. aeruginosa*, but it has less activity against other Gram-negative organisms or against Gram-positive bacteria. Phenoxyethanol is stable to autoclaving and is compatible with anionic and cationic surfactants, but it shows reduced activity in the presence of polysorbate 80. It is used as a preservative, typical concentration 1% (Denyer & Wallhäusser, 1990).

11.8 Chlorbutanol (chlorbutol)

Chlorbutol is an antibacterial and antifungal agent. It has been used, at a concentration of 0.5% w/v, as a bactericide in injections. One drawback to its employment is its instability, since at acid pH it decomposes at the high temperature used in sterilization processes into hydrochloric acid, and at alkaline pH it is unstable at room temperature.

Chlorbutanol is incompatible with some non-ionic surfactants. Its typical in-use concentration as a pharmaceutical preservative is 0.3–0.5% w/v (Denyer & Wallhäusser, 1990).

11.9 2,4-Dichlorobenzyl alcohol

This substance is a white powder, soluble in water to 1% and readily soluble in alcohols. Its ionization is negligible for all practical purposes and it is thus active over a wide pH range. It has a broad spectrum of activity, but both pseudomonads and *S. aureus* show some resistance to it (Toler, 1985).

12 Peroxygens

12.1 Hydrogen peroxide

Hydrogen peroxide (H_2O_2) is a familiar household antiseptic. It was discovered in 1818 and was early recognized as possessing antibacterial properties. These were extensively investigated in 1893 by Traugott.

Hydrogen peroxide is available as a solution designated as 20- or 10-volume, a means of indicating its strength by describing the volume (20 or 10, respectively) of oxygen evolved from 1 volume of the peroxide solution. Strengths for industrial use of 35, 50 or 90% are available. Hydrogen peroxide solutions are unstable, and benzoic acid or another suitable substance is added as a stabilizer.

Hydrogen peroxide solutions possess disinfectant, antiseptic and deodorant properties. When in contact with living tissue and many metals they decompose, evolving oxygen. Hydrogen peroxide is bactericidal and sporicidal (Russell, 1982, 1990a,b, 1991a,b; Baldry, 1983; Baldry & Fraser, 1988) and is believed to act as a generator of free hydroxyl radicals, which can cause DNA strand breakage. It is an oxidizing agent and reacts with oxidizable material, for example alkali nitrites used in anticorrosion solutions. It is environmentally friendly because its decomposition products are oxygen and water (Miller, 1996).

Hydrogen peroxide has been used in aseptic packaging technology and for disinfecting contact lenses.

Microbial inactivation is more rapid with liquid peroxide than with vapour generated from that liquid acting at the same temperature (Sintim-Damoa, 1993). However, the vapour can be used for the purposes of sterilization, where, at a concentration of 1–5 mg/l, it generally shows good penetration.

Attention has recently been devoted to developing a plasma-activated peroxide vapour process, in which radio waves produce the plasma. This is believed to be microbicidal by virtue of the hydroxyl ions and other free radicals that are generated (Groschel, 1995; Lever & Sutton, 1996).

The use of hydrogen peroxide as a contact-lens disinfectant has been reviewed (Miller, 1996).

12.2 Peracetic acid

Peracetic acid, $CH_3{\cdot}COOOH$, was introduced as an antibacterial agent in 1955. It is available commercially as a 15% aqueous solution, in which an equilibrium exists between peracetic acid and its decomposition products acetic acid ($CH_3{\cdot}COOH$) and hydrogen peroxide.

Peracetic acid solution has a broad spectrum of activity, including bacteria and their spores, moulds, yeasts, algae and viruses. It finds extensive use in the food industry and for disinfecting sewage sludge. It is a powerful oxidizing agent and in certain situations can be corrosive. The great advantage of peracetic acid is that its final decomposition products, oxygen and water, are innocuous.

More comprehensive data on peracetic acid are provided by Baldry (1983), Fraser (1986), Baldry & Fraser (1988), Coates (1996) and Russell & Chopra (1996).

13 Chelating agents

This section will deal briefly with chelating agents based on EDTA. Ethylenediamine tetraacetic acid has been the subject of intensive investigation for many years, and its antibacterial activity has been reviewed by Russell (1971a), Leive (1974) and Wilkinson (1975). The chemical nature of its complexation with metals has been well considered by West (1969).

The chemical structures of EDTA, ethylenedioxybis(ethyliminodi(acetic acid)) (EGTA), *N*-hydroxyethylethylenediamine-*NN′N′*-triacetic acid (HDTA), *trans*-1,2-diaminocyclohexane-*NNN′N′*-tetra-acetic acid (CDTA), iminodiacetic acid (IDA) and nitrilotriacetic acid (NTA) are provided in Fig. 2.26. Table 2.13 lists their chelating and antibacterial activities.

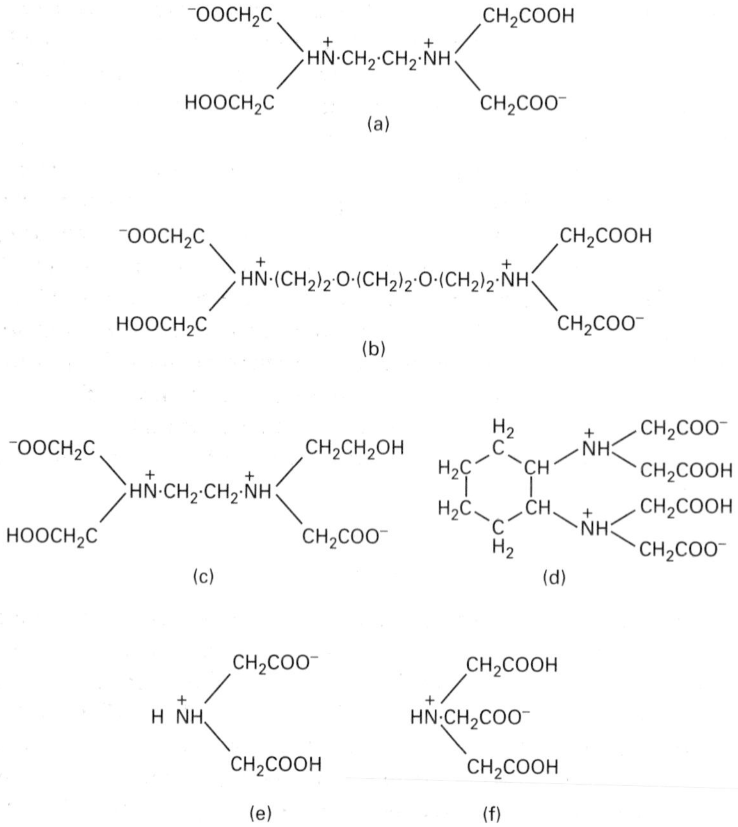

Fig. 2.26 Chelating agents. (a) Ethylenediamine tetraacetic acid (EDTA); (b) ethylenedioxybis (ethyliminodi(acetic acid)) (EGTA); (c) *N*-hydroxyethylenediamine-*NN′N′*-triacetic acid (HDTA); (d) *trans*-1,2-diaminocyclohexane-*NNN′N′*-tetraacetic acid (CDTA); (c) iminodiacetic acid (IDA); (f) nitrilotriacetic acid (NTA).

Table 2.13 Properties of chelating agents.

Property	EDTA	EGTA	HDTA	CDTA	IDA	NTA
Log stability constant*						
Ba	7.76	8.41	5.54	7.99	1.67	4.82
Ca	10.70	11.0	8.0	12.5	2.59	6.41
Mg	8.69	5.21	5.2	10.32	2.94	5.41
Zn	16.26	14.5	14.5	18.67	7.03	10.45
Antibacterial activity†						
Alone	Good	Good	Good	Low	Low	
As a potentiating agent for disinfectants	Yes		Yes	Yes	Somewhat	Somewhat

*Abstracted from the information supplied by West (1969).
†Based on the activity against *P. aeruginosa* described by Roberts *et al.* (1970) and Haque & Russell (1974a,b).

13.1 Ethylendiamine tetraacetic acid

In medicine, EDTA is commonly employed as the sodium or calcium–sodium salts. Sodium calcium edetate is used in the treatment of chronic lead poisoning, and the sodium salts are used clinically to chelate calcium ions, thereby decreasing serum calcium. Also EDTA is used as a stabilizing agent in certain injections and eye-drop preparations (Russell *et al.*, 1967).

The most important early findings, in a microbiological context, were made by Repaske (1956, 1958), who showed that certain Gram-negative bacteria became sensitive to the enzyme lysozyme in the presence of EDTA in tris buffer and that EDTA alone induced lysis of *P. aeruginosa*. The importance of tris itself has also been recognized (Leive & Kollin, 1967; Neu, 1969), since it appears to affect the permeability of the wall of various Gram-negative bacteria, as well as the nucleotide pool and RNA, which may be degraded. A lysozyme–tris–EDTA system in the presence of sucrose is a standard technique for producing spheroplasts/protoplasts in Gram-negative bacteria (McQuillen, 1960). During this conversion, several enzymes are released into the surrounding medium. A technique known as 'cold shock', which involves treating *E. coli* with EDTA + tris in hypertonic sucrose, followed by rapid dispersion in cold magnesium chloride—thus producing a sudden osmotic shift—again results in the release of enzymes, but without destroying the viability of the cells.

In the context of disinfection, EDTA is most important in that it will potentiate the activity of many antibacterial agents against many types of Gram-negative but not Gram-positive bacteria. This was clearly shown by Gray & Wilkinson (1965) and has since been confirmed and extended (Russell, 1971a; Wilkinson, 1975). An interesting offshoot was the development of Dettol Chelate, which consists of chloroxylenol and EDTA in a suitable formulation; unlike chloroxylenol alone, this new product has significant activity against *P. aeruginosa* strains (Russell & Furr, 1977). Ethylemediamine tetraacetic acid induces a non-specific increase in the permeability of the outer envelope of Gram-negative cells (Leive, 1974), thereby allowing more penetration of non-related agents. Ayres *et al.* (1993) reported on the permeabilizing activity of EDTA and other agents against *P. aeruginosa* in a rapid test method, the principle of which was the rapid lysis induced in this organism on exposure to the presumed permeabilizing agent plus lysozyme, an enzyme normally excluded in whole cells from its peptidoglycan target.

The mechanism of action of EDTA is dealt with in Chapter 9.

13.2 Other chelating agents

Chelating agents other than EDTA are described chemically in Fig. 2.26, and some of their properties (based in part on the excellent book of West, 1969) are listed in Table 2.13. While EGTA forms a stronger complex with Ca than does EDTA, for most other metals, except Ba and Hg, it is a weaker complexing agent than EDTA.

Notably, there is a divergency of 5.79 log K units between the stability constants of the Ca and Mg complexes with EGTA (West, 1969). Compared with EDTA, CDTA has superior complexing powers and it is better than all the other chelating agents listed in complexing Mg^{2+} ions. From a microbiological point of view, CDTA was found by Roberts *et al.* (1970) and Haque & Russell (1974a,b) to be the most toxic compound to *P. aeruginosa* and other Gram-negative bacteria in terms of leakage, lysis and loss of viability and in extracting metal ions from isolated cell envelopes (Haque & Russell, 1976).

The chelating agent HDTA corresponds to EDTA, one acetic acid of the latter molecule being replaced by a hydroxyethyl group. Its complexes are invariably less stable than those of EDTA. In a microbiological context, HDTA was found (Haque & Russell, 1976) to be rather less effective than EDTA.

Iminodiacetic acid forms weak complexes with most metal ions, whereas NTA is more reactive. Both have little activity against *P. aeruginosa*, although both, to some extent, potentiate the activity of other agents (disinfectants) against this organism.

14 Permeabilizers

Permeabilizers (permeabilizing agents) are chemicals that increase bacterial permeability to biocides (Vaara, 1992). Such chemicals include chelating agents, described above in Section 13, polycations, lactoferrin, transferrin and the salts of certain acids.

14.1 Polycations

Polycations such as poly-L-lysine (lysine$_{20}$; PLL) induce lipopolysaccharide (LPS) release from the outer membrane of Gram-negative bacteria. Organisms treated with PLL show greatly increased sensitivity to hydrophobic antibiotics (Vaara & Vaara, 1983a,b; Viljanen, 1987) but responses to biocides do not appear to have been studied.

14.2 Lactoferrin

Lactoferrin is an iron-binding protein that acts as a chelator, inducing partial LPS loss from the outer membrane of Gram-negative bacteria (Ellison *et al.*, 1988).

Lactoferricin B is a peptide produced by gastric peptic digestion of bovine lactoferrin. It is a much more potent agent than lactoferrin, binds rapidly to the bacterial cell surface and damages the outer membrane but has reduced activity in the presence of divalent cations (Jones *et al.*, 1994).

14.3 Transferrin

This iron-binding protein is believed to have a similar effect to lactoferrin (Ellison *et al.*, 1988). All are worthy of further studies as potentially important permeabilizers.

14.4 Citric and other acids

Used at alkaline pH, citric, gluconic and malic acids all act as permeabilizers (Ayres *et al.*, 1993). They perform as chelating agents and activity is reduced in the presence of divalent cations.

15 Heavy-metal derivatives

The historical introduction (Chapter 1) has already described the early use of high concentrations of salt employed empirically in the salting process as a preservative for meat, and the use of copper and silver vessels to prevent water from becoming fouled by microbial growth. Salting is still used in some parts of the world as a meat preservative and salts of heavy metals, especially silver, mercury, copper and, more recently, organotin, are still used as antimicrobial agents. The metal derivatives of copper, mercury, silver and tin, which find use as antiseptics and preservatives, will be discussed in this chapter. Kushner (1971) has reviewed the action of solutes other than heavy metal derivatives on microorganisms.

In addition to possessing antimicrobial activity in their own right, many metal ions are necessary for the activity of other drugs. A typical example is 8-hydroxyquinoline (Section 10.1), which needs Fe^{2+} for activity. The interesting relationship between antimicrobial compounds and metal cations has been reviewed by Weinberg (1957).

15.1 Copper compounds

Although the pharmacopoeias list a number of recipes containing copper salts (sulphate, actetate, citrate) as ingredients of antiseptic astringent lotions, the main antimicrobial use of copper derivatives is in algicides and fungicides. The copper(II) ion Cu^{2+} is pre-eminently an algicidal ion and at a final concentration of 0.5–2.9 μg/ml, as copper sulphate, it has been used to keep swimming-pools free from algae. Copper is thought to act by the poisoning effect of the copper(II) ion on thiol enzymes and possibly other thiol groups in microbial cells.

Copper sulphate and copper sulphate mixed with lime, Bordeaux mixture, introduced in 1885, are used as fungicides in plant protection. The latter formulation proved especially efficacious, as it formed a slow-release copper complex which was not easily washed from foliage. It was said to be first used as a deterrent to human predators of the grape crop and its antifungal properties emerged later. Copper metal, in powder form, finds an interesting application as an additive to cements and concretes. Its function is to inhibit microbial attack on the ingredients of these artificial products. The uses of copper metal here, and as vessels for drinking-water in the ancient world, illustrate a phenomenon which has been called the oligodynamic action of metals (Langwell, 1932). Metals are slightly soluble in water and in the case of copper, and also silver (q.v.), a sufficient concentration of ions in solution is achieved to inhibit microbial growth. Copper complexes, e.g. copper naphthenate and copper-7-hydroxyquinolate, have been particularly successful in the preservation of cotton fabrics. Wood, paper and paint have also been successfully preserved with copper compounds. As the preservation of paints, timber, etc. will be dealt with elsewhere in this volume (see Chapter 18), this chapter will merely summarize, by means of Table 2.14, some copper compounds and their application.

Table 2.14 Copper compounds used as preservatives and some examples of their application.

Compound	Example(s) of application
Copper metal	Concrete
Copper sulphate	Wood, water
Cuprammonium hydroxide	
Cuprammonium carbonate	
Cuprammonium fluoride	Fabrics, especially cellulosics
Copper chromate	
Copper borate	
Cuprous oxide	Paints, dark shades
Copper acetoarsenite	Paints, green shades
Copper oleate	
Copper stearate	Fabrics
Copper formate	
Copper naphthenate	Wood, fabric
Copper-8-hydroxyquinolate	Paint, papers
Copper phenylsalicylate	
Copper pentachlorphenate	Fabric

15.2 Silver compounds

Silver and its compounds have found a place in antimicrobial application from ancient times to the present day (Weber & Rutala, 1995). Apart from the use of silver vessels to maintain water in a potable state, the first systematic use of a silver compound in medicine was its use in the prophylaxis of ophthalmia neonatorum by the installation of silver nitrate solution into the eyes of newborn infants. Silver compounds have been used in recent years in the prevention of infection in burns, but are not very effective in treatment. An organism frequently associated with such infections is *P. aeruginosa*, and Brown & Anderson (1968) have discussed the effectiveness of Ag^+ in the killing of this organism. Among the Enterobacteriaceae, plasmids may carry genes specifying resistance to antibiotics and to metals. Plasmid-mediated resistance to silver salts is of particular importance in the hospital environment, because silver nitrate and silver sulphadiazine (AgSu) may be used topically for preventing infections in severe burns (Russell, 1985).

As might be imagined, silver nitrate is a somewhat astringent compound, below 10^{-4} mol/l a protein precipitant, and attempts to reduce this undesirable propensity while maintaining antimicrobial potency have been made. A device much used in pharmaceutical formulation to promote slow release of a potent substance is to combine it with a high-molecular-weight polymer. By mixing silver oxide or silver nitrate with gelatin or albumen, a water-soluble adduct is obtained, which slowly releases silver ions but lacks the caustic astringency of silver nitrate. A similar slow-release compound has been prepared by combining silver with disodiumdinaphthylmethane disulphate (Goldberg *et al.*, 1950).

The oligodynamic action of silver (Langwell, 1932), already referred to in the historical introduction (Chapter 1) and above, has been exploited in a water purification system employing what is called katadyn silver. Here, metallic silver is coated on to sand used in filters for water purification. Silver-coated charcoal has been used in a similar fashion (Bigger & Griffiths, 1933; Gribbard, 1933; Brandes, 1934; Moiseev, 1934). The activity of a silver-releasing surgical dressing has been described by Furr *et al.* (1944), who used a neutralization system to demonstrate that Ag^+ ions releases were responsible for its antibacterial effects.

Russell & Hugo (1994) have reviewed the antimicrobial activity and action of silver compounds. At a concentration of 10^{-9} to 10^{-6} mol/l, Ag^+ is an extremely active biocide. Originally considered to act as a 'general protoplasmic poison', it is now increasingly seen that this description is an oversimplification. It reacts strongly with structural and functional thiol groups in microbial cells, induces cytological changes and interacts with the bases in DNA.

Silver sulphadiazine is essentially a combination of two antibacterial agents, Ag^+ and sulphadiazine. It has a broad spectrum of activity, produces surface and membrane blebs and binds to various cell components, especially DNA (reviewed by Russell & Hugo, 1994), although its precise mode of action has yet to be elucidated. Silver sulphadiozine has been reinvestigated by Hamilton-Miller *et al.* (1993).

15.3 Mercury compounds

Mercury, long a fascination for early technologists (alchemists, medical practitioners, etc.), was used in medicine by the Arabian physicians. In the 1850s, mercury salts comprised, with phenol, the hypochlorites and iodine, the complement of topical antimicrobial drugs at the physician's disposal. Mercuric chloride was used and evaluated by Robert Koch and by Geppert. Nowadays its use in medicine has decreased, although a number of organic derivatives of mercury (Fig. 2.27) are used as bacteriostatic and fungistatic agents and as preservatives and bactericides in injections; examples include mercurochrome, nitromersol, thiomersal and phenylmercuric nitrate (Fig. 2.27). Salts such as the stearate, oleate and naphthenate were, until much more recently, extensively employed in the preservation of wood, textiles, paints and leather, to quote a few examples (Table 2.15). With the advent of a major health disaster in Japan due to mercury waste, feeling is hardening all over the world against the use of mercury in any form where it might pollute the environment, and it is unlikely that the inclusion of mercury in any product where environmental pollution may ensue will be countenanced by regulatory authorities.

Mercury resistance is inducible and is not the result of training or tolerance. Plasmids conferring resistance are of two types: (i) 'narrow-spectrum', encoding resistance to Hg(II) and to a few specified

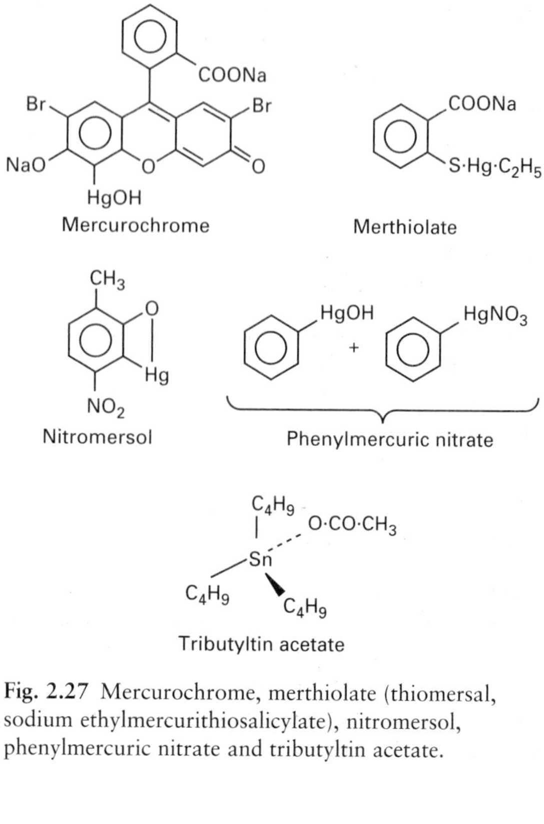

Mercurochrome

Merthiolate

Nitromersol

Phenylmercuric nitrate

Tributyltin acetate

Fig. 2.27 Mercurochrome, merthiolate (thiomersal, sodium ethylmercurithiosalicylate), nitromersol, phenylmercuric nitrate and tributyltin acetate.

Table 2.15 Derivatives of mercury and their uses as preservatives.

Compound	Use(s)
Phenylmercuric stearate	Leather
Phenylmercuric oleate	Leather
Mercuric naphthenate	Paint
Phenylmercuric acetate	Papers, textiles, pharmaceuticals*
Phenylmercuric nitrate	Pharmaceuticals*

*For additional information, see Chapter 16.

organomercurials; and (ii) 'broad-spectrum', encoding resistance to those in (i) plus other organomercury compounds (Foster, 1983). In (i) there is enzymatic reduction of mercury to Hg metal and its vaporization, and in (ii) there is enzymatic hydrolysis of an organomercurial to inorganic mercury and its subsequent reduction as in (i) (Silver & Misra, 1988). Further details are provided in Chapter 10B and by Russell & Chopra (1996).

Mercury is an environmental pollutant of considerable concern because it is very toxic to living cells. Ono *et al.* (1988) showed that the yeast cell wall acted as an adsorption filter for Hg^+. Later (Ono *et al.*, 1991) they demonstrated that methylmercury-resistant mutants of *S. cerevisiae* overproduced hydrogen sulphide, with an accumulation of hydrosulphide (HS^-) ions intracellularly, which was responsible for detoxification of methylmercury.

15.3.1 Mercurochrome (disodium-2,7-dibromo-4-hydroxymercurifluorescein)

This is now only of historical interest; it was the first organic mercurial to be used in medicine and an aqueous solution enjoyed a vogue as a substitute for iodine solutions as a skin disinfectant.

15.3.2 Nitromersol (anhydro-2-hydroxymercuri-6-methyl-3-nitrophenol)

A yellow powder, it is not very soluble in water or organic solvents but will dissolve in aqueous alkali, and is used as a solution of the sodium salt. It is active against vegetative microorganisms but ineffective against spores and acid-fast bacteria. It is mostly used in the USA.

*15.3.3 Thiomersal (merthiolate; sodium-*o*-(ethylmercurithio)-benzoate)*

This derivative was used as a skin disinfectant, and is now employed as a fungicide and as a preservative (0.01–0.02%) for biological products, for example, bacterial and viral vaccines. It possesses antifungal properties but is without action on spores.

Solutions are stable when autoclaved but less stable when exposed to light or to alkaline conditions, and they are incompatible with various chemicals, including heavy-metal salts (Denyer & Wallhäusser, 1990).

15.3.4 Phenylmercuric nitrate (PMN)

This organic derivative is used as a preservative in multidose containers of parenteral injections and eye-drops at a concentration of 0.001% and 0.002% w/v, respectively (Brown & Anderson, 1968). It was formerly employed in the UK as an adjunct to heat in the now-discarded process of 'heating with a bactericide'.

Phenylmercuric nitrate is incompatible with various compounds, including metals. Its activity is reduced by anionic emulsifying and suspending agents (Denyer & Wallhäusses, 1990). Sulphydryl agents are used as neutralizers in bactericidal studies and in sterility testing (Russell *et al.*, 1979; Sutton, 1996). Phenylmercuric nitrate is a useful preservative and is also employed as a spermicide.

Phenylmercuric nitrate solutions at room temperature are ineffective against bacterial spores, but they possess antifungal activity and are used as antifungal agents in the preservation of paper, textiles and leather. Voge (1947) has discussed PMN in a short review. An interesting formulation

Table 2.16 Tin compounds used as preservatives and some examples of their uses.

Compound	Chemical formula	Use(s)
Tributyltin oxide	$((C_4H_9)_3\ Sn)_2O$	Antifouling paints Wallpaper adhesives Wood preservatives Antislime agents
Tributyltin fluoride	$(C_4H_9)_3\ SnF$	Antifouling paints
Tributyltin acetate	$(C_4H_9)_3\ SnOCOCH_3$	Antifouling paints
Tributyltin benzoate	$(C_4H_9)_3\ SnOCOC_6H_5$	Germicide: usually used with formaldehyde or a QAC
Triphenyltin acetate	$(C_6H_5)_3SnOCOCH_3$	Agricultural fungicides
Triphenyltin hydroxide	$(C_6H_5)_3SnOH$	Agricultural pesticides Disinfectants

of PMN with sodium dinaphthylmethanedisulphonate has been described, in which enhanced activity and greater skin penetration is claimed (Goldberg *et al.*, 1950).

15.3.5 *Phenylmercuric acetate (PMA)*

This has the same activity, properties and general uses as PMN (Denyer & Wallhäusser, 1990) and finds application as a preservative in pharmaceutical and other fields.

15.4 Tin and its compounds (organotins)

Tin, stannic or tin(IV) oxide was at one time used as an oral medicament in the treatment of superficial staphylococcal infections. Tin was claimed to be excreted via sebaceous glands and thus concentrated at sites of infection. More recently, organic tin derivatives (Table 2.16, Fig. 2.27) have been used as fungicides and bactericides and as textile and wood preservatives (Smith & Smith, 1975).

The organotin compounds which find use as biocides are derivatives of tin(IV). They have the general structure R_3SnX where R is butyl or phenyl and X is acetate, benzoate, fluoride, oxide or hydroxide. In structure–activity studies, activity has been shown to reside in the R group; the nature of X determines physical properties such as solubility and volatility (Van der Kerk & Luijten, 1954; Rose & Lock, 1970). The R_3SnX compounds, with R = butyl or phenyl, combine high biocidal activity with low mammalian toxicity. Samples of the range of R_3SnX compounds and their use as biocides are shown in Tables 2.16 and 2.17. Tin differs significantly from copper, silver and mercury salts in being intrinsically much less toxic. It is used to coat cans and vessels used to prepare food or boil water. Organotin compounds have some effect on oxidative phosphorylation (Aldridge & Threlfall, 1961) and act as ionophores for anions (Chapter 9). Possible environmental toxicity should be borne in mind when tin compounds are used.

Table 2.17 Minimum inhibitory concentrations (MICs) of tributyltin oxide towards a range of microorganisms.

Organism	MIC (μg/ml)
Aspergillus niger	0.5
Chaetomium globosum	1.0
Penicillium expansum	1.0
Aureobasidium pullulans	0.5
Trichoderma viride	1.0
Candida albicans	1.0
Bacillus mycoides	0.1
Staphylococcus aureus	1.0
Bacterium ammoniagenes	1.0
Pseudomonas aeruginosa	> 500
Enterobacter aerogenes	> 500

16 Anilides

Anilides (Fig. 2.28) have the general structure $C_6H_5.NH.COR$. Two derivatives—salicylanilide, where $R = C_6H_4OH$, and diphenylurea (carbanilide), where $R = C_6H_5.NH$—have formed the basis for antimicrobial compounds.

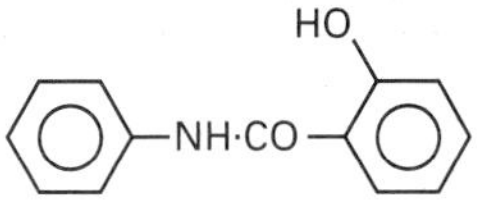

Salicylanilide

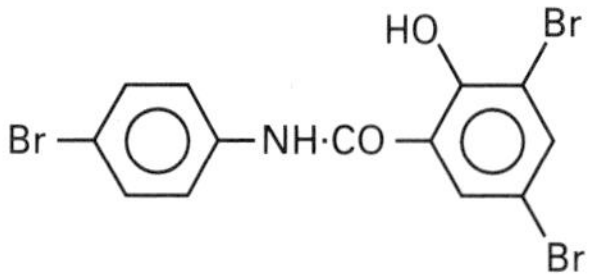

3,4',5-Tribromosalicylanilide (Tribromsalan)

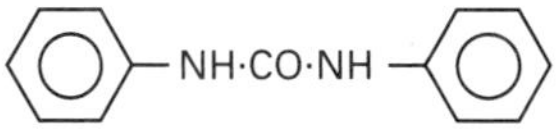

Diphenylurea (Carbanilide)

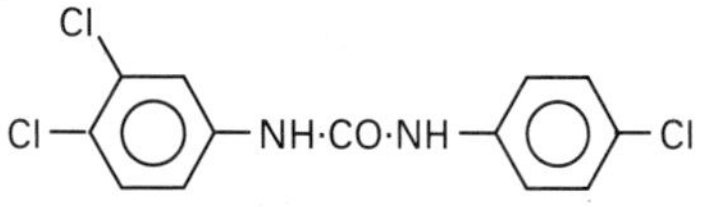

Trichlorocarbanilide

Fig. 2.28 Anilides.

16.1 Salicylanilide

The parent compound, salicylanilide, was introduced in 1930 as a fungistat for use on textiles (Fargher *et al.*, 1930). It occurs as white or slightly pink crystals, m.p. 137°C, which are soluble in water and organic solvents. It has also been used in ointment form for the treatment of ringworm, but concentrations above 5% should not be used in medicinal products because of skin irritancy. Minimum inhibitory concentrations (μg/ml) for a number of fungi were: *Trichophyton mentagrophytes*, 12; *Trichophyton tonsurans*, 6; *Trichophyton rubrum*, 3; *Epidermophyton floccosum*, 6; *Microsporum adovini*, 1.5. Despite the effectiveness of the parent compound, attempts were made to improve on its performance by the usual device of adding substituents, notably halogens, to the benzene residues; these are considered below.

16.1.1 Substituted salicylanilides

Lemaire *et al.* (1961) investigated 92 derivatives of salicylanilide and related compounds, i.e. benzanilides and salicylaldehydes. The intrinsic antimicrobial activity was obtained from literature values and was usefully summarized as follows. One ring substituent would give an MIC value for *S. aureus* of 2 μg/ml, but this value could be decreased to 1 μg/ml if substitution occurred in both rings.

The researchers were particularly interested in the role of these compounds as antiseptics for addition to soaps, and went on to evaluate them in this role. They were also interested to find to what extent they remained on the skin (skin substantivity) after washing with soaps containing them. They found that di- to pentachlorination or bromination with more or less equal distribution of the substituent halogen in both rings gave the best results both for antimicrobial activity and skin substantivity. However, it was also found that skin photosensitization was caused by some analogues.

Of the many compounds tested, the 3,4′,5-tribromo, 2,3,5,3′- and 3,5,3′,4′-tetrachloro salicylanilides have been the most widely used as antimicrobial agents; however, their photosensitizing properties have tended to restrict their use in any situation where they may come in contact with human skin.

Over and above this, many workers who have investigated germicidal soaps, i.e. ordinary soap products with the addition of a halogenated salicylanilide, carbanilide, or for that matter phenolic compounds such as hexachlorophane (2.9.1) or DCMX (2.6.5), have doubted their value in this role, although some may act as deodorants by destroying skin organisms which react with sweat to produce body odour.

16.2 Diphenylureas (carbanilides)

16.2.1 3,4,4′-Trichlorocarbanilide (TCC, triclocarban)

From an extensive study by Beaver *et al.* (1957), the above emerged as one of the most potent of this family of biocides. It inhibits the growth of many Gram-positive bacteria at concentrations from 0.1 to 1.0 μg/ml. Fungi were found to be more resistant, since 1000 μg/ml failed to inhibit *A. niger, Penicillium notatum, C. albicans* and

Fusarium oxysporium. *Trichophyton gypseum* and *Trichophyton inguinale* were inhibited at 50 μg/ml.

It occurs as a white powder, m.p. 250°C; it is very slightly soluble in water.

Like the salicylanilides, it has not found favour in products likely to come in contact with human skin, despite the fact that it had been extensively evaluated as the active ingredient of some disinfectant soaps.

16.3 Mode of action

The mode of action of salicylanilides and carbanilides (diphenylureas) has been studied in detail by Woodroffe & Wilkinson (1966a,b) and Hamilton (1968). The compounds almost certainly owe their bacteriostatic action to their ability to discharge part of the proton-motive force, thereby inhibiting processes dependent upon it, i.e. active transport and energy metabolism. Further general details will be found by consulting Chapter 9 and Russell & Chopra (1996).

17 Miscellaneous preservatives

Included in this section are those chemicals which are useful preservatives but which do not form part of the biocidal groups already discussed.

17.1 Derivatives of 1,3-dioxane

17.1.1 6-Acetoxy-2,4-dimethyl-1,3-dioxane (dimethoxane) (Dioxin: registered trade mark, Sindar Corporation, New York, USA)

Dioxin (Fig. 2.29) is a liquid, colourless when pure and soluble in water and organic solvents. It has a marked odour. It is active against a wide range of microorganisms at concentrations ranging from 300 to 2500 μg/ml (Anon., 1962). It should be noted that the name 'dioxin' is also used for a reaction product, 2,3,7-8-tetrachlorodibenzo-*p*-dioxin (TCDD), which may be formed during the manufacture of trichlorophenol. The MIC values (μg/ml) for representative microorganisms are: *S. cerevisiae*, 2500; *A. niger*, 1250; *S. aureus*, 1250; *P. aeruginosa*, 625; *Salmonella cholerae-suis*, 312.

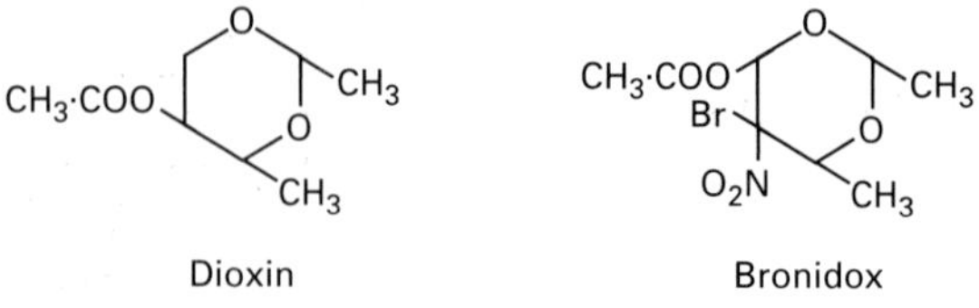

Dimethoxane is not affected by changes in pH but it is slowly hydrolysed in aqueous solution, producing ethanal (acetaldehyde). It is compatible with non-ionic surface-active agents but may cause discoloration in formulations that contain amines or amides.

Dimethoxane finds application as a preservative for cosmetics, emulsion paints and cutting oils. A detailed study of the components of the commercial preparation Giv Gard DXN (Givaudan & Co. Ltd., Whyteleafe, Surrey, UK) showed that the acetoxy group may be either 6-α (74%) or 6-β (22%) to the 1,3-dioxane ring. Small amounts of acetaldehyde may also be present (Woolfson & Woodside, 1976). Later, in a bacteriological study, Woolfson (1977) attributed the action of the commercial product partially to its aldehyde content and partially to the 1,3-dioxane components.

$CH_3{\cdot}COO$, O, CH_3, O, CH_3

Dioxin

$CH_3{\cdot}COO$, Br, O_2N, O, CH_3, O, CH_3

Bronidox

Fig. 2.29 Dioxanes: dioxin and bronidox.

17.1.2 5-Bromo-5-nitro-1,3-dioxane (Bronidox: Henkel Chemicals Ltd, Tretol House, London NW9 0HT, UK)

This nitro–bromo derivative of dioxane is available as a 10% solution in propylene glycol as Bronidox L. It is used as a preservative for toiletries and has been described in some detail by Potokar *et al.* (1976) and Lorenz (1977). Its stability at various pH values is tabulated by Croshaw (1977).

It is active against bacteria and fungi and does not show a *Pseudomonas* gap. Minimum inhibitory concentrations of the active ingredient (μg/ml) were: *E. coli*, 50; *P. aeruginosa*, 50; *P. vulgaris*, 50; *P. fluorescens*, 50; *S. typhi*, 50; *Serratia marcescens*, 25; *S. aureus*, 75; *S. faecalis*, 75; *C. albicans*, 25; *S. cerevisiae*, 10; *A. niger*, 10.

Its activity is not affected between pH 5 and 9 and it probably acts as an oxidizing agent, oxidizing –SH to –S–S– groups in essential enzymes. It does not act as a formaldehyde releaser.

It is recommended for use as a preservative for a variety of toiletries, including shampoos and hand lotions.

17.2 Derivatives of imidazole

Imidazolines (Fig. 2.30) are 2,3-dihydroimidazoles; 2-heptadecyl-2-imidazoline was introduced as an agricultural fungicide as far back as 1946. Other derivatives containing the imidazole ring have recently found successful application as preservatives. Two are derivatives of 2,4-dioxotetrahydroimidazole, the imidazolidones; the parent diketone is hydantoin.

17.2.1 1,3-Di(hydroxymethyl)-5,5-dimethyl-2,4-dioxoimidazole; 1,3-Di-hydroxymethyl)-5,5-dimethylhydantoin (Dantoin)

A 55% solution of this compound (Fig. 2.30) is available commercially as Glydant (Glyco Chemicals Inc., Greenwich, Conn., USA). This product is water-soluble, stable and non-corrosive, with a slight odour of formaldehyde. It is active over a wide range of pH and is compatible with most ingredients used in cosmetics. It has a wide spectrum of activity against bacteria and fungi, being active at concentrations of between 250 and 500 μg/ml. The moulds *Microsporum gypseum* and *Trichophyton asteroides*, however, are particularly susceptible, being inhibited at 32 μg/ml. Its mode of action is attributed to its ability to release formaldehyde, the rate of release of which is more rapid at high pH values, 9–10.5, than low, 3–5. Its optimum stability lies in the range pH 6–8. It has an acceptable level of toxicity and can be used as a preservative over a wide field of products. It has been evaluated by Schanno *et al.* (1980).

17.2.2 N,N″-methylene bis [5′[1-hydroxymethyl] -2,5-dioxo-4-imidazolidinyl urea] (Germall 115: Sutton Laboratories Inc., Roselle, N.J., USA)

In 1970 a family of imidazolidinyl ureas for use as preservatives was described (Berke & Rosen, 1970). One of these, under the name Germall 115, has been studied extensively (Rosen & Berke, 1973; Berke & Rosen, 1978). Germall 115 is a white powder very soluble in water, and hence tends to remain in the aqueous phase of emulsions. It is non-toxic, non-irritating and non-sensitizing. It is compatible with emulsion ingredients and with proteins.

A claimed property of Germall 115 has been its ability to act synergistically with other preservatives (Jacobs *et al.*, 1975; Rosen *et al.*, 1977; Berke & Rosen, 1980). Intrinsically it is more active against bacteria than fungi. Most of the microbiological data are based on challenge tests in cosmetic formulations, data which are of great value to the cosmetic microbiologist. An investigation of its activity against a series of *Pseudomonas* species and strains (Berke & Rosen, 1978) showed that in a challenge test 0.3% of the compound cleared all species but *P. putida* and *P. aureofaciens* in 24 h. The latter species were killed between 3 and 7 days. In an agar cup-plate test, 1% solution gave the following size inhibition zones (mm): *S. aureus*, 7,6; *S. aureus*, penicillin sensitive, 15.5; *Staphylococcus albus*, 9.0; *B. subtilis*, 15.0; *Corynebacterium. acne*, 5.0; *E. coli*, 3.6; *Pseudomonas ovale*, 2.0.

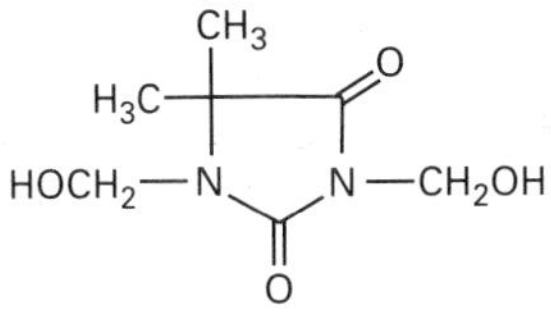

CH_3, H_3C, O, $HOCH_2$—N, N—CH_2OH, O

Glydant DMDMH–55

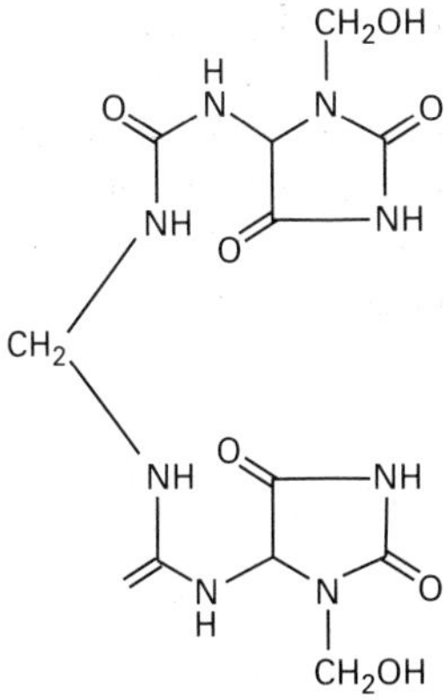

CH_2OH, H, O, N, N, O, NH, O, NH, CH_2, NH, O, NH, N, H, N, O, CH_2OH

Germall 115

Fig. 2.30 Dantoin or Glydant DMDMH-55 and Germall 115.

17.3 Isothiazolones

Ponci *et al.* (1964) studied the antifungal activity of a series of 5-nitro-1,2-dibenzisothiazolones and found many of them to possess high activity. Since this publication a number of isothiazolones (Fig. 2.31) have emerged as antimicrobial preservatives. They are available commercially, usually a suspensions rather than as pure compounds, and find use in a variety of industrial situations. Nicoletti *et al.* (1993) have described their activity.

17.3.1 5-Chloro-2-methyl-4-isothiazolin-3-one (CMIT)

17.3.2 2-Methyl-4-isothiazolin-3-one (MIT)

A mixture of these two derivatives, known as Kathon 886 MW (Rohm and Haas (UK) Ltd., Croydon, CR9 3NB, UK), containing about 14% of active ingredients is available as a preservative for cutting oils and as an in-can preservative for emulsion paints. This mixture is active at concentrations of 2.25–9 μg/ml active ingredient against a wide range of bacteria and fungi and does not show a *Pseudomonas* gap. It is also a potent algastat. Kathon CG, containing 1.5% active ingredients and magnesium salts, has been suggested as a preservative for cosmetic products up to a final concentration of 25 μg/ml active ingredients.

It possesses the additional advantage of being biodegradable to non-toxic metabolites and is non-irritating at normal in-use concentrations. It is water-soluble and compatible with most emulgents. The stability of Kathon 886 at various pH values is described by Croshaw (1977).

17.3.3 2-n-Octyl-4-isothiazolin-3-one (Skane M8: ICI)

This is available as a 45% solution in propylene glycol and is active against bacteria over a range of 400–500 μg/ml active ingredient. To inhibit the growth of one strain of *P. aeruginosa* required 500 μg/ml. Fungistatic activity was shown against a wide number of species over the range 0.3–8.0 μg/ml. It is also effective at preventing algal growth at concentrations of 0.5–5.0 μg/ml. It is biodegradable but shows skin and eye irritancy. As might be expected from its *n*-octyl side-chain, it is not soluble in water.

17.3.4 1,2-Benzisothiazolin-3-one (BIT). (Proxel CRL, GXL, AB: Imperial Chemical Industries Ltd., Blackley, Manchester M9 3DA)

This is available commercially in various formulations and is recommended as a preservative for industrial emulsions, adhesives, polishes, glues and paper products. It possesses a low mammalian toxicity but is not recommended for medicinal and cosmetic use for it exhibits marked skin irritancy.

17.3.5 Mechanism of action

As growth-inhibitory concentrations, BIT has little effect on the membrane integrity of *Staph. aureus*, but significantly inhibits active transport and oxidation of glucose and has a marked effect on thiol-containing enzymes.

Thiol-containing compounds quench the activity of BIT, CMIT and MIT against *E. coli*, which suggests that these isothiazolones interact strongly with –SH groups. The activity of CMIT is also overcome by non-thiol amino acids, so that this compound might thus react with amines as well as with essential thiol groups (Collier *et al.*, 1990a,b).

17.4 Derivatives of hexamine

Hexamine (hexamethylene tetramine; 1,3,5,7-triaza-1-azonia-adamantane) has been used as a

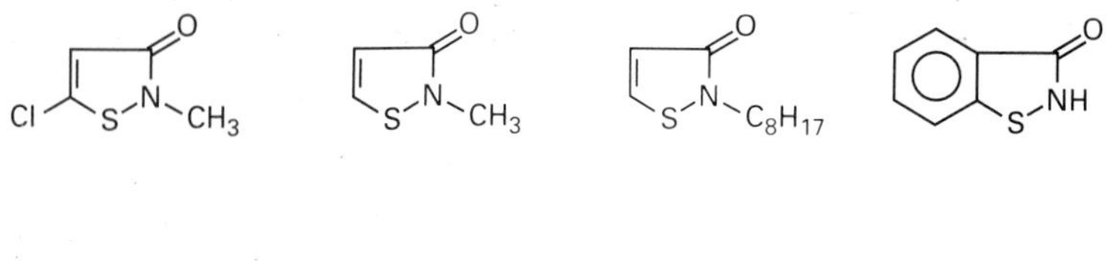

Cl S N CH_3 O — S N CH_3 O — S N C_8H_{17} O — S NH O

Fig. 2.31 Isothiazolones. From left to right: 5-chloro-2-methyl-4-isothiazolin-3-one (CMIT, Section 17.3.1 in text), 2-methyl-4-isothiazolin-3-one (MIT; 17.3.2), 2-*n*-octyl-4-isothiazolin-3-one (17.3.3) and 1,2-benzisothiazolin-3-one (BIT; 17.3.4).

Table 2.18 Inhibitory concentrations for hexamine quaternized with $-CH_2Cl{=}CHCl$ compared with values for hexamine and formaldehyde.

	MIC* against					
Inhibitor	*Staph. aureus*	*Sal. typhi*	*K. aerogenes*	*Ps. aeruginosa*	*B. subtilis*	*D. desulphuricans*
Hexamine quaternized with $-CH_2-CH{=}CHCl$	4×10^{-4} (100)	2×10^{-4} (50)	2×10^{-4} (50)	2×10^{-3} (500)	4×10^{-4} (100)	2.9×10^{-2} (7250)
Hexamine	3.5×10^{-2} (5000)	3.5×10^{-3} (500)	–	–	–	5.3×10^{-2} (7500)
Formaldehyde	1.6×10^{-3} (50)	3.3×10^{-3} (100)	1.6×10^{-3} (50)	–	–	–

*Molar values (in parentheses μg/ml).

Table 2.19 Properties of the most commonly used gaseous disinfectants.

Gaseous disinfectant	Molecular weight	Boiling point (°C)	Solubility in water	Sterilizing concn (mg/l)	Relative humidity requirements (%)	Penetration of materials	Microbidical activity*	Best application as gaseous disinfectant†
Ethylene oxide	44	10.4	Complete	400–1000	Non-desiccated 30–50; large load 60	Moderate	Moderate	Sterilization of plastic medical supplies
Propylene oxide	58	34	Good	800–2000	Non-desiccated 30–60	Fair	Fair	Decontamination
Formaldehyde	30	90°C/ Formalin‡	Good	3.10	75	Poor (surface sterilant)	Excellent	Surface sterilant for rooms
β-Propiolactone	72	162	Moderate	2–5	>70	None (surface sterilant)	Excellent	Surface sterilant for rooms
Methyl bromide	95	4.6	Slight	3500	30–50	Excellent	Poor	Decontamination

*Based on an equimolar comparison.
†See later also, Chapter 21.
‡Formalin contains formaldehyde plus methanol.

urinary antiseptic since 1894. Its activity is attributed to a slow release of formaldehyde. Other formaldehyde-releasing compounds are considered in Sections 7.2.4, 17.2, 17.5 and 17.6. Wohl in 1886 was the first to quaternize hexamine, and in 1915–16 Jacobs and co-workers attempted to extend the antimicrobial range of hexamine by quaternizing one of its nitrogen atoms with halo-hydrocarbons (Jacobs & Heidelberger, 1915a,b; Jacobs *et al.*, 1916a,b). These workers did not consider that their compounds acted as formaldehyde releasers but that activity resided in the whole molecule.

The topic was taken up again by Scott & Wolf (1962). These workers re-examined quaternized hexamine derivatives with a view to using them as preservatives for toiletries, cutting oils and other products. They looked at 31 such compounds and compared their activity also with hexamine and formaldehyde. As well as determining their inhibitory activity towards a staphylococcus, enterobacteria and a pseudomonad, they also assessed inhibitory activity towards *Desulphovibrio desulphuricans*, a common contaminant of cutting oils.

Polarographic and spectroscopic studies of formaldehyde release were made on some of the derivatives; this release varied with the substituent used in forming the quaternary salt. A typical set of data for the antimicrobial activity (MIC) of one derivative compared with hexamine and formaldehyde is shown in Table 2.18. In general, the quaternized compounds were found to be more active w/w than hexamine but less active than formaldehyde. Although chemically they contain a quaternized nitrogen atom, unlike the more familiar antimicrobial quaternized compounds (Section 6.1), they are not inactivated by lecithin or protein. The compounds are not as surface-active as conventional QACs. Thus an average figure for the surface tension, dyne cm^{-1}, for 0.1% solutions of the quaternized hexamines was 54; that for 0.1% cetrimide (Section 6.1) was 34.

One of these derivatives of hexamine, i.e. that quaternized with *cis*-1,3-dichloropropene, is being used as a preservative under the name Dowicil 200 (Dow Chemical Co., Wilmslow, Cheshire, UK). *Cis*-1-(3-cis-chloroallyl)-3,5,7-triaza-1-azonia-admantane chloride *N*-(3-chloroallyl) hexamine (Dowicil 200; Fig. 2.32) is a highly water-soluble hygroscopic white powder; it has a low oil solubility. It is active against bacteria and fungi. Typical MIC (μg/ml) were: *E. coli*, 400; *P. vulgaris*, 100; *S. typhi*, 50; *Alcaligenes faecalis*, 50; *P. aeruginosa*, 600; *S. aureus*, 200; *B. subtilis*, 200; *A. niger*, 1200; *T. interdigitale*, 50.

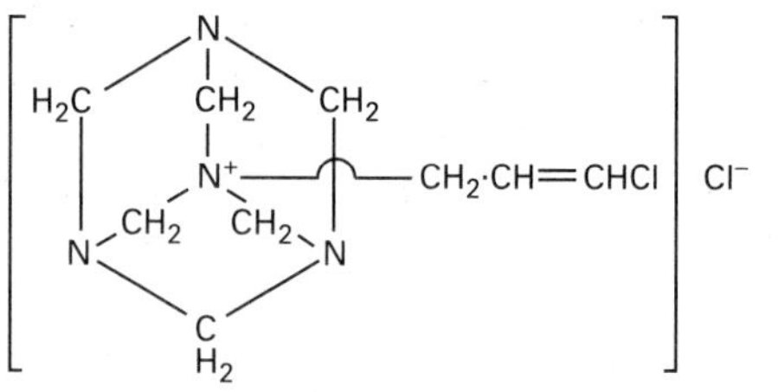

Fig. 2.32 Dowicil 200 (*N*-(3-*cis*-chloroallyl)hexamine).

It is recommended for use as a preservative for cosmetic preparations at concentrations of from 0.1 to 0.2%. Because of its high solubility, it does not tend to concentrate in the oil phase of these products, but remains in the aqueous phase, where contamination is likely to arise. It is not inactivated by the usual ingredients used in cosmetic manufacture. Its activity is not affected over the usual pH ranges found in cosmetic or cutting oil formulations. For further information, see Rossmore & Sondossi (1988).

17.5 Triazines

The product, theoretically from the condensation of three molecules of ethylamine with three of formaldehyde, is hexahydro-1,3,5-triethyl-*s*-triazine (Bactocide THT: Cochrane and Keene (Chemicals), Rochdale, UK; Fig. 2.33a). This is a clear white or slightly yellow viscous liquid, readily soluble in water, acetone, ethanol and ether. It is bactericidal and fungicidal and inhibits most bacteria, including *P. aeruginosa* and *D.*

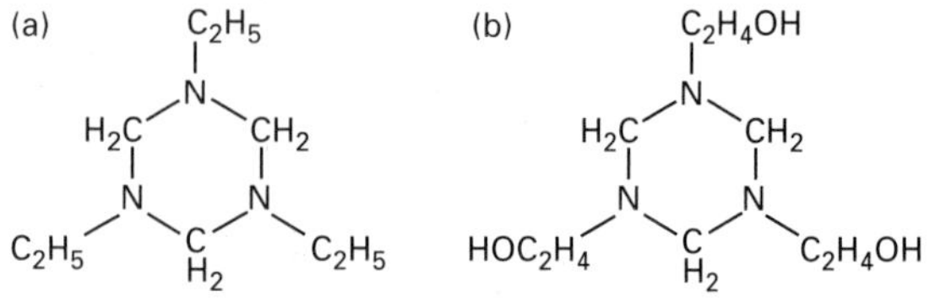

Fig. 2.33 (a) Hexahydro-1,3,5-triethyl-*s*-triazine (Bactocide THT): (b) 1,3,5-tris(2-hydroxyethyl)-*s*-triazine (Grotan).

desulphuricans at concentrations of 0.3 mg/ml. Fungi, such as *A. niger*, *Penicillium glaucum* and *P. notatum* are inhibited at 0.1 mg/ml, and *Sacch. cerevisiae* at 0.05 mg/ml. It owes its activity to a release of formaldehyde. It has been used as a preservative for cutting oils, for the 'in-can' preservation of emulsion paints for proteinaceous adhesives and to control slime in paper and cardboard manufacture, and to prevent the growth of microorganisms in water-cooling systems. It has a low intrinsic toxicity and at use dilutions is not irritant to the skin.

If formaldehyde is reacted with ethanolamine, the compound 1,3,5-tris(2-hydroxyethyl)-*s*-triazine can be formed (Grotan: Stirling Industrial, Sheffield, UK; Fig. 2.33b). This has both antibacterial and antifungal activity and is recommended as a preservative for cutting oils. Despite the figures for fungal inhibition, it is often found, in practical preservation situations, that, although this triazine will inhibit microbial growth, a fungal superinfection is often established; a total preservation system which includes a triazine might well have to contain an additional antifungal compound (Rossmore *et al.*, 1972; Paulus, 1976). This situation may be compared with that found with imidazole derivatives (Section 17.2).

Rossmore (1979) has discussed the uses of heterocyclic compounds as industrial biocides, and Rossmore & Sondossi (1988) have reviewed formaldehyde condensates in general.

17.6 Oxazolo-oxazoles

By reacting formaldehyde with tris(hydroxymethyl)-methylamine, a series of derivatives is obtained. The commercial product (Nuosept 95: Tenneco Organics Ltd., Avonmouth, Bristol, UK; Fig. 2.34) contains the molecules species: 5-hydroxymethoxymethyl-1-aza-3,7-dioxabicyclo (3.3.0) octane, 24.5%; 5-hydroxymethyl-1-aza-3,7-dioxabicyclo (3.3.0) octane, 17.7%; 5-hydroxypolymethylenoxy (74% C_2, 21% C_3, 4% C_4, 1% C_5) methyl-1-aza-3,7-dioxabicyclo (3.3.0) octane, 7.8%, and acts as a biostat by virtue of being a formaldehyde releaser.

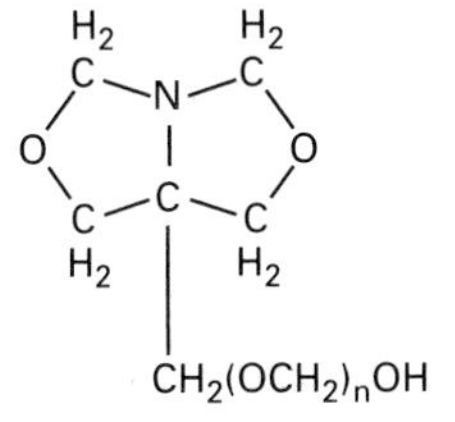

It is obtained as a clear, pale-yellow liquid, which is miscible with water, methanol, ethanol, chloroform and acetone in all proportions, and is recommended as a preservative for cutting oils, water treatment, plants, emulsion (latex) paints, industrial slurries and starch- and cellulose-based products. It is slightly irritant to intact and abraded skin and is a severe eye irritant.

$CH_2(OCH_2)_nOH$

Fig. 2.34 Nuosept 95 (n = 0–5).

17.7 Methylene bisthiocyanate

This is available commercially as a 10% solution and is recommended for the control of slime in paper manufacture, where it provides a useful alternative to mercurials. The compound (Fig. 2.35) is a skin and eye irritant and thus care is required in its use. Its toxicity is low enough to enable it to be used in the manufacture of papers destined for the packaging of food. At in-use dilutions, it is unlikely to cause corrosion of materials used in the construction of paper-manufacturing equipment.

17.8 Captan

Captan is *N*-(trichloromethylthio)cyclohex-4-ene-1,2-dicarboximide (Fig. 2.36). It is a white crystalline solid, insoluble in water and only slightly

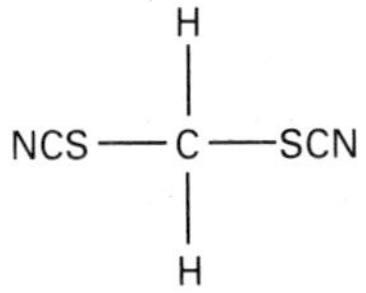

NCS—CH_2—SCN

Fig. 2.35 Methylene bisthiocyanate.

N—S·CCl_3

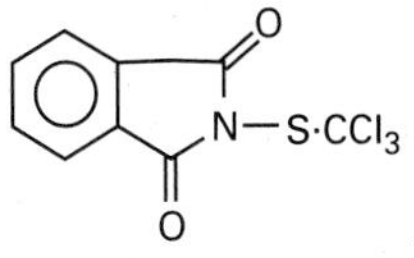

Fig. 2.36 Captan.

soluble in organic solvents. It is decomposed in alkaline solution. Despite its low solubility, it can be shown to be an active biocide, being active against both Gram-negative and Gram-positive bacteria, yeasts and moulds. It has been used as an agricultural fungicide, being primarily employed against diseases of fruit trees. It has also been used to prevent spoilage of stored fruit and in the treatment of skin infections due to fungi in humans and animals.

17.9 Essential oils

Essential oils have been used empirically throughout history as preservatives. Their re-examination as antimicrobial agents has received attention from many workers, as their use as natural preservatives has contemporary appeal. Their antibacterial properties have been reviewed by Deans & Ritchie (1987).

17.10 General statement

Many of these compounds are relatively new in the preservation field and much of the information concerning their properties and uses is found in the manufacturers' information brochures. Any person wishing to explore their use should consult the manufacturers. An ever-present problem with cosmetics preservation is that of contact sensitization. This is discussed in some detail by Marzulli & Maibach (1973) and is a point which must be carefully checked before a preservative is committed to a product. Another hazard which may arise is that of an induced change in the skin microflora during continuous use of products containing antimicrobial preservatives; this is discussed by Marples (1971).

18 Vapour-phase disinfectants

Gaseous sterilization is the subject of a later chapter (Chapter 21) and thus only a few comments will be made here. It is only comparatively recently that a scientific basis for using gases as sterilizing or disinfecting agents has been established. Factors influencing the activity of gaseous formaldehyde were described by Nordgren (1939) and later by a Committee on Formaldehyde Disinfection (Anon., 1958). The possible uses of gaseous formaldehyde in the disinfection of hospital bedding and blankets and, in conjunction with low-temperature steam, for disinfection of heat-sensitive material, are considered in Section 18.2.1 (see also Chapter 21).

Phillips & Kaye (1949) reviewed the earlier work which had taken place with ethylene oxide, which has bactericidal, mycobactericidal, sporicidal, fungicidal and viricidal activity (Ernst, 1974). A later review is by Richards *et al.* (1984).

Other gases of possible value include β-propiolactone, propylene oxide, ozone, methyl bromide and glycidaldehyde (Russell, 1976). Physical and chemical properties of these and the two most important ones (ethylene oxide and formaldehyde) are listed in Table 2.19 and their chemical structures are given in Fig. 2.37.

Gaseous hydrogen peroxide and gas plasmas are likely to play an important role as sterilizing agents in the future.

18.1 Ethylene oxide

This is discussed in detail later (Chapter 21) and will not be considered here in detail. Its antibicrobial activity is affected by concentration, temperature, relative humidity and the water content of microorganisms. It acts, by virtue of its alkylating properties, on proteins and nucleic acids. A consideration of its antimicrobial activity with compounds of a similar chemical structure (Figs 2.37 and 2.38) demonstrates that cyclopropane, which is not an alkylating agent, is not antimicrobial whereas those that have the ability to alkylate are potent antimicrobials.

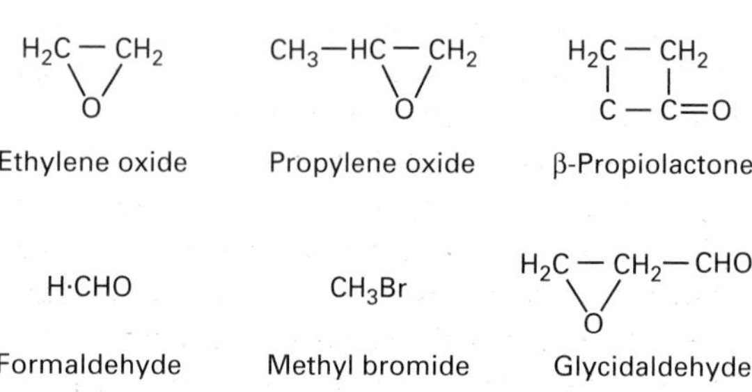

Fig. 2.37 Chemical structures of gaseous disinfectants.

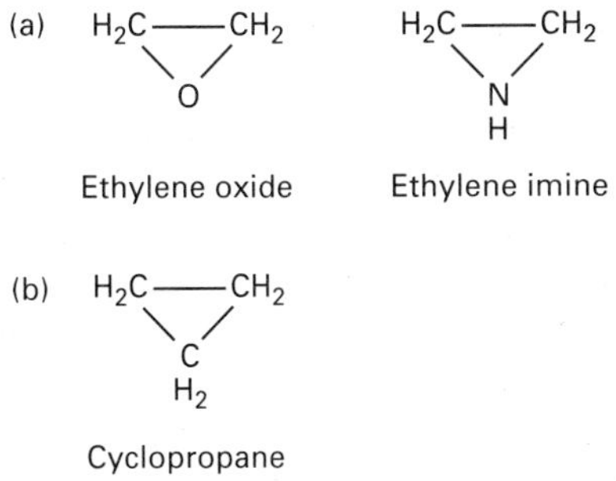

(a) H_2C—CH_2 with O: Ethylene oxide; H_2C—CH_2 with NH: Ethylene imine

(b) H_2C—CH_2 with CH_2: Cyclopropane

Fig. 2.38 Compounds similar to ethylene oxide: (a) alkylating and antimicrobial compounds; (b) non-alkylating, non-antimicrobial agent.

Useful reviews are those by Hoffman (1971), Phillips (1977), Richards *et al.* (1984), Burgess & Reich (1993), Jorkasky (1993), Page (1993) and Sintim-Damoa (1993).

18.2 Formaldehyde-releasing agents

Paraformaldehyde ($HO(CH_2O)_n.H$, where n = 8–100) is a polymer of formaldehyde and is produced by evaporating aqueous solutions of formaldehyde. Although it was considered originally to be of little practical use (Nordgren, 1939) paraformaldehyde has since been shown to depolymerize rapidly when heated, to produce formaldehyde (Taylor *et al.*, 1969). Paraformaldehyde is considered by Tulis (1973) to be an excellent source of monomeric formaldehyde gas, because it can be produced in a temperature-controlled reaction, and there are no contaminating residues (methanol and formic acid) produced during evaporation of formalin solutions, in contrast to the method of evaporating formalin solutions containing 10% methanol to prevent polymerization.

Other formaldehyde-releasing agents are melamine formaldehyde and urea formaldehyde (Fig. 2.39). The former is produced from formaldehyde and melamine under alkaline conditions and the latter is a mixture of monomethyloyl urea and dimethyloyl urea. When exposed to elevated temperatures these agents release potentially sterilizing amounts of gaseous formaldehyde, the rate of release being a function of time and temperature. These formaldehyde-releasing agents are, however, much less effective as disinfecting or sterilizing sources than paraformaldehyde. The

Melamine formaldehyde

HO—CH_2—NH—CO—NH—CH_2—OH: Urea formaldehyde

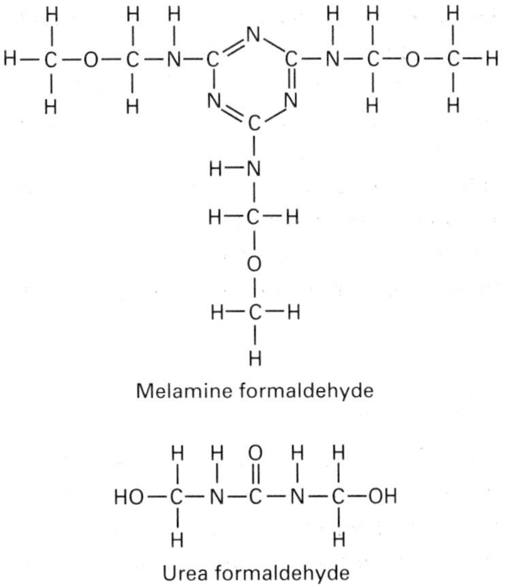

Fig. 2.39 Melamine formaldehyde and urea formaldehyde.

reason for this is that there is a much greater release of formaldehyde from paraformaldehyde than from the resins at various temperatures, and the microbicidal process is strictly a function of the available formaldehyde gas.

Applications and mode of action of formaldehyde-condensate biocides have been reviewed by Rossmore & Sondossi (1988) and Rossmore (1995).

18.2.1 Uses of formaldehyde vapour

Formaldehyde vapour has found use as a disinfectant in the following situations (Russell, 1976).

1 In combination with low-temperature steam (70–90°C) as a method for disinfecting heat-sensitive materials (Alder *et al.*, 1971, 1990). This will be discussed later (Chapter 19A); however, some recent studies (Wright *et al.*, 1996) have cast doubt on the efficacy of this process as a sterilization method because it has been possible by means of a post-heating shock to revive some treated spores.

2 Rarely, in the disinfection of hospital bedding and blankets, when formaldehyde solutions are used in the penultimate rinse of laundering blankets to give a residual bactericidal activity because of the slow evolution of formaldehyde

vapour (Dickinson & Wagg, 1967; Alder *et al.*, 1971, 1990).

3 In the terminal disinfection of premises, although this is considered to be of limited value (Kelsey, 1967).

4 As a fumigant in poultry houses after emptying and before new stock is introduced (Nicholls *et al.*, 1967; Anon., 1970) and in the hatcher to prevent bacterial contamination of shell eggs (Harry, 1963).

5 In the disinfection of safety cabinets.

18.3 Betapropiolactone

Betapropiolactone (BPL) requires heating to produce the vapour form, has weak penetrating powers (Table 2.19) and hydrolyses readily in water to give hydracrylic acid (β-hydroxypropionic acid). Its antimicrobial activity depends primarily on its concentration and the temperature and r.h. at which it is used. Its antibacterial activity is maximal at r.h. levels of 75–80%, although, as with ethylene oxide, it is not so much the environmental moisture content that is important but the content and location of water within the bacterial cell (Hoffman & Warshowsky, 1958). The possibility of BPL being carcinogenic (Walpole *et al.*, 1954) has obviously limited its applications, although BPL vapour may have a use in the decontamination of premises (Spiner & Hoffman, 1960).

18.4 Propylene oxide

Propylene oxide requires only mild heating to produce the vapour form and has a fair penetration of materials (Table 2.19). It hydrolyses slowly in the presence of only a small amount of moisture to give the non-toxic propylene glycol (Kereluk, 1971) and there is no need to remove it from exposed materials (Sykes, 1965). Antibacterial activity decreases with an increase in r.h. (Bruch & Koesterer, 1961), although with desiccated organisms the reverse applies (Himmelfarb *et al.*, 1962). Propylene oxide has been shown to be suitable for treating powdered or flaked foods (Bruch & Koesterer, 1961).

18.5 Methyl bromide

Methyl bromide is a gas at normal temperatures. It is considerably less active as an antibacterial agent than ethylene oxide (Kelsey, 1967; Kereluk, 1971) or propylene oxide (Kelsey, 1967) but has good penetrative ability (Table 2.19). Methyl bromide is listed by Kereluk (1971) as being suitable for some types of fumigation.

18.6 Glycidaldehyde

Glycidaldehyde vapour inactives sporing and nonsporing bacteria; the inactivation rate depends on concentration, temperature and inversely on r.h. (Dawson, 1962). There is little information as to its possible usefulness as a disinfecting or sterilizing agent.

18.7 Ozone

Ozone, O_3, is an allotropic form of oxygen. It has powerful oxidizing properties, inhibits bacterial growth (Ingram & Haines, 1949; Baird-Parker & Holbrook, 1971) and is bactericidal, viricidal and sporicidal, although spores are 10–15 times more resistant than non-sporing bacteria (Gurley, 1985; Rickloff, 1985). Gaseous ozone reacts with amino acids, RNA and DNA. It is unstable chemically in water, but activity persists because of the production of free radicals, including $HO^{\bullet}$. A synergistic effect has been shown with the simultaneous use of sonication (Burleson *et al.*, 1975).

18.8 Carbon dioxide

Carbon dioxide in soft drinks inhibits the development of various types of bacteria (Dunn, 1968). The growth of psychrotolerant, slime-producing bacteria is markedly inhibited by CO_2 gas in the atmosphere (Clark & Lentz, 1969).

18.9 Mechanism of action

Only a few brief comments will be made, and the interested reader is directed to the reviews of Bruch & Bruch (1970), Hoffman (1971), Russell (1976) Richards *et al.* (1984) and Russell & Chopra (1996) for further information. As noted above

(Section 18.1, Figs. 2.37 and 2.38), there is strong evidence that ethylene oxide acts by virtue of its alkylating properties; this gaseous agent reacts with proteins and amino acids, and with nucleic acid guanine (to give 7-(2′-hydroxyethyl) guanine), with alkylation of phosphated guanine possibly being responsible for its activity (Michael & Stumbo, 1970). The N-7 guanine position may also be a primary reaction site for BPL (Troll *et al.*, 1969). Formaldehyde is an extremely reactive chemical, which interacts with cell protein, RNA and DNA (Russell & Hopwood, 1976).

19 Aerial disinfectants

An early procedure for aerial disinfection was the employment of sulphur dioxide, obtained by burning sulphur, or of chlorine for fumigating sickrooms.

An effective aerial disinfectant should be capable of being dispersed in the air so that complete and rapid mixing of infected air and disinfectant ensues. Additionally, an effective concentration should be maintained in the air, and the disinfectant must be highly and rapidly effective against airborne microorganisms at different relative humidities. To these microbiological properties must be added the property of no toxicity or irritancy.

The most important means of using aerial disinfectants is by aerosol production. Aerosols consist of a very fine dispersed liquid phase in a gaseous (air) disperse phase. The lethal action of aerosols is believed to be due to condensation of the disinfectant on to the microbial cell (Sykes, 1965). Thus, the disinfectant must be nebulized in a fine spray to enable it to remain airborne and thereby come into contact, by random collision, with any microorganisms present in the air. Aerosol droplets of $< 1\ \mu m$ tend to be the accepted standard. Relative humidity has an important bearing on activity and at low r.h. inadequate condensation of disinfectant on to the microbial cell occurs. This means that dust-borne organisms are less susceptible to aerial disinfectants than are those enclosed in droplets; the optimum r.h. is usually 40–60%. In practice, chemical aerosols may be generated by spraying liquid chemicals into the air from an atomizer; solids may be vaporized by heat from a thermostatically controlled hotplate or dissolved in an appropriate solid and atomized.

Various chemicals have been employed for disinfecting air, including the following.

1 Hexylresorcinol: this phenolic substance is active against a wide range of bacteria, but not spores, in air. It is vaporized from a thermostatically controlled hotplate, and the vapour is odourless and non-toxic.

2 Lactic acid: this is an effective bactericidal aerial agent, but is unfortunately irritant at high concentrations.

3 Propylene glycol: this may be employed as a solvent for dissolving a solid disinfectant prior to atomization, but is also a fairly effective and non-irritating antimicrobial agent in its own right (Baird-Parker & Holbrook, 1971).

4 Formaldehyde: in summary of previous information, formaldehyde gas may be generated by:

(a) evaporating commercial formaldehyde solution (formalin);

(b) adding formalin to potassium permanganate;

(c) volatilizing paraformaldehyde (Taylor *et al.*, 1969);

(d) exposing certain organic resins or polymers, such as melamine formaldehyde or urea formaldehyde, to elevated temperatures (Tulis, 1973; see Russell, 1976).

Fumigation by formaldehyde has found considerable use in poultry science (Anon., 1970).

20 Disinfectants in the food, dairy, pharmaceutical and cosmetic industries

The effectiveness of many disinfectants is reduced in the presence of organic matter in its various forms, such as blood, serum pus, dirt, earth, milkstone, food residues and faecal material (Chapter 3). This decreased activity has an important bearing on disinfectant use in the cosmetic (Davis, 1972a), pharmaceutical (Bean, 1967), food (Kornfeld, 1966; Goldenberg & Relf, 1967; Olivant & Shapton, 1970; Banner, 1995) and dairy (Clegg, 1967, 1970; Davis, 1972b; Anon., 1977) industries. The principles in all cases are the same, namely either adequate precleaning before use of the disinfectant or a combination of the disinfectant with a suitable detergent.

Organic matter may reduce activity either as a result of a chemical reaction between it and the compound, thus leaving a smaller antimicrobial concentration for attacking microorganisms, or through a protection of the organisms from attack (Sykes, 1965). Phospholipids in serum, milk and faeces will reduce the antimicrobial activity of QACs.

The nature of the surface being disinfected and the protection afforded by soiling film are of considerable importance, and invisible milkstone in the dairy industry may protect microorganisms against disinfection (Clegg, 1967). Rapid removal of soiling film may be achieved by use of high pH, for example the use of a combined hypochlorite-detergent at pH 11 (Clegg, 1967). Notwithstanding the lower activity of chlorine disinfectants at alkaline pH, an enhanced effect is observed because of the greater contact between microorganisms and disinfectant. Of course, under certain circumstances caustic soda solutions are themselves sporicidal (Clegg, 1970). Detergents themselves have a killing effect on some microorganisms and are frequently, if not invariably, used hot. Some disinfectants may exert a detergent action.

Cosmetic and pharmaceutical creams may pose several problems, since remnants of production batches may remain in relatively inaccessible orifices and crevices in apparatus and machinery used in their preparation. Such remnants could form foci for the infection of future production batches, which in turn could influence the activity of the preservative selected for incorporation into the product. Bean (1967) recommends cleaning of apparatus and machinery, after use, with hot water and detergent, followed by an appropriate disinfectant or steam.

Davis (1972a) recommends four ways of chemically sterilizing/disinfecting equipment in the cosmetic industry.

1 Detergent, such as alkali, followed by a hypochlorite or a QAC.

2 Cleaning by a stronger concentration of detergent–disinfectant and then sterilization/disinfection by a weaker concentration.

3 Cleaning and sterilizing/disinfecting with a detergent–disinfectant (such as alkali and QAC), followed by a 'sterile rinse' with a QAC or a hypochlorite.

4 Using a single substance, such as sodium hydroxide or nitric acid, which has powerful cleaning and sterilizing properties, followed by a sterile rinse.

A publication by the British Standards Institute (Anon., 1977) is worthy of comment. This deals with recommended methods for sterilizing plant and equipment used in the dairy industry; the term 'sterilization' as used in this report means 'a process which reduces the number of bacteria in dairy plant and utensils to a level consistent with acceptable quality control and hygienic standards'. Thus, while some of the processes recommended might achieve sterilization in the normally accepted sense of the word, the present authors consider that the terms 'disinfection' and 'disinfectant' are more logical. The chemical agents described are: chlorine (see Section 9.2 in the present chapter); iodophors (Section 9.1.2); QACs (Section 6.1); amphoteric surface-active agents (Section 6.4); anionic surface-active agents (Section 6.2) with an inorganic acid, usually phosphoric acid, to give highly acid solutions for removing and preventing milkstone; sodium hydroxide; and formaldehyde (Section 7.2). The report provides useful information on the inclusion of detergents into the formulation to provide balanced products which clean, which are microbicidal and which can be employed below 60°C. At temperatures of 70°C and above, the detergents alone are able to kill most spoilage and pathogenic bacteria. Of prime importance are the compatibility of the two ingredients (in particular, the fact that activity of a microbicidal agent may be enhanced or reduced by a detergent; see Chapter 3) and the need to avoid an increase in the risk of corrosion of the plant or equipment. In the latter context, it is of interest to note that the incorporation of suitable alkaline agents reduces the risks of corrosion induced by chlorine-releasing agents.

Ultrahigh-temperature (UHT) plant in the dairy industry requires true sterilization (as opposed to disinfection see above) and for this pressurized hot water at 140–150°C is recommended in the report.

Finally, mention should be made of some studies by Muys *et al.* (1978), who investigated hydrochloric acid vapour as a sterilizing agent for heat-sensitive food containers. The aim of this work was to obtain a rapid low-temperature method in which no toxic residues remained, as occurred with other vapour-phase chemicals, such as ethylene oxide, hydrogen peroxide, methyl bromide and propylene oxide. Such residues are unacceptable because they could contaminate food packed in the treated containers. The sporicidal activity of hydrochloric acid vapour in this investigation suggests that it is worthy of further study.

21 Disinfectants in recreational waters

The growing popularity of public and private swimming-pools has led to the inevitable problems of maintaining adequate hygienic standards, notably in relation to the possible transmission of infective microorganisms from one person to another. At the same time, control measures must ensure that the swimming-pool water has no toxic or irritant effects on the users of the pool. Various microorganisms have been associated with infections arising from hydrotherapy pools, swimming-pools and whirlpools, but the most frequently implicated organism is *Ps. aeruginosa*, the source of which is often the pool pumps (Friend & Newsom, 1986; Aspinall & Graham, 1989). For many years, chlorine disinfectants have been employed as a sanitary control measure. In 1959, the effectiveness of iodine in the disinfection of swimming-pool water was described (Black *et al.*, 1959) and since then two important papers which compare the relative effectiveness of chlorine and iodine have been published by Black and his colleagues (Black *et al.*, 1970a,b). Iodine scored over chlorine in the following ways: free chlorine and iodine were effective pool sanitizers, but chlorine is more expensive, and iodine is more stable in dilute aqueous solution. Chlorine employment involves the drawback of maintaining adequate residual concentrations when the pool is heavily used, and its eye toxicity is another factor that must be considered; in contrast, its instability can be considered advantageous in terms of keeping a pool free from organic matter and free available chlorine is active in controlling algae. Iodine is ineffective against algae, and thus cannot be recommended for the disinfection of swimming-pool water until suitable formulations can be developed which overcome this disadvantage. Another useful agent used for the disinfection of swimming-pools is the polymeric biguanide, Baquacil SB (Imperial Chemical Industries, Manchester M9 3DA). The properties of this type of compound have been described in Section 5.3.

Warren *et al.* (1981) have published a comparative assessment of swimming-pool disinfectants. Problems arising from the increasing use of whirlpools are referred to in Report (1989).

Hydrotherapy pools are the subject of a later chapter (Chapter 15).

22 Other uses of antimicrobial agents

Antimicrobial agents are used widely as disinfectants and antiseptics in the hospital and domestic enviroments, as preservatives or bactericides in sterile or non-sterile pharmaceutical or cosmetic products (Hodges & Denyer, 1996), and as preservatives in certain foodstuffs. Additionally, they are employed in certain specialized areas, such as cutting oils, fuels, paper, wood, paint, textiles and the construction industry. Some of these aspects are considered in detail in later chapters.

23 Which antimicrobial agent?

23.1 Regulatory requirements

The Federal Drug Administration (FDA) in the USA, the EU for the European community and most other countries publish information on the permitted use and concentration of preservatives. Current regulations should be consulted and complied with when manufacturing in these countries and exporting to them.

The situation from the American point of view has been reviewed by Eirmann (1984). Greenwood (1990) has provided a very comprehensive overview for preservative use over a wide range of countries.

Cosmetic preservatives allowed in the EU are described by Hill (1995), who also considers what percentage, if any, of each is permitted for use in US cosmetic formulations. In the UK, the Ministry of Agriculture, Fisheries and Food (MAFF) publishes information on food additives and E-numbers.

23.2 Which preservative?

Because of the many variables which affect the activity of antimicrobial agents, it is almost impossible from a mere scrutiny of the literature to select a preservative that will be optimal in a particular product. Legislation passed in the USA by the FDA required the manufacturers of cosmetics to declare the ingredients in their products and to state their function or purpose. This information was computerized and the data relating to declared preservatives published (Richardson, 1981). In this survey 19 584 formulae from 902 companies were included. This list of the 10 most used antimicrobial agents, with the number of times they appeared in the 19 584 submissions processed, was as follows:

Methyl *p*-hydroxybenzoate	6785
Propyl *p*-hydroxybenzoate	6174
Imidazolidinyl urea	1684
N-(3-*cis*-chlorallyl)hexamine	1001
Formaldehyde	874
Butyl *p*-hydroxybenzoate	668
2-Bromo-2-nitropropan-1,3-diol	566
Sorbic acid	393
Sodium dehydroacetate	191
Ethyl *p*-hydroxybenzoate	159

Although this is a statistical, rather than a scientific, survey, it does represent the combined expertise of a large number of organizations. Unfortunately, this list did not indicate if and where combinations of preservatives were used.

As regards combinations, an appraisal of the literature seems to suggest that a combination of one of the more water-soluble esters of *p*-hydroxybenzoic acid, probably the methyl ester, together with one of the water-soluble urea derivatives or a sulphydryl reactive compound, might be a good combination to start with. Denyer *et al.* (1985) have discussed synergy in preservative combinations.

If the product is a water-in-oil emulsion, and it is felt that the oily phase needs protection, especially from mould infestation, then a third component, one of the oil-soluble esters of *p*-hydroxybenzoic acid, e.g. the butyl ester, or an oil-soluble phenol, such as *o*-phenylphenol, might well be added. Over and above this, there remains the question-begging proviso 'providing other criteria such as compatibility, stability, toxicity and regulatory requirements are satisfied'.

23.3 New concepts

In recent years, 'natural antimicrobial agents' have increasingly been considered by food microbiologists as potential preservatives for food products. These agents may be associated with immune systems and have been examined in mammals, insects and amphibians. As pointed out by Board (1995), an agent active against prokaryotic but not mammalian cells is of obvious interest. Although Board (1995) was discussing natural antimicrobials from animals as potential food preservatives, it is clear that their possible use in other areas should also be investigated.

Likewise, natural antimicrobials from plants (Nychas, 1995) merit further consideration. It is of interest to note here that 'natural and physical preservative systems' are also being considered as an important part of the production of cosmetic and non-sterile pharmaceutical products (Leech, 1988). Such systems refer to the utilization of pH, natural antimicrobial agents or antimicrobial formulation components. Aspects have already been discussed in this chapter or will be considered in Chapter 3, which presents data about the influence of various factors on antimicrobial activity.

24 The future

New biocidal agents are unlikely to be produced in the foreseeable future, although it might be possible to modify chemically some of the existing compounds with the aim of enhancing their activity. Such a procedure has worked well with chemotherapeutic drugs.

With the emergence of 'new' pathogenic entities, such as the prions, glycopeptide-resistant enterococci and multidrug-resistant mycobacteria, as well as biocide-resistant mycobacteria, it is clear that better usage of existing biocides is necessary. This has been discussed by Russell & Russell (1995) and Russell & Chopra (1996). In brief, future policies might well be to examine combinations of biocides, or of a biocide with a permeabilizer, to re-evaluate older, perhaps discarded, molecules, to consider whether physical procedures can enhance antimicrobial activity and, where relevant, to determine how natural antimicrobial systems can be better utilized.

A long-term goal should be the achievement of a better understanding of the ways in which microorganisms are inactivated and of the mechanisms whereby they circumvent the action of a biocide.

Current knowledge about these aspects will be found in the subsequent chapters that form Part I of this book.

25 References

Aalto, T.R., Firman, M.C. & Rigler, N.E. (1953) *p*-Hydroxybenzoic acid esters as preservatives. 1. Uses, antibacterial and antifungal studies, properties and determination. *Journal of the American Pharmaceutical Association*, **42**, 449–457.

Akamatsu, T., Tabata, K., Hironago, M. & Uyeda, M. (1997) Evaluation of the efficacy of a 3.2% glutaraldehyde product for disinfection of fibreoptic endoscopes with an automatic machine. *Journal of Hospital Infection*, **35**, 47–57.

Akers, M.J. (1984) Considerations in selecting antimicrobial preservative agents for parenteral product development. *Pharmaceutical Technology*, **8**, 36–46.

Albert, A. (1966) *The Acridines: Their Preparation, Properties and Uses*, 2nd edn. London: Edward Arnold.

Albert, A. (1979) *Selective Toxicity: The Physico-Chemical Basis of Therapy*, 6th edn. London: Chapman and Hall.

Alder, V.G., Boss, E., Gillespie, W.A. & Swann, A.J. (1971) Residual disinfection of wool blankets treated with formaldehyde. *Journal of Applied Bacteriology*, **34**, 757–763.

Alder, V.G., Brown, A.M. & Gillespie, W.A. (1990) Disinfection of heat-sensitive material by low-temperature steam and formaldehyde. *Journal of Clinical Pathology*, **19**, 83–89.

Aldridge, W.N. & Threlfall, C.J. (1961) Trialkyl tins and oxidative phosphorylation. *Biochemical Journal*, **79**, 214–219.

Alexander, A.E. & Tomlinson, A.J.H. (1949) *Surface Activity*, p. 317. London: Butterworth.

Alfa, M.J. & Sitter, D.L. (1994) In-hospital evaluation of ortho-phthalaldehyde as a high level disinfectant for flexible endoscopes. *Journal of Hospital Infection*, **26**, 15–26.

Allawala, N.A. & Riegelman, S. (1953) The properties of iodine in solutions of surface-active agents. *Journal of the American Pharmaceutical Association, Scientific Edition*, **42**, 396–401.

Allwood, M.C. & Myers, E.R. (1981) Formaldehyde-releasing agents. *Society for Applied Bacteriology Technical Series 16*, pp. 69–76. London: Academic Press.

Anderson, R.A. & Chow, C.E. (1967) The distribution and activity of benzoic acid in some emulsified systems. *Journal of the Society of Cosmetic Chemists*, **18**, 207–214.

Anon. (1958) Disinfection of fabrics with gaseous formaldehyde. Committee on formaldehyde disinfection. *Journal of Hygiene, Cambridge*, **56**, 488–515.

Anon. (1962) Dimethoxane, a new preservative effective with non-ionic agents. *American Perfumer and Cosmetics*, 77, 32–38.

Anon. (1965) Report of the Public Health Laboratory Service Committee on the Testing and Evaluation of Disinfectants. *British Medical Journal*, **i**, 408–413.

Anon. (1970) *The Disinfection and Disinfestation of Poultry Houses*. Ministry of Agriculture, Fisheries and Food: Advisory Leaflet 514, revised 1970. London: HMSO.

Anon. (1977) Recommendations for sterilisation of plant and equipment used in the dairying industry. BS 5305. London: British Standards Institution.

Ascenzi, J.M. (1996a) *Handbook of Disinfectants and Antiseptics*. New York: Marcel Dekker.

Ascenzi, J.M. (1996b) Antiseptics and their role in infection control. In *Handbook of Disinfectants and Antiseptics* (ed. Ascenzi, J.M.), pp. 63–72. New York: Marcel Dekker.

Ascenzi, J.M. (1996c) Glutaraldehyde-based disinfectants. In *Handbook of Disinfectants and Antiseptics* (ed. Ascenzi, J.M.), pp. 111–132. New York: Marcel Dekker.

Aspinall, S.T. & Graham, R. (1989) Two sources of contamination of a hydrotherapy pool by environmental organisms. *Journal of Hospital Infection*, **14**, 285–292.

Ayliffe, G.A.J., Collins, B.J. & Lowbury, E.J.L. (1966) Cleansing and disinfection of hospital floors. *British Medical Journal*, **ii**, 442–445.

Ayres, H.M., Furr, J.R. & Russell, A.D. (1993) A rapid method of evaluating permeabilizing activity against *Pseudomonas aeruginosa. Letters in Applied Microbiology*, **17**, 149–151.

Babb, J.R. (1993) Disinfection and sterilization of endoscopes. *Current Opinion in Infectious Diseases*, **6**, 532–537.

Babb, J.R., Bradley, C.R. & Ayliffe, G.A.J. (1980) Sporicidal activity of glutaraldehyde and hypochlorites and other factors influencing their selection for the treatment of medical equipment. *Journal of Hospital Infection*, **1**, 63–75.

Babb, J.R. & Bradley, C.R. (1995) A review of glutaraldehyde alternatives. *British Journal of Theatre Nursing*, **5**, 20–24.

Baillie, L. (1987) Chlorhexidine resistance among

bacteria isolated from urine of catheterized patients. *Journal of Hospital Infection*, **10**, 83–86.

Baird-Parker, A.C. & Holbrook, R. (1971) The inhibition and destruction of cocci. In *Inhibition and Destruction of the Microbial Cell* (ed. Hugo, W.B.), pp. 369–397. London: Academic Press.

Baldry, M.G.C. (1983) The bactericidal, fungicidal and sporicidal properties of hydrogen peroxide and peracetic acid. *Journal of Applied Bacteriology*, **54**, 417–423.

Baldry, M.G.C. & Fraser, J.A.L. (1988) Disinfection with peroxygens. In *Industrial Biocides* (ed. Payne, K.R.), Critical Reports on Applied Chemistry, Vol. 22, pp. 91–116. Chichester: John Wiley & Sons.

Bandelin, F.J. (1950) The effects of pH on the efficiency of various mould inhibiting compounds. *Journal of the American Pharmaceutical Association, Scientific Edition*, **47**, 691–694.

Bandelin, F.J. (1977) Antibacterial and preservative properties of alcohols. *Cosmetics and Toiletries*, **92**, 59–70.

Banner, M.J. (1995) The selection of disinfectants for use in food hygiene. In *Handbook of Biocide and Preservative Use* (ed. Rossmore, H.W.), pp. 315–333. London: Blackie Academic & Professional.

Barrett, M. (1969) Biocides for food plant. *Process Biochemistry*, **4**, 23–24.

Barrett-Bee, K., Newboult, L. & Edwards, S. (1994) The membrane destabilising action of the antibacterial agent chlorhexidine. *FEMS Microbiology Letters*, **119**, 249–254.

Bartoli, M. & Dusseau, J.Y. (1995) Aldéhydes. In *Antisepsie et Désinfection* (eds Fleurette, J., Freney, J. & Reverdy, M.-E.), pp. 292–304. Paris: Editions ESKA.

Bassett, D.C.J. (1971) The effect of pH on the multiplication of a pseudomonad in chlorhexidine and cetrimide. *Journal of Clinical Pathology*, **24**, 708–711.

Bean, H.S. (1967) The microbiology of topical preparations in pharmaceutical practice. 2. Pharmaceutical aspects. *Pharmaceutical Journal*, **199**, 289–292.

Bean, H.S. & Berry, H. (1950) The bactericidal activity of phenols in aqueous solutions of soap. Part I. The solubility of water-insoluble phenol in aqueous solutions of soap. *Journal of Pharmacy and Pharmacology*, **2**, 484–490.

Bean, H.S. & Berry, H. (1951) The bactericidal activity of phenols in aqueous solutions of soap. Part II. The bactericidal activity of benzylchlorophenol in aqueous solutions of potassium laurate. *Journal of Pharmacy and Pharmacology*, **3**, 639–655.

Bean, H.S. & Berry, H. (1953) The bactericidal activity of phenols in aqueous solutions of soap. Part III. The bactericidal activity of chloroxylenol in aqueous solutions of potassium laurate. *Journal of Pharmacy and Pharmacology*, **5**, 632–639.

Beath, T. (1943) The suppression of infection in recent wounds by the use of antiseptics. *Surgery*, **13**, 667–676.

Beaver, D.J., Roman, D.P. & Stoffel, P.J. (1957) The preparation and bacteriostatic activity of substituted ureas. *Journal of the American Chemical Society*, **79**, 1236–1245.

Beckett, A.H. & Robinson, A.E. (1958) The inactivation of preservatives by non-ionic surface active agents. *Soap, Perfumery and Cosmetics*, **31**, 454–459.

Bell, T.A., Etchells, J.L. & Borg, A.F. (1959) Influence of sorbic acid on the growth of certain species of bacteria, yeasts and filamentous fungi. *Journal of Bacteriology*, **77**, 573–580.

Bellamy, K. (1995) A renew of the test methods used to establish virucidal activity. *Journal of Hospital Infection*, **30** (Suppl.), 389–396.

Beneke, E.S. & Fabian, F.W. (1955) Sorbic acid as a fungistatic agent at different pH levels for moulds isolated from strawberries and tomatoes. *Food Technology*, **9**, 486–488.

Bergan, T. & Lystad, A. (1972) Evaluation of disinfectant inactivators. *Acta Pathologica et Microbiologica Scandinavica, Section B*, **80**, 507–510.

Berke, P.A. & Rosen, W.E. (1970) Germall, a new family of antimicrobial preservatives for cosmetics. *American Perfumer and Cosmetics*, **85**, 55–60.

Berke, P.A. & Rosen, W.E. (1978) Imidazolidinyl urea activity against *Pseudomonas*. *Journal of the Society of Cosmetic Chemists*, **29**, 757–766.

Berke, P.A. & Rosen, W.E. (1980) Are cosmetic emulsions adequately preserved against *Pseudomonas*? *Journal of the Society of Cosmetic Chemists*, **31**, 37–40.

Berry, H. (1944) Antibacterial values of ethylene glycol monophenyl ether (phenoxetol). *Lancet*, **ii**, 175–176.

Berry, H. & Briggs, A. (1956) The influence of soaps on the bactericidal activity of sparingly water soluble phenols. *Journal of Pharmacy and Pharmacology*, **8**, 1143–1154.

Berry, H. & Stenlake, J.B. (1942) Variations in the bactericidal value of Lysol BP. *Pharmaceutical Journal*, **148**, 112–113.

Berry, H., Cook, A.M. & Wills, B.A. (1956) Bactericidal activity of soap–phenol mixtures. *Journal of Pharmacy and Pharmacology*, **8**, 425–441.

Beveridge, E.G. & Hart, A. (1970) The utilisation for growth and the degradation of *p*-hydroxybenzoate esters by bacteria. *International Biodeterioration Bulletin*, **6**, 9–12.

Beveridge, E.G. & Hope, I.A. (1967) Inactivation of benzoic acid in sulphadimidine mixture for infants B.P.C. *Pharmaceutical Journal*, **198**, 457–458.

Bigger, J.W. & Griffiths, L.I. (1933) The disinfection of water by the Katadyn system. *Irish Journal of Medical Sciences*, **85**, 17–25.

Black, A.P., Lackey, J.B. & Lackey, E.W. (1959) Effectiveness of iodine for the disinfection of swimming pool water. *American Journal of Public Health*, **49**, 1061–1068.

Black, A.P., Kinman, R.N., Keirn, M.A., Smith, J.J. & Harlan, W.E. (1970a) The disinfection of swimming pool water. Part 1. Comparison of iodine and chlorine as swimming pool disinfectants. *American Journal of Public Health*, **60**, 535–545.

Black, A.P., Keirn, M.A., Smith, J.J., Dykes, G.M. & Harlan, W.E. (1970b) The disinfection of swimming pool water. Part II. A field study of the disinfection of public swimming pools. *American Journal of Public Health*, **60**, 740–750.

Blatt, R. & Maloney, J.V. (1961) An evaluation of the iodophor compounds as surgical germicides. *Surgery, Gynaecology & Obstetrics*, **113**, 699–704.

Blaug, S.M. & Ahsan, S.S. (1961) Interaction of parabens with non-ionic macromolecules. *Journal of Pharmaceutical Sciences*, **50**, 441–443.

Block, S.S. (1983) Surface-active agents: amphoteric compounds. In *Disinfection, Sterilisation and Preservation* (ed. Block, S.S.), 3rd edn, pp. 335–345. Philadelphia: Lea & Febiger.

Bloomfield, S.F. (1974) The effect of the antibacterial agent Fentichlor on energy coupling in *Staphylococcus aureus*. *Journal of Applied Bacteriology*, **37**, 117–131.

Bloomfield, S.F. (1996) Chlorine and iodine formulations. In *Handbook of Disinfectants and Antiseptics* (ed. Ascenzi, J.M.), pp. 133–158. New York: Marcel Dekker.

Bloomfield, S.F. & Arthur, M. (1994) Mechanisms of inactivation and resistance of spores to chemical biocides. *Journal of Applied Bacteriology Symposium Supplement*, **76**, 91S–104S.

Bloomfield, S.F. & Miles, G.A. (1979a) The antibacterial properties of sodium dichloroisocyanurate and sodium hypochlorite formulations. *Journal of Applied Bacteriology*, **46**, 65–73.

Bloomfield, S.F. & Miles, G.A. (1979b) The relationship between residual chlorine and disinfection capacity of sodium hypochlorite and sodium dichloroisocyanurate solutions in the presence of *Escherichia coli* and of milk. *Microbios Letters*, **10**, 33–43.

Bloomfield, S.F. & Miller, E.A. (1989) A comparison of hypochlorite and phenolic disinfectants for disinfection of clean and soiled surfaces and blood spillages. *Journal of Hospital Infection*, **13**, 231–239.

Bloomfield, S.F. & Uso, E.E. (1985) The antibacterial properties of sodium hypochlorite and sodium dichloroisocyanurate as hospital disinfectants. *Journal of Hospital Infection*, **6**, 20–30.

Bloomfield, S.F., Smith-Burchnell, C.A. & Dalgleish, A.G. (1990) Evaluation of hypochlorite-releasing agents against the human immunodeficiency virus (HIV). *Journal of Hospital Infection*, **15**, 273–278.

Board, R.G. (1995) Natural antimicrobials from animals. In *New Methods of Food Preservation* (ed. Gould, G.W.), pp. 40–57. London: Blackie Academic and Professional.

Bond, W.W. (1995) Activity of chemical germicides against certain pathogens: human immunodeficiency virus (HIV), hepatitis B virus (HBV) and *Mycobacterium tuberculosis* (MTB). In *Chemical Germicides in Health Care* (ed. Rutala, W.), pp. 135–148. Morin Heights: Polyscience Publications.

Booth, I.R. & Kroll, R.G. (1989) The preservation of foods by low pH. In *Mechanisms of Action of Food Preservation Procedures* (ed. Gould, G.W.), pp. 119–160. London: Elsevier Applied Science.

Borick, P.M. (1968) Chemical sterilizers (Chemosterilizers). *Advances in Applied Microbiology*, **10**, 291–312.

Borick, P.M. & Pepper, R.E. (1970) The spore problem. In *Disinfection* (ed. Benarde, M.), pp. 85–102. New York: Marcel Dekker.

Bosund, I. (1962) The action of benzoic and salicylic acids on the metabolism of microorganisms. *Advances in Food Research*, **11**, 331–353.

Boucher, R.M.G. (1974) Potentiated acid 1.5-pentanedial solution—a new chemical sterilizing and disinfecting agent. *American Journal of Hospital Pharmacy*, **31**, 546–557.

Bradley C.R., Babb, J.R. & Aycliffe, G.A.J. (1995) Evaluation of the Steris System 1 peracetic acid endoscope processor. *Journal of Hospital Infection*, **29**, 143–151.

Brandes, C.H. (1934) Ionic silver sterilisation. *Industrial and Engineering Chemistry*, **26**, 962–964.

British Pharmacopoeia (1993) London: HMSO.

British Standards (BS) relating to disinfectants (date in parentheses at end of an entry means that the Standard was confirmed on that date without further revision).

(1950) Specification for QAC Based Aromatic Disinfectant Fluids. BS 6424: 1984 (1990).

(1976) Aromatic Disinfectant Disinfectant Fluids. BS 5197: 1976 (1991).

(1984) Method for Determination of the Antimicrobial Activity of QAC Disinfectant Formulations. BS 6471: 1984 (1994).

(1985) Method for Determination of the Rideal–Walker Coefficient of Disinfectants. BS 541: 1985 (1991).

(1986) Method for Assessing the Efficacy of Disinfectants by the Modified Chick–Martin Test. BS 808: 1986 (1991).

(1986) Specification for Black and White Disinfectants. BS 2462: 1986 (1991).

(1986) Glossary of Terms Relating to Disinfectants. BS 5283: 1986 (1991).

(1997a) *Chemical Disinfectants and Antiseptics—Basic Bactericidal Activity—Test Method and Requirements (Phase 1)*. BS EN 1040: 1997.

(1997b) *Chemical Disinfectants and Antiseptics—Basic Fungicidal Activity—Test Method and Requirements (Phase 1)*. BS EN 1275: 1997.

(1997c) *Chemical Disinfectants and Antiseptics—Hygienic Handwash—Test Method and Requirements (Phase 2/Step 2)*. BS EN 1499: 1997.

Broadley, S.J., Jenkins, P.A., Furr, J.R. & Russell, A.D. (1991) Antimycobacterial activity of biocides. *Letters in Applied Microbiology*, **13**, 118–122.

Brown, M.R.W. (1975) The role of the cell envelope in resistance. In *Resistance of Pseudomonas aeruginosa* (ed. Brown, M.R.W.), pp. 71–107. London: John Wiley & Sons.

Brown, M.R.W. & Anderson, R.A. (1968) The bacterial effect of silver ions on *Pseudomonas aeruginosa*. *Journal of Pharmacy and Pharmacology*, **20**, 1S–3S.

Browne, M.K. & Stoller, J.L. (1970) Intraperitoneal noxythiolin in faecal peritonitis. *British Journal of Surgery*, **57**, 525–529.

Browne, M.K., Leslie, G.B. & Pfirrman, R.W. (1976) Taurolin, a new chemotherapeutic agent. *Journal of Applied Bacteriology*, **41**, 363–368.

Browne, M.K., Leslie, G.B., Pfirrman, R.W. & Brodhage, H. (1977) The *in vitro* and *in vivo* activity of Taurolin against anaerobic pathogenic organisms. *Surgery, Gynaecology and Obstetrics*, **145**, 842–846.

Browne, M.K., MacKenzie, M. & Doyle, P.J. (1978) A controlled trial of Taurolin in establishing bacterial peritonitis. *Surgery, Gynaecology and Obstetrics*, **146**, 721–724.

Browning, C.H. (1964) Chemotherapy of antibacterial dyestuffs. In *Experimental Chemotherapy*, Vol. 2 (eds Schnitzer, R.T. & Hawkins, F.), pp. 1–136. London: Academic Press.

Browning, C.H., Gulbransen, R. & Kennaway, E.L. (1919–20) Hydrogen-ion concentration and antiseptic potency, with special references to the action of acridine compounds. *Journal of Pathology and Bacteriology*, **23**, 106–108.

Broxton, P., Woodcock, P.M. & Gilbert, P. (1983) A study of the antibacterial activity of some polyhexamethylene biguanides towards *Escherichia coli* ATCC 8739. *Journal of Applied Bacteriology*, **54**, 345–353.

Broxton, P., Woodcock, P.M., Hearley, F. & Gilbert, P. (1984a) Interaction of some polyhexamethylene biguanides and membrane phospholipids in *Escherichia coli*. *Journal of Applied Bacteriology*, **57**, 115–124.

Broxton, P., Woodcock, P.M. & Gilbert, P. (1984b) Binding of some polyhexamethylene biguanides to the cell envelope of *Escherichia coli* ATCC 8739. *Microbios*, **41**, 15–22.

Bruch, C.W. (1991) Role of glutaraldehyde and other liquid chemical sterilants in the processing of new medical devices. In *Sterilization of Medical Products* (eds Morrissey, R.F. & Prokopenko, Y.I.) Vol. V, pp. 377–396. Morin Heights, Canada: Polyscience Pulications Inc.

Bruch, C.W. & Bruch, M.K. (1970) Gaseous disinfection. In *Disinfection* (ed. Benarde, M.), pp. 149–206. New York: Marcel Dekker.

Bruch, C.W. & Koesterer, M.G. (1961) The microbicidal activity of gaseous propylene oxide and its application to powdered or flaked foods. *Journal of Food Science*, **26**, 428–435.

Bruch, M.K. (1996) Chloroxylenol: an old–new antimicrobial. In *Handbook of Disinfectants and Antiseptics* (ed. Ascenzi, J.M.), pp. 265–294. New York: Marcel Dekker.

Bryce, D.M., Croshaw, B., Hall, J.E., Holland, V.R. & Lessel, B. (1978) The activity and safety of the antimicrobial agent bronopol (2-bromo-2-nitropropan-1,3-diol). *Journal of the Society of Cosmetic Chemists*, **29**, 3–24.

Burgess, D.J. & Reich, R.R. (1993) Industrial ethylene oxide sterilization. In *Sterilization Technology. A Practical Guide for Manufacturers and Uses of Health Care Products* (eds Morrissey, R.F. & Briggs Phillips, G.), pp. 152–195. New York: Van Nostrand Reinhold.

Burleson, G.R., Murray, T.M. & Pollard, M. (1975) Inactivation of viruses and bacteria by ozone, with and without sonication. *Applied Microbiology*, **29**, 340–344.

Chawner, J.A. & Gilbert, P. (1989a) A comparative study of the bactericidal and growth inhibitory activities of the bisbiguanides, alexidine and chlorhexidine. *Journal of Applied Bacteriology*, **66**, 243–252.

Chawner, J.A. & Gilbert, P. (1989b) Interaction of the bisbiguanides chlorhexidine and alexidine with phospholipid vesicles: evidence for separate modes of action. *Journal of Applied Bacteriology*, **66**, 253– 258.

Cherrington, C.A., Hinton, M. & Chopra, I. (1990) Effect of short-chain organic acids on macromolecular synthesis in *Escherichia coli*. *Journal of Applied Bacteriology*, **68**, 69–74.

Cherrington, C.A., Hinton, M., Mead, G.C. & Chopra, I. (1991) Organic acids: chemistry, antibacterial activity and practical applications. *Advances in Microbial Physiology*, **32**, 87–108.

Clark, D.S. & Lentz, C.P. (1969) The effect of carbon dioxide on the growth of slime producing bacteria on fresh beef. *Canadian Institute of Food Technology Journal*, **2**, 72–75.

Clegg, L.F.L. (1967) Disinfectants in the dairy industry. *Journal of Applied Bacteriology*, **30**, 117–140.

Clegg, L.F.L. (1970) Disinfection in the dairy industry. In *Disinfection* (ed. Bernarde, M.A.), pp. 311–375. New York: Marcel Dekker.

Coal Tar Data Book (1965) 2nd edn. Leeds: The Coal Tar Research Association.

Coates, D. (1985) A comparison of sodium hypochlorite and sodium dichloroisocyanurate products. *Journal of Hospital Infection*, **6**, 31–40.

Coates, D. (1988) Comparison of sodium hypochlorine and sodium dichloroisocyanurate disinfectants: neutralization by serum. *Journal of Hospital Infection*, **11**, 60–67.

Coates, D. (1996) Sporicidal activity of sodium dichloroisocyanurate, peroxygen and glutaraldehyde disinfectants against *Bacillus subtilis*. *Journal of Hospital Infection*, **32**, 283–294.

Coates, D. & Death, J.E. (1978) Sporicidal activity of mixtures of alcohol and hypochlorite. *Journal of Clinical Pathology*, **31**, 148–152.

Coates, D. & Wilson, M. (1989) Use of sodium dichloroisocyanurate granules for spills of body fluids. *Journal of Hospital Infection*, **13**, 241–251.

Coates, D. & Hutchinson, D.N. (1994) How to produce a hospital disinfection policy. *Journal of Hospital Infection*, **26**, 57–68.

Colebrook, L. (1941) Disinfection of the skin. *Bulletin of War Medicine*, **2**, 73–79.

Colebrook, L. & Maxted, W.R. (1933) Antiseptics in midwifery. *Journal of Obstetrics and Gynaecology of the British Empire*, **40**, 966–990.

Collier, H.O.J., Cox, W.A., Huskinson, P.L. & Robinson, F.A. (1959) Further observations on the biological properties of dequalinium (Dequadin) and hedaquinium (Teoquil). *Journal of Pharmacy and Pharmacology*, **11**, 671–680.

Collier, P.J., Ramsey, A.J., Austin, P. & Gilbert, P. (1990a) Growth inhibitory and biocidal activity of some isothiazolone biocides. *Journal of Applied Bacteriology*, **69**, 569–577.

Collier, P.J., Ramsey, A., Waight, K.T., Douglas, N.T., Austin, P. & Gilbert, P. (1990b) Chemical reactivity of some isothiazolone biocides. *Journal of Applied Bacteriology*, **69**, 578–584.

Collins, J. (1986) The use of glutaraldehyde in laboratory discard jars. *Letters in Applied Microbiology*, **2**, 103–105.

Corner, T.R., Joswick, H.L., Silvernale, J.N. & Gerhardt, P. (1971) Antimicrobial actions of hexachlorophane: lysis and fixation of bacterial protoplases. *Journal of Bacteriology*, **108**, 501–507.

Cottone, J.A. & Molinari, J.A. (1996) Disinfectant use in dentistry. In *Handbook of Disinfectants and Antiseptics* (ed. Ascenzi, J.M.), pp. 73–82. New York: Marcel Dekker.

Cousins, C.M. & Allan, C.D. (1967) Sporicidal properties of some halogens. *Journal of Applied Bacteriology*, **30**, 168–174.

Cox, W.A. & D'Arcy, P.F. (1962) A new cationic antimicrobial agent. *N*-dodecyl-4-amino quinaldinium acetate (Laurolinium acetate). *Journal of Pharmacy and Pharmacology*, **15**, 129–137.

Craven, D.E., Moody, B., Connolly, M.G., Kollisch, N.R., Stottmeier, K.D. & McCabe, W.R. (1981) Pseudobacteremia caused by povidone-iodine solution contaminated with *Pseudomonas cepacia*. *New England Journal of Medicine*, **305**, 621–623.

Crewther, W.G. & McQuade, A.B. (1964) Disinfection of woollen blankets. *Journal of Hygiene, Cambridge*, **62**, 29–37.

Croshaw, B. (1971) The destruction of mycobacteria. In *Inhibition and Destruction of the Microbial Cell* (ed. Hugo, W.B.), pp. 419–449. London: Academic Press.

Croshaw, B. (1977) Preservatives for cosmetics and toiletries. *Journal of the Society of Cosmetic Chemists*, **28**, 3–16.

Croshaw, B. & Holland, V.R. (1984) Chemical preservatives: use of bronopol as a cosmetic preservative. In *Cosmetic and Drug Preservation. Principles and Practice* (ed. Kabara, J.J.), pp. 31–62. New York: Marcel Dekker.

Cruess, W.V. & Richert, P. (1929) Effects of hydrogen ion concentration on the toxicity of sodium benzoate to microorganisms. *Journal of Bacteriology*, **17**, 363–371.

Curd, F.H.S. & Rose, F.L. (1946) Synthetic antimalarials. Part X. Some aryl-diaguanide ('-biguanide') derivatives. *Journal of the Chemical Society*, 729–737.

Dancer, B.N., Power, E.G.M. & Russell, A.D. (1989) Alkali-induced revival of *Bacillus* spores after inactivation by glutaraldehyde. *FEMS Microbiology Letters*, **57**, 345–348.

Dankert, J. & Schut, I.K. (1976) The antibacterial activity of chloroxylenol in combination with ethylenediamine tetraacetic acid. *Journal of Hygiene, Cambridge*, **76**, 11–22.

D'Arcy, P.F. (1971) Inhibition and destruction of moulds and yeasts. In *Inhibition and Destruction of the Microbial Cell* (ed. Hugo, W.B.), pp. 613–686. London: Academic Press.

D'Arcy, P.F. & Taylor, E.P. (1962a) Quaternary ammonium compounds in medicinal chemistry. I. *Journal of Pharmacy and Pharmacology*, **14**, 129–146.

D'Arcy, P.F. & Taylor, E.P. (1962b) Quaternary ammonium compounds in medicinal chemistry. II. *Journal of Pharmacy and Pharmacology*, **14**, 193–216.

Davies, A., Bentley, M. & Field, B.S. (1968) Comparison of the action of Vantocil, cetrimide and chlorhexidine on *Escherichia coli* and the protoplasts of Gram-positive bacteria. *Journal of Applied Bacteriology*, **31**, 448–461.

Davies, D.J.G. (1980) Manufacture and supply of contact lens products. I. An academic's view. *Pharmaceutical Journal*, **225**, 343–345.

Davies, G.E. (1949) Quaternary ammonium compounds. A new technique for the study of their bactericidal action and the results obtained with Cetavlon (cetyltrimethyl ammonium bromide). *Journal of Hygiene, Cambridge*, **47**, 271–277.

Davies, G.E., Francis, J., Martin, A.R., Rose, F.L. & Swain, G. (1954) 1:6-Di-4′-chlorophenyl-diguanidinohexane ('Hibitane'): a laboratory investigation of a new antibacterial agency of high potency. *British Journal of Pharmacology*, **9**, 192–196.

Davis, J.G. (1960) Methods for the evaluation of the antibacterial activity of surface active compounds: technical aspects of the problem. *Journal of Applied Bacteriology*, **23**, 318–344.

Davis, J.G. (1962) Idophors as detergent-sterilizers. *Journal of Applied Bacteriology*, **25**, 195–201.

Davis, J.G. (1972a) Fundamentals of microbiology in relation to cleansing in the cosmetics industry. *Journal of the Society of Cosmetic Chemists*, **23**, 45–71.

Davis, J.G. (1972b) Problems of hygiene in the dairy industry. Parts 1 and 2. *Dairy Industries*, **37**, 212–215; (5) 251–256.

Dawson, F.W. (1962) Glycidaldehyde vapour as a disinfectant. *American Journal of Hygiene*, **76**, 209–215.

Deans, S.G. & Ritchie, G. (1987) Antibacterial properties of plant essential oils. *International Journal of Food Microbiology*, **5**, 165–180.

Death, J.E. & Coates, D. (1979) Effect of pH on sporicidal and microbicidal activity of buffered mixtures of alcohol and sodium hypochlorite. *Journal of Clinical Pathology*, **32**, 148–153.

Denyer, S.P. & Wallhäusser, K.H. (1990) Antimicrobial preservatives and their properties. In *Guide to Microbial Control in Pharmaceutical* (eds Denyer, S.P. & Baird, R.M.), pp. 251–273. Chichester: Ellis Horwood.

Denyer, S.P., Hugo, W.B. & Harding, V.D. (1985) Synergy in preservative combinations. *International Journal of Pharmaceutics*, **25**, 245–253.

Dickinson, J.C. & Wagg, R.E. (1967) Use of formaldehyde for the disinfection of hospital woollen blankets on laundering. *Journal of Applied Bacteriology*, **33**, 566–573.

Domagk, G. (1935) Eine neue Klasse von Disinfektionsmitteln. *Deutsche Medizinische Wochenschrift*, **61**, 829–932.

Dunning, F., Dunning, B. & Drake, W.E. (1931) Preparation and bacteriological study of some symmetrical organic sulphides. *Journal of the American Chemical Society*, **53**, 3466–3469.

Dychdala, G.R. (1983) Chlorine and chlorine compounds. In *Disinfection, Sterilization and Preservation* (ed. Block, S.S.), 3rd edn, pp. 157–182. Philadelphia: Lea & Febiger.

Eager, R.C., Leder, J. & Theis, A.B. (1986) Glutaraldehyde: factors important for microbicidal efficacy. *Proceedings of the 3rd Conference on Progress in Chemical Disinfection*, pp. 32–49. Binghamton, New York.

Eirmann, H.J. (1984) Cosmetic product preservation. Safety and regulatory issues. In *Cosmetic and Drug Preservation: Principles and Practice* (ed. Kabara, J.J.), pp. 559–569. New York: Marcel Dekker.

Eklund, T (1980) Inhibition of growth and uptake processes in bacteria by some chemical food preservatives. *Journal of Applied Bacteriology*, **48**, 423–432.

Eklund, T. (1985) Inhibition of microbial growth at different pH levels by benzoic and propionic acids and esters of *p*-hydroxybenzoic acid. *International Journal of Food Microbiology*, **2**, 159–167.

Eklund, T. (1989) Organic acids and esters. In *Mechanisms of Action of Food Preservation Procedure* (ed. Gould, G.W.), pp. 161–200. London: Elsevier Applied Science.

El-Falaha, B.M.A., Russel, A.D. & Furr, J.R. (1983) Sensitivities of wild-type and envelope-defective strains of *Escherichia coli* and *Pseudomonas aeruginosa* to antibacterial agents. *Microbios*, **38**, 99–105.

Ellison, R.T., Giehl, T.J. & LaForce, F.M. (1988) Damage of the outer membrane of enteric Gram-negative bacteria by lactoferrin and transferrin. *Infection and Immunity*, **56**, 2774–2781.

Elsmore, R. (1993) Practical experience of the use of bromine based biocides in cooling towers. *Biodeterioration and Biodegradation*, **9**, 114–122.

Elsmore, R. (1995) Development of bromine chemistry in controlling microbial growth in water systems. *International Biodeterioration and Biodegradation*, **36**, 245–253.

Elworthy, P.H. (1976) The increasingly clever micelle. *Pharmaceutical Journal*, **217**, 566–570.

Ernst, R.R. (1974) Ethylene oxide sterilization kinetics. *Biotechnology and Bioengineering Symposium*, No. 4, pp. 865–878.

Fargher, R.G., Galloway, L.O. & Roberts, M.E. (1930) The inhibitory action of certain substances on the growth of mould fungi. *Journal of Textile Chemistry*, **21**, 245–260.

Farkas-Himsley, H. (1964) Killing of chlorine-resistant bacteria by chlorine-bromide solutions. *Applied Microbiology*, **12**, 1–6.

Favero, M.S. (1985) Sterilization, disinfection and antisepsis in the hospital. In *Manual of Clinical Microbiology* (eds Lennette, E.H., Balows, A., Hausler, W.J., Jr & Shadomy, H.J.), 4th edn, pp. 129–137. Washington, DC: American Society for Microbiology.

Favero, M.S. (1995) Chemical germicides in the health care field: the perspective from the Centers for Disease Control and Prevention. In *Chemical Germicides in Health Care* (ed. Rutala, W.A.), pp. 33–42. Morin Heights: Polyscience Publications.

Favero, M.S. & Bond, W.W. (1991) Chemical disinfection of medical and surgical materials. In *Disinfection, Sterilization and Preservation* (ed. Block, S.S.), 4th edn, pp. 617–641. Philadelphia: Lea & Febiger.

Fels, P., Gay, M., Kabay, A. & Urban, S. (1987) Antimicrobial preservation. Manufacturers' experience with pharmaceuticals in the efficacy test and in practice. *Pharmaceutical Industry*, **49**, 631–637.

Finch, W.E. (1953) A substitute for Lysol. *Pharmaceutical Journal*, **170**, 59–60.

Finch, W.E. (1958) *Disinfectants – Their Value and Uses.* London: Chapman & Hall.

Fitzgerald, K.A., Davies, A. & Russell, A.D. (1989) Uptake of ^{14}C-chlorhexidine diacetate to *Escherichia coli* and *Pseudomonas aeruginosa* and its release by azolectin. *FEMS Microbiology Letters*, **60**, 327–332.

Fitzgerald, K.A., Davies, A. & Russell, A.D. (1992a) Sensitivity and resistance of *Escherichia coli* and *Staphylococcus aureus* to chlorhexidine. *Letters in Applied Microbiology*, **14**, 33–36.

Fitzgerald, K.A., Davies, A. & Russell, A.D. (1992b) Effect of chlorhexidine and phenoxyethanol on cell surface hydrophobicity of Gram-positive and Gram-negative bacteria. *Letters in Applied Microbiology*, **14**, 91–95.

Fleurette, J., Freney, J. & Reverdy, M.-E. (1995) *Antisepsie et Désinfection.* Paris: Editions ESKA.

Foster, J.H.S. & Russell, A.D. (1971) Antibacterial dyes and nitrofurans. In *Inhibition and Destruction of the Microbial Cell* (ed. Hugo, W.B.), pp. 185–208. London: Academic Press.

Foster, T.J. (1983) Plasmid-determined resistance to antimicrobial drugs and toxic metal ions in bacteria. *Microbiological Reviews*, **47**, 361–409.

Fraenkel-Conrat, H., Cooper, M. & Alcott, H.S. (1945) The reaction of formaldehyde with proteins. *Journal of the American Chemical Society*, **67**, 950–954.

Frank, M.J. & Schaffner, W. (1976) Contaminated aqueous benzalkonium chloride: an unnecessary hospital infection hazard. *Journal of the American Medical Association*, **236**, 2418–2419.

Fraser, J.A.L. (1986) Novel applications of peracetic acid. *Chemspec '86: BACS Symposium*, pp. 65–69.

Frederick, J.F., Corner, T.R. & Gerhardt, P. (1974) Antimicrobial actions of hexachlorophane: inhibition of respiration in *Bacillus megaterium. Antimicrobial Agents and Chemotherapy*, **6**, 712–721.

Freese, E. & Levin, B.C. (1978) Action mechanisms of preservatives and antiseptics. *Developments in Industrial Microbiology*, **19**, 207–227.

Freese, E., Sheu, W. & Galliers, E. (1973) Function of lipophilic acids as antimicrobial food additives. *Nature, London*, **241**, 321–325.

Freney, J. (1995) Composés phénoliques. In *Antisepsie et Désinfection* (eds Fleurette, J., Freney, J. & Reverdy, M.-E.), pp. 90–134. Paris: Editions ESKA.

Friend, P.A. & Newsom, S.W.B. (1986) Hygiene for hydrotherapy pools. *Journal of Hospital Infection*, **8**, 213–216.

Frier, M. (1971) Derivatives of 4-amino-quinaldinium and 8-hydroxyquinoline. In *Inhibition and Destruction of the Microbial Cell* (ed. Hugo, W.B.), pp. 107–120. London: Academic Press.

Furr, J.R. & Russell, A.D. (1972a) Some factors influencing the activity of esters of *p*-hydroxybenzoic acid against *Serratia marcescens. Microbios*, **5**, 189–198.

Furr, J.R. & Russell, A.D. (1972b) Uptake of esters of *p*-hydroxy benzoic acid by *Serratia marcescens* and by fattened and non-fattened cells of *Bacillus subtilis. Microbios*, **5**, 237–346.

Furr, J.R. & Russell, A.D. (1972c) Effect of esters of *p*-hydroxybenzoic acid on spheroplasts of *Serratia marcescens* and protoplasts of *Bacillus megaterium. Microbios*, **6**, 47–54.

Furr, J.R., Russell, A.D., Turner, T.D. & Andrews, A. (1994) Antibacterial activity of Actisorb, Actisorb Plus and silver nitrate. *Journal of Hospital Infection*, **27**, 201–208.

Galbraith, H., Miller, T.B., Paton, A.M. & Thompson, J.K. (1971) Antibacterial activity of long chain fatty acids and the reversal with calcium, magnesium, ergocalciferol and cholesterol. *Journal of Applied Bacteriology*, **34**, 803–813.

Galland, R.B., Saunders, J.H., Mosley, J.G. & Darrell, J.C. (1977) Prevention of wound infection in abdominal operations by per-operative antibiotics or povidone-iodine. *Lancet*, **ii**, 1043–1045.

Gardner, J.F. & Peel, M.M. (1986) *Introduction to Sterilization and Disinfection.* Edinburgh: Churchill Livingstone.

Gardner, J.F. & Peel, M.M. (1991) *Introduction to Sterilization, Disinfection and Infection Control.* Edinburgh: Churchill Livingstone.

Gavin, J., Button, N.F., Watson-Craik, I.A. & Logan, N.A. (1996) Efficacy of standard disinfectant test methods for contact lens-care solutions. *International Biodeterioration and Biodegradation*, **36**, 431–440.

Gershenfeld, L. (1956) A new iodine dairy sanitizer. *American Journal of Pharmacy*, **128**, 335–339.

Gershenfeld, L. (1962) Povidone-iodine as a sporicide. *American Journal of Pharmacy*, **134**, 78–81.

Gilbert, P., Pemberton, D. & Wilkinson, D.E. (1990a) Barrier properties of the Gram-negative cell envelope towards high molecular weight polyhexamethylene biguanides. *Journal of Applied Bacteriology*, **69**, 585–592.

Gilbert, P., Pemberton, D. & Wilkinson, D.E. (1990b) Synergism within polyhexamethylene biguanide biocide formulations. *Journal of Applied Bacteriology*, **69**, 593–598.

Gillespie, E.H. & Robinson, W. (1959) Blanket laundering and sterilization. *Journal of Clinical Pathology*, **12**, 351.

Gjermo, P., Rolla, G. & Arskaug, L. (1973) The effect on dental plaque formation and some *in vitro* properties of 12 bis-biguanides. *Journal of Periodontology*, **8**, 81–88.

Goldberg, A.A., Shapero, M. & Wilder, E. (1950) Antibacterial colloidal electrolytes: the potentiation of the activities of mercuric, phenylmercuric and silver ions by a colloidal and sulphonic anion. *Journal of Pharmacy and Pharmacology*, **2**, 20–26.

Goldenberg, N. & Relf, C.J. (1967) Use of disinfectants in the food industry. *Journal of Applied Bacteriology*, **30**, 141–147.

Gooding, C.M., Melnick, D., Lawrence, R.L. & Luckmann, F.H. (1955) Sorbic acid as a fungistatic agent for foods. IX. Physico-chemical considerations in using sorbic acid to protect foods. *Food Research*, **20**, 639–648.

Gorman, S.P. & Scott, E.M. (1985) A comparative evaluation of dental aspirator cleansing and disinfectant solutions. *British Dental Journal*, **158**, 13–16.

Gorman, S.P., Scott, E.M. & Russell, A.D. (1980) Antimicrobial activity, uses and mechanism of action of glutaraldehyde. *Journal of Applied Bacteriology*, **48**, 161–190.

Gottardi, W. (1985) The influence of the chemical behaviour of iodine on the germicidal action of disinfection solutions containing iodine. *Journal of Hospital Infection*, **6** (Suppl. A), 1–11.

Gould, G.W. & Jones, M.V. (1989) Combination and synergistic effects. In *Mechanisms of Action of Food Preservation Procedures* (ed. Gould, G.W.), pp. 401–421. London: Elsevier Applied Science.

Gould, G.W. & Russell, N.J. (1991) Sulphite. In *Food Preservatives* (eds Russell, N.J. & Gould, G.W.) pp. 72–88. Glasgow: Blackie.

Gray, G.W. & Wilkinson, S.G. (1965) The action of ethylenediamine tetraacetic acid on *Pseudomonas aeruginosa*. *Journal of Applied Bacteriology*, **28**, 153–164.

Greenwood, R.K. (1990) Preservatives: registration and regulatory affairs. In *Guide to Microbiology Control in Pharmaceuticals* (eds Denyer, S.P. & Baird, R.M.), pp. 313–340. Chichester: Ellis Horwood.

Gribbard, J. (1933) The oligodynamic action of silver in the treatment of water. *Canadian Journal of Public Health*, **24**, 96–97.

Groschel, D.H.M. (1995) Emerging technologies for disinfection and sterilization. In *Chemical Germicides in Health Care* (ed. Rutala, W.), pp. 73–82. Morin Heights: Polyscience Publications.

Grossgebauer, K. (1970) Virus disinfection. In *Disinfection* (ed. Benarde, M.), pp. 103–148. New York: Marcel Dekker.

Gueklhorn, I.R. (1970) Antimicrobials in cosmetics. Parts 1–7. *Manufacturing Chemist and Aerosol News*, **41** (6) 44–45; (7) 51–52; (8) 28–29; (10) 49–50; (11) 48–49; (12) 50–51.

Gueklhorn, I.R. (1971) Antimicrobials in cosmetics. Parts 8 and 9. *Manufacturing Chemist and Aerosol News*, **42** (1) 35–37; (2) 35–39.

Gump, W.S. & Walter, G.R. (1960) Chemical and antimicrobial activity of bis phenols. *Journal of the Society of Cosmetic Chemists*, **11**, 307–314.

Gump, W.S. & Walter, G.R. (1963) Chemical structure and antimicrobial activity of bis phenols. III. Broad spectrum evaluation of hexachlorophane and its isomers. *Journal of the Society of Cosmetic Chemists*, **14**, 269–276.

Gump, W.S. & Walter, G.R. (1964) Chemical structure and antimicrobial activity of bis phenols. IV. Broad spectrum evaluation of 2,2′-methylene bis (dichlorophenols). *Journal of the Society of Cosmetic Chemists*, **15**, 717–725.

Gurevich, I., Rubin, R. & Cunha, B.A. (1996) Dental instrument and device sterilization and disinfection practices. *Journal of Hospital Infection*, **32**, 295–304.

Gurley, B. (1985) Ozone: pharmaceutical sterilant of the future? *Journal of Parenteral Science and Technology*, **39**, 256–261.

Haag, T.E. & Loncrini, D.F. (1984) Esters of *para*-hydroxybenzoic acid. In *Cosmetic and Drug Preservation. Principles and Practice* (ed. Kabara, JJ.), pp. 63–77. New York: Marcel Dekker.

Haler, D. (1974) The effect of 'Noxyflex' (Noxythiolin), on the behaviour of animals which have been infected intraperitoneally with suspensions of faeces. *International Journal of Clinical Pharmacology*, **9**, 160–164.

Hamilton, W.A. (1968) The mechanism of the bacteriostatic action of tetrachlorosalicylanide: a membrane-active antibacterial compound. *Journal of General Microbiology*, **50**, 441–458.

Hamilton, W.A. (1971) Membrane-active antibacterial compounds. In *Inhibition and Destruction of the Microbial Cell* (ed. Hugo, W.B.), pp. 77–106. London: Academic Press.

Hamilton-Miller, J.M.T., Shah, S. & Smith, C. (1993) Silver sulphadiazine: a comprehensive *in vitro* reassessment. *Chemotherapy*, **39**, 405–409.

Hammond, S.M. & Carr, J.G. (1976) The antimicrobial activity of SO_2. In *Inhibition and Inactivation of Vegetative Microbes* (eds Skinner, F.A. & Hugo, W.B.), Society for Applied Bacteriology Symposium Series No. 5, pp. 89–110. London: Academic Press.

Haque, H. & Russell, A.D. (1974a) Effect of ethylenediamine tetraacetic acid and related chelating agents on whole cells of Gram-negative bacteria. *Antimicrobial Agents and Chemotherapy*, **5**, 447–452.

Haque, H. & Russell, A.D. (1974b) Effect of chelating agents on the susceptibility of some strains of Gram-negative bacteria to some antibacterial agents. *Antimicrobial Agents and Chemotherapy*, **6**, 200–206.

Haque, H. & Russell, A.D. (1976) Cell envelopes of Gram-negative bacteria: composition, response to chelating agents and susceptibility of whole cells to antibacterial agents. *Journal of Applied Bacteriology*, **40**, 89–99.

Harry, E.G. (1963) The relationship between egg spoilage and the environment of the egg when laid. *British Poultry Science*, **4**, 91–100.

Hatch, E. & Cooper, P. (1948) Sodium hexametaphosphate in emulsions of Dettol for obstetric use. *Pharmaceutical Journal*, **161**, 198–199.

Heinzel, M. (1988) The phenomena of resistance to disinfectants and preservatives. In *Industrial Biocides* (ed. Payne, K.R.), Critical Reports on Applied Chemistry, Vol. 22, pp. 52–67. Chichester: John Wiley & Sons.

Hernández, A., Belda, F.J., Dominguez, J. *et al.* (1996) Evaluation of the disinfectant effect of Solprogel against human immunodeficiency virus type 1 (HTV-1). *Journal of Hospital Infection*, **34**, 223–228.

Hernández, A., Belda, F.J., Dominguez, J. *et al.* (1997) Inactivation of hepatitis B virus: evaluation of the efficacy of the disinfectant 'Solprogel' using a DNA-polymerase assay. *Journal of Hospital Infection*, **36**, 305–312.

Hill, G. (1995) Preservation of cosmetics and toiletries. In *Handbook of Biocide and Preservative Use* (ed. Rossmore, H.W.), pp. 349–415. London: Blackie Academic & Professional.

Himmelfarb, P., El-Bis, H.M., Read, R.B. & Litsky, W. (1962) Effect of relative humidity on the bactericidal activity of propylene oxide vapour. *Applied Microbiology*, **10**, 431–435.

Hiom, S.J., Hann, A.C., Furr, J.R. & Russell, A.-D. (1995a) X-ray microanalysis of chlorhexidine-treated cells of *Saccharomyces cerevisiae*. *Letters in Applied Microbiology*, **20**, 353–356.

Hiom, S.J., Furr, J.R. & Russell, A.-D. (1995b) Uptake of ^{14}C-chlorhexidine gluconate by *Saccharomyces cerevisiae, Candida albicans* and *Candida glabrata*. *Letters in Applied Microbiology*, **21**, 20–22.

Hodges, N.A. & Denyer, S.P. (1996) Preservative testing. In *Encyclopedia of Pharmaceutical Technology* (eds Swarbrick, J. & Boylen, J.C.), pp. 21–37. New York: Marcel Dekker.

Hoffman, H.-P., Geftic, S.M., Gelzer, J., Heymann, H. & Adaire, F.W. (1973) Ultrastructural alterations associated with the growth of resistant *Pseudomonas aeruginosa* in the presence of benzalkonium chloride. *Journal of Bacteriology*, **113**, 409–416.

Hoffman, R.K. (1971) Toxic gases. In *Inhibition and Destruction of the Microbial Cell* (ed. Hugo, W.B.), pp. 225–258. London: Academic Press.

Hoffman, R.K. & Warshowsky, B. (1958) Beta-propiolactone vapour as a disinfectant. *Applied Microbiology*, **6**, 358–362.

Holloway, P.M., Bucknall, R.A. & Denton, G.W. (1986) The effects of sub-lethal concentrations of chlorhexidine on bacterial pathogenicity. *Journal of Hospital Infection*, **8**, 39–46.

Hopwood, D. (1975) The reactions of glutaraldehyde with nucleic acids. *Histochemical Journal*, **7**, 267–276.

Hopwood, D., Allen, C.R. & McCabe, M. (1970) The reactions between glutaraldehyde and various proteins. An investigation of their kinetics. *Histochemical Journal*, **2**, 137–150.

Hugo, W.B. (1971) Amidines. In *Inhibition and Destruction of the Microbial Cell* (ed. Hugo, W.B.), pp. 121–136. London: Academic Press.

Hugo, W.B. (1978) Membrane-active antimicrobial drugs—a reappraisal of their mode of action in the light of the chemiosmotic theory. *International Journal of Pharmaceutics*, **1**, 127–131.

Hugo, W.B. (1979) Phenols: a review of their history and development as antimicrobial agents. *Microbios*, **23**, 83–85.

Hugo, W.B. (1991) The degradation of preservatives by microorganisms. *International Biodeterioration*, **27**, 185–194.

Hugo, W.B. & Beveridge, E.G. (1964) The resistance of gallic acid and its alkyl esters to attack by bacteria able to degrade aromatic ring compounds. *Journal of Applied Bacteriology*, **27**, 304–311.

Hugo, W.B. & Bloomfield, S.F. (1971a) Studies on the mode of action of the phenolic antibacterial agent Fentichlor against *Staphylococcus aureus* and *Escherichia coli*. 1. The absorption of Fentichlor by the bacterial cell and its antibacterial activity. *Journal of Applied Bacteriology*, **34**, 557–567.

Hugo, W.B. & Bloomfield, S.F. (1971b) Studies on the mode of action of the phenolic antimicrobial agent Fentichlor against *Staphylococcus aureus* and *Escherichia coli*. II. The effects of Fentichlor on the bacterial membrane and the cytoplasmic constituents of the cell. *Journal of Applied Bacteriology*, **34**, 569–578.

Hugo, W.B. & Bloomfield, S.F. (1971c) Studies on the mode of action on the antibacterial agent Fentichlor on *Staphylococcus aureus* and *Escherichia coli*. III. The effect of Fentichlor on the metabolic activities of *Staphylococcus aureus* and *Escheria coli*. *Journal of Applied Bacteriology*, **34**, 579–591.

Hugo, W.B. & Bowen, J.G. (1973) Studies on the mode of action of 4-ethylphenol. *Microbios*, **8**, 189–197.

Hugo, W.B. & Foster, J.H.S. (1964) Growth of *Pseudomonas aeruginosa* in solutions of esters of *p*-hydroxy benzoic acid. *Journal of Pharmacy and Pharmacology*, **16**, 209.

Hugo, W.B. & Longworth, A.R. (1964a) Some aspects of the mode of action of chlorhexidine. *Journal of Pharmacy and Pharmacology*, **16**, 655–662.

Hugo, W.B. & Longworth, A.R. (1964b) Effect of chlorhexidine on 'protoplasts' and spheroplasts of *Escherichia coli*, protoplasts of *Bacillus megaterium* and the Gram staining reaction of *Staphylococcus aureus*. *Journal of Pharmacy and Pharmacology*, **16**, 751–758.

Hugo, W.B. & Longworth, A.R. (1965) Cytological aspects of the mode of action of chlorhexidine. *Journal of Pharmacy and Pharmacology*, **17**, 28–32.

Hugo, W.B. & Longworth, A.R. (1966) The effect of chlorhexidine on the electrophoretic mobility, cytoplasmic constituents, dehydrogenase activity and cell walls of *Escherichia coli* and *Staphyloccus aureus*. *Journal of Pharmacy of Pharmacology*, **18**, 569–578.

Ikeda, T., Tazuke, S., Bamford, C.H. & Ledwith, A. (1984) Interaction of a polymeric biguanide biocide with phospholipid membranes. *Biochimica et Biophysica Acta*, **769**, 57–66.

Imperial Chemical Industries (n.d.) *'Hibitane'/ Chlorhexidine*. Manufacturer's Handbook.

Ingram, M. (1959) Benzoate-resistant yeasts. *Journal of Applied Bacteriology*, **22**, vi.

Ingram, M. & Haines, R.B. (1949) Inhibition of bacterial growth by pure ozone in the presence of nutrients. *Journal of Hygiene, Cambridge*, **47**, 146–168.

Isenberg, H.D. (1985) Clinical laboratory studies on disinfection with sporicidin. *Journal of Clinical Microbiology*, **22**, 735–739.

Ismaeel, N., El-Moug, T., Furr, J.R. & Russel, A.D. (1986a) Resistance of *Providencia stuartii* to chlorhexidine: a consideration of the role of the inner membrane. *Journal of Applied Bacteriology*, **60**, 361–367.

Ismaeel, N., Furr, J.R. & Russell, A.D. (1986b) Reversal of the surface effects of chlorhexidine diacetate on cells of *Providencia stuartii*. *Journal of Applied Bacteriology*, **61**, 373–381.

Jacobs, G., Henry, S.M. & Cotty, Y.F. (1975) The influence of pH, emulsifier and accelerated ageing upon preservative requirements of o/w emulsions. *Journal of the Society of Cosmetic Chemists*, **26**, 105–117.

Jacobs, W.A. (1916) The bactericidal properties of the quaternary salts of hexamethylenetetramine. I. The problem of the chemotherapy of experimental bacterial infections. *Journal of Experimental Medicine*, **23**, 563–568.

Jacobs, W.A. & Heidelberger, M. (1915a) The quaternary salts of hexamethylenetetramine. I. Substituted benzyl halides and the hexamethylene tetramine salts derived therefrom. *Journal of Biological Chemistry*, **20**, 659–683.

Jacobs, W.A. & Heidelberger, M. (1915b) The quaternary salts of hexamethylenetetramine. VIII. Miscellaneous substances containing aliphatically bound halogen and the hexamethylenetetramine salts derived therefrom. *Journal of Biological Chemistry*, **21**, 465–475.

Jacobs, W.A., Heidelberger, M. & Amoss, H.L. (1916a) The bactericidal properties of the quaternary salts of hexamethylenetetramine. II. The relation between constitution and bactericidal action in the substituted benzylhexamethylenetetraminium salts. *Journal of Experimental Medicine*, **23**, 569–576.

Jacobs, W.A., Heidelberger, M. & Bull, C.G. (1916b) The bactericidal properties of the quaternary salts of hexamethylenetetramine. III. The relation between constitution and bactericidal action in the quaternary salts obtained from halogenacetyl compounds. *Journal of Experimental Medicine*, **23**, 577–599.

James, A.M. (1965) The modification of the bacterial surface by chemical and enzymic treatment. In *Cell Electrophoresis* (ed. Ambrose, E.J.), pp. 154–170. London: J. & A. Churchill.

Joly, B. (1995) La résistance microbienne à l'action des antiseptiques et désinfectants. In *Antisepsie et Désinfection* (eds Fleurette, J., Freney, J. & Reverdy, M.-E.), pp. 52–65. Paris: Editions ESKA.

Jones, E.M., Smart, A., Bloomberg, G., Burgess, L. & Millar, M.R. (1994) Lactoferricin, a new antimicrobial peptide. *Journal of Applied Bacteriology*, **77**, 208–214.

Jorkasky, J.F. (1993) Special considerations for ethylene oxide: chlorofluorocarbons (CFCs). In *Sterilization Technology. A Practical Guide for Manufacturers and Users of Health Care Products* (eds Morrissey, R.F. & Briggs Phillips, G.), pp. 391–401. New York: Van Nostrand Reinhold.

Joswick, H.L., Corner, T.R., Silvernale, J.N. & Gerhardt, P. (1971) Antimicrobial actions of hexachlorophane: release of cytoplasmic materials. *Journal of Bacteriology*, **168**, 492–500.

Kabara, J.J. (1978) Fatty acids and derivatives as antimicrobial agents—a review. In *The Pharmacological Effects of Lipids* (ed. Kabara, J.J.), pp. 1–14. Champaign, Illinois: The American Oil Chemists' Society.

Kabara, J.J. (1980) GRAS antimicrobial agents for cosmetic products. *Journal of the Society of Cosmetic Chemists*, **31**, 1–10.

Kabara, J.J. (1984) Medium chain fatty acids and esters as antimicrobial agents. In *Cosmetic and Drug Preservation: Principles and Practice* (ed. Kabara, J.J.), pp. 275–304. New York: Marcel Dekker.

Kabara, J.J. & Eklund, T. (1991) Organic acids and esters. In *Food Preservatives* (eds Russell, N.J. & Gould, G.W.), pp. 44–71. Glasgow and London: Blackie.

Kaslow, R.A., Mackel, D.C. & Mallison, G.F. (1976) Nosocomial pseudobacteraemia: positive blood cultures due to contaminated benzalkonium antiseptic. *Journal of the American Medical Association*, **236**, 2407–2409.

Kay, J.B. (1980) Manufacture and supply of contact lens products. 2. An industrial view. *Pharmaceutical Journal*, **225**, 345–348.

Kelsey, J.C. (1967) Use of gaseous antimicrobial agents with special reference to ethylene oxide. *Journal of Applied Bacteriology*, **30**, 92–100.

Kelsey, J.C. & Maurer, I.M. (1972) *The Use of Chemical Disinfectants in Hospitals*. Public Health Laboratory Service Monography Series No. 2. London: HMSO.

Kelsey, J.C., Mackinnon, I.H. & Maurer, I.M. (1974) Sporicidal activity of hospital disinfectants. *Journal of Clinical Pathology*, **27**, 632–638.

Kereluk, K. (1971) Gaseous sterilization: methyl bromide, propylene oxide and ozone. In *Progress in Industrial Microbiology* (ed. Hockenhull, D.J.D.), Vol. 10, pp. 105–128. Edinburgh: Churchill Livingstone.

Khunkitti, W., Lloyd, D., Furr, J.R. & Russell, A.D. (1996) The lethal effects of biguanides on cysts and trophozoites of *Acanthamoeba castellanii*. *Journal of Applied Bacteriology*, **81**, 73–77.

Khunkitti, W., Lloyd, D., Furr, J.R. & Russell, A.D. (1997) Aspects of the mechanisms of action of biguanides: on trophozoites and cysts of *Acanthamoeba castellanii*. *Journal of Applied Microbiology*, **82**, 107–114.

Khunkitti, W., Lloyd, D., Furr, J.R. & Russell, A.D. (1998) *Acanthamoeba castellanii*: growth, encystment, excystment and biocide susceptibility. *Journal of Infection* **36**, 43–48.

Kingston, D. (1965) Release of formaldehyde from polynoxyline and noxythiolin. *Journal of Clinical Pathology*, **18**, 666–667.

Klarmann, E.G. & Shternov, V.A. (1936) Bactericidal value of coal-tar disinfectants. Limitation of the *B. typhosus* phenol coefficient as a measure. *Industrial and Engineering Chemistry, Analytical Edition*, **8**, 369–372.

Klarmann, E.G. & von Wowern, J. (1929) The preparation of certain chloro- and bromo-derivatives of 2,4-dihydroxydiphenylmethane and ethane and their germicidal action. *Journal of the American Chemical Society*, **51**, 605–610.

Klarmann, E.G., Shternov, V.A. & von Wowern, J. (1929) The germicidal action of halogen derivatives of phenol and resorcinol and its impairment by organic matter. *Journal of Bacteriology*, **17**, 423–442.

Klarmann, E.G., Gates, L.W. & Shternov, U.A. (1932) Halogen derivatives of monohydroxydiphenylmethane and their antibacterial activity. *Journal of the American Chemical Society*, **54**, 3315–3328.

Klarmann, E.G., Shternov, V.A. & Gates, L.W. (1933) The alkyl derivatives of halogen phenols and their bactericidal action. I. Chlorphenols. *Journal of the American Chemical Society*, **55**, 2576–2589.

Knott, A.G., Russell, A.D. & Dancer, B.N. (1995) Development of resistance to biocides during sporulation of *Bacillus subtilis*. *Journal of Applied Bacteriology*, **79**, 492–498.

Kornfeld, F. (1966) Properties and techniques of application of biocidal ampholytic surfactants. *Food Manufacture*, **41**, 39–46.

Krebs, H.A., Wiggins, D., Stubbs, M., Sols, A. & Bedoya, F. (1983) Studies on the mechanism of the antifungal action of benzoate. *Biochemical Journal*, **214**, 657–663.

Kushner, D.J. (1971) Influence of solutes and ions on microorganisms. In *Inhibition and Destruction of the Microbial Cell* (ed. Hugo, W.B.), pp. 259–283. London: Academic Press.

Kuyyakanond, T. & Quesnel, L.B. (1992) The mechanism of action of chlorhexidine. *FEMS Microbiology Letters*, **100**, 211–216.

Lacey, R.W. (1979) Antibacterial activity of povidone iodine towards non-sporing bacteria. *Journal of Applied Bacteriology*, **46**, 443–449.

Langwell, H. (1932) Oligodynamic action of metals. *Chemistry and Industry*, **51**, 701–702.

Lawrence, C.A. (1948) Inactivation of the germicidal action of quaternary ammonium compounds. *Journal of the American Pharmaceutical Association, Scientific Edition*, **37**, 57–61.

Lawrence, C.A. (1950) *Surface-active Quaternary Ammonium Germicides*. London and New York: Academic Press.

Laycock, H.H. & Mulley, B.A. (1970) Application of the Ferguson principle to the antibacterial activity of mono- and multi-component solutions of quaternary ammonium surface-active agents. *Journal of Pharmacy and Pharmacology*, **22**, 157S–162S.

Leach, E.D. (1981) A new synergized glutaraldehyde-phenate sterilizing solution and concentrated disinfectant. *Infection Control*, **2**, 26–30.

Lee, C.R. & Corner, T.R. (1975) Antimicrobial actions of hexachlorophane: iron salts do not reverse inhibition. *Journal of Pharmacy and Pharmacology*, **27**, 694–696.

Leech, R. (1988) Natural and physical preservative systems. In *Microbial Quality Assurance in Pharmaceuticals, Cosmetics and Toiletries* (eds Bloomfield, S.F., Baird, R., Leak, R. & Leech, R.), pp. 77–93. Chichester: Ellis Horwood.

Leclaporn, A., Paulsen, I.T., Tennent, J.M., Littlejohn, T.G. & Skurray, R.A. (1994) Multidrug resistance to antiseptics and disinfectants in coagulase-negative staphylococci. *Journal of Medical Microbiology*, **40**, 214–220.

Leive, L, (1974) The barrier function of the

Gram-negative envelope. *Annals of the New York Academy of Sciences*, **235**, 109–127.

Leive, L. & Kollin, V. (1967) Controlling EDTA treatment to produce permeable *E. coli* with normal metabolic process. *Biochemical and Biophysical Research Communications*, **28**, 229–236.

Lemaire, H.C., Sehramm, C.H. & Cahn, A. (1961) Synthesis and germicidal activity of halogenated salicylanilides and related compounds. *Journal of Pharmaceutical Sciences*, **50**, 831–837.

Lesher, R.J., Bender, G.R. & Marquis, R.E. (1977) Bacteriolytic action of fluoric ions. *Antimicrobial Agents and Chemotherapy*, **12**, 339–345.

Lever, A.M. & Sutton, S.V.W. (1996) Antimicrobial effects of hydrogen peroxide as an antiseptic and disinfectant. In *Handbook of Disinfectants and Antiseptics* (ed. Ascenzi, J.M.), pp. 159–176. New York: Marcel Dekker.

Lilley, B.D. & Brewer, J.H. (1953) The selective antibacterial activity of phenylethyl alcohol. *Journal of the American Pharmaceutical Association, Scientific Edition*, **42**, 6–8.

Littlejohn, T.G., Paulsen, I.T., Gillespie, M.T. *et al.* (1992) Substrate specificity and energetics of antiseptic and disinfectant resistance in *Staphylococcus aureus*. *FEMS Microbiology Letters*, **95**, 259–266.

Lloyd, A.G. & Drake, J.J.P. (1975) Problems posed by essential food preservatives. *British Medical Journal*, **iii**, 214–219.

Loffer, F.D. (1990) Disinfection vs. sterilization of gynecologic laparoscopy equipment. The experience of the Phoenix Surgicenter. *Journal of Reproductive Medicine*, **25**, 263–266.

Longworth, A.R. (1971) Chlorhexidine. In *Inhibition and Destruction of the Microbial Cell* (ed. Hugo, W.B.), pp. 95–106. London: Academic Press.

Lorenz, P. (1977) 5-Bromo-5-nitro-1, 3-dioxane: a preservative for cosmetics. *Cosmetics and Toiletries*, **92**, 89–91.

Lovelock, J.E. (1948) Aliphatic-hydroxycarboxylic acids as air disinfectants. In *Studies in Air Hygiene*, Medical Research Council Special Report Series No. 262, pp. 89–104. London: HMSO.

Lovelock, J.E., Lidwell, O.M. & Raymond, W.F. (1944) Aerial disinfection. *Nature, London*, **153**, 20–21.

Lowbury, E.J.L. (1951) Contamination of cetrimide and other fluids with *Pseudomonas aeruginosa*. *British Journal of Industrial Medicine*, **8**, 22–25.

Lowbury, E.J.L. & Lilley, H.A. (1960) Disinfection of the hands of surgeons and nurses. *British Medical Journal*, **i**, 1445–1450.

Lowbury, E.J.L., Lilley, H.A. & Bull, J.P. (1964) Methods of disinfection of hands. *British Medical Journal*, **ii**, 531–536.

Lueck, E. (1980) *Antimicrobial Food Additives*. Berlin: Springer-Verlag.

Lynch, M., Lund, W. & Wilson, D.A. (1977) Chloroform as a preservative in aqueous systems. Losses under 'in-use' conditions and antimicrobial effectiveness. *Pharmaceutical Journal*, **219**, 507–510.

McCoy, W.F. & Wireman, J.W. (1989) Efficacy of bromochlorodimethylhydantoin against *Legionella pneumophila* in industrial cooling water. *Journal of Industrial Microbiology*, **4**, 403–408.

Mackinnon, I.H. (1974) The use of inactivators in the evaluation of disinfectants. *Journal of Hygiene, Cambridge*, **73**, 189–195.

McQuillen, K. (1960) Bacterial protoplasts. In *The Bacteria*, Vol. I (eds Gunsalus, I.C. & Stanier, R.Y.), pp. 249–349. London: Academic Press.

Malek, J.R. & Speier, J.L. (1982) Development of an organosilicone antimicrobial agent for the treatment of surfaces. *Journal of Coated Fabrics*, **12**, 38–45.

Marouchoc, S.R. (1979) Classical phenol derivatives and their uses. *Developments in Industrial Microbiology*, **20**, 15–24.

Marples, R.R. (1971) Antibacterial cosmetics and the microflora of human skin. *Developments in Industrial Microbiology*, **12**, 178–187.

Marzulli, F.N. & Maibach, H.J. (1973) Antimicrobials: experimental contact sensitization in man. *Journal of the Society of Cosmetic Chemists*, **24**, 399–421.

Mathews, C., Davidson, J., Bauer, E., Morrison, J.L. & Richardson, A.P. (1956) *p*-Hydroxybenzoic acid esters as preservatives. II. Acute and chronic toxicity in dogs, rats and mice. *Journal of the American Pharmaceutical Association*, **45**, 260–267.

Mbithi, J.N., Springthorpe, V.S., Sattar, S.A. & Pacquette, M. (1993) Bactericidal, virucidal and mycobacterial activities of reused alkaline glutaraldehyde in an endoscopy unit. *Journal of Clinical Microbiology*, **31**, 2933–2995.

Merianos, J.J. (1991) Quaternary ammonium compounds. In Disinfection, Sterilisation and Preservation (ed Block, S.S.) 4th edn, pp. 225–255. Philadelphia: Lea and Febiger.

Michael, G.T. & Stumbo, C.R. (1970) Ethylene oxide sterilisation of *Salmonella senftenberg* and *Escherichia coli*: death kinetics and mode of action. *Journal of Food Science*, **35**, 631–634.

Miller, M.J. (1996) Contact lens disinfectants. In *Handbook of Disinfectants and Antiseptics* (ed. Ascenzi, J.M.), pp. 83–110. New York: Marcel Dekker.

Mitchell, A.G. (1964) Bactericidal activity of chloroxylenol in aqueous solutions of ectomacrogol. *Journal of Pharmacy and Pharmacology*, **16**, 533–537.

Moats, W.A. & Maddox, S.E., Jr (1978) Effect of pH on the antimicrobial activity of some triphenylmethane dyes. *Canadian Journal of Microbiology*, **24**, 658–661.

Moiseev, S. (1934) Sterilization of water with silver coated sand. *Journal of the American Water Works Association*, **26**, 217–222.

Molinari, J.A. (1995) Disinfection and sterilization strategies for dental instruments. In *Chemical Germicides in Health Care* (ed. Rutala, W.), pp. 129–134. Morin Heights: Polyscience Publications.

Moore, O. & Walker, J.N. (1939) Selective action in germicidal preparations containing chlorinated phenols. *Pharmaceutical Journal*, **143**, 507–509.

Morgan, D.A. (1989) Chlorinated solutions: E (useful) or (E) useless? *Pharmaceutical Journal*, **243**, 219–220.

Morris, E.J. & Darlow, H.M. (1971) Inactivation of viruses. In *Inhibition and Destruction of the Microbial Cell* (ed. Hugo, W.B.), pp. 687–702. London: Academic Press.

Morton, H.E. (1950) Relationship of concentration and germicidal efficiency of ethyl alcohol. *Annals of the New York Academy of Sciences*, **53**, 191–196.

Morton, H.E. (1977) Alcohols. In *Disinfection, Sterilization and Preservation* (ed. Block, S.S.), 2nd edn, pp. 301–308. Philadelphia: Lea & Febiger.

Muys, G.T., van Rhee, R. & Lelieveld, H.L.M. (1978) Sterilization by means of hydrochloric acid vapour. *Journal of Applied Bacteriology*, **45**, 213–217.

Myers, J.A., Allwood, M.C., Gidley, M.J. & Sanders, J.K.M. (1980) The relationship between structure and activity of Taurolin. *Journal of Applied Bacteriology*, **48**, 89–96.

Neu, H.C. (1969) The role of amine buffers in EDTA toxicity and their effect on osmotic shock. *Journal of General Microbiology*, **57**, 215–220.

Newcastle Regional Hospital Board Working Party (1962) Blankets and air hygiene: a report of a trial of blanket disinfection. *Journal of Hygiene, Cambridge*, **60**, 85–94.

Nicholls, A.A., Leaver, C.W.E. & Panes, J.J. (1967) Hatchery hygiene evaluation as measured by microbiological examination of samples of fluff. *British Poultry Science*, **8**, 297.

Nicoletti, G., Boghossian, V., Gurevitch, F., Borland, R. and Morgenroth, P. (1993) The antimicrobial activity *in vitro* of chlorhexidine, a mixture of isothiazolines ('Kathon' CG) and cetyltrimethylammonium bromide (CTAB). *Journal of Hospital Infection*, **23**, 87–111.

Nordgren, C. (1939) Investigations on the sterilising efficacy of gaseous formaldehyde. *Acta Pathologica et Microbiologica Scandinavica, Supplement* XL, pp. 1–165.

Nychas, G.J.E. (1995) Natural antimicrobials from plants. In *New Methods of Food Preservation* (ed. Gould, G.W.), pp. 58–89. London: Blackie Academic and Professional.

Olivant, D.J. & Shapton, D.A. (1970) Disinfection in the food processing industry. In *Disinfection* (ed. Benarde, M.A.), pp. 393–428. New York: Marcel Dekker.

O'Neill, J.J., Peelor, P.L., Peterson, A.F. & Strube, C.H. (1979) Selection of parabens as preservatives for cosmetics and toiletries. *Journal of the Society of Cosmetic Chemists*, **30**, 25–39.

Ono, B.-I., Ishii, N., Fujino, S. & Aoyama, I. (1991) Role of hydrosulfide ions (HS) in methylmercury resistance in *Saccharomyces cerevisiae. Applied and Environmental Microbiology*, **57**, 3183–3186.

Ono, B., Ohwe, H. & Ishihara, F. (1998) Role of the cell wall in *Saccharomyces cerevisae* mutants resistant to Hg^{2+}, *Journal of Bacteriology*, **170**, 5877–5882.

Owens, R.G. (1969) Organic sulphur compounds. In *Fungicides* (ed. Torgeson, D.C.), Vol. 2, pp. 147–301. New York: Academic Press.

Page, B.F.J. (1993) Special considerations for ethylene oxide: product residues. In *Sterilization Technology* (ed. Morrissey, R.F. & Phillips, G.B.), pp. 402–420. New York: Van Nostrand Reinhold.

Palfreyman, D. (1977) *John Jeyes... the Making of a Household Name*. Thetford: Jeyes.

Palleroni, N.J. & de Prinz, M.J.R. (1960) Influence of sorbic acid on acetate oxidation by *Saccharomyces cerevisae* var. *ellipsoideus. Nature, London*, **185**, 688–689.

Patel, W.K. & Kostenbauder, H.B. (1958) Binding of *p*-hydroxybenzoic acid esters by polyoxyethylene 21 sorbitan mono-oleate. *Journal of the American Pharmaceutical Association*, **47**, 289–293.

Paulsen, I.T., Brown, M.H., Littlejohn, T.A., Mitchell, B.A. & Skurray, R.A. (1996a) Multidrug resistance proteins qacA and qacB from *Staphylococcus aureus*. Membrane topology and identification of residues involved in substrate specificity. *Proceedings of the National Academy of Sciences, US*, **93**, 3630–3635.

Paulsen, I.T., Skurray, R.A., Tam, R. *et al.* (1996b) The SMR family: a novel family of multidrug efflux proteins involved with the efflux of lipophilic drugs. *Molecular Microbiology*, **19**, 1167–1175.

Paulus, W. (1976) Problems encountered with formaldehyde-releasing compounds used as preservatives in aqueous systems, especially lubricoolants—possible solutions to the problems. In *Proceedings of the 3rd International Biodegradation Symposium* (eds Shaply, J.M. & Kaplan, A.M.), pp. 1075–1082. London: Applied Science Publishers.

Pepper, R.E. (1980) Comparison of the activities and stabilities of alkaline glutaraldehyde sterilizing solutions. *Infection Control*, **1**, 90–92.

Pepper, R.E. & Chandler, V.L. (1963) Sporicidal activity of alkaline alcoholic saturated dialdehyde solutions. *Applied Microbiology*, **11**, 384–388.

Pfirrman, R.W. & Leslie, G.B. (1979) The anti-endotoxic activity of Taurolin in experimental animals. *Journal of Applied Bacteriology*, **46**, 97–102.

Pfleger, R., Schraufstatter, E., Gehringer, F. & Sciuk, J. (1949) Zur Chemotherapie der Pilzimfektionen. I. Mitteilung: *In vitro* Untersuchungen aromatischer sulphide. *Zeitschrift für Naturforschung*, **4b**, 344–350.

Pharmaceutical Codex (1979) London: Pharmaceutical Press.

Phillips, C.R. (1977) Gaseous sterilization. In *Disinfection, Sterilization and Preservation* (ed. Block, S.S.), 2nd edn, pp. 529–611. Philadelphia: Lea & Febiger.

Phillips, C.R. & Kaye, S. (1949) The sterilizing action of gaseous ethylene oxide. I. Review. *American Journal of Hygiene*, **50**, 270–279.

Phillips, I., Lobo, A.Z., Fernandes, R. & Gundara, N.S. (1968) Acetic acid in the treatment of superficial wounds infected by *Pseudomonas aeruginosa. Lancet*, **i**, 11–12.

Philpott-Howerd, J.H. & Casewell, M. (1994) *Hospital Infection Control. Policies and Practical Procedures*. London: W.B. Saunders.

Pickard, R.G. (1972) Treatment of peritonitis with per and post-operative irrigation of the peritoneal cavity with noxythiolin solution. *British Journal of Surgery*, **59**, 642–648.

Pisano, F.D. & Kostenbauder, H.B. (1959) Correlation of binding data with required preservative concentrations of *p*-hydroxybenzoates in the presence of Tween 80. *Journal of the American Pharmaceutical Association*, **48**, 310–314.

Pollard, J.A. (1991) Legislative aspects. In *Food Preservation* (eds Russell, N.J. & Gould, G.W.) pp. 235–266. Glasgow: Blackie.

Ponci, R., Baruffini, A. & Gialdi, F. (1964) Antifungal activity of 2′,2′-dicarbamino-4′,4-dinitrodiphenyl-disulphides and 5-nitro-1,2-benzisothiazolones. *Farmaco, Edizione Scientifica*, **19**, 121–136.

Potokar, M., Greb, W., Ippen, H., Maibach, H.I., Schulz, K.H. & Gloxhuber, C. (1976) Bronidox, ein neues Konservierungsmittel fur die Kosmetic Eigenschaften und toxikologisch-dermatologische Prufergebnisse. *Fette, Seife, Anstrichmittel*, **78**, 269–276.

Power, E.G.M. (1997) Aldehydes as biocides. *Progress in Medicinal Chemistry*, **34**, 149–201.

Power, E.G.M. & Russell, A.D. (1988) Studies with Cold Sterilog, a glutaraldehyde monitor. *Journal of Hospital Infection*, **11**, 376–380.

Power, E.G.M. & Russell, A.D. (1989) Glutaraldehyde: its uptake by sporing and non-sporing bacteria, rubber, plastic and an endoscope. *Journal of Applied Bacteriology*, **67**, 329–342.

Power, E.G.M. & Russell, A.D. (1990) Sporicidal action of alkaline glutaraldehyde: factors influencing activity and a comparison with other aldehydes. *Journal of Applied Bacteriology*, **69**, 261–268.

Power, E.G.M., Dancer, B.N. & Russell, A.D. (1988) Emergence of resistance to glutaraldehyde in spores of *Bacillus subtilis* 168. *FEMS Microbiology Letters*, **50**, 223–226.

Power, E.G.M., Dancer, B.N. & Russell, A.D. (1989) Possible mechanisms for the revival of glutaraldehyde-treated spores of *Bacillus subtilis* NCTC 8236. *Journal of Applied Bacteriology*, **67**, 91–98.

Power, E.G.M., Dancer, B.N. & Russell, A.D. (1990) Effect of sodium hydroxide and two proteases on the revival of aldehyde-treated spores of *Bacillus subtilis. Letters in Applied Microbiology*, **10**, 9–13.

Price, P.B. (1950) Re-evaluation of ethyl alcohol as a germicide. *Archives of Surgery*, **60**, 492–502.

Prince, D.L., Prince, H.N., Thraenhart, O., Muchmore, E., Bonder, E. & Pugh, J. (1993) Methodological approach to disinfection of human hepatitis B virus. *Journal of Clinical Microbiology*, **31**, 3296–3304.

Quack, J.M. (1976) Quaternary ammonium compounds in cosmetics. *Cosmetics and Toiletries*, **91** (2), 35–52.

Quinn, P.J. (1987) Evaluation of veterinary disinfectants and disinfection processes. In *Disinfection in Veterinary and Farm Animal Practice* (eds Linton, A.H., Hugo, W.B. & Russell, A.D.), pp. 66–116. Oxford: Blackwell Scientific Publications.

Rackur, H. (1985) New aspects of the mechanism of action of povidone-iodine. *Journal of Hospital Infection*, **6** (Suppl. A), 13–23.

Ramos-Nino, M.E., Clifford, M.N. & Adams, M.R. (1996) Quantitative structure activity relationship for the effect of benzoic acids, cinnamic acids and benzaldehydes on *Listeria monocytogenes. Journal of Applied Bacteriology*, **80**, 303–310.

Ranganathan, N.S. (1996) Chlorhexidine. In *Handbook of Disinfectant and Antiseptics* (ed. Ascenzi, J.M.), pp. 235–264. New York: Marcel Dekker.

Rapps, N.F. (1933) The bactericidal efficiency of chlorocresol and chloroxylenol. *Journal of the Society of Chemical Industry*, **52**, 175T–176T.

Reeves, D.S. & Schweitzer, F.A.W. (1973) Experimental studies with an antibacterial substance, Taurolin. *Proceedings of the 8th International Congress of Chemotherapy* (Athens), pp. 583–586. Athens, Hellenic.

Repaske, R. (1956) Lysis of Gram-negative bacteria by lysozyme. *Biochimica et Biophysica Acta*, **22**, 189–191.

Repaske, R. (1958) Lysis of Gram-negative organism and the role of versene. *Biochimica et Biophysica Acta*, **30**, 225–232.

Report (1989) Expert Advisory Committee on Biocides, p. 32. London: HMSO.

Resnick, L., Veren, K., Zaki, S.S., Tondreau, S.S. & Markham, P.D. (1986) Stability and inactivation of HTLV-III/LAV under clinical and laboratory conditions. *Journal of the American Medical Association*, **255**, 1887–1891.

Reverdy, M.-E. (1995a) La chlorhexidine. In *Antisepsie et Désinfection* (eds Fleurette, J., Freney, J. & Reverdy, M.-E.), pp. 135–168. Paris: Editions ESKA.

Reverdy, M.-E. (1995b) Les ammonium quaternaires. In *Antisepsie et Désinfection* (eds Fleurette, J., Freney, J.

& Reverdy, M.-E.), pp. 174–198. Paris: Editions ESKA.

Richards, C., Furr, J.R. & Russell, A.D. (1984) Inactivation of micro-organisms by lethal gases. In *Cosmetic and Drug Preservation: Principles and Practice* (ed. Kabara, J.J.), pp. 209–222. New York: Marcel Dekker.

Richards, R.M.E. & McBride, R.J. (1973) Enhancement of benzalkonium chloride and chlorhexidine acetate activity against *Pseudomonas aeruginosa* by aromatic alcohols. *Journal of Pharmaceutical Sciences*, **62**, 2035–2037.

Richardson, E.L. (1981) Update: frequency of preservative use in cosmetic formulas as disclosed to FDA. *Cosmetics and Toiletries*, **96**, 91–92.

Richardson, G. & Woodford, R. (1964) Incompatibility of cationic antiseptics with sodium alginate. *Pharmaceutical Journal*, **192**, 527–528.

Rickloff, J.R. (1985) An evaluation of the sporicidal activity of ozone. *Applied and Environmental Microbiology*, **53**, 683–686.

Roberts, N.A., Gray, G.W. & Wilkinson, S.G. (1970) The bactericidal action of ethylenediamine tetraacetic acid on *Pseudomonas aeruginosa*. *Microbios*, **2**, 189–208.

Rose, A.H. & Pilkington, B.J. (1989) Sulphite. In *Mechanisms of Action of Food Preservation Procedures* (ed. Gould, G.W.), pp. 201–223. London: Elsevier Applied Science.

Rose, F.L. & Swain, G. (1956) Bisguanides having antibacterial activity. *Journal of the Chemical Society*, 4422–4425.

Rose, M.S. & Lock, E.A. (1970) The interaction of triethyltin with a component of guinea-pig liver supernatant. *Biochemical Journal*, **190**, 151–157.

Rosen, W.E. & Berke, P.A. (1973) Modern concepts of cosmetic preservation. *Journal of the Society of Cosmetic Chemists*, **24**, 663–675.

Rosen, W.E., Berke, P.A., Matzin, T. & Peterson, A.F. (1977) Preservation of cosmetic lotions with imidazolidinyl urea plus parabens. *Journal of the Society of Cosmetic Chemists*, **28**, 83–87.

Rossmore, H.W. (1979) Heterocyclic compounds as industrial biocides. *Developments in Industrial Microbiology*, **20**, 41–71.

Rossmore, H.W. (1995) *Handbook of Biocide and Preservative Use*. London: Blackie.

Rossmore, H.W. & Sondossi, M. (1988) Applications and mode of action of formaldehyde condensate biocides. *Advances in Applied Microbiology*, **33**, 223–277.

Rossmore, H.W., DeMare, J. & Smith, T.H.F. (1972) Anti- and pro-microbial activity of hexahydro-1,3,5-tris(2-hydroxyethyl)-*s*-triazine in cutting fluid emulsion. In *Biodeterioration of Materials* (eds Walters, A.H. & Hueek-van der Plas, E.H.), Vol. 2, pp. 266–293. London: Applied Science Publishers.

Rubbo, S.D., Gardner, J.F. & Webb, R.L. (1967) Biocidal activities of glutaraldehyde and related compounds. *Journal of Applied Bacteriology*, **30**, 78–87.

Russell, A.D. (1971a) Ethylenediamine tetraacetic acid. In *Inhibition and Destruction of the Microbial Cell* (ed. Hugo, W.B.), pp. 209–224. London: Academic Press.

Russell, A.D. (1971b) The destruction of bacterial spores. In *Inhibition and Destruction of the Microbial Cell* (ed. Hugo, W.B.), pp. 451–612. London: Academic Press.

Russell, A.D. (1976) Inactivation of non-sporing bacteria by gases. *Society for Applied Bacteriology Symposium No. 5: Inactivation of Vegetative Micro-organisms* (eds Skinner, F.A. & Hugo, W.B.), pp. 61–88. London: Academic Press.

Russell, A.D. (1982) *The Destruction of Bacterial Spores*. London: Academic Press.

Russell, A.D. (1985) The role of plasmids in bacterial resistance to antiseptics, disinfectants and preservatives. *Journal of Hospital Infection*, **6**, 9–19.

Russell, A.D. (1986) Chlorhexidine: antibacterial action and bacterial resistance. *Infection*, **14**, 212–215.

Russell, A.D. (1990a) The bacterial spore and chemical sporicides. *Clinical Microbiology Reviews*, **3**, 99–119.

Russell, A.D. (1990b) The effects of chemical and physical agents on microbes: Disinfection and sterilization. In *Topley & Wilson's Principles of Bacteriology, Virology and Immunity* (eds Dick, H.M. & Linton, A.H.), 8th edn, Vol. 1, pp. 71–103. London: Edward Arnold.

Russell, A.D. (1991a) Principles of antimicrobial activity. In *Disinfection, Sterilization and Preservation* (ed. Block, S.S.), 4th edn. Philadelphia: Lea & Febiger.

Russell, A.D. (1991b) Chemical sporicidal and sporistatic agents. In *Disinfection, Sterilization and Preservation* (ed. Block, S.S.), 4th edn. Philadelphia: Lea & Febiger.

Russell, A.D. (1994) Glutaraldehyde: its current status and uses. *Infection Control and Hospital Epidemiology*, **15**, 724–733.

Russell, A.D. (1995) Mechanisms of microbial resistance to disinfectant and antiseptic agents. In *Chemical Germicides in Health Care* (ed. Rutala, W.A.), pp. 256–269. Morin Heights: Polyscience.

Russell, A.D. (1996) Activity of biocides against mycobacteria. *Journal of Applied Bacteriology, Symposium Supplement*, **81**, 87S–101S.

Russell, A.D. (1997) Plasmids and bacterial resistance to biocides. *Journal of Applied Microbiology*, **82**, 155–165.

Russell, A.D. & Chopra, I. (1996) *Understanding Antibacterial Action and Resistance*, 2nd edn. Chichester: Ellis Horwood.

Russell, A.D. & Day, M.J. (1993) Antibacterial activity

of chlorhexidine. *Journal of Hospital Infection*, **25**, 229–238.

Russell, A.D. & Day, M.J. (1996) Antibiotic and biocide resistance in bacteria. *Microbios*, **85**, 45–65.

Russell, A.D. & Furr, J.R. (1977) The antibacterial activity of a new chloroxylenol preparation containing ethylenediamine tetraacetic acid. *Journal of Applied Bacteriology*, **43**, 253–260.

Russell, A.D. & Furr, J.R. (1986a) The effects of antiseptics, disinfectants and preservatives on smooth, rough and deep rough strains of *Salmonella typhimurium*. *International Journal of Pharmaceutics*, **34**, 115–123.

Russell, A.D. & Furr, J.R. (1986b) Susceptibility of porin- and lipopolysaccharide-deficient strains of *Escherichia coli* to some antiseptics and disinfectants. *Journal of Hospital Infection*, **8**, 47–56.

Russell, A.D. & Furr, J.R. (1987) Comparative sensitivity of smooth, rough and deep rough strains of *Escherichia coli* to chlorhexidine, quaternary ammonium compounds and dibromopropamide isethionate. *International Journal of Pharmaceutics*, **36**, 191–197.

Russell, A.D. & Hopwood, D. (1976) The biological uses and importance of glutaraldehyde. In *Progress in Medicinal Chemistry* (eds Ellis, G.P. & West, G.B.), Vol. 13, pp. 271–301. Amsterdam: North-Holland Publishing Company.

Russell, A.D. & Hugo, W.B. (1987) Chemical disinfectants. In *Disinfection in Veterinary and Farm Animal Practice* (eds Linton, A.H., Hugo, W.B. & Russell, A.D.), pp. 12–42. Oxford: Blackwell Scientific Publications.

Russell, A.D. & Hugo, W.B. (1994) Antibacterial action and activity of silver. *Progress in Medicinal Chemistry*, **31**, 351–371.

Russell, A.D. & Munton, T.J. (1974) Bactericidal and bacteriostatic activity of glutaraldehyde and its interaction with lysine and proteins. *Microbios*, **11**, 147–152.

Russell, A.D. & Russell, N.J. (1995) Biocides: activity, action and resistance. In *Fifty Years of Antimicrobials: Past Perspectives and Future Trends* (ed. Hunter, P.A., Darby, G.K. & Russell, N.J.), 53rd Symposium of the Society for General Microbiology, pp. 327–365. Cambridge: Cambridge University Press.

Russell, A.D., Jenkins, J. & Harrison, I.H. (1967) Inclusion of antimicrobial agents in pharmaceutical products. *Advances in Applied Microbiology*, **9**, 1–38.

Russell, A.D., Ahonkhai, I. & Rogers, D.T. (1979) Microbiological applications of the inactivation of antibiotics and other antimicrobial agents. *Journal of Applied Bacteriology*, **46**, 207–245.

Russell, A.D., Yarnych, V.S. & Koulikouskii, A.U. (1984) *Guidelines on Disinfection in Animal Husbandry for Prevention and Control of Zoonotic Diseases*. WHO/UPH/84.4. Geneva: World Health Organization.

Russell, A.D., Furr, J.R. & Pugh, W.J. (1985) Susceptibility of porin- and lipopolysaccharide-deficient mutants of *Escherichia coli* to a homologous series of esters of *p*-hydroxybenzoic acid. *International Journal of Pharmaceutics*, **27**, 163–173.

Russell, A.D., Hammond, S.A. & Morgan, J.R. (1986) Bacterial resistance to antiseptics and disinfectants. *Journal of Hospital Infection*, **7**, 213–225.

Russell, A.D., Furr, J.R. & Pugh, W.J. (1987) Sequential loss of outer membrane lipopolysaccharide and sensitivity of *Escherichia coli* to antibacterial agents. *International Journal of Pharmaceutics*, **35**, 227–232.

Russell, J.B. (1992) Another explanation for the toxicity of fermentation acids at low pH: anion accumulation versus uncoupling. *Journal of Applied Bacteriology*, **73**, 363–370.

Russell, N.J. & Gould, G.W. (1991a) *Food Preservatives*. Glasgow and London: Blackie.

Russell, N.J. & Gould, G.W. (1991b) Factors affecting growth and survival. In *Food Preservatives* (eds Russell, N.J. & Gould, G.W.), pp. 13–21. Glasgow and London: Blackie.

Rutala, W.A. (1990) APIC Guidelines for infection control practice. *American Journal of Infection Control*, **18**, 99–117.

Rutala, W.A. (1995a) *Chemical Germicides in Health Care*. Morin Heights: Polyscience Publications.

Rutala, W.A. (1995b) Use of chemical germicides in the United States: 1994 and beyond. In *Chemical Germicides in Health Care* (ed. Rutala, W.A.), pp. 1–22. Morin Heights: Polyscience Publications.

Rutala, W.A. & Weber, D.J. (1995) FDA labeling requirements for disinfection of endoscopes: a counterpoint. *Infection Control and Hospital Epidemiology*, **16**, 231–235.

Rutala, W.A., Gergen, M.F. & Weber, D.J. (1993a) Inactivation of *Clostridium difficile* spores by disinfectants. *Infection Control and Hospital Epidemiology*, **14**, 36–39.

Rutala, W.A., Gergen, M.F. & Weber, D.J. (1993b) Sporicidal activity of chemical sterilants used in hospitals. *Infection Control and Hospital Epidemiology*, **14**, 713–718.

Sabalitschka, T. (1924) Chemische Konstitution und Konservierungsvermögen. *Pharmazeutisch Monatsblatten*, **5**, 235–327.

Sabalitschka, T. & Dietrich, R.K. (1926) Chemical constitution and preservative properties. *Disinfection*, **11**, 67–71.

Sabalitschka, T., Dietrich, K.R. & Bohm, E. (1926) Influence of esterification of carbocyclic acids on inihibitive action with respect to micro-organisms. *Pharmazeutische Zeitung*, **71**, 834–836.

Salmond, C.V., Kroll, R.H. & Booth, I.R. (1984) The effect of food preservatives on pH homeostasis in

Escherichia coli. Journal of General Microbiology, **130**, 2845–2850.

Salton, M.R.J. (1986) Lytic agents, cell permeability and monolayer penetratability. *Journal of General Physiology*, **52**, 2275–2825.

Sattar, S.A. & Springthorpe, V.S. (1991) Survival and disinfectant inactivation of the human immunodeficiency virus: a critical review. *Reviews of Infectious Diseases*, **13**, 430–447.

Sattar, S.A. & Springthorpe, V.S. (1995) Methods under development for evaluating the antimicrobial activity of chemical germicides. In *Chemical Germicides in Health Care* (ed. Rutala, W.), pp. 237–254. Morin Heights: Polyscience Publications.

Schaeufele, P.J. (1986) Advances in quaternary ammonium biocides. *Proceedings of the 3rd Conference on Progress in Chemical Disinfection*, pp. 508–519. Binghamton, New York.

Schanno, R.J., Westlund, J.R. & Foelsch, D.H. (1980) Evaluation of 1.3-dimethylol-5,5-dimethylhydantoin as a cosmetic preservative. *Journal of the Society of Cosmetic Chemists*, **31**, 85–96.

Schmolka, I.R. (1973) The synergistic effects of non ionic surfactants upon cationic germicidal agents. *Journal of the Society of Cosmetic Chemists*, **24**, 577–592.

Schwabacher, H., Salsburgy, A.J. & Fincham, W.J. (1958) Blankets and infection: wool, terylene or cotton? *Lancet*, **ii**, 709–712.

Scott, C.R. & Wolf, P.A. (1962) The antibacterial activity of a series of quaternaries prepared from hexamethylene tetramine and halohydrocarbons. *Applied Microbiology*, **10**, 211–216.

Scott, E.M. & Gorman, S.P. (1987) Chemical disinfectants, antiseptics and preservatives. In *Pharmaceutical Microbiology* (eds Hugo, W.B. & Russell, A.D.), 4th edn, pp. 226–252. Oxford: Blackwell Scientific Publications.

Seevers, H.M., Shideman, F.E., Woods, L.A., Weeks, J.R. & Kruse, W.T. (1950) Dehydroactic acid (DHA). II. General pharmacology and mechanism of action. *Journal of Pharmacology and Experimental Therapeutics*, **99**, 69–83.

Seiler, D.A.L. & Russell, N.J. (1991) Ethanol as a food preservative. In *Food Preservatives* (eds Russell, N.J. & Gould, G.W.), pp. 153–171. Glasgow and London: Blackie.

Shaker, L.A., Russell, A.D. & Furr, J.R. (1986) Aspects of the action of chlorhexidine on bacterial spores. *International Journal of Pharmaceutics*, **34**, 51–56.

Shaker, L.A., Furr, J.R. & Russell, A.D. (1988a) Mechanism of resistance of *Bacillus subtilis* spores to chlorhexidine. *Journal of Applied Bacteriology*, **64**, 531–539.

Shaker, L.A., Dancer, B.N., Russell, A.D. & Furr, J.R. (1988b) Emergence and development of chlorhexidine resistance during sporulation of *Bacillus subtilis* 168. *FEMS Microbiology Letters*, **51**, 73–76.

Sheu, C.W., Salomon, J.L., Simmons, J.L., Sreevalsan, T. & Freese, E. (1975) Inhibitory effect of lipophilic fatty acids and related compounds on bacteria and mammalian cells. *Antimicrobial Agents and Chemotherapy*, **7**, 349–363.

Shibasaki, I. & Kato, N. (1978) Combined effects on antibacterial activity of fatty acids and their esters against Gram-negative bacteria. In *The Pharmacological Effects of Lipids* (ed. Kabara, J.J.), pp. 15–24. Champaign, Illinois, American Oil Chemists' Society.

Silver, S. & Misra, S. (1988) Plasmid-mediated heavy metal resistances. *Annual Review of Microbiology*, **42**, 717–743.

Silvernale, J.N., Joswick, H.L., Corner, T.R. & Gerhardt, P. (1971) Antimicrobial action of hexachlorophene: cytological manifestations. *Journal of Bacteriology*, **108**, 482–491.

Simon, E.W. (1953) Mechanisms of dinitrophenol toxicity. *Biological Reviews*, **28**, 453–479.

Simon, E.W. & Beevers, H. (1952a) The effect of pH on the biological activities of weak acids and bases. I. The most usual relationship between pH and activity. *New Phytologist*, **51**, 163–190.

Simon, E.W. & Beevers, H. (1952b) The effect of pH on the biological activities of weak acids and bases. II. Other relationships between pH and activity. *New Phytologist*, **51**, 191–197.

Simon, E.W. & Blackman, G.E. (1949) *The Significance of Hydrogen Ion Concentration in the Study of Toxicity*, Symposium of the Society of Experimental Biology No. 3, pp. 253–265. Cambridge: Cambridge University Press.

Simpson, R.A. (1986) Systemic and topical antimicrobial agents in the prevention of catheter-associated bacteriuria and its consequences. *Infection Control*, **7**, 100–103.

Sintim-Damoa, K. (1993) Other gaseous sterilization methods. In *Sterilization Technology* (eds Morrissey, R.F. & Phillips, G.B.), pp. 335–347. New York: Van Nostrand Reinhold.

Smith, C.R. (1968) Mycobactericidal agents. In *Disinfection, Sterilization and Preservation* (eds Lawrence, C.A. & Block, S.S.), 2nd edn, pp. 504–514. Philadelphia: Lea & Febiger.

Smith, P.J. & Smith, L. (1975) Organotin compounds and applications. *Chemistry in Britain*, **11**, 208–212, 226.

Sofos, J.N., Pierson, M.D., Blocher, L.C. & Busta, F.F. (1986) Mode of action of sorbic acid on bacterial cells and spores. *International Journal of Food Microbiology*, **3**, 1–17.

Sokol, H. (1952) Recent developments in the preservation of pharmaceuticals. *Drug Standards*, **20**, 89–106.

Speier, J.L. & Malek, J.R. (1982) Destruction of

microorganisms by contact with solid surfaces. *Journal of Colloid and Interfacial Science*, **89**, 68–76.

Spicher, G. & Peter, J. (1976) Microbial resistance to formaldehyde. I. Comparative quantitative studies in some selected species of vegetative bacteria, bacterial spores, fungi, bacteriophages and viruses. *Zentralblatt für Bakteriologie und Hygiene I, Abteilung Originale*, **B163**, 486–508.

Spicher, G. & Peter, J. (1981) Heat activation of bacterial spores after inactivation by formaldehyde: dependence of heat activation on temperature and duration of action. *Zentralblatt für Bakteriologie und Hygiene 1, Abteilung Originale*, **B173**, 188–196.

Spiner, D.R. & Hoffman, R.K. (1960) Method of disinfecting large enclosures with BPL vapour. *Applied Microbiology*, **8**, 152–155.

Springthorpe, V.S., Mbithi, J.N. & Sattar, S.A. (1995) Microbiocidal activity of chemical sterilants under reuse conditions. In *Chemical Germicides in Health Care* (ed. Rutala, W.A.), pp. 181–202. Morin Heights: Polyscience Publications.

Staehelin, M. (1958) Reaction of tobacco mosaic virus nucleic acid with formaldehyde. *Biochimica et Biophysica Acta*, **29**, 410–417.

Stanier, R.Y. & Orston, L.N. (1973) The ketoadipic pathway. In *Advances in Microbial Physiology* (eds Rose, A.H. & Tempest, D.W.), Vol. 9, pp. 89–151. London: Academic Press.

Stanier, R.Y., Sleeper, B.P., Tsuchida, M. & Macdonald, D.L. (1950) The bacterial oxidation of aromatic compounds. III. The enzymic oxidation of catechol and proto-catechuic acid to β-ketoadipic acid. *Journal of Bacteriology*, **59**, 137–151.

Stevenson, A.F. (1915) *An Efficient Liquid Disinfectant*. Public Health Reports 30, pp. 3003–3008. Washington, DC: US Public Health Service.

Stickler, D.J., Thomas, B., Clayton, C.L. & Chawala, J.C. (1983) Studies on the genetic basis of chlorhexidine resistance. *British Journal of Clinical Practice*, Symposium No. 25, pp. 23–28.

Suter, G.M. (1941) Relationships between the structure and bactericidal properties of phenols. *Chemical Reviews*, **28**, 269–299.

Sutton, S.V.W. (1996) Neutralizer evaluations as control experiments for antimicrobial efficacy tests. In *Handbook of Disinfectants and Antiseptics* (ed. Ascenzi, J.M.), pp. 43–62. New York: Marcel Dekker.

Sykes, G. (1965) *Disinfection and Sterilization*, 2nd edn. London: E. & F.N. Spon.

Taylor, L.A., Barbeito, M.S. & Gremillion, G.G. (1969) Paraformaldehyde for surface sterilization and detoxification. *Applied Microbiology*, **17**, 614–618.

Te Giffel, M.C., Beumer, R.R., Van Dam, W.F., Slaghuis, B.A. & Rombouts, F.M. (1996) Sporicidal effect of disinfectants on *Bacillus cereus* isolated from the milk processing environment. *International Biodeterioration and Biodegradation*, **36**, 421–430.

Thampuran, N. & Surendran, P.K. (1996) Effect of chemical agents on swarming of *Bacillus* species. *Journal of Applied Bacteriology*, **80**, 296–302.

Thomas, C.G.A., West, B. & Besser, H. (1959) Cleansing and sterilization of hospital blankets. *Guy's Hospital Reports*, **108**, 446–463.

Thornley, M.J. & Yudkin, J. (1959a) The origin of bacterial resistance to proflavine. I. Training and reversion in *Escherichia coli*. *Journal of General Microbiology*, **20**, 355–364.

Thornley, M.J. & Yudkin, J. (1959b) The origin of bacterial resistance to proflavine. 2. Spontaneous mutation to proflavine resistance in *Escherichia coli*. *Journal of General Microbiology*, **20**, 365–372.

Thrower, W.R. & Valentine, F.C.O. (1943) Propamidine in chronic wound sepsis. *Lancet*, **i**, 133.

Tilbury, R. (ed.) (1980) *Developments in Food Preservatives*. London: Applied Science Publishers.

Tilley, F.W. & Schaffer, J.M. (1925) Germicidal efficiency of coconut oil and linseed oil soaps and their mixtures with cresol. *Journal of Infectious Diseases*, **37**, 359–367.

Tjøtta, E., Hungnes, O. & Grinde, B. (1991) Survival of HIV-1 activity after disinfection, temperature and pH changes, or drying. *Journal of Medical Virology*, **35**, 223–227.

Toler, J.C. (1985) Preservative stability and preservative systems. *International Journal of Cosmetic Sciences*, **7**, 157–164.

Troll, W., Rinde, E. & Day, P. (1969) Effect on N-7 and C-8 substitution of guanine in DNA on T_m buoyant density and RNA polymerase primary. *Biochimica et Biophysica Acta*, **174**, 211–219.

Trueman, J.R. (1971) The halogens. In *Inhibition and Destruction of the Microbial Cell* (ed. Hugo, W.B.), pp. 135–183. London: Academic Press.

Tulis, J.J. (1973) Formaldehyde gas as a sterilant. In *Industrial Sterilization*, International Symposium, Amsterdam, 1972 (eds Phillips, G.B. & Miller, W.S.), pp. 209–238. Durham, North Carolina: Duke University Press.

Tyler, R., Ayliffe, G.A.J. & Bradley, C. (1990) Virucidal activity of disinfectants: studies with the poliovirus. *Journal of Hospital Infection*, **15**, 339–345.

Vaara, M. (1992) Agents increase the permeability of the outer membrane. *Microbiological Reviews*, **56**, 395–411.

Vaara, M. & Vaara, T. (1983a) Polycations sensitise enteric bacteria to antibiotics. *Antimicrobial Agents and Chemotherapy*, **24**, 107–113.

Vaara, M. & Vaara, T. (1983b) Polycations as outer membrane-disorganizing agents. *Antimicrobial Agents and Chemotherapy*, **24**, 114–122.

van Bueren, J. (1995) Methodology for HIV disinfectant testing. *Journal of Hospital Infection*, **30** (Suppl.), 383–388.

van Bueren, J., Larkin, D.P. & Simpson, R.A. (1994) Inactivation of human immunodeficiency virus type 1 by alcohols. *Journal of Hospital Infection*, **28**, 137–148.

Van der Kerk, H.J.M. & Luijten, J.G.A. (1954) Investigations on organo-tin compounds. III. The biocidal properties of organo-tin compounds. *Journal of Applied Chemistry*, **4**, 314–319.

Viljanen, P. (1987) Polycations which disorganize the outer membrane inhibit conjugation in *Escherichia coli*. *Journal of Antibiotics*, **40**, 882–886.

Viljanen P. & Borakynski, J. (1991) The susceptibility of conjugative resistance transfer in Gram-negative bacteria to physicochemical and biochemical agents. *FEMS Microbiology Reviews*, **88**, 43–54.

Voge, C.I.B. (1947) Phenylmercuric nitrate and related compounds. *Manufacturing Chemist and Manufacturing Perfumer*, **18**, 5–7.

Wallhäusser, K.H. (1984) Antimicrobial preservatives used by the cosmetic industry. In *Cosmetic and Drug Preservation: Principles and Practice* (ed. Kabara, J.J.), pp. 605–745. New York: Marcel Dekker.

Walpole, A.L., Roberts, D.C., Rose, F.L., Hendry, J.A. & Homer, R.F. (1954) Cytotoxic agents. IV. The carcinogenic actions of some monofunctional ethylene amine derivatives. *British Journal of Pharmacology*, **9**, 306–323.

Walter, G.R. & Gump, W.S. (1962) Chemical structure and antimicrobial activity of bisphenols. II. Bactericidal acitivity in the presence of an anionic surfactant. *Journal of the Society of Cosmetic Chemists*, **13**, 477–482.

Warren, I.C., Hutchinson, M. & Ridgway, J.W. (1981) Comparative assessment of swimming pool disinfectants. In *Disinfectants: Their Use and Evaluation of Effectiveness* (eds Collins, C.H., Allwood, M.C., Bloomfield, S.F. & Fox, A.), Society for Applied Bacteriology Technical Series No. 16, pp. 123–139. London: Academic Press.

Watanabe, T. (1963) Infective heredity of multiple drug resistance in bacteria. *Bacteriological Reviews*, **27**, 87–115.

Weber, D.J. & Rutala, W.A. (1995) Use of metals as microbicides for the prevention of nosocomial infections. In *Chemical Germicides in Health Care* (ed. Rutala, W.), pp. 271–286. Morin Heights: Polyscience Publications.

Weber, G.R. & Black, L.A. (1948) Laboratory procedure for evaluating practical performance of quaternary ammonium and other germicides proposed for sanitizing food utensils. *American Journal of Public Health*, **38**, 1405–1417.

Weber, G.R. & Levine, M. (1944) Factors affecting germicidal efficiency of chlorine and chloramine. *American Journal of Public Health*, **32**, 719–728.

Wedzicha, B.C. (1984) *Chemistry of Sulphur Dioxide in Foods*. London: Elsevier Applied Science Publishing.

Weinberg, E.D. (1957) The mutual effect of antimicrobial compounds and metallic cations. *Bacteriological Reviews*, **21**, 46–68.

Weiner, N.D., Hart, F. & Zografi, G. (1965) Application of the Ferguson principle to the antimicrobial activity of quaternary ammonium salts. *Journal of Pharmacy and Pharmacology*, **17**, 350–355.

West, T.S. (1969) *Complexometry with EDTA and Related Agents*, 3rd edn. Poole: BDH Chemicals.

Westwood, N. & Pin-Lim, B. (1972) Survival of *E. coli, Staph. aureus, Ps. aeruginosa* and spores of *B. subtitlis* in BPC mixtures. *Pharmaceutical Journal*, **208**, 153–154.

Wien, R., Harrison, J. & Freeman, W.A. (1948) Diamidines as antibacterial compounds. *British Journal of Pharmacology*, **3**, 211–218.

Wilkins, K.M. & Board, R.G. (1989) Natural antimicrobial systems. In *Mechanisms of Action of Food Preservation Systems* (ed. Gould, G.W.), pp. 285–362. London: Elsevier Applied Science.

Wilkinson, S.G. (1975) Sensitivity to ethylenediamine tetra-acetic acid. In *Resistance of* Pseudomonas aeruginosa (ed. Brown, M.R.W.), pp. 145–188. London: John Wiley & Sons.

Williams, D.E., Worley, S.D., Barnela, S.B. & Swango, L.J. (1987) Bactericidal activities of selected organic *N*-halamines. *Applied and Environmental Microbiology*, **53**, 2082–2089.

Williams, D.E., Elder, E.D. & Worley, S.D. (1988) Is free halogen necessary for disinfection? *Applied and Environmental Microbiology*, **54**, 2583–2585.

Williams, N.D. & Russell, A.D. (1991) The effects of some halogen-containing compounds on *Bacillus subtilis* endospores. *Journal of Applied Bacteriology*, **70**, 427–436.

Williams, N.D. & Russell, A.D. (1992) The nature and site of biocide-induced sublethal injury in *Bacillus subtilis* spores. *FEMS Microbiology Letters*, **99**: 277–280.

Williams, N.D. & Russell, A.D. (1993a) Injury and repair in biocide-treated spores of *Bacillus subtilis*. *FEMS Microbiology Letters*, **106**, 183–186.

Williams, N.D. & Russell, A.D. (1993b) Revival of biocide-treated spores of *Bacillus subtilis*. *Journal of Applied Bacteriology*, **75**, 69–75.

Williams, N.D. & Russell, A.D. (1993c) Revival of *Bacillus subtilis* spores from biocide-induced injury in germination processes. *Journal of Applied Bacteriology*, **75**, 76–81.

Wolf, P.A. (1950) Dehydroacetic acid, a new microbiological inhibitor. *Food Technology*, **4**, 294–297.

Wolf, P.A. & Westveer, W.M. (1950) The antimicrobial

activity of several substituted pyrones. *Archives of Biochemistry*, **28**, 201–206.

Woodcock, P.M. (1988) Biguanides as industrial biocide. In *Industrial Biocides* (ed. Payne, K.R.), pp. 19–36. Chichester: Wiley.

Woodroffe, R.C.S. & Wilkinson, B.E. (1966a) The antibacterial action of tetrachlorosalicylanilide. *Journal of General Microbiology*, **44**, 343–352.

Woodroffe, R.C.S. & Wilkinson, B.E. (1966b) Location of the tetrachlorosalicylanilide taken in by *Bacillus megaterium*. *Journal of General Microbiology*, **244**, 353–358.

Woolfson, A.D. (1977) The antibacterial activity of dimethoxane. *Journal of Pharmacy and Pharmacology*, **29**, 73P.

Woolfson, A.D. & Woodside, W. (1976) Analysis of the constituents of commercial dimethoxane. *Journal of Pharmacy and Pharmacology*, **28**, 28P.

Working Party (1985) Acquired immune deficiency syndrome: recommendations of a Working Party of the Hospital Infection Society. *Journal of Hospital Infection*, **6** (Suppl. C), 67–80.

Worley, S.D., Williams, D.E. & Barnela, S.B. (1987) The stabilities of new *N*-halamine water disinfectants. *Water Research*, **21**, 983–988.

Wright, A.M., Hoxey, E.V., Soper, C.J. & Davies, D.J.G. (1996) Biological indicators for low temperature steam and formaldehyde sterilization: investigation of the effect of the change in temperature and formaldehyde concentration on spores of *Bacillus stearothermophilus* NCIMB 8224. *Journal of Applied Bacteriology*, **80**, 259–265.

Wright, C.J. & McAllister, T.A. (1967) Protective action of noxythiolin in experimental endotoxaemia. *Clinical Trials Journal*, **4**, 680–681.

York, G.K. & Vaughan, R.H. (1955) Site of microbial inhibition by sorbic acid. *Bacteriological Proceedings*, **55**, 20.

CHAPTER 3

Factors Influencing the Efficacy of Antimicrobial Agents

1 Introduction

The activity of biocides (antiseptics, disinfectants and preservatives) against microorganisms depends on:

1 the external physical environment;

2 the nature, structure, composition and condition of the organism itself;

3 the ability of the organism to degrade or inactivate the particular substance converting it to an inactive form (Russell, 1991a).

It has long been known that a modification of the concentration of the antimicrobial agent, or the temperature or pH at which it is acting, can have profound influence on activity. The practical value of a knowledge of these effects in terms of antisepsis, disinfection or preservation, or as an aid in certain thermal sterilization processes, may be considerable. However, many other parameters must also be considered. While many of these may be of academic value only, taken *in toto* they may lead to a better understanding of the reasons for the sensitivity or resistance of microorganisms to biocides, as well as to possible means of improving, or potentiating, the activity of such agents.

For these reasons as many factors as possible will be considered, but those antimicrobial substances which will be dealt with will be biocides (disinfectants, antiseptics and preservatives) and not antibiotics, which are outside the scope of this chapter. Antibiotics were considered in an earlier paper (Russell, 1974).

Three main aspects will be examined, namely how pretreatment, in-treatment and post-treatment factors influence activity. Wherever possible, practical implications as well as theoretical ones will be discussed; in this context, Rutala (1990) and Russell & Gould (1988, 1991) should be consulted for further information.

As pointed out above, the activity of an antimicrobial compound depends on the external environment and on the organism itself; additionally, its ability to degrade or inactivate the particular compound by converting it to an inactive form must also be considered. While there is much evidence for the enzymatic inactivation of antibiotics, there is far less information available as to the inactivation of biocides (Hugo, 1991; Beveridge, 1998). This aspect will be considered briefly later (Section 3.8). Of increasing importance is the existence of bacteria as biofilms and the possible decreased susceptibility to biocides and antibiotics. This is discussed in Section 5.

2 Pretreatment conditions

Investigators have, over the years, used a variety of techniques with the result that a considerable amount of useful information has accrued. Basically, techniques of growing bacteria have been either by means of continuous, or of batch, culture, with the latter predominating. The main criticism of batch culture is, of course, that cells of different physiological ages will be present, whereas continuous cultures, e.g. those grown in a chemostat, overcome this criticism. Farewell & Brown (1971) have reviewed pretreatment procedures on subsequent sensitivity of microbes to inimical treatments.

2.1 Chemostat-grown cultures

Bacterial cell walls are highly variable structures, which can change in response to the growth environment. Chemostat cultures of *Aerobacter aerogenes* grown under conditions of Mg^{2+}, glycerol or phosphate limitation produce cells with wide variation in wall composition (Tempest & Ellwood, 1969). Cells of a *Bacillus subtilis* suspension showed differing responses to the enzyme lysozyme, which acts on peptidoglycan, depending on whether they had been chemostat-grown under conditions of Mg^{2+}, phosphate or ammonia limitation. Thus, phenotypic variation in bacterial cell walls is achieved under a rigidly controlled chemical environment in the chemostat. Investigations into the effect of antibacterial agents on chemostat-grown cultures have been made by Melling *et al.* (1974) and Dean *et al.* (1976), who showed that *Pseudomonas aeruginosa* exhibited different degrees of sensitivity, when grown under magnesium-limited conditions and at varying dilution rates, to ethylenediamine tetraacetic acid (EDTA) and various antibiotics.

2.2 Batch-grown cultures

Far more extensive investigations have been undertaken with batch-grown cultures, and thus these will be examined in greater detail.

2.2.1 Growth medium

Growth-medium composition may markedly influence the subsequent sensitivity of cells to antibacterial agents, e.g. the leakage of 260-nm-absorbing material from hexachlorophane-treated *Bacillus megaterium* (Joswick *et al.* 1971).

'Fattened' cells of Gram-positive bacteria are produced when cultures are grown in glycerol glycerol-containing broth. Alteration in the cell wall lipid of these cells may profoundly affect their sensitivity to antibacterial agents (Vaczi, 1973), notably phenols (Hugo & Franklin, 1968) and esters of *p*-hydroxbenzoic acids. (Furr & Russell, 1972). Growth of an *Escherichia coli* strain in a medium containing L-alanine or L-cystine resulted in cells which differed greatly from broth-grown cells in their response to biocides (Hugo & Ellis, 1975). The L-alanine-grown cells had a structural deformity, which rendered them more permeable, and hence more susceptible, to these antibacterial agents, whereas the comparative response of L-cystine-grown and broth-grown cells could be correlated with the differences in the composition of the cell walls.

Magnesium-limited batch cultures of *Ps. aeruginosa* produce cells that are highly resistant to EDTA (Brown & Melling, 1969), to chloroxylenol (Cowen, 1974) and to a combination of chloroxylenol and EDTA (Dankert & Schut, 1976). Profound changes occur in the walls of Mg^{2+}-limited cells of this organism (Eagon *et al.*, 1975) and these alterations are intimately linked with sensitivity and resistance of the whole cells to antiseptics and other antibacterial agents.

It seems likely that, in the envelopes of Mg-limited cells, the normal outer membrane-stabilizing Mg^{2+} bridges are replaced by polyamides, thereby reducing sensitivity to ion chelators and to biocides that promote their own uptake by displacing cations (Gilbert & Wright, 1987).

The sensitivity of *B. megaterium* cells to chlorhexidine and phenoxyethanol alters when changes in growth rate and nutrient limitation are made (Russell & Chopra, 1996). Nevertheless, lysozyme-induced protoplasts remain sensitive to these membrane-active agents; thus the cell wall is responsible for the modified response in whole cells.

There is little published information that deals with the effect of changes in sporulation medium on the subsequent sensitivity of bacterial spores to antibacterial agents. Chlorocresol has been found (Purves & Parker, 1973) to have a greater inhibitory effect on the germination of spores produced on a complex medium, where absorption of spore coats occurred, than on the germination of those produced on a synthetic medium, where emergence was by rupture of the coats.

It has been recommended that, since the composition of the sporulation medium can influence the response of spores to antibacterial agents, spores should be prepared in chemically defined media (Hodges *et al.*, 1980). This is obviously of importance where standardization of test methods is concerned. It has recently been demonstrated (Knott *et al.*, 1997) that different types of water used in preparing culture media can have a profound influence on germination, outgrowth and sporulation of *B. subtilis* and this is a factor that should be taken into account in assessing sensitivity or otherwise to antibacterial agents.

2.2.2 *pH of culture medium*

There is surprisingly little information as to the effect of variations in the pH of the culture medium on subsequent sensitivity of bacteria to antimicrobial agents. Differences in the phospholipid contents of batch-grown cells of *B. megaterium* and *Staphylococcus aureus* grown at different pH values have been observed, but cell wall changes have not been examined (Houtsmuller & Van Deenen, 1964; Op den Kamp *et al.*, 1965).

Changes in cell walls of bacteria grown in media of different pH values might be expected to lead to variations in response of the organisms to biocides. It must, however, be added that changes in pH value of the medium will occur during growth of the organism as a result of its metabolic activity.

2.2.3 *Temperature of incubation*

Again, there is surprisingly little information on the effect of incubation temperature of the culture medium in which the cells are grown and their sensitivity when later exposed to a non-antibiotic antimicrobial agent. Studies have been carried out with antibiotics, e.g. the effect of antibiotics on methicillin-resistant *Staph. aureus* (MRSA), and the effect of nystatin on the yeast, *Saccharomyces cerevisiae*, grown at different temperatures. Quite significant changes may occur in cells grown at different temperatures, notably the phospholipid content (de Siervo, 1969).

There is no doubt that a comparison of the response to antimicrobial agents of microorganisms grown at different temperatures could provide much useful information, especially if quantitative studies on cell-wall composition are made simultaneously.

Changes in sporulation conditions have been shown to influence not only the composition of spores but also their responses to heat and radiation (Russell, 1971b, 1982). *Bacillus subtilis* spores produced at 37°C are rather more sensitive to inhibition by chlorocresol of their germination than are spores produced at 50°C (Bell & Parker, 1975). However, there is a dearth of information in this area, and no conclusions can as yet be reached.

2.2.4 *Anaerobiosis*

Data about the effect of antibacterial agents on bacteria grown under anaerobic conditions are sparse. In a review of those factors influencing the antimicrobial activity of phenols, Bennett (1959) pointed out that aerobic organisms were more resistant than anaerobes, and that faculative aerobes were sensitive under aerobic, but much less so under anaerobic, conditions. The basis of this response is unknown.

2.3 Condition of organism

2.3.1 *Gaseous disinfectants*

The state of hydration of the microorganisms under test may be an important factor in determining their sensitivity or resistance to an antimicrobial agent. Pretreatment equilibration of bacterial spores, *E. coli* and *Staph. aureus*, to low relative humidity (r.h.) values, 1%, increases their resistance to ethylene oxide at 33% r.h., whereas under 'optimum' conditions, i.e. with 'naked' spores placed on filter-paper, the antibacterial activity is most rapid at this r.h. (Gilbert *et al.*, 1964). Once bacterial cells have been dried beyond a certain critical point, they must be physically wetted or placed in an environment of 100% r.h. to become rehydrated. This factor is of paramount importance in ensuring sterilization by ethylene oxide.

It has also been shown that organisms predried from different media vary in their subsequent sensitivity to ethylene oxide. Bacterial spores dried from saline, serum and broth are more resistant than those dried from water or methanol, and those dried from saline always have a small proportion of cells which are not killed, even after prolonged exposure to the gas (Beeby & Whitehouse, 1965). Bacteria trapped inside crystals are protected from the action of ethylene oxide, which is unable to penetrate crystalline materials. *Staphylococcus aureus* cells grown in tryptose broth, washed with water, placed on filter discs and exposed to ethylene oxide at 'optimum' (33%) r.h. are more readily killed than similarly grown but unwashed cells of this organism (Gilbert *et al.*, 1964). Adsorption of organic matter, represented by tryptose broth, to the cells is the probable reason for the reduced effect of the gas.

The nature of the surface on which organisms are dried before exposure to ethylene oxide may have a considerable effect on response to the gas. Bacteria dried on hard or non-hygroscopic surfaces are more resistant on subsequent exposure than are the same organisms dried on absorbent or hygroscopic surfaces (Kereluk *et al.*, 1970).

The inactivation of microorganisms by ethylene oxide and other gases has been the subject of several reviews, notably those by Hoffman (1971), Ernst (1974), Russell (1976) and Richards *et al.* (1984). Chapter 21 in the present volume should also be consulted.

2.3.2 *Liquid biocides*

Dried bacteria are considerably more resistant than bacteria in liquid suspension. In experiments with glutaraldehyde, A.D. Russell (unpublished data) found that concentrations of 50 times those needed to kill liquid suspensions of non-sporulating bacteria were necessary to kill the same strains dried on to syringe needles. This is by no means an isolated occurrence. In practice, bacteria are frequently found in dry conditions, and simulated tests can provide useful information. In this context, the publication detailing the Association of Official Analytical Chemists (AOAC) test methods for evaluating disinfectant activity is a valuable document (AOAC, 1998).

2.4 Pretreatment with chemical agents

Some significant findings, especially from an understanding of the nature of bacterial permeability or impermeability to biocides, have resulted from investigations involving pre-exposure of microorganisms to chemical agents before treatment of cells with antimicrobial compounds. This section will thus deal with the following pretreatment environments.

1 Growth of microorganisms in a specified medium containing a specified chemical agent.

2 Growth in a specified medium, followed by washing the cells, and exposing them to a specified chemical agent.

3 Exposure of cells to a specified mutagen.

2.4.1 *Pretreatment with polysorbate*

Polysorbates (tweens) are non-ionic surface-active agents which find importance in the formulation of certain pharmaceutical products (see Chapter 16). Polysorbate 80-treated *Ps. aeruginosa* cells, in which organisms were grown in broth containing up to 0.175% polysorbate, became permeable to the dye, anilinonaphthalene-8-sulphonate (Brown & Winsley, 1969). It is possible that polysorbate alters the permeability of the cells, since it has been found that polysorbate 80-treated bacteria leak intracellular constituents and become susceptible to changes in pH, temperature or sodium chloride (NaCl) concentration (Brown & Winsley, 1969; see also Brown, 1975). Support for this comes from the findings (Brown & Richards, 1964) that pretreatment of *Ps. aeruginosa* with polysorbate 80 renders the cells more sensitive to benzalkonium chloride and chlorhexidine diacetate.

2.4.2 *Pretreatment with cationic surface-active agents*

Pretreatment of *Ps. aeruginosa* with benzalkonium chloride produced cells sensitive to polysorbate 80, which adversely affected the cell envelope, and to phenethyl alcohol, which had an enhanced effect on the membrane (Hoffman *et al.*, 1973; Richards & Cavill, 1976). In this context it is of interest to note that the cationic agent, cetyltrimethylammonium bromide (CTAB), is believed to unmask a subunit of the carrier protein in the outer layer of the cytoplasmic membrane, thereby allowing the transport of β-galactoside into permease-less *E. coli* mutants (Ulitzer, 1970). However, pretreatment of *Proteus* spp. with cationic agents did not increase their sensitivity to unrelated agents (Chapman & Russell, 1978).

2.4.3 *Pretreatment with permeabilizers*

Permeabilizers are chemical agents that increase bacterial permeability to antimicrobial agents. To date, permeabilizers have been most widely studied with Gram-negative bacteria and include chelating agents, polycations, lactoferrin and transferrin, triethylene tetramine and specific cationic compounds (Smith, 1975; Vaara & Vaara, 1983a, b; Hukari *et al.*, 1986; Viljanen, 1987; Modha *et al.*, 1989, Ayres *et al.*, 1993; Russell & Chopra, 1996).

Leive (1965) found that, whereas *E. coli* cells were normally insensitive to the antibiotic actinomycin D, pretreatment of the cells with EDTA rendered them susceptible to the antibiotic. This is probably the result of a non-specific increase in permeability as a consequence of treatment with the chelating agent, since cells of many Gram-negative strains pretreated with EDTA or a related chelating agent become sensitive to many unrelated antibacterial agents, including chlorhexidine, benzalkonium chloride and cetrimide (for reviews, see Russell, 1971a, 1990a, 1991a; Wilkinson, 1975; Hart, 1984; Russell & Gould, 1988; Russell & Chopra, 1996.

Ethylenediaminetetra-acetic acid is believed to remove cations, especially Mg^{2+} and Ca^{2+}, from the outer envelope layers of Gram-negative bacteria. Additionally, a considerable amount of lipopolysaccharide is removed, although generally the cells remain viable.

In some experiments, permeabilizers are included with test inhibitor in the growth medium. Properties of these permeabilizing agents are considered in Table 3.1. Other permeabilizers used in the laboratory for increasing bacterial spore sensitivity to biocides include urea in combination with dithiothreitol and sodium lauryl sulphate (UDS; Russell, 1990b, 1991b). Few, if any, significant studies have been made about ways of increasing the permeability to biocides of mycobacteria or fungi.

2.4.4 *Pretreatment with cross-linking agents*

Pretreatment of Gram-negative bacteria with glutaraldehyde (Munton & Russell, 1972; Russell & Haque, 1975) or other cross-linking agents (Schmalreck & Teuber, 1976) renders the cells more resistant to lysis by osmotic shock, EDTA-lysozyme or sodium lauryl sulphate. Glutaraldehyde-treated cells of *Staph. aureus* became more resistant to lysis by lysostaphin (Russell & Vernon, 1975). Such findings are of potential value in studying the mechanism of action of cross-linking agents, which appear to act on the bacterial cell wall or envelope.

Type of agent	Example	Action
Some organic acids	Citric, malic acids	Chelate Mg^{2+} ions in outer membrane
Chelating agent	EDTA (and similar agents)	Leakage (and lysis in *Ps. aeruginosa*); removal of some outer membrane Mg^{2+} and LPS
Polycations	Polylysine	Displacement of outer membrane Mg^{2+} and release of LPS
Iron-binding proteins	Lactoferrin, transferrin	Partial LPS loss

LPS, lipopolysaccharide.

Table 3.1 Permeabilizing agents (based on Russell & Chopra, 1996).

Pretreatment of bacterial spores with glutaraldehyde reduces the permeabilizing-induced sensitivity lysozyme (Thomas & Russell, 1974), providing evidence for a binding of the aldehyde at the spore surface but not ruling out penetration into the spore.

2.4.5 Exposure of cells to mutagenic agents

Methods of using mutagenic agents, such as *N*-methyl-*N*′-nitro-*N*-nitrosoguanidine (NTG), to produce mutants of bacteria of fungi have been described by Adelberg *et al.* (1965) and Hopwood (1970). Novobiocin-supersensitive (NS) mutants of *E. coli* have been produced by exposure of the parent cells to NTG (Tamaki *et al.*, 1971; Ennis & Bloomstein, 1974). These NS mutants were more sensitive than the parent cells to EDTA, lysozyme and tris, as well as to deoxycholate (Singh & Reithmeier, 1975), and were shown to be heptose-deficient mutants with associated alterations in the protein component of the outer membrane.

The response of antibiotic-supersensitive strains of *Ps. aeruginosa* and *E. coli* to biocides has been studied (El-Falaha *et al.*, 1983; Russell & Furr, 1986; Russell *et al.*, 1985, 1986, 1987). All *E. coli* strains showed a similar degree of sensitivity to chlorhexidine, but deep rough mutants were much more sensitive to quaternary ammonium compounds (QACs) and parabens.

2.4.6 Induction of spheroplasts, protoplasts and mureinoplasts

Spheroplasts are osmotically fragile forms of bacteria which retain at least some of their outer envelope material. They are usually induced in hypertonic media by antibiotics, such as penicillins, cephalosporins or D-cycloserine, which inhibit a specific stage in the biosynthesis of the bacterial cell wall, or by exposure of cells to EDTA, tris, lysozyme and sucrose. If the latter treatment is used, however, it is pertinent to note that the outer membrane of stationary-phase cells may be more resistant to 'destabilizers', such as tris and EDTA, than are exponentially growing cells, i.e. the outer membrane of the former may be more stable than that of the latter cells (Witholt *et al.*, 1976).

Protoplasts are osmotically fragile forms of bacteria which contain no cell wall material. Sensitive bacteria, such as *Micrococcus lysodeikticus*, *Sarcina lutea* and *B. megaterium*, can be converted into protoplasts by means of the enzyme lysozyme.

Mureinoplasts are osmotically fragile forms of Gram-negative bacteria which have lost the outer lipoprotein and lipopolysaccharide layers by repeated washing of the cells with hypertonic sucrose (Gorman & Scott, 1977; see also Weiss, 1976). Mureinoplasts which retain the original peptidoglycan may be converted to protoplasts by treatment with lysozyme.

Treatment of spheroplasts, protoplasts or mureinoplasts with biocides may be of value in assessing the influence of the outer cell layers on the penetration of the antibacterial compounds. It must, however, be recognized that in these forms there may be stretching of the remaining outside layers, as in spheroplasts, or of the cytoplasmic membrane itself (as in all three forms), which could distort the conclusions reached. For this reason, effects of biocides on such morphological variants should only be considered in relation to other techniques (Russell & Chopra, 1996).

3 Factors during treatment

Several parameters influence the in-use activity of biocides. These include the concentration of agent; the number, type and location of microorganisms; the temperature and pH of treatment; and the presence of extraneous material, such as organic or other interfering matter. These have important effects on the actual performance of disinfectants, antiseptics and preservatives, and consequently will be considered at some length.

3.1 Kinetics of microbial inactivation

Kinetics of the inactivation of a microbial population by a biocide (Jacobs, 1960) can be determined from the inactivation (rate) constant, k. The rate of change of the population is given by

$$\frac{-dN}{dt} = kt \qquad (3.1)$$

or

$$\frac{N_t}{N_0} = \exp^{-kt} \qquad (3.2)$$

in which N_0 and N_t represent the numbers of viable cells (colony-forming units (cfu)) per ml at zero time and at time t, respectively.

From eqn. (3.2),

$$-kt = \ln \frac{N_t}{N_0}$$

or

$$k = \frac{1}{t} \ln \frac{N_0}{N_t} \qquad (3.3)$$

or

$$k = \frac{1}{t}\, 2.303 \log_{10} \frac{N_0}{N_t} \qquad (3.4)$$

The rate of biocide-induced inactivation of a microorganism will depend markedly on the biocide concentration (Section 3.2) as well as on the temperature of exposure (Section 3.4), as also possibly on pH (Section 3.5) and the presence of organic matter (Section 3.6.1).

3.2 Concentration of biocide

Kinetic studies involving the effect of concentration on the lethal activity of microbicidal substances have employed a symbol, η, termed the concentration exponent (dilution coefficient), which is a measure of the effect of changes in concentration (or dilution) on cell death rate. To determine η, it is necessary to measure the time necessary to produce a comparable degree of death of a bacterial suspension at two different concentrations of the antimicrobial agent. Death rates may be determined in different ways, including an assessment of decimal reduction times (D-values) (Hurwitz & McCarthy, 1985).

Then, if C_1 and C_2 represent the two concentrations and t_1 and t_2 the respective times to reduce the viable population to a similar degree

$$C_1^{\eta} t_1 = C_2^{\eta} t_2 \qquad (3.5)$$

or

$$\eta = \frac{\log t_2 - \log t_1}{\log C_1 - \log C_2} \qquad (3.6)$$

A decrease in concentration of substances with high η values results in a marked increase in the time necessary to achieve a comparable kill, other conditions remaining constant. In contrast, compounds with low η values are much less influenced (Table 3.2; see also Table 3.3).

A knowledge of the effect of concentration on antimicrobial activity is essential in the following situations:

1 in the evaluation of biocidal activity;

Table 3.2 Concentration exponents (η values) of various antimicrobial agents (based, in part, on Bean, 1967).

Substance(s)	η Value	Increased time factor (x ...) when concentrated reduced to: One-half	One-third
Phenolics	6	2^6, i.e. $64x$	3^6, i.e. $729x$
Alcohol	10	2^{10}, i.e. $1024x$	3^{10}, i.e. $59000x$
Parabens	2.5	$2^{2.5}$, i.e. $5.7x$	$3^{2.5}$, i.e. $15.6x$
Chlorhexidine	2	$4x$	$8x$
Mercury compounds	1	$2x$	$3x$
Quaternary ammonium compounds	1	$2x$	$3x$
Formaldehyde	1	$2x$	$3x$

2 in the sterility testing of pharmaceutical and medical products (*British Pharmacopoeia* 1998)
3 in ensuring adequate preservative levels in pharmaceutical products;
4 in deciding what dilution instructions are reasonable in practice.

Other factors, which will be considered later, may also influence the effective ('free') available concentration of an antimicrobial agent.

3.3 Numbers and location of microorganisms

It is obviously easier for an antimicrobial agent to be effective when there are few microorganisms against which it has to act. This is particularly important in the production of various types of pharmaceutical and cosmetic products, and is discussed in detail later (Chapter 16). Likewise, the location of microorganisms must be considered in assessing activity (Scott & Gorman, 1998). An example of this occurs in the cleaning of equipment used in the large-scale production of creams (Bean, 1967), where difficulties may arise in the penetration of a disinfectant to all parts of the equipment.

3.4 Temperature

The activity of a disinfectant or preservative is usually increased when the temperature at which it acts is increased. Useful formulae to measure the effect of temperature on activity are given by

$$\theta^{(T_2 - T_1)} = k_2/k_1 \quad (3.7)$$

or

$$\theta^{(T_2 - T_1)} = t_1/t_2 \quad (3.8)$$

in which k_2 and k_1 are the rate (velocity) constants at temperatures T_2 and T_1, respectively (eqn 3.7) and t_2 and t_1 are the respective times to bring about a complete kill at T_2 and T_1 (eqn 3.8).

The temperature coefficient, θ, refers to the

Table 3.3 Possible relationship between concentration exponents and mechanisms of action of biocides (based on Hugo & Denyer, 1987 and Russell & Chopra, 1996).

Group	Examples	Mechanism of action
A (η1–2)	Chlorhexidine	Membrane disrupter
	QACs	Membrane disrupter
	Mercury components	–SH reactors
	Glutaraldehyde	$-NH_2$ groups and nucleic acids
B (η2–4)	Parabens	Concentration-dependent effects: transport inhibited (low), membrane integrity affected (high)
	Sorbic acid	Transport inhibitor (effect on proton-motive force); another unidentified mechanism?
C (η>4)	Aliphatic alcohols, Phenolics	Membrane disrupters

effect of temperature per 1°C rise, and is nearly always between 1.0 and 1.5 (Bean, 1967). Consequently, it is more usual to specify the θ^{10} (or Q_{10}) value, which is the change in activity per 10°C rise in temperature (Table 3.4).

The relationship between θ and Q_{10} is given by

$$\theta = \sqrt[10]{Q_{10}} \tag{3.9}$$

i.e. θ is the 10th root of Q_{10} (or θ^{10}).

The activity of isoascorbic acid increases markedly at elevated temperatures (Mackey & Seymour, 1990). Other examples are provided by phenolics and organomercurials (chlorocresol and phenylmercuric nitrate were at one time used at 98–100°C as a means of sterilizing certain parenteral and ophthalmic solutions in the UK) and by formaldehyde when employed in a low-temperature steam and formaldehyde (LTSF) system (Wright *et al.*, 1997).

The potent microbicidal agent, glutaraldehyde, shows a very marked temperature-dependent activity. The alkalinized, or 'potentiated', form of this dialdehyde is a far more powerful agent at 20°C than the more stable acid formulation (Section 3.5). However, at temperatures of about 40°C and above there is little, if any, difference in activity (Boucher, 1975), although the alkaline formulation is less stable at higher temperatures (Gorman *et al.*, 1980; Russell, 1994).

3.5 Environmental pH

pH can influence biocidal activity in the following ways.

1 Changes may occur in the molecule. Substances such as phenol, benzoic acid, sorbic acid and dehydroacetic acid are effective only or mainly in the un-ionized form (see also Chapter 2) and as the pH rises an increase takes place in their degree of dissociation. Glutaraldehyde is more stable at acid pH but is considerably more potent at alkaline pH, and it has been postulated that its interaction with amino groups, which occurs most rapidly above pH 7, may be responsible for its lethal effect (Russell & Hopwood, 1976; Gorman *et al.*, 1980; Power & Russell, 1990; Russell, 1994).

2 Changes may occur in the cell surface. As pH increases, the number of negatively charged groups on the bacterial cell surface increases, with the result that positively charged molecules have an enhanced degree of binding, e.g. QACs (Hugo, 1965, 1991) and dyes, such as crystal violet and ethyl violet (Moats & Maddox, 1978), which remain essentially in their ionized form over the pH range 5–9.

3 Partitioning of a compound between a product in which it is present and the microbial cell may be influenced by pH (Bean, 1972).

Table 3.5 summarizes the effects of pH on antimicrobial activity and lists some postulated reasons for these modifications. The sporicidal activity of sodium hypochlorite is potentiated in the presence of alcohols, especially methanol (Coates & Death, 1978), although there is no simple explanation between activity, stability and pH change of the mixture. Maximal sporicidal activity and stability are achieved by buffering hypochlorite alone or a hypochlorite/methanol mixture to within a pH range of 7.6–8.1 (Death & Coates, 1979).

3.6 Interfering substances

3.6.1 *Organic matter*

Organic matter occurs in various forms: serum, blood, pus, earth, food residues, milkstone (dried residues of milk), faecal material. Organic matter

Table 3.4 Temperature coefficient (Q_{10} values) of various antimicrobial agents (based, in part, on Bean, 1967).

Substance(s)	Q_{10} Value	Special application
Phenols and cresols	3–5	Bactericides in some injections*
Formaldehyde	1.5	
Aliphatic alcohols	30–50	
Ethylene oxide	2.7	Sterilization (may be used at 60°C)
β-Propiolactone	2–3	Sterilization (but carcinogenic?)

*Heating with a bactericide, a process no longer official (*British Pharmacopoeia*, 1998).

Table 3.5 Effect of pH on antimicrobial activity.

Activity as environmental pH increases	Comments
Decreased activity	
Phenols Organic acids (e.g. benzoic, sorbic)*	Increase in degree of dissociation of molecule
Hypochlorites	Active factor is undissociated hypochlorous acid (see Chapter 2)
Iodine	Most active form is diatomic iodine, I_2 (see Chapter 2)
Increased activity	
Quaternary ammonium compounds Biguanides Diaminidines	Increase in degree of ionization of bacterial surface groups
Acridines Triphenylmethane dyes	Basic nature: competition with H+ ions
Glutaraldehyde	Interaction with $-NH_2$ groups? (Increases with increasing pH)

*It is now considered that the anion also plays some role in antimicrobial activity; see Eklund (1980, 1983, 1985a,b), Salmond *et al.* (1984) and Sofos *et al.* (1986).

may interfere with the microbicidal activity of disinfectants and other antimicrobial compounds. This interference generally takes the form of a 'reaction' between the biocide and the organic matter, thus leaving a reduced concentration of antimicrobial agent for attacking microorganisms. This reduced activity is notably seen with highly reactive compounds, such as chlorine disinfectants. An alternative possibility is that organic material protects microorganisms from attack.

Organic soil (as also yeast) has been incorporated into various testing procedures, such as the Chick–Martin procedure and the 'dirty conditions' of the modified Kelsey–Sykes test (Kelsey & Maurer, 1974; Coates, 1977; Cowen, 1978), which at least give some indication of the likely usefulness of the disinfectant in actual practice.

Organic matter decreases the effect of hypochlorites against bacteria (including mycobacteria and spores), viruses and fungi (Grossgebauer, 1970; Russell, 1971b; Trueman, 1971; Croshaw, 1977; Russell & Hugo, 1987; Scott & Gorman, 1987). Because of their lower chemical reactivity, iodine and iodophors are influenced to a rather lesser extent (Sykes, 1965). Phenols may also show a reduced activity in the presence of organic matter, although Lysol will retain much of its activity in the presence of faeces and sputum. Because of its reactivity with–NH_2 groups, it would be expected that the antimicrobial activity of glutaraldehyde would be reduced in the presence of serum; this does not, however, appear to be the case (Borick, 1968; A.D. Russell, unpublished), although conflicting data have been reported (Bergan & Lystad, 1971a,b).

Disinfectant use in the cosmetic, pharmaceutical, food and dairy industries is influenced by the reduction of activity that may occur in the presence of organic soil (Bean, 1967; Clegg, 1967; Goldenberg & Relf, 1967; Davis, 1972a,b). Adequate precleaning before employment of a disinfectant or a combination of disinfectant with a suitable detergent may overcome the problem. The nature of the surface and the protection afforded by soiling film are of considerable importance; in the dairy industry, invisible milkstone may protect microorganisms against disinfection. For further information, Chapter 2 should be consulted.

Detergents themselves may have a lethal effect on microorganisms and are frequently, if not invariably, used hot. Some disinfectants may exert a detergent action. Cosmetic and pharmaceutical creams may pose a disinfection problem, since remnants of production batches may remain in relatively inaccessible orifices and crevices in apparatus and machinery used for their preparation; the likely outcome is that such remnants would form foci for the infection of future production batches. Cleaning of all apparatus with hot water and detergent, followed by an appropriate disinfectant or steam, has been recommended (Bean, 1967).

3.6.2 *Surface-active agents*

The antimicrobial activity of methyl and propyl *p*-hydrozybenzoates and of quaternary ammonium compounds is reduced markedly by macromolecular polymers and by non-ionic agents. Significant increases in concentration of these antimicrobial compounds are needed to inhibit growth of microorganisms in the presence of polysorbates (tweens) (Patel & Kostenbauder, 1958; Kostenbauder, 1983). Nevertheless, although the *total* inhibitory concentration increases with increasing polysorbate concentration, the concentration of *free* preservative required for microbial inhibition is a constant, which is independent of the polysorbate concentration, and which is considerably less than the total concentration (Figs 3.1 and 3.2).

The amount of preservative bound to a non-ionic surfactant may be obtained from the following equation:

$$R = SC + 1 \qquad (3.10)$$

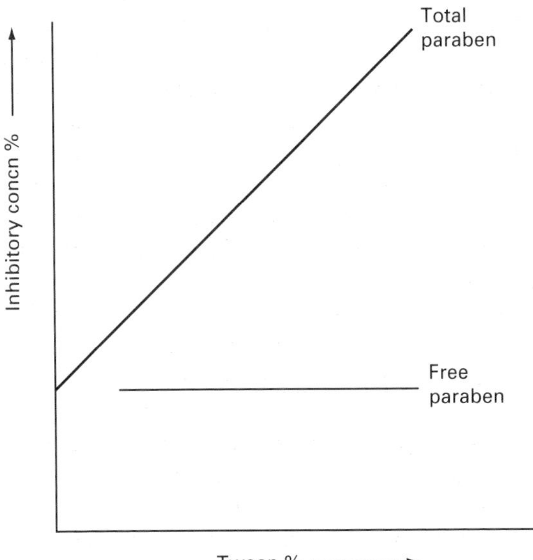

Fig. 3.1 Effect of polysorbate (tween) 80 concentration on the inhibitory concentration of methyl-*p*-hydroxybenzoate (methyl paraben).

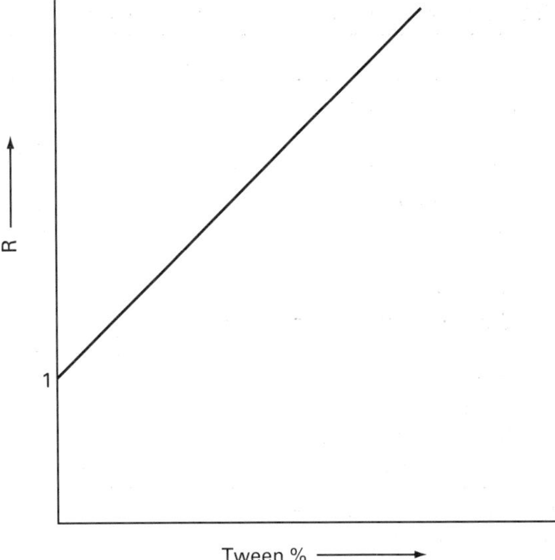

Fig. 3.2 Relationship between polysorbate (tween) 80 concentration and *R* (ratio of total : free drug).

in which *R* is the ratio of total to free preservative concentration, *S* is the surfactant concentration and *C* is a constant, which has a unique value for each surfactant–preservative mixture and which increases in value as the lipid solubility of the preservative increases.

The interaction (considered briefly below) of preservatives with non-ionic surface-active agents has important repercussions in the preservation of various types of pharmaceutical and cosmetic products, notably creams and emulsions. This aspect is considered in detail in Chapter 16. Interaction of preservatives with non-ionic surfactants could be the result of either micellar solubilization or complex formation between the two molecules.

Interaction between a preservative and a macromolecule does not necessarily mean that the preservative has no effect. Provided that compensation is made for the amount of bound preservative, an appropriate preservative concentration may be included in a product. This implies that an adequate concentration of free preservative exists in the aqueous phase outside the micelle or complex. However, other problems could also arise, including possible difficulties in formulation and toxicity to the user.

A seemingly paradoxical result is the observation that non-ionic surfactants can increase the efficacy of antimicrobial agents. Low concentrations of polysorbates, tritons and tergitols have been shown to increase the microbicidal potency of esters of *p*-hydroxybenzoic acid and of benzalkonium chloride and chlorhexidine (Allwood, 1973). The antagonistic and synergistic effects of non-ionic surfactants on the antibacterial activity of cationic surface-active agents have been well documented by Schmolka (1973). Below the critical micelle concentration (CMC) of the non-ionic agent, it is believed that potentiation occurs by an effect of this agent on the surface layers of the bacterial cell, resulting in an increased cellular permeability to the antimicrobial compound; above the CMC of the non-ionic agent, the germicide is distributed between the aqueous and micellar phases, or complexes with the non-ionic surfactant. However, it is only the concentration of germicide in the aqueous phase that is available for attacking microorganisms.

Because of their inactivation of various types of antimicrobial preservatives, non-ionic surfactants are frequently employed as neutralizing agents (Russell *et al.*, 1979; Russell, 1981) and this aspect is considered in more detail in Section 4.1.

Other surface-active agents that influence the activity of antimicrobial compounds include the soaps. Soap is employed as a solubilizing agent, whereby 'solutions' of phenols with a low aqueous solubility may be prepared. Several phenols have a low aqueous solubility; however, bactericidal activity depends on the proportion of soap to phenol. A considerable amount of research has been carried out on the effect of the anionic agent, potassium laurate, on the bactericidal potency of benzylchlorphenol (Cook, 1960). Below the CMC of the soap, there is only low solubility of the phenol; at the CMC, solubility increases rapidly. There is an initial rapid increase in bactericidal activity until just beyond the CMC. As the soap concentration increases, the solubility of the phenol increases until a second critical concentration is reached and then remains constant. The bactericidal activity decreases until this second critical point is reached and subsequently increases. Several interpretations of these findings are possible and have been put forward by various authors. However, there are three important points that must be considered in any final analysis.

1 Low soap concentrations modify the bacterial surface, whose permeability is thereby modified with a resultant increased entry of the phenol.
2 High soap concentrations are themselves bactericidal.
3 It is the concentration of benzylchlorphenol in the aqueous (non-micellar) phase that is responsible for the bactericidal effect.

It is generally agreed that in concentrated solutions of Lysol (solution of cresol with soap) the cresol is solubilized within the micelles and that dilution below the CMC releases the cresol to produced a highly active solution. Further information has been provided in Chapter 2.

3.6.3 *Partitioning between oil and water*

A problem encountered in the formulation of pharmaceutical and cosmetic creams is that, whereas the preservatives employed may have a good antimicrobial activity in aqueous conditions, their biological activity may be decreased considerably when an oil is present. The reason for this is that the preservative is partitioned between the oil and aqueous phases of the cream; since microorganisms may live and multiply in the aqueous phase, it is necessary that an adequate preservative concentration should be maintained in this phase.

Bean and his co-workers (see Bean, 1972) have derived the following equation whereby the concentration of preservative in the aqueous phase may be obtained:

$$C_w = C\,(\Psi + 1) \,/\, (K_w^o\,\Psi + 1) \qquad (3.11)$$

In this equation, C_w represents the concentration of preservative in the aqueous phase, C the total preservative concentration and Ψ the oil/water ratio. The partition coefficient, K_w^o, may vary widely for a single preservative, depending on the type of oil used. If K_w^o is high, then an adequate aqueous phase concentration of preservative can be achieved only by means of an excessive total concentration.

Other significant contributions in this field have been made by Mitchell & Kazmi (1975) Kazmi & Mitchell (1978a,b) and Parker (1978), and these are considered in greater detail in Chapter 16.

It does not necessarily follow that the total

amount of preservative in the aqueous phase is available for attacking microorganisms, because the nature of the emulgent must be taken into account (Section 3.6.2). Likewise, the pH of the cream must be considered, since pH may affect the partition coefficient, may cause dissociation of the preservative molecule or may, in its own right, inhibit growth.

3.6.4 *Partitioning between rubber and water*

Two important types of sterile pharmaceutical products are injections and eye-drops. Multiple-dose formulations are prepared with rubber closures for the former and with silicone rubber closures for the latter. Such formulations require the presence of suitable antimicrobial agents, which act as preservatives and (in some instances in Britain) as an aid to the sterilization process. A major problem, however, is the partitioning of the antimicrobial agent that occurs between the rubber closure and the aqueous product (Wiener, 1955; Wing, 1955, 1956a,b). The distribution between rubber and water for phenol is 25 : 75; for chlorocresol 85 : 15; chlorbutanol 80–90 : 10–20; phenylmercuric nitrate 95 : 5.

This problem and the means of, at least partially, overcoming it are described in greater detail by Allwood (1978).

3.6.5 *Metal ions*

The activity of antimicrobial agents may be reduced or enhanced or remain unchanged in the presence of cations. Mn^{2+} and Zn^{2+} ions reduce and enhance, respectively, the antipseudomonal activity of salicylaldehyde, whereas Ca^{2+} and Mg^{2+} have no effect. The antistaphylococcal potency of anionic surfactants is increased in the presence of low concentrations of divalent cations, whereas the bactericidal activity of long-chain fatty acids is diminished greatly in the presence of Mg^{2+}, Ca^{2+} or Ba^{2+} ions (Galbraith & Miller, 1973).

The antibacterial activity of many antibacterial compounds is potentiated against Gram-negative bacteria when EDTA is present (Russell, 1971a; Wilkinson, 1975; Hart, 1984), and one disinfectant/antiseptic product incorporated chloroxylenol and EDTA in a suitable formulation. The antibacterial activity of this product against *Ps. aeruginosa* is reduced in the presence of Mg^{2+} or Ca^{2+} ions (Dankert & Schut, 1976) or of artificial hard water, prepared to the specifications of the World Health Organization, at various pH levels (Dankert & Schut, 1976; Russell & Furr, 1977). Obviously, hard water should be widely employed in microbicidal tests on disinfectants and antiseptics.

3.7 Humidity

Ideally, r.h. should be considered from two points of view, namely the effect of prehumidification of the cells, and the effect of humidity during treatment. Prehumidification was discussed earlier (Section 2.3.1) and thus only humidity during treatment will be dealt with here, since the subject is considered in depth later (Chapter 21).

Relative humidity has a profound influence on the activity of gaseous disinfectants, such as ethylene oxide, β-propiolactone and formaldehyde (Anon., 1958; Hoffman, 1971; Russell, 1976, 1982, 1990b). With bacterial spores dried on cotton patches as test pieces, ethylene oxide is most active at r.h. of 28–32%, β-propiolactone at r.h. above 70% and formaldehyde at about 60%. This is, in fact, an oversimplification of the effect of r.h., which is the single most important factor influencing the activity of vapour-phase disinfectants (Chapter 21).

3.8 Type of organism

Different organisms show varying responses to biocides. The reasons are not always clear but progress continues to be made (Russell, 1995). In this section, the effects of biocides on bacterial cells and spores, moulds and yeasts, viruses and prions will be examined. In addition, because of the current interest in genetically engineered microorganisms as potential biopesticides and frost-protection agents in agriculture, the effects of biocides on such organisms will also be considered briefly. Information on the efficacy of biocides against rickettsiae, *Chlamydia* and *Mycoplasma* is open lacking, although Quinin (1987) has provided some preliminary data. Protozoa are described in detail elsewhere in the book (Chapter 8A, B).

3.8.1 *Gram-positive bacteria*

This subsection deals with Gram-positive bacteria other than mycobacteria and bacterial spores, which are considered in Sections 3.8.2 and 3.8.4, respectively. As well as being important pathogens, Gram-positive bacteria may also be associated with spoilage of pharmaceutical and cosmetic products. Generally, however, they are more sensitive to biocides than are Gram-negative bacteria. Probably the main reason for this difference in sensitivity resides in the relative composition of the cell envelope. In general terms, the cell wall of Gram-positive bacteria is composed basically of peptidoglycan, which forms a thick, fibrous layer. Interspersed with this basal structure may be other molecules, such as teichoic and teichuronic acids (Rogers *et al.*, 1978) and lipids, although the latter usually occur to a much smaller extent than in the wall of Gram-negative bacteria. Many antibacterial agents (see Chapter 9) must penetrate the outer and cytoplasmic membranes to reach their site of action. It is unlikely that the wall of Gram-positive bacteria presents a barrier to entry of antibacterial substances as does the lipid-rich envelope of Gram-negative organisms.

The effects of various disinfectants, antiseptics and preservatives on Gram-positive bacteria have been well documented (Baird-Parker & Holbrook, 1971). Cocci are readily killed by halogens, but staphylococci are generally more resistant than streptococci to alcohols and glycols; staphylococci tend to be less susceptible than other non-sporing bacteria to ethylene oxide. Cocci are generally sensitive to phenols, especially the bisphenols. Gram-positive bacteria are considerably more sensitive than Gram-negative bacteria to quaternary ammonium compounds and salicylanilides (Hamilton, 1971). Plasmid-encoded resistance of some *S. aureus* strains to mercuric chloride and to organomercury compounds has been well documented (Lyon & Skurray, 1987; Silver & Misca, 1988; Silver *et al.*, 1989). The susceptibility of enterococci, in particular antibiotic-resistant strains, to biocides has not been widely studied. There is some evidence to show that vancomycin- and gentamicin-resistant *Enterococcus faecalis* and *Enterococcus faecium* are susceptible to chlorhexidine and Alquarashi *et al.* (1996).

A particular problem might be found with MRSA strains, which, in addition to being antibiotic-resistant, may also be less sensitive than methicillin-sensitive (MSSA) strains to some biocides. Antibiotic-resistant cocci are considered more fully in Chapter 10F.

Although resistance to antibiotics, notably the β-lactam group, is frequently associated with the ability of the organism to destroy the drug, the development of resistance to a biocide, i.e. during 'training' of an organism by repeated exposure to gradually increasing concentrations of that agent, is not necessarily associated with any increased destruction of the compound. Chaplin (1951) was the first to associate this type of resistance with the increased lipid content found in Gram-negative bacteria, and it thus seems likely that this extra lipid acts as an additional barrier to the entry of an antibacterial compound. Staphylococcal walls normally have a low wall-lipid content; however, an increase in this wall lipid leads to an enhanced resistance of staphylococci (or of vegetative cells of *B. subtilis*) to phenols and to other agents (Hugo & Franklin, 1968; Hugo & Davidson, 1973). Conversely, a decrease in the lipid content of walls of staphylococci renders the cells more sensitive to antibacterial agents (Hugo & Davidson, 1973). Vaczi (1973) provides an excellent account of the role of lipid in bacterial resistance.

3.8.2 *Mycobacteria*

For convenience, mycobacteria are considered separately from other Gram-positive bacteria.

Croshaw (1971) reviewed the mycobactericidal activity of chemical disinfectants. At that time, however, reliable information was still somewhat lacking, and it is only comparatively recently that it has been possible to describe accurately the response of mycobacteria to biocides (Russell, 1996). The sensitivity of such acid-fast bacteria is considered to be intermediate between that of vegetative bacteria and that of bacterial spores (Spaulding *et al.*, 1977; Favero & Bond, 1991, 1993). Different types of mycobacteria vary in their responses to biocides, however, and *Mycobacterium chelonae* (*M. chelonci*) is a particularly resistant species (Russell, 1996).

Resistance of mycobacteria to many disinfectants is undoubtedly linked to the composition of the cell walls of these organisms.

Mycobacteria possess an unusually high wall-lipid content, and the resultant hydrophobic nature of the wall may be responsible, at least in part, for their high resistance, which is more or less proportional to the content of waxy material (Croshaw, 1971). Quaternary ammonium compounds and dyes are inhibitory to *Mycobacterium tuberculosis* but are not tuberculocidal, and this organism is also resistant to chlorhexidine, acids and alkalis but moderately sensitive to ampholytic surface-active agents, including the 'Tego' compounds. Of the phenols, *o*-phenylphenol is particularly effective, but the bisphenols are inactive. Alcohols, formaldehyde (liquid and vapour forms), formaldehyde-alcohol, iodine-alcohol and ethylene oxide are tuberculocidal agents (Newman *et al*., 1955; Anon., 1958; Spaulding, 1977; Rubin, 1983). Glutaraldehyde is generally considered to be a good mycobactericidal agent (see review by Russell & Hopwood, 1976), although slow tuberculocidal action has also been observed (Bergan & Lystad, 1971a,b). F.M. Collins (1986) and J. Collins (1986) have now confirmed that glutaraldehyde is mycobactericidal.

Susceptibility and resistance to biocides, together with the possible underlying mechanisms, are discussed in Chapter 10D; see also Rubin (1991).

3.8.3 Gram-negative bacteria

Gram-negative bacteria, especially *E. coli*, *Klebsiella* spp., *Proteus* spp., *Ps. aeruginosa* and *Serratia marcescens* are common hospital pathogens. *Pseudomonas aeruginosa*, in particular, has long been considered an extremely troublesome organism, with above-average resistance to many antibiotics and other antibacterial agents (Brown, 1975). Russell *et al.* (1986) have examined the responses of hospital isolates of Gram-negative bacteria to various biocides.

The control of legionellae, especially in recirculating water systems, may present a problem (Report, 1989; see also Chapter 10E). *Acinetobacter* spp. are becoming of increasing significance (Bergogne-Bérézin, 1995) and more efficient control measures may be needed to contain outbreaks. More information about the biocide susceptibility of epidemic, multiple-antibiotic-resistant strains of *Stenotrophomonas* (formerly *Pseudomonas*, *Xanthomonas*) *maltophilia* and *Burkholderia* (formerly *Pseudomonas*) *cepacia* is also needed (Spencer, 1995).

Gram-negative are often less sensitive than Gram-positive bacteria to biocides (Baird-Parker & Holbrook, 1971). This may reflect the considerable differences in the composition, notably the lipid content, of the cell envelopes of the two types of organisms (Russell & Chopra, 1996).

Resistance of Gram-negative bacteria to many antibiotics is linked to R-plasmid-mediated enzymatic inactivation or to intrinsic resistance. Likewise, R^+ strains of Gram-negative bacteria may destroy mercury compounds (Smith, 1967; Summers & Silver, 1972; Foster, 1983; Silver & Misra, 1988). Some R-plasmids may be associated with sensitivity and resistance to sodium deoxycholate (Hesslewood & Smith, 1974). The role of plasmids in bacterial resistance to biocides has been described by Russell, (1985, 1996) and Russell & Chopra (1996); see also Chapter 10B.

3.8.4 Bacterial spores

Comprehensive reviews of the resistance of bacterial spores to chemical and physical agents have been published (Russell, 1971b, 1982, 1983, 1990b, 1991b; Bloomfield & Arthur, 1994; Setlow, 1994; Russell & Russell, 1995; Russell & Chopra, 1996). Many antibacterial compounds are not sporicidal but are sporistatic, inhibiting germination or outgrowth, e.g. phenols, QACs, mercury compounds, biguanides, alcohols, parabens. For example, depending on its concentration, phenol will retard or inhibit germination (Parker, 1969; Russell *et al.*, 1985), whereas QACs allow germination to proceed but inhibit outgrowth (Russell *et al.*, 1985). Non-sporicidal concentrations of ethylene oxide also inhibit outgrowth (Marletta & Stumbo, 1970).

Bacterial spores are considerably more resistant than vegetative cells. The stages during sporulation at which resistance develops air gradually being elucidated (Knott & Russell, 1995; Knott *et al.*, 1995).

Examples of sporicides include glutaraldehyde, formaldehyde, halogens, ethylene oxide and acid alcohol (Anon., 1958; Sykes, 1970; Hoffman, 1971; Russell, 1971b; Trueman, 1971; Kelsey *et al.*, 1974; Russell & Hopwood, 1976).

The resistance to biocides of bacterial spores is considered in more detail in Chapter 10C.

3.8.5 *Moulds and yeasts*

Several species of moulds and yeasts are pathogenic. Others are important spoilage organisms of foods and pharmaceutical and cosmetic products. Thus, a brief discussion of their sensitivity and resistance will be made.

Many compounds show both antibacterial and antifungal activity. These include phenolics (notably the halogenated members and hexachlorophane), QACs (D'Arcy, 1971), oxine, diamidines, organic mercury derivatives (including penotrane) and esters of *p*-hydroxybenzoic acids, the parabens. Sorbic acid shows significant antifungal activity at low pH values, when it occurs in solution mainly in the undissociated form. At higher pH values, it dissociates and activity is lost. Glutaraldehyde possesses significant fungicidal activity.

Comparatively little is known about the mechanisms of fungal inactivation or of fungal resistance, but steady progress is being made (Hiom *et al.*, 1995a,b, 1996; Russell & Furr, 1996).

The antifungal activity of biocides is discussed in detail in Chapter 5.

3.8.6 *Viruses*

Several bactericidal agents possess viricidal properties, although antibacterial activity does not necessarily imply antiviral potency. For a comprehensive treatise of virus disinfection, the excellent review of Grossgebaeur (1970) should be consulted. Mechanisms of antiviral activity of biocides are well discussed by Thurman & Gerba (1988, 1989). Stagg (1982), Springthorpe & Sattar (1990), Sattar *et al.* (1994), Bellamy (1995), van Bueren (1995) and Anderson *et al.* (1997) have considered methods of estimating viricidal activity.

Some antimicrobial agents are much less active in destroying non-lipid-enveloped viruses (e.g. enteroviruses, such as polio, Coxsackie and Echo) than lipid-enveloped ones. On the other hand, the latter are quite sensitive to disinfectants with a lipophilic character. Into this category come certain phenol derivatives, such as *o*-phenylphenol, isopropanol, cationic detergents (although viruses are more resistant to these compounds than are bacteria or fungi), ether and chloroform (Grossgebauer, 1970; Klein & Deforest, 1983). Chlorine disinfectants are considered to be effective in killing all virus types (Dychdala, 1983) and to be useful in preventing the spread of foot-and-mouth disease (Trueman, 1971). Mercury compounds are inactive against viruses.

Formaldehyde, which is often used in the preparation of viral vaccines, may require an extensive period in order to be viricidal (Grossgebauer, 1970) and in the vapour state it has a low power of penetration. β-Propiolactone vapour acts similarly, but the liquid form is strongly viricidal. Ethylene oxide is viricidal when employed in both the liquid and gaseous states (Sykes, 1965).

Glutaraldehyde is a compound with considerable activity against most types of microorganisms (Chapter 2). It is, in addition, a viricidal agent with activity against many types of viruses (Chambon *et al.*, 1992; Russell, 1994).

Viruses that have, in recent years, caused a considerable degree of concern are hepatitis B virus (HBV) and human immunodeficiency virus (HIV). The former is now believed to be less resistant than at first thought, and both it and HIV (Spire *et al.*, 1984) can be readily inactivated by glutaraldehyde and chlorine-releasing agents (Bloomfield *et al.*, 1990; Committee, 1990; see also Russell, 1990b). The responses of various animal viruses to biocides were discussed by Russell & Hugo (1987).

Increasing interest is also being shown about the manner in which viruses are being inactivated, including changes in their morphological structure (Taylor & Butler, 1982). Bacteriophages have an important role to play here, although they should ideally be regarded as models for human and animal viruses (Maillard *et al.*, 1995, 1996a,b).

Viral inactivation is discussed at length in Chapter 6A–D; see also Maillard & Russell (1997).

3.8.7 Prions

Unconventional agents are believed to be highly resistant to many chemical disinfection and physical sterilization processes (Committee, 1986), including ultraviolet and ionizing radiations, high temperatures, glutaraldehyde and chlorine. Sodium hydroxide is, however, considered to be an effective decontaminant (Brown *et al.*, 1984). The subject is discussed in more detail later (Chapter 7).

Little is known at present about the mechanisms of inactivation of or mechanisms of resistance by these unconventional agents by/to biocides.

3.8.8 Protozoa

An increasing amount of information has become available about the sensitivity of protozoa to biocides, with considerable attention paid to the trophozoite and cyst forms of organisms belonging to the genus *Giardia*. An excellent review on the sensitivity of *Giardia* cysts has been published by Jarroll (1988). Additionally, the effects of biocides on the trophozoite and cyst forms of *Acanthamoeba* spp. are becoming clearer (Khunkitti *et al.*, 1997; 1998).

Further information about the biocidal inactivation of protozoa is provided in Chapter 8A, B.

3.8.9 Genetically engineered microorganisms

The potential risks associated with releasing genetically engineered microbes (GEMs) into the environment mean that appropriate containment methods have to be considered (Jackman *et al.*, 1992).

Such general methods include chemical disinfection, physical procedures (e.g. burning), biological agents, such as bacteriophages or protozoa, and suicide plasmids. Of these, chemical and physical methods are the most important.

Blackburn *et al.* (1994) and Weir *et al.* (1994, 1996) have described the use of QACs and hypochlorites in containing and destroying GEMs, not only in the laboratory but also in the environment. The authors emphasized that it was unrealistic to expect chemical agents to control released bacteria on a large scale, but stated that accidental spills into soil at a specific site might require the use of a chemical biocide. Not surprisingly, organisms were more resistant in soil than in broth, and alginate encapsulation increased survival. It was concluded that killing GEMs in soil could prove difficult unless a 'powerful' biocide, such as formaldehyde, was used.

4 Post-treatment factors

Several factors influence the recovery of microorganisms exposed to antimicrobial compounds. These include the composition and pH of the recovery medium, removal of the antimicrobial agent, the temperature and period of incubation and the composition of the diluent used for serial dilution in the carrying out of viable counts. However, there is very little information as to the actual repair of injury suffered by damaged but still-viable microorganisms (in contrast to the increasingly interesting data pertaining to the repair of bacteria damaged by exposure to ionizing or ultraviolet radiation or to heat). This point will be returned to later.

4.1 Neutralization of biocides

To prevent an inhibitory concentration of an antimicrobial agent from being transferred to the recovery medium, it is essential that the activity of the antimicrobial compound be nullified. This may be achieved by means of a neutralizing agent (inactivator, neutralizer, antidote), which overcomes the activity of the inhibitory (antimicrobial) agent. The neutralizer must itself be non-toxic to microorganisms and any product resulting from neutralization must likewise be non-toxic. Examples of suitable neutralizers are provided in Table 3.6.

Biocides that have high dilution coefficients (Section 3.1) rapidly lose their activity on dilution and this may be sufficient to overcome any residual activity, i.e. dilution to a subinhibitory value in the recovery medium. Neutralizing agents such as tweens may, however, provide a suitable alternative (Table 3.6). Neutralizing agents may be included in the first diluent tube (Section 4.2) or recovery medium (Section 4.3) or both.

Table 3.6 Neutralizing agents for some antimicrobial agents.*

Antimicrobial agent	Possible neutralizing agent(s)	Comments
Phenols and cresols	None (dilution) Tweens (polysorbates)	High dilution coefficient (see Table 3.2)
Parabens	None (dilution) Tweens	
Iodine and related compounds	Sodium thiosulphate	Sodium thiosulphate may be inhibitory to some bacteria, e.g. staphylococci
Chlorine and hypochlorites	Nutrient media Sodium thiosulphate	See Kelsey *et al.* (1974) Also, sodium thiosulphate may be toxic to some bacterial species
Glutaraldehyde	Sodium sulphite Glycine Dilution	Sodium sulphite is not recommended because of toxicity Glycine provides optimum neutralization
Quaternary ammonium compounds, chlorhexidine	Lubrol + lecithin Lecithin + tween (Letheen)	Culture media containing neutralizer system can be purchased
Mercury compounds	–SH compounds	Thioglycollate may be toxic to bacteria
Silver compounds	–SH compounds	–SS and other S-containing compounds inactive
Organic arsenicals	–SH compounds	
Bronopol	–SH compounds	

*For further details, see Russell *et al.* (1979), Russell (1981) and Russell and Hugo (1994).
Note that non-ionic surface-active agents may themselves adversely affect microorganisms. A 'universal neutralizing solution' is available, but it is unclear whether it neutralizes all types of biocides.

A third technique is one involving membrane filtration. In this the mixture of disinfectant plus microorganisms is filtered through a membrane filter; this is then washed *in situ*, so that the organisms are retained on the membrane and traces of antimicrobial agent are removed. Transfer of the membrane to an appropriate agar medium enables any surviving cells to produce colonies. This method was originally devised for sterility testing and has since been applied to disinfectant evaluation (Prince *et al.*, 1975).

The microbiological importance of overcoming the activity of various classes of antibiotics and other antimicrobial compounds has been discussed in detail by Russell *et al.* (1979) and Russell (1981).

4.2 Diluent in viable counting procedures

Sterile-glass distilled water, one-quarter-strength Ringer's solution, 0.9% w/v saline, peptone water and nutrient broth have been employed as diluents by various investigators; for their possible toxic effects, see King & Hurst (1963). Some bacteria, e.g. *Ps. aeruginosa* (Brown, 1975) and some strains of *Proteus* spp., are affected by water, and viable counts in which water is the diluent may be lower than when another diluent is employed. It must be remembered that bacteria exposed to a chemical agent may already be in a stressed state (if not already dead) before a viable count of survivors is undertaken. Use of an 'incorrect' diluent could exacerbate this condition and lead to inaccurate conclusions as to the potency of the bactericide.

4.3 Recovery media

The composition of the recovery medium may influence the counts of cells exposed to chemical antimicrobial compounds. Surprisingly, the subject has been comparatively little studied. It is, however, known that nutrient broth containing activated charcoal (Norit) or various cations will reduce both the rate and extent of damage of phenol-treated bacteria (Harris, 1963). Likewise, there is a dearth of information as to the effects of recovery-medium pH on viable counts.

The composition of the recovery medium was of no great significance in determining survivor levels of *B. subtilis* spores treated with iodine preparations, chlorine-releasing agents or glutaraldehyde (Williams & Russell, 1993d). The addition to recovery media of various supplements usually had no beneficial effect on colony counts, except that soluble starch significantly increased survivor counts for iodine-treated spores.

The possible value of varying the composition of the recovery medium when studies of the mechanism of action of a chemical agent are being carried out is demonstrated clearly in Table 3.7, which is based on the studies of Michael & Stumbo (1970). An interesting finding was that of Durant & Higdon (1987), who showed that the numbers of colonies from *Ps. aeruginosa* cells previously treated with bronopol were several-hundredfold higher on recovery media containing catalase than on unsupplemented agar. This was attributed to the presence of sublethally injured bacteria, but the mechanism of this repair has not been elucidated.

4.4 Incubation temperature

Bacteria which survive an inimical treatment may recover better at a temperature below the optimum for undamaged bacteria. Harris (1963) has shown that the optimum temperature for phenol-damaged bacteria is 28°C. This may be analogous to the minimal medium repair (MMR) sometimes found with heat-stressed bacteria (Pierson *et al.*, 1978), although there is no evidence that MMR occurs with bactericide-injured cells.

Chemical-treated spores may require long incubation periods before germination and growth occur (Williams & Russell, 1993a). An optimum incubation temperature of 30–37°C has been found to be necessary for halogen- or glutaraldehyde-treated spores (Williams & Russell, 1993a–d).

An interesting phenomenon has been observed with spores exposed to formaldehyde, where it has been shown that a postheating process enables the organisms to revive (Spicher & Peters, 1981). Such a finding has now cast doubt on what had originally appeared to be a useful sterilization process in LTSF (Wright *et al.*, 1997).

4.5 Repair of injury

Studies on the repair of thermally injured organisms have been made by several investigators, notably Ordal and his colleagues (see Tomlins & Ordal, 1976). One aspect that has yielded much useful information is to determine colony formation of aliquots of heated suspensions of

Table 3.7 Growth of *Salmonella senftenberg* after exposure to ethylene oxide† (after Michael & Stumbo, 1970).*

Cells	Recovery medium	Result
Unexposed	1 TSY broth	Growth
	2 MS broth	Growth (rate less than TSY)
EO-exposed	1 TSY broth	Slight lag, then growth
	2 MS broth	Very long lag
EO-exposed	1 MS broth + guanine	Repair and reproduction
	2 MS broth + GTP	(Repair and reproduction)
	3 MS broth + other supplements†	No repair or reproduction
	4 MS broth + EO-exposed guanine	Repair and reproduction
	5 MS broth + EO-exposed GTP	No repair or reproduction

* The use of MS broth containing various supplements demonstrates the importance of guanine and GTP in repair and reproduction and further shows that GTP, in particular, is a likely cellular target for ethylene oxide action.

† Other supplements tested: amino acids, organic acids, base components of DNA and RNA, vitamins, nucleic-acid sugars.

EO, ethylene oxide; TSY broth, trypticase soy broth + 0.5% yeast extract; MS broth, a minimal salts + glucose liquid medium; GTP, guanosine triphosphate; DNA, deoxyribonucleic acid; RNA, ribonucleic acid.

Staph. aureus on an agar medium and on the same medium containing sodium chloride, to which the thermally injured cells are susceptible; for further information see Busta (1978).

The principles of this method can certainly be adapted to a study of cells stressed after treatment with an antimicrobial compound. Following exposure, the cells are transferred to a suitable liquid medium and incubated; during intervals thereafter, the surviving cells do not increase in numbers, as shown by the constancy of viable counts on 'optimal composition' agar. Counts on agar containing a high concentration of NaCl (or any other appropriate medium to which the stressed cells become sensitive (Corry *et al.*, 1977)) increase until they reach the level attained on the 'optimal composition' agar. At this point, repair of injury is considered to be complete. This method has been adopted by M.C. Allwood and colleagues (personal communication) for studying the repair of chlorhexidine-injured *E. coli* cells, and by Corry *et al.* (1977), who investigated the repair of damage of bacteria following treatment with some antibiotics and other antimicrobial agents. Table 3.7 should also be consulted in this context.

Further information on revival after chemical injury or in general can be obtained by consulting Gilbert (1984) and Andrew & Russell (1984), respectively. An interesting concept of repair would be to consider the sensitivity and revival of the well-defined deoxyribonucleic acid (DNA) repair mutants so widely employed in studies of ultraviolet and ionizing radiation.

Sublethal spore injury may be manifested by an increased susceptibility to various types of stressing agents, i.e. to chemicals that are not inhibitory or lethal towards untreated spores. Repair of injury in damaged spores can then be monitored by a decreased susceptibility to stressing agents. These principles have been utilized by Williams & Russell (1993b–d) in studying the repair processes in *B. subtilis* spores treated with various types of biocides.

5 Bacterial biofilms

The interaction of bacteria with surfaces is initially reversible but eventually irreversible. Such irreversible adhesion is initiated by bacteria binding by means of expolysaccharide glycocalyx polymers (Costerton *et al.*, 1987). The sister cells produced as a result of cell division are then bound within this matrix and eventually there is a continuous biofilm on the colonized surface. Bacteria enclosed in this biofilm exist in a specific microenvironment that differs from cells grown in batch culture under ordinary laboratory conditions.

Bacteria within biofilms are much more resistant to antibacterial agents (both biocides and antibiotics) than are batch-grown cells, e.g. to chlorine (LeChevalier *et al.*, 1988), chlorhexidine (Marrie & Costerton, 1981) and iodine (Pyle & McFeters, 1990). Interestingly, hydrogen peroxide, at concentrations well below those required for total disinfection, has been found to remove biofilms (Christensen *et al.*, 1990).

There are several possible reasons for the reduced sensitivity of sessile bacteria within a biofilm, compared with planktonic cells in a laboratory culture.

1 Exclusion or reduced access of a biocide to an underlying cell, which depends upon the nature of the biocide, the binding capacity of the glycocalyx for that biocide and the rate of growth of a microcolony relative to the diffusion rate of the biocide.

2 Modulation of the microenvironment, associated with nutrient limitation and bacterial growth rate.

3 Increased production of degradative enzymes by attached cells.

Highly reactive chemicals, such as iodine, iodine-releasing agents and isothiazolones, react chemically with the glycocalyx, so that their antibacterial efficacy is reduced. In contrast, the dialdehyde glutaraldehyde not only penetrates a biofilm but also kills cells protected by that biofilm and accelerates the natural detachment of organisms, termed an enhanced erosion-rate mechanism.

Further comprehensive details of biofilms are provided by Brown & Gilbert (1993) and Poxton (1993). Russell & Chopra (1996) have provided information about the role of biofilms in conferring intrinsic resistance in various industrial, clinical and food microbiology contexts.

Biofilms associated with legionellae are discussed in Chapter 10E and in a wider context in Chapter 10A.

6 Conclusions

It is important to have a sound knowledge of those factors that may influence the antimicrobial activity of chemical agents. Different chemicals are influenced to varying degrees by concentration, pH, temperature and the presence of extraneous matter. The effects of concentration, in particular, are often poorly understood (Hugo & Denyer, 1987), but failure to appreciate that some compounds lose activity on dilution much more than others could have serious repercussions. The type, nature and condition of a microorganism and its previous history and post-treatment handling can all influence the response to a biocidal agent.

Several of the factors outlined here will be further emphasized in subsequent chapters.

7 References

Adelberg, E.A., Mandel, M. & Chen, G.C.C. (1965) Optimal conditions for mutagenesis by N-methyl-N′-N-nitrosoguanidine in *Escherichia coli*. *Biochemical and Biophysical Research Communications*, **18**, 788–795.

Allwood, M.C. (1973) Inhibition of *Staphylococcus aureus* by combinations of non-ionic surface-active agents and anti-bacterial substances. *Microbios*, 7, 209–214.

Allwood, M.C. (1978) Antimicrobial agents in single- and multi-dose injections. *Journal of Applied Bacteriology*, **44**, Svii–Sxvii.

Alqurashi, A.M., Day, M.J. & Russell, A.D. (1996) Susceptibility of some strains of enterococci and staphylococci to antibiotics and biocides. *Journal of Antimicrobial Chemotherapy*, **38**, 745.

Anderson, D.A., Grgacic, E.V.L., Luscombe, C.A., Gu, X. & Dixon, R. (1997) Quantification of infectious duck hepatitis B virus by radioimmunofocus assay. *Journal of Medical Virology*, **52**, 354–361.

Andrew, M.H.E. & Russell, A.D. (eds) (1984) *The Revival of Injured Microbes*. Society for Applied Bacteriology Symposium Series No. 12. London: Academic Press.

Anon. (1958) Disinfection of fabrics with gaseous formaldehyde. Committee on Formaldehyde Disinfection. *Journal of Hygiene, Cambridge*, **56**, 488–515.

AOAC (1998) *Official Methods of Analysis of AOAC International*, 16th edn, 4th revision. Gaithersburg, USA: AOAC International.

Ayres, H.M., Furr, J.R. & Russell, A.D. (1993) A rapid method of evaluating permeabilizing activity against *Pseudomonas aeruginosa*. *Letters in Applied Microbiology*, **17**, 149–151.

Baird-Parker, A.C. & Holbrook, R. (1971) The inhibition and destruction of cocci. In *Inhibition and Destruction of the Microbial Cell* (ed. Hugo, W.B.), pp. 369–397. London: Academic Press.

Bean, H.S. (1967) Types and characteristics of disinfectants. *Journal of Applied Bacteriology*, **30**, 6–16.

Bean, H.S. (1972) Preservatives for pharmaceuticals. *Journal of the Society of Cosmetic Chemists*, **23**, 703–720.

Beeby, M.M. & Whitehouse, C.E. (1965) A bacterial spore test piece for the control of ethylene oxide sterilization. *Journal of Applied Bacteriology*, **28**, 349–360.

Bell, N.D.S. & Parker, M.S. (1975) The effect of sporulation temperature on the resistance of *Bacillus subtilis* to a chemical inhibitor. *Journal of Applied Bacteriology*, **38**, 295–299.

Bellamy, K. (1995) A review of the test methods used to establish virucidal activity. *Journal of Hospital Infection*, **30** (Suppl.), 389–396.

Bennett, E.O. (1959) Factors affecting the antimicrobial activity of phenols. *Advances in Applied Microbiology*, **1**, 123–140.

Bergan, T, & Lystad, A. (1971a) Disinfectant evaluation by a capacity use-dilution test. *Journal of Applied Bacteriology*, **34**, 741–750.

Bergan, T. & Lystad, A. (1971b) Antitubercular action of disinfectants. *Journal of Applied Bacteriology*, **34**, 751–756.

Bergogne-Bérézin, E. (1995) The increasing significance of outbreaks of *Acinetobacter* spp.: the need for control and new agents. *Journal of Hospital Infection*, **30** (Suppl.), 441–452.

Beveridge, E.G. (1998) Microbial spoilage and preservation of pharmaceutical products. In *Pharmaceutical Microbiology*, 6th edn, (eds Hugo, W.B. & Russell, A.D.), pp. 355–373. Oxford: Blackwell Scientific Publications.

Blackburn, N.T., Seech, A.G. & Trevors, J.T. (1994) Survival and transport of *lac–lux* marked *Pseudomonas fluorescens* strain in uncontaminated and chemically contaminated soils. *Systematic and Applied Microbiology*, **17**, 574–580.

Bloomfield, S.F. & Arthur, M. (1994) Mechanisms of inactivation and resistance of spores to chemical biocides. *Journal of Applied Bacteriology, Symposium Supplement*, **76**, 91S–104S.

Bloomfield, S.F., Smith-Burchnell, C.A. & Dalgleish, A.G. (1990) Evaluation of hypochlorite-releasing disinfectants against the human immunodeficiency virus. *Journal of Hospital Infection*, **15**, 273–278.

Borick, P.M. (1968) Chemical sterilizers (Chemosterilizers). *Advances in Applied Microbiology*, **10**, 291–312.

Boucher, R.M.G. (1975) On biocidal mechanisms in the aldehyde series. *Canadian Journal of Pharmaceutical Sciences*, **10**, 1–7.

British Pharmacopoeia. (1998) London: Pharmaceutical Press.

Brown, M.R.W. (1975) The role of the cell envelope in resistance. In *Resistance of Pseudomonas aeruginosa* (ed. Brown, M.R.W.), pp. 71–107. London: John Wiley & Sons.

Brown, M.R.W. & Gilbert, P. (1993) Sensitivity of biofilms to antimicrobial agents. *Journal of Applied Bacteriology, Symposium Supplement*, **74**, 87S–97S.

Brown, M.R.W. & Melling, J. (1969) Loss of sensitivity to EDTA by *Pseudomonas aeruginosa* grown under conditions of Mg-limitation. *Journal of General Microbiology*, **54**, 439–444.

Brown, M.R.W. & Richards, R.M.E. (1964) Effect of polysorbate (Tween) 80 on the resistance of *Pseudomonas aeruginosa* to chemical inactivation. *Journal of Pharmacy and Pharmacology*, **16** (Suppl.) 51T-55T.

Brown, M.R.W. & Winsley, B.E. (1969) Effect of polysorbate 80 on cell leakage and viability of *Pseudomonas aeruginosa* exposed to rapid changes of pH, temperature and toxicity. *Journal of General Microbiology*, **56**, 99–107.

Brown, P., Rohwer, R.G. & Gajdusek, D.C. (1984) Sodium hydroxide decontamination of Creutzfeldt-Jakob disease virus. *New England Journal of Medicine*, **310**, 727.

Busta, F.F. (1978) Introduction to injury and repair of microbial cells. *Advances in Applied Microbiology*, **20**, 185–201.

Chambon, M., Bailly, J.-L. and Peigue-Lafeuille, H. (1992) Activity of glutaraldehyde at low concentrations against capsid proteins of poliovirus type 1 and echovirus type 25. *Applied and Environmental Microbiology*, **58**, 3517–3521.

Chaplin, C.E. (1951) Observations on quaternary ammonium disinfectants. *Canadian Journal of Botany*, **29**, 373–382.

Chapman, D.G. & Russell, A.D. (1978) Pretreatment with colistin and *Proteus* sensitivity to other agents. *Journal of Antibiotics*, **31**, 124–130.

Christensen, B.E., Trønnes, H.N., Vollan, K., Smidsrød, O. & Bakke, R. (1990) Biofilm removal by low concentrations of hydrogen peroxide. *Biofouling*, **2**, 165–175.

Clegg, L.F.L. (1967) Disinfectants in the dairy industry. *Journal of Applied Bacteriology*, **30**, 117–140.

Coates, D. (1977) Kelsey–Sykes capacity test: origin, evolution and current status. *Pharmaceutical Journal*, **219**, 402–403.

Coates, D. & Death, J.E. (1978) Sporicidal activity of mixtures of alcohol and hypochlorite. *Journal of Clinical Pathology*, **31**, 148–152.

Collins, F.M. (1986) Kinetics of the tuberculocidal response by alkaline glutaraldehyde in solution and on an inert surfce. *Journal of Applied Bacteriology*, **61**, 87–93.

Collins, J. (1986) The use of glutaraldehyde in laboratory discard jars. *Letters in Applied Microbiology*, **2**, 103–105.

Committee (1986) Committee on Health Care Issues, American Neurological Association. Precautions in handling tissues, fluids and other contaminated materials from patients with documented or suspected Creutzfeldt–Jakob disease. *Annals of Neurology*, **19**, 75–77.

Committee (1990) Advisory Committee on Dangerous Pathogens. *HIV—the Causative Agent of AIDS and Related Conditions.*

Cook, A.M. (1960) Phenolic disinfectants. *Journal of Pharmacy & Pharmacology*, **12**, 19T–28T.

Corry, J.E.L., Van Doornf, H. & Mossel, D.A.A. (1977) Recovery and revival of microbial cells, especially those from environments containing antibiotics. In *Antibiotics and Antibiosis in Agriculture* (ed. Woodbine, M.), pp. 174–196. London: Butterworth.

Costerton, J.W., Cheng, K.-J., Geesey, G.G. *et al.* (1987) Bacterial biofilms in nature and disease. *Annual Review of Microbiology*, **41**, 435–464.

Cowen, R.A. (1974) Relative merits of 'in use' and laboratory methods for the evaluation of antimicrobial products. *Journal of the Society of Cosmetic Chemists*, **25**, 307–323.

Cowen, R.A. (1978) Kelsey–Sykes capacity test: a critical review. *Pharmaceutical Journal*, **220**, 202–204.

Croshaw, B. (1971) The destruction of mycobacteria. In *Inhibition and Destruction of the Microbial Cell* (ed. Hugo, W.B.), pp. 419–449. London: Academic Press.

Croshaw, B. (1977) Preservatives for cosmetics and toiletries. *Journal of the Society of Cosmetic Chemists*, **28**, 3–16.

Dankert, J. & Schut, I.K. (1976) The antibacterial activity of chloroxylenol in combination with ethylenediamine tetra-acetic acid. *Journal of Hygiene, Cambridge*, **76**, 11–22.

D'Arcy, P.F. (1971) Inhibition and destruction of moulds and yeasts. In *Inhibition and Destruction of the Microbial Cell* (ed. Hugo, W.B.), pp. 613–686. London: Academic Press.

Davis, J.G. (1972a) Fundamentals of microbiology in relation to cleansing in the cosmetic industry. *Journal of the Society of Cosmetic Chemists*, **23**, 45–71.

Davis, J.G. (1972b) Problems of hygiene in the dairy industry, Parts 1 and 2. *Dairy Industries*, **37** (4), 212–215; (5), 251–256.

Dean, A.C.R., Ellwood, D.C., Melling, J. & Robinson, A. (1976) The action of antibacterial agents on bacteria grown in continuous culture. In *Continuous Culture—Applications and New Techniques* (eds

Dean, A.C.R., Ellwood, D.C., Evans, C.G.T. & Melling, J.), pp. 251–261. London: Ellis Horwood.

Death, J.E. & Coates, D. (1979) Effect of pH on sporicidal and microbicidal activity of buffered mixtures of alcohol and sodium hypochlorite. *Journal of Clinical Pathology*, **32**, 148–153.

de Siervo, A.J. (1969) Alterations in the phospholipid composition of *Escherichia coli* during growth at different temperatures. *Journal of Bacteriology*, **100**, 1342–1349.

Durant, C. & Higdon, P. (1987) Preservation of cosmetic and toiletry products. In *Preservatives in the Food, Pharmaceutical and Environmental Industries* (eds Board, R.G., Allwood, M.C. & Banks, J.G.), Society for Applied Bacteriology Technical Series No. 22, pp. 231–253. Oxford: Blackwell Scientific Publications.

Dychdala, G.R. (1983) Chlorine and chlorine compounds. In *Disinfection, Sterilization and Preservation* (ed. Block, S.S.), 3rd edn, pp. 157–182. Philadelphia: Lea & Febiger.

Eagon, R.G., Stinnett, J.D. & Gilleland, H.E. (1975) Ultrastructure of *Pseudomonas aeruginosa* as related to resistance. In *Resistance of* Pseudomonas aeruginosa (ed. Brown, M.R.W.), pp. 109–143. London: John Wiley & Sons.

Eklund, T. (1980) Inhibition of growth and uptake processes in bacteria by some chemical food preservatives. *Journal of Applied Bacteriology*, **48**, 423–432.

Eklund, T. (1983) The antimicrobial effect of dissociated and undissociated sorbic acid at different pH levels. *Journal of Applied Bacteriology*, **54**, 383–389.

Eklund, T. (1985a) The effect of sorbic acid and esters of *p*-hydroxybenzoic acid on the protonmotive force in *Escherichia coli* membrane vesicles. *Journal of General Microbiology*, **131**, 73–76.

Eklund, T. (1985b) Inhibition of microbial growth at different pH levels by benzoic and propionic acids and esters of *p*-hydroxybenzoic acid. *International Journal of Food Microbiology*, **2**, 159–167.

El-Falaha, B.M.A., Russell, A.D. & Furr, J.R. (1983) Sensitivities of wild-type and envelope-defective strains of *Escherichia coli* and *Pseudomonas aeruginosa* to antibacterial agents. *Microbios*, **38**, 99–105.

Ennis, H.L. & Bloomstein, M.I. (1974) Antibiotic-sensitive mutants of *Escherichia coli* possess altered outer membranes. *Annals of the New York Academy of Sciences*, **235**, 593–600.

Ernst, R.R. (1974) Ethylene oxide sterilisation kinetics. In *Biotechnology and Bioengineering Symposium No. 4*, pp. 858–878.

Farewell, J.A. & Brown, M.R.W. (1971) The influence of inoculum history on the response of micro-organisms to inhibitory and destructive agents. In *Inhibition and Destruction of the Microbial Cell* (ed. Hugo, W.B.), pp. 703–752. London: Academic Press.

Favero, M.S. Bond, W.W. (1991) Sterilization, disinfection and antisepsis in the hospital. In *Manual of Clinical Microbiology*, 5th edn (eds Balows, A., Hausler, W.J., Jr, Herrman, K.I., Isenber, H.D. and Shadomy, H.J.), pp. 183–200. Washington, DC: American Society for Microbiology.

Favero, M.S. & Bond, W.W. (1993) The use of liquid chemical germicides. In *Sterilization Technology: A Practical Guide for Manufacters* (eds Morrissey, R.F. & Phillips, G.B.), pp. 309–334. New York: Van Nostrand Reinhold.

Foster, T.J. (1983) Plasmid-determined resistance to antimicrobial drugs and toxic metal ions in bacteria. *Microbiological Reviews*, **47**, 361–409.

Furr, J.R. & Russell, A.D. (1972) Uptake of esters of *p*-hydroxybenzoic acid by *Serratia marcescens* and by fattened and non-fattened cells of *Bacillus subtilis*. *Microbios*, **5**, 237–246.

Galbraith, H. & Miller, T.B. (1973) Effect of metal cations and pH on the antibacterial activity and uptake of long chain fatty acids. *Journal of Applied Bacteriology*, **36**, 635–646.

Gilbert, G.L., Gambill, D.M., Spiner, D.R., Hoffman, R.K. & Phillips, C.R. (1964) Effect of moisture on ethylene oxide sterilization. *Applied Microbiology*, **12**, 496–503.

Gilbert, P. (1984) The revival of micro-organisms sublethally injured by chemical inhibitors. In *The Revival of Injured Microbes* (eds Andrew, M.H.E. & Russell, A.D.), Society for Applied Bacteriology Symposium Series No. 12, pp. 175–197. London: Academic Press.

Gilbert, P. & Wright, N. (1987) Non-plasmidic resistance towards preservatives of pharmaceutical products. In *Preservatives in the Food, Pharmaceutical and Environmental Industries* (eds Board, R.G., Allwood, M.C. & Banks, J.G.), Society for Applied Bacteriology Technical Series No. 22, pp. 255–279. Oxford: Blackwell Scientific Publications.

Goldenberg, N. & Relf, C.J. (1967) Use of disinfectants in the food industry. *Journal of Applied Bacteriology*, **30**, 141–147.

Gorman, S.P. & Scott, E.M. (1977) Preparation and stability of mureinoplasts of *Escherichia coli*. *Microbios*, **18**, 123–130.

Gorman, S.P., Scott, E.M. & Russell, A.D. (1980) Antimicrobial activity, uses and mechanism of action of glutaraldehyde. *Journal of Applied Bacteriology*, **48**, 161–190.

Grossgebauer, K. (1970) Virus disinfection. In *Disinfection* (ed. Benarde, M.A.), pp. 103–148. New York: Marcel Dekker.

Hamilton, W.A. (1971) Membrane-active antibacterial compounds. In *Inhibition and Destruction of the Microbial Cell* (ed. Hugo, W.B.), pp. 77–93. London: Academic Press.

Harris, N.D. (1963) The influence of recovery medium

and incubation temperature on the survival of damaged bacteria. *Journal of Applied Bacteriology*, **26**, 387–397.

Hart, J.R. (1984) Chelating agents as preservative potentiators. In *Cosmetic and Drug Preservation: Principles and Practice* (ed. Kabara, J.J.), pp. 323–337. New York: Marcel Dekker.

Hesslewood, S.R. & Smith, J.T. (1974) Envelope alterations produced by R-factors in *Proteus mirabilis*. *Journal of General Microbiology*, **85**, 146–152.

Hiom, S.J., Furr, J.R. & Russell, A.D. (1995a) Uptake of ^{14}C-chlorhexidine gluconate by *Saccharomyces cerevisiae*, *Candida albicans* and *Candida glabrata*. *Letters in Applied Microbiology*, **21**, 20–22.

Hiom, S.J., Hann, A.C., Furr, J.R. & Russell, A.D. (1995b) X-ray microanalysis of chlorhexidine-treated cells of *Saccharomyces cerevisiae*. *Letters in Applied Microbiology*, 353–356.

Hiom, S.J., Furr, J.R., Russell, A.D. & Hann, A.C. (1996) The possible role of yeast cell walls in modifying cellular response to chlorhexidine diacetate. *Cytobios*, **86**, 123–135.

Hodges, N.A., Melling, J. & Parker, S.J. (1980) A comparison of chemically defined and complex media for the production of *Bacillus subtilis* spores having reproducible resistance and germination characteristics. *Journal of Pharmacy and Pharmacology*, **32**, 126–130.

Hoffman, H.P., Geftic, S.G., Gelzer, J., Heyman, H. & Adair, F.W. (1973) Ultrastructural observations associated with the growth of resistant *Pseudomonas aeruginosa* in the presence of benzalkonium chloride. *Journal of Bacteriology*, **113**, 409–416.

Hoffman, R.K. (1971) Toxic gases. In *Inhibition and Destruction of the Microbial Cell* (ed. Hugo, W.B.), pp. 225–258. London: Academic Press.

Hopwood, D.A. (1970) The isolation of mutants. In *Methods of Microbiology* (eds Norris, J.R. & Ribbons, D.W.), Vol. 3A, pp. 363–433. London: Academic Press.

Houtsmuller, U.M.T. & Van Deenen, L.L.M. (1964) Identification of a bacterial phospholipid as an *o*-ornithine ester of phosphatidyl glycerol. *Biochimica et Biophysica Acta*, **70**, 211–213.

Hugo, W.B. (1965) Some aspects of the action of cationic surface-active agents on microbial cells with special reference to their action on enzymes. In *Surface Activity and the Microbial Cell*, SCI Monograph 19, pp. 67–82. London: Society of Chemical Industry.

Hugo, W.B. (1991) The degradation of preservatives by microorganisms. *International Biodeterioration*, **27**, 185–194.

Hugo, W.B. & Davidson, J.R. (1973) Effect of cell lipid depletion in *Staphylococcus aureus* upon its resistance to antimicrobial agents. II. A comparison of the response of normal and lipid depleted cells of *S. aureus* to antibacterial drugs. *Microbios*, **8**, 63–72.

Hugo, W.B. & Denyer, S.P. (1987) The concentration exponent of disinfectants and preservatives (biocides). In *Preservatives in the Food, Pharmaceutical and Environmental Industries* (eds Board, R.G., Allwood, M.C. & Banks, J.G.), Society for Applied Bacteriology Technical Series No. 22, pp. 281–291. Oxford: Blackwell Scientific Publications.

Hugo, W.B. & Ellis, J.D. (1975) Cell composition and drug resistance in *Escherichia coli*. In *Resistance of Microorganisms to Disinfectants* (ed. Kedzia, W.B.), 2nd International Symposium, pp. 43–45. Poznan, Poland: Polish Academy of Sciences.

Hugo, W.B. & Franklin, I. (1968) Cellular lipid and the antistaphylococcal activity of phenols. *Journal of General Microbiology*, **52**, 365–373.

Hukari, R., Helander, I.M. & Vaara, M. (1986) Chain length heterogencity of lipopolysaccharide released from *Salmonella typhimurium* by ethylene-diaminetetraacetic acid or polycations. *Journal of Biological Chemistry*, **154**, 673–676.

Hurwitz, S.J. & McCarthy, T.J. (1985) Dynamics of disinfection of selected preservatives against *Escherichia coli*. *Journal of Pharmaceutical Sciences*, **74**, 892–894.

Jackman, S.C., Lee, H. & Trevors, J.T. (1992) Survival, detection and containment of bacteria. *Microbial Releases*, **1**, 125–154.

Jacobs, S.E. (1960) Some aspects of the dynamics of disinfection. *Journal of Pharmacy and Pharmacology*, **12**, 9T–18T.

Jarroll, E.L. (1988) Effect of disinfectants on *Giardia* cysts. *CRC Critical Review in Environmental Control*, **18**, 1–28.

Joswick, H.L., Corner, T.R., Silvernale, J.N. & Gerhardt, P. (1971) Antimicrobial actions of hexachorophane: release of cytoplasmic materials. *Journal of Bacteriology*, **108**, 492–500.

Kazmi, S.J.A. & Mitchell, A.G. (1978a) Preservation of solubilized and emulsified systems. I. Correlation of mathematically predicted preservative availability with antimicrobial activity. *Journal of Pharmaceutical Sciences*, 7, 1260–1266.

Kazmi, S.J.A. & Mitchell, A.G. (1978b) Preservation of solubilized and emulsified systems. II. Theoretical development of capacity and its role in antimicrobial activity of chlorocresol in cetomacrogol-stabilized systems. *Journal of Pharmaceutical Sciences*, **67**, 1266–1271.

Kelsey, J.C. & Maurer, I.M. (1974) An improved Kelsey–Sykes test for disinfectants. *Pharmaceutical Journal*, **213**, 528–530.

Kelsey, J.C., Mackinnon, I.H. & Maurer, I.M. & (1974) Sporicidal activity of hospital disinfectants. *Journal of Clinical Pathology*, **27**, 632–638.

Kereluk, K., Gammon, R.A. & Lloyd, R.S. (1970) Microbiological aspects of ethylene oxide sterilization. II. Microbial resistance to ethylene oxide. *Applied Microbiology*, **19**, 152–156.

Khunkitti, W., Lloyd, D., Furr, J.R. & Russell, A.D. (1997) Aspects of the mechanisms of action of biguanides on trophozoites and cysts of *Acanthamoeba castellanii. Journal of Applied Microbiology*, **82**, 107–114.

Khunkitti, W., Lloyd, D., Furr, J.R. & Russell, A.D. (1998) *Acanthamoeba castellanii*: growth encystment, excystment and biocide susceptibility. *Journal of Infection*, **36**, 43–48.

King, W.L. & Hurst, A. (1963) A note on the survival of some bacteria in different diluents. *Journal of Applied Bacteriology*, **26**, 504–506.

Klein, M. & Deforest, A. (1983) Principles of viral inactivation. In *Disinfection, Sterilization and Preservation* (ed. Block, S.S.), 3rd edn, pp. 422–434. Philadelphia: Lea & Febiger.

Knott, A.G. & Russell, A.D. (1995) Effects of chlorhexidine gluconate on the development of spores of *Bacillus subtilis. Letters in Applied Microbiology*, **21**, 117–120.

Knott, A.G., Russell, A.D. & Dancer, B.N. (1995) Development of resistance to biocides during sporulation of *Bacillus subtilis. Journal of Applied Bacteriology*, **79**, 492–498.

Knott, A.G., Dancer, B.N., Hann, A.C. & Russell, A.D. (1997) Non-variable sources of pure water and the germination and outgrowth of *Bacillus subtilis* spores. *Journal of Applied Microbiology*, **82**, 267–272.

Kostenbauder, H.B. (1983) Physical factors influencing the activity of antimicrobial agents. In *Disinfection, Sterilization and Preservation* (ed. Block, S.S.), 3rd edn, pp. 811–828. Philadelphia: Lea & Febiger.

LeChevalier, M.W., Cawthorn, C.D. & Lee, R.G. (1988) Inactivation of biofilm bacteria. *Applied and Environmental Microbiology*, **54**, 2492–2499.

Leive, L. (1965) A non-specific increase in permeability in *Escherichia coli* produced by EDTA. *Proceedings of the National Academy of Sciences, USA*, **53**, 745–750.

Lyon, B.R. & Skurray, R.A. (1987) Antimicrobial resistance of *Staphylococcus aureus:* genetic base. *Microbiology Reviews*, **51**, 88–135.

Mackey, B.M. & Seymour, D.A. (1990) The bactericidal effect of isoascorbic acid combined with mild heat. *Journal of Applied Bacteriology*, **67**, 629–638.

Maillard, J.-Y. & Russell, A.D. (1997) Viricidal activity and mechanisms of action of biocides. *Science Progress* (in press).

Maillard, J.-Y., Beggs, T.S., Day, M.J., Hudson, R.A. & Russell, A.D. (1995) Electronmicroscopic investigation of the effect of biocides on *Pseudomonas aeruginosa* PAO bacteriophage F116. *Journal of Medical Microbiology*, **42**, 415–420.

Maillard, J.-Y., Beggs, T.S., Day, M.J., Hudson, R.A. & Russell, A.D. (1996a) Damage to *Pseudomonas aeruginosa* PA101 bacteriophage F116 DNA by biocides. *Journal of Applied Bacteriology*, **80**, 540–544.

Maillard, J.-Y., Beggs, T.S., Day, M.J., Hudson, R.A. & Russell, A.D. (1996b) The effect of biocides on proteins of *Pseudomonas aeruginosa* PAO bacteriophage F116. *Journal of Applied Bacteriology*, **80** 605–610.

Marletta, J. & Stumbo, C.R. (1970) Some effects of ethylene oxide on *Bacillus subtilis. Journal of Food Science*, **35**, 627–631.

Marrie, T.J. & Costerton, J.W. (1981) Prolonged survival of *Serratia marcescens* in chlorhexidine. *Applied and Environmental Microbiology*, **42**, 1093–1102.

Melling, J., Robinson, A. & Ellwood, D.C. (1974) Effect of growth environment in a chemostat on the sensitivity of *Pseudomonas aeruginosa* to polymyxin B sulphate. *Proceedings of the Society for General Microbiology*, **1**, 61.

Michael, G.I. & Stumbo, C.R. (1970) Ethylene oxide sterilization of *Salmonella senftenberg* and *Escherichia coli:* death kinetics and mode of action. *Journal of Food Science*, **35**, 631–634.

Mitchell, A.G. & Kazmi, S.J.A. (1975) Preservative availability in emulsified systems. *Canadian Journal of Pharmaceutical Sciences*, **10**, 67–68.

Moats, W.A., Kinner, J.A. & Maddox, S.E., Jr (1974) Effect of heat on the antimicrobial activity of brilliant green dye. *Applied Microbiology*, **27**, 844–847.

Modha, J., Berrett-Bee, K.J. & Rowbury, R.J. (1989) Enhancement by cationic compounds of the growth inhibitory effect of novobiocin on *Escherichia coli. Letters in Applied Microbiology*, **8**, 219–222.

Munton, T.J. & Russell, A.D. (1972) Effect of glutaraldehyde on the outer layers of *Escherichia coli. Journal of Applied Bacteriology*, **35**, 193–199.

Newman, L.B., Colwell, C.A. & Jameson, A.L. (1955) Decontamination of articles made by tuberculous patients in physical medicine and rehabilitation. *American Review of Tuberculosis and Pulmonary Diseases*, **71**, 272–278.

Op den Kamp, J.A.F., Houtsmueller, U.M.T. & Van Deenen, L.L.M. (1965). On the phospholipids of *Bacillus megaterium. Biochimica et Biophysica Acta*, **106**, 438–441.

Parker, M.S. (1969) Some effects of preservatives on the development of bacterial spores. *Journal of Applied Bacteriology*, **32**, 322–328.

Parker, M.S. (1978) The preservation of cosmetic and pharmaceutical creams. *Journal of Applied Bacteriology*, **44**, Sxxix–Sxxiv.

Patel, N.K. & Kostenbauder, H.B. (1958) Interaction of preservatives with macromolecules. I. *Journal of the American Pharmaceutical Association, Scientific Edition*, **47**, 289–293.

Pierson, M.D., Gomez, R.F. & Martin, S.E. (1978)

The involvement of nucleic acids in bacterial injury. In *Advances in Applied Microbiology* (ed. Perlman, D.), Vol. 23, pp. 263–284. New York: Academic Press.

Power, E.G.M. & Russell, A.D. (1990) Uptake of L-(^{14}C)-alanine by glutaraldehyde-treated and untreated spores of *Bacillus subtilis*. *FEMS Microbiology Letters*, **66**, 271–276.

Poxton, I.R. (1993) Prokaryote envelope diversity. *Journal of Applied Bacteriology, Symposium Supplement*, **74**, 1S-11S.

Prince, J., Deverill, C.E.A. & Ayliffe, G.A.J. (1975) A membrane filter technique for testing disinfectants. *Journal of Clinical Pathology*, **28**, 71–76.

Purves, J. & Parker, M.S. (1973) The influence of sporulation and germination media on the development of spores of *Bacillus megaterium* and their inhibition by chlorocresol. *Journal of Applied Bacteriology*, **36**, 39–45.

Pyle, B.H. & McFeters, G.A. (1990) Iodine susceptibility of pseudomonads grown attached to stainless steel surfaces. *Biofouling*, **2**, 113–120.

Quinn, P.J. (1987) Evaluation of veterinary disinfectants and veterinary processes. In *Disinfection in Veterinary and Farm Animal Practice* (eds Linton, A.H., Hugo, W.B. & Russell, A.D.), pp. 66–116. Oxford: Blackwell Scientific Publications.

Report (1989) *Report of the Expert Advisory Committee on Biocides*. Department of Health. London: HMSO.

Richards, C., Furr, J.R. & Russell, A.D. (1984) Inactivation of micro-organisms by lethal gases. In *Cosmetic and Drug Preservation: Principles and Practice* (ed. Kabara, J.J.), pp. 209–222. New York: Marcel Dekker.

Richards, R.M.E. & Cavill, R.H. (1976) Electron microscope study of effect of benzalkonium chloride and edetate disodium on cell envelope of *Pseudomonas aeruginosa*. *Journal of Pharmaceutical Sciences*, **65**, 76–80.

Rogers, H.J., Ward, J.B. & Burdett, I.D.J. (1978) Structure and growth of the walls of Gram-positive bacteria. In *Relations between Structure and Function in the Prokaryotic Cell* (eds Stanier, R.Y., Rogers, H.J. & Ward, J.B.), 28th Symposium of the Society for General Microbiology, pp. 139–175. Cambridge: Cambridge University Press.

Rubin, J. (1983) Agents for disinfection and control of tuberculosis. In *Disinfection, Sterilization and Preservation* (ed. Block, S.S.), 3rd edn, pp. 414–421. Philadelphia: Lea & Febiger.

Rubin, J. (1991) Mycobacterial disinfection and control. In *Disinfection, Sterilization and Preservation* (ed. Block, S.S.), 4th edn, pp. 377–385. Philadelphia: Lea & Febiger.

Russell, A.D. (1971a) Ethylenediamine tetraacetic acid. In *Inhibition and Destruction of the Microbial Cell* (ed. Hugo, W.B.), pp. 209–225. London: Academic Press.

Russell, A.D. (1971b) The destruction of bacterial spores. In *Inhibition and Destruction of the Microbial Cell* (ed. Hugo, W.B.), pp. 451–612. London: Academic Press.

Russell, A.D. (1974) Factors influencing the activity of antimicrobial agents: an appraisal. *Microbios*, **10**, 151–174.

Russell, A.D. (1976) Inactivation of non-sporing bacteria by gases. In *The Inactivation of Vegetative Bacteria* (eds Skinner, F.A. & Hugo, W.B.), pp. 61–88. Society for Applied Bacteriology Symposium Series No. 5. London: Academic Press.

Russell, A.D. (1981) Neutralization procedures in the evaluation of bactericidal activity. Society for Applied Bacteriology, Technical Series No. 15. London: Academic Press.

Russell, A.D. (1982) *The Destruction of Bacterial Spores* London: Academic Press.

Russell, A.D. (1983) Mechanism of action of chemical sporicidal and sporistatic agents. *International Journal of Pharmaceutics*, **16**, 127–140.

Russell, A.D. (1985) The role of plasmids in bacterial resistance to antiseptics, disinfectants and preservatives. *Journal of Hospital Infection*, **6**, 9–19.

Russell, A.D. (1990a) The bacterial spore and chemical sporicidal agents. *Clinical Microbiology Reviews*, **3**, 99–119.

Russell, A.D. (1990b) The effect of chemical and physical agents on microbes: disinfection and sterilization. In *Topley & Wilson's Principles of Bacteriology and Immunity* (eds Dick, H.M. & Linton, A.H.), 8th edn, pp. 71–103. London: Edward Arnold.

Russell, A.D. (1991a) Principles of antimicrobial activity. In *Disinfection, Sterilization and Preservation* (ed. Block, S.S.), 4th edn, (29–58) Philadelphia: Lea & Febiger.

Russell, A.D. (1991b) Chemical sporicidal and sporistatic agents. In *Disinfection, Sterilization and Preservation* (ed. Block, S.S.), 4th edn, (365–376)) Philadelphia: Lea & Febiger.

Russell, A.D. (1994) Glutaraldehyde: its current status and uses. *Infection Control and Hospital Epidemiology*, **15**, 724–733.

Russell, A.D. (1995) Mechanisms of bacterial resistance to biocides. *International Biodeterioration and Biodegradation*, **36**, 247–265.

Russell, A.D. (1996) Activity of biocides against mycobacteria. *Journal of Applied Bacteriology, Symposium Supplement*, **81**, 87S–101S.

Russell, A.D. & Chopra, I. (1996) *Understanding Antibacterial Action and Resistance*, 2nd edn, Chichester: Ellis Horwood.

Russell, A.D. & Furr, J.R. (1977) The antibacterial activity of a new chloroxylenol preparation containing ethylenediamine tetraacetic acid. *Journal of Applied Bacteriology*, **45**, 253–260.

Russell, A.D. & Furr, J.R. (1986) The effects of antiseptics, disinfectants and preservatives on smooth, rough and deep rough strains of *Salmonella typhimurium. International Journal of Pharmaceutics*, **34**, 115–123.

Russell, A.D. & Furr, J.R. (1996) Biocides: mechanisms of antifungal action and antifungal resistance. *Science Progress*, **79**, 27–48.

Russell, A.D. & Gould, G.W. (1988) Resistance of Enterobacteriaceae to preservatives and disinfectants. *Journal of Applied Bacteriology, Symposium Supplement*, **65**, 167S–195S.

Russell, A.D. & Haque, H. (1975) Inhibition of EDTA-lysozyme lysis of *Pseudomonas aeruginosa* by glutaraldehyde. *Microbios*, **13**, 151–153.

Russell, A.D. & Hopwood, D. (1976) The biological uses and importance of glutaraldehyde. In *Progress in Medicinal Chemistry* (eds Ellis, G.P. & West, G.B.), Vol. 13, pp. 271–301. Amsterdam: North-Holland Publishing.

Russell, A.D. & Hugo, W.B. (1987) Chemical disinfectants. In *Disinfection in Veterinary and Farm Animal Practice* (eds Linton, A.H., Hugo, W.B. & Russell, A.D.), pp. 12–42. Oxford: Blackwell Scientific Publications.

Russell, A.D. & Hugo, W.B. (1994) Antimicrobial activity and action of silver. *Progress in Medicinal Chemistry*, **31**, 351–371.

Russell, A.D. & Russell, N.J. (1995) Biocides: activity, action and resistance. In *Fifty Years of Antimicrobials: Past Perspectives and Future Trends* (eds Hunter, P.A., Darby, G.K. & Russell, N.J.), 53rd Symposium of the Society for General Microbiology, pp. 327–365. Cambridge: Cambridge University Press.

Russell, A.D. & Vernon, G.N. (1975) Inhibition by glutaraldehyde of lysostaphin-induced lysis of *Staphylococcus aureus. Microbios*, **13**, 147–149.

Russell, A.D., Ahonkhai, I. & Rogers, D.T. (1979) Microbiological applications of the inactivation of antibiotics and other antimicrobial agents. *Journal of Applied Bacteriology*, **46**, 207–245.

Russell, A.D., Furr, J.R. & Pugh, W.J. (1985) Susceptibility of porin- and lipopolysaccharide-deficient mutants of *Escherichia coli* to a homologous series of esters of *p*-phydroxybenzoic acid. *International Journal of Pharmaceutics*, **27**, 163–173.

Russell, A.D., Hammond, S.A. & Morgan, J.R. (1986) Bacterial resistance to antiseptics and disinfectants. *Journal of Hospital Infection*, **7**, 213–225.

Russell, A.D., Furr, J.R. & Pugh, W.J. (1987) Sequential loss of outer membrane lipopolysaccharide and sensitivity of *Escherichia coli* to antibacterial agents. *International Journal of Pharmaceutics*, **35**, 227–232.

Russell, N.J. & Gould, G.W. (1991) Factors affecting growth and survival. In *Food Preservatives* (eds Russell, N.J. & Gould, G.W.), pp. 13–21. Glasgow & London: Blackie.

Rutala, W.A. (1990) API guideline for selection and use of disinfectants. *American Journal of Infection Control*, **18**, 99–117.

Salmond, C.V., Kroll, R.G. & Booth, I.R. (1984) The effect of food preservatives on pH homeostasis in *Escherichia coli. Journal of General Microbiology*, **130**, 2845–2850.

Sattar, S.A. Springthorpe, V.S., Conway, B. & Xu, Y. (1994) Inactivation of the human immunodeficiency virus: an update. *Reviews of Medical Microbiology*, **5**, 139–150.

Schmalreck, A.F. & Teuber, M. (1976) Effect of chemical modification by (di)imidoesters on cells and cell envelope components of *Escherichia coli and Salmonella typhimurium. Microbios*, **17**, 93–101.

Schmolka, I.R. (1973) The synergistic effects of non-ionic surfactants upon cationic germicidal agents. *Journal of the Society of Cosmetic Chemists*, **24**, 577–592.

Scott, E.M. & Gorman, S.P. (1998) Chemical disinfectants, antiseptics and preservatives. In *Pharmaceutical Microbiology* (eds Hugo, W.B. & Russell, A.D.), 6th edn, pp. 201–228. Oxford: Blackwell Scientific Publications.

Setlow, P. (1994) Mechanisms which contribute to the long-term survival of spores of *Bacillus* species. *Journal of Applied Bacteriology, Symposium Supplement*, **76**, 49S–60S.

Silver, S. & Misra, S. (1988) Plasmid-mediated heavy metal resistances. *Annual Review of Microbiology*, **42**, 717–743.

Silver, S., Nucifora, G., Chu, L. & Misra, T.K. (1989) Bacterial ATPases: primary pumps for exporting toxic cations and anions. *Trends in Biochemical Sciences*, **14**, 76–80.

Singh, A.P. & Reithmeier, A.F. (1975) Leakage of periplasmic enzymes from cells of heptose-deficient mutants of *Escherichia coli* associated with alterations in the protein component of the outer membrane. *Journal of General and Applied Microbiology*, **21**, 109–118.

Smith, D.H. (1967) R-factors mediate resistance to mercury, nickel and cobalt. *Science*, **156**, 1114–1115.

Smith, G. (1975) Triethylene tetramine, a new potentiator of antibiotic activity. *Experientia*, **31**, 84–85.

Sofos, J.N., Pierson, M.D., Blocher, J.C. & Busta, F.F. (1986) Mode of action of sorbic acid on bacterial cells and spores. *International Journal of Food Microbiology*, **3**, 1–17.

Spaulding, E.H., Cundy, K.R. & Turner, F.J. (1977) Chemical disinfection of medical and surgical materials. In *Disinfection, Sterilization and Preservation* (ed. Block, S.S.), 2nd edn, pp. 654–684. Philadelphia: Lea & Febiger.

Spencer, R.C. (1995) The emergence of epidemic, multiple-antibiotic-resistant *Stenotrophomonas (Xanthomonas) maltophilia* and *Burkholderia (Pseudomonas) cepacia*. *Journal of Hospital Infection*, **30**, (Suppl.), 453–464.

Spicher, G. & Peters, J. (1981) Heat activation of bacterial spores after inactivation by formaldehyde: dependance of heat activation on temperature and duration of action. *Zentralblatt für Bakteriologie, Parasitenkunde, Infektionskrankheiten und Hygiene, I. Abteilung Originale, Reihe B*, **173**, 188–196.

Spire, B., Barré-Sinoussi, F., Montagnier, L. & Chermann, J.C. (1984) Inactivation of lymphadenopathy associated virus by chemical disinfectants. *Lancet*, **ii**, 899–901.

Springthorpe, V.S. & Sattar, S.A. (1990) Chemical disinfection of virus-contaminated surfaces. *CRC Critical Reviews in Environmental Control*, **20**, 169–229.

Stagg, C.H. (1982) Evaluating chemical disinfectants for virucidal activity. In *Methods in Environmental Virology* (eds Gerba, C.P. & Goyal, S.M.), pp. 331–348. New York: Marcel Dekker.

Summers, A.O. & Silver, S. (1972) Mercury resistance in a plasmid-bearing strain of *Escherichia coli*. *Journal of Bacteriology*, **112**, 1228–1236.

Sykes, G. (1965) *Disinfection and Sterilization*, 2nd edn, London: E. & F.N. Spon.

Sykes, G. (1970) The sporicidal properties of chemical disinfectants *Journal of Applied Bacteriology*, **33**, 147–156.

Tamaki, S., Sato, T. & Matsuhashi, M. (1971) The role of lipopolysaccharides in antibiotic resistance and bacteriophage adsorption of *Eschericha coli* K-12. *Journal of Bacteriology*, **105**, 968–975.

Taylor, G.R. & Butler, M. (1982) A comparison of the virucidal properties of chlorine, chlorine dioxide, bromine chloride and iodine. *Journal of Hygiene, Cambridge*, **89**, 321–328.

Tempest, D.W. & Ellwood, D.C. (1969) The influence of growth conditions on the composition of some cell wall components of *Aerobacter aerogenes*. *Biotechnology and Bioengineering*, **11**, 775–783.

Thomas, S. & Russell, A.D. (1974) Temperature-induced changes in the sporicidal activity and chemical properties of glutaraldehyde. *Applied Microbiology*, **28**, 331–335.

Thurman, R.B. & Gerba, C.P. (1988) Molecular mechanisms of viral inactivation by water disinfectants. *Advances in Applied Microbiology*, **33**, 75–105.

Thurman, R.B. & Gerba, C.P. (1989) The molecular mechanisms of copper and silver ion disinfection of bacteria and viruses. *CRC Critical Reviews in Environmental Control*, **18**, 295–315.

Tomlins, R.I. & Ordal, Z.J. (1976) Thermal injury and inactivation in vegetative bacteria. In *The Inactivation of Vegetative Bacteria* (eds Skinner, F.A. & Hugo, W.B.), pp. 153–190. Society for Applied Bacteriology Symposium Series No. 5. London: Academic Press.

Trueman, J.R. (1971) The halogens. In *Inhibition and Destruction of the Microbial Cell* (ed. Hugo, W.B.), pp. 135–183. London: Academic Press.

Tyler, R. & Ayliffe, G.A.J. (1987) A surface test for virucidal activity of disinfectants: preliminary study with herpes virus. *Journal of Hospital Infection*, **9**, 22–29.

Ulitzer, S. (1970) The transport of β-galactosides across the membrane of permeaseless *Escherichia coli* ML 35 cells after treatment with cetyltrimethylammonium bromide. *Biochimica et Biophysica Acta*, **211**, 533–541.

Vaara, M. & Vaara, T. (1983a) Polycations sensitize enteric bacteria to antibiotics. *Antimicrobial Agents and Chemotherapy*, **24**, 107–113.

Vaara, M. & Vaara, T. (1983b) Polycations as outer membrane disorganizing agents. *Antimicrobial Agents and Chemotherapy*, **24**, 114–122.

Vaczi, L. (1973) *The Biological Role of Bacterial Lipids*. Budapest: Akademiai Kiadó.

van Bueren, J. (1995) Methodology for HIV disinfectant testing. *Journal of Hospital Infection*, **30** (Suppl.), 383–388.

Vaughan, J.M., Chen, Y.S., Lindburg, K. & Morales, D. (1987) Inactivation of human and simian rotaviruses by ozone. *Applied and Environmental Microbiology*, **53**, 2218–2221.

Viljanen, P. (1987) Polycations which disorganize the outer membrane inhibit conjugation in *Escherichia coli*. *Journal of Antibiotics*, **40**, 882–886.

Wade, J.J. (1995) The emergence of *Enterococcus faecium* resistant to glycopeptides and other standard agents: preliminary report. *Journal of Hospital Infection*, **30** (Suppl.), 483–493.

Weir, S.C., Lee, H. & Trevors, J.T. (1994) Survival and respiratory activity of genetically engineered *Pseudomonas* spp. exposed to antimicrobial agents in broth and soil. *Microbial Releases*, **2**, 239–245.

Weir, S.C., Lee, H. & Trevors, J.T. (1996) Survival of free and alginate-encapsulated *Pseudomonas aeruginosa* UG2Lr in soil treated with disinfectants. *Journal of Applied Bacteriology*, **80**, 19–25.

Weiss, R.L. (1976) Protoplast formation in *Escherichia coli*. *Journal of Bacteriology*, **128**, 668–670.

Wiener, S. (1955) The interference of rubber with the bacteriostatic action of thiomersalate. *Journal of Pharmacy and Pharmacology*, **7**, 118–125.

Wilkinson, S.G. (1975) Sensitivity to ethylenediamine tetraacetic acid. In *Resistance of Pseudomonas aeruginosa* (ed. Brown, M.R.W.), pp. 145–188. London: John Wiley & Sons.

Williams, N.D. & Russell, A.D. (1993a) Injury and

repair in biocide-treated spores of *Bacillus subtilis*. *FEMS Microbiology Letters*, **106**, 183–186.

Williams, N.D. & Russell, A.D. (1993b) Revival of biocide-treated spores of *Bacillus subtilis*. *Journal of Applied Bacteriology*, 75, 69–75.

Williams, N.D. & Russell, A.D. (1993c) Revival of *Bacillus subtilis* spores from biocide-induced injury in germination processes. *Journal of Applied Bacteriology*, 75, 76–81.

Williams, N.D. & Russell, A.D. (1993d) Conditions suitable for the recovery of biocide-treated spores of *Bacillus subtilis*. *Microbios*, **74**, 121–129.

Wing, W.T. (1955) An examination of rubber used as a closure for containers of injectable solutions. Part I. Factors affecting the absorption of phenol. *Journal of Pharmacy and Pharmacology*, 7, 648–658.

Wing, W.T. (1956a) An examination of rubber used as a closure for containers of injectable solutions. Part II. The absorption of chlorocresol. *Journal of Pharmacy and Pharmacology*, **8**, 734–737.

Wing, W.T. (1956b) An examination of rubber used as a closure for containers of injectable solutions. Part III. The effect of the chemical composition of the rubber mix on phenol and chlorocresol absorption. *Journal of Pharmacy and Pharmacology*, 7, 738–743.

Witholt, B., Van Heerikhuizen, H. & De Leij, L. (1976) How does lysozyme penetrate through the bacterial outer membrane? *Biochimica et Biophysica Acta*, **443**, 534–544.

Wright, A.M., Hoxey, E.V., Soper, C.J. & Davies, D.J.G. (1997) Biological indicators for low temperature steam and formaldehyde sterilization: effect of variations in recovery conditions on the responses of spores of *Bacillus stearothemophilus* NCIMB 8224 to low temperature steam and formaldehyde. *Journal of Applied Bacteriology*, **82**, 552–556.

CHAPTER 4

Evaluation of Antibacterial and Antifungal Efficacy

A. EVALUATION OF THE ANTIBACTERIAL AND ANTIFUNGAL ACTIVITY OF DISINFECTANTS

1 Introduction

There is no general agreement on what disinfection really means, as it is a domain that is situated between cleaning (removal of dirt and, as a result, removal or dilution of microorganisms) and sterilization (killing of all microorganisms). Although there are many definitions of disinfection, it is common to all that the main purpose is the elimination of the hazard of contamination or infection. In consequence, the purpose of testing disinfectants is to check if these products fulfil their objective or, more usually, to determine whether microorganisms are killed or eliminated by the action of the disinfectant. The principle of evaluation of disinfectants is simple: microbial cells are added to the test dilution of the disinfectant, and, after a specified exposure period, it is then checked to determine whether they have been killed. Developing tests of this kind, however, is difficult and complex because many factors have to be incorporated: choice of the test organisms, preparation of the cell suspensions, neutralization of the disinfectant residues in the subculture (Chapter 3), determination of the end-point, etc.

Although antiseptics and disinfectants were tested early in the history of microbiology, even before the 'golden age' of bacteriology (Hugo, 1978), a general internationally accepted test scheme does not exist (Reybrouck, 1975, 1986, 1991). Originally, experiments were directed mainly towards the kinetics of disinfection. It was considered sufficient to examine whether microorganisms were killed by a disinfectant in terms of a stated concentration (or a range of concentrations) or times of exposure, in suspension tests, such as the determination of the phenol coefficient, or in carrier tests. Later on, capacity tests and practical tests were developed in order to simulate real-life situations, and the results give more precise information on the effective use dilution for a given field of application. According to the specific purpose for which the product is used, other test organisms and other exposure times are tested, and the influence of water hardness and other factors can be included. In some European countries, it was realized that not only disinfectants themselves, but also their use in a given field of application or disinfection procedure should be tested (Borneff *et al.*, 1975). Nevertheless, the real situation is that every country has its own testing methods, and different professions (food, human medicine, veterinary medicine, water) within a country also use different techniques.

It is unusual, with some few exceptions, for a manual to describe a complete test scheme with detailed testing methods which have to be followed rigorously for registration purposes, or are at least generally accepted. The best-known examples are those of the American Association of Official Analytical Chemists (AOAC), the German Society for Hygiene and Microbiology (*Deutsche Gesellschaft für Hygiene und Mikrobiologie* (DGHM)) and the French Association of Normalization (Association française de normalisation (AFNOR)). The American association publishes the *Official Methods of Analysis* (AOAC, 1990), in which one chapter is concerned with disinfectants. From 1959, the German society edited the *Richtlinien für die Prüfung chemischer Desinfektionsmittel* (Guidelines for the Evaluation of Chemical Disinfectants) (Kliewe *et al.,* 1959). These were revised several times, and the last edition, which is still incomplete, is based on the *Empfehlungen für die Prüfung und Bewertung der Wirksamkeit chemischer Desinfektionsverfahren* (Recommendations for the testing and the evaluation of the efficacy of chemical disinfectant procedures), produced by a working group of German hygienists (Beck *et al.,* 1977). The present edition (DHGM, 1991) refers to a previous edition, which will hereinafter be referred to as DGHM Guidelines (Borneff *et al.,* 1981). The French association, AFNOR, has collected the official methods into a bilingual (French–English) manual (AFNOR, 1989). The German Veterinary Society (*Deutsche Veterinärmedizinische Gesellschaft*), (DVG, 1988) and the British Standards Institution (BSI) have also published some test methods.

The most important evolution in the domain of disinfectant testing is the founding, in 1990, by the CEN (European Committee for Standardization/ *Comité Européen de Normalisation/Europäisches Komitee für Normung*) of the Technical Committee (TC) 216 Chemical Disinfectants and Antiseptics. The scope of TC 216 is:

> the standardization of the terminology, requirements, test methods including potential efficacy under in-use conditions, recommendations for use and labelling in the whole field of chemical disinfection and antisepsis. Areas of activity include agriculture (but not crop protection chemicals), domestic service, food hygiene and other industrial fields, institutional, medical, and veterinary applications.

The CEN covers not only the European Community but also the six partners of the European Free Trade Association. The following countries are members: Austria, Belgium, Denmark, Finland, France, Germany, Greece, Iceland, Ireland, Italy, Luxemburg, the Netherlands, Norway, Portugal, Spain, Sweden, Switzerland and the UK. The member states of the CEN have undertaken not to publish a new national standard that does not completely conform to a European standard (*Norme européenne, europäische Norm*) (EN) or a harmonization document. Consequently, most scientific work on disinfectant testing in these 18 countries concentrates on the development of new European standards. Three main working groups (WG) are active in the CEN/TC 216: WG1 covers human medicine, WG2 veterinary use and WG3 food hygiene and domestic and institutional use; their work is supervised by a horizontal working group and by the Technical Committee itself. A draft of a standard can be submitted to CEN enquiry and then becomes a proposal for a European standard (prEN). When the prEN is accepted by a sufficient number of member states, it becomes an EN. It takes many years before a proposal of a standard is developed and implemented as an EN. There is an agreement (the so-called Vienna agreement from 1991) on close technical cooperation between the CEN and the International Organization for Standardization (ISO). The task assigned to the CEN/TC 216 was very ambitious; it will cover the complete domain of disinfectant testing, and much work is in progress, but until now only a few standards are in the prEN stage. One peculiarity must be borne in mind. The intention of a standards institution is not to test disinfectants in a scientific way and to cover all conditions (i.e. testing concentrations of a product and exposure periods from completely inactive to active), but only to check whether a specified requirement is fulfilled (e.g. minimal decimal log reduction of 5 attained after an exposure time of 5 min).

There also exists an almost incalculable number

of other methods, some of which are more or less successful, but most are only of local importance. In this survey, an attempt will be made to make some sense out of the present multiplicity of methods and to discuss the problems as clearly as possible. However, only the more widely used techniques will be considered, omitting those which have not yet been subjected to the criteria of wide use and critique. Attention will be drawn especially to the techniques followed in the evaluation of disinfectants for use in hospitals and medicine. More detailed reviews may be found elsewhere (Ayliffe, 1989; Reuter, 1989; Cremieux & Fleurette, 1991; Mulberry, 1995).

2 Classification of disinfectant tests

Although all disinfectant tests have the same final purpose, namely measuring the antimicrobial activity of a chemical substance or preparation, a large number of testing methods have been described. In order to clarify these tests, it is helpful to subdivide them, and this can be done in different ways (Table 4.1). In addition, rapid testing methods are considered briefly in Chapter 4B.

First, the antimicrobial efficiency of a disinfectant can be examined at three stages of testing. The first stage concerns laboratory tests, in which it is verified whether a chemical compound or a preparation possesses antimicrobial activity. These are the preliminary screening tests. The second stage is still carried out in the laboratory but in conditions simulating real-life situations. In these tests, disinfection procedures and not disinfectants are examined. It is determined in which conditions and at which use dilution the preparation is active. The last stage takes place in the field, and comprises the *in loco* or *in situ* tests. These are less popular, since complete standardization is impossible in the field. Variants of these *in loco* tests are in-use tests, which examine whether, after a normal period of use, germs in the disinfectant solution are still killed.

The CEN/TC 216 follows the same classification principle. In phase 1, only suspension tests are considered, and even so in a restrained way: only two test organisms are tested in the basic bactericidal and in the basic fungicidal suspension test. In phase 2, it is determined whether the disinfectant can be active for a given application. In phase 2/step 1, the basic suspension test is extended with other test organisms, more exposure periods are included or interfering substances are added, whereas, in phase 2/step 2, practical tests are performed. Phase 3 tests are tests in the field.

Most simple tests, such as suspension and phenol coefficient tests, are first stage preliminary tests. The use dilution of the disinfectant is determined by another method, usually a more practical test, but in some instances the use dilutions of surface disinfectants are determined by simple tests. In the UK the Kelsey–Sykes test, which is a capacity test, and in the USA the AOAC use-dilution method, which is a carrier test, were the recommended or official tests. For convenience, we shall designate as an *in vitro* test all methods with a simple structure that are not carried out under practical conditions or in the field. Schematically, they may be divided into suspension, capacity and carrier tests. The main second-stage tests are the practical tests, which are also carried out in the laboratory. If a disinfectant is intended for floor disinfection, its activity is determined on the different kinds of surface which may be encountered in a hospital, such as tiles, stainless-steel surfaces, polyvinyl chloride (PVC) sheets, etc. These are contaminated artificially and, after exposure to the product, they are examined for surviving microorganisms. This is a practical test, whereas an in-use test is carried out in the hospital environment.

Hence we shall distinguish between *in vitro*, practical and in-use tests. This classification is followed in the examination of disinfectants active against vegetative bacteria (bactericidal tests), bacterial spores (sporicidal), mycobacteria (tuberculocidal) and fungi (fungicidal). Viricidal testing methods are considered in Chapter 6. The suffix-static means that the growth of the microorganisms is only inhibited, whereas -cidal refers to the killing of the organisms.

3 Tests determining the activity of disinfectants against vegetative bacteria

3.1 *In vitro* tests

No chemical substance or preparation can be

Table 4.1 Classification of disinfectant tests.

A *Classification according to test organism*
1 Determination of antibacterial activity
Non-acid-fast vegetative bacteria: bactericidal tests
Acid-fast bacteria: tuberculocidal (mycobactericidal) tests
Bacterial spores: sporicidal tests
2 Determination of antifungal activity: fungicidal tests
3 Determination of antiviral activity: viricidal tests

B *Classification according to the type of action: 'static' versus -'cidal' tests*
Bacteriostatic and bactericidal, tuberculostatic and tuberculocidal, sporistatic and sporicidal, fungistatic and fungicidal, viristatic and viricidal tests

C *Classification according to the test structure*
1 *In vitro* tests
Test cells in suspension: suspension tests
Several additions of cell suspension: capacity tests
Test organisms on carrier: carrier tests
2 Practical tests
Tests determining the efficacy of the disinfection of surfaces, rooms, instruments, fabrics, excreta, the hands, the skin
3 In-use tests

D *Classification according to the aim of the test*
1 First testing stage: preliminary tests, screening tests
Tests determining whether a chemical substance or preparation possesses antibacterial properties
Tests determining the relationship between exposure periods and disinfectant dilutions
Tests determining the influence of organic matter, serum, etc.
2 Second testing stage
Tests determining the use dilution of a disinfectant for a specific application
3 Third testing stage
Tests in the field, *in loco* or *in situ*, determining the usability of the disinfectant in practice
Clinical effectiveness studies

E *Classification according to CEN/TC 216*
1 Phase 1
Tests determining whether a preparation possesses antimicrobial properties: basic suspension tests
2 Phase 2/step 1
Tests determining whether a preparation possesses antimicrobial properties specific for a defined application: extended suspension tests
3 Phase 2/step 2
Tests determining whether a preparation possesses antimicrobial properties in practice-mimicking conditions: practical tests
4 Phase 3
Tests in the field

regarded as a disinfectant if it is not active against vegetative bacteria; this is the first and main requirement. Therefore, disinfectant testing always starts with the determination of antibacterial activity. As stated above, *in vitro* tests can be classified as suspension tests, capacity tests or carrier tests. Bacterial cells exposed to the action of the disinfectant are, as the name implies, suspended in a medium or diluent in suspension tests, whereas in carrier tests they are fixed and dried on a vehicle. In capacity tests, the test dilution of the disinfectant is loaded with several addition of a bacterial suspension, and after each addition the reaction mixture is subcultured for survivors to determine whether the capacity of the agent has been exhausted by successive additions of bacteria. Tests for the determination of bacteriostatic properties will be treated separately.

3.1.1 *Tests for determining bacteriostatic activity*

The bacteriostatic activity of a disinfectant is determined by an evaluation of the minimum inhibitory concentration (MIC). This is the simplest method of measuring inhibition of bacterial growth, and is similar to the test-tube serial dilution method for determining susceptibility to antibiotics. The disinfectant is mixed with nutrient broth in decreasing concentrations and the tubes are inoculated with a culture of the bacterium to be tested; after a suitable period of incubation, the lowest concentration that inhibits the growth of the organisms is the MIC value. It is important to ensure the absence of any antagonist (neutralizer or inactivator) which might further inhibit the bacteriostatic activity of the disinfectant or its residues in the subculture. The structure of such a test is shown in Fig. 4.1. These tests are rarely used in the evaluation of disinfectants, since a disinfectant is required to have bactericidal rather than bacteriostatic activity. Nevertheless, in the DGHM Guidelines (Borneff *et al.*, 1981) and the DVG Guidelines (DVG, 1988), this technique is used for determining the efficacy of the neutralizer used in bactericidal tests, and Kelsey & Sykes (1969; see also Kelsey & Maurer, 1974) apply it for the selection of the most resistant test organism for inclusion in their capacity test.

3.1.2 *Suspension tests*

Suspension tests have the following features in common: an appropriate volume of bacterial suspension, the inoculum, is added to the disinfectant

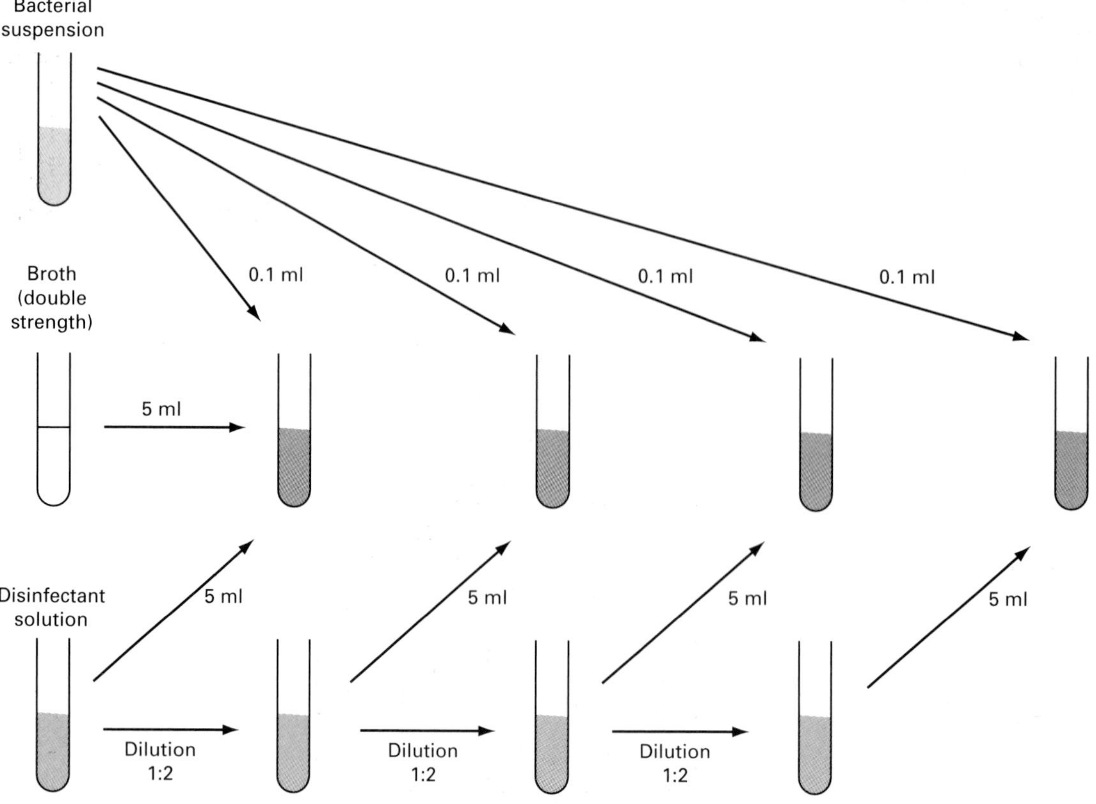

Fig. 4.1 A test for the determination of the minimum inhibitory concentration: the DGHM test.

in the concentration to be tested and, after a predetermined exposure (reaction, disinfection, medication) time, an aliquot is examined to determine whether the inoculum is killed or not. This can be done in a qualitative way (presence or absence of growth in the subculture) or quantitatively (counting the number of surviving organisms in order to compare them with the original inoculum size). The simple structure enables the test to be easily extended: several concentrations or additional exposure periods can be examined, potentially inhibitory substances, such as organic matter or soap, can be added and the influence of water hardness or other factors can be determined. The influence of such interfering substances is determined separately in the French test schedule by the AFNOR tests NF T 72-170 and NF T 72-171 (determination of bactericidal activity in the presence of specific interfering substances—dilution–neutralization method and membrane-filtration method, respectively) (AFNOR, 1989), whereas most other prescriptions include these substances in the basic tests (e.g. the European suspension test, the Kelsey–Sykes test) or in the practical tests (e.g. the DGHM Guidelines).

Qualitative suspension tests. The procedure in a qualitative suspension test is as follows: after a fixed exposure period a sample is withdrawn from the disinfectant/bacterial-cell mixture and added to nutrient broth; the presence of macroscopically observable growth after incubation indicates a failure of the disinfectant activity. An example is given in Fig. 4.2. The main disadvantage of these extinction tests is that survival of a single bacterial cell gives the same final result as an inoculum that is not affected at all by the disinfectant. Results are reproducible as long as completely active or completely inactive use dilutions are tested, but in the critical concentration both negative and positive cultures will appear. The difficulty of interpreting such results can be partially overcome by subculturing more samples; if only a small number of cells survive, not all subculture tubes will show

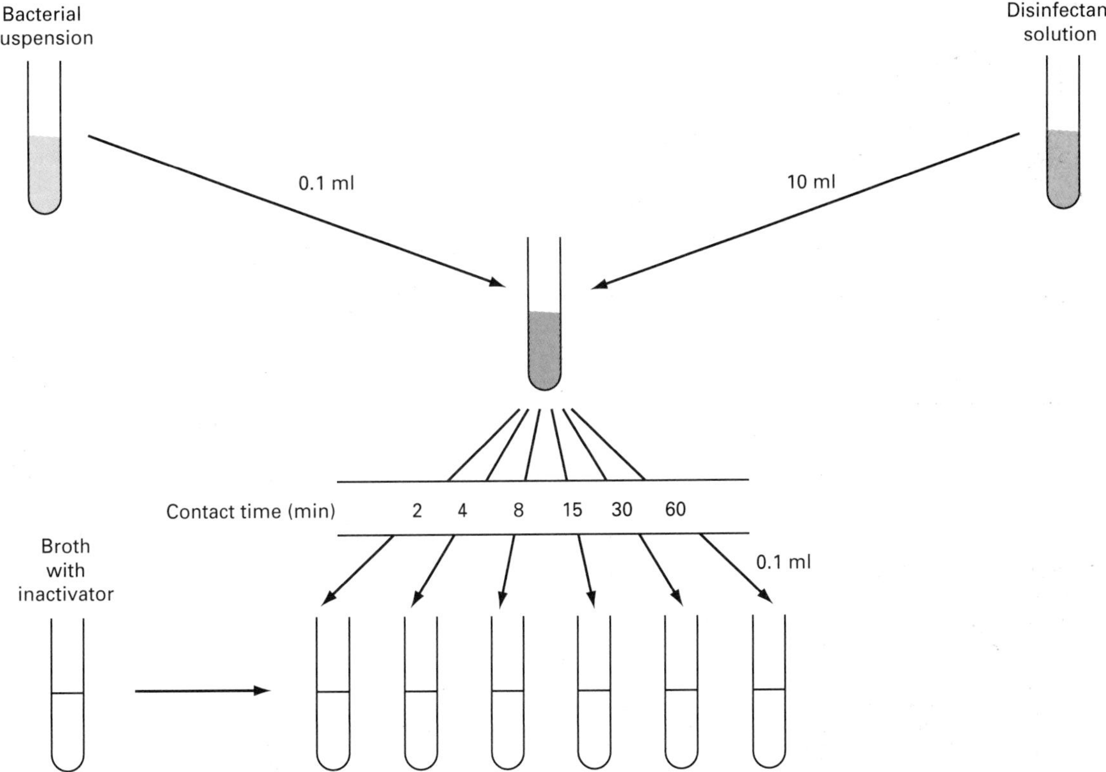

Fig. 4.2 A qualitative suspension test: the DGHM test.

growth and the proportion of negative cultures gives a semiquantitative indication of the activity of the disinfectant.

Qualitative suspension tests are still found in the German prescriptions. Four test organisms are used in the DGHM Guidelines (Borneff *et al.*, 1981); they are *Staphylococcus aureus* ATCC 6538, *Escherichia coli* ATCC 11229, *Proteus mirabilis* ATCC 14153 and *Pseudomonas aeruginosa* ATCC 15442. The DVG Guidelines (DVG, 1988) use the same organisms, but *E. coli* is substituted by *Enterococcus faecium* DSM 2918. Several exposure periods between 5 min (in former editions, 2 min) and 60 min (or 30 s, 1, 2 and 5 min for hand disinfectants) are examined. The results show the concentration/time relationship of a disinfectant, but, although it is possible to quantify the germicidal activity from extinction data, if multiple tubes are inoculated (Reybrouck, 1975), these tests remain without any practical value.

Determination of the phenol coefficient. Tests for determining the phenol coefficient are essentially qualitative suspension tests, in which the activity of the disinfectant under test is compared with that of phenol. By introducing this standard disinfectant in the same experiment, Rideal and Walker in 1903 tried to resolve the major difficulty of reproducibility; all casual factors influencing the resistance of the organisms were thus eliminated, since the same test suspension was used for the standard and the unknown disinfectant. Originally the test organism was *Salmonella typhi*, which is rather sensitive to phenolics. More exposure times,

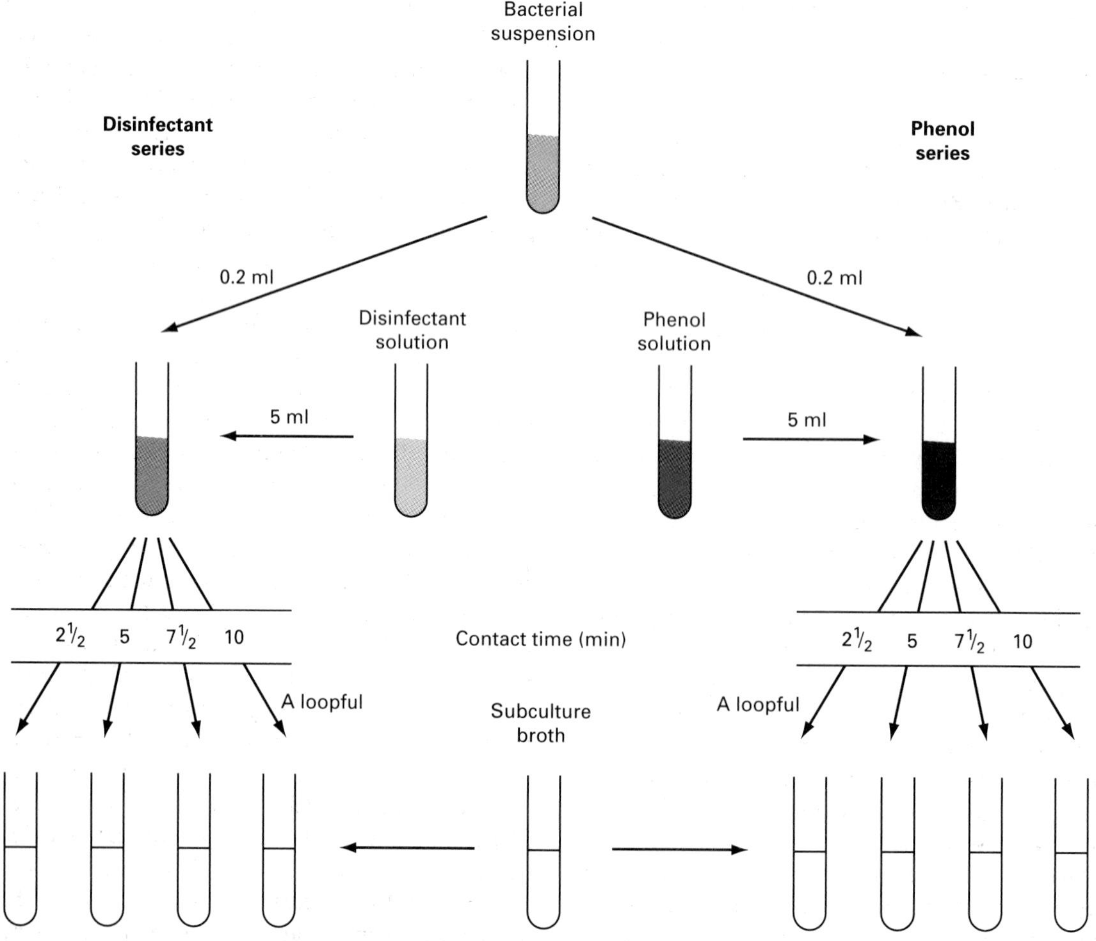

Fig. 4.3 A test for the determination of the phenol coefficient: the Rideal–Walker test.

e.g. $2^1/_2$, 5, $7^1/_2$ and 10 min, were included and dividing the highest dilution of the test disinfectant showing a negative culture after $7^1/_2$ min but growth after 5 min by the phenol dilution gives the phenol coefficient, as shown in Fig. 4.3. The Rideal–Walker test was adapted by the British Standards Institution (BSI, 1985). In the modification by Chick and Martin (BSI, 1986), the bacterial cells are mixed with a yeast suspension before exposure to the disinfectant, thereby increasing the organic load. The manual of the *Official Methods of Analysis* (AOAC, 1990; Beloian, 1993) also describes a very detailed test procedure for the Rideal–Walker test, using *Sal. typhi* ATCC 6539 and *Staph. aureus* ATCC 6538 as test organisms. The phenol coefficient is applicable only to phenolic preparations and has the same defects as the qualitative tests, especially the presence of skips or wild pluses (Croshaw, 1981). It would be better if these tests were replaced by quantitative suspension tests.

Quantitative suspension tests. Many quantitative suspension tests have been described in the last four decades (Reybrouck, 1980). After the exposure of bacterial cells to the disinfectant, surviving organisms can be counted by two techniques, either by direct culture or by membrane filtration.

The basic principle of the quantitative suspension tests using direct culture is as follows: after contact with the disinfectant a sample of the reaction mixture is inoculated on a solid nutrient medium; after incubation the number of survivors is counted and compared with the initial inoculum size. The decimal log-reduction rate, microbicidal effect (ME) or germicidal effect (GE) can be calculated, using the formula GE = log N_C − log N_D (N_C being the number of colony-forming units developed in the control series in which the disinfectant is replaced by distilled water, and N_D being the number of colony-forming units counted after exposure to the disinfectant). The pour-plate technique as well as surface plates may also be used for subculturing. Figure 4.4 shows the basic structure of such a test.

Most of the bactericidal tests used for routine, as well as research, purposes are quantitative suspension tests, in which the number of survivors is determined by direct culture. One of the first tests to be published was the *Method for Laboratory Evaluation of Disinfectant Activity of Quaternary Ammonium Compounds* (BSI, 1960). It describes only the outline of the testing procedure, however, and omits details of type of culture media, fixed reaction times, etc. These different elements can be varied depending on the aim of the test, e.g. as a test for the influence of organic matter or as a test in the presence of milk. The AOAC test for the determination of the sanitizing action of germicidal and detergent disinfectants for food-contact surfaces (AOAC, 1990) is, on the contrary, more detailed.

Several tests with detailed methods are now widely in use in Europe. The Dutch standard suspension test (Van Klingeren *et al.*, 1977) is based on a modification of the technique by Mossel (1963) in the Central Institute for Nutrition Research and the Committee on Phytopharmacy (Reybrouck, 1975). Originally this test was designed for the food industry, which explains why the bacterial cells are suspended in an albumin solution before exposure to the disinfectant. The organic load renders the test more severe than other similar tests. The exposure period is 5 min, pour plates are used for culturing after exposure to disinfectants and the incubation temperature is 32°C. There are separate versions for hospitals, for the food industry and for veterinary use, which differ only in details, e.g. the choice of test organisms. The common name for the standard suspension test is the 5–5–5 test, because five test organisms (*Ps. aeruginosa, E. coli, Staph. aureus, Bacillus cereus* and *Saccharomyces cerevisiae*) were originally tested, the exposure time was 5 min and the criterion for activity was a germicidal effect of 5 log. In the last version of the hospital test, the bacteria are *Ps. aeruginosa* ATCC 15442, *P. mirabilis* ATCC 14153, *Salmonella typhimurium* ATCC 13311 and *Staph. aureus* ATCC 6538.

A new test was developed on the basis of the food industry edition of the standard suspension test: it is the so-called European suspension test (Council of Europe, 1987). The test organisms are *Staph. aureus* ATCC 6538, *E. faecium* DVG 8582, *Ps. aeruginosa* ATCC 15442, *P. mirabilis* ATCC 14153 and *Sacch. cerevisiae* ATCC 9763. The disinfectant concentration is prepared in hard water. The version for clean conditions prescribes

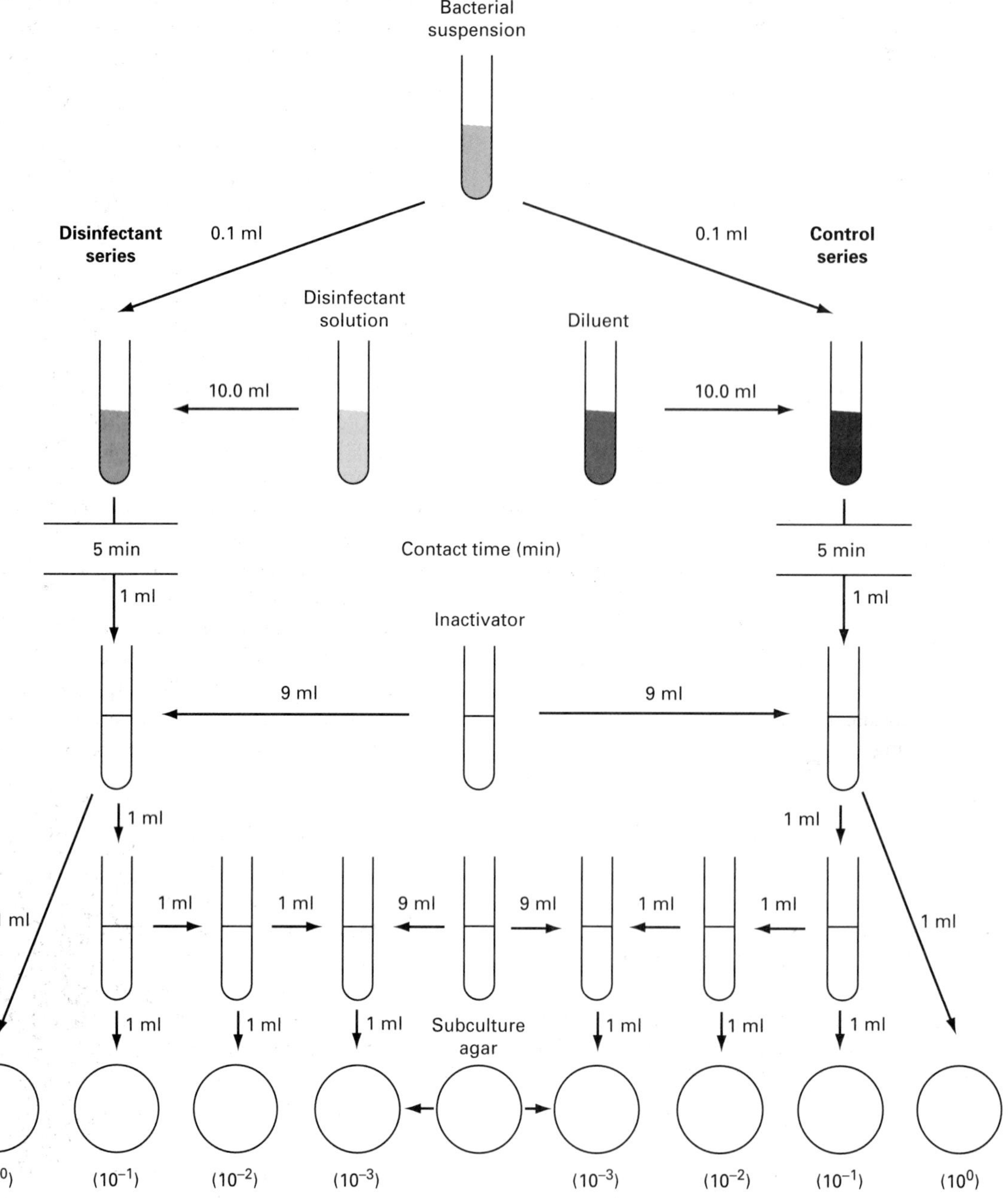

Fig. 4.4 A quantitative suspension test: the *in vitro* test.

an organic load of 0.03% bovine albumin in the preparation of the bacterial suspension; the organic load for dirty conditions is 1.0% bovine albumin. The criterion is a reduction of at least 5 log after 5 min.

The other widely propagated quantitative suspension tests are those of AFNOR and DGHM (Reybrouck, 1980). The criterion of the French AFNOR test NF T 72-150 (determination of bactericidal activity; dilution–neutralization method) (AFNOR, 1989) is also a reduction of 5 log after a reaction time of 5 min. The following test organisms are proposed: *Ps. aeruginosa* CIP A 22, *E. coli* ATCC 10536, *Staph. aureus* ATCC 9144 and *E. faecium* ATCC 10541; the incubation temperature is 37°C and also the pour-plate technique is followed. Under the auspices of the Committee of the International Colloquium on the Evaluation of Disinfectants in Europe, a new *in vitro* test was developed in 1975 (Reybrouck & Werner, 1977; Reybrouck *et al.*, 1979), which served as a basis for the quantitative suspension test of the DGHM Guidelines (Borneff *et al.*, 1981).

It is not surprising that all these quantitative suspension tests differ only in details; their structure and most of the items (test organisms, nutrient media, diluents, etc.) are identical (Reybrouck, 1980). This is also true for the proposal of the new basic bactericidal test of the CEN, which could replace the preceding tests, namely prEN 1040 (CEN, 1996a). There are only two test organisms, *Ps. aeruginosa* ATCC 15442 and *Staph. aureus* ATCC 6538. The contact time can be 1, 5, 15, 30, 45 or 60 min. Also the pour-plate technique is followed, but, if no suitable neutralizer is found, the membrane filtration technique is applied for determining the number of survivors after disinfection. In this case, the reaction mixture is filtered through the membrane filter, which retains the bacteria on its surface, whereafter it is rinsed with large volumes of sterile physiological saline to remove all disinfectant residues. The main advantage of this procedure is that neutralization by inactivators becomes unnecessary. Nevertheless, this technique is rather sensitive and some disinfectants, such as surface-active agents, are difficult to remove. It was developed by AFNOR in the test NF T 72-151 (AFNOR, 1989).

3.1.3 *Capacity tests*

Each time a mop is soaked in a bucket containing a disinfectant solution or a soiled instrument is placed in a container of disinfectant, a certain quantity of dirt and bacteria is added to the solution. The ability to retain activity in the presence of an increasing load is the capacity of the disinfectant. Capacity tests simulate the practical situations of housekeeping and instrument disinfection. The scheme is as follows (Fig. 4.5): a predetermined volume of bacterial suspension is added to the use dilution of the agent, and after a given exposure time the mixture is sampled for survivors, mostly in a semiquantitative way, by inoculating several culture broths. After a certain period, a second addition of the bacterial suspension is made and a new subculture is made after the same reaction time; several additions with subcultures are carried out. Although capacity tests are *in vitro* tests, they closely resemble real-life situations, and in most instances are used as tests confirming the use dilution.

The most widely used capacity test, not only in the UK, but also elsewhere in Europe, is the Kelsey–Sykes test: the original method of 1965 (Kelsey *et al.*, 1965) was modified in 1969 (Kelsey & Sykes, 1969) and improved in 1974 (Kelsey & Maurer, 1974). The bacteria in these tests are suspended in standard hard water for the test under clean conditions, and in a yeast suspension for the test under dirty conditions. The latter was revised as a British standard (BSI, 1987) to estimate the concentration of disinfectants which may be recommended for use under dirty conditions in hospitals. This version is as follows: there are four test organisms, *Ps. aeruginosa* NCTC 6749, *Proteus vulgaris* NCTC 4635, *E. coli* NCTC 8196 and *Staph. aureus* NCTC 4163; the bacteria are suspended in a yeast suspension and the disinfectant is diluted in hard water, the initial volume being 3 ml. The reaction time is 8 min and a new addition of 1 ml of bacterial suspension is carried out 2 min after the subculture of the preceding addition; subculture is done by transferring a 0.02 ml aliquot portion to each of five subculture tubes. Generally, this test is more severe for disinfectants than suspension tests, and is affected by organic matter or by the hardness of the water (Reybrouck, 1975, 1992); it does, however, give a valuable evaluation of the efficacy of agents for floor disinfection (Croshaw, 1981) and instrument disinfection. The AOAC test for the determination of the chlorine germicidal equivalent concentration (AOAC, 1990) is also a capacity test.

3.1.4 *Carrier tests*

It seems logical that, for evaluating the efficacy of

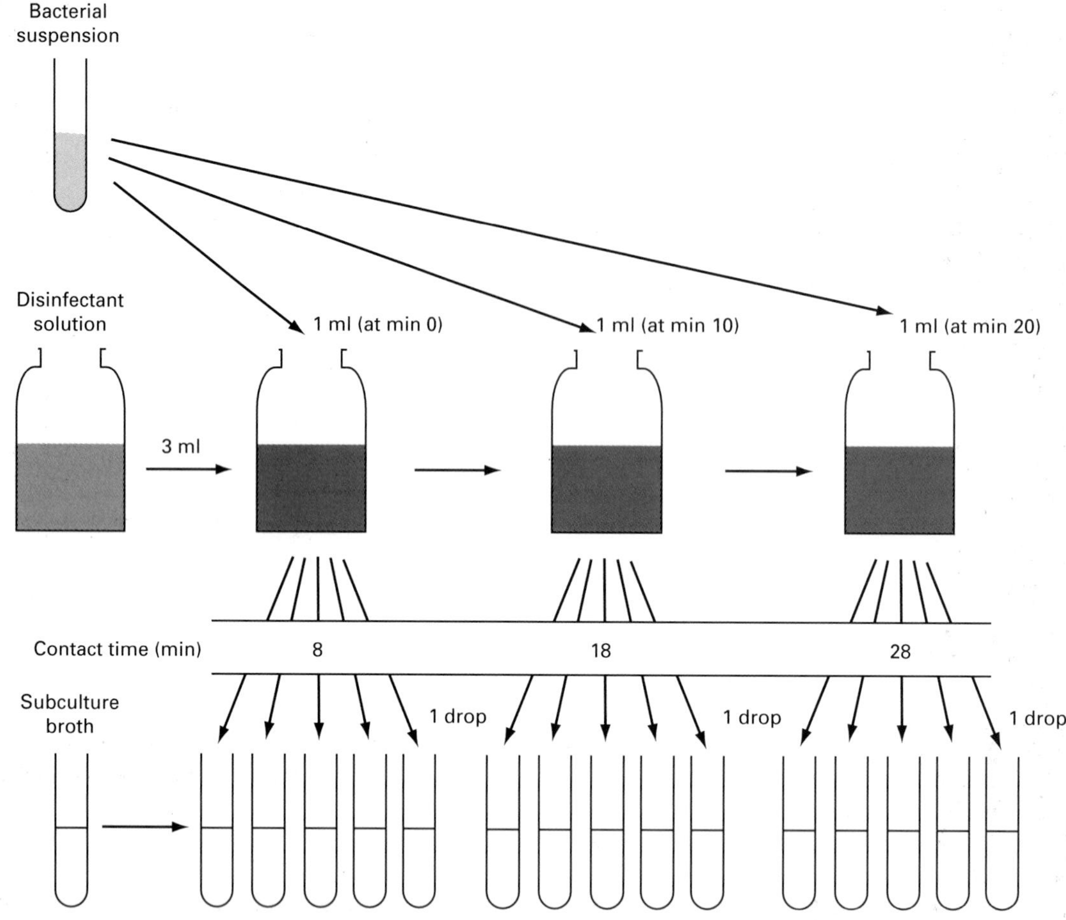

Fig. 4.5 A capacity test: the Kelsey–Sykes test.

preparations intended for instrument disinfection, pieces of metal or catheters should be contaminated artificially and then immersed in the use dilution; thereafter it is checked to determine whether all germs are killed. In tests on pieces of cloth or other textiles, they can be soaked in the disinfectant. Although such techniques may be considered to be practical tests, the situation is different when the carriers to be disinfected are abstracted and standardized into non-realistic objects, e.g. a porcelain cylinder, or when conclusions are applied to other fields. Therefore, these tests are treated as *in vitro* tests. The structure of a carrier test is very simple (Fig. 4.6): the carrier is transferred to the use dilution of the disinfectant, and after a fixed reaction time it is transferred to nutrient broth for subculture; usually a minimum of 10 carriers are used in a test.

The most widely reported carrier tests are those of the DGHM and the use-dilution method of the AOAC. In the carrier test of the DGHM Guidelines (Borneff *et al.*, 1981), the carriers, pieces of a standard cotton cloth each 1 cm^2, are contaminated by soaking for 15 min in a suspension of one of the five test bacteria; the wet pieces of cloth are placed in a dish, and 10 ml of the disinfectant solution is added. After each exposure time, ranging from 5 to 120 min, one carrier is transferred to broth with neutralizer for rinsing and then into another for final culture. This German carrier test serves only as an *in vitro* test, giving an indication of potentially active concentration/time relationships.

In the use-dilution method of the AOAC (1990), the test organisms are *Salmonella cholerae-suis* ATCC 10708, *Staph. aureus* ATCC 6538 and *Ps.*

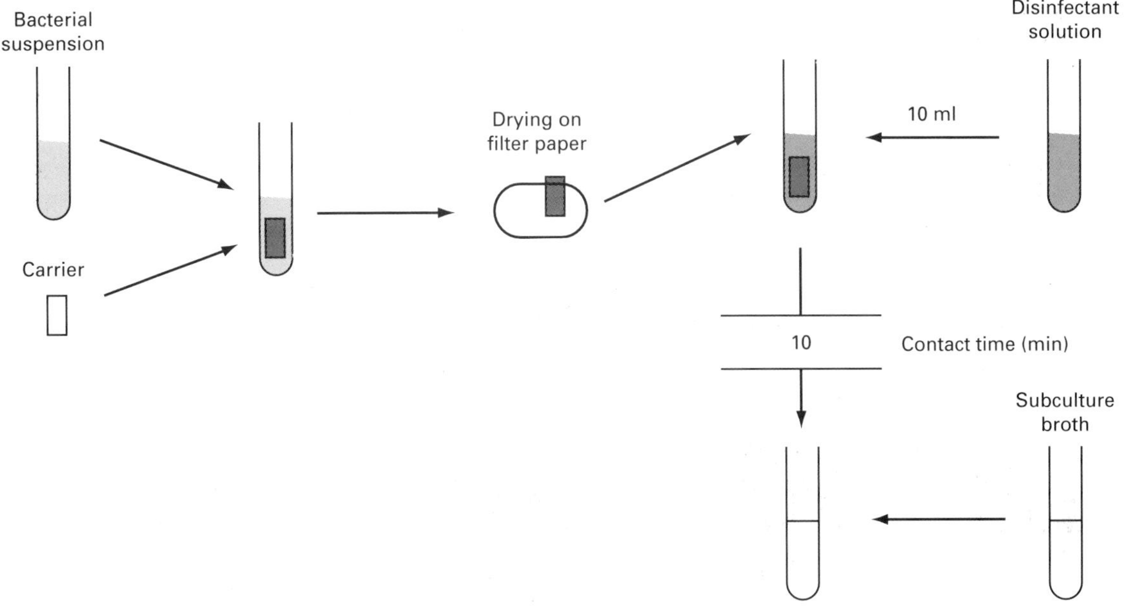

Fig. 4.6 A carrier test: the AOAC use-dilution test.

aeruginosa ATCC 15442; in each test, 10 stainless-steel penicillin cups are contaminated and immersed for 10 min in 10 ml of use dilution of the disinfectant under test, and then they are subcultured. This test confirms the phenol coefficient results and determines the maximum dilution that is still effective for practical disinfection. In this sense, it is also an *in vitro* test, although it is much more severe than the suspension tests or the Kelsey–Sykes test (Reybrouck & Van de Voorde, 1975; Reybrouck, 1992). An extreme variability of the test results obtained by the use-dilution method among different laboratories, especially in the case of *Ps. aeruginosa*, was observed, even when the methodology was modified and more standardized in 32 instances (Cole *et al.*, 1988). As it was impossible to abandon it in favour of a suspension test, the best solution was to develop a new test (Mulberry, 1995). The AOAC hard-surface carrier test (HSCT) has now replaced the use-dilution method (Beloian, 1993), but the greater part of the test procedure is identical. The main differences are that glass penicylinders are substituted for the stainless steel and that the inoculum is more standardized (Rubino *et al.*, 1992; Hamilton *et al.*, 1995). The incorporation of standard hard water and of an organic load will approximate actual use conditions (Beloian, 1995).

3.2 Practical tests

The practical tests under real-life conditions belong to the second testing stage. After measuring the time/concentration relationship of the disinfectant in the *in vitro* test, these practical tests are performed to verify if the proposed use dilution is still adequate in these real-life conditions. In this way, these tests are adapted to present a picture of the microbicidal efficacy of a preparation in the conditions under which it would be used, but have the advantage that the experiments still take place in the laboratory and can be better standardized.

The formation and elaboration of such tests is not difficult, but most of them have a limited application since they are found to be poorly reproducible. Factors influencing the resistance of the test bacteria to a disinfectant are more easily recognized in *in vitro* tests, but in the practical tests it can be difficult, if not impossible, to standardize some of them. Drying of organisms on carriers, hands or fabrics results not only in a decrease in the number of test bacteria, but probably also in the viability of the cell. The changes will be influenced by many factors, such as the drying time, the temperature and relative humidity of the air, the intrinsic humidity of the carrier itself, the suspending medium of the cells and the growth phase of the organisms. Although repeatability in one laboratory may be reasonable, collaborative trials in different laboratories show that reproducibility is not easily attained. That is the reason why in some countries the use dilution is determined in tests classified as *in vitro* tests.

In the countries where these practical tests are used, several tests are described for each field of application, including the assessment of disinfection of instruments and surfaces, cubicles and rooms, the air, sputum and faeces, hands and skin, swimming-pools, effluents and others. The most elaborate and complete review can be found in the methods of the DGHM. This chapter deals only with those fields of application for which typical tests are described and which are generally accepted and practised in the countries concerned.

3.2.1 Tests for instrument disinfection

The technique that is most likely to be followed for the assessment of instrument disinfection is a carrier test with standardized pieces of metal or of catheters. The use-dilution method of the AOAC (1990) is such a test. In the DGHM Guidelines (DGHM, 1991), specific instrument-disinfection tests, which are different from the carrier tests, are described; a broth culture of the same test organisms as used in the suspension tests is mixed with bovine blood to a final concentration of 20% and the disinfectant is diluted in standard hard water, to which 0.5% bovine albumin is added; rubber hoses of standardized composition and dimensions are soaked in the culture/blood mixture and then dried for 4 h at 36°C; thereafter they are immersed in the disinfectant solution for 15, 30, 45 and 60 min, respectively. After this exposure period, one carrier is withdrawn, rinsed in a culture broth with neutralizer and subcultured in another tube of broth for 7 days. In this way, the lower limit of the active concentration is determined. These tests differ from the carrier tests mainly by the higher load of organic matter and the dilution of the disinfectant in hard water.

3.2.2 Tests for surface disinfection

The assessment of disinfectants for surface disinfection is done in some countries by methods that have been classified under the *in vitro* tests: in the Netherlands by the standard suspension test, in the UK by the Kelsey–Sykes test and in the USA by the use-dilution method of the AOAC.

In Germany in particular, preparations for surface disinfection are evaluated by a test under practical conditions. These tests are based on the work of Heicken (1949), who studied the efficacy of different agents on suspensions of *Salmonella paratyphi* and on infected stools dried on different carriers, such as wood, lacquered or painted wood, glass, linoleum, etc. These tests were modified several times; the most recent DGHM Guidelines (DGHM, 1991) are based on the technique of the Hygiene Institute of Mainz (Borneff & Werner, 1977). The test schedule is as follows (Fig. 4.7): a 30 mm × 30 mm area of standard operating-theatre tiles or PVC floor covering measuring 50 mm × 50 mm is contaminated with a standardized inoculum of the following test bacteria: *Staph. aureus* ATCC 6538, *E. coli* ATCC 11229 and *Ps. aeruginosa* ATCC 15442; after a drying time of 90 min at room temperature, a definite volume of the disinfectant solution is distributed over the carrier; exposure lasts for 15 min, 30 min, 1 h, 2 h and 4 h; the number of survivors is determined by a rinsing technique, in which the carrier is rinsed in a diluent and the number of bacteria is determined in the rinsing fluid. In order to determine the spontaneous dying rate of the organisms caused by drying on the carrier, a control series is included and, from the comparison of the survivors in this with the test series, the reduction is determined quantitatively.

Another practical test for surface disinfection is the AFNOR test NF T 72-190 (determining bactericidal, fungicidal and sporicidal action, germ-carrier method) (AFNOR, 1989). In this test, skim milk is added to the bacterial suspension (*Ps. aeruginosa* CIP A 22, *E. coli* ATCC 10536, *Staph. aureus* ATCC 9144, *E. faecium* ATCC 10541); the mixture is spread over the carrier (watch-glasses, stainless steel, plastic supports) and dried on it; disinfection is performed by spreading 0.2 ml disinfectant solution over the carrier and, after the

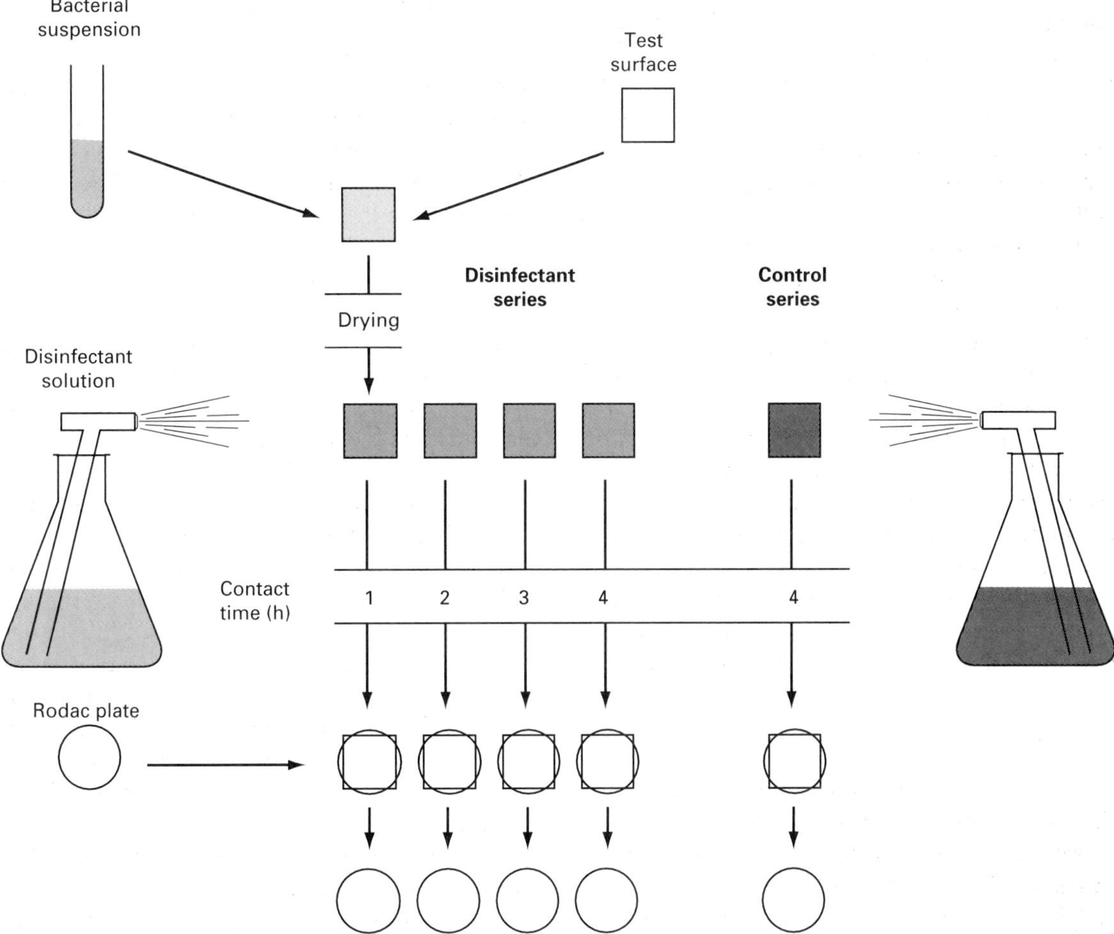

Fig. 4.7 A practical test: the DGHM surface-disinfection test.

chosen contact time, the support is immersed in a rinsing fluid; after shaking, the carrier is withdrawn, put on a solid nutrient medium and covered by a thin layer of melted agar; the rinsing fluid is cultured by membrane filtration. Other tests are the Dutch quantitative carrier test (Van Klingeren, 1978), the Leuven test (Reybrouck, 1990a) and the quantitative surface disinfectant test, QSDT (Reybrouck, 1990b).

It is logical that the above-mentioned testing techniques, which differ, not only in details, but in essential and important elements, should give varying results (Reybrouck, 1986, 1990c). On the basis of this experience, a working group of the CEN/TC 216 developed a new surface-disinfectant test. The carriers are small circular stainless-steel surfaces (2 cm diameter); they are inoculated with a drop of 0.05 ml bacterial suspension; after 1 h drying at 37°C, the inoculum is covered with 0.1 ml disinfectant solution; after the defined exposure time, the carrier is submerged in neutralizing fluid and shaken and the surviving cells are counted, using a standard pour-plate technique. Although a collaborative study gave satisfying results (Bloomfield *et al.*, 1993, 1994), further refining of the technique seems necessary.

3.2.3 Tests for textile disinfection

The assessment of preparations for laundry

disinfection exemplifies clearly that the three stages of disinfectant testing are necessary. By a suspension test it can be stated whether the laundry additive possesses bactericidal properties. A carrier test, using fabrics that are treated in an experimental washing-machine at the same temperature and with the same disinfectant concentration as in the washing cycle, is used in the second stage. In such tests it can be proved that some preparations act on the washing fluid but not the textile, whereas others show the reverse phenomenon. These differences cannot be demonstrated by an *in vitro* test. In practice, it is found that the third testing stage is also necessary, since the peculiarities of a washing system cannot necessarily be reproduced on a laboratory scale. This is particularly true for continuous washing-machines.

The practical tests for textile disinfection of the DGHM Guidelines (DGHM, 1991) are the most detailed. The test for chemical laundry disinfection differs basically from the carrier test in two respects: the disinfectant is diluted in standard hard water, to which 0.2% bovine albumin is added, and the exposure lasts 4, 6 and 12 h at 12–14 °C. This test only gives a clear picture of the disinfection of fabrics by immersion at room temperature and for a long time. In another test for chemothermal laundry disinfection, the contaminated test pieces are washed with other hospital laundry in a washing-machine at 90 °C. Thereafter, the test pieces, as well as 500 ml of the washing fluid, are examined qualitatively for survivors. If the disinfectant is adopted for continuous washing-machines, then a washing cycle in such machines has to be performed, i.e. an *in loco* test.

3.2.4 *Other practical tests*

Since, in most countries, preparations for hand and skin disinfection are regulated by the legislation on drugs, their testing is performed mostly in other laboratories and often not by those dealing with other fields of disinfection. Antiseptics are not treated in, for example, the manual of the AOAC. Tests for hand and skin disinfection will be considered in the chapter on antisepsis (Chapter 13). In addition to the above-mentioned practical tests, there exist tests for many other fields of application, e.g. for swimming-pool water, in the manual of the AOAC (1990). The discussion of all such tests is beyond the scope of this chapter and most are not generally acceptable outside the country of origin.

3.3 In-use tests

The only valid test of a bactericidal product is its evaluation in the field under actual conditions of use, and preferably by assessing its performance in the prevention of the transmission of infection (or contamination). Nevertheless, today it is practically impossible to evaluate the effectiveness of a disinfectant using this criterion. The occurrence of infection is influenced by many factors, of which only a few are identified and can be evaluated. We are now unable to measure the value of hand antisepsis by a decrease of the infection rate, as Semmelweis did more than a century ago.

An indirect method of measuring the efficacy of a disinfectant is by a microbiological monitoring of the environment. Although a decrease in bacterial contamination in the environment does not automatically result in a drop of the infection rate, the inverse relationship is more likely, i.e. no decrease in the number of infections might be expected without improved hygiene measures. In this sense, the degree of contamination of the surfaces after disinfection can be used to assess the effectiveness of the procedure.

A technique that can detect the failure of a disinfection procedure in a more direct way is the in-use test. This type of test is based on the principle that the use dilution of an effective preparation for surface or instrument disinfection should not retain surviving bacteria after use; the solution should be sufficiently bactericidal, despite the load of dirt, blood or serum, for it to continue to kill the germs within a short time. An in-use test is performed in the following way (Kelsey & Maurer, 1966; Prince & Ayliffe, 1972): A sample is taken from bucket contents after cleaning, from liquid wrung from mops, from containers for contaminated instruments, etc. It is diluted 1 to 10 in an inactivating solution to neutralize the action of the disinfectant and five or 10 drops of this dilution are placed on to the surface of an agar plate; if after incubation growth of non-sporulating bacteria occurs, then the use dilution of the disinfectant tested was certainly too low. The membrane-filtration technique can also be applied for isolation of survivors in the disinfectant solution (Prince & Ayliffe, 1972). Another technique consists in the monitoring of the disinfected and cleaned surfaces by means of culture on Rodac plates (Scott *et al.*, 1984). In-use tests are very helpful in the monitoring of disinfection practice in a hospital, but they are not usually applied routinely.

4 Tests determining the activity of disinfectants against mycobacteria

Tuberculocidal (or mycobactericidal) tests are considered separately from the methods for the determination of the general bactericidal properties of disinfectants. Mycobacteria are more resistant to the influence of external factors, such as desiccation and chemical disinfection, than are other vegetative bacteria (see Chapter 3). Although comparatively few substances show tuberculocidal characteristics, this property gains in importance in the light of the emergence of multidrug-resistant strains (see Chapter 10D). Most pathogenic mycobacteria grow slowly, so that definitive results are only available after months. Rapid-growing mycobacteria, such as *Mycobacterium smegmatis*, are therefore taken as test organisms, certainly for preliminary tests. As with the other bactericidal test, a distinction can be drawn between suspension test, capacity test, carrier tests and tests under practical conditions. Some of the *in vitro* tests mentioned above have been adapted as tuberculocidal tests. Most AFNOR tests can be performed using *M. smegmatis* CIP 7326 as the test organism.

The *Official Methods of Analysis* (AOAC, 1990) only mentions carrier tests, namely a presumptive screening test, using *M. smegmatis* PRD 1 and a confirmative test using *Mycobacterium bovis* (Bacillus Calmette-Guérin (BCG)). The carriers are porcelain penicylinders, 10 of which are tested per trial. After contamination they are submitted to the action of the disinfectant under test for 10 min. In the confirmatory test, each carrier is transferred to a tube with 10 ml of serum or neutralizer, followed by transfer of the cylinder and two 2 ml amounts of serum to subculture broth. The maximum dilution of the disinfectant which kills the test organisms in the 10 carriers and shows no growth in each of the two additional subcultures, represents the maximum safe use dilution for practical tuberculocidal disinfection. As in the case of other carrier tests, a revision of this test has been undertaken, since it lacks precision and accuracy (Ascenzi *et al.*, 1986). At present the Environmental Protection Agency (EPA) tuberculocidal activity test method, which is based on the work of Ascenzi (Ascenzi *et al.*, 1987; Ascenzi, 1991), is utilized in the USA. It is a quantitative suspension test. There is doubt about the reproducibility of the resistance of the suspension of the test organism, *M. bovis* (Robison *et al.*, 1996).

The most extensive test schedule is found in the DGHM methods (Borneff *et al.*, 1981; DGHM, 1991). The first-stage tests are qualitative suspension test and carrier test, using small pieces of cotton cloth, as described in the bactericidal tests; the test organism is *Mycobacterium tuberculosis* ATCC 25618. The contaminated carriers are submerged in the disinfectant solution for times ranging from 5 to 120 min; they are then rinsed twice in a neutralizer and transferred to the surface of a Loewenstein–Jensen agar plate for subculture. The second-stage tests are practical tests for the disinfection of fabrics and instruments. Since the strain *M. tuberculosis* ATCC 25618 has at least two variants, which differ in resistance towards disinfectants, it is now usual to use *Mycobacterium terrae* for determining the tuberculocidal potential of disinfectants (Gundermann, 1987; Van Klingeren & Pullen, 1987). *Mycobacterium terrae* ATCC 15755 is used at present in the newly developed suspension and carrier test (Hingst *et al.*, 1990), the quantitative suspension test of the DGHM (1996) and the tests for the surface and for instrument disinfection of the German Federal Health Office (BGA, 1994; Robert Koch Institute, 1995). For this test organism also, a difference in resistance between test cultures is found (Bansemir *et al.*, 1996).

There is an urgent need for more precise and reliable mycobactericidal tests to be developed (Sattar *et al.*, 1995). One possibility is the Bactec method, which relies upon the release of carbon dioxide-14 ($^{14}CO_2$) from a radiolabelled amino acid.

5 Tests determining the activity of disinfectants against bacterial spores

The determination of the sporicidal properties of disinfectants is very important. Since bacterial spores are more resistant to the action of chemical substances than any other living organisms (Chapters 3 and 10C), a disinfectant prossessing sporicidal activity is by definition a sterilant. In this sense procedure of a sporicidal test should be so stringent that in practice the most resistant spores should be used and, after the exposure to the disinfectant, surviving spores should be capable of resuscitation under optimal conditions.

Some bactericidal suspension tests have been modified to a sporicidal test. In the Dutch standard suspension test (Van Klingeren *et al.*, 1977), *B. cereus* ATCC 9139 is taken as the test organism. The spores are suspended in distilled water and heated up at 80°C for 60 s. Whereas the general criterion for a bactericidal disinfectant is a lethal effect of 5 log within 5 min, in this case a microbicidal effect of only 1 log after the same reaction period is required. This criterion does not correspond to any realistic condition, and it is imposed on every disinfectant; in this context the test does not determine sporicidal properties of any practical value.

The best-known sporicidal test is the carrier test of the AOAC (1990). The carriers are porcelain penicylinders or silk-suture loops. Spores of *Bacillus subtilis* ATCC 19659 or *Clostridium sporogenes* ATCC 3584 are standardized with regard to their resistance towards a 2.5 mol/l solution of hydrochloric acid; in each experiment 30 carriers are tested and the exposure period is not fixed. A preparation is considered to be sporicidal if at least 59 out of 60 replicates do not show growth. This test also shows some inconsistencies in the results, probably due to the microbial load of the carriers (Danielson, 1993; Miner *et al.*, 1995).

The tests proposed in France, AFNOR tests NF T 72-230 and NF T 72-231 (determination of sporicidal activity; dilution–neutralization method and membrane filtration method, respectively) (AFNOR, 1989), are quantitative suspension tests using *B. cereus* CIP 7803, *B. subtilis* var. *niger* ATCC 9372 and *Cl. sporogenes* 51 CIP 7939 as the test organisms. It is worth mentioning that none of the German scientific societies describes any sporicidal test, although their range of tests is the most extensive; some of the existing German techniques have been modified to, and proposed as, a sporicidal test (Stockinger *et al.*, 1989).

Some other sporicidal tests have been described, but there is doubt about attaching the designation 'sporicidal' to a disinfectant, and such tests are less frequently made. Since the consequences of the use of sterile objects in medicine, and in the pharmaceutical and food industries, are so far-reaching (Chapter 19C,D), the user is unlikely to be satisfied by a single sporicidal test applied to the proposed chemosterilizing procedure. Regular sterility controls are needed to monitor the technique and the preparation. These, as well as the biological sterilization-control procedures using test spores, are in fact *in loco* tests.

6 Tests determining the activity of disinfectants against fungi

Since, in clinical microbiology, mycology is possibly less important than bacteriology or virology, there is little medical interest in fungicidal tests. In most instances, they are confined to an adaptation of the bactericidal test, using *Candida albicans* as the test organism. An example of such an adaptation is the Dutch standard suspension test for hospital disinfectants (Van Klingeren *et al.* 1977), although in the original description (Mossel, 1963), and in the version for the food industry, *Sacch. cerevisiae* is taken as test organism. The DGHM Guidelines (Borneff *et al.*, 1981) also use *C. albicans* ATCC 10231 in both the fungistatic and the fungicidal suspension tests and in the practical tests for textile and instrument disinfection. In the test for surface disinfection, *C. albicans* ATCC 10231 and *Trichophyton mentagrophytes* ATCC 9533 are used as test organisms (DGHM, 1991); small pieces of beech wood measuring 5×20×2 mm are contaminated by a suspension of these organisms; exposure lasts 5, 15 and 30 min and 1, 2 and 4 h; after disinfection and neutralization the wooden pieces are inoculated on Sabouraud nutrient agar, and growth is assessed semiquantitatively.

The best-known and probably the most widely

used fungicidal test is that of the AOAC (1990), which is an adaptation of the phenol-coefficient test and is thus a qualitative suspension test. The organism used is *T. mentagrophytes*. After exposure of the standardized suspension to the disinfectant solution for 5, 10 and 15 min, a sample is taken and, after neutralization, is inoculated into glucose broth. The highest dilution that kills the test cells in 10 min is considered to be the highest dilution that could be expected to disinfect inanimate surfaces contaminated with pathogenic fungi.

Both French tests, the AFNOR tests NF T 72-200 and NF T 72-201 (determination of fungicidal activity; dilution–neutralization method and membrane-filtration method, respectively) (AFNOR, 1989) are quantitative suspension tests; the test organisms are *Absidia corymbifera*, *Cladosporium cladosporioides*, *Penicillium verricosum* var. *cyclopium* and *C. albicans* ATCC 2091. The proposal for a basic fungicidal test of the CEN resembles the AFNOR tests (CEN, 1996b); there are two test organisms: *C. albicans* ATCC 10231 and *Aspergillus niger* ATCC 16404. Other fungicidal tests have been published and different varieties of testing methods are followed in the preservation of wood and paints (see Chapter 18).

Generally, it can be stated that, in medicine, tests with *C. albicans* serve as fungicidal tests, and that even an extension of the test strains to *Trichophyton* spp. does not make the test of representative value. Other fungi, e.g. the conidiospores of *Aspergillus* species, can be more resistant (Lensing & Oei, 1985). In addition to this, it should be remembered that tests on inanimate surfaces and clinical studies with preparations for medical or veterinary use are two different aspects, and that today the interest in antifungal drugs is greater than that in antifungal disinfectants. In this sense, it appears difficult to prove the fungicidal properties of a disinfectant in an accepted scientific way.

7 Conclusion

It may cause some surprise that the evaluation of the microbiological activity of disinfectants cannot be summarized in a few pages. In theory, disinfectant testing is very easy: test organisms (bacteria, spores, fungi or viruses) in suspension, fixed on carriers, or dried on test surfaces for the practical tests, are exposed to the disinfectant solution under test and, after a predetermined exposure period, it is checked to determine whether and to what extent the microorganisms have been killed. The number of tests described and their diversity show that there is a lack of agreement among workers on the standardization of all the components of a testing method, and that all these factors influence the resistance, the survival and the recovery of test organisms. Since the performance of different testing procedures yields such a diversity of results for the same disinfectant, it is not surprising that some preparations are applied at a lower use concentration in one country than in another. Agreement can probably be more easily reached as to the requirements a disinfectant should satisfy for a certain field of application; deciding on criteria of reduction rates after a given exposure is more difficult. Disagreement is still apparent on the testing methods themselves; even the necessity to test disinfectants in three stages is not generally accepted. So long as there is absence of agreement on such principles, different testing methods will be used and varying results will be obtained. In this sense, harmonization of the testing schedule and of disinfectant tests will not occur in the immediate future.

8 References

AFNOR, (Association Française de Normalisation) (1989) *Recueil de normes françaises. Antiseptiques et désinfectants*, 2nd edn. Paris La Défense: Association Française de Normalisation.

AOAC (Association of Official Analytical Chemists) (1990) *Official Methods of Analysis*, 15th edn. Arlington: Association of Official Analytical Chemists.

Ascenzi, J.M. (1991) Standardization of tuberculocidal testing of disinfectants. *Journal of Hospital Infection*, **18** (Suppl. A), 256–263.

Ascenzi, J.M., Ezzell, R.J. & Wendt, T.M. (1986) Evaluation of carriers used in the test methods of the Association of Official Analytical Chemists. *Applied and Environmental Microbiology*, **51**, 91–94.

Ascenzi, J.M., Ezzell, R.J. & Wendt, T.M. (1987) A more accurate method for measurement of tuberculocidal activity of disinfectants. *Applied and Environmental Microbiology*, **53**, 2189–2192.

Ayliffe, G.A.J. (1989) Standardization of disinfectant

testing. *Journal of Hospital Infection*, **13**, 211–216.

Bansemir, K., Goroncy-Bermes, P., Kirschner, U., Ostermeyer, C., Pfeiffer, M. & Rödger, H.-J. (1966) Efficacy testing of disinfectants against mycobacteria in the quantitative suspension test. *Hygiene und Medizin*, **21**, 381–388.

Beck, E.G., Borneff, J., Grün, L. *et al.* (1977) Empfehlungen für die Prüfung und Bewertung der Wirksamkeit chemischer Desinfektionsverfahren. *Zentralblatt für Bakteriologie, Parasitenkunde, Infektionskrankheiten und Hygiene, I. Abteilung Originale, Reihe B*, **165**, 335–380.

Beloain, A. (1993) General Referee Reports. Disinfectants. *Journal of AOAC International*, **76**, 97–98.

Beloian, A. (1995) General Referee Reports. Disinfectants. *Journal of AOAC International*, **78**, 179.

BGA (1994) BGA guideline on testing the efficacy of surface disinfectants in disinfecting for tuberculosis. *Hygiene und Medizin*, **19**, 474–478.

Bloomfield, S.F., Arthur, M., Begun, K. & Patel, H. (1993) Comparative testing of disinfectants using proposed European surface test methods. *Letters in Applied Microbiology*, **17**, 119–125.

Bloomfield, S.F., Arthur, M., Van Klingeren, B., Pullen, W., Holah, J.T. & Elton, R. (1994) An evaluation of the repeatability and reproducibility of a surface test for the activity of disinfectants. *Journal of Applied Bacteriology*, **76**, 86–94.

Borneff, J. & Werner, H.-P. (1977) Entwicklung einer neuen Prüfmethode für Flächendesinfektionsverfahren. VII. Mitteilung: Vorschlag der Methodik. *Zentralblatt für Bakteriologie, Parasitenkunde, Infektionskrankheiten und Hygiene, I. Abteilung Originale, Reihe B*, **165**, 97–101.

Borneff, J., Werner, H.-P., Van De Voorde, H. & Reybrouck, G. (1975) Kritische Beurteilung der Prüfmethoden für chemische Desinfektionsmittel und Verfahren. *Zentralblatt für Bakteriologie, Parasitenkunde, Infektionskrankheiten und Hygiene. I. Abteilung, Originale, Reihe B*, **160**, 590–600.

Borneff, J., Eggers, H.-J., Grün, L. *et al.* (1981) *Richtlinien für die Prüfung und Bewertung chemischer Desinfektionsverfahren.* Erster Teilabschnitt. Stuttgart: Gustav Fischer Verlag.

BSI (British Standards Institution) (1960) *Method for Laboratory Evaluation of Disinfectant Activity of Quaternary Ammonium Compounds.* BS 3286: 1960, London: BSI.

BSI (British Standards Institution) (1985) *Determination of the Rideal–Walker Coefficient of Disinfectants.* BS 541: 1985, London: BSI.

BSI (British Standards Institution) (1986) *Assessing the Efficacy of Disinfectants by the Modified Chick–Martin Test.* BS 808: 1986, London: BSI.

BSI (British Standards Institution) (1987) *Estimation of Concentration of Disinfectants Used in 'Dirty' Conditions in Hospitals by the Modified Kelsey–Sykes Test.* BS 6905: 1987, London: BSI.

CEN (European Committee for Standardization, Comité Européen de Normalisation, Europäisches Komitee für Normung) (1996a) *Chemical Disinfectants and Antiseptics—Basic Bactericidal Activity—Test Method and Requirements (Phase 1).* prEN 1040: 1996.

CEN (European Committee for Standardization, Comité Européen de Normalisation, Europäisches Komitee für Normung) (1996b) *Chemical Disinfectants and Antiseptics—Basic Fungicidal Activity—Test Method and Requirements (Phase 1).* prEN 1275: 1996.

Cole, E.C., Rutala, W.A. & Samsa, G.P. (1988) Disinfectant testing using a modified use-dilution method: collaborative study. *Journal of the Association of Official Analytical Chemists*, **71**, 1187–1194.

Council of Europe (1987) *Test Methods for the Antimicrobial Activity of Disinfectants in Food Hygiene.* Strasbourg: Council of Europe.

Cremieux, A. & Fleurette, J. (1991) Methods of testing disinfectants. In *Disinfection, Sterilization and Preservation* (ed. Block, S.S.), 4th edn, pp. 1009–1027. Philadelphia: Lea & Febiger.

Croshaw, B. (1981) Disinfectant testing—with particular reference to the Rideal–Walker and Kelsey–Sykes tests. In *Disinfectants: Their Use and Evaluation of Effectiveness* (eds Collins, C.H., Allwood, M.C., Bloomfield, S.F. & Fox, A.), pp. 1–15. London: Academic Press.

Danielson, J.W. (1993) Evaluation of microbial loads of *Bacillus subtilis* spores on penicylinders. *Journal of AOAC International*, **76**, 355–360.

DGHM (Deutsche Gesellschaft für Hygiene und Mikrobiologie) (1991) *Prüfung und Bewertung chemischer Desinfektionsverfahren. Stand: 12.7.1991.* Wiesbaden: mhp-Verlag.

DGHM (Deutsche Gesellschaft für Hygiene und Mikrobiologie) (1996) Quantitative suspension test with *Mycobacterium terrae* for testing instruments disinfectants. *Hygiene und Medizin*, **21**, 375–380.

DVG (Deutsche Veterinärmedizinische Gesellschaft) (1988) *Richtlinien für die Prüfung chemischer Desinfektionsmittel*, 2nd edn. Giessen: Deutsche Veterinärmedizinische Gesellschaft.

Gundermann, K.O. (1987) Zur Frage der Empfindlichkeit der verschiedenen Mykobakterienstämme gegen Desinfektionsmittel unterschiedlicher Zusammensetzung. *Das Ärztliche Laboratorium*, **33**, 327–330.

Hamilton, M.A., De Vries, T.A. & Rubino, J.R. (1995) Hard surface carrier test as a quantitative test of disinfection: a collaborative study. *Journal of AOAC International*, **78**, 1102–1109.

Heicken, K. (1949) Die Prüfung und Wertbestimmung chemischer Desinfektionsmittel für die Zimmerdesinfektion. *Zeitschrift für Hygiene*, **129**, 538–569.

Hingst, V., Wurster, C. & Sonntag, H.-G. (1990) A quantitative test method for the examination of antimycobacterial disinfection procedures. *Zentralblatt für Hygiene und Umweltmedizin*, **190**, 127–140.

Hugo, W.B. (1978) Early studies in the evaluation of disinfectants. *Journal of Antimicrobial Chemotherapy*, **4**, 489–494.

Kelsey, J.C. & Maurer, I.M. (1966) An in-use test for hospital disinfectants. *Monthly Bulletin of the Ministry of Health and the Public Health Laboratory Service*, **25**, 180–184.

Kelsey, J.C. & Maurer, I.M. (1974) An improved (1974) Kelsey–Sykes test for disinfectants. *Pharmaceutical Journal*, **207**, 528–530.

Kelsey, J.C. & Sykes, G. (1969) A new test for the assessment of disinfectants with particular reference to their use in hospitals. *Pharmaceutical Journal*, **202**, 607–609.

Kelsey, J.C., Beeby, M.M. & Whitehouse, C.W. (1965) A capacity use-dilution test for disinfectants. *Monthly Bulletin of the Ministry of Health and the Public Health Laboratory Service*, **24**, 152–160.

Kliewe, H., Heicken, K., Schmidt, B. *et al.* (1959) *Richtlinien für die Prüfung chemischer Desinfektionsmittel*. Deutsche Gesellschaft für Hygiene und Mikrobiologie. Stuttgart. Gustav Fischer Verlag.

Lensing, H.H. & Oei, H.L. (1985) Investigations on the sporicidal and fungicidal activity of disinfectants. *Zentralblatt für Bakteriologie, Parasitenkunde, Infektionskrankheiten und Hygiene, I. Abteilung Originale, Reihe B*, **181**, 487–495.

Miner, N.A., Mulberry, G.K., Starks, A.N. *et al.* (1995) Identification of possible artifacts in the Association of Official Analytical Chemists sporicidal test. *Applied and Environmental Microbiology*, **61**, 1658–1660.

Mossel, D.A.A. (1963) The rapid evaluation of disinfectants intended for use in food processing plants. *Laboratory Practice*, **12**, 898–890.

Mulberry, G.K. (1995) Current methods of testing disinfectants. In *Chemical Germicides in Health Care* (ed. Rutala, W.A.), pp. 224–235. Washington: Association for Professionals in Infection Control.

Prince, J. & Ayliffe, G.A.J. (1972) In-use testing of disinfectants in hospitals. *Journal of Clinical Pathology*, **25**, 586–589.

Reuter, G. (1989) Anforderungen an die Wirksamkeit von Desinfektionsmitteln für den lebensmittelverarbeitenden Bereich. *Zentralblatt für Bakteriologie, Parasitenkunde, Infektionskrankheiten und Hygiene, I. Abteilung Originale, Reihe B*, **187**, 564–577.

Reybrouck, G. (1975) A theoretical approach of disinfectant testing. *Zentralblatt für Bakteriologie, Parasitenkunde, Infektionskrankheiten und Hygiene, I. Abteilung Originale, Reihe B*, **160**, 342–367.

Reybrouck, G. (1980) A comparison of the quantitative suspension tests for the assssment of disinfectants. *Zentralblatt für Bakteriologie, Parasitenkunde, Infektionskrankheiten und Hygiene, I. Abteilung Originale, Reihe B*, **170**, 449–456.

Reybrouck, G. (1986) Uniformierung der Prüfung von Desinfektionsmitteln in Europa. *Zentralblatt für Bakteriologie, Parasitenkunde, Infektionskrankheiten und Hygiene, I. Abteilung Originale Reihe B*, **182**, 485–498.

Reybrouck, G. (1990a) The assessment of the bactericidal activity of surface disinfectants. 1. A comparison of three practical tests. *Zentralblatt für Hygiene und Umweltmedizin*, **190**, 479–491.

Reybrouck, G. (1990b) The assessment of the bactericidal activity of surface disinfectants. II. Two other practical tests. *Zentralblatt für Hygiene und Umweltmedizin*, **190**, 492–499.

Reybrouck, G. (1990c) The assessment of the bactericidal activity of surface disinfectants. III. Practical tests for surface disinfection. *Zentralblatt für Hygiene und Umweltmedizin*, **190**, 500–510.

Reybrouck, G. (1991) International standardization of disinfectant testing: is it possible? *Journal of Hospital Infection*, **18** (Suppl. A), 280–288.

Reybrouck, G. (1992) The assessment of the bactericidal activity of surface disinfectants. IV. The AOAC use-dilution method and the Kelsey–Sykes test. *Zentralblatt für Hygiene und Umweltmedizin*, **192**, 432–437.

Reybrouck, G. & Van de Voorde, H. (1975) Aussagekraft der Ergebnisse von vier nationalen Methoden zur Wertbestimmung von Desinfektionsmitteln. *Zentralblatt für Bakteriologie, Parasitenkunde, Infektionskrankheiten und Hygiene, I. Abteilung Originale, Reihe B*, **160**, 541–550,

Reybrouck, G. & Werner, H.-P. (1977) Ausarbeitung eines neuen quantitativen *in-vitro*-Tests für die bakteriologische Prüfung chemischer Desinfektionsmittel. *Zentralblatt für Bakteriologie, Parasitenkunde, Infektionskrankheiten und Hygiene, I. Abteilung Originale, Reihe B*, **165**, 126–137.

Reybrouck, G, Borneff, J., Van De Voorde, H. & Werner, H.-P. (1979) A collaborative study on a new quantitative suspension test, the *in vitro* test, for the evaluation of the bactericidal activity of chemical disinfectants. *Zentralblatt für Bakteriologie, Parasitenkunde, Infektionskrankheiten und Hygiene, I. Abteilung Originale, Reihe B*, **168**, 463–479.

Robert Koch Institute (1995) Guideline of the Robert Koch Institute on validation of the efficacy of disinfectants for chemical disinfection of instruments in the case of tuberculosis. *Hygiene und Medizin*, **20**, 80–84.

Robison, R.A., Osguthorpe, R.J., Carroll, S.J., Leavitt, R.W., Schaalje, G.B. & Ascenzi, J.M. (1996) Culture variability associated with the US Environmental Protection Agency tuberculocidal activity test method. *Applied and Environmental Microbiology*, **62**, 2681–2686.

Rubino, J.R., Bauer, J.M., Clarke, P.H., Woodward, B.B., Porter, F.C. & Hilton, H.G. (1992) Hard surface carrier test for efficiency testing of disinfectants: collaborative study. *Journal of AOAC International*, **75**, 635–645.

Sattar, S.A., Best, M., Springthorpe, V.S. & Sanani, G. (1995) Mycobactericidal testing of disinfectants: an update. *Journal of Hospital Infection*, **30** (Suppl.), 372–382.

Scott, E., Bloomfield, S.F. & Barlow, C.G. (1984) Evaluation of disinfectants in the domestic environment under 'in-use' conditions. *Journal of Hygiene, Cambridge*, **92**, 193–203.

Stockinger, H., Böhm, R. & Strauch, D. (1989) Die vergleichende experimentelle Prüfung zweier verschiedener Desinfektionsmittelwirkstoffe auf Sporozidie im Modellversuch mit Sporen pathogener und apathogener Clostridienarten sowie von *Bacillus cereus*. *Zentralblatt für Hygiene und Umweltmedizin*, **188**, 166–178.

Van Klingeren, B. (1978) Experience with a quantitative carrier test for the evaluation of disinfectants. *Zentralblatt für Bakteriologie, Parasitenkunde, Infektionskrankheiten und Hygiene, I. Abteilung Originale, Reihe B*, **167**, 514–527.

Van Klingeren, B. & Pullen, W. (1987) Comparative testing of disinfectants against *Mycobacterium tuberculosis* and *Mycobacterium terrae* in a quantitative suspension test. *Journal of Hospital Infection*, **10**, 292–298.

Van Klingeren, B., Leussink, A.B. & Van Wijngaarden, L.J. (1977) A collaborative study on the repeatability and the reproducibility of the Dutch standard-suspension test for the evaluation of disinfectants. *Zentralblatt für Bakteriologie, Parasitenkunde, Infektionskrankheiten und Hygiene, I. Abteilung Originale, Reihe B*, **164**, 521–548.

B. EVALUATION OF BIOCIDAL ACTIVITY BY RAPID METHODS

1 Introduction

The words 'viable' and 'viability' and their converse have long exercised microbiologists. Nowhere is this more apposite than when experiments are designed to evaluate the microbicidal activity of a test compound (Sykes, 1965). By tradition, such tests have invariably involved treatment of the test organism, quenching or other neutralization (Russell *et al.*, 1979) of residual activity and either transfer of an aliquot to a liquid medium to detect if turbidity is/is not produced after incubation (qualitive method) or to a solid recovery medium for colony production after incubation (quantitative procedure). In the former technique, one cell (theoretically) or many cells will be ultimately responsible for visible growth, whereas in the latter it is assumed that each surviving cell is eventually responsible for a colony and conversely that each colony has arisen from a single cell and not from, say, a clump of cells. Full details were provided in Chapter 4A.

Such methods can be laborious and time-consuming, with incubation at an appropriate temperature for 24 h (and preferably longer) adding to the length of time needed to determine whether, and to what extent, a microbidical effect has been achieved. Further, bacterial spores have to germinate and grow into vegetative cells before cell division takes place (Russell, 1990), and many mycobacterial species are notoriously slow growers (Grange, 1996).

It is, therefore, an attractive idea to consider whether viability can be detected far more rapidly than by these conventional procedures (Lloyd & Hayes, 1995). Here, we consider briefly: (i) some classical techniques that have been in existence for many years, although not necessarily used to detect viability after exposure of a microorganism to an inimical agent; and (ii) more modern procedures, together with their perceived advantages and limitations.

2 Historical aspects

2.1 Biochemical methods

Rapid methods for determining bacterial presence, for example on a surface in a food factory or in a microbicidal system, are a much published research field and the subject of many recent symposia. However, many experimental approaches were undertaken several years ago, sometimes as early as the last century. A few examples will be given below.

Extensive studies on bacterial metabolism were proceeding in the 1920s in the Department of Biochemistry at Cambridge University. One paper of interest described the action of chemicals on the dehydrogenases of *Bacterium (Escherichia) coli*

(Quastel & Whetham, 1925), which led to further studies in this field (Sykes, 1939).

Using molecular oxygen rather than methylene blue as hydrogen acceptor, Baker *et al.* (1941) studied the action of synthetic detergents on bacterial metabolism. An alternative hydrogen acceptor, triphenyltetrazolium bromide, was examined by Hugo (1952).

None of these biochemical methods involving bacterial enzyme inhibition has been adopted for evaluating biocidal activity (Hugo, 1952). One biochemical method that has been adopted, however, is that which seeks to determine adenosine triphosphate (ATP) as an indicator or reporter in bacteria. The procedure utilizes a reaction between the luciferin–luciferase enzyme complex and ATP to give light, the intensity of which can be measured (Stewart, 1990). It is interesting to note that luminous bacteria were used as early as 1942 as a rapid method for determining antibiotic activity.

2.2 Physical methods

When bacteria grow, they produce metabolites which alter the conductivity of the medium, a property first observed in 1898. With the use of modern electrical measuring equipment, this nineteenth-century observation has been put to use as a rapid impedance microbiology technique (Silley & Forsythe, 1996). Equally, when bacteria metabolize, they produce heat. Microcalorimetry has consequently been investigated as a rapid method (Beezer, 1980).

3 Rapid methods and their possible uses

3.1 Direct epifluorescent filtration technique (DEFT)

The principle of this procedure is that viable microorganisms fluoresce (orange-red) when stained with acridine orange, whereas non-viable cells do not (Denyer *et al.*, 1989; Pettipher *et al.*, 1989). Thus, examination and counting of cells under a fluorescent microscope can provide a quantitative assessment of the number of viable cells present. In practice (Pettipher, 1986; Pettipher *et al.*, 1989), the liquid to be tested is filtered through a membrane filter, which is then stained with acridine orange and examined microscopically.

The method has been used in microbiological quality control, for the rapid estimation of microbial counts in foods, beverages, meat and poultry and for detecting organisms in urine and in intravenous fluids.

3.2 Flow cytometry

Several reviews have appeared that discuss the principles of flow cytometry (Lloyd, 1993; McSherry, 1994; Davey & Kell, 1996). The method has been used to evaluate antibacterial and antiprotozoal activity, as discussed below. In a typical flow cytometer, individual particles pass through an illumination zone at the rate of several thousand cells per second; appropriate detectors measure the magnitude of a pulse representing the extent of light scattered. By 'labelling' the cells with fluorescent molecules, e.g. an appropriate dye, that have high specificity to one particular cellular constituent, it is possible to measure the content of that constituent (Shapiro, 1990).

Flow cytometry can be used to detect viable and dead bacterial cells, and has been employed to assess the lethal effects of biguanides and other biocides on spores and trophozoites of *Acanthamoeba castellanii* (Khunkitti *et al.*, 1997) and the damaging effects of antibiotics on bacteria (Suller *et al.*, 1997).

3.3 Microcalorimetry

Microcalorimetry is based upon the principle that bacteria and other microorganisms produce heat when they metabolize. Microcalorimeters can detect the small amount of heat produced (Beezer, 1980).

The technique can be applied to evaluating the effects of inimical treatments on microorganisms. Following biocidal exposure and quenching of residual biocidal activity, organisms are transferred to a nutrient medium. Any surviving cells will, during subsequent incubation, metabolize and generate heat.

3.4 Bioluminescence

Some marine bacteria can emit light. A segment of

deoxyribonucleic acid (DNA) was isolated from *Photobacterium (Vibrio) fischeri* and cloned into *E. coli*, which was thereby provided with a bioluminescent phenotype (Engebrecht *et al.*, 1983). Bioluminescence provides a direct measure of viability (Stewart *et al.*, 1991; 1996) and a rapid means of measuring bacterial response to inimical treatments (Stewart *et al.*, 1991). The procedure has been used to measure the effects of phenol (Stewart *et al.*, 1991) and other biocides (Walker *et al.*, 1992) on bioluminescent *E. coli* and to compare the rsults with those obtained by conventional plating experiments. Decimal reduction times (*D*-values) obtained by the two methods were identical, and both procedures could be used for determining concentration exponents (dilution coefficients, η-values) with equal confidence. Bioluminescence thus provides a rapid method for evaluating biocidal activity and can detect a 5 $\log_{10}$ reduction in viability from a starting inoculum of around 10^7 colony-forming units (cfu)ml.

The system has now been expanded to bacterial spores and sporicidal activity (Hill *et al.*, 1994). Dark spores of *Bacillus* spp. are produced from phenotypically bioluminescent vegetative cells, since spores do not possess the energy to drive the light reaction (Carmi *et al.*, 1987). During germination of lux-containing spores, however, bioluminescence is produced. Highly luminescent *Bacillus subtilis* cells have been constructed that can express a *luxAB* fusion gene from vegetative or sporulation-specific promoters. These *B. subtilis* spores have been used to monitor ethylene oxide sterilization and the use of a germination-specific promoter element, rather than a vegetative cell-specific promoter element, is claimed to enable sublethally injured spores to be detected (Hill *et al.*, 1994).

3.5 Triphenyltetrazolium chloride (TTC) reduction

Triphenyltetrazolium chloride (TTC) reduction by bacteria has long been recognized (Section 2). This principle was utilized by Hurwitz & McCarthy (1986) in developing a rapid test for evaluating biocidal activity against *E. coli*. In essence, cells exposed to a biocide are removed by filtrate, excess biocide quenched and the filter transferred to a growth medium containing TTC. During subsequent incubation at 37°C, formazan is extracted and colour development measured spectrophotometrically.

The method permits a 2–3 $\log_{10}$ reduction cycle to be followed and inactivation kinetics to be calculated. The incubation period takes about 4–5 h to provide a minimum detection level of *c.* 10^5 cfu/ml.

4 Conclusions

The development of rapid methods for evaluating biocidal activity provides an exciting element in the current evolution of biocides as increasingly important infection-control and preservative agents. To date, no rapid method has replaced a traditional one, but bioluminescence in particular offers scope for further investigation.

The possibility that damaged, but not inactivated, microbial cells require additional periods of time and other appropriate recovery conditions for repair has not always been addressed and needs to be considered in further studies.

5 References

Baker, Z., Harrison, R.H. & Miller, B.F. (1941) Action of synthetic detergents on the metabolism of bacteria. *Journal of Experimental Medicine*, **73**, 249–271.

Beezer, A.E. (1980) *Biological Microcalorimetry*. London: Academic Press.

Carmi, O.A., Stewart, S.G.A.B., Ulitzer, S. & Kuhn, J. (1987) Use of bacterial luciferase to establish a promoter probe vehicle capable of nondestructive real-time analysis of gene expression in *Bacillus* spp. *Journal of Bacteriology*, **169**, 2165–2170.

Davey, H.M. & Kell, D.B. (1996) Flow cytometry and cell sorting of heterogeneous microbial populations: the importance of single-cell analayses. *Microbiology Reviews*, **60**, 641–696.

Denyer, S.P., Lynn, R.A.P & Proves, P.S. (1989) Medical and pharmaceutical applications of the direct epifluorescent filter technique (DEFT). In *Rapid Microbiological Methods for Foods, Beverages and Pharmaceuticals* (eds Stannard, C.J., Petitt, S.B. & Skinner, F.A.), Society for Applied Bacteriology, Technical Series No. 25, pp. 59–71. Oxford: Blackwell Scientific Publications.

Engebrecht, J., Nealson, K. & Silverman, M. (1983) Bacterial bioluminescence—isolation and generic analysis of functions from *Vibrio fischeri*. *Cell*, **32**, 773–781.

Grange, J.M. (1996) The biology of the genus *Mycobacterium*. *Journal of Applied Bacteriology Symposium Supplement* **81**, 1S–9S.

Hill, P.J., Hall, L, Vinicombe, D.A. *et al.* (1994) Bioluminescence and spores as biological indicators of inimical processes. *Journal of Applied Bacterioogy Symposium Supplement*, **76**, 129S–134S.

Hugo, W.B. (1952) Observations on the manometric estimation of bactericidal activity. *Proceedings of the Society for Applied Bacteriology*, **15**, 31–33.

Hurwitz, S.J. & McCarthy, T.J. (1986) 2,3,5-Triphenyltetrazolium chloride as a novel tool in germicide dynamics. *Journal of Pharmaceutical Sciences*, **75**, 912–916.

Khunkitti, W., Avery, S.K., Lloyd, D., Furr, J.R. & Russell, A.D. (1997) Effects of biocides on *Acanthamoeba castellanii* as measured by flow cytometry and plaque assay. *Journal of Antimicrobial Chemotherapy*, **40**, 227–233.

Lloyd, D. (1993) *Flow Cytometry in Microbiology*. London: Springer Verlag.

Lloyd, D. & Hayer, A.J. (1995) Vigour, vitality and viability of microorganisms. *FEMS Microbiology Letter*, **133**, 1–7.

McSherry, J.J. (1994) Uses of flow cytometry in microbiology. *Clinical Microbiology Reviews*, **7**, 576–604.

Pettipher, G.L. (1986) Review: the direct epifluorescent filter technique. *Journal of Food Technology*, **21**, 535–546.

Pettipher, G.L., Kroll, R.G., Farr, L.J. & Betts, R.P. (1989) DEFT: recent developments for foods and beverages. In *Rapid Microbiological Methods for Foods, Beverages and Pharmaceuticals* (eds Stannard, C.J., Petitt, S.B. & Skinner, F.A.), Society for Applied Bacteriology, Technical Series No. 25, pp. 33–45. Oxford: Blackwell Scientific Publications.

Quastel, J.H. & Whetham, M.D. (1925) Dehydrogenases produced by resting bacteria. *Biochemical Journal*, **19**, 520–531.

Russell, A.D. (1990) Bacterial spores and chemical sporicidal agents. *Clinical Microbiology Reviews*, **3**, 99–119.

Russell, A.D., Ahonkai, I. & Rogers, D.T. (1979) Microbiological applications of the inactivation of antibiotics and other antimicrobial agents. *Journal of Applied Bacteriology*, **46**, 207–245.

Shapiro, H.M. (1990) Flow cytometry in laboratory technology: new directions. *ASM News*, **56**, 584–586.

Silley, P. & Forsythe, S. (1996) Impedance microbiology—a rapid change for microbiologists. *Journal of Applied Bacteriology*, **80**, 233–243.

Stewart, G.S.A.B. (1990) *In vivo* bioluminescence: new potentials for microbiology. *Letters in Applied Microbiology*, **10**, 1–8.

Stewart, G.S.A.B., Jassim, S.A.A. & Denyer, S.P. (1991) Mechanisms of action and rapid biocide testing. In *Mechanisms of Action of Chemical Biocides* (eds Denyer, S.P. & Hugo, W.B.), Society for Applied Bacteriology, Technical Series No. 27, pp. 319–329.

Stewart, G.S.A.B., Loessner, M.J. & Scherer, S. (1996) The bacterial lux gene bioluminescent biosensor. *ASM News*, **62**, 297–301.

Suller, M.T.E., Stark, J.M. & Lloyd, D. (1997) A flow cytometric study of antibiotic-induced damage and the development of a rapid antibiotic susceptibility test. *Journal of Antimicrobial Chemotherapy*, **40**, 77–83.

Sykes, G. (1939) The influence of germicides on the dehydrogenases of *Bact. coli*. *Journal of Hygiene, Cambridge*, **39**, 463–469.

Sykes, G. (1965) *Disinfection and Sterilization*, 2nd edn. London: E. & F.N. Spon.

Walker, A.J., Holah, J.T., Denyer, S.P. & Stewart, G.S.A.B. (1992) The antibacterial activity of Virkon measured by colony growth and bioluminescence of *lux* recombinant *Listeria monocytogenes*. *Letters in Applied Microbiology*, **15**, 80–82.

CHAPTER 5

Antifungal Activity of Biocides

1 Introduction

Yeasts and moulds comprise important groups of microorganisms that are responsible for various types of infections and for causing spoilage of foods, pharmaceutical products and cosmetic products. Some fungal species are of agricultural and industrial importance and many cause disease in plants. Yeasts are unicellular ovoid or spherical cells that reproduce by bud formation, sexual spores not being formed. Moulds grow as branching filaments or hyphae, which form a mass of intertwining strands, the mycelium. Yeast-like fungi grow as round or ovoid cells or as non-branching filaments (pseudohyphae), which unlike true hyphae, do not form spores but reproduce by budding. The best-known example of a yeast-like fungus is *Candida*, with *Candida albicans* a particularly important organism because of its association with oral thrush in infants and with intestinal and vaginal candidiasis. *Candida glabrata* is one type of *Candida* that does not produce pseudohyphae.

Fungal infections (mycoses) in humans or animals are essentially of two types: superficial, involving skin, nails or hair and readily transmissible, and deep (or systemic). It is noticeable that comparatively few chemotherapeutic drugs are available for treating deep mycoses; the most important drugs are polyenic antibiotics, imidazoles and flucytosine, with griseofulvin suitable for superficial mycoses. These will not be described *per se*, except to consider how studies with such drugs could point the way for investigations with biocides.

The effects of biocides on bacteria and bacterial spores have been widely studied. A vast literature provides information about sensivity and mechanisms of action and, to some extent, of resistance. This is not true with fungi. Data are comparatively sparse and scattered throughout many types of publication, and there have been few advanced studies of the modes of antifungal action of biocides or of the mechanisms of fungal resistance. Some of these aspects will be considered here, and suggestions made about possible ways of obtaining additional information.

Reviews that deal, in part, with antifungal activity of antiseptics, disinfectants and preservatives have been published by Torgeson (1969), D'Arcy (1971), Hugo (1971), Russell (1971, 1994), Trueman (1971), Dawes (1976), Lueck (1980), Croshaw

& Holland (1984), Haag & Loncrini (1984), Hall (1984), Kabara (1984), Report (1984), Wallhäusser (1984), Gardner & Peel (1986), Chapman (1987), Quinn (1987), Baldry & Fraser (1988), Eigener (1988), Heinzel (1988), Lehmann (1988), Woodcock (1988), Russell & Gould (1991), Koller (1992), Russell & Hugo (1994), Russell & Russell (1995) and Russell & Furr (1996).

2 Fungi: composition and structure

Fungi, as distinct from bacteria, are classified as eukaryotic organisms. They differ from bacteria, the prokaryotes, in many important respects (Wilkinson, 1986). Chiefly, fungi possess a nuclear membrane and mitochondria and contain more than the one chromosome characteristic of bacteria. Their cell wall chemistry also differs profoundly. These facts must be borne in mind when conducting mode of action studies. Fungal structure will now be considered in more detail.

The outermost region, as in bacteria, is the cell wall. This surrounds the delicate plasma (cytoplasmic) membrane, internal to which is the cytoplasm. The fungal cell wall demonstrates mechanical strength and a close relationship exists between wall composition and taxonomic classification (Bartnicki-Garcia, 1968; Table 5.1). Some 80–90% of the dry weight of fungal cell walls is made up of polysaccharides. Skeletal polysaccharides consist of chitin, cellulose and glucans, and are composed mainly of glucose and *N*–acetylglucosamine (GlcNAc), as demonstrated in Fig. 5.1. Chitin is a linear polymer of β (1–4)-

Table 5.1 Chemical composition of fungal cell walls.

Principal cell-wall polymers	Taxonomic class	Example
Chitin, chitosan	Zygomycetes	*Mucor rouxii*
Chitin, glucan	Ascomycetes (mycelial forms)	*Neurospora crassa*
	Deuteromycetes (mycelial forms)	*Aspergillus niger*
Glucan, mannan	Ascomycetes (yeast forms)	*Saccharomyces cerevisiae*
	Deuteromycetes (yeast forms)	*Candida utilis*

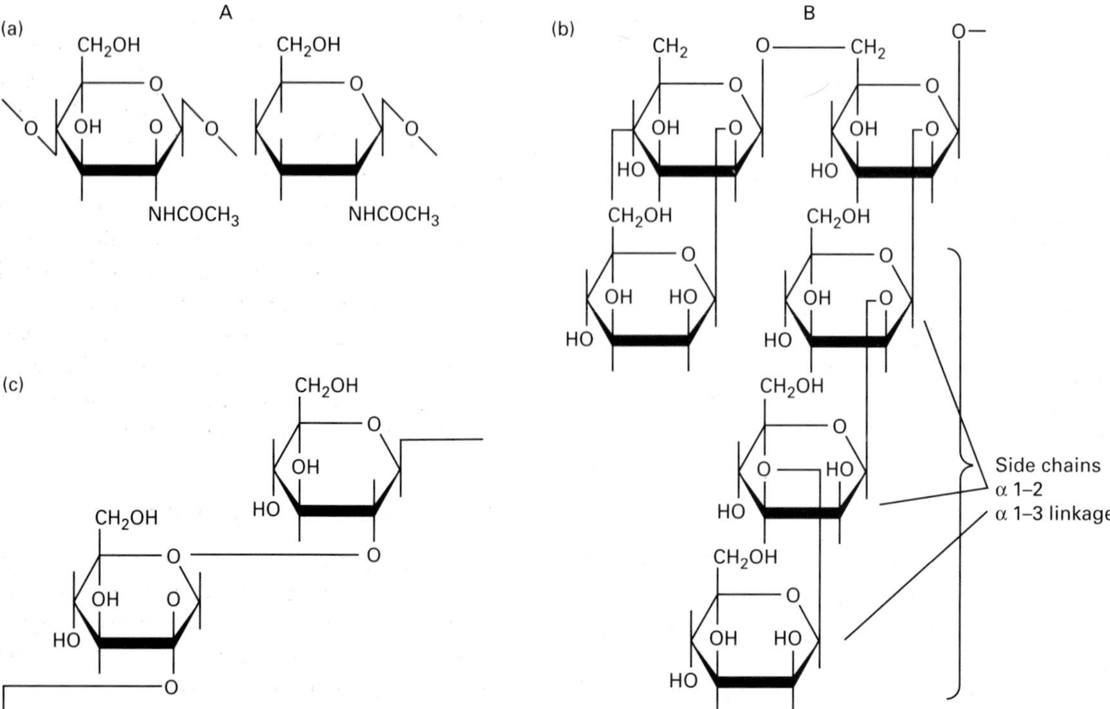

Fig. 5.1 Polysaccharides found in fungal cell walls: (a) chitin; (b) mannan; (c) glucan.

linked *N*-acetylglucosamine molecules and is a universal component of fungal cell walls. In the yeast cell wall, it exists in the α form, where chains are antiparallel in alignment and orientated so that hydrogen bonding is maximal, thereby producing a strong, rigid structure which is highly resistant to chemicals (Gooday, 1979). Chitin appears to be closely associated with other wall polysaccharides, especially glucan, to which it is linked by β (1–6) linkages (Wessels, 1990).

Chitin and β-glucans are responsible for the mechanical strength of the wall. Other sugars, often in chemical complexes with proteins, consist of homo- and heteropolysaccharides, which act as cementing substances (Farkas, 1979). In *Saccharomyces cerevisiae*, the glucan is composed mainly of a high-molecular-weight β(1–3) fraction containing a small proportion of β (1–6) linkages (Balint *et al.*, 1976). Ballou (1976) has described the structure and biosynthesis of the mannan component of fungal cell walls. A small amount of lipid may also be present. For comprehensive details of *Candida* spp., see Odds (1988).

Differences have been noted in the appearance of fungal cell walls in cells of different ages (Farkas, 1979). An interesting aspect of this has been the finding that stationary-phase cells of *C. albicans* are several others more resistant to the polyene antibiotic, amphotericin, than are exponential-phase cells (Gale *et al.*, 1980; Notario *et al.*, 1982). The walls of the former are thicker and more likely, therefore, to act as a barrier to the antibiotic.

The fungal cell wall should not, however, be regarded as a compact structure, since some large molecules can pass through the wall in both directions. This suggests that a certain number of pores must be present (Farkas, 1979) or that a reorganization of the wall structure occurs to produce openings that will allow the passage of these molecules (Scherer *et al.*, 1974).

A schematic design of the cell wall of *S. cerevisiae* and *C. albicans* is presented in Fig. 5.2.

Beneath, and protected by, the cell wall is the plasma membrane (cytoplasmic membrane), which is lipoprotein in nature and in which sterols, notably ergosterol, are present, interrelated with phospholipids, with phosphatidylcholine, phosphatidylethanolamine and phosphatidylinositol

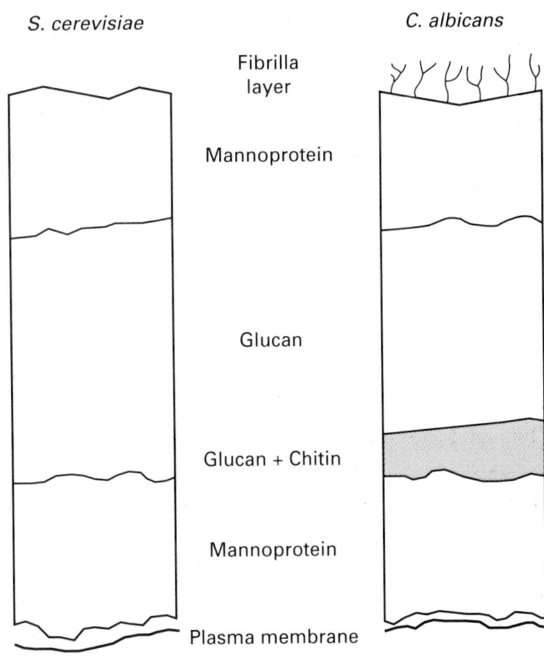

Fig. 5.2 Possible structure of the cell walls of *Saccharomyces cerevisiae* and *Candida albicans*.

forming 70–85% of the total phospholipids. Small amounts of phosphatidylserine have also been reported in certain species (Bowman *et al.*, 1987). Sterols are essential for the stability of fungal membranes; ergosterol is the main sterol detected (Bowman *et al.*, 1987) and is a target site for some chemotherapeutic antifungal drugs.

Fungi are eukaryotes and contain a wide range of membrane-bound organelles, including endoplasmic reticula, mitochondria and well-defined nuclei. The nucleus and other internal organelles (the mitochondria and chloroplasts) are enclosed in membranes within the cytosol, and ribosomes are 80S (40S and 60S subunits), as opposed to the 70S (30S and 50S) found in prokaryotes.

3 Fungal sensitivity to biocides

The chemical and biological properties of a range of antimicrobial agents were considered earlier in this volume (Chapters 2 and 3). In this section, the inhibitory and lethal effects of some of those compounds on fungi will be assessed and a comparison made, where possible, with activity against bacteria and their spores.

3.1 Inhibitory and lethal effects of biocides

Tables 5.2 and 5.3 provide a list of minimum inhibitory concentrations (MICs) and minimum fungicidal concentrations of some antiseptics, disinfectants and preservatives against some commonly found or medically important fungi. From these tables it is possible to reach the following conclusions.

1 Fungicidal concentrations are often much higher than those needed to inhibit growth.
2 Moulds are sometimes, but not invariably, more resistant than yeasts; see, for example, data on chlorhexidine and the organomercury compounds.
3 The parabens show the classical response of increasing activity with ascension of the homologous series from methyl to butyl ester.

More quantitative data with some of these

Table 5.2 Inhibitory concentrations of biocides towards some common fungi (based on data in Wallhäusser, 1984, and D'Arcy, 1971). Quantities are in μg/ml, except for ethanol (% v/v).

	Yeasts		Moulds		
Antimicrobial agent	*C. albicans*	*Sacch. cerevisiae*	*Trichophyton* spp.	*Penicillium* spp.	*Aspergillus* spp.
Organic acids					
Benzoic	500–1000	750		500–1000	500–1000
Dehydroacetic		300			
Propionic	2000			2000	2000
Sorbic	25–50	200–500		200–500	200–500
Parabens					
Methyl	1000	1000	160	500	600
Ethyl	800	500	80	250	400
Propyl	250	125	40	125	200
Butyl	125	63	20	100	150
QACs					
Benzalkonium chloride		20		50	50
Cetrimide/CTAB	12.5	50		100	50
Dequalinium chloride	0.63–5				
Biguanides					
Chlorhexidine	10–20	20		200	200
Phenols					
Chlorocresol	2500	2500			2500
Chloroxylenol	2000	1000			2000
Alcohols					
Benzyl alcohol	2500				5000
Bronopol	200–1000		50–200	200–1000	200–1000
Chlorbutanol		2000			
Ethanol	10%			10%	10%
Phenoxyethanol	5000	5000			5000
Phenylethanol	2500	5000		5000	5000
Mercurials					
PMN/PMA	8	8		16	16
Thiomersal	32	32		128	128

QACs, quaternary ammonium compounds; CTAB, cetyltrimethylammonium bromide, PMA, phenylmercuric acetate; PMN, phenylmercuric nitrate.

Table 5.3 Lethal concentration of biocides towards some fungi (derived from information provided by Wallhäusser, 1984). Quantities are in μg/ml.

Group	Antimicrobial agent	Yeast *Candida albicans*	Moulds *Penicillium chrysogenum*	*Aspergillus niger*
Organic acids	Benzoic	1200	1000	1000
Parabens	Methyl	5000	5000	5000
	Ethyl	2500	2500	5000
	Propyl	625	1250	2500
	Butyl	625	1250	1250
QACs	Benazalkonium chloride	10	100–200	100–200
	Cetrimide/CTAB	25	100	250
Biguanides	Chlorhexidine	20–40	400	200
Alcohols	Chlorbutanol	2500		5000
Mercurials	Thiomersal	128	2048	4096

biocides have been published by Brown & Bullock (1960), Gerrard *et al.* (1960), Chauhan & Walters (1961, 1962), Chauhan *et al.* (1963) and Rivers & Walters (1966). As would be expected, activity depended on concentration, time of exposure and temperature. For example, a 99% kill of *Penicillium notatum* spores at 20°C was achieved in 20 min by 1.125% and in 80 min by 1% phenol (Chauhan & Walters, 1961); as temperature increased, the time to produce this 2-log kill cycle was reduced, being 1 min at 45°C (Chauhan & Walters, 1962). Inhibition of oxygen uptake does not provide a quantitative measure of the fungicidal activity of phenol (Chauhan *et al.*, 1963; Rivers & Walters, 1966) or of other inhibitors (Rivers & Walters, 1966). Fungicidal test methods are described by Czerkowicz (1983) and in Chapter 4.

Chlorhexidine salts are less active against yeasts and moulds than non-sporing bacteria. Inactivation of *C. albicans*, *C. glabrata* and *Sacch. cerevisiae* depends on chlorhexidine concentration, with a tailing off in the rate of kill noted at lower biguanide concentrations (Hiom *et al.*, 1992, 1993).

Glutaraldehyde is a bactericidal, sporicidal and viricidal agent (Gorman *et al.*, 1980). It also shows fungistatic (Dabrowa *et al.*, 1972) and fungicidal activity (Stonehill *et al.*, 1963; Dabrowa *et al.*, 1972; Gorman & Scott, 1977; Gorman *et al.*, 1980; Gray, 1980). Formaldehyde is equally effective in killing *C. albicans* as in killing vegetative Gram-negative bacteria; the conidia of *Aspergillus niger* are more resistant but not more so than *Staphylococcus aureus* (Spicher & Peters, 1976).

Various organic acids, e.g. benzoic, sorbic (Bandelin, 1950; Gooding *et al.*, 1955; Bell *et al.*, 1959; Balatsouras & Polymenacos, 1963; Hunter & Segal, 1973; Krebs *et al.*, 1983; Kabara, 1984; Cole & Keenan, 1987) and the esters of *p*-(4)-hydroxybenzoic acid (Aalto *et al.*, 1953; Maddox, 1982; Haag & Loncrini, 1984; Report, 1984) are effective antifungal agents. Environmental pH markedly affects the activity of the former, but not the antifungal efficacy of the latter.

Peracetic acid is an excellent bactericide, sporicide and fungicide (Baldry, 1983; Baldry & Fraser, 1988), but its activity decreases with increasing pH.

Pospisil (1989) has examined the efficacy of various antiseptic and disinfectant preparations against potentially pathogenic micromycetes, and Berger *et al.* (1976) have described the antifungal properties of electrically generated metallic ions.

The antimicrobial properties of sulphur dioxide (SO_2) depend upon the degree of ionization of the molecule and on pH (Hammond & Carr, 1976; Babich & Stotzky, 1978). When dissolved in water, SO_2 or its salts (sulphite (SO^{2-}), bisulphite (HSO_3^-) and metabisulphite) set up a pH-dependent equilibrium mixture and SO_2 activity is maximal at acid pH. At these low pH values, the proportion of SO_3^{2-} ions decreases and that of SO_2 molecules increases at the expense of bisulphate (HSO_3^-) ions. The active principle is the unbound (free) SO_2 concentration, and molecular SO_2, i.e. the molecules of SO_2 existing in aqueous solution at low pH (Hammond & Carr, 1976), is *c.* 100 and 500 times more active against *A. niger* and yeasts, respectively, than sulphite or bisulphite ions.

Organic sulphur compounds, such as dithiocarbamates, for plant-disease control, and thiram (tetramethylthiuram disulphide), are highly active fungicides, but mercaptans and alkyl sulphides have a low order of fungicidal activity (Owens, 1969). Bent (1979) has described the wide variety of chemical structures that are used as agricultural fungicides. Chlorine compounds are used for killing aspergilli in buildings.

3.2 Comparative responses of bacteria and fungi

Spaulding (1972) has listed the following categories of biocidal activity.

1 High level — a biocide inactivating bacterial spores, vegetative bacteria, fungi, lipid-enveloped and non-lipid-enveloped viruses.
2 Intermediate level — a biocide inactivating all those listed in 1 except bacterial spores.
3 Low level — a biocide inactivating vegetative bacteria, lipid enveloped viruses and fungi only.

From this it can be seen that antifungal activity is perceived as being of a low level, i.e. that fungi are not particularly resistant to biocides. This point of view is substantiated in Favero's (1985) important contribution. Nevertheless, instances abound where activity of a biocide is shown to be considerably less against yeasts and moulds than against non-sporulating bacteria. Some examples are provided in Table 5.4, from which it can be seen that *C. albicans* and (especially) *A. niger* are much more resistant than *Escherichia coli*, *Pseudomonas aeruginosa* and *Staph. aureus* (surprisingly the most resistant bacterial strain) to phenol, two alcohols and a quaternary ammonium compound (QAC). Quaternary ammonium compounds have also been found to be less effective vs. *C. albicans* by Weiner *et al.* (1965).

The kinetic approach to the testing of preservative efficacy is a useful one, since it provides important information about the rate of kill, often measured as the decimal reduction time (*D*-value). This is the time of exposure necessary for a specific concentration at defined pH and temperature to reduce the viable population by one log cycle. This is the approach adopted in Table 5.4, thereby enabling a direct comparison to be made with different organisms. This procedure is based on the work of Orth (1979, 1980, 1984), who developed this method for evaluating preservative efficacy in cosmetics, but it is equally applicable to pharmaceutical products. It is noticeable that Orth pointed out the much higher resistance of *A. niger* and *Aspergillus flavus* to several preservatives than that shown by non-sporulating bacteria. This kinetic assessment can be used to determine the time necessary to inactivate an appropriate fraction of a microbial inoculum added to a test pharmaceutical (or other) product, e.g. as ex-

Table 5.4 Kinetic approach: D values at 20°C of biocides against bacteria and fungi (abstracted from the work of Karabit *et al.*, 1985, 1986, 1988, 1989).

Antimicrobial agent	pH	Concentration (%)	*D*-values (h) vs.				
			A. niger	*C. albicans*	*E. coli*	*Ps. aeruginosa*	*Staph. aureus*
Phenol	5.1	0.5	20	13.5	0.94	–*	0.66
	6.1	0.5	32.4	18.9	1.72	0.166	1.9
Benzyl alcohol	5.0	1.0	28.8	39	0.37	0.16	5.48
	6.1	1.0	76.8	92.1	8.53	1.48	7.2
Benzalkonium	6.1	0.001	–†	9.66	0.06	3.01	3.12
chloride	6.1	0.002	–†	5.5	–*	0.054	0.67
Ethanol	7.1	20	58	1.31	0.03	–*	1.05

*Inactivation so rapid that *D*-values could not be measured.
† No inactivation; fungistatic effect only.

emplified in the British (1998) and United States pharmacopoeias. Table 5.5 compares the requirements of these two official volumes; while there are differences between the compendia, it is again clear that inactivation of bacteria is more rapid than that of yeasts and moulds.

3.3 Uses of antifungal agents

Fungal infections are not usually life-threatening, although some can be serious, particularly in patients with depressed immunity. Chemotherapeutic considerations are outside the scope of this chapter, but it is important to discuss biocides predominantly as: (i) preservatives to prevent contamination or spoilage of formulated products; (ii) disinfectants for those occasions where yeasts and moulds might prove to be an environmental problem or hazard, and (iii) as industrial and agricultural fungicides.

Fungal contamination of food, pharmaceutical and cosmetic products can be a problem, particularly if these are of high water activity (A_w) and stored in warm conditions. Apart from such obvious measures as quality control of all raw materials, including water, the inclusion of a suitable preservative may be necessary. This aspect is covered more fully in Chapters 16 and 17.

Disinfectants specifically for use against yeasts and moulds are not often required, although it is as well to re-emphasize that fungi are often more resistant than non-sporulating bacteria but less so than bacterial spores. Hypochlorites are very effective fungicidal agents.

Agricultural fungicides make up 10–15% of total pesticide sales in the USA. Such fungicides include the most widely used type, the dithiocarbamates (see also Owens, 1969), heterocyclic nitrogen compounds, e.g. captan, quinones, such as chloranil and dichlone, and heavy metals, in particular Bordeaux mixture, a copper salt mixed with lime, which is the most widely used fungicide for control of foliar disease (Bent, 1979; Lukens, 1983). Properties of these were considered in Chapter 2. Industrially important products that may require the presence of an appropriate antifungal-type preservative include wool, cotton, wood and leather (Block, 1983). Further aspects of these are dealt with in the various sections of Chapter 17; see also Lyr (1987a,b).

Benzoic and salicylic acids are used for treating skin infections, and copper 8-quinolonate for treating room surfaces following outbreaks of *Aspergillus* in immunocompromised patients (Barnes & Rogers, 1989). Sulphur dioxide, in the form of appropriate salts, is often applied to foods (Hammond & Carr, 1976).

4 Mechanisms of antifungal action

4.1 Biocide penetration into fungal cells

Comparatively little is known about the ways in which fungi are killed by biocides. It is often assumed that they are inactivated in a similar or identical fashion to vegetative bacteria. While such a proposition has undoubted attractions, the different structural and chemical properties of bacteria and fungi mean that this concept may not necessarily or always be true. Nevertheless, it is probably correct to state that in both the prokaryotic (bacterial) and eukaryotic (fungal)

Table 5.5 Pharmacopoeial requirements in antimicrobial agent tests for preservative efficiency.

	BP (1993)		USP (XXIII)	
Pharmaceutical	Bacteria	Yeasts and moulds	Bacteria	Yeasts and moulds
Sterile products	Not less than a 3-log reduction in 24 h, and no survivors at 28 days	Not less than a 2-log reduction in 7 days, and no increase thereafter	A 3-log reduction in 14 days	No increase after 14 and 28 days

BP, *British Pharmacopoeia*; USP (XXI), *United States Pharmacopoeia*, edn XXIII.

cells the first interaction between biocide and organisms occurs at the cell surface, followed by passage of the biocide across the cell wall (or outer membrane) to reach its target site(s) within the cell. Some biocides are likely to have a predominant effect on the outer layers (Section 4.2). In Gram-positive cocci, simple diffusion across the cell wall is likely to occur; in Gram-negative bacteria, passage occurs either via the hydrophilic or hydrophobic routes, or possibly via a self-promoted entry mechanism (Hancock, 1984). The obvious question arises as to how biocides enter yeasts and moulds, but at present there is little information available. However, Gerston *et al.* (1966) considered that pores in fungal cell walls were too small for the entrance of very large molecules.

The porosity of the yeast cell wall is affected by its chemical composition, the wall acting as a barrier or modulator to the entry and exit of various compounds. According to Scherer *et al.* (1974), compounds with molecular weights not greater than 700 Da can diffuse freely through the yeast wall; these are however, many examples of the secretion of much larger molecules into the medium.

De Nobel *et al.* (1989, 1990a,b) have used the uptake of fluorescein isothiocyanurate (FITC) dextrans and the release of the periplasmic enzyme, invertase, as indicators of yeast cell-wall porosity. Intact *Sacch. cerevisiae* cells were able to endocytose FITC-dextrans of 70 kDA but not of 150 kDa. Subsequently, these authors developed an assay to determine relative cell wall porosity in yeast based upon polycation-induced leakage of ultraviolet (UV)-absorbing compounds.

As the age of a *Sacch. cerevisiae* culture increases, there is a significant increase in the thickness of the cell wall (Hiom *et al.*, 1996) Conversely, the relative porosity decreases with increasing culture age (Hiom *et al.*, 1996). Older cultures also take up less ^{14}C-chlorhexidine gluconate from solution (Hiom *et al.*, 1995a). It is likely that these events are interrelated; since mannan mutants of *Sacch. cerevisiae* show a similar order of sensitivity to the parent strain with regard to chlorhexidine (Hiom *et al.*, 1992), it is possible that the glucan component of the yeast wall has an important role to play in limiting the entry of the biguanide. The glucan layer is shielded from β-glucuronidase by mannoproteins, but this effect is overcome by 2-mercaptoethanol (Zlotnick *et al.*, 1984). The mannoprotein consists of two fractions, namely sodium dodecyl sulphate (SDS)-soluble mannoproteins and SDS-insoluble, glucanase-soluble ones. The latter are known to limit cell-wall porosity (De Nobel *et al.*, 1990a,b). The significance of glucan is further shown by the fact that yeast protoplasts prepared by β-glucuronidase–mecaptoethanol treatment are lysed by concentrations of chlorhexidine well below those active against normal cells (Hiom *et al.*, 1993).

Adsorption of biocides by yeasts and moulds has not been widely studied, although, as with bacteria, it is a phenomenon that has been known for several years. Knaysi & Gordon (1930), for example, described the adsorption of iodine by yeast, and this was later examined in greater detail (Hugo & Newton, 1964). An unusual pattern of uptake, Z-curve adsorption, was noted by Gilbert *et al.* (1978) in their studies on the uptake of 2-phenoxyethanol by *E. coli* and *Candida lipolytica*;

Table 5.6 Postulated mechanisms of action of antifungal agents.

Target	Antifungal	Comment
Fungal cell wall	Glutaraldehyde	Cross-linking agent
Plasma membrane	Chlorhexidine QACs	Leakage of intracellular constituents; probably cause generalized increase in permeability
	Organic acids	Undissociated form is most active Intracellular shift in pH
	Parabens	Not fully understood

interestingly, a C-type adsorption uptake pattern was observed with *Ps. aeruginosa*. The Z-pattern is interpreted as being produced by a concentration of phenoxylethanol that promotes a breakdown in structure of the adsorbing species, i.e. the microorganism, leading to the production of new adsorption sites, whereas the C-pattern is believed to indicate a more ready penetration of biocide into the adsorbate (here the microorganism) than of the solvent. Adsorption of dyes by fixed yeast cells was described by Giles & Mackay (1965).

Chlorhexidine binds strongly to whole cells and isolated cell walls of *Sacch. cerevisiae*; furthermore, it causes a reduction in electrophoretic mobility at biguanide concentrations up to 50 µg/ml, but much higher concentrations (>700 µg/ml) cause reversal of net surface charge (Walters *et al.*, 1983). As with bacteria (Fitzgerald *et al.*, 1989), this interaction takes place very rapidly, but it is not possible to correlate this with the rate of cell inactivation (Hiom *et al.*, 1995a). However, the organism (*Sacch. cerevisiae*) most sensitive to the biguanide took up significantly more chlorhexidine than did other organisms (Hiom *et al.*, 1995a). Norris & Kelley (1979), Gadd & White (1989) and Gadd (1990) have described the accumulation of metals by yeasts and other organisms.

Useful though they are, however, adsorption studies and effects on electrophoretic mobility (surface-charge changes) provide only preliminary data about the site and mechanism of action of a biocide acting on bacteria or fungi. While it would be inadvisable to omit studies on adsorption from any investigation, it would be equally irresponsible to base conclusions about the mode of action solely on whole-cell interactions. Large numbers of microbes are invariably needed (but may be reduced if a radioactive compound is available) and, certainly with some bacterial studies, it may be difficult to relate adsorption of a biocide with cellular sensitivity or resistance. Insufficient is known about adsorption by fungi of differing sensitivities to reach a similar conclusion. Furthermore, ^{14}C-chlorhexidine gluconate is rapidly taken up by yeast cells, as pointed out above, but might be evenly distributed within the organisms (Hiom *et al.*, 1995b).

A most interesting paper dealing with mechanisms for fungitoxicants reaching their site of action was published more than 20 years ago by Miller (1969). Other important reviews are those of Somers (1962), Owens (1963, 1969), Owens & Hayes (1964), Lukens (1971, 1983), Bent (1979) and Lyr (1987b). Hansch & Lien (1971) have surveyed structure–activity relationships in antifungal agents, and information on selective toxicity mechanisms can be obtained from Albert's (1979) extensive work. Lyr (1987a) has edited a comprehensive work on the mechanisms of action of modern selective fungicides.

4.2 Fungal cell walls as targets

Few antimicrobial agents are likely to have the fungal cell wall as a major, or sole, target. Compounds that would be assumed to have at least some effect include cross-linking agents, such as glutaraldehyde and formaldehyde, and cationic biocides, such as QACs and chlorhexidine. It was shown above that biocides do, indeed, adsorb to yeasts, although this in itself does not necessarily explain their mechanism of action.

Glutaraldehyde is an important 'chemosterilizing' agent that combines strongly with $-NH_2$ groups at the microbial cell surface and elsewhere within the cell (Gorman *et al.*, 1980). Glutaraldehyde inhibits spore germination and sporulation, and the presence of polymers (e.g. chitin) in the cell walls of fungi that resemble bacterial peptidoglycan demonstrates a potentially reactive site (Gorman & Scott, 1977). As would be expected from antibacterial studies, the activity of the dialdehyde on *C. lipolytica* increases with concentration, pH and period of contact (Navarro & Monsan, 1976). These authors demonstrated that glutaraldehyde agglutinated the cells of this organism, of *Saccharomyces carisbergensis* and of some bacterial species and increased their settling rate, as a consequence of an effect on the outer cell layers.

4.3 Membrane-active biocides

The plasma membrane is likely to be a major target site for many antifungal agents, as it is for several antibacterial agents (Russell & Hugo, 1988; Kuyyakanond & Quesnel, 1992;

Bassett-Bee *et al.*, 1994; Russell & Chopra, 1996). This section will concentrate on the activity towards fungi of chlorhexidine, QACs, organic acids and ethanol, although other compounds will be considered briefly: see also Table 5.6.

4.3.1 *Chlorhexidine*

Only few studies of any significance have been made on the mechanism of action of chlorhexidine against yeasts. Elferink & Booij (1974) described the effects of chlorhexidine on baker's yeast and found that the biguanide induced the rapid release of K^+ ions, indicative of membrane damage. Similar findings were made by Walters *et al.* (1983), who observed that pentose release from *Sacch. cerevisiae* was induced maximally at a concentration of 50 μg/ml (exposure time 3 h, temperature 30°C), as opposed to an MIC of 7 μg/ml. There was no evidence of lysis, but the highest chlorhexidine level (1000 μg/ml) induced some clumping.

Chlorhexidine and the QAC, cetylpyridinium chloride (CPC), induced leakage and caused protoplast lysis, as well as interacting with crude cell sap (Hiom *et al.*, 1993). However, the diphasic effect noted above with chlorhexidine was not seen with CPC when protoplast lysis was determined. Differing effects were also observed with cell-sap interactions (Hiom *et al.*, 1993). It was also found with chlorhexidine that death preceded leakage.

Bobichon & Bouchet (1987) investigated the action of chlorhexidine, at a sublethal concentration, on the ultrastructure of budding *C. albicans* and observed a loss of cytoplasmic components, indicative of plasma membrane damage, together with coagulation of 'nucleoproteins' and wall modification.

4.3.2 *Quaternary ammonium compounds*

Like chlorhexidine, QACs are known to induce leakage of intracellular material from yeasts (Armstrong, 1957, 1958; Scharff & Beck, 1959; Elferink & Booij, 1974). Armstrong (1957, 1958) studied the effects of six cationic compounds on baker's yeast with a view to exploring any relationship between cytolytic damage, as determined by phosphorus release from treated cells, and metabolism (measured by the conversion of glucose to acid and carbon dioxide). He concluded that the initial toxic effect on the cell was a disorganization of the cell membrane, followed by inactivation of cell enzymes. It has been suggested that one QAC, cetyltrimethylammonium bromide (CTAB), disrupts organized lipid structures in lipid bilayers and in the yeast membrane (Elferink & Booij, 1974).

Low concentrations of benzalkonium chloride stimulated oxygen consumption in baker's yeasts, while inhibiting the Pasteur effect, but without causing appreciable alterations in membrane permeability; higher concentrations, however, induced K^+ loss (Scharff & Beck, 1959). Sevag & Ross (1944), studying the effect of QACs on enzyme systems in yeasts, noted an inhibition of glucose oxidation.

4.3.3 *Organic acids and esters*

Organic acids, such as benzoic and sorbic acids, are rapidly taken up by yeasts (Macris, 1974; Warth, 1977, 1985, 1986, 1988; Krebs *et al.*, 1983). They act as lipophilic acids, which damage the plasma membrane, and at the acid pH at which they are employed the anion is concentrated in the cytoplasm. Hunter & Segal (1973) provided evidence for an inhibition of active transport in *Penicillium chrysogenum*. Cole & Keenan (1987) proposed that *Zygosaccharomyces bailii* increased its cytoplasmic buffering capacity and secreted organic acids during normal metabolism, and thus concluded that acid tolerance in this organism was based on an ability to withstand large falls in intracellular pH. Krebs *et al.* (1983) showed that, in *Sacch. cerevisiae*, benzoic acid enters the cell in its undissociated form and that the neutralization of the acid within the cell caused an intracellular pH shift of more than one pH unit.

Mitchell's chemiosmotic theory (considered in greater detail in Chapter 9) is a mechanism whereby, during metabolism, protons are extruded, with acidification of the external environment. Hunter & Segal (1973), in their studies on the effects of weak acids on amino acid transport in *P. chrysogenum*, have demonstrated the existence of a proton or charge gradient as the driving force. Organic acids and esters produce inhibition of Δ pH across the bacterial cytoplasmic membrane, and a similar effect may be produced in fungi.

4.3.4 Alcohols

Ethanol induces leakage of intracellular material from *Sacch. cerevisiae* and ethanol tolerance has been claimed to be associated with reduced leakage (Salueiro *et al.*, 1988). Lipid composition and plasma-membrane fluidity also play a role in the susceptibility of yeasts to alcohol (Alexandre *et al.*, 1994). Ethanol transport in the bacterium, *Zymomonas mobilis*, has been measured *in vivo* by using nuclear magnetic resonance spin transfer (Schoberth *et al.*, 1996), a technique that would be useful with yeasts under different conditions.

4.3.5 Other agents

Heavy metals, e.g. copper salts and organomercury compounds, may act by binding to key functional groups of enzymes in fungi (Lukens, 1983). Quinones, such as chloranil and dichlone, may produce alkylation of $-NH_2$ groups in enzymes. Simon (1953a,b,c) found that 3,5-dinitro-*o*-cresol acted as an uncoupling agent in yeast, stimulating oxygen uptake. Ethylenediamine tetraacetate (EDTA) affects fungal membranes (Indge, 1968a,b), inducing K^+ leakage (Elferink, 1974) and decreasing protoplast resistance to osmotic lysis (Diamond & Rose, 1970). Sulphur dioxide interacts with enzyme systems (Hammond & Carr, 1976). A particularly sensitive target site for the action of sulphite in *Sacch. cerevisiae* appears to be glyceraldehyde-3-phosphate dehydrogenase, although it is unclear whether the enzyme *per se*, its substrate or its cofactor is inactivated, since all contain sensitive groups (Gould & Russell, 1991).

4.4 Other target sites

Other potential target sites in fungi include the ribosomes, nucleic acids and structural and functional (enzymes) proteins. It is difficult to state the role of ribosomes, structural protein, ribonucleic acid (RNA) and deoxyribonucleic acid (DNA) as targets for fungicidal attack, since so few relevant studies have been made.

In contrast, some investigations (considered in Section 4.3.2) have examined effects of antifungal agents on specific enzyme systems, at least some of which are associated with the plasma membrane. However, as pointed out by Hugo (1981), it is difficult to envisage a situation in which inhibition and/or cell death can be accounted for by inhibition of a specific enzyme, unless this reaction is essential for the metabolism of the cell. Thus enzyme inactivation must be considered as being only one of many inhibited reactions, and it is unlikely to be the primary mechanism of action of an antifungal agent.

Sulphur dioxide interacts with disulphide bridges in proteins, e.g., cystine sulphitolysis is responsible for cleavage of the disulphide bond in cystine, producing cysteine and cysteine sulphonate. Interaction of sulphur dioxide with nucleic acids is responsible for mutagenic effects in yeasts (Hammond & Carr, 1976).

5 Possible mechanisms of fungal resistance to biocides

5.1 Theoretical concepts

Two basic mechanisms of fungal resistance to biocides can be envisaged (Table 5.7). In the first, natural (intrinsic) resistance is associated with the innate ability of a fungal cell to present a permeability barrier to one or more biocides, or to inactivate a biocide by virtue of constitutively present enzymes. In the second, acquired resistance to a biocide could ensue as a result of mutation or via the acquisition of genetic material. While a considerable amount of information is available about these two major aspects of bacterial resistance to antibiotics and there is a steadily accumulating fund of knowledge of resistance to biocides (Russell & Chopra, 1996), data on the mechanisms of fungal resistance to non-antibiotic agents are sparse. Fungal resistance to agricultural fungicides is discussed by Dekker (1987) and Georgopoulos (1987), and Hector (1993) describes compounds active against fungal cell walls.

5.2 Intrinsic biocide resistance

The structure of the fungal cell wall (see Table 5.1

Table 5.7 Possible mechanisms of fungal resistance to biocides.

Type of resistance	Possible mechanisms
Intrinsic	Exclusion of biocide, thereby limiting uptake into cell Enzymatic inactivation Phenotypic modulation
Acquired	Mutation Inducible elimination system Plasmid-mediated response

and Fig. 5.1) suggests that there is ample opportunity for a cell to exclude biocide molecules. No significant investigations have been made to date with biocides, but some evidence accumulated from studies on the sensitivity of *C. albicans* to the polyenic antibiotic, amphotericin (Gale, 1986; Kerridge, 1986), points the way towards a more fundamental approach. It should be possible to determine the component(s) of cell walls responsible for limiting biocide entry by the use of appropriate cell wall-degrading enzymes and specific wall-acting antibiotics or other drugs, by using cells of different physiological ages and by the utilization of mutant strains that are defective in a cell wall component. Some studies with *Sacch. cerevisiae* (Hiom *et al.*, 1992, 1993, 1995a,b) have likewise shown that the culture age influences the response to chlorhexidine. When these results are considered in conjunction with the findings discussed in Section 4.2, it is possible to examine those parameters that might influence the susceptibility of this organism to the biguanide (Table 5.8).

Yeasts grown under different conditions show different levels of sensitivity to ethanol. Cells with linoleic acid-enriched membranes are more resistant than cells with oleic acid-enriched membranes, from which it has been inferred (Gomez & Herrero, 1983; Rose, 1987) that a more fluid membrane enhances ethanol resistance, as pointed out above.

Production of hydrogen sulphide (H_2S) by microorganisms can reduce heavy-metal toxicity, because H_2S combines with heavy metals to form insoluble sulphides. Consequently, H_2S-producing microbes may demonstrate tolerance to such metals. For example, strains of *Sacch. cerevisiae* that produce H_2S are more tolerant to copper and mercury than are non-tolerant strains, because in the tolerant strains the metals are precipitated as insoluble sulphides (Gadd & Griffiths, 1978; Gadd, 1990). Inactivation of an organomercury compound, phenylmercuric acetate, by *Penicillium roqueforti* Thom has been observed (Russell, 1955), although reduced permeability to the phenylmercury ion has also been proposed as a mechanism of resistance or tolerance (Greenaway, 1972; Greenaway *et al.*, 1978). Tolerance to organomercury has been found in *Pyrenophora avenae* (Crosier *et al.*, 1970).

Inactivation of other fungitoxic agents has also been described. Yanagita (1980), Kato *et al.* (1982, 1983) and Heinzel (1988) have all reported the

Table 5.8 Possible parameters influencing susceptibility of *Saccharomyces cerevisiae* to chlorhexidine (Based on Hiom *et al.*, 1996).

Parameter	Possible role in chlorhexidine (CHA) susceptibility
Cell wall composition	
Mannan	Unlikely to be of significance
Glucan	Possible significance: yeast protoplasts are lysed by CHA concentrations below those active vs. 'ordinary' cells
Cell wall thickness	Increases in cells in older cultures Possible significance in reducing CHA uptake
Relative porosity	Decreases in cells in older cultures Possible significance in reducing CHA uptake

role of formaldehyde dehydrogenase in resistance to formaldehyde, and the degradation of potassium sorbate by a *Penicillium* species has also been observed. The ability of certain fungi to reduce toxic metallic arsenic derivatives to the volatile and dispersible arsine has been known from the time when these compounds were used as wallpaper colourants.

5.3 Acquired biocide resistance

There appears to be no evidence linking the presence of plasmids in fungal cells and the ability of the organisms to acquire resistance to fungicidal or fungistatic agents. However, acquired resistance to organic acids has been described. Starved cells of *Saccharomyces bailii* concentrate benzoic and sorbic acids intracellularly, whereas in the presence of glucose their intracellular concentration is reduced considerably. The effect of glucose can be quenched by means of metabolic inhibitors (Warth, 1977). Pitt (1974) had previously shown that growth of this organism in the presence of subinhibitory concentrations of a preservative greatly increased its resistance when exposed to higher concentrations, higher resistance levels being found in the presence of higher glucose levels. Thus, this organism possesses an inducible preservative elimination system. In subsequent studies, Warth (1985, 1986, 1988) demonstrated that a major effect of benzoic acid on yeasts of various levels of susceptibility in the presence of glucose was the energy requirement for the reduction in cytoplasmic benzoate concentration and the maintenance of internal pH (pH_i). Hydrogen ions arising from the dissociation of benzoic acid inside the cell must be exported, hence the need for the energy requirement to maintain the alkaline pH. Benzoate in energized cells is considered to be eliminated by flowing down the electrochemical gradient (Warth, 1988). A similar model may apply to explain the resistance of acid-tolerant yeasts to acetate (Moon, 1983). However, Cole & Keenan (1987) consider that resistance of *Zygosacch. bailii* to weak acids is not the consequence of a simple pH_i-independent extrusion pumping mechanism, but that it includes an ability of the cell to tolerate significant pH_i falls with a consequent compensation by a re-establishment of a 'normal' pH_i value. Warth (1989a,b,c) has since demonstrated that organic acids, but not methyl paraben, are continuously removed from the cell. The prime permeability barrier to propanoic acid in *Zygosacch. bailii* is the plasma membrane and not the cell wall (Warth, 1989a).

6 Conclusions

A considerable variation exists in the response of various yeasts and moulds to biocides. Generally, fungi are more resistant than non-sporulating bacteria (except mycobacteria) to these agents, but more susceptible than bacterial spores. Consequently, sporicidal compounds, such as glutaraldehyde and chlorine-based disinfectants, will also be fungicidal. The mechanisms of action of fungitoxic compounds are often poorly understood, as are reasons for differing sensitivities shown by fungi. Nevertheless, some progress is now being made in understanding the uptake of chemical agents by fungal cells and of the components of the cell wall that might present a barrier (Table 5.8).

Antifungal agents are important in product preservation, as disinfectants and as agricultural and industrial fungicides. Bent's (1979) review describes the range of chemical compounds investigated for use as agricultural fungicides, and illustrates the chemical structures of many of them.

7 References

Aalto, T.R., Firman, M.C. & Rigler, N.E. (1953) *p*-Hydroxybenzoic acid esters as preservatives. I. Uses, antibacterial and antifungal studies, properties and determination. *Journal of the American Pharmaceutical Association, Scientific Edition*, **42**, 449–457.

Albert, A. (1979) *Selective Toxicity: the Physicochemical Basis of Therapy*, 6th edn. London: Chapman & Hall.

Alexandre, H., Rousseaux, I. & Charpentier, C. (1994) Relationship between ethanol tolerance, lipid composition and plasma membrane fluidity in *Saccharmoyces cerevisiae* and *Koleckera apiculata*. *FEMS Microbiology Letters*, **124**, 17–22.

Armstrong, W.M. (1957) Surface-active agents and cellular metabolism. I. The effect of cationic detergents on the production of acid and carbon dioxide by baker's yeast. *Archives of Biochemistry and Biophysics*, **71**, 137–147.

Armstrong, W.M. (1958) The effect of some synthetic dyestuffs on the metabolism of baker's yeast. *Archives of Biochemistry and Biophysics*, **73**, 153–160.

Babich, H.L. & Stotzky, S. (1978) Influence of pH on inhibition of bacteria, fungi and coliphages by bisulphite and sulphite. *Environmental Research*, **15**, 405–417.

Balatsouras, G.D. & Polymenacos, N.G. (1963) Chemical preservatives as inhibitors of yeast growth. *Journal of Food Science*, **28**, 267–275.

Baldry, M.G.C. (1983) The bactericidal, fungicidal and sporicidal properties of hydrogen peroxide and peracetic acid. *Journal of Applied Bacteriology*, **54**, 417–423.

Baldry, M.G.C. & Fraser, J.A.L. (1988) Disinfection with peroxygens. In *Industrial Biocides* (ed. Payne, K.R.), Critical Reports on Applied Chemistry, Vol. 22, pp. 91–116. Chichester: John Wiley & Sons.

Balint, S., Farkas, V. & Bauer, S. (1976) Biosynthesis of β-glucans catalyzed by a particulate enzyme preparation from yeast. *FEBS Letters*, **64**, 44–47.

Ballou, C.E. (1976) Structure and biosynthesis of the mannan component of the yeast cell envelope. *Advances in Microbial Physiology*, **14**, 93–158.

Bandelin, F.J. (1950) The effects of pH on the efficiency of various mould inhibiting compounds. *Journal of the American Pharmaceutical Association, Scientific Edition*, **47**, 691–694.

Barnes, R.A. & Rogers, T.R.F. (1989) Control of an outbreak of nosocomial aspergillosis by laminar air-flow isolation. *Journal of Hospital Infection*, **14**, 89–94.

Barrett-Bee, K., Newboult, L. & Edwards, S. (1994) The membrane destabilising action of the antibacterial agent chlorhexidine. *FEMS Microbiology Letters*, **119**, 249–254.

Bartnicki-Garcia, S. (1968) Cell wall chemistry, morphogenesis and taxonomy of fungi. *Annual Review of Microbiology*, **22**, 87–108.

Bell, T.A., Etchells, J.L. & Borg, A.F. (1959) Influence of sorbic acid on the growth of certain species of bacteria, yeasts and filamentous fungi. *Journal of Bacteriology*, **77**, 573–580.

Bent, K.J. (1979) Fungicides in perspective: 1979. *Endeavour*, **3** (1), 7–14.

Berger, T.J., Spadaro, J.A., Bierman, R., Chapin, S.E. & Becker, R.O. (1976) Antifungal properties of electrically generated metallic ions. *Antimicrobial Agents and Chemotherapy*, **10**, 856–860.

Block, S.S. (1983) Preservatives for industrial products. In *Disinfection, Sterilization and Preservation* (ed. Block, S.S.), 3rd edn, pp. 608–655. Philadelphia: Lea & Febiger.

Bobichon, H. & Bouchet, P. (1987) Action of chlorhexidine on budding *Candida albicans*: scanning and transmission electron microscopic study. *Mycopathologia*, **100**, 27–35.

Bowman, B.J., Borgeson, C.E. & Bowman, E.J. (1987) Composition of *Neurospora crassa* vacuolar membranes and comparison to endoplasmic reticulum, plasmalemmas and mitochondrial membranes. *Experimental Mycology*, **11** 197–205.

British Pharmacopoeia (1998) London: Pharmaceutical Press.

Brown, M.R.W. & Bullock, K. (1960) Mould spore suspensions and powders for use in fungicidal kinetic studies. Part I. Preliminary experiments with *Rhizopus nigricans* and *Penicillium digitatum*. *Journal of Pharmacy and Pharmacology*, **12**, 119T–126T.

Chapman, D.G. (1987) Preservatives available for use. In *Preservatives in the Food, Pharmaceutical and Environmental Industries* (eds Board, R.G., Allwood, M.C. & Banks, J.G.), Society for Applied Bacteriology Technical Series No. 22, pp. 177–195. Oxford: Blackwell Scientific Publications.

Chauhan, N.M. & Walters, V. (1961) Studies on the kinetics of fungicidal action. Part I. The effect of concentration and time on the viability of *Penicillium notatum* spores in solutions of phenol. *Journal of Pharmacy and Pharmacology*, **13**, 470–478.

Chauhan, N.M. & Walters, V. (1962) Studies on the kinetics of fungicidal action. Part II. The effect of temperature on the viability of *Penicillium notatum* spores in water and solutions of phenol. *Journal of Pharmacy and Pharmacology*, **14**, 605–610.

Chauhan, N.M., Rivers, S.M. & Walters, V. (1963) On the relationship between the effect of phenol on the oxygen uptake and the viability of *Penicillium notatum* spores. *Journal of Pharmacy and Pharmacology*, **15**, 143T–147T.

Cole, M.B. & Keenan, M.H.J. (1987) Effects of weak acids and external pH on the intracellular pH of *Zygosaccharomyces bailii*, and its implications in weak-acid resistance. *Yeast*, **3**, 23–32.

Croshaw, B. & Holland, V.R. (1984) Chemical preservatives: use of bronopol as a cosmetic preservative. In *Cosmetic and Drug Preservation: Principles and Practice* (ed. Kabara, J.J.), pp. 31–62. New York: Marcel Dekker.

Crosier, W.F., Waters, E.C. & Crosier, D.C. (1970) Development of tolerance to organic mercurials by *Pyrenophora avenae*. *Plant Disease Reporter*, **54**, 783–785.

Czerkowicz, T.J. (1983) Methods of testing fungicides. In *Disinfection, Sterilization and Preservation* (ed. Block, S.S.), 3rd edn, pp. 998–1008. Philadelphia: Lea & Febiger.

Dabrowa, N., Landau, J.W. & Newcomer, V.D. (1972) Antifungal activity of glutaraldehyde *in vitro*. *Archives of Dermatology*, **105**, 555–557.

D'Arcy, P.F. (1971) Inhibition and destruction of moulds and yeasts. In *Inhibition and Destruction of the Microbial Cell* (ed. Hugo, W.B.), pp. 613–686. London: Academic Press.

Dawes, I.W. (1976) The inactivation of yeasts. In *Inhibition and Inactivation of Vegetative Microbes* (eds Skinner, F.A. & Hugo, W.B.), Society for Applied Bacteriology Symposium Series No. 5, pp. 279–304. London: Academic Press.

Dekker, J. (1987) Development of resistance to modern fungicides and strategies for its avoidance. In *Modern Selective Fungicides* (ed. Lyr, H.), pp. 39–52. Harlow, Essex: Longman.

De Nobel, J.G., Dijkers, C., Hooijberg, E. & Klis, F.M. (1989) Increased cell wall porosity in *Saccharomyces cerevisiae* after treatment with dithiothreitol or EDTA. *Journal of General Microbiology*, **135**, 2077–2084.

De Nobel, J.G., Klis, F.M., Munnik, T. & Van Den Ende, H. (1990a) An assay of relative cell porosity in *Saccharomyces cerevisiae, Kluyveromyces lactis* and *Schizosaccharomyces pombe. Yeast*, **6**, 483–490.

De Nobel, J.G., Klis, F.M., Munnik, T. & Van Den Ende, H. (1990b) The glucanase-soluble mannoproteins limit cell wall porosity in *Saccharomyces cerevisiae. Yeast*, **6**, 491–499.

Diamond, R.J. & Rose, A.H. (1970) Osmotic properties of spheroplasts from *Saccharomyces cerevisiae* grown at different temperatures. *Journal of Bacteriology*, **102**, 311–319.

Eigener, U. (1988) Disinfectant testing and relevance in practical application. In *Industrial Biocides* (ed. Payne, K.R.), Critical Reports on Applied Chemistry, Vol. 22, pp. 37–51. Chichester: John Wiley & Sons.

Elferink, J.G.R. (1974) The effect of ethylenediaminetetra-acetic acid on yeast cell membranes. *Protoplasma*, **80**, 261–268.

Elferink, J.G.R. & Booij, H.L. (1974) Interaction of chlorhexidine with yeast cells. *Biochemical Pharmacology*, **23**, 1413–1419.

Farkas, V. (1979) Biosynthesis of cell walls of fungi. *Microbiological Reviews*, **43**, 117–144.

Favero, M.S. (1985) Sterilization, disinfection and antisepsis in the hospital. In *Manual of Clinical Microbiology* (eds Lennette, E.H., Balows, A., Hausler, W.J., Jr & Shadomy, H.J.), 4th edn, pp. 129–137. Washington, DC: American Society for Microbiology.

Fitzgerald, K.A., Davies, A. & Russell, A.D. (1989) Uptake of ^{14}C-chlorhexidine diacetate to *Escherichia coli* and *Pseudomonas cerevisiae* and its release by azolectin. *FEMS Microbiology Letters*, **60**, 327–332.

Gadd, G.M. (1990) Metal tolerance. In *Microbiology of Extreme Environments* (ed. Edwards, C.), pp. 178–210. Milton Keynes: Open University Press.

Gadd, G.M. & Griffiths, A.J. (1978) Microorganisms and heavy metal toxicity. *Microbial Ecology*, **4**, 303–317.

Gadd, G.M. & White, C. (1989) Heavy metal and radionuclide accumulation and toxicity in fungi and yeasts. In *Metal–Microbe Interactions* (eds Poole, R.K. & Gadd, G.M.), Special Publications of the Society for General Microbiology, No. 26, pp. 19–38. Oxford: Oxford University Press.

Gale, E.F. (1986) Nature and development of phenotypic resistance to amphotericin B in *Candida albicans. Advances in Microbial Physiology*, **27**, 277–320.

Gale, E.F., Ingram, H., Kerridge, D., Notario, V. & Wayman, F. (1980) Reduction of amphotericin resistance in stationary phase cultures of *Candida albicans* by treatment with enzymes. *Journal of General Microbiology*, **117**, 383–391.

Gardner, J.F. & Peel, M.M. (1986) *Introduction to Sterilization and Disinfection.* Edinburgh and London: Churchill Livingstone.

Georgopoulos, S.G. (1987) The genetics of fungicide resistance. In *Modern Selective Fungicides* (ed. Lyr, H.), pp. 53–63. Harlow, Essex: Longman.

Gerrard, H.N., Harkiss, A.V. & Bullock, K. (1960) Mould spore suspensions and powders for use in fungicidal kinetic studies. Part II. Preparations using *Penicillium spinulosum. Journal of Pharmacy and Pharmacology*, **12**, 127T–133T.

Gerston, H., Parmegiana, R., Weiner, A. & D'Ascoli, R. (1966) Fungal spore walls as a possible barrier against potential antifungal agents of the group copper (II) complexes of 5-halogeno- and 5-nitro-8-quinolinols. *Contributions of the Boyce Thompson Institute*, **23**, 219–228.

Gilbert, P., Beveridge, E.G. & Sissons, I. (1978) The uptake of some membrane-active agents by bacteria and yeast: possible microbiological examples of Z-curve adsorption. *Journal of Colloid and Interfacial Science*, **64**, 377–379.

Giles, C.H. & McKay, R.B. (1965) The adsorption of cationic (basic) dyes by fixed yeast cells. *Journal of Bacteriology*, **89**, 390–397.

Gomez, R.F. & Herrero, A.A. (1983) Chemical preservation of foods. In *Economic Microbiology* (ed. Rose, A.H.), Vol. 8: *Food Microbiology*, pp. 77–116. London: Academic Press.

Gooday, G.W. (1979) Chitin synthesis and differentiation in *Coprinus cinereus.* In *Fungal Walls and Hyphal Growth* (eds Burnett, J.H. & Trinci, A.P.J.), pp. 203–223. Cambridge: Cambridge University Press.

Gooding, C.M., Melnick, D., Lawrence, R.L. & Luckmann, F.H. (1955) Sorbic acid as a fungistatic agent for foods. IX. Physico-chemical considerations in using sorbic acid to protect foods. *Food Research*, **20**, 639–648.

Gorman, S.P. & Scott, E.M. (1977) A quantitative evaluation of the antifungal properties of glutaraldehyde. *Journal of Applied Bacteriology*, **43**, 83–89.

Gorman, S.P., Scott, E.M. & Russell, A.D. (1980) Antimicrobial activity, uses and mechanism of action of glutaraldehyde. *Journal of Applied Bacteriology*, **48**, 161–190.

Gould, G.W. & Russell, N.J. (1991). Sulphite. In *Food Preservatives* (eds Russell, N.J. & Gould, G.W.), pp. 72–88. Glasgow and London: Blackie.

Gray, K.G. (1980) The microbiology of glutaraldehyde. *Australian Journal of Hospital Pharmacy*, **10**, 139–141.

Greenaway, W. (1972) Permeability of phenyl-Hg^+-resistant and phenyl-Hg^+-susceptible isolates of *Pyrenophora avenae* to the phenyl-Hg^+ ion. *Journal of General Microbiology*, **73**, 251–255.

Greenaway, W., Ward, S., Rajan, A.K. & Whatley, F.R. (1978) A spectrophotometric technique for recording uptake of an organomercurial by mycelial fungi. *Journal of General Microbiology*, **107**, 31–35.

Haag, T.E. & Loncrini, D.F. (1984) Esters of *para*-hydroxy-benzoic acid. In *Cosmetic and Drug Preservation: Principles and Practice* (ed. Kabara, J.J.), pp. 63–67. New York: Marcel Dekker.

Hall, A.L. (1984) Cosmetically acceptable phenoxy-ethanol. In *Cosmetic and Drug Preservation: Principles and Practice* (ed. Kabara, J.J.), pp. 79–108. New York: Marcel Dekker.

Hammond, S.M. & Carr, J.G. (1976) The antimicrobial activity of SO_2 with particular reference to fermented and non-fermented fruit juices. In *Inhibition and Inactivation of Vegetative Microbes* (eds Skinner, F.A. & Hugo, W.B.), Society for Applied Bacteriology Symposium Series No. 5, pp. 89–110. London: Academic Press.

Hancock, R.E.W. (1984) Alterations in outer membrane permeability. *Annual Review of Microbiology*, **38**, 237–264.

Hansch, C. & Lien, E.J. (1971) Structure–activity relationships in antifungal agents: a survey. *Journal of Medicinal Chemistry*, **14**, 653–669.

Hector, R.F. (1993) Compounds active against cell walls of medically important fungi. *Clinical Microbiology Reviews*, **6**, 1–21.

Heinzel, M. (1988) The phenomena of resistance to disinfectants and preservatives. In *Industrial Biocides* (ed. Payne, K.R.), Critical Reports on Applied Chemistry, Vol. 22, pp. 52–67. Chichester: John Wiley & Sons.

Hiom, S.J., Furr, J.R., Russell, A.D. & Dickinson, J.R. (1992) Effects of chlorhexidine diacetate on *Candida albicans, C. glabrata* and *Saccharomyces cerevisiae*. *Journal of Applied Bacteriology*, **72**, 335–340.

Hiom, S.J., Furr, J.R., Russell, A.D. & Dickinson, R.J. (1993) Effects of chlorhexidine diacetate and cetyl-pyridinium chloride on whole cells and protoplasts of *Saccharomyces cerevisiae*. *Microbios*, **74**, 111–120.

Hiom, S.J., Furr, J.R. & Russell, A.D. (1995a) Uptake of ^{14}C-chlorhexidine gluconate by *Saccharomyces cerevisiae, Candida albicans* and *Candida glabrata*. *Letters in Applied Microbiology*, **21**, 20–22.

Hiom, S.J., Hann, A.C., Furr, J.R. & Russell, A.D. (1995b) X-ray microanalysis of chlorhexidine-treated cells of *Saccharomyces cerevisiae*. *Letters in Applied Microbiology*, 353–356.

Hiom, S.J., Furr, J.R., Russell, A.D. & Hann, A.C. (1996) The possible role of yeast cell walls in modifying cellular response to chlorhexidine diacetate. *Cytobios*, **86**, 123–135.

Hugo, W.B. (1971) Amidines. In *Inhibition and Destruction of the Microbial Cell* (ed. Hugo, W.B.), pp. 121–136. London: Academic Press.

Hugo, W.B. (1981) The mode of action of antiseptics. In *Handbuch der Antiseptik* (eds Weuffen, W., Kramer, A., Gröschel, D., Berencsi, G. & Bulka, E.), Band I, Teil 2, pp. 39–77. Berlin: VEB Verlag Volk un Gesundheit.

Hugo, W.B. & Newton, J.M. (1964) The adsorption of iodine from solution by microorganisms and by serum. *Journal of Pharmacy and Pharmacology*, **16**, 48–55.

Hunter, D.R. & Segal, I.H. (1973) Effect of weak acids on amino acid transport by *Penicillium chrysogenum*: evidence for a proton or charge gradients as the driving force. *Journal of Bacteriology*, **113**, 1184–1192.

Indge, K.J. (1968a) The effect of various anions and cations on the lysis of yeast protoplasts by osmotic shock. *Journal of General Microbiology*, **41**, 425–432.

Indge, K.J. (1968b) Metabolic lysis of yeast protoplasts. *Journal of General Microbiology*, **41**, 433–440.

Kabara, J.J. (1984) Composition and structure of microorganisms. In *Cosmetic and Drug Preservation: Principles and Practice* (ed. Kabara, J.J.), pp. 21–27. New York: Marcel Dekker.

Karabit, M.S., Juneskans, O.T. & Lundgren, P. (1985) Studies on the evaluation of preservative efficacy. I. The determination of antimicrobial characteristics of phenol. *Acta Pharmaceutica Suecica*, **22**, 281–290.

Karabit, M.S., Juneskans, O.T. & Lundgren, P. (1986) Studies on the evaluation of preservative efficacy. II. The determination of antimicrobial characteristics of benzyl alcohol. *Journal of Clinical and Hospital Pharmacy*, **11**, 281–289.

Karabit, M.S., Juneskans, O.T. & Lundgren, P. (1988) Studies on the evaluation of preservative efficacy. III. The determination of antimicrobial characteristics of benzalkonium chloride. *International Journal of Pharmaceutics*, **46**, 141–147.

Karabit, M.S., Juneskans, O.T. & Lundgren, P. (1989) Factorial designs in the evaluation of preservative efficacy. *International Journal of Pharmaceutics*, **56**, 169–174.

Kato, N., Miyawaki, N. & Sakasawa, C. (1982) Oxidation of formaldehyde by resistant yeasts *Debaryomyces vanriji* and *Trichosporon penicil-*

latum. *Agricultural and Biological Chemistry*, **46**, 655–661.

Kato, N., Miyawaki, N. & Sakasawa, C. (1983) Formaldehyde dehydrogenase from formaldehyde-resistant *Debaryomyces vanriji* FT-1 and *Pseudomonas putida* F61. *Agricultural and Biological Chemistry*, **47**, 415–416.

Kerridge, D. (1986) Mode of action of clinically important antifungal drugs. *Advances in Microbial Physiology*, **27**, 1–72, 321.

Knaysi, G. & Gordon, M. (1930) The manner of death of certain bacteria and yeast when subjected to mild chemical and physical agents. *Journal of Infectious Diseases*, **47**, 303–317.

Koller, W. (1992) Antifungal agents with target sites in sterol functions and biosynthesis. In *Target Sites of Fungicides Action* (ed. Koller, W.), pp. 119–206. Boca Raton: CRC Press.

Krebs, H.A., Wiggins, D., Stubbs, M., Sols, A. & Bedoya, F. (1983) Studies on the antifungal action of benzoate. *Biochemical Journal*, **214**, 657–663.

Kuyyakanond, T. & Quesnel, L.B. (1992) The mechanism of action of chlorhexidine. *FEMS Microbiology Letters*, **100**, 211–216.

Lehmann, R.H. (1988) Synergisms in disinfectant formulations. In *Industrial Biocides* (ed. Payne, K.R.), Critical Reports on Applied Chemistry, Vol. 22, pp. 68–90. Chichester: John Wiley & Sons.

Lueck, E. (1980) *Antimicrobial Food Additives*. New York: Springer-Verlag.

Lukens, R.J. (1971) *Chemistry of Fungicidal Action*. Molecular Biology, Biochemistry and Biophysics, No. 10. London: Chapman & Hall.

Lukens, R.J. (1983) Antimicrobial agents in crop production. In *Disinfection, Sterilization and Preservation* (ed. Block, S.S.), 3rd edn, pp. 695–713. Philadelphia: Lea & Febiger.

Lyr, H. (ed.) (1987a) *Modern Selective Fungicides*. Harlow, Essex: Longman.

Lyr, H. (1987b) Selectivity in modern fungicides and its basis. In *Modern Selective Fungicides* (ed. Lyr, H.), pp. 31–88. Harlow, Essex: Longman.

Macris, B.J. (1974) Mechanism of benzoic acid uptake by *Saccharomyces cerevisiae*. *Applied Microbiology*, **30**, 503–506.

Maddox, D.N. (1982) The role of *p*-hydroxybenzoates in modern cosmetics. *Cosmetics & Toiletries*, **97**, (11), 85–88.

Marth, E.H., Capp, C.M., Hasenzahl, L., Jackson, H.W. & Hussong, R.V. (1966) Degradation of potassium sorbate by *Penicillium* species. *Journal of Dairy Science*, **49**, 1197–1205.

Miller, L.P. (1969) Mechanisms for reaching the site of action. In *Fungicides: An Advanced Treatise* (ed. Torgeson, D.C.), Vol. 2, pp. 1–58. New York: Academic Press.

Moon, N.J. (1983) Inhibition of the growth of acid tolerant yeasts by acetate, lactate and propionate and their synergistic mixtures. *Journal of Applied Bacteriology*, **55**, 453–460.

Navarro, J.M. & Monsan, P. (1976) Étude du mécanisme d'interaction du glutaraldéhyde avec les microorganismes. *Annales Microbiologie (Institut Pasteur)*, **127B**, 295–307.

Norris, P.R. & Kelley, D.P. (1979) Accumulation of metals by bacteria and yeasts. *Developments in Industrial Microbiology*, **20**, 299–308.

Notario, V., Gale, E.F., Kerridge, D. & Wayman, F. (1982) Phenotypic resistance to amphotericin B in *Candida albicans*: relationship to glucan metabolism. *Journal of General Microbiology*, **128**, 761–777.

Odds, F.C. (1988) *Candida and Candidosis: A Review and Bibliography*. London: Baillière Tindall.

Orth, D.S. (1979) Linear regression method for rapid determination of cosmetic preservative efficacy. *Journal of the Society of Cosmetic Chemists*, **30**, 321–332.

Orth, D.S. (1980) Establishing cosmetic preservative efficacy by use of D-values. *Journal of the Society of Cosmetic Chemists*, **31**, 165–172.

Orth, D.S. (1984) Evaluation of preservatives in cosmetic products. In *Cosmetic and Drug Preservation: Principles and Practice* (ed. Kabara, J.J.), pp. 403–421. New York: Marcel Dekker.

Owens, R.G. (1963) Chemistry and physiology of fungicidal action. *Annual Review of Phytopathology*, **1**, 77–100.

Owens, R.G. (1969) Organic sulfur compounds. In *Fungicides: An Advanced Treatise* (ed. Torgeson, D.C.), Vol. 2, pp. 147–301. New York: Academic Press.

Owens, R.G. & Hayes, A.D. (1964) Biochemical action of thiram and some dialkyl dithiocarbamates. *Contributions of the Boyce Thompson Institute*, **22**, 227–240.

Pitt, J.I. (1974) Resistance of some food spoilage yeasts to preservatives. *Food Technology in Australia*, **26**, 238–241.

Pospisil, J. (1989) Efficacy of selected disinfectants and antiseptic preparations against potentially pathogenic micromycetes. *Cs. Epidemiologie, Mikrobiologie, Immunologie*, **38**, 180–187.

Quinn, P.J. (1987) Evaluation of veterinary disinfectants and disinfection processes. In *Disinfection in Veterinary and Farm Animal Practice* (eds Linton, A.H., Hugo, W.B. & Russell, A.D.), pp. 66–116. Oxford: Blackwell Scientific Publications.

Report (1984) Final report on the safety assessment of methylparaben, ethylparaben, propylparaben and butylparaben. *Journal of the American College of Toxicology*, **3**, 147–209.

Rivers, S.M. & Walters, V. (1966) The effect of benzoic

acid, phenol and hydroxybenzoates on the oxygen uptake and growth of some lipolytic agents. *Journal of Pharmacy and Pharmacology*, **18**, 45S–51S.

Rose, A.H. (1987) Responses to the chemical environment. In *The Yeasts* (ed. Rose, A.H. & Harrison, J.S.), 2nd edn, Vol. 2: *Yeasts and the Environment*, pp. 5–40. London: Academic Press.

Russell, A.D. (1971) Ethylenediamine tetraacetic acid. In *Inhibition and Destruction of the Microbial Cell* (ed. Hugo, W.B.), pp. 209–224. London: Academic Press.

Russell, A.D. (1994) Glutaraldehyde: its current status and uses. *Infection Control and Hospital Epidemiology*, **15**, 724–733.

Russell, A.D. & Chopra, I. (1996) *Understanding Antibacterial Action and Resistance*, 2nd edn. Chichester: Ellis Horwood.

Russell, A.D. & Furr, J.R. (1996) Biocides: mechanisms of antifungal action and fungal resistance. *Science Progress*, **79**, 27–48.

Russell, A.D. & Hugo, W.B. (1988) Perturbation of homeostatic mechanisms in bacteria by pharmaceuticals. In: *FEMS Symposium No. 44*, pp. 206–219. Bath: Bath University Press.

Russell, A.D. & Hugo, W.B. (1994) Antibacterial activity and resistance. *Progress in Medicinal Chemistry*, **31**, 351–371.

Russell, A.D. & Russell, N.J. (1995) Biocides: activity, action and resistance. In *Fifty Years of Antimicrobials: Past Perspectives and Future Trends* (eds Hunter, P.A., Darby, G.K. & Russell, N.J.), 53rd Symposium of the Society for General Microbiology, pp. 327–365. Cambridge: Cambridge University Press.

Russell, N.J. & Gould, G.W. (eds) (1991) *Food Preservatives*. Glasgow & London: Blackie.

Russell, P. (1955) Inactivation of phenylmercuric acetate in ground wood pulp by a mercury-resistant strain of *Penicillium roqueforti* Thom. *Nature, London*, **176**, 1123–1124.

Salueiro, S.P., Sa-Correia, I. & Novias, J.M. (1988) Ethanol-induced leakage in *Saccharomyces cerevisiae*: kinetics and relationship to yeast ethanol tolerance and alcohol fermentation productivity. *Applied and Environmental Microbiology*, **54**, 903–909.

Scharff, T.G. & Beck, J.L. (1959) Effects of surface-active agents on carbohydrate metabolism in yeast. *Proceedings of the Society of Experimental Biology and Medicine*, **100**, 307–311.

Scherer, R., Loudon, L. & Gerhardt, P. (1974) Porosity of the yeast cell wall and membrane. *Journal of Bacteriology*, **118**, 534–540.

Schoberth, S.M., Chapman, B.E., Kuchel, P.W. *et al.*: (1996) Ethanol transport in *Zymomonas mobilis* measured by using *in vivo* nuclear magnetic resonance spin transfer. *Journal of Bacteriology*, **178**, 1756–1761.

Sevag, M.G. & Ross, O.A. (1944) Studies on the mechanism of the inhibitory action of zephiran on yeasts cells. *Journal of Bacteriology*, **48**, 677–682.

Simon, E.W. (1953a) The action of nitrophenols in respiration and glucose assimilation in yeasts. *Journal of Experimental Botany*, **4**, 377–392.

Simon, E.W. (1953b) Dinitrocresol, cyanide and the Pasteur effect in yeast. *Journal of Experimental Botany*, **4**, 393–402.

Simon, E.W. (1953c) Mechanisms of dinitrophenol toxicity. *Biological Reviews*, **28**, 453–479.

Somers, E. (1962) Mechanisms of toxicity of agricultural fungicides. *Science Progress*, **198**, 218–234.

Spaulding, E.H. (1972) Chemical disinfection and antisepsis in the hospital. *Journal of Hospital Research*, **9**, 5–31.

Spicher, G. & Peters, J. (1976) Microbial resistance to formaldehyde. I. Comparative quantitative studies in some selected species of vegetative bacteria, bacterial spores, fungi, bacteriophages and viruses [in German]. *Zentralblatt für Bakteriologie, Parasitenkunde, Infektionskrankheiten und Hygiene, I. Abteilung Originale Reihe B*, **163**, 486–508.

Splittstoesser, D.F., Queale, D.T. & Mattick, L.R. (1978) Growth of *Saccharomyces bisporus* var. *bisporus*, a yeast resistant to sorbic acid. *American Journal of Enology and Viticology*, **29**, 272–276.

Stonehill, A.A., Krop, S. & Borick, P.M. (1963) Buffered glutaraldehyde, a new chemical sterilizing solution. *American Journal of Hospital Pharmacy*, **20**, 458–465.

Tadeusiak, B. (1976) Fungicidal activity of glutaraldehyde. *Roczniki Panstwowego Zakladu Higieny* (Poland), **27**, 689–695.

Torgeson, D.C. (ed.) (1969) *Fungicides: An Advanced Treatise*, Vol. 2. London: Academic Press.

Trueman, J.R. (1971) The halogens. In *Inhibition and Destruction of the Microbial Cell* (ed. Hugo, W.B.), pp. 137–183. London: Academic Press.

United States Pharmacopoeia (1995) Edition XXIII. Rockville, MD: US Pharmacopoeia Convention.

Wallhäusser, K.H. (1984) Antimicrobial preservatives used by the cosmetic industry. In *Cosmetic and Drug Preservation: Principles and Practice* (ed. Kabara, J.J.), pp. 605–745. New York: Marcel Dekker.

Walters, T.H., Furr, J.R. & Russell, A.D. (1983) Antifungal action of chlorhexidine. *Microbios*, **38**, 195–204.

Warth, A.D. (1977) Mechanism of resistance of *Saccharomyces bailii* to benzoic, sorbic and other weak acids used as food preservatives. *Journal of Applied Bacteriology*, **43**, 215–230.

Warth, A.D. (1985) Resistance of yeast species to benzoic and sorbic acids and to sulfur dioxide. *Journal of Food Protection*, **48**, 564–569.

Warth, A.D. (1986) Effect of nutrients and pH on the resistance of *Zygosaccharomyces bailii* to benzoic acid. *International Journal of Food Microbiology*, **3**, 263–271.

Warth, A.D. (1988) Effect of benzoic acid on growth yield of yeasts differing in their resistance to preservatives. *Applied and Environmental Microbiology*, **54**, 2091–2095.

Warth, A.D. (1989a) Transport of benzoic and propanoic acids by *Zygosaccharomyces bailii*. *Journal of General Microbiology*, **135**, 1383–1390.

Warth, A.D. (1989b) Relationships among cell size, membrane permeability and preservative resistance in yeast species. *Applied and Environmental Microbiology*, **55**, 2995–2999.

Warth, A.D. (1989c) Relationships between the resistance of yeasts to acetic, propanoic and benzoic acids and to methyl paraben and pH. *International Journal of Food Microbiology*, **8**, 343–349.

Weiner, N.D., Hart, F. & Zografi, G. (1965) Application of the Ferguson principle to the antimicrobial activity of quaternary ammonium salts. *Journal of Pharmacy and Pharmacology*, **17**, 350–355.

Wessels, J.G.H. (1990) Gene expression during fruiting in *Schizophyllum commune*. *Mycological Research*, **98**, 609–620.

Wilkinson, J.F. (1986) *Introduction to Microbiology*, 3rd edn. Oxford: Blackwell Scientific Publications.

Woodcock, P.M. (1988) Biguanides as industrial biocides. In *Industrial Biocides* (ed. Payne, K.R.), Critical Reports on Applied Chemistry, Vol. 22, pp. 19–36. Chichester: John Wiley & Sons.

Yanagita, T. (1980) Studies on the formaldehyde resistance of *Aspergillus* fungi attacking the silkworm larvae. II. Aldehyde dehydrogenase of *Aspergillus* spp. *Journal of Sericultural Science of Japan*, **49**, 45–50.

Zlotnick, H., Fenadez, H.P., Bowers, B. & Cabib, E. (1984) *Saccharomyces cerevisiae* mannoproteins form an external cell wall layer that determines wall porosity. *Journal of Bacteriology*, **159**, 1018–1026.

CHAPTER 6

Viricidal Activity of Biocides

A. ACTIVITY AGAINST HUMAN VIRUSES

1 Introduction

In spite of the low infective dose reported for many human pathogenic viruses (Westwood & Sattar, 1976; Ward *et al.*, 1986), the speed with which virus infections can spread and the enormous economic impact of virus infections (Springthorpe & Sattar, 1990), relatively little is known about interrupting the spread of viral diseases with biocides.

Biocides used against viruses are variously termed disinfectants, germicides, viricides (virucides) or, if they are used on skin, topicals or antiseptics. Relatively few systematic studies have been performed on the potency of biocides against viruses; information is scattered through the scientific literature over many years. The importance of biocidal inactivation of viruses was re-emphasized only after the advent of human immunodeficiency virus (HIV) (Sattar & Springthorpe, 1991; Sattar *et al.*, 1994; Druce *et al.*, 1995; van Bueren, 1995) and the recognition of the spread of viruses through blood, blood products and tissues. Ideally, this chapter should present data on the viricidal potency of biocides in a format to provide easy answers for the reader. However, the wide disparity in test conditions and methods precludes easy summarization, because comparisons between studies are generally difficult.

This chapter will focus on understanding the potential for biocides to interrupt the transmission of viruses and the potency of different classes of biocides, and will pinpoint the issues to be aware of in interpreting studies of virus inactivation by biocides.

2 The importance of human viral infections

Nearly 1000 different types of viruses are known to infect humans, and it has been estimated that they account for approx. 60% of human infections (Horsfall, 1965). Many virus infections are subclinical, and viruses which are already recognized are now being implicated in a variety of chronic diseases where their role was not previously suspected (Shah & Buscema, 1988; Yousef *et al.*, 1988). An increased association between viral agents and malignancies is also likely (Darcel, 1994); Epstein–Barr, hepatitis B, herpes and papilloma viruses are already implicated in this regard. Furthermore, newly discovered viruses are known to be associated with serious or highly contagious diseases (Schmaljohn, 1985; Piot *et al.*, 1988; Saif & Theil, 1989). Increased international travel and trade in foodstuffs, animals and animal products continue to enhance the danger of importing exotic viruses and of rapid worldwide spread during epidemics of viral disease. As techniques for virus detection and identification improve, these agents may become implicated in diseases with as yet unknown etiology. Continued virus evolution may also alter virus host range and/or the spectrum of disease for which viruses are responsible.

The social and economic impact of viral disease on families, in the workplace and in health care is considerable, and often underestimated (Springthorpe & Sattar, 1990). Poor socio-economic status, leading to crowded and unhygienic living, favours transmission of viral infections. Burgeoning population growth in urban centres can also lead to crowding in institutional settings, such as day-care centres, schools, hospitals and nursing homes. Rapid spread of viral disease in school (Papaevangelou, 1984), day-care establishments (Storch *et al.*, 1979; Pickering *et al.*, 1981; Pass *et al.*, 1984), nursing homes (Fauvel *et al.*, 1980; Halvorsrud & Orstavik, 1980; Mathur *et al.*, 1980), business offices (Friedman *et al.*, 1983) and crowded working and living conditions all contribute to health-care costs, and days lost from work decrease the economic output (Haskins & Kotch, 1986).

Young, elderly and immunocompromised individuals are particularly susceptible to virus infections, and sometimes a virus infection can explain the atypical symptoms presented by a concomitant bacterial pathogen (Dagan *et al.*, 1985). Many viral infections in healthy adults and/or children are asymptomatic. Such infections may represent a particular hazard in the hospital setting (Champsaur *et al.*, 1984), because proper precautions, including disinfection, are not taken. Respiratory and enteric infections appear to account for the majority of nosocomially acquired virus diseases (Wenzel *et al.*, 1977; Valenti *et al.*, 1980a,b; Welliver & McLaughlin, 1984). In one study (Valenti *et al.*, 1980a), viruses were found to be responsible for 71.4%, 58.6% and 19.7% of the total nosocomially acquired gastrointestinal, upper respiratory and lower respiratory infections, respectively.

Lack of both vaccines and safe and effective chemotherapeutic agents against the majority of viruses, together with successful control and prevention of many important bacterial diseases, has increased the relative importance of diseases caused by viruses. Proper isolation of virus-infected individuals is often difficult or impractical, and heavy reliance is usually placed on chemical disinfection and antisepsis as means by which the spread of viral infections can be limited. Therefore, it is extremely important both to select suitable viricidal agents and to apply them effectively in order to reduce transmission of viral diseases.

3 Effective use of disinfectants against viruses

Figure 6.1 summarizes the cycle for transmission of infections. Infected hosts shed viruses into the environment through body secretions and excretions. Virus survival in or on contaminated vehicles is a requirement for transmission, whether the vehicle is a toy, a telephone, a glass of water or a piece of fruit. Cellular and other debris present can protect the viral agents from degradation outside the host, and the chances of virus transmission increase in direct proportion to the extent of virus survival. A detailed discussion of the extent of virus survival and the factors which affect it is beyond the scope of this chapter and the reader is referred to other sources (Sattar & Springthorpe,

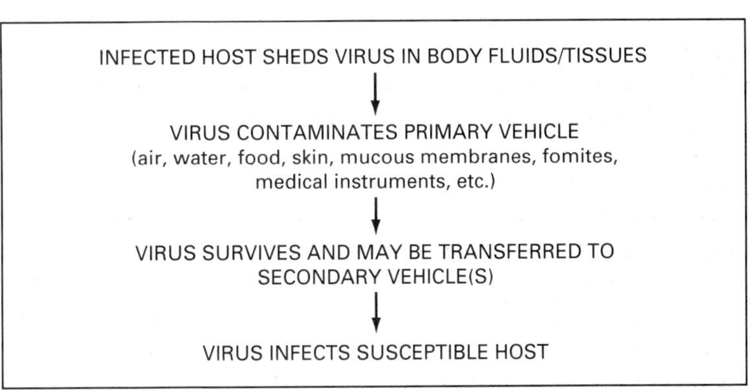

Fig. 6.1 Environmental transmission of virus infections.

1991; Sattar *et al.*, 1991). The low minimal infectious dose for many viruses implies that, even when viruses survive rather poorly, vehicles contaminated with them may act as sources of viruses for several hours. At the other extreme, viruses may remain infectious for weeks, months and, in rare cases, years.

Clearly biocides are only one potential barrier, but to interrupt virus transmission effectively they must be applied to virus-contaminated vehicles. Viral infections that spread primarily through air or food or by parenteral or venereal routes are usually less amenable to control by biocides than those that spread through the faecal–oral route via fomites and hands. However, in addition to the normal environmental transmission of viral infections, the increasing use of therapeutic blood and tissue products and tissues for transplantation has raised the profile of virus disinfection for certain viruses that would normally only be transmitted by parenteral routes. In such cases, biocides may be only one of many strategies employed during production to eliminate viruses from the product (Burstyn & Hageman, 1996; Horowitz & Ben-Hur, 1996; Manabe, 1996), but validation of virus removal is a crucial part of the product-quality assurance (Walter *et al.*, 1996). A detailed treatment of this subject is beyond the scope of this chapter, but the reader is urged to consult current databases for further information.

The concentrations of biocides to which humans can be exposed is limited. Only low levels of disinfectant chemicals can be permitted in air, water and food; of these, water is the vehicle most amenable to disinfection. The kinetics and efficacy of water disinfection have been extensively studied, and the mechanisms of viral inactivation in water have been reviewed (Thurman & Gerba, 1988). Chemicals are also frequently used in the preparation of inactivated viral vaccines, blood products and medical devices of animal origin for implantation. As these are administered directly, the levels of disinfectants therein must be limited, and products must be properly treated to prevent parenteral transmission of pathogens. In these situations, it is important to study thoroughly the kinetics of disinfectant action, because contact time is not a limiting factor, and prolonged contact may be necessary in view of the low levels of chemicals used. For disinfection of water, vaccines and blood products, physical methods of virus removal or inactivation are frequently employed in addition to chemical treatment.

The kinetics of virus inactivation is often quite different from that of bacteria. With the exception of certain slow-acting biocides, virus inactivation generally occurs rapidly or not at all. This is important to remember when developing a strategy for virus control by biocides and selecting the product, concentration and contact time for its use.

For disinfection of virus-contaminated surfaces, practical considerations limit the available contact time for soaks (minutes to hours) and wipes (1 min/or less); the kinetics of disinfection is usually less important than whether the concentration of the particular chemical can effectively decontaminate a surface during an appropriate contact time. Moreover, although the types of chemicals used may be restricted, depending on the nature of the surface material and considerations of toxicity, the disinfectant concentration is usually considerably higher than that permitted for water disinfection.

Heat-sensitive medical instruments require biocide treatment as critical or semicritical medical devices (Rutala, 1996), i.e. biocide concentrations and exposure conditions should be capable of providing chemosterilization or high-level disinfection, respectively. Environmental surfaces in clinical settings are generally considered important only if they are in areas where highly susceptible individuals are housed, e.g. neonatal intensive-care units, burn units, operating suites, etc. In other areas of hospitals, and in other institutions, environmental surfaces are generally considered to be less important as vehicles of virus transmission, and only low-level disinfection is practised. Animate surfaces, especially hands, present a particularly difficult problem. They are frequently contaminated with viruses (Hendley *et al.*, 1973; Keswick *et al.*, 1983; Samadi *et al.*, 1983; Hutto *et al.*, 1986), which may remain infectious for several hours (Ansari *et al.*, 1988, 1991), and, because of skin sensitivity, they can only be treated with certain types of chemicals. The importance of hands in the transmission of virus infections is well recognized, but scant attention is paid to the possible (re)contamination of hands by contact with other contaminated surfaces, although it may be demonstrated to occur readily (Ansari *et al.*, 1988; Mbithi *et al.*, 1992). Therefore, any infection control strategy should address both hands and contaminated surfaces. Failures of infection control are usually attributed to lack of compliance with established protocols rather than inadequacy of biocides. However, there is reason to believe (Favero, 1985) that many currently marketed biocides perform inadequately under field conditions, and use of such products, even with perfect compliance to procedures, would not necessarily prevent the occurrence of viral infections.

Although certain viruses can be identified as problems in particular settings (e.g. rotaviruses and hepatitis A virus in day care, hepatitis viruses and HIV in blood products), in general, biocide use takes place in an environmental where the specific microbial targets are unknown. Therefore, products that exhibit a wide spectrum of activity may be the most desirable. On the other hand, such products can be very potent chemicals and the safety of biocides for their intended purpose is also extremely important. When viruses are considered in conjunction with other microbial pathogens, a hierarchy of susceptibility or resistance to biocides can be given (Rutala, 1996). Such a hierarchy should be treated very much as a guide only; considerable overlap in susceptibility among microbial classes occurs (Fig. 6.2), and comparisons between specific pathogens that may be valid for one biocide may not hold for other formulations. It is generally accepted that most enveloped viruses are inactivated relatively easily and that many non-enveloped viruses offer greater resistance to chemical inactivation. While this is generally correct, we would suggest that, under natural or simulated environmental conditions,

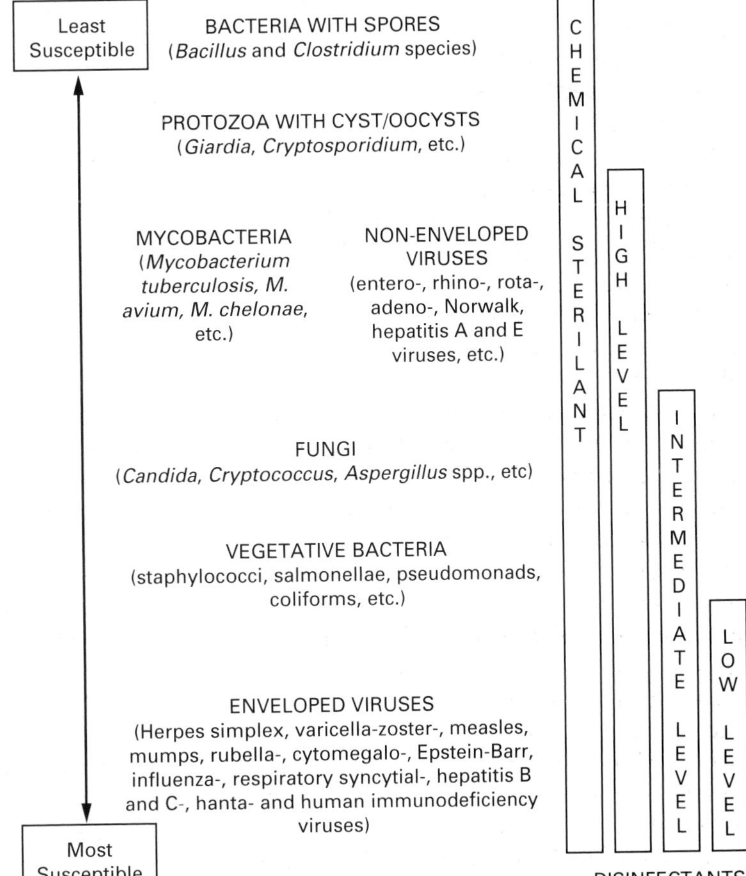

Fig. 6.2 Comparative susceptibility of microorganisms to biocides (see also Section 4.1).

enveloped viruses are often more refractory to disinfectant inactivation than is realized (Sattar *et al.*, 1989) and that, although non-enveloped viruses are generally more resistant, chemical disinfectants can be identified to which even the hardiest viruses are sensitive.

The potential of biocides to control viral transmission can only be realized when there is direct contact for an adequate time between an appropriate concentration of disinfectant and the target agent(s). When contaminated surfaces are treated, then the nature and properties of the surface also become factors in the disinfection process. The presence of other substances with which the disinfectant reacts influences both the degree of disinfectant contact with the intended target(s) and the effective disinfectant concentration. Such material may be deposited on the surface before, during or after contamination with the target agent, or it may be inherent to the surface itself. Furthermore, the diluent used for preparing the working concentration of disinfectant and the disinfectant applicator, if one is used, can sometimes contain components that react with the disinfectant. In addition, the natures of both the contaminating agent and the disinfectant chemical play an important role in determining disinfectant efficacy, and the whole process is influenced by environmental parameters, such as temperature and relative humidity.

There is insufficient information to be able to evaluate the effectiveness of virus disinfection. Even when laboratory-based studies indicate the viricidal potential of biocides, tests often fail to examine the disinfectant under simulated use conditions, and clinical trials necessary to establish effectiveness (Haley *et al.*, 1985) are invariably lacking. However, in one experimental setting, environmental surface disinfection has been shown to prevent viral disease spread (Ward *et al.*, 1991).

4 Virus disinfection in detail

The factors affecting disinfection have been reviewed elsewhere (Springthorpe & Sattar, 1990; see also Chapter 3). However, the nature of the virus, the nature of the virus-contaminated vehicle and the composition and concentration of the disinfectant deserve further discussion here because of their importance in the contact made between virus and biocide.

4.1 The target virus

Because of their extremely small size (approx. 20–300 nm in diameter), virus particles have a huge surface-to-mass ratio, approximately 10^7 greater than that of a human being (Pollard, 1953). Therefore, a large proportion of the virion is in direct contact with its immediate surroundings and is greatly influenced by their physical and chemical nature. The molecular mechanism(s) of disinfectant action are not fundamentally different between bacteria and viruses. There can be many potential points of attack for disinfectants in the mature virion (see also Chapter 6D), and most disinfectants are not sufficiently specific to react with only one virus component or functional group. Mature infectious virions of conventional viruses contain a nucleoprotein core and a structural protein coat. This macromolecular structure is either naked, or surrounded by a lipid-containing envelope, which is usually essential for virus infection. Since enveloped viruses are more readily inactivated by most chemical disinfectants than are non-enveloped viruses (Klein & Deforest, 1983; Sattar *et al.*, 1989), lipophilic disinfectants and chaotropic agents should have little difficulty in breaching a normal lipid bilayer. It is probable, therefore, that the infectivity of enveloped viruses could be destroyed with little or no direct damage to the protein or nucleic acid of the virus. However, it is not known how such damage must be done to the virus envelope before virus infection is prevented. At high disinfectant concentrations, damage to the proteins and nucleic acids of the virion is also likely. Non-enveloped viruses appear to differ markedly from one another in their sensitivity to many disinfectants (Klein and Deforest, 1983; Mahnel, 1979; Sattar *et al.*, 1989). Inactivation of these viruses by chemical disinfectants is assumed to involve damage to either the structural or functional proteins of the virion, which are necessary for infection and replication, or to the nucleic acid, or both. The first contact of disinfectant and non-enveloped viruses is made with the protein coat, which usually forms 60–90% of the total virus mass. There are obviously many specific sites in virion protein components that are critical for virus integrity, infectivity or replication. For example, the site on the virus capsid that interacts with the cellular surface is obviously important in all viruses, because damage to it may interfere with virus infectivity. However, the symmetry of virus structure often means that such sites are present in multiple copies and, because of this redundancy, damage to the majority or all of these sites may be necessary before virus infectivity is destroyed.

Apart from this, virus types containing several functionally active proteins, such as replication enzymes, may be more vulnerable to the action of biocides than those viruses which depend largely on cellular functions for their replication. The secondary and tertiary structure of proteins and nucleic acids leaves specific areas of the molecules more exposed to biocide attack. The vulnerability of these regions is governed not only by their location in the virion, but also by the hydrophobicity and other aspects of the immediate molecular environment which control biocide access.

In many viruses, the nucleic acid core of the virus may be well protected from biocides by overlying protein. However, damage to the nucleic acid core may account for virus inactivation in cases where the coat protein is relatively refractory to damage and is permeable to particular disinfectants, or where prolonged access to the virus allows penetration of the disinfectant into the virion. The ease with which disinfectants can penetrate the virus capsid is unknown and probably varies dramatically between viruses and between disinfectants. The number of potential sites for attack within the target virus increases with the use of disinfectants containing multiple active ingredients with different modes of action; either additive or synergistic effects may be observed (Hugo, 1992; see also Chapter 9).

Larger non-enveloped viruses are often more readily disinfected than smaller ones (Klein & Deforest, 1983), although there are exceptions to this (Raphael *et al.*, 1987). In some cases, this may be related to structural considerations in the virion itself which protect the nucleic acid from certain types of disinfectant; in others, it may be because the smaller the particle, the more easily it is shielded from disinfectant action by other contaminating materials.

Within their target cells, viruses are often produced as close-packed crystalline-like arrays. Enveloped viruses are often individually budded from the membrane of their host cells, but many may remain as clumps associated with cellular debris in sloughed cells. Non-enveloped viruses may be released when the host cell bursts, and, although some can be found dispersed singly, many remain clumped and/or associated with cellular debris (Williams, 1985; Hoff & Akin, 1986; Thurman & Gerba, 1988). Furthermore, individual virus particles often have a tendency to adhere to other particulate matter and surfaces. Therefore, viruses in body fluids and on naturally contaminated surfaces are often found as clumps or aggregates (Thurman & Gerba, 1988).

Viruses located at the centre of such clumps will be more inaccessible to disinfectants by virtue of their protection by virions or particulates in the outer layer(s). For spherical viruses, 16 spheres identical in diameter to the virion at the centre are required to protect a central virion (Thurman & Gerba, 1988), and so clumps of viruses containing more than 16 virions will probably show some resistance to disinfectants. Further protection of the target virus on contaminated surfaces may be afforded by the secretions or excretions in which viruses are invariably embedded when they are shed from the infected host; very rarely would viruses be the only microorganisms present, although they may be the only pathogen. Natural virus suspensions may be somewhat viscous and not readily penetrable to disinfectants, especially when dried on to the surface. In addition to the physical protection provided to viruses contaminating surfaces, the matrix of organic molecules and inorganic salts that comprises the body fluids, together with the cellular debris from virus-infected or uninfected cells, is likely to react chemically with most disinfectants. This will tend to neutralize the disinfectant and reduce its effective working concentration. The mass of protective material may considerably exceed the mass of the contaminating virus and present a severe challenge to the biocide.

Disinfectant efficacy against a target virus must be measured in terms of the degree of lost infectivity, usually in cell culture. Although this is usually equated to *in vivo* infectivity of the same virus preparation, it is not necessarily so. In view of the above discussion, tests conducted to assess biocide potency and potential for field application should use virus preparations similar to those that would be naturally shed, rather than highly purified preparations. The latter are suited only for detailed kinetic studies, in particular applications of biocides.

Klein & Deforest (1963) made their original deductions regarding virus susceptibility to disinfectants from the study of relatively few virus–disinfectant pairs, and, in general, their conclusions are still valid. More definite patterns of disinfectant efficacy can be seen to emerge during systematic study involving several disinfectants with the same or similar active ingredients and one or more viruses (Lloyd-Evans *et al.*, 1986; Springthorpe *et al.*, 1986; Sattar *et al.*, 1989). It is possible, therefore, to make some general statements regarding the viricidal efficacy of different disinfectant classes, although finer distinctions between different formulations of the same type of disinfectant may be more unpredictable, particularly at high biocide dilutions.

The difficulty of predicting the viricidal efficacy of disinfectants against a variety of viruses is partly due to the unrecognized differences in susceptibility and partly due to variation in the overall properties of the virus preparations. Virus preparations obtained from natural infections differ in the target organs in which the viruses were produced, the clonal composition from the immunological pressure exerted, in the composition of the medium in which the viruses were shed, in the degree of cell association of the virus and in the numbers of infectious virus particles. Even in virus pools produced in the laboratory for the express purpose of disinfectant testing, where the same cell strain has been used for growing the different viruses and the number of infectious virus particles has been standardized, differences can be expected in the degree of virus–cell association and possible clonal differences in susceptibility.

When doing comparative testing of disinfectants against viruses, it is often thought desirable to maintain a constant disinfectant-to-virus ratio. However, should this be for the total numbers of virions, or only the infectious particles? It is usually and logically taken to be the latter, and it would be practically more difficult to determine and standardize the former. For different viruses, and even for the same virus grown under different conditions, there will be varying proportions of infectious to non-infectious viruses in a prepared pool. Obviously, all viruses, whether infectious or not, will react chemically with disinfectants. In some virus preparations, only very few of the virions may be infectious when measured using cell culture techniques; for example, about 1 in 40 000 rotavirus particles may be infectious (Ward *et al.*, 1984). If a comparison were to be made between such a pool and that of another virus where 1 in 4 viruses was infectious in cell culture, then it is obvious that the disinfectant would have to react with 10 000 times more viruses in the one case in order to achieve the same reduction in infectious virus titre in both preparations. In practical terms, the differences in ratios of infectious to non-infectious viruses and even the absolute virus numbers may not be as important as the level of contaminating material which the biocide must overcome. Sublethal damage to viruses in aggregates and clumps could permit a productive infection through complementation (Thurman & Gerba, 1988).

Repeated exposures to inadequate levels of disinfectants could provide a selective pressure and give rise to virus isolates with altered susceptibility (Bates *et al.*, 1977). Although changes in susceptibility could be manifested through physical alterations of the virion macromolecular structure, altered interaction with the host cell(s) and virion protection could be an equally probable reason. It is important, however, not to equate disinfectant failure with microbial resistance; it is more probably due to the improper use of biocides (Russell *et al.*, 1986). If sublethal damage to viruses results in strains with increased resistance to disinfectants, then these changes must maintain or increase the infectivity of the virus in order to be selected for. A genetic, rather than an environmental, basis for virus resistance to disinfectants has not yet been established. Even if the selection of viruses which are genetically more resistant to disinfectants is subsequently shown to be a common phenomenon, it is unlikely to be more important for virus protection against disinfectants than is the nature and protection of the surrounding organic and particulate matter.

4.2 The contaminated carrier

Surfaces contaminated by viruses can be of many different types, and can be broadly classified into non-porous inanimate, porous inanimate and animate. Whatever the type of surface, however, it is recognized as having a characteristic composition, wettability and structural microtopography (Springthorpe & Sattar, 1990). Since viruses are usually between 20 and 300 nm in diameter, even scratches and imperfections on 'smooth' surfaces can usually accommodate both individual viruses and virus clumps. In addition, no surface is completely 'clean'; there is always some adherent organic matter. Any surface that touches human or animal skin will acquire microorganisms, sebum components and other molecules from the skin surface. Any surface exposed to air, particularly when it is horizontal, will become coated with dust particles, oily emulsions and aqueous aerosols. Depending on the surface and the use to which it is put, one can envisage a layered structural soil containing bacterial cells and spores, fungal spores, dirt and grease. Viruses will also be incorporated in such soil, as they contaminate surfaces by: (i) direct contact deposition from the contaminated secretion or excretion of an infected host; (ii) transfer via other animate or inanimate surfaces; (iii) deposition from contaminated fluids in contact with the surface; or (iv) deposition from large- or small-particle aerosols. The organic material likely to be present in virus contamination has already been discussed, but bacteria themselves, the matrices in which they are suspended and many other soiling compounds will also react with and neutralize disinfectant solutions. Under natural conditions of soiling, therefore, virus-contaminated surfaces represent a complex challenge to disinfectants, which might be compared to dried or aged bacterial biofilms (Costerton *et al.*, 1987). It is important, therefore, that biocides contain 'surface-active' components which permit them to readily wet the surfaces and the accumulated soil. It should also be noted that repeated use of disinfectants that act as fixatives (e.g. alcohols, aldehydes) may help to build up residual soil on surfaces. Some products, particularly cationic surfactants, such as the quaternary ammonium compounds (QACs), which are readily neutralized by organic soil, carry warnings that they should be applied only to precleaned surfaces; such procedures could carry risks for untrained personnel (Springthorpe & Sattar, 1990). Furthermore, precleaning of contaminated surfaces must be done in a manner compatible with the subsequent disinfectant to be applied; soaps and detergent residues on surfaces may interfere with the subsequent action of certain disinfectants. It is thus necessary to rinse the surface well before applying the disinfectant. The precleaning and rinsing steps are necessary to ensure proper disinfection of critical items, such as endoscopes, and this is done by fully trained personnel. However, practical and staffing considerations preclude this as a routine for all disinfectant uses. Biocides intended for use on surfaces against viruses should be examined for potency in a carrier test rather than in suspension.

There are special problems with residues which may be present on human skin. Normal skin harbours a large population of resident and transient flora and is subject to continuous natural secretions. All soaps and disinfectant solutions have a tendency to dry the skin, and the use of hand lotions is common among personnel who wash their hands frequently. The effects of these skin residues on the efficacy of antiseptic products is largely unknown. Some antiseptics are selected not just for their immediate efficacy, but for the deliberate residual activity remaining on the hands after use (e.g. chlorhexidine salts).

Hands, in particular, may be the single most important vehicle in the transmission of human and, to some extent, animal virus diseases. Contaminated hands can result in inoculation of self or others by contact with portals of entry on a susceptible host, and, because of frequent contacts with food, water and other animate or inanimate surfaces, they can transfer infectious virus to other potential vehicles (Pancic *et al.*, 1980; Cliver & Kostenbader, 1984; Ansari *et al.*, 1988). In institutions housing infants and young children, the numbers of hand–hand and hand-object contacts are inevitably high. Children frequently suck their fingers and put toys and other objects in their mouths; in one study, these activities were noted as often as every 2–3 min (Black *et al.*, 1981). Biocides intended for topical application should be tested on virus-contaminated skin in either an *in vivo* system (Ansari *et al.*, 1989) or an *ex vivo* model (Graham *et al.*, 1996).

The extent to which virus transfer to food and beverages can occur during meal preparation is unknown, but food handlers are known to be involved in the transmission of a variety of virus diseases. Cliver & Kostenbader (1984) have demonstrated transfer from contaminated hands to foods under experimental conditions. Transfer of viruses between skin and inanimate surfaces has been documented for several viruses (Hall *et al.*, 1980; Pancic *et al.*, 1980; Cliver & Kostenbader, 1984; Ansari *et al.*, 1988). In one study which quantitated experimental transfer of rotavirus from contaminated to clean surfaces (Ansari *et al.*, 1988), using realistic levels of contaminating virus, transfer between contaminated finger pads and surfaces and their clean counterparts was recorded at each contact made.

Much of the contamination of surfaces by viruses is not apparent. Obvious contamination may, in fact, be the least hazardous, because it is more likely to be cleaned and disinfected promptly. Although proper attention to disinfection of critical-care items is the most essential focus of disinfection for the hospital community at the present time, improper use of general purpose low-level disinfectants may also contribute significantly to the transmission of virus diseases. Perhaps the best example of this is the acquisition of viral infections within day-care centres and their focus for disease transmission in the general community (Denny *et al.*, 1986; Henderson & Giebink, 1986; Klein, 1986; Pass & Hutto, 1986 Pickering *et al.*, 1986).

Even though airborne viruses are not generally amenable to biocide control, because of the hazards of widespread biocide use in ambient air, use of biocidal sprays may be considered desirable in special circumstances. Under these conditions, the prevailing ambient relative humidity (r.h.) would be an important factor in the survival of both aerosolized viruses (Sattar & Ijaz, 1987) and viral aerosols deposited on to surfaces (Sattar *et al.*, 1986). In theory, r.h. should be considered from two viewpoints, prehumidification of the contaminated surface before disinfectant treatment and humidification during treatment. Although high r.h. will favour survival of some viruses, it is likely that prehumidification will enhance the action of almost all disinfectants by increasing the ease of penetration of dried organic residues and improving accessibility to the target organisms. It is also likely to promote a higher degree of wettability of the surface structure. Humidification during disinfection will probably have similar but probably much smaller effects in this regard; however, it may help prevent rapid evaporation of water and volatile disinfectant products.

4.3 The biocide

Under most in-use conditions, it is not practical to use different products for different viruses, and therefore caution should mandate the choice of infection control product to be one that will potentially inactivate all viruses of concern in a particular setting. Hepatitis A is one of the most difficult viruses to disinfect, based on *in vitro* data (Mbithi *et al.*, 1990, 1993a,b), and may require relatively potent biocides for its elimination as naturally shed (Thraenhart, 1991). However, safety and choice of biocides for other purposes often restricts those available for virus control. Table 6.1 gives a summary of the classes of biocides, indicating their potential for virus control. The literature cited in Table 6.1 is not a complete listing of all the studies available, and the reader is urged to examine current databases for the most recent information. While this chapter is not focused on specifying biocides for particular viruses, some general information is available (Springthorpe & Sattar, 1990; Bellamy, 1995) and on hepatitis viruses in particular (Thraenhart, 1991; Deva *et al.*, 1996).

Certain biocides clearly have a broad spectrum of biocidal activity and can, at a suitable concentration, inactivate all conventional viral agents. Sodium hypochlorite is often the biocide of choice in conditions where hazardous agents are known to be, or suspected of being, present. The World Health Organization (WHO) *Laboratory Biosafety Manual* (WHO, 1993) recommends its use at concentrations of 1000 parts/10^6 for general use and 5000 parts/10^6 for blood spills or when organic material is present. It is also recommended at 5000 parts/$10^6$for emergency use when agents such as Lassa or Ebola may be present.

Table 6.1 Disinfectants used for the control of human pathogenic viruses.

Disinfectant class	Uses	Properties	Activity	References
Halogens				
Chlorine	Water disinfection General purpose disinfection General sanitation in food service and manufacture Often recommended as the standard disinfectant for inactivation of viral pathogens	Used as chlorine gas or sodium hypochlorite solution Relatively low residual toxicity Stability of hypochlorite solutions affected by chlorine concentration and pH Hypochlorous acid, favoured at low pH, is most active germicidal species Oxidizing agent	Wide-spectrum viricide at sufficient concentration Activity affected by presence of reducing agents, temperature Readily neutralized by exposure to organic material or UV radiation Many studies on chlorine inactivation of viruses have ignored the organic material which is naturally present in the field Increased levels needed in the presence of hard water and of organic matter	Clarke *et al.* (1956); Herniman *et al.* (1973); Wright (1970); Bates *et al.* (1977); Evans *et al.* (1977); Engelbrecht *et al.* (1980); Gowda *et al.* (1981); Fauris *et al.* (1982); Peterson *et al.* (1983); Berman and Hoff (1984); Churn *et al.* (1984); Grabow *et al.* (1984); Harakeh (1984); Harakeh and Butler (1984); Lloyd-Evans *et al.* (1986); Springthorpe *et al.* (1986); Raphael *et al.* (1987); Dychdala (1991); Sobsey *et al.* (1991); Krilov & Harkness (1993); Ceisel *et al.* (1995); Rutala (1996)
Monochloramine	Water disinfection	Formed by the addition of ammonia after the chlorine gas	Reacts only slowly with organic material; generally poor viricide May have some advantages in areas where residual needs to be maintained	Sobsey *et al.* (1991); Chepurnov *et al.* (1995)
Chlorine dioxide	Water disinfection General-purpose disinfectant, sporicide	Suggested to have advantages over chlorine for some applications Prepared on site	May be similar in activity to sodium hypochlorite for many viruses	Springthorpe *et al.* (1986)
Organochlorines	General-purpose disinfection Disinfection of swimming-pools (sodium dichlorodiisocyanurate) Sanitizers in food and dairy industry (chloramine T)	Act as demand-type disinfectants	Reacts more slowly with biological material and therefore less efficient as disinfectant May have some advantages in areas where considerable organic soil exists	Springthorpe *et al.* (1986); Gottardi and Bock (1988); Sattar *et al.* (1989)

(Continued on p. 178)

Table 6.1 (*Continued.*)

Disinfectant class	Uses	Properties	Activity	References
Bromine and mixed halides	Limited use	Addition to chlorine-based products improves efficiency		Keswick *et al.* (1981); Taylor and Butler (1982)
Iodine/ iodophores	Regarded as essential 'drug' by World Health Organization for its disinfection properties As a topical antiseptic In acidic solution as a sanitizer	Analogous to chlorine but reactions more complex Inorganic iodine mostly replaced by iodophores, in which iodine is a loose complex with a carrier molecule (usually a neutral organic polymer) This permits greater solubility and sustained release of the active germicidal species Surface-active properties of carrier may improve wetting and soil-penetrating properties Oxidizes –SH groups, unsaturated carbon bonds Tend to stain skin	Although affected, iodine compounds are less inhibited by organic matter than other halogens In dilute solution, may act like free iodine, whereas, in a more concentrated solution, it behaves as a demand-type disinfectant Neutralized by reducing agents Addition of alcohol can improve viricidal properties	Hsu *et al.* (1966); Jordan and Nassar (1973); Wallbank *et al.* (1978); Taylor and Butler (1982); Lloyd-Evans *et al.* (1986); Springthorpe *et al.* (1986); Gottardi (1991); Krilov & Harkness, 1993
Phenolics	General purpose germicides Some selective phenolics (e.g. trichlosan) used as topical antiseptics	Complex group of chemicals Not systematically studied as viricides	Activity very formulation-dependent Also depends on temperature, concentration, pH, level of organic matter, etc. Cationic and non-ionic surfactants neutralize activity Enveloped viruses more susceptible Need to test against specific viruses because it is difficult to generalize	Klein and Deforest (1983); Drulak *et al.* (1984); Springthorpe *et al.* (1986); Krilov & Harkness (1993);
Alcohols	Used alone or in formulations to potentiate the activity of other active ingredients	As length of aliphatic chain increases, there is increased activity on lipophilic virus, but the reverse is generally true	Acts on envelope and denatures proteins Not markedly affected by contaminating organic matter	Wright (1970); Hendley *et al.* (1978); Kurtz (1979); Kurtz *et al.* (1980); Brade *et al.* (1981); Klein and

(Continued)

Table 6.1 (*Continued.*)

Disinfectant class	Uses	Properties	Activity	References
	General purpose disinfectant Antiseptic in topical preparations and waterless hand washes	for the non-enveloped hydrophilic viruses Ethanol is the most commonly used alcohol	Affected by dilution Ethanol at least 70% is wide-spectrum viricide Surface-active agents may improve penetration on dried material	Deforest (1983); Lloyd-Evans *et al.* (1986); Sattar *et al.* (1986); Springthorpe *et al.* (1986); Ansari *et al.* (1989); Larson & Morton (1991); Bellamy *et al.* (1993); Krilov & Harkness (1993); van Bueren *et al.* (1994); Ceisel *et al.* (1995)
Aldehydes	Production of inactivated viral vaccines Fumigation (formaldehyde, paraformaldehyde) Sterilization of tissues and medical devices (glutaraldehyde) Topicals which release formaldehyde Disinfection of medical instruments, notably endoscopes, before reuse (glutaraldehyde)	Glutaraldehyde is a dialdehyde which acts more rapidly than formaldehyde and is capable of cross-linking molecules Stable in acid solution but more active at alkaline pH Binds to proteins through amide and amino groups Most glutaraldehyde used at approx. 2% for high-level disinfection	Activity increases with temperature React readily with proteins Wide spectrum of activity against viruses when used at appropriate concentration Activity decreases rapidly as product diluted on reuse Prolonged contact needed at lower concentrations Activity improved by addition of surface active agents or inorganic cations	Sidwell *et al.* (1970); Saitanu & Lund (1975); Thraenhart & Kuwert (1975); Mahnel & Kunz (1976a,b); Drulak *et al.* (1978a,b); Gorman *et al.* (1980); Brade *et al.* (1981); Lloyd-Evans *et al.* (1986); Springthorpe *et al.* (1986); Sattar *et al.* (1989); Scott & Gorman (1991); Hanson *et al.* (1994); Chepurnov *et al.* (1995); Deva *et al.* (1996)
Acids	Mainly used for pH modulation in formulations Toilet-bowl cleaners Constituents of anionic surfactant or iodophore preparations Organic acids in food and pharmaceuticals	Use limited by corrosion Phosphoric acid often used because deposits resist corrosion Organic acids are potentially more important than generally recognized	Many viruses susceptible to low pH; small variations can affect results Nature of acid affects activity Nature of diluent can affect activity Can be affected by residuals from prior cleaning by alkaline cleaners	Wright (1970); Herniman *et al.* (1973); Hendley *et al.* (1978); Kuhrt *et al.* (1984); Hayden *et al.* (1985); Dick *et al.* (1986); Springthorpe *et al.* (1986)
Alkalis	Used mainly to modulate pH of formulations Domestic and industrial sanitizers and cleaners	Use limited by corrosion pH levels up to 13 or higher are used	Many viruses susceptible to high pH	Lloyd-Evans *et al.* (1986); Springthorpe *et al.* (1986); Sattar *et al.* (1989)

(Continued on p. 180)

Table 6.1 (*Continued.*)

Disinfectant class	Uses	Properties	Activity	References
Anionic surfactants	Used in phenolic disinfectants and acidic anionic-surfactant sanitizers Often not considered disinfectants	Primary effects on lipid envelope Often used in conjunction with phosphoric acid	Active against enveloped but not non-enveloped viruses Nature of acids in formulation can affect activity	Fellowes (1965); Herniman *et al.* (1973); Springthorpe *et al.* (1986); Sattar *et al.* (1989)
Cationic surfactants	More widely used in North America than in Europe Constituents of many consumer products Dilute aqueous solutions used as topicals for skin and mucous membranes Hard-surface disinfectants Can be used in alcoholic solution	Quaternary ammonium group, with hydrogen groups replaced by alkyl or aryl substituents Most active are those with single long hydrocarbon chain (C8–C16) Surface-active properties Concentrations of up to 20 000 parts/10^6 used, but concentrations of 400–800 parts/10^6 more common because of costs	Efficiency reduced by soap Readily neutralized by proteins Should be applied to chemically clean surfaces unless formulated as disinfectant cleaners Mainly useful against enveloped viruses; non-enveloped viruses refractory Activity of alcoholic solutions similar to alcohols	Fellowes (1965); Kirchhoff (1968); Wright (1970); Oxford *et al.* (1971); Poli *et al.* (1978); Anderson & Winkler (1979); Lloyd-Evans *et al.* (1986); Springthorpe *et al.* (1986); Ansari *et al.* (1989); Sattar *et al.* (1989); Merianos (1991); Krilov & Harkness (1993); Kennedy *et al.* (1995)
Amphoteric compounds	More widely used in Europe than in North America	Amphoteric surfactants with amino acids substituted with long-chain alkyl amine groups	Activity mainly against enveloped viruses Activity poor against most non-enveloped viruses	Springthorpe *et al.* (1986); Block (1991b)
Peroxides and peracids				
Hydrogen peroxide	Long known as disinfectant/ antiseptic; formerly unstable, new preparations highly stabilized Many potential uses Disinfection of plastics and implants Food industry lines Some experimental use in water disinfection	Potent oxidant which is usually considered to act through the formation of hydroxyl radicals Very formulation-dependent, acts slowly as pure chemical 3–6% used for disinfection 6–25% used for sterilization; care needed in handling higher concentrations	Not widely studied as viricide Synergism with ultrasound reported for bacteria, not studied for viruses	Mentel & Schmidt (1973); Turner (1983); Lloyd-Evans *et al.* (1986); Block (1991a)
Peracids	Similar to peroxides Many uses, from sewage disinfection	Contain varying amounts of hydrogen peroxide; peracetic acid	Generally considered as potent viricide in appropriate	Kline & Hull (1960); Sprossig (1975); Sporkenbach *et al.*

(*Continued*)

Table 6.1 (*Continued.*)

Disinfectant class	Uses	Properties	Activity	References
	to sterilization in health care, use in dialysis machines and on food-contact surfaces	is the most common Oxidizer, pungent odour; hazardous to handle Tumour promoter and possible cocarcinogen	concentrations Powdered preparations less potent than liquids Not as affected by organic material as some other disinfectants	(1981); Lloyd-Evans *et al.* (1986); Block (1991a)
Ozone	Water disinfection	Powerful and fast-acting oxidizing agent Unstable; therefore, must be generated on site	Strong and broad-spectrum viricidal activity	Wickramanayake (1991); Helmer & Finch (1993)
Chlorhexidine and polymeric biguanides	Widely used in aqueous solution as topical in hygenic hand wash preparations In alcoholic solution used as waterless hand wash or preoperative skin preparation Alcoholic solution useful in critical care Sometimes used for general purpose disinfection	Available as dihydrochloride, diacetate or gluconate Gluconate most soluble and most common Low oral and percutaneous toxicity	Activity reduced in presence of anions; often contains cationic surfactants to avoid such effects Acts at level of envelope; viricidal activity poor in aqueous solution, and confined to enveloped viruses Alcoholic solutions inactivate similar viruses to alcohols	Bailey & Longson (1972); Springthorpe *et al.* (1986); Ansari *et al.* (1989); Wickramanayake (1991)
β-*Propiolactone*	Has been used for production of inactivated viral vaccines Possible value when hazardous agents are known to be present	As lactone, it alkylates nucleic acids In aqueous solution, lactone hydrolysed to inactive products Possible carcinogen Purity and storage history important	Rate and extent of activity dependent on concentration and temperature Higher concentrations needed when proteins present	Dawson *et al.* (1959, 1960); Lloyd *et al.* (1982)
Ethylene oxide		Alkylation of –SH groups		Parisi and Young (1991)

UV, ultraviolet.

5 Concluding remarks

The selection and use of biocides for virus control require a clear understanding of the potency and limitations of individual chemical formulations. They also require a knowledge of the material that has to be decontaminated and assurance that its treatment with the selected chemical will not compromise its subsequent safety and integrity. It must also be re-emphasized that the mass of individual viruses is very small and that contamination of surfaces with organic or inorganic soils or the presence of organic materials in solution will tend to interfere with and limit the viricidal potential of many biocides, as well as shielding contaminating viruses from biocide contact. Finally, the reader is cautioned about extrapolating potential for biocide effectiveness in the field from *in vitro* studies conducted on relatively pure virus preparations. Similarly, the effectiveness of topical agents should be assessed under clinically relevant conditions, using *in vivo* or *ex vivo* systems whenever possible.

6 References

Anderson, L.J. & Winkler, W.G. (1979) Aqueous quaternary ammonium compounds and rabies treatment. *Journal of Infectious Diseases*, **139**, 494–495.

Ansari, S.A., Sattar, S.A., Springthorpe, V.S., Wells, G.A. & Tostowaryk, W. (1988) Rotavirus survival on human hands and transfer of infectious virus to animate and non-porous inanimate surfaces. *Journal of Clinical Microbiology*, **26**, 1513–1518.

Ansari, S.A., Sattar, S.A., Springthorpe, V.S., Wells, G.A. & Tostowaryk, W. (1989) *In vivo* protocol for testing efficacy of handwashing agents against viruses and bacteria: experiments with rotavirus and *Escherichia coli*. *Applied and Environmental Microbiology*, **55**, 3113–3118.

Ansari, S.A., Springthorpe, V.S. & Sattar, S.A. (1991) Survival and vehicular spread of human rotavirus: possible relation to seasonality of outbreaks. *Reviews in Infectious Diseases*, **13**, 448–461.

Bailey, A. & Longson, M. (1972) Virucidal activity of chlorhexidine on strains of Herpesvirus hominis, poliovirus and adenovirus. *Journal of Clinical Pathology*, **25**, 76–78.

Bates, R.C., Shaffer, P.T.B. & Sutherland, S.M. (1977) Development of poliovirus having increased resistance to chlorine inactivation. *Applied and Environmental Microbiology*, **34**, 849–853.

Bellamy, K. (1995). A review of the test methods used to establish virucidal activity. *Journal of Hospital Infection*, **30** (Suppl.), 389–396.

Bellamy, K., Alcock, R., Babb, J.R., Davies, J.G. & Ayliffe, G.A.J. (1993) A test for the assessment of 'hygienic' hand disinfection using rotavirus. *Journal of Hospital Infection*, **24**, 201–210.

Berman, D. & Hoff, J.C. (1984) Inactivation of simian rotavirus SA-11 by chlorine, chlorine dioxide and monochloramine. *Applied and Environmental Microbiology*, **48**, 317–323.

Black, R.E., Dykes, A.C., Anderson, K.E. *et al.* (1981) Handwashing to prevent diarrhia in day-care centres. *American Journal of Epidemiology*, **113**, 445–451.

Block, S.S. (1991b) Surface active agents: amphoteric compounds. In *Disinfection, Sterilization and Preservation*, 4th edn (ed. Block, S.S.), pp. 263–273. Philadelphia: Lea & Febiger.

Block, S.S. (1991a) Peroxygen compounds. In *Disinfection, Sterilization and Preservation*, 4th edn (ed. Block, S.S.), pp. 167–181. Philadelphia: Lea & Febiger.

Brade, L., Schmidt, W.A.K. & Gattert, I. (1981) Zur relativen Wirksam keit von Desinfektion-mitteln gegenuber Rotaviren. *Zentralblatt für Bakteriologie, Mikrobiologie und Hygiene* (Orig. B), **174**, 151–159.

Burstyn, D.G. & Hageman, T.C. (1996) Strategies for viral removal and inactivation. *Developments in Biological Standardization*, **88**, 73–79.

Ceisel, R.J., Osetek, E.M., Turner, D.W. & Spear , P.G. (1995) Evaluating chemical inactivation of viral agents in handpiece splatter. *Journal of the American Dental Association*, **126**, 197–202.

Champsaur, H., Questiaux, E., Prevot, J. *et al.* (1984) Rotavirus carriage, asymptomatic infection and disease in the first two years of life. *Journal of Infectious Disease*, **149**, 667–674.

Chepurnov, A.A., Chuev, Y.P., P'yankov, O.V. & Efimova, I.V. (1995) Effects of some physical and chemical factors on inactivation of ebola virus. *Russian Progress in Virology*, **2**, 40–43.

Churn, C.C., Boardman, G.D. & Bates, R.C. (1984). The inactivation kinetics of H-1 parvovirus by chlorine. *Water Research*, **18** 195–203.

Clarke, N.A., Stevenson, R.E. & Kabler, P.W. (1956) The inactivity of purified type 3 adenovirus in water by chlorine. *American Journal of Hygiene*, **64**, 314–319.

Cliver, D.O. & Kostenbader, K.D., Jr (1984) Disinfection of virus on hands for the prevention of food-borne disease. *International Journal of Food Microbiology*, **1** 75–87.

Costerton, J.W., Cheng, K.J., Geesey, G.G. *et al.* (1987) Bacterial biofilms in nature and disease. *Annual Reviews of Microbiology*, **41**, 435–464.

Dagan, R., Hall, C.B. & Menegus, M.A. (1985) Atypical bacterial infections explained by a concomitant virus infection. *Pediatrics*, **76**, 411–414.

Darcel, C. (1994) Reflections on viruses and cancer. *Veterinary Research Communications*, **18**, 43–61.

Dawson, F.W., Hearn, H.J. & Hoffman, R.K. (1959) Virucidal activity of beta-propiolactone vapour. I. Effect of beta-propiolactone on Venezuelan equine encephalitis virus. *Applied Microbiology*, **7**, 199–201.

Dawson, F.W., Janssen, R.J. & Hoffman, R.K. (1960) Virucidal activity of beta-propiolactone vapor. II. Effect on the etiological agents of smallpox, yellow fever, psittacosis and Q fever. *Applied Microbiology*, **8** 39–41.

Denny, F.W., Collier, A.M. & Henderson, F.W. (1986) Acute respiratory infections in day care. *Reviews of Infectious Diseases*, **8**, 527–532.

Deva, A.K., Vickery, K., Zou, J., West, R.H., Harris, J.P. & Cossart, Y.E. (1996) Establishment of an in-use testing method for evaluating disinfection of surgical instruments using the duck hepatitis B model. *Journal of Hospital Infection*, **33**, 119–130.

Dick, E.C., Hossain, S.U., Mink, K.A. *et al.* (1986)

Interruption of transmission of rhinovirus colds among human volunteers using virucidal paper handkerchiefs. *Journal of Infectious Diseases*, **153**, 352–356.

Druce, J.D., Jardine, D., Locarnini, S.A. & Birch, C.J. (1995) Susceptibility of HIV to inactivation by disinfectants and ultraviolet light. *Journal of Hospital Infection*, **30**, 167–180.

Drulak, M.W., Wallbank, A.M. & Lebtag, I. (1984) The effectiveness of six disinfectants in the inactivation of reovirus 3. *Microbios*, **41**, 31–38.

Drulak, M., Wallbank, A.M. & Lebtag, I. (1978a) The relative effectiveness of commonly used disinfectants in inactivation of echovirus 11. *Journal of Hygiene*, **81**, 77–87.

Drulak, M., Wallbank, A.M., Lebtag, I., Werboski, L. & Poffenroth, L. (1978b) The relative effectiveness of commonly used disinfectants in inactivation of coxsackievirus B_5. *Journal of Hygiene*, **81**, 389–397.

Dychdala, G.R. (1991) Chlorine and chlorine compounds. In *Disinfection, Sterilization and Preservation*, 4th edn (ed. Block, S.S. pp. 131–151, Philadelphia: Lea & Febiger.

Engelbrecht, R.S., Weber, M.J., Salter, B.L. & Schmidt, C.A. (1980) Comparative inactivation of viruses by chlorine. *Applied and Environmental Microbiology*, **40**, 249–256.

Evans, D.H., Stuart, P. & Roberts, D.H. (1977) Disinfection of animal viruses. *British Veterinary Journal*, **133**, 356–359.

Fauris, C., Danglot, C. & Vilagines, R. (1982) Parameters influencing poliovirus inactivation by chlorine. *Comptes Rendu de l'Académie des Sciences (Paris)*, **295**, 73–76.

Fauvel, M., Chagnon, A. & Svorc-Ranco, R. (1980) Rotavirus gastroenteritis outbreak in a senior citizen's home—Quebec. *Canada Diseases Weekly Reports*, **6**, 205–206.

Favero, M.S. (1985) Sterilization, disinfection and antisepsis in the hospital. In *Manual of Clinical Microbiology* (ed. in chief Lennette, E.H.) pp. 129–137. Washington, DC: American Society for Microbiology.

Fellowes, O.N. (1965) Some surface-active agents and their virucidal effect on foot-and-mouth disease virus. *Applied Microbiology*, **13**, 694–697.

Friedman, S.M., Schultz, S., Goodman, A., Millian, S. & Cooper, L.Z. (1983) Rubella outbreak among office workers—New York City. *Morbidity Mortality Weekly Reports*, **32**, 349–352.

Gorman, S.P., Scott, E.M. & Russell, A.D. (1980) Antimicrobial activity, uses and mechanism of action of glutaraldehyde. *Journal of Applied Bacteriology*, **48**, 161–190.

Gottardi, W. (1991) Iodine and iodine compounds. In *Disinfection, Sterilization and Preservation*, 4th edn (ed. Block, S.S.), pp. 152–166. Philadelphia: Lea & Febiger.

Gottardi, W. & Bock, V. (1988) The reaction of chloramine T (CAT) with protein constituents: model experiments on the halogen demand during the disinfection of biological material. In *Proceedings of the 4th Conference on Progress in Chemical Disinfection*, Binghamton, New York, April 1988, p. 35.

Gowda, N.M.M., Trieff, N.M. & Stanton, G.J. (1981) Inactivation of poliovirus by chloramine-T. *Applied and Environmental Microbiology*, **42**, 469–476.

Grabow, W.O.K., Coubrough, P., Hilner, C. & Bateman, B.W. (1984) Inactivation of hepatitis A virus, other enteric viruses and indicator organisms in water by chlorination. *Water Science and Technology*, **17**, 657–664.

Graham, M.L., Springthorpe, V.S. & Sattar, S.A. (1996) *Ex vivo* protocol for testing virus surival on human skin: experiments on herpes virus 2. *Applied and Environmental Microbiology*, **62**, 4252–4255.

Haley, R.W., Culver, D.H., White, J.W. *et al.* (1985) The efficacy of infection surveillance and control programs in preventing nosocomial infections in US hospitals. *American Journal of Infection Control*, **121**, 182–205.

Hall, C.B., Douglas, G., Jr & Geiman, J.M. (1980) Possible transmission by fomites of respiratory syncytial virus. *Journal of Infectious Diseases*, **141**, 98–102.

Halvorsrud, J. & Orstavik, I. (1980) An epidemic of rotavirus-associated gastroenteritis in a nursing home for the elderly. *Scandinavian Journal of Infectious Diseases*, **12**, 161–164.

Hanson, P.J.V., Bennett, J., Jeffries, D.J. & Collins, J.V. (1994) Enteroviruses, endoscopy and infection control: an applied study. *Journal of Hospital Infection*, **27**, 61–67.

Harakeh, M.S. (1984) Inactivation of enteroviruses, rotaviruses and bacteriophages by peracetic acid in a municipal sewage effluent. *FEMS Microbiology Letters*, **23**, 27–30.

Harakeh, M. & Butler, M. (1984) Inactivation of human rotavirus, SA-11 and other enteric viruses in effluent by disinfectants. *Journal of Hygiene*, **93**, 157–163.

Haskins, R. & Kotch, J. (1986) Day care and illness: evidence, costs, and public policy. *Pediatrics*, **77**, 951–982.

Hayden, G.F., Gwaltney, J.M., Jr., Thacker, D.F. & Hendley, J.O. (1985) Rhinovirus inactivation by nasal tissues treated with virucide. *Antiviral Research*, **5**, 103–109.

Helmer, R.D. & Finch, G.R. (1993) Use of MS2 coliphage as a surrogate for enteric viruses in surface waters disinfected with ozone. *Ozone Science and Engineering*, **15**, 279–293.

Henderson, F.W. & Giebink, G.S. (1986) Otitis media among children in day care: epidemiology and pathogenesis. *Reviews of Infectious Diseases*, **8**, 533–538.

Hendley, J.O., Mika, L.A. & Gwaltney, J.M. (1978) Evaluation of virucidal compounds for inactivation of rhinovirus on hands. *Antimicrobial Agents and Chemotherapy*, **14**, 690–694.

Hendley, J.O., Wenzel, R.P. & Gwaltney, J.M., Jr (1973) Transmission of rhinovirus colds by self-inoculation. *New England Journal of Medicine*, **288**, 1361–1364.

Herniman, K.A.J., Medhurst, P.M., Wilson, J.N. & Sellers, R.F. (1973) The action of heat, chemicals and disinfectants on swine vesicular disease virus. *Veterinary Record*, **93**, 620–624.

Hoff, J.C. & Akin, E.W. (1986) Microbial mechanisms of resistance to disinfectants: mechanisms and significance. *Environmental Health Perspectives*, **69**, 7–13.

Horowitz, B. & Ben-Hur, E. (1996) Viral inactivation of blood components: recent advances. *Transfusion clinique et biologique*, **3**, 75–77.

Horsfall, F.L., Jr (1965) General principles and historical aspects. In *Viral and Rickettsial Infections of Man* (eds Horsfall, F.L., Jr & Tamm, I.), pp. 1–10. New York: Lippincott.

Hsu, Y.-C., Nomura, S. & Kruse, C.W. (1966) Some bactericidal and virucidal properties of iodine not affecting infectious RNA and DNA. *American Journal of Epidemiology*, **82**, 317–328.

Hugo, W.B. (1992) Disinfection mechanisms. In *Principles and Practice of Disinfection, Preservation and Sterilization* (eds Russell, A.D., Hugo, W.B. & Ayliffe, G.A.J.), 2nd edn, pp. 187–210. Oxford: Blackwell Scientific Publications.

Hutto, C., Little, E.A., Ricks, R., Lee, J.D. & Pass, R.F. (1986) Isolation of cytomegalovirus from toys and hands in a day care center. *Journal of Infectious Diseases*, **154**, 527–530.

Jordan, F.T.W. & Nassar, T.J. (1973) The survival of infectious bronchitis (IB) virus in an iodophor disinfectant and the influence of certain components. *Journal of Applied Bacteriology*, **36**, 335–341.

Kennedy, M.A., Mellon, V.S., Caldwell, G. & Potgieter, L.N.D. (1995) Virucidal efficacy of the newer quaternary ammonium compounds. *Journal of the American Animal Hospital Association*, **31**, 254–258.

Keswick, B.H., Fujioka, R.S. & Loh, P.C. (1981) Mechanism of poliovirus inactivation by bromine chloride. *Applied and Environmental Microbiology*, **42**, 824–829.

Keswick, B.H., Pickering, L.K., DuPont, H.L. & Woodward, W.E. (1983) Survival and detection of rotaviruses on environmental surfaces in day-care centers. *Applied and Environmental Microbiology*, **46**, 813–816.

Kirchhoff, H. (1968) The effect of quaternary ammonium compounds on Newcastle disease virus and parainfluenza virus. *Deutsche Tierarztliche Wochenschrift*, **75**, 160–165.

Klein, J.O. (1986) Infectious diseases and day care. *Reviews of Infectious Diseases*, **8**, 521–526.

Klein, M. & Deforest, A. (1963) The inactivation of viruses by germicides. In *Proceedings of the 49th Midyear Meeting of the Chemical Specialties Manufacturers Association*, Chicago, Illinois, pp. 116–118.

Klein, M. & Deforest, A. (1983) Principles of viral inactivation. In *Disinfection, Sterilization and Preservation* (ed. Block, S.S.), pp. 422–434. Philadelphia: Lea & Febiger.

Kline, L.B. & Hull, R.N. (1960) The virucidal properties of peracetic acid. *American Journal of Clinical Pathology*, **33**, 30–33.

Krilov, L.R. & Harkness, S.H. (1993) Inactivation of respiratory syncytial virus by detergents and disinfectants. *Pediatric Infectious Diseases Journal*, **12**, 582–584.

Kuhrt, M.F., Fancher, M.J., McKinlay, M.A. & Lennert, S.D. (1984) Virucidal activity of glutaric acid and evidence for dual mechanism of action. *Antimicrobial Agents and Chemotherapy*, **26**, 924–927.

Kurtz, J.B. (1979) Virucidal effects of alcohols against echovirus 11. *Lancet*, **i**, 496–497.

Kurtz, J.B., Lee, T.W. & Parsons, A.J. (1980) The action of alcohols on rotavirus, astrovirus and enterovirus. *Journal of Hospital Infection*, **1**, 321–325.

Larson, E.L. & Morton, H.E. (1991) Alcohols. In *Disinfection, Sterilization and Preservation*, 4th edn (ed. Block, S.S.), pp. 191–203. Philadelphia: Lea & Febiger.

Lloyd, G., Bowen, E.T.W. & Slade, J.H.R. (1982) Physical and chemical methods of inactivating Lassa virus. *Lancet*, **i**, 1046–1048.

Lloyd-Evans, N., Springthorpe, V.S. & Sattar, S.A. (1986) Chemical disinfection of human rotavirus-contaminated surfaces. *Journal of Hygiene*, **97**, 163–173.

Mahnel, H. (1979) Variations in resistance of viruses from different groups to chemico-physical decontamination methods. *Infection*, **7**, 240–246.

Mahnel, H. & Kunz, W. (1976a) Suitability of carriers for the examination of disinfectants against viruses. *Berliner und Münchener Tierarztliche Wocheschrift*, **89**, 138–142.

Mahnel, H. & Kunz, W. (1976b) Suitability of carriers for the examination of disinfectants against viruses. *Berliner und Münchener Tierarztliche Wochenscrift*, **89**, 149–152.

Manabe, S. (1996) Removal of virus through novel membrane filtration method. *Developments in Biological Standardization*, **88**, 81–90.

Mathur, U., Bentley, D.W. & Hall, C.B. (1980) Concurrent respiratory syncytial virus and influenza A infections in the institutionalized elderly and chronically ill. *Annals of Internal Medicine*, **93**, 49–52.

Mbithi, J.N., Springthorpe, V.S. & Sattar, S.A. (1990) Chemical disinfection of hepatitis A virus on environmental surfaces. *Applied and Environmental Microbiology*, **56**, 3601–3604.

Mbithi, J.N., Springthorpe, V.S., Boulet, J.R. & Sattar, S.A. (1992) Survival of hepatitis A virus on human hands and its transfer on contact with animate and inanimate surfaces. *Journal of Clinical Microbiology*, **30**, 757–763.

Mbithi, J.N., Springthorpe, V.S., Sattar, S.A. &

Pacquette, M. (1993a) Bactericidal, virucidal and mycobactericidal activity of alkaline glutaraldehyde under reuse in an endoscopy unit. *Journal of Clinical Microbiology*, **31**, 2988–2995.

Mbithi, J.N., Springthorpe, V.S. & Sattar, S.A. (1993b) Comparative *in vivo* efficiency of hand-washing agents against hepatitis A virus (HM-175) and poliovirus type 1 (Sabin). *Applied and Environmental Microbiology*, **59**, 3463–3469.

Mentel, R. & Schmidt, J. (1973) Investigations on rhinovirus inactivation by hydrogen peroxide. *Acta Virologica*, **17**, 351–354.

Merianos, J.J. (1991) Quaternary ammonium antimicrobial compounds. In *Disinfection, Sterilization and Preservation*, 4th edn (ed. Block, S.S.), pp. 225–255. Philadelphia: Lea & Febiger.

Oxford, J.S., Potter, C.W., MaLaren, C. & Hardy, W. (1971) Inactivation of influenza and other viruses by a mixture of virucidal compounds. *Applied Microbiology*, **21**, 606–610.

Pancic, F., Carpenter, D.C. & Came, P.E., (1980) Role of infectious secretions in the transmission of rhinovirus. *Journal of Clinical Microbiology*, **12**, 467–471.

Papaevangelou, G.J. (1984) Global epidemiology of hepatitis A. In *Hepatitis A* (ed. Gerety, R.J.), p. 101. Orlando, Florida: Academic Press.

Parisi, A.N. & Young, W.E. (1991) Sterilization with ethylene oxide and other gases. In *Disinfection, Sterilization and Preservation*, (ed. Block, S.S.) 4th edn, pp. 580–595. Philadelphia: Lea & Febiger.

Pass, R.F. & Hutto, S.C. (1986) Group daycare and cytomegalovirus infections of mothers and children. *Reviews of Infectious Disease*, **8**, 599–605.

Pass, R.F., Hutto, S.C., Reynolds, D.W. & Polhill, R.B. (1984) Increased frequency of cytomegalovirus infection in children in group day care. *Pediatrics*, **74**, 121–126.

Peterson, D.A., Hurley, T.R., Hoff, J.C. & Wolfe, L.G. (1983) Effect of chlorine treatment on infectivity of hepatitis A virus. *Applied and Environmental Microbiology*, **45**, 223–227.

Pickering, L.K., Evans, D.G., Dupont, H.L. & Vollet, J.J. III (1981) Diarrhea caused by *Shigella*, rotavirus and *Giardia* in day-care centers. *Journal of Pediatrics*, **99**, 51–56.

Pickering, L.K., Bartlett, A.V. & Woodward, W.E. (1986) Acute infectious diarrhea among children in day care: epidemiology and control. *Reviews of Infectious Diseases*, **8**, 539–547.

Piot, P., Plummer, F.A., Mhalu, F.S., Lamboray, J.-L., Chin, J. & Mann, J.M. (1988) AIDS: an international perspective. *Science*, **239**, 573–579.

Poli, G., Ponti, W., Micheletti, R. & Cantoni, C. (1978) Virucidal activity of some quaternary ammonium compounds. *Drug Research*, **28**, 1672–1675.

Pollard, E.C. (1953) *The Physics of Viruses*. Academic Press, New York, p. 122.

Raphael, R.A., Sattar, S.A. & Springthorpe, V.S. (1987) Lack of human rotavirus inactivation by residual chlorine in municipal drinking water systems. *Revue Internationale de Science de l'Eau*, **3**, 67–69.

Russell, A.D., Hammond, S.A. & Morgan, J.R. (1986) Bacterial resistance to antiseptics and disinfectants. *Journal of Hospital Infection*, **7**, 213–225.

Rutala, W.A. (with 1994, 1995 and 1996 APIC Guidelines Committee) (1996) APIC guideline for the selection and use of disinfectants. *American Journal of Infection Control*, **24** (Suppl.), 313–342.

Saif, L.J. & Theil, K.W. (1989) *Viral Diarrheas of Man and Animals*. Boca Raton, Florida: CRC Press.

Saitanu, K. & Lund, E. (1975) Inactivation of enterovirus by glutaraldehyde. *Applied Microbiology*, **29**, 571–574.

Samadi, A.R., Huq, M.I. & Ahmed, Q.S. (1983) Detection of rotavirus in the handwashings of attendants of children with diarrhea. *British Medical Journal*, **286**, 188.

Sattar, S.A. & Ijaz, M.K. (1987) Spread of viral infections by aerosols. *CRC Critical Reviews in Environmental Control*, **17** (2), 89–131.

Sattar, S.A. & Springthorpe, V.S. (1991) Survival and disinfectant inactivation of the human immunodeficiency virus: a critical review. *Reviews in Infectious Diseases*, **13**, 430–447.

Sattar, S.A., Lloyd-Evans, N., Springthorpe, V.S. & Nair, R.C. (1986) Institutional outbreaks of rotavirus diarrhea: possible role of fomites and environmental surfaces as vehicles for virus transmission. *Journal of Hygiene*, **96**, 277–289.

Sattar, S.A., Springthorpe, V.S., Karim, Y. & Loro, P. (1989) Chemical disinfection of non-porous inanimate surfaces experimentally-contaminated with four human pathogenic viruses. *Epidemiology and Infection*, **102**, 493–505.

Sattar, S.A., Springthorpe, V.S., Conway, B. & Xu, Y. (1994) Inactivation of the human immunodeficiency virus: an update. *Reviews in Medical Microbiology*, **5** (3), 139–150.

Schmaljohn, C.S., Hasty, S.E., Dalrymple, J.M. *et al.* (1985) Antigenic and genetic properties of viruses linked to hemorrhagic fever with renal syndrome. *Science*, **227**, 1041–1044.

Scott, E.M. & Gorman, S.P. (1991) Sterilization with glutaraldehyde. In *Disinfection, Preservation and Sterilization*, (ed. Block, S.S.) 4th edn, pp. 596–614. Philadelphia: Lea & Febiger.

Shah, K.V. & Buscema, J. (1988) Genital warts, papillomaviruses and genital malignancies. *Annual Reviews of Medicine*, **39**, 371–379.

Sidwell, R.W., Westbrook, L., Dixon, G.J. & Happich, W.F. (1970) Potentially infectious agents associated with shearling bedpads. I. Effect of laundering with detergent-disinfectant combinations on polio and vaccinia viruses. *Applied Microbiology*, **19**, 53–59.

Sobsey, M.D., Fuji, T. & Hall, R.M. (1991) Inactivation of cell-associated and dispersed hepatitis A virus in water. *Journal of the American Water Works Association*, **83**, 64–67.

Sporkenbach, J., Wiegers, K.J. & Dernick, R. (1981) The virus inactivating efficacy of peracids and peracidous disinfectants. *Zentralblatt für Bakteriologie, Mikrobiologie und Hygiene (Orig. B)*, **173**, 425–439.

Springthorpe, V.S. & Sattar, S.A. (1990) Chemical disinfection of virus-contaminated surfaces. *Critical Reviews in Environmental Control*, **20** (3), 169–229.

Springthorpe, V.S., Grenier, J.L., Lloyd-Evans, N. & Sattar, S.A. (1986) Chemical disinfection of human rotaviruses: efficacy of commercially-available products in suspension tests. *Journal of Hygiene*, **97**, 139–161.

Sprossig, M. (1975) Peracetic acid and resistant microorganisms. In *Resistance of Microorganisms of Disinfectants*, 2nd International Symposium, Poznan (ed. Kedzia, W.B.), pp. 89–91. Warsaw: Polish Academy of Sciences.

Storch, G., McFarland, L.M., Kelso, K., Heilman, C.J. & Caraway, C.T. (1979) Viral hepatitis associated with daycare centers. *Journal of the American Medical Association*, **242**, 1514–1518.

Taylor, G.R. & Butler, M. (1982) A comparison of the virucidal properties of chlorine, chlorine dioxide, bromine chloride and iodine. *Journal of Hygiene*, **89**, 321–328.

Thraenhart, O. (1991) Measures for disinfection and control of viral hepatitis. In *Disinfection, Preservation and Sterilization*, (ed. Block, S.S.) 4th edn, pp. 445–471. Philadelphia: Lea & Febiger.

Thraenhart, O. & Kuwert, E. (1975) Virucidal activity of the disinfectant 'Gigasept' against different enveloped and non-enveloped RNA- and DNA-viruses pathogenic for man. I. Investigation in the suspension test. *Zentralblatt für Bakteriologie und Hygiene, I. Abt. Orig. B*, **161**, 209–232.

Thurman, R.B. & Gerba, C.P. (1988) Molecular mechanisms of viral inactivation by water disinfectants. *Advances in Applied Microbiology*, **33**, 75–105.

Turner, F.J. (1983) Hydrogen peroxide and other oxidant disinfectants. In *Disinfection, Sterilization and Preservation*, (ed. Block, S.S.), pp. 240–250. Philadelphia: Lea & Febiger.

Valenti, W.M., Hall, C.B., Douglas, R.G., Menegus, M.A. & Pincus, P.H. (1980a) Nosocomial viral infections: I. Epidemiology and significance. *Infection Control*, **1**, 33–37.

Valenti, W.M., Betts, R.F., Hall, C.B., Hruska, J.F. & Douglas, R.G. (1980b) Nosocomial viral infections: II. Guidelines for prevention and control of respiratory viruses, herpesviruses, and hepatitis viruses. *Infection Control*, **1**, 165–178.

van Bueren, J. (1995) Methodology for HIV disinfectant testing. *Journal of Hospital Infection*, **30** (Suppl.), 383–388.

van Bueren, J., Larkin, D.P. & Simpson, R.A. (1994) Inactivation of human immunodeficiency virus type 1 by alcohols. *Journal of Hospital Infection*, **28**, 137–148.

Wallbank, A.M., Drulak, M., Poffenroth, L., Barnes, C., Kay, C. & Lebtag, I. (1978) Wescodyne: lack of activity against poliovirus in the presence of organic matter. *Health Laboratory Science*, **15**, 133–137.

Walter, J.K., Werz, W. & Berthold, W. (1996) Process scale considerations in evaluation studies and scale up. *Developments in Biological Standardization*, **88**, 99–108.

Ward, R.L., Knowlton, D. & Pierce, M.J. (1984) Efficiency of human rotavirus propagation in cell culture. *Journal of Clinical Microbiology*, **19**, 748– 753.

Ward, R.L., Bernstein, D.I., Young, E.C., Sherwood, J.R., Knowlton, D.R. & Schiff, G.M. (1986) Human rotavirus studies in volunteers: determination of infectious dose and serological response to infection. *Journal of Infectious Diseases*, **154**, 871–880.

Ward, R.L., Bernstein, D.I., Knowlton, D.R. *et al.* (1991) Prevention of surface to human transmission of rotaviruses by treatment with a disinfectant spray. *Journal of Clinical Microbiology*, **29**, 1991–1996.

Welliver, R.C. & McLaughlin, S. (1984) Unique epidemiology of nosocomial infection in a children's hospital. *American Journal of Diseases of Children*, **138**, 131–135.

Wenzel, R.P., Deal, E.C. & Hendley, J.O (1977) Hospital-acquired viral respiratory illness on a pediatric ward. *Pediatrics*, **60**, 367–371.

Westwood, J.C.N. & Sattar, S.A. (1976) The minimal infective dose. In *Viruses in Water*. (eds Berg, G. *et al.*), pp. 61–69. Washington, DC: American Public Health Association.

Wickramanayake, G.B. (1991) Disinfection and sterilization by ozone. In *Disinfection, Preservation and Sterilization*, (ed. Block, S.S.) 4th edn, pp. 182–190. Philadelphia: Lea & Febiger.

Williams, F.P. (1985) Membrane-associated viral complexes observed in stools and cell cultures. *Applied and Environmental Microbiology*, **50**, 523–526.

World Health Organization (WHO) (1993) *Laboratory Biosafety Manual*, 2nd edn, Chapter 9. Geneva: WHO.

Wright, H. (1970) Inactivation of vesicular stomatitis virus by disinfectants. *Applied Microbiology*, **19**, 96–98.

Young, D.C. & Sharp, D.G. (1979) Partial reactivation of chlorine-treated echovirus. *Applied and Environmental Microbiology*, **37**, 766–773.

Yousef, G.E., Bell, E.J., Mann G.F. *et al.* (1988). Chronic enterovirus infection in patients with postviral fatigue syndrome. *Lancet*, **i**, 146–150.

Chapter 6

B. ACTIVITY AGAINST VETERINARY VIRUSES

1 Introduction

The development of intensive systems of livestock production, the increased value of individual animals and the emergence of new or recently recognized diseases have created many challenges for the veterinary profession, particularly in the area of disease control. Measures applied for the prevention or control of viral disease are aimed at lessening the possibility of infection in susceptible populations. The control of viral infections relies on a range of specific measures appropriate for each virus family. Decisions relating to individual viruses are usually determined by their importance in animal or human populations, their mode of spread and their disease-producing capacity. In the case of endemic viral diseases, measures range from vaccination and disinfection to effective management strategies, while some exotic diseases are currently controlled by test and slaughter policies followed by thorough disinfection. Despite steady progress in vaccine development, many economically important viral diseases still cannot be controlled through immunization. Several viral diseases of animals are transmissible to humans and disinfection is used to limit the spread of zoonotic agents during the production phase of food-producing animals and subsequently in meat plants and dairies.

Infected animals shed viruses, often in large numbers, and environmental contamination frequently follows. Inanimate surfaces can play an important role in the transmission of viral infections. Contaminated biological materials, such as faeces, urine and exudates, and contaminated transport vehicles or buildings may harbour infectious agents for long periods and perpetuate infections in groups of animals unless the cycle of infection is interrupted by effective control measures. Disinfection plays an important role in the destruction of infectious agents in contaminated biological products, transport vehicles, equipment, footware and clothing of personnel, as well as in successful implementation of test and slaughter policies (Table 6.2). Increased reliance on disinfection procedures for the control of infectious diseases in animals derives in part from the trend towards intensive rearing of livestock, with the consequent build-up of infectious agents. The necessity to have expensive buildings restocked soon after completion of a production cycle reinforces the need for efficient disinfection programmes to deal with the residual infectious agents, especially when dealing with diseases of complex aetiology. These considerations apply particularly to the intensive factory-farming practices of the pig and poultry industries. Viral infections usually spread rapidly indoors among intensively-reared animals, and

Table 6.2 Applications of disinfection in the control of viral diseases of veterinary importance.

Preventing disease transmission by lateral spread—animals to humans and humans to animals
Elimination of build-up of viruses in farm buildings and lairages
Decontamination of transport vehicles
Maintaining farm buildings or animal production units free from viral disease by the use of foot-baths and wheel baths
Maintaining boarding kennels, catteries and laboratory-animal units free of infection by strategic disinfection of equipment and by the use of foot-baths
Decontamination of water systems
Facilitating the safe operation of quarantine stations, aircraft and ships used for importing animals

often result in a high incidence of disease. In addition, viral diseases in intensively-reared animals tend to be more severe than in animals under extensive systems of husbandry. The financial losses incurred by producers through clinical and subclinical disease, the cost of vaccination and the lack of effective drugs for treating viral infections emphasize the continuing need for thorough cleaning, disinfection and isolation procedures to prevent transmission of viral diseases. Disinfection plays an important role in eradication programmes for a number of viral diseases, classed as List A diseases by the Office International des Epizooties, including foot-and-mouth disease, African swine fever and rinderpest (Fotheringham, 1995).

2 Disinfection

Effective disinfection can only be achieved when there is direct contact between an appropriate concentration of an effective biocide and the target virus for sufficient time. The type of virus and the chemical composition of the biocide play an important part in determining the outcome of disinfection programmes. In addition, the success of the procedure is strongly influenced by environmental factors, such as the presence of organic matter, pH, temperature and relative humidity (see also Chapters 2 and 3).

2.1 The target virus

Klein & Deforest (1983) extended the classification system of Noll & Younger (1959) based on the lipophilic properties of viruses, proposing that the lipid content and the size of a virus were useful for predicting the susceptibility of a virus to biocides. These workers described three groups:

> Group A viruses, which possess lipoprotein envelopes, are highly susceptible to most biocides.
> Group B viruses, containing no lipid and among the smallest in size, are resistant to lipophilic biocides.
> Group C viruses, containing no lipid but which adsorb some lipids, are intermediate in their susceptibility patterns.

However, predictions about the susceptibility pattern of a virus to disinfectants based on the pattern displayed by another member of the same family are not always valid. For example, within the *Picornaviridae*, foot-and-mouth disease virus, which is a member of the genus aphthovirus, is unstable at pH values below 6.5, while swine vesicular disease, which is a member of the genus enterovirus, is stable at low pH values.

Viruses released from cells, whether by budding or following rupture, frequently remain clumped or associated with cellular debris. In addition, individual virions usually have a tendency to adhere to other particulate matter and surfaces. As a result, in aggregations on contaminated surfaces or in body fluids, virions in the centre of such clumps may be afforded physical protection by particles in the outer layers. The number of particles will also influence the quantity of active biocide required to inactivate all the virions present. Virus suspensions can be rather viscous and impede penetration by biocides. In addition, the matrix of organic molecules and inorganic salts in body fluids, along with cellular debris associated with viruses shed from infected hosts, provides physical protection for the viruses, as well as reacting chemically with most biocides (Springthorpe & Sattar, 1990).

2.2 The disinfectant

A large range of active biocides are available, and may be grouped according to chemical structure into about a dozen categories. Only about one-third of the available biocides are commonly used in the veterinary field (Jeffrey, 1995). The choice of disinfectant will be influenced by several factors. The microbiocidal attributes of the disinfectant are obviously important and few compounds are capable of killing all types of microorganisms. Many commercial products contain a number of active ingredients with different modes of biocidal action, resulting in additive or sometimes synergistic antimicrobial effects. Soaps or detergents are frequently combined with an active biocide. The speed of action of biocides varies and this must be considered in the context of particular disinfection programmes and the contact time with targeted viruses. Within limits, the longer the contact time the more effective the biocide. The chemical and physical properties of the biocide may render it unsuitable for use in particular circumstances. For example, sodium hydroxide reacts with and corrodes materials containing tin, zinc or aluminium, hypochlorites corrode metals and oxidizing agents are neutralized by the presence of reducing substances. Toxicity, tainting or staining properties also influence the selection of a biocide. Only a limited range of biocides can be used for antisepsis because of the sensitivity of animal skin to certain chemicals. The method of application of the biocide is an important consideration. Fumigation is labour-saving and, in many instances, more effective for disinfection of buildings than the application of chemical solutions by spraying. However, it can be used only if the building can be sealed securely. The cost of disinfectants is a significant factor affecting choice, and consideration must also be given to the method of disposal, in order to minimize the risk of environmental pollution.

2.3 Environmental factors

Organic material can dilute, neutralize and prevent penetration of many biocidal chemicals and its presence may therefore be critical in determining the outcome of any disinfection programme. The type, extent and nature of organic contamination will affect the efficacy of a biocide. The most frequently encountered organic contaminants are blood, urine, faeces, fats and dust. The presence of inorganic material, such as lime scale, accumulated salt deposits and soil, may reduce the efficacy of biocides. Adherent organic material is commonly encountered on inanimate surfaces in buildings where animals are housed. Any surface in contact with animal skin will acquire microorganisms, sebum and other organic material. Horizontal surfaces exposed to air quickly become coated with dust, oily emulsions and aerosols. Bacteria, fungi and non-pathogenic viruses on surfaces effectively inactivate biocides and reduce their effective working concentration against pathogenic viruses. Vigorous precleaning must therefore precede the application of biocides unless there are human health or other risks which require immediate application of a disinfectant. Halogen disinfectants, particularly sodium hypochlorite, are readily inactivated by organic matter, whereas phenolic disinfectants retain much of their activity in similar circumstances.

The rate of chemical reactions increases as temperature increases. In general, the higher the temperature of the disinfectant, subject to thermal stability, the more effective it is. The hardness of the water used to dilute a biocide may affect its activity. Biocides are also affected by pH, some requiring a defined pH for stability and optimum activity. Traces of inhibitory substances, such as soaps and detergents, may interfere with the viricidal activity of quaternary ammonium compounds (QACs) or biguanides. High relative humidity favours the survival of many viruses and is also an important requirement for the use of some biocides, such as formaldehyde gas. Prehumidification of surfaces, before disinfectant treatment commences, enhances the action of most biocides by facilitating penetration of dried organic residues and promoting improved adherence of biocide to the surfaces.

3 Design of disinfection programmes

Intensive animal-production units contain high numbers of animals occupying the same air space and often there are problems associated with overcrowding and competition for floor and trough space. The environment in intensive-production units is frequently dusty and contains airborne viruses. In such systems, it is unrealistic to expect a disinfection programme to compensate for poor management, poor building design or construction, inadequate ventilation and low standards of hygiene. Disinfection programmes must complement good animal management, which should take into account the species and age of the animals and the aims of the production system. An environment in which the animals' health can be maintained and productivity sustained at a reasonable cost is the main objective. The design and implementation of an effective disinfection programme requires evaluation of the disease status of the farm, consideration of the buildings involved and review of isolation facilities for replacement animals. Consideration should also be given to the water supply, use of foot-baths and wheel baths, the cleaning equipment and the existing management policy regarding disinfection.

Building design features may militate against the implementation of an effective disinfection programme. Uneven, cracked, unplastered or pitted surfaces are difficult to disinfect, as are old wooden fittings. Houses with slatted floors, buildings with open-ridge ventilation and ill-fitting doors or windows make fumigation inefficient. Calf pens with wooden pallets used as slats or with earth floors are extremely difficult to clean and disinfect. The design of particular drainage and ventilation systems may also present special difficulties for thorough disinfection. The absence of electricity, a power hose and a mains water-supply on remote farms or 'out farms' may make efficient cleaning impossible. The selection of a particular chemical biocide for individual situations must relate to the environmental conditions in which it is being used and to the infectious agents present. It is difficult to clean all parts of an animal house equally well and it is generally advisable to select disinfectants that remain active in the presence of organic matter.

3.1 Cleaning prior to disinfection

Surfaces should be thoroughly cleaned before application of disinfectants. This process, if properly carried out, removes most microorganisms. Adequate training of the responsible personnel is required for a proper understanding of the specific needs of the entire procedure. Electricity should be disconnected before washing commences. All portable equipment and movable items should be removed, soaked in detergent solution and cleaned separately by brushing or hosing before disinfection. All organic material, including manure, litter, bedding and feed, should be removed and disposed of in a suitable manner. Small amounts of bedding and litter may be burned or composted. Gross dirt should be removed manually or if possible by mechanical means. To avoid the generation of dust, which may harbour viruses, and also to remove dried faeces, urine, milk and other adherent material, walls and other surfaces in the premises should be sprayed with water, preferably containing detergent. A non-foaming detergent or 4% sodium carbonate (washing-soda) is suitable. Pressure hosing, preferably using a high-pressure, low-volume system, should be employed to clean all surfaces capable of withstanding the pressure. Steam cleaners are particularly effective for cleaning greasy areas, but rapid cooling on surfaces tends to limit their antimicrobial effect. Cleaning should commence at the highest parts of the building and at points furthest from the main drain. In a large building with separate divisions, it is important to ensure that newly cleaned areas are not recontaminated as cleaning proceeds. Particular attention should be paid to feeding equipment and drinking bowls. The tanks supplying drinking-water should be emptied and cleaned, prior to disinfection of the entire water system with sodium hypochlorite. When the building is visibly clean, it can be disinfected. If disinfection has to be carried out in buildings still occupied by animals, complete cleaning is impossible and the biocides used must be non-toxic. All-in/all-out management practices with disinfection of unoccupied buildings are more effective.

3.2 Disinfection procedure

Surfaces of a building may be treated with a disinfectant solution by brushing or by spraying under low or high pressure. Portable items should be soaked in a tank of disinfectant. In buildings of suitable design, fumigation is an extremely useful and effective option. The building, with clean bedding and fittings in place, can be fumigated, using either formaldehyde or methyl bromide. Both chemicals are potentially dangerous, and experienced operators are essential to ensure safety and success. The building should be sealed to prevent the escape of gas, the ambient temperature should be close to 20°C and relative humidity should be above 70%, without pools of water forming on the floors. Fumigation can be carried out by heating paraformaldehyde (5–10 g/m^3), by adding formalin to potassium permanganate (20 ml formalin added to 10 g potassium permanganate crystals/m^3) or by producing a formalin aerosol using a generator (10–60 ml/m^3). Trials with aerosol generators indicate that this method may give variable results (Scarlett & Mathewson, 1977; Ide, 1979). Formaldehyde gas is pungent and irritating to mucous membranes even at low concentrations. Personnel should wear respirators and should not be exposed to concentrations above 2 parts/10^6. At higher concentrations, the gas is rapidly toxic and the long-term effects of constant exposure to low doses may present some health risks. Methyl bromide has greater penetrating power than formaldehyde but is extremely toxic and should be used by fully trained and equipped personnel only. The building should be left sealed for 24 h before being thoroughly ventilated. Drinking bowls and food containers should be rinsed with water before use.

3.3 Foot-baths

Foot-baths should be located at suitable entry points to the unit or farm. Suggested dimensions for a foot-bath are 50 cm × 50 cm with a depth of 25 cm. Suitable biocides include phenols, cresols and iodophors. Foot-baths are only likely to be effective if all staff wear waterproof footwear, which should be immersed, after thorough cleaning, in disinfectant to a depth of 15 cm for at least 1min. The disinfectant in a foot-bath should be changed at regular intervals (1–3 days), depending on the frequency of use and level of contamination with organic matter. In circumstances where gross soiling of footwear is unavoidable, a second foot-bath containing dilute detergent for preliminary washing should be positioned alongside the disinfectant foot-bath. Footwear design, such as angled corrugations on the soles and heels, may permit retention of organic matter, even after routine washing. Parallel corrugations are more easily cleaned than complex patterns. Foot-baths should be protected from flooding by surface water or heavy rainfall. Foot-baths serve to alert staff to the risk of human transfer of infectious agents. Waterproof protective clothing, which can be easily hosed down, should be worn when dealing with exotic or highly infectious viral diseases.

3.4 Wheel baths

Vehicles visiting successive farms may inadvertently transfer infection on the body of the vehicle or on its wheels. Wheel baths should only be installed if their use and cost can be justified in the context of the overall disinfection programme. The large volume of diluted disinfectant required (approximately 5000 l) and the cost of maintaining the biocide in an active state are serious limitations to their routine use. Other limiting factors are the need for a vacuum tanker (slurry tanker) for routine filling and emptying of the bath and the difficulty of disposing of large volumes of biocide in an environmentally-acceptable manner. Disposal of used biocide into a large slurry tank, followed by agitation of the slurry, is one possible solution. Phenolic-based biocides are comparatively cheap but may be difficult to dispose of in large volumes. Iodophor disinfectants are more environmentally safe, more readily neutralized than phenolic biocides and more stable than hypochlorite-based biocides. Iodine-based biocides, used at a concentration of 0.5%, changed at frequent intervals and replenished if diluted by heavy rain, have a wide spectrum of activity and are usually non-toxic for humans and animals.

The siting of a wheel bath requires careful planning so that it cannot be bypassed by vehicles entering the farm. The design of the wheel bath should allow for thorough immersion of one complete revolution of the largest-circumference wheel. Suggested dimensions are 7 m × 3.5 m, with a depth of 60 cm (Quinn, 1991). The slope at the entrance and exit to the bath should be 1 in 12. A depth of 20 cm of biocide is required in the bath. Ramps should be placed at the entrance to and exit from the bath to slow the passage of vehicles. The bath should be constructed to the highest specifications to ensure that no leaks of disinfectant occur.

3.5 Slurry disposal

The disinfection of slurry is generally considered difficult and is rarely attempted. Haas *et al.* (1995) have recently published a comprehensive review of the inactivation of viruses in liquid manure. A number of viruses, such as those causing Aujeszky's disease, foot-and-mouth disease and African swine fever, are capable of surviving for extended periods in liquid manure or slurry. Unlike farmyard manure, slurry does not normally compost and generate the type of self-heating processes which could destroy pathogens. The titre of some viruses will reduce by 1–2 $\log_{10}$ units/month at 4°C. Therefore, the minimum time required for inactivation of all viruses in stored slurry is probably of the order of 6 months. During this period, no new slurry should be added to the storage tanks.

Following an outbreak of a notifiable disease, it is often necessary to ensure inactivation of viruses in slurry. This is possible using physical, biological or chemical methods. The use of physical methods, such as pasteurization, or biological methods, such as anaerobic digestion, is often impractical because of the need for specialist equipment. Several biocides, including aldehydes, acids, oxidizing agents and alkalis, are considered suitable for chemical disinfection of slurry. Aldehydes, such as formalin (25–40 l/m^3 for more than 4 days), are economical, biodegradable, minimally corrosive and highly effective. Their main disadvantages are the irritating smell and unsuitability for use below 10°C. Inorganic acids are generally too corrosive for use, while organic acids are significantly affected by the high organic content of slurry. Oxidizing agents, such as peracetic acid (25–40 l/m^3 for more than 1 h), are effective but have a tendency to cause strong foaming following mixing with slurry. Alkalis, such as slaked lime (40% solution, 40–60 l/m^3 for more than 4 days) and sodium hydroxide (50% solution, 16–30 l/m^3 for more than 4 days), are cheap and effective but rather corrosive. The large volumes of lime required can also be a disadvantage. Treatment for 4 days is usually considered the minimum period for effective disinfection but exposure for 7 days is advisable. Storage tanks should not be full in order to allow for the addition of a sufficient quantity of the chemical. The biocide must be thoroughly dissolved and evenly distributed in the slurry by adding it to the tank at several points simultaneously. An aqueous suspension of biocide should be used rather than powder or granules, which are difficult to dissolve in slurry. Vigorous agitation of the slurry, using high-performance stirring equipment, is required before, during and for 6 h after the addition of the biocide. Stirring for at least 2 h/day should also be carried out during the treatment period. The disinfection of slurry tanks located under occupied animal houses should be avoided. Following treatment, the slurry should be spread on arable land and ploughed into the soil.

3.6 Activity of biocides against viruses of veterinary importance

Although disinfection is an important method for controlling viral diseases, remarkably few systematic studies have been carried out to evaluate the ability of different biocides to inactivate viruses of veterinary importance. A summary of relevant, published information is given in Table 6.3. Most of the studies published have evaluated disinfectants under laboratory conditions and the conclusions drawn may not be valid when applied to field situations. In addition, researchers frequently use different efficacy tests and test conditions. As a result, the findings of different studies are not always directly comparable. Demonstration of virus survival in efficacy tests requires either tissue culture, chick embryo or animal inoculation. The sensitivity of each system for detection of virus viability is dependent on the specific test virus and the method of demonstrating viability. A minimum number of virus particles is required to produce disease in susceptible animals or to induce cytopathic effects in tissue culture. The toxicity of

Table 6.3 The viricidal spectrum of disinfectants.

Viruses*	Acids	Alkalis	Alcohols	Aldehydes	Biguanides	QACs	Halogens: Chlorine	Halogens: Iodine	Phenolic compounds	Peroxygens
Group A Lipid-containing viruses										
Coronaviridae										
Canine coronavirus[1]	NT	NT	+	+	–	+	+	+	+	NT
Transmissible gastroenteritis virus[2,3]	–	+	+	+	+	+	+	+	V	+
Herpesviridae										
Aujeszky's disease virus[2]	NT	+	+	+	+	+	+	+	+	NT
Feline viral rhinotracheitis virus[4]	NT	NT	+	+	+	+	+	+	+	NT
Infectious bovine rhinotracheitis virus[3,5]	+	NT	NT	+/–	NT	NT	+	+	V	+
Paramyxoviridae										
Canine distemper virus[6]	NT	NT	+	+	NT	+	+	+	+	NT
Newcastle disease virus[7,8]	NT	+	NT	+	NT	+	+	+	–	NT
Parainfluenza virus[3,5]	+/–	NT	NT	+	NT	NT	+	+	+/–	+
Poxviridae										
Orf virus[3]	NT	NT	NT	+	NT	NT	+	+/–	+	+
Retroviridae										
Equine infectious anaemia virus[9]	NT	+	+	+	+	NT	+	+	+	NT
Flaviviridae										
Bovine virus diarrhoea virus[3]	NT	NT	NT	+	NT	NT	+	+/–	+/–	+

(Continued p. 194)

disinfectants for tissue cultures is an additional difficulty.

The virus of foot-and-mouth disease was rapidly inactivated in the presence of acid or alkali (Sellers, 1968). Sodium hypochlorite was equally effective, provided organic matter was not present. The rate of virus inactivation was slow with phenolic disinfectants. Of 10 commercially available biocides tested for their ability to inactivate African swine fever virus, only one containing *o*-phenylphenol (2-phenylphenol) had viricidal activity when virus–biocide mixtures were tested in pigs (Stone & Hess, 1973). Blackwell *et al.* (1975) tested 13 compounds against swine vesicular disease virus. Sodium hydroxide, sodium hypochlorite, formaldehyde and tincture of iodine inactivated the virus completely after 30 min at 25°C. Ten biocides were tested for viricidal activity against porcine enterovirus 1 (Talfan disease) and a porcine adenovirus (Derbyshire & Arkell, 1971). Sodium hypochlorite and ethyl alcohol were the most efficient, while formaldehyde inactivated the

Table 6.3 (*Continued.*)

Viruses*	Acids	Alkalis	Alcohols	Aldehydes	Biguanides	QACs	Halogens Chlorine	Halogens Iodine	Phenolic compounds	Peroxygens
Group B Small, non-lipid-containing viruses										
Parvoviridae										
Feline panleucopenia virus[4]	NT	NT	–	+	–	–	+	+/–	–	+
Canine parvovirus[1,8]	NT	+	–	+	–	–	+	+	–	NT
Picornaviridae										
Porcine enterovirus 1[3,5,10]	–	+	+	+	–	–	+	+/–	–	+
Foot-and-mouth disease virus[11]	+	+	NT	NT	NT	NT	+	NT	+/–	NT
Swine vesicular disease virus[12]	–	+	NT	+	–	NT	+	+/–	–	NT
Group C Non-lipid-containing viruses										
Adenoviridae										
Canine adenovirus 1[7,13]	NT	+	+/–	+	NT	+/–	V	V	V	NT
Porcine adenovirus[10]	NT	+	+	+	–	+/–	+	+/–	+	NT
Calciviridae										
Feline calicivirus[4]	NT	NT	+/–	+	–	–	+	+/–	+	+
Reoviridae										
Bovine rotavirus[14,15]	NT	NT	+	+	NT	+	+	NT	+	NT

*The viruses are grouped in categories according to their susceptibility to disinfectants.

1 Saknimit *et al.* (1988);
2 Brown (1981);
3 Evans *et al.* (1977);
4 Scott (1980);
5 Slavin (1973);
6 Watanabe *et al.* (1989);
7 Mahnel and Herlyn (1976);
8 McGavin (1987);
9 Shen *et al.* (1977);
10 Derbyshire and Arkell (1971);
11 Sellers (1968);
12 Blackwell *et al.* (1975);
13 Nomura *et al.* (1991);
14 Ferrari *et al.* (1986);
15 Kurtz *et al.* (1980).

QACs quaternary ammonium compounds; NT, not tested; +, effective; –, ineffective; +/–, limited efficacy; V, variable (published data inconsistent).

viruses slowly. Cetrimide and a phenolic disinfectant were active against the adenovirus but not against the enterovirus.

Each of the 12 biocides tested by Shen *et al.* (1977) succeeded in inactivating 4 $\log_{10}$ of equine infectious anaemia virus within 5 min at 23°C. Canine distemper virus was shown to be inactivated by alcohols, formalin, halogen compounds, QACs and cresol (Watanabe *et al.*, 1989). Canine coronavirus was inactivated by ethanol,

Table 6.4 Factors contributing to the failure of disinfection programmes.

Disinfectant	Environmental factors	Apparent failure
Selection of disinfectant ineffective against the infectious agent(s)	Presence of organic matter due to inadequate cleaning	Reintroduction of viruses via infected animals, fomites, vehicles, personnel, water, wildlife or carrier animals
Disinfectant too dilute	Inactivation of QACs and biguanides by residual soaps and detergents	
Insufficient contact time	Incorrect application and inadequate disinfectant penetration or coverage	
Temperature too low	Inadequate treatment of water supply	
Relative humidity too low for gaseous disinfectants	Interference with the activity of QACs and biguanides by synthetic materials and plastics	

QACs, quaternary ammonium compounds.

isopropanol, halogen compounds, cresol soap, formaldehyde and QACs, while canine parvovirus was inactivated by formaldehyde and halogen compounds (Saknimit *et al.*, 1988). McGavin (1987) showed that halogen compounds, aldehydes and sodium hydroxide are highly effective against canine parvovirus. More than 20 commercial biocides were evaluated by Scott (1980) for their viricidal activity against feline viral rhinotracheitis virus (FVRV), feline calicivirus (FCV) and feline panleucopenia virus (FPV). Of 22 biocides tested against FVRV, all were viricidal, while 11 of 35 were effective against FCV. Only three of the 27 tested were effective against FPV.

The efficacy of nine biocides against viruses representative of eight virus families was assessed by Evans *et al.* (1977). Formalin, glutaraldehyde, hypochlorite and peracetic acid were effective against all the viruses selected. Slavin (1973) evaluated the activity of several phenolic compounds and hypochlorite against infectious bovine rhinotracheitis (IBR) virus, bovine parainfluenza virus 3 (PI-3) and porcine enterovirus. The phenolic compounds and hypochlorite were effective against IBR virus and PI-3, while only hypochlorite inactivated the porcine enterovirus. Fourteen biocides were evaluated against porcine parvovirus, transmissible gastroenteritis (TGE) virus and Aujeszky's disease virus by Brown (1981). Aujeszky's disease virus and TGE virus were inactivated by all the biocides tested, whereas only sodium hypochlorite, sodium hydroxide and aldehyde compounds were effective against porcine parvovirus. Nine biocides were tested for viricidal activity against several veterinary viruses by Nomura *et al.* (1991). Phenolic compounds were shown to be the most active group of compounds. Mahnel and Herlyn (1976) tested formalin, phenol, sodium hydroxide and halogen compounds against porcine enterovirus 1 (Teschen disease), infectious canine hepatitis virus, Newcastle disease virus and vaccinia virus. The halogen compounds were the most effective, while phenol had almost no viricidal effect. The effect of several different biocides on bovine rotavirus has been evaluated (Kurtz *et al.*, 1980; Ferrari *et al.*, 1986). Formaldehyde, phenol, sodium hypochlorite, alcohol and a commercial product containing a QAC, amphoteric salts and propylene glycol were all shown to be effective. In contrast, Snodgrass & Herring (1977) failed to inactivate lamb rotavirus in intestinal contents using sodium hypochlorite.

3.7 Failure of a disinfection programme

Factors contributing to the failure of a disinfection programme can be divided into those that relate to the biocide itself, the environment and apparent failure when viral disease is re-introduced by restocking with infected animals (Table 6.4).

4 References

Blackwell, J.H., Graves, J.H. & McKercher, P.D. (1975) Chemical inactivation of swine vesicular disease virus. *British Veterinary Journal*, **131**, 317–322.

Brown, T.T. (1981) Laboratory evaluation of selected disinfectants as virucidal agents against porcine parvovirus, pseudorabies virus, and transmissible gastroenteritis virus. *American Journal of Veterinary Research*, **42**, 1033–1036.

Derbyshire, J.B. & Arkell, S. (1971) The activity of some chemical disinfectants against Talfan virus and porcine adenovirus type 2. *British Veterinary Journal*, **127**, 137–142.

Evans, D.H., Stuart, P. & Roberts, D.H. (1977) Disinfection of animal viruses. *British Veterinary Journal*, **133**, 356–359.

Ferrari, M., Gualandi, G.L. & Minelli, M.F. (1986) A study on the sensitivity of bovine rotavirus to some chemical agents. *Microbiologica*, **9**, 147–150.

Fotheringham, V.J.C. (1995) Disinfection of livestock production premises. *Revue scientifique et technique de l'Office International des Épizooties*, **14**, 191–205.

Haas, B., Ahl, R., Bohm, R. & Strauch, D. (1995) Inactivation of viruses in liquid manure. *Revue scientifique et technique de l'Office International des Épizooties*, **14**, 435–445.

Ide, P.R. (1979) The sensitivity of some avian viruses to formaldehyde fumigation. *Canadian Journal of Comparative Medicine*, **106**, 4–7.

Jeffrey, D.J. (1995) Chemicals used as disinfectants: active ingredients and enhancing additives. *Revue scientifique et technique de l'Office International des Épizooties*, **14**, 57–74.

Klein, M. & Deforest, A. (1983) Principles of viral inactivation. In *Disinfection, Sterilization and Preservation*, 3rd edn (ed. Block, S.S.), pp. 422–434. Philadelphia: Lea and Febiger.

Kurtz, J.B., Lee, T.W. & Parsons, A.J. (1980) The action of alcohols on rotavirus, astrovirus and enterovirus. *Journal of Hospital Infection*, **1**, 321–325.

McGavin, D. (1987) Inactivation of canine parvovirus by disinfectants and heat. *Journal of Small Animal Practice*, **28**, 523–535.

Mahnel, H. & Herlyn, M. (1976) Stability of Teschen, HCC, ND and vaccinia viruses against five disinfectants. *Journal of Veterinary Medicine B*, **23**, 403–411.

Noll, H. & Younger, J.S. (1959) Virus lipid interactions: the mechanism of adsorption of lipophilic viruses to water insoluble polar lipids. *Virology*, **8**, 319–343.

Nomura, Y., Ohita, C., Shirahata, T. & Goto, H. (1991) Virucidal effect of disinfectants on several animal viruses. *Research Bulletin of Obihiro University*, **17**, 103–107.

Quinn, P.J. (1991) Disinfection and disease prevention in veterinary medicine. In *Disinfection, Sterilization, and Preservation*, 4th edn (ed. Block, S.S.), pp. 846–870. Philadelphia: Lea and Febiger.

Saknimit, M., Inatsuki, I., Sugiyama, Y. & Yagami, K. (1988) Virucidal efficacy of physico-chemical treatments against coronaviruses and parvoviruses of laboratory animals. *Experimental Animals*, **37**, 341–345.

Scarlett, C.M. & Mathewson, G.K. (1977) Terminal disinfection of calf houses by formaldehyde fumigation. *Veterinary Record*, **101**, 7–10.

Scott, F.W. (1980) Virucidal disinfectants and feline viruses. *American Journal of Veterinary Research*, **41**, 410–414.

Sellers, R.F. (1968) The inactivation of foot-and-mouth disease virus by chemicals and disinfectants. *Veterinary Record*, **83**, 504–506.

Shen, D.T., Crawford, T.B., Gorham, J.R. & McGuire, T.C. (1977) Inactivation of equine infectious anaemia virus by chemical disinfectants. *American Journal of Veterinary Research*, **38**, 1217–1219.

Slavin, G. (1973) A reproducible surface contamination method for disinfectant tests. *British Veterinary Journal*, **129**, 13–18.

Snodgrass, D.R. and Herring, A.J. (1977) The action of disinfectants on lamb rotavirus. *Veterinary Record*, **101**, 81.

Springthorpe, V.S. & Sattar, S.A. (1990) Chemical disinfection of virus-contaminated surfaces. *Critical Reviews in Environmental Control*, **20**, 169–229.

Stone, S.S. & Hess, W.R. (1973) Effects of some disinfectants on African swine fever virus. *Applied Microbiology*, **25**, 115–122.

Watanabe, Y., Miyata, H. & Sato, H. (1989) Inactivation of laboratory animal RNA-viruses by physicochemical treatment. *Experimental Animals*, **38**, 305–311.

C. EVALUATION OF VIRICIDAL ACTIVITY

1 Introduction

Chemical disinfectants are used extensively in disease-control programmes to prevent the spread of infectious agents. The bactericidal, fungicidal or viricidal activity of particular chemical compounds cannot be reliably predicted from their chemical composition alone and standardized testing procedures are required to evaluate their efficacy. There are few internationally-accepted tests for the evaluation of viricides, reflecting the complexity of testing procedures and the difficulty of standardizing the many variables involved. Although there is a substantial body of scientific literature on the bactericidal properties of disinfectants (see Chapters 2 and 3), corresponding reports relating to viricides are uncommon and there are few definitive studies published on this topic. Because viruses are more resistant to disinfectants than vegetative bacteria, recommendations based on bactericidal testing methods are inappropriate for viral pathogens in many instances.

Viruses are divided into families on the basis of size, symmetry, type of nucleic acid genome (ribonucleic acid (RNA) or deoxyribonucleic acid (DNA)), form of nucleic acid genome and mode of replication (Murphy *et al.*, 1995). The enormous diversity among virus families permits few generalizations relating to their susceptibility to chemical agents to be made. Viruses of different families vary in their resistance to chemical disinfectants, enveloped viruses usually being more sensitive than non-enveloped viruses. The viral diseases of animals and humans, which are spread mainly through contact with virus-contaminated surfaces, are those which are more likely to be controlled by disinfection procedures. In disinfection programmes employing chemical substances, many factors, some relating to the number and accessibility of viruses and others to the presence of organic matter or other interfering compounds in the environment, determine the success or failure of the procedure. Viricidal testing methods should be designed to simulate the conditions that prevail in practical circumstances. Even if laboratory-based studies confirm the viricidal activity of a disinfectant, field trials are required to confirm its efficacy in situations where uncontrollable factors, such as virus concentration, the presence of organic matter, contact time and temperature, may determine the outcome.

2 Cultivation of viruses

Viruses replicate only within living cells. Replication of some viruses is restricted to specific cell types and a few viruses have not yet been cultivated. Most viruses can replicate in cultured cells, in embryonated hens' eggs or in laboratory animals. In veterinary virology, the natural host animal can also be used for the cultivation of viruses. Human volunteers have been used for Norwalk virus and other fastidious viruses that produce enteric disease in humans. *In vitro* cultivation of viruses in cells is routinely used for diagnostic and research purposes and for the evaluation of viricides. Many cell types cultured *in vitro* from human or animal tissues undergo only a few divisions before dying off; others can survive for many generations and some can be propagated indefinitely.

There are three basic types of cell culture: primary cultures, diploid cell lines and continuous cell lines. Primary cultures are prepared by dispersing cells, often from fetal organs or tissues, with trypsin. Although they are unable to grow for more than a few passages in culture, they contain several cell types and are thus sensitive to many viruses. Diploid cell lines are secondary cultures which have undergone a change that allows limited culture that roughly correlates to the lifespan of the species of origin: up to 50 passages for fetal human cells and approximately 10 passages for fetal cells from cattle and horses. Continuous cell lines are cells of a single type that are capable of indefinite propagation *in vitro*. They often originate from malignant tissues or by spontaneous transformation of a diploid cell line. No single cell line is appropriate for the wide range of viruses encountered in human and veterinary medicine. The type of cell used for virus cultivation depends on its suitability for the particular virus.

Embryonated eggs have been used for many years for the cultivation of viruses. Although largely replaced by tissue-culture methods, they are still used for the isolation and cultivation of many avian viruses. Eggs for virological investigations should be selected from specific pathogen-free poultry and the vaccination programme of the flock must be known, since passive antibody transmission via the yolk-sac may interfere with the isolation of some avian viruses.

Susceptible experimental animals are still essential for some procedures in virology, involving viral pathogens that cannot be cultured *in vitro*, and for vaccine development.

3 Virus quantitation

Quantitation of virus is not easily achieved, as many viruses are either cell-associated or adsorbed to tissue debris. To ensure reproducibility and to facilitate standardization, viricidal systems should contain a defined number of virus particles. The number of virions in suspension can be counted directly by electron microscopy. This can be achieved by mixing the virus suspension with a known number of latex particles, viewing a droplet of the mixture by electron microscopy and counting the two types of particles present.

To allow enumeration, viruses can be deposited on a grid by ultracentrifugation or allowed to diffuse into agar on the underside of an ultrathin carbon-coated plastic film on a copper grid. A relatively concentrated preparation of virus is necessary for these procedures. However, these methods do not distinguish infectious from non-infectious particles. Procedures for assaying infectivity of viruses include the plaque method, the production of lesions on the chorioallantoic membrane of embryonated eggs and the quantal assay. In the plaque method, a series of 10-fold dilutions of a viral suspension is inoculated on to monolayers of cultured cells. The virions are allowed time to attach to the cells and the monolayers are overlaid with agar or methylcellulose gel to ensure that viral progeny are restricted to the immediate vicinity of infected cells. As each infectious virus produces a plaque, a localized focus of infected and lysed cells is visible after the monolayer is stained. The infectivity titre of the original suspension is expressed in terms of plaque-forming units (pfu/ml). Viruses, such as herpesviruses and poxviruses, will produce plaques in cell monolayers maintained in liquid medium.

Some viruses, such as vaccinia, form pocks when inoculated onto the chorioallantoic membrane of an embryonated egg. By relating the number of pocks formed to the virus dilution, the concentration of viable virions can be calculated.

Data produced by quantal assay relate to the visible effects of dilution of the virus suspension and include features such as death of cells in culture and death of a chick embryo or experimental animal. The end-point of a quantal titration is the dilution of virus which infects or kills 50% of inoculated hosts (infective dose (ID_{50}) for animals or $TCID_{50}$ in tissue culture). The number of infectious particles in the inoculum is not determined by this method.

4 Detection of viral growth in cell culture

The growth of viruses in cell culture can be monitored by visible effects, such as cell death, or by a number of biochemical procedures which demonstrate an increase in intracellular viral macromolecules. For tissue-culture procedures, several dilution series of the recovered virus should be employed and, in addition, a number of subpassages should be carried out before final interpretation of the data.

The most easily recognized effects of infection with lytic viruses are cytopathic effects (CPE), which can be observed both macroscopically and microscopically. Virus-induced CPE include lysis or necrosis and the formation of inclusion bodies or syncytia. Some viruses produce obvious CPE that are characteristic of the virus group. Cells infected with viruses that bud from cytoplasmic membranes, such as orthomyxoviruses and paramyxoviruses, acquire the ability to adsorb suitable erythrocytes to their cell membranes. This phenomenon is referred to as haemadsorption and, in some cases, occurs in the absence of cytopathic effects. Haemagglutination is a different but related phenomenon, in which erythrocytes are agglutinated by free virus particles, such as influenza virus. Although haemagglutination is not a sensitive indicator of small numbers of virions, it provides a simple and convenient assay if large amounts of virus are present.

Some viruses replicate in cell culture without producing CPE. These non-cytopathic viruses can be detected by interference, i.e. their ability to prevent the entry and subsequent CPE of cytopathic strains of the same virus which are added later to the cell culture. Oncogenic viruses may induce morphological transformation, accompanied by loss of contact inhibition and piling up of cells at discrete foci on the monolayer.

Newly synthesized viral antigen can be detected by adding antibody, labelled or conjugated with material that can be visualized with either the light or the electron microscope, to the fixed-cell monolayer. Antibody labelled with fluorescein or peroxidase is commonly used for light microscopy. For electron microscopy, antibody tagged with large particles, such as ferritin, is often used.

Virus growth in embryonated eggs may result in dwarfing of the embryo, pocks on the chorioallantoic membrane, development of haemagglutinins in the embryonic fluids or death of the embryo. The particular effects relate to the type of virus under test.

5 Viricidal tests

Viruses exhibit considerable heterogeneity not only in their morphological features but also in their susceptibility to chemical disinfectants. The viricidal activity of chemical disinfectants cannot be reliably predicted from their composition. Variations in activity arising from dilution, pH changes and interactions with organic matter or other interfering substances must be considered in the design and interpretation of viricidal tests. The characteristics of the test virus, number of virions present, concentration of viricide, hydrogen ion concentration, temperature, duration of exposure and methods used to avoid cytotoxic effects of the viricide are important variables in tests to evaluate the activity of disinfectants (Fig. 6.3). The sensitivity of the test method for assessing virus survival or inactivation may determine the reliability of the results obtained. A particularly important factor, which may influence the interpretation of test results, is the degree of aggregation of virus particles in the test system (Thurman & Gerba, 1988).

5.1 Mechanisms of viral inactivation

Inactivation of a virus implies that, as a consequence of the disinfection procedure, there is permanent loss of infectivity. Any released nucleic acid must also be destroyed before a virus can be considered truly inactivated. Exposure of a

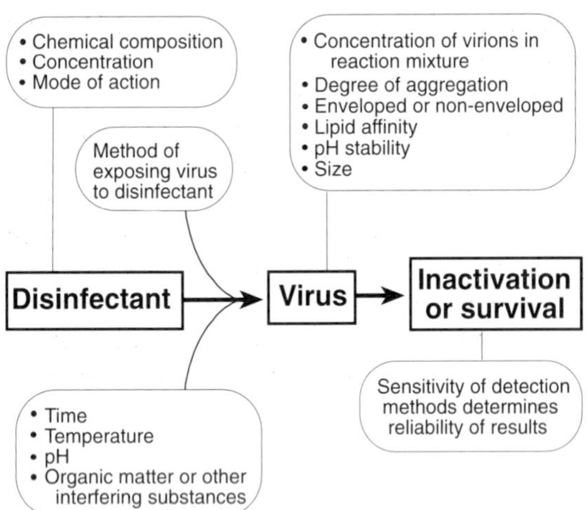

Fig. 6.3 Factors that influence disinfectant–virus interactions.

population of virions to physical or chemical inactivation procedures for a limited time results in the inactivation of a proportion of virions, while others retain infectivity. When a microbial population, particularly a bacterial one, is exposed to a lethal agent such as a disinfectant, the kinetics of inactivation are usually exponential. The rate of killing of bacteria following exposure to lethal agents such as heat or chemical disinfectants follows the kinetics of a first-order reaction, in which the logarithm of the number of survivors decreases as a linear function of time of exposure. With viruses, the shape of the survival curve can be used to evaluate the possible mechanism of inactivation and the dose of the agent required to achieve a defined degree of inactivation. Inactivation of viruses should, ideally, follow a similar pattern. For this to happen, viruses should occur as discrete units equally susceptible to the disinfection procedure; both viruses and disinfectant must be uniformly dispersed in the fluid phase; the disinfectant should be stable in its chemical composition; and it is imperative that organic matter or other interfering substances be absent from the reaction. Survival curves for viruses may follow a linear pattern (single-hit curve), exhibiting the kinetics of a first-order reaction, or they may exhibit multiple-hit or multicomponent patterns, which are non-linear (Thurman & Gerba, 1988). Errors in interpretation may occur when the survival curve is of either the multiple-hit or the multicomponent type. In viricidal tests, any aggregation of virus, alteration in disinfectant stability or change in the experimental methodology, which alters the kinetics of disinfection, is likely to cause deviation from ideal exponential inactivation.

Different types of viruses have varying susceptibilities to disinfectants and, in addition, the susceptibility of a given virus will vary with the type of disinfectant employed. There can be many potential points of interaction between disinfectants and viruses. Most disinfectants are not sufficiently specific to react with one virus component or functional group. Viricidal compounds may bring about their effects by denaturing protein, including specific enzymes, lipid or nucleic acid. Inactivation may result from changes in virus conformation or damage to the envelope, capsid proteins or the nucleic acid. Other changes may relate to alteration in the overall charge of virus particles or alteration in the surface components at, or adjacent to, the attachment site, which interacts with the receptor on the surface of a host cell. Virus clumping or aggregation may prevent contact with disinfectant, as some virions in the centre of aggregated masses may not be acted on by the disinfectant.

These mechanisms are considered further in Chapter 6D.

5.2 Factors influencing viricidal testing procedures

Although laboratory testing of viricidal compounds is undoubtedly useful, such testing should be regarded as a preliminary step prior to field testing. The testing protocol should be designed to evaluate disinfectants in a realistic manner, so that results can be correlated with practical in-use conditions, where methods of application may be difficult to standardize. The extent of viral environmental contamination of equipment may vary widely and the testing protocol should allow for the presence of high concentrations of virus. The criterion set for viricidal efficacy is somewhat arbitrary. A number of investigators have proposed a $3\log_{10}$ reduction in titre as being adequate (Springthorpe & Sattar, 1990; Prince *et al.*, 1991).

5.3 Elimination of cytotoxic effects of disinfectants for mammalian cells

Chemical disinfectants are not selectively toxic for microorganisms; they also kill mammalian cells and therefore the disinfectant must be removed, diluted to non-toxic levels or neutralized before testing for virus survival (Fig. 6.4).

Dilution is an appropriate method for overcoming toxicity but requires a high titre of test virus. Neutralization of the disinfectant is an alternative to dilution, but neutralizing compounds must themselves be free of cytotoxic effects. Viricidal testing employing neutralizing compounds requires the following protocol: (i) virus alone; (ii) virus and disinfectant; (iii) disinfectant alone; (iv) virus, disinfectant and neutralizer; (v) neutralizer alone; and (vi) virus and neutralizer. Samples from each of these preparations should be tested in cell cultures or by inoculation into embryonated eggs. The significance of any cytopathic effects should be interpreted with reference to the changes induced by disinfectant or neutralizer alone or in combination with virus.

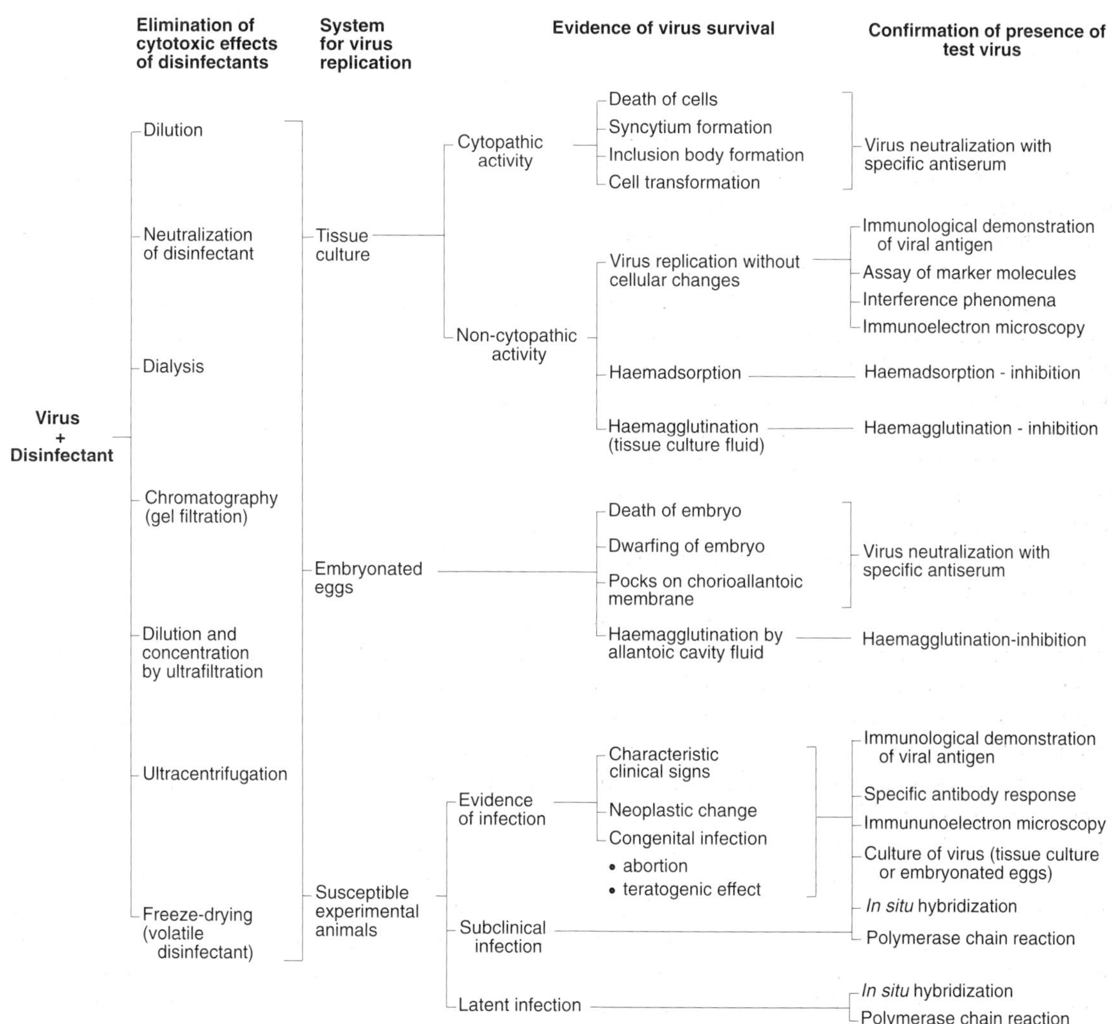

Fig. 6.4 Procedures for evaluating the efficacy of chemicals with viricidal activity.

Dialysis has been proposed as a method for removing or reducing the concentration of disinfectant in viricidal tests to a level that would not interfere with the growth of cell cultures. Gel filtration, using a cross-linked dextran gel, has been employed for the separation of virus and disinfectant (Blackwell & Chen, 1970).

Ultrafiltration has been used as a method of overcoming the limitations of dilution of the disinfectant (Boudouma *et al.*, 1984). In this procedure, the virus suspension and disinfectant are mixed, and the mixture is sampled after specified incubation intervals. The sample aliquot is diluted in phosphate-buffered saline to stop the reaction, concentrated at 4°C by ultrafiltration and titrated for virus survival. The disinfectant is removed during ultrafiltration and its possible cytotoxic effects on cell cultures thus avoided.

Other possible methods of separating virus from disinfectant include density-gradient ultracentrifugation, preparative isoelectric focusing and a range of electrophoretic procedures, using support media of appropriate pore size. Volatile disinfectants, such as alcohols, can be removed by freeze-drying the virus–disinfectant mixtures (P.J. Quinn & M.P. Scanlon, 1996, unpublished observations).

Figure 6.4 illustrates procedures for evaluating viricides, including methods appropriate for confirming survival of test viruses.

5.4 Viricidal testing methods

There are no standardized procedures agreed internationally for assessing the viricidal activity of chemical disinfectants. Methods used include suspension tests and carrier methods (Springthorpe & Sattar, 1990; Prince *et al.*, 1991). Plaque-suppression tests and bacteriophage test systems have also been used to a lesser extent.

5.4.1 Suspension methods

Some viruses may be inactivated by drying, and suspension tests are appropriate for such viruses. These tests usually employ a virus suspension of specified concentration and dilutions of disinfectant. Serum or other sources of organic matter may be added to simulate practical conditions of use. The virus–disinfectant mixture is usually incubated at room temperature for fixed intervals and residual virus infectivity is determined in cell cultures, embryonated eggs or susceptible animals. Appropriate controls for each reagent used should be included in each test. The cytotoxicity produced by some chemical compounds can be eliminated by the methods outlined in Fig. 6.4. It is recommended that the virus titre used in suspension experiments be at least 10^4 and that the protocol should allow for replicate sampling. Test results should be reported as the reduction in virus titre, expressed as $\log_{10}$, attributed to the activity of disinfectant and should be calculated by an accepted statistical method.

Establishing the number of infective units in suspension tests is hampered by the possibility of aggregate formation. Aggregation may even be caused by the disinfectant used, especially if it precipitates protein. Clusters of more than 100 infective virions, which are not uncommon in enterovirus preparations, may register as only a single infective unit after 99% infectivity reduction (Moldenhauer, 1984). Suspension tests generally only furnish the minimum requirements for virus inactivation, and for practical recommendations carrier methods should be employed.

5.4.2 Carrier methods

Viricides that are intended for use on dry environmental surfaces should be tested under simulated-use conditions. Carrier methods are used to test the activity of disinfectants against viruses dried on surfaces. A particular difficulty with these methods is that some viruses may be inactivated by drying.

Carrier rings, cylinders, discs of stainless steel, glass, plastic and the surface of hands of a volunteer have been used in carrier methods. To simulate in-use conditions, the test virus is inoculated on to a hard, non-porous surface, allowed to dry and then treated with the disinfectant at different dilutions. Alternatively, the carriers may be immersed in virus suspension and then dried. It is generally recommended that a recoverable virus titre of at least 10^4 be used on the test surface and at least a $3\log_{10}$ reduction in viral titre, without cytotoxicity, be obtained.

Lorenz & Jann (1964) described a carrier

method using Newcastle disease virus, a paramyxovirus. Carrier rings were immersed in virus suspensions and then dried. They were then transferred to dilutions of disinfectant and subsequently to broth. Ten-day-old embryonated eggs were inoculated with a small aliquot (0.1 ml) of this broth into the allantoic sac. If none of the inoculated embryos died within 5 days after inoculation, the disinfectant was judged to be effective at the dilution tested. An obvious limitation of this method is its restriction to viruses causing death of the chick embryo.

Slavin (1973) described a surface-disinfectant test (carrier test) using stainless-steel discs suitable for both bacteria and viruses. A 15% solution of gelatin containing 2.5% yeast suspension, Tween 80 and the test virus at a suitable density was placed in a cavity on the disc and cooled at 4°C. Three viruses, a bovine herpesvirus, a bovine paramyxovirus and a porcine enterovirus, were used. The discs were placed in disinfectant for the required time and transferred to distilled water and then into nutrient broth containing 5% horse serum. The nutrient broth was held at 37°C to allow the gelatin to liquefy, and titrations of the virus were added to cell cultures. The effective concentration of disinfectant was taken as that which gave a $4\log_{10}$ drop in virus titre.

A suspension test using 11 viruses was compared with a carrier test (Schürmann & Eggers, 1983) using the surface of both hands and the individual fingertips of a single volunteer. It was concluded that the hand test was a useful model and that the suspension test was less realistic in the data it provided.

Discs of stainless steel, glass and two types of plastic were used to evaluate the viricidal activity of 27 disinfectants against human rotavirus (Lloyd-Evans *et al.*, 1986). A volume of 20 µl of this rotavirus, containing 10^7 PFU, was air-dried on each disc. An equal volume of disinfectant was applied over the surface of each virus-contaminated disc and, after 1min, the reaction was stopped by the addition of tryptose phosphate broth. Virus was eluted from the discs using a sonic bath, diluted in Earle's balanced salt solution and plaque-assayed. A disinfectant was considered effective if it reduced the plaque titre by $3\log_{10}$ or greater.

A carrier method employing virus dried on coverslips under vacuum in the cold was developed by Allen *et al.* (1988). Virus titres remained high for up to 3 weeks at −70°C. Coverslips with dried virus were exposed to disinfectant in a cuvette. Cytotoxicity of disinfectant was determined by exposing the coverslip without virus to disinfectant and then placing it in medium with indicator cells.

Stainless steel discs contaminated with Coxsackie virus, adenovirus and parainfluenza virus were air-dried under ambient conditions and treated with 16 disinfectant formulations for 1 min, eluted into tryptose phosphate broth and plaque-assayed (Sattar *et al.*, 1989). A $3\log_{10}$ or greater reduction in virus infectivity was considered effective for the viricides used.

A number of workers have found that some carriers, such as porcelain and stainless steel penicylinders, fail to carry sufficient titre of virus for viricidal tests (Chen & Koski, 1983). In addition, considerable variation in recovered virus titres can be attributed to washing off of virus by disinfectant. This variation appears to be inherent in this type of testing procedure (Allen *et al.*, 1988).

5.4.3 *Plaque-suppression tests*

The principle of this method is that a layer of host cells on a suitable agar medium is infected with virus. Small discs of filter-paper treated with disinfectant are applied. After a designated incubation period, the discs are removed and the agar is stained with a suitable dye in order to observe plaque suppression and also possible toxicity to host cells (Sykes, 1965). This method can be applied to a range of viruses, including vaccinia, herpes and Newcastle disease viruses (Tyler & Ayliffe, 1987; Tyler *et al.*, 1990).

5.4.4 *Assessment of viricidal activity with bacteriophages*

Bacteriophages have been used in place of animal and human viruses to test the viricidal activity of disinfectants. The coliphages T2, MS2 and ØX 174 were used by Lepage & Romond (1984) to test the viricidal activity of iodophor, aldehyde, hypochlorite, quaternary ammonium and amphoteric compounds. The coliphage ØX 174 has been used in both suspension and carrier tests to determine the viricidal activity of disinfectants (Bydžovská & Kneiflová, 1983). Bacteriophages, particularly coliphages, such as MS2, have been used as indicators for enteroviruses in waste water and polluted water, but they are more resistant than enteroviruses to adverse environmental conditions and to disinfection (Kott, 1981). The bacteriophage MS2 has been used as a test virus for evaluating the viricidal activity of disinfectants in hand-washing procedures (Davies *et al.*, 1993). Because this bacteriophage has some characteristics in common with poliovirus, it has been used as an alternative for poliovirus in viricidal testing procedures (Jones *et al.*, 1991).

The bacteriophage B40-8 of *Bacteroides fragilis* has been used to assess the viricidal activity of disinfectants. The survival of B40-8 equalled or exceeded that of certain animal viruses in testing procedures (Pinto *et al.*, 1991).

5.4.5 Approved tests for viricidal activity

A limited number of tests are recognized by professional groups or governments for approval of viricides. The German Society for Veterinary Medicine has issued a defined protocol for testing the viricidal activity of disinfectants (Schliesser, 1979). The test procedure employs a virus suspension of 10^6 ID_{50} in 20% bovine serum. Four test viruses, two enveloped and two non-enveloped, are used: enteric cytopathogenic bovine orphan virus (picornavirus), infectious canine hepatitis virus (adenovirus), Newcastle disease virus (paramyxovirus) and vaccinia virus (poxvirus). A suspension test in the presence and absence of 20% bovine serum is employed, and a carrier test using wood and gauze is also specified (virus dried at 37°C for 90 min). Appropriate dilutions of disinfectant are added for 15, 30, 60 and 120 min; test samples are inoculated into cell cultures and embryonated eggs. Toxicity of the disinfectant alone for the cell cultures and embryonated eggs must be assessed. Disinfectants are rated according to the effective concentration that achieves complete inactivation or limited viricidal activity.

In the UK, the Ministry of Agriculture, Fisheries and Food (1970) has published the protocol of a test for the approval of disinfectants for use against fowl pest (Newcastle disease virus and fowl plague virus—avian influenza). Two separate tests are employed: a toxicity test, to determine if the disinfectant under test is toxic for embryonated eggs, and a virus test system to assess the degree of inactivation of the test virus (Newcastle disease virus), using 9-day-old embryonated eggs inoculated into the allantoic cavity. The disinfectant under test must give a reduction of at least 10^4 in virus titre.

5.4.6 Virus survival or inactivation

Evidence for virus survival or inactivation requires inoculation of either tissue culture, embryonated eggs or susceptible animals (Fig. 6.4). When animal inoculation is employed it is essential that the animals used are: (i) susceptible to the virus or infectious agent; (ii) immunologically naïve; and (iii) in the appropriate age category or physiological state to show clinical signs of the replicating agent. For diseases with long incubation periods, the lifespan of the animal species selected is another important consideration.

Methods for assessing the survival or inactivation of a test virus must be based on its cultural characteristics or its ability to induce either clinical, subclinical or latent disease in a susceptible animal. Demonstration of a latent infection may require the use of immunosuppressive drugs, such as corticosteroids. Pregnant animals are required to test the survival of viral agents that attack the developing fetus. Re-isolation of the infectious agent is an essential part of the laboratory procedure. As there is a minimal infective dose for most viruses, the amount of virus surviving following chemical treatment may determine the outcome of animal inoculation. Experimental animals (chimpanzees and gibbons) have been used for those human viruses such as hepatitis B virus (HBV) which are difficult to culture *in vitro* (Bond *et al.*, 1983). Animals for HBV investigations should be kept in quarantine for at least 3 months and their health status monitored. Their transaminase values should be in the normal range and, if necessary, liver biopsy can be carried out. It may be necessary to monitor exposed animals for at least 6 months, as the incubation period can vary with the virus content of the challenge dose. Duck hepatitis B virus has also been used as a model to test the efficacy of disinfectants against hepadnavirus activity (Murray *et al.*, 1991).

Confirmation of the presence of test virus in tissue culture, in tissues of experimental animals or in embryonated eggs requires the use of appropriate detection systems (see Fig. 6.4). A range of immunodetection systems can be applied to demonstrate virus replication in cell cultures. Where appropriate, DNA probing, with or without amplification, may be used. Assay of marker molecules may also be employed, and virus replication can be detected by *in situ* hybridization, using a radioactive genomic probe.

Direct and indirect tests are also available for human immunodeficiency virus (HIV), and these include reverse-transcriptase assay, viral-antigen enzyme-linked immunosorbent assays, radioimmunoassay, indirect immunofluorescence and *in situ* hybridization (Levy, 1988). Human immunodeficiency virus can also be cultured in phytohaemagglutinin-stimulated leucocytes from seronegative donors. In some human T-cell lines, HIV will induce plaque and syncytium formation.

6 Concluding remarks

Development of an ideal testing procedure for viricidal disinfectants presents many technical problems. A suitable test virus, easily grown to high titres and representative of a given family, with appropriate attributes of stability and safety, is not easily identifiable. Because of the diversity of viruses encountered in human and veterinary medicine, test viruses representing the more important families should be included in a standardized protocol. Virus concentration, contact time, temperature, presence of organic matter and the method of exposing virus to disinfectant should be clearly specified. A well-defined test procedure would remove uncertainty from an area of biology where microbiology and pharmacology interact, and it could contribute to the development of more effective measures for the control of viral diseases in human and animal populations.

7 References

Allen, L.B., Kehoe, M.J., Hsu, S.C., Barfield, R., Holland, C.S. & Dimitrijevich, S.D. (1988) A simple method of drying virus on inanimate objects for virucidal testing. *Journal of Virological Methods*, **19**, 239–248.

Blackwell, J.H. & Chen, J.H.S. (1970) Effects of various germicidal chemicals on H.Ep.2 cell cultures and herpes simplex virus. *Journal of the Association of Official Analytical Chemists*, **53**, 1229–1236.

Bond, W.W., Favero, M.S., Petersen, N.J. & Ebert, J.W. (1983) Inactivation of hepatitis B virus by intermediate-to-high level disinfectant chemicals. *Journal of Clinical Microbiology*, **18**, 535–538.

Boudouma, M., Enjalbert, L. & Didier, J. (1984) A simple method for the evaluation of antiseptic and disinfectant virucidal activity. *Journal of Virological Methods*, **9**, 271–276.

Bydžovská, O. & Kneiflová, J. (1983) Assessment of viral disinfection by means of bacteriophage ØX 174. *Journal of Hygiene, Epidemiology, Microbiology and Immunology*, **27**, 60–68.

Chen, J.H.S. & Koski, T.A. (1983) Methods of testing virucides. In *Disinfection, Sterilization and Preservation*, (ed. Block, S.S.) 3rd edn, pp. 981–997. Philadelphia: Lea and Febiger.

Davies, J.G., Babb, J.R., Bradley, C.R. & Ayliffe, G.A. (1993) Preliminary study of test methods to assess the virucidal activity of skin disinfectants using poliovirus and bacteriophages. *Journal of Hospital Infection*, **25**, 125–131.

Jones, M.V., Bellamy, K., Alcock, R. & Hudson, R. (1991) The use of bacteriophage MS2 as a model system to evaluate virucidal hand disinfectants. *Journal of Hospital Infection*, **17**, 279–285.

Kott, Y. (1981) Viruses and bacteriophages. *Science of the Total Environment*, **18**, 13–23.

Lepage, Ch. & Romond, Ch. (1984) Détermination de l'activité virucide: intérêt du bactériophage comme modèle viral. *Pathologie Biologie*, **32**, 631–635.

Levy, J.A. (1988) Retroviridae: human immunodeficiency virus. In *Laboratory Diagnosis of Infectious Disease* (eds Lennette, E.H., Halonen, P. & Murphy, F.A.), Vol. II, pp. 677–691. New York: Springer-Verlag.

Lloyd-Evans, N., Springthorpe, V.S. & Sattar, S.A. (1986) Chemical disinfection of human rotavirus-contaminated inanimate surfaces. *Journal of Hygiene, Cambridge*, **97**, 163–173.

Lorenz, D.E. & Jann, G.J. (1964) Use-dilution test and Newcastle disease virus. *Applied Microbiology*, **12**, 24–26.

Ministry of Agriculture, Fisheries and Food (1970) *Protocol of test for Approval of Disinfectants for Use Against Fowl Pest (Newcastle Disease Virus, Fowl Plague Virus)*. Weybridge: Central Veterinary Laboratory, MAFF.

Moldenhauer, D. (1984). Quantitative evaluation of the

effects of disinfectants against viruses in suspension experiments. *Zentralblatt für Bakteriologie und Hygiene, I Abteilung Originale*, B **179**, 544–554.

Murphy, F.A., Fauquet, C.M., Bishop, D.H.L. *et al.*, (1995) Virus taxonomy: classification and nomenclature of viruses. *Archives of Virology*, Suppl. 10.

Murray, S.M., Freiman, J.S., Vickery, K., Lim, D., Cossart, Y.E. & Whiteley, R.K. (1991) Duck hepatitis B virus: a model to assess efficacy of disinfectants against hepadnavirus activity. *Epidemiology and Infection*, **106**, 435–443.

Pinto, R.M., Abad, F.X., Riera, J.M. & Bosch, A. (1991) The use of bacteriophages of *Bacteroides fragilis* as indicators of the efficiency of virucidal products. *FEMS Microbiology Letters*, **66**, 61–65.

Prince, H.N., Prince, D.L. & Prince, R.N. (1991) Principles of viral control and transmission. In *Disinfection, Sterilization and Preservation*, (ed. Block, S.S.) 4th edn, pp. 411–444. Philadelphia: Lea and Febiger.

Sattar, S.A., Springthorpe, V.S., Karim, Y. & Loro, P. (1989) Chemical disinfection of non-porous inanimate surfaces experimentally contaminated with four human pathogenic viruses. *Epidemiology and Infection*, **102**, 493–505.

Schliesser, T. (1979) Testing of chemical disinfectants for veterinary medicine. *Hygiene und Medizin*, **4**, 51–56.

Schürmann, W. & Eggers, H.J. (1983) Anitviral activity of an alcoholic hand disinfectant. Comparison of the *in vitro* suspension test with the *in vivo* experiments on hands, and on individual fingertips. *Antiviral Research*, **3**, 25–41.

Slavin, G. (1973) A reproducible surface contamination method for disinfectant tests. *British Veterinary Journal*, **129**, 13–18.

Springthorpe, V.S. & Sattar, S.A. (1990) Chemical disinfection of virus-contaminated surfaces. *Critical Reviews in Environmental Control*, **20**, 169–229.

Sykes, G. (1965) *Disinfection and Sterilization*, pp. 291–308. London: Chapman and Hall.

Thurman, R.B. & Gerba, C.P. (1988) Molecular mechanisms of viral inactivation by water disinfectants. *Advances in Applied Microbiology*, **33**, 75–105.

Tyler, R. & Ayliffe, G.A.J. (1987) A surface test for virucidal activity: preliminary study with herpesvirus. *Journal of Hospital Infection*, **9**, 22–29.

Tyler, R., Ayliffe, G.A.J. & Bradley, C.R. (1990) Virucidal activity of disinfectants. *Journal of Hospital Infection*, **15**, 339–345.

D. MECHANISMS OF VIRICIDAL ACTION

1 Introduction

Viricidal activity is an important property of several but not all biocides, i.e. disinfectants, antiseptics and preservatives. The viricidal properties of such agents often depend on: (i) the nature of the virus (e.g. morphology, size); (ii) several parameters inherent to the biocide, such as concentration, pH, contact time and temperature; and (iii) the manner in which a viral particle is exposed to the biocide, e.g. presence or absence of organic matter. Those factors influencing the microbicidal activity of biocides have been described in Chapter 3.

Although the viricidal activity of biocides is now becoming well documented (Chapter 6A), the viricidal mechanisms of action of biocides have been poorly studied. In consequence information obtained with other microorganisms, such as bacteria, yeasts and spores, will be used as the basis of explaining the activity of biocides against viruses. The viricidal mechanisms of action of biocides will be considered in the following sections.

2 Viral structure and targets

2.1 Viral structure

With the exception of prions, viruses are smaller than other microorganisms and usually have a simpler structure. Therefore, viruses present fewer target sites to biocides. Furthermore, they do not show any metabolic activity, which further reduces the number of target sites available to biocides, especially those that affect the proton-motive force (e.g. 2,4-dinitrophenol, carbanilides, salicylanilides) and the electron-transport system (e.g. hexachlorophane) of other microorganisms.

Conventional viral classification is based on the chemical and physical properties and structure of viruses (Prince *et al.*, 1991). However, when susceptibility to disinfection is considered, three groups of viruses can be distinguished (Klein & Deforest, 1983): (i) enveloped viruses, which are the most sensitive to chemical disinfection, due to their large size and lipophilic nature (e.g. human immunodeficiency virus (HIV)); (ii) large non-enveloped viruses (e.g. adenovirus), more resistant than the former group; and (iii) small naked viruses (e.g. picornavirus and parvovirus), the most resistant to disinfection. However, this classification has its limitations, since viruses belonging to the same group sometimes show different sensitivities to a particular biocide under the same disinfection conditions. Furthermore, complex viruses, such as rhabdoviruses, have to be classified separately due to their unusual structure (i.e. the presence of several envelopes). However, most of them do contain a lipid coat, which makes them as susceptible to disinfection as large enveloped viruses. Tailed bacteriophages, having a well-defined structure, with an icosahedral head attached to a helical tail, show different sensitivity to disinfection. Their complex structure and other characteristics are an advantage when mechanisms of action of biocides are investigated (Maillard, 1996).

2.2 Viral targets

Generally, viruses present only a few structural targets to biocides: (i) the envelope (when present); (ii) glycoproteinic receptors; (iii) the capsid; and (iv) the viral genome (Fig. 6.5).

2.2.1 *Viral envelope*

Envelopes are generally derived from the host-cell cytoplasmic membrane (e.g. influenza virus) but also from the nuclear membrane (e.g. herpes simplex virus). The viral envelope is a typical unit membrane, containing lipids in high quantity (Fig. 6.5). This might account for the sensitivity of enveloped viruses to compounds such as phenols, chloroform and ether. The activity of biocides against the viral envelope has not been documented but it might be expected that membrane-active agents, such as quaternary ammonium compounds (QACs), and bibiguanides, such as chlorhexidine, will act in the same way against viral envelopes as on the bacterial cytoplasmic membrane.

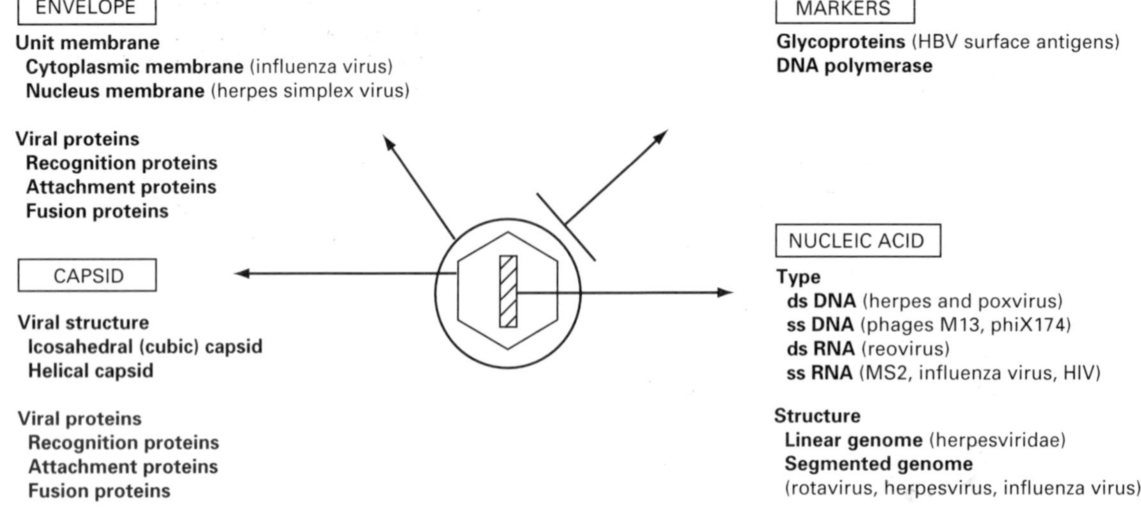

Fig. 6.5 Viral target sites for biocidal activity.

Furthermore, host-cell proteins are excluded from the viral envelope and proteins encoded by the viral genome are usually present. These serologically important proteins often serve as host-cell receptors and can have a predominant role in viral infection (e.g. fusion proteins). The alteration of these proteins might decrease or stop viral infections (Fig. 6.6). Finally, the destruction of the viral envelope only would release an intact nucleocapsid, which could remain infectious (Fig. 6.6).

2.2.2 *Capsid*

One of the main target sites of biocides is the viral capsid (see Fig. 6.5). The capsid is responsible for the shape of the virus and the protection of the viral nucleic acid from external factors, such as disinfection. The size of the capsid might influence biocidal activity, since large capsids present more target sites to the biocides. Capsid constituents are principally protein in nature. Any biocides reacting

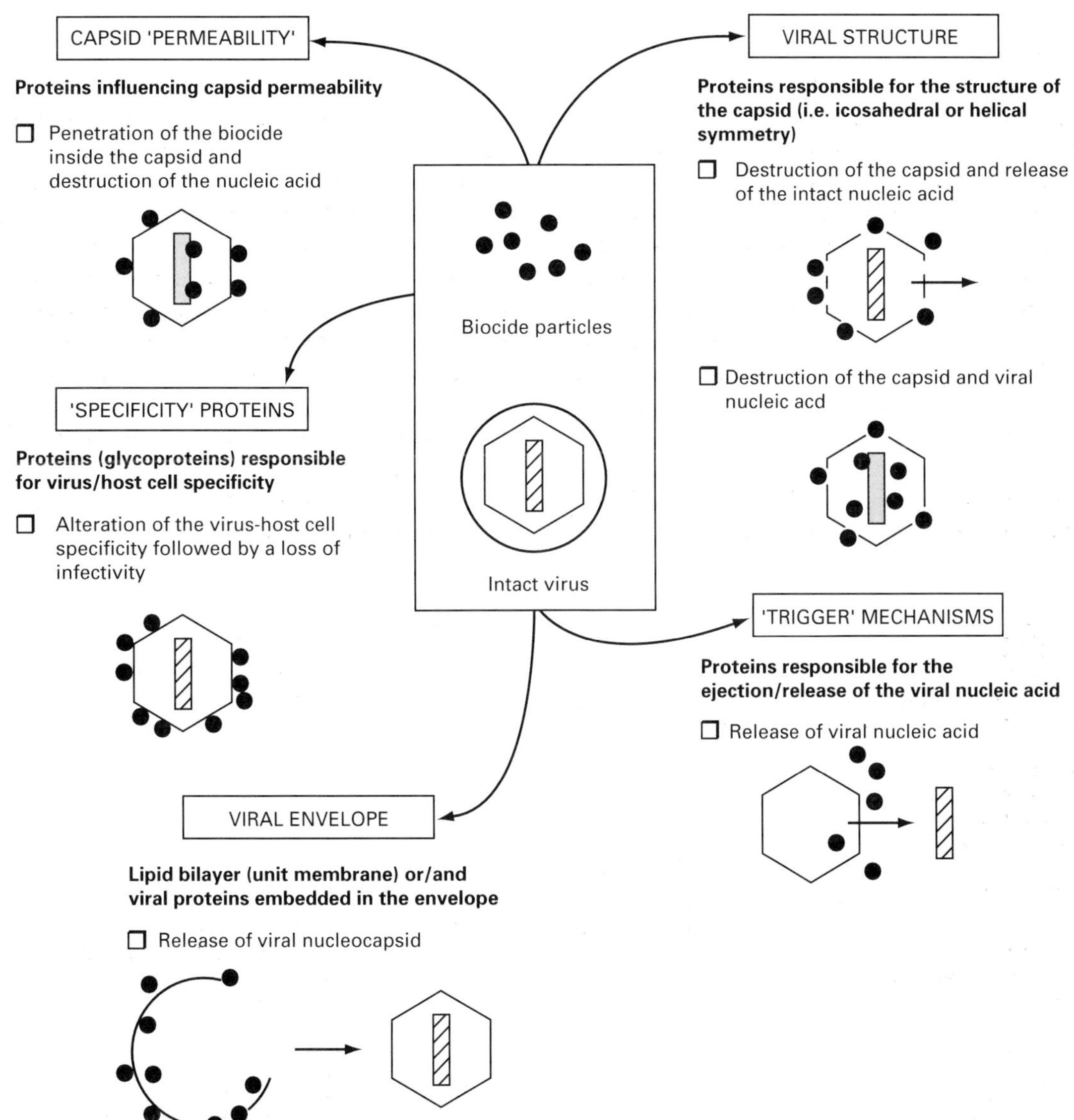

Fig. 6.6 Possible interaction between biocides and viruses.

strongly with protein $-NH_2$ groups (e.g. glutaraldehyde (GTA), ethylene oxide) or –SH groups (e.g. hypochlorite, iodine, ethylene oxide, hydrogen peroxide) might possess viricidal activity.

The capsid also contains proteins, often protruding outwards, with a particular function, such as host-cell specificity, release of viral genome or guidance of viral nucleic acid within the host-cell cytoplasm. As an example, the A protein of the bacteriophage MS2 and the H protein of the ØX174 coliphage (McKenna *et al.*, 1992) act as a 'pilot protein' with multiple functions, such as adsorption, penetration and the early intracellular stages of viral chromosome expression (Quinn, 1978). A biocide specifically active against these proteins will result in loss of infectivity of the virus (Fig. 6.6).

2.2.3 *Viral genome*

The viral nucleic acid is the infectious part of the virus. Releasing an intact viral nucleic acid into the environment following the destruction of the capsid might be cause for concern, since some nucleic acids are known to remain infectious when liberated from the capsid. It should be noted that viral inactivation will be complete only if the viral nucleic acid is destroyed (Fig. 6.6).

The size and nature of the genome certainly play a role in the sensitivity of a virus to disinfection. The viral genome is extremely diversified among viruses, in size, in content (double-stranded (ds) deoxyribonucleic acid (DNA), single-stranged (ss) DNA, ds ribonucleic acid (dsRNA), ssRNA) and in appearance (circle or linear particle or several linear particles (see Fig. 6.5). Furthermore, the relationship of the genome with the capsid (e.g. helical structure) is also important when disinfection is considered. It has been noticed that nucleocapsids with a helical symmetry are more closely linked with the viral nucleic acid than nucleocapsids with an icosahedral capsid and therefore are more susceptible to alteration caused by biocides because of shearing forces.

The effects of biocides and radiations against the viral nucleic acid outside its protective capsid are probably similar to those against the bacterial genome. This particular aspect is described in Chapters 9 and 20A, B.

3 Viricidal mechanisms of action of biocides

3.1 Aldehydes

Glutaraldehyde has been extensively studied (Eagar *et al.*, 1986; Bruch, 1991) and is widely used for high-level disinfection. Glutaraldehyde has been shown to react with the α-amino groups of amino acids, the N-terminal amino groups of some peptides and the sulfhydryl group of cysteine. With other proteins, such as bovine serum albumin, GTA was shown to react with the ε-amino groups of lysine to form mainly intermolecular cross-linkages (Habeeb & Hiramoto, 1968). Not surprisingly, GTA has a broad range of viricidal activity against enveloped viruses (Brown, 1981), large non-enveloped viruses (Gorman *et al.*, 1980; Bond *et al.*, 1983; Kobayashi & Tsuzuki, 1984; Kobayashi *et al.*, 1984; Springthorpe *et al.*, 1986; Springthorpe & Sattar, 1990) and small naked viruses (Brown, 1981; Mbithi *et al.*, 1990; Tyler *et al.*, 1990; Bailly *et al.*, 1991, Best *et al.*, 1994; Maillard *et al.*, 1994).

The effects of GTA on viruses can be considered according to viral target sites and structural markers of virus inactivation. However, the relationship between viral inactivation and alteration of a particular target site remains unclear.

3.1.1 *Interaction of glutaraldehyde with viral structures*

Used as a fixative, 4% GTA was shown to change both the appearance and the physical properties of the foot-and-mouth disease virus. Larger viral particles were observed following treatment, but it is unclear whether the change of appearance is due to the viral RNA contained within the viral capsid (Sangar *et al.*, 1973). Prolonged exposure to GTA or formaldehyde was shown to increase the buoyant density of the poliovirus and its permeability to phosphotungstic acid (Wouters *et al.*, 1973); however, shorter exposure to 4% GTA did not affect its physical properties (Baltimore & Huang, 1968). In an attempt to develop a system (morphological alteration and disintegration test (MADT)) to measure the viricidal activity of biocides against the hepatitis B virus (HBV), Thraenhart *et al.*

(1977) showed that the morphology of Dane particles was severely altered by succinaldehyde (Gigasept). Disintegration of the outer membrane and asymmetric enlargement of the space between the outer membrane and the HBV core resulted eventually, with longer exposure, to a loss of the characteristic substructure. The severity of damage caused to the structure of HBV Dane particles challenged with different disinfectants was classified by: (i) an alteration of the outer shell; (ii) an alteration of all substructures; and (iii) loss of all substructures. Although a longer exposure with Gigasept did produce a disintegration of the majority of the Dane particles, a combination of formaldehyde and Gigasept left virus particles undamaged. Furthermore, the relationship between virus infectivity and alteration to the virus substructure remains unknown.

A study involving the *Pseudomonas aeruginosa* PAO F116 bacteriophage showed that 1% GTA was the only biocide tested that produced a higher number of empty heads, i.e. intact structures with no material packaged inside (Maillard *et al.*, 1995a). It was suggested that GTA triggered the mechanism, causing the genome to be ejected from the phage particles. A study of sodium dodecyl sulphate (SDS)-polyacrylamide gel electrophoresis of F116 proteins (Maillard *et al.*, 1996a) showed that two protein bands, Pp4 (mol.wt 59100) and Pp8 (mol.wt 10900), were possibly associated with the release of F116 nucleic acid.

3.1.2 Interaction of glutaraldehyde with viral antigens

It has been shown that 2% alkaline GTA (Cidex), 2% alkaline GTA with surface-active ingredients (Cidex Formula 7) and formaldehyde (2.02%) alter the HBV surface (HBsAg) and core antigens (HBcAg) (Adler-Storthz *et al.*, 1983). A decrease in HBV antigens following treatment with formaldehyde has also been described (Frösner *et al.*, 1982). Although the exact physical and chemical mechanism of action of GTA was not explained, it was suggested that GTA probably reacted chemically with HbsAg and HBcAg sites containing lysine residues. In fact, GTA is known for its ability to cross-link proteins (Richards & Knowles, 1968), the reaction involving lysine and hydroxylysine residues and GTA in the relative amounts of 4 mol GTA to 1 mol lysine (Korn *et al.*, 1972). Similarly, GTA was shown to affect the antigenicity of hepatitis A virus (HAV) (Passagot *et al.*, 1987). However, it was noted that reduction in viral antigenicity and reduction in infectivity were different.

3.1.3 Interactions of glutaraldehyde with capsid proteins

Chambon *et al.* (1992) showed that low concentrations of GTA (0.005–0.10%) caused the formation of high-molecular-weight complexes between capsid proteins of the poliovirus type 1 and echovirus type 25. It was suggested that cross-linkages between capsid polypeptides of the poliovirus were caused by accessibility to GTA of lysine residues of VP1 and VP3. It was shown elsewhere that the capsid proteins of the poliovirus, VP1, VP2 and VP3, contained respectively 15, 5 and 10 lysine residues (Racaniello & Baltimore, 1981). The aldehyde groups of GTA cross-link essentially with the ε-amino groups of lysine residues of proteins (Korn *et al.*, 1972). Furthermore, the three-dimensional structure of the poliovirus showed that two top loops, one in VP1 and the other in VP3, exposed lysine residues immediately accessible to GTA (Hogle *et al.*, 1985), which might account for the intermolecular cross-linkage of the two polypeptides (Chambon *et al.*, 1992). Similarly the amino acid sequence of the HAV structural protein VP1 was shown to contain lysine (Linemeyer *et al.*, 1985) and is also likely to react with GTA.

3.1.4 Interactions of glutaraldehyde with other viral markers

Howard *et al.* (1983) showed that a GTA-based disinfectant (Kohrsolin) reduced the activity of HBV DNA polymerase and possibly denatured HBcAg. The aldehyde-based compound was also shown to affect the structure of HBV particles. It was suggested that chemical changes of markers (e.g. DNA polymerase, HBcAg) may precede gross morphological changes. It was, however, stated that experiments using markers do not necessarily reflect a loss in virus infectivity.

3.1.5 Interactions of glutaraldehyde with viral nucleic acid

Bailly *et al.* (1991) showed that 1% GTA was ineffective against the poliovirus type 1 RNA. Similarly, Maillard *et al.* (1996b) showed that the nucleic acid extracted from the capsid of the *Ps. aeruginosa* F116 bacteriophage after a challenge with 1% GTA was undamaged. However, another study demonstrated that low concentrations of GTA (0.05–1%) were sufficient to inhibit the transduction ability of the phage (Maillard *et al.*, (1995c). It is possible that the inhibition of transduction was due to the alteration of a protein target responsible for the event, rather than an undetected alteration of the phage genome.

3.2 Halogen-releasing agents

3.2.1 Chlorine compounds

Olivieri *et al.* (1975) showed that chlorine inactivated naked f2 RNA at the same rate as it did RNA in the intact phage, whereas f2 capsid proteins were still able to adsorb to the host following a chlorine treatment. Similarly, poliovirus type 1 RNA was shown to be degraded into fragments within the capsid and then released after a challenge with chlorine (1mg/l). Similarly, it has been suggested that chlorine dioxide and bromine chloride act preferentially on the viral nucleic acid, since poliovirus challenged with these biocides remained structurally unaltered (Taylor & Butler, 1982). It was also noticed that poliovirus inactivation preceded any severe morphological changes after being challenged with high concentrations of chlorine (Taylor & Butler, 1982). Interestingly, in another study, chlorine was found to have no effect on RNA extracted from poliovirus before treatment with chlorine (O'Brien & Newman, 1979), and Floyd *et al.* (1979) showed that the capsid of the poliovirus type 1 was broken following challenge with similar concentrations of chlorine. Furthermore, chlorine was shown to alter the HBV structure severely (Thraenhart *et al.*, 1977). Similarly, Tenno *et al.* (1979) suggested that the mechanism of action of chlorine against the poliovirus was via slight structural alteration of the capsid, since viral RNA remained infectious after virus inactivation by the biocide. Alvarez & O'Brien (1982) showed that poliovirus RNA was released from the capsid as a result, and not as a cause, of virus inactivation by chlorine. They suggested that the apparent discrepancy in results was due to variations in chlorine concentrations used in the different studies. This rapid activity achieved by low concentrations of chlorine and sodium hypochlorite against viral nucleic acid before or after structural damage might explain the viricidal activity against enveloped viruses, such as HIV (Resnick *et al.*, 1986; Bloomfield *et al.*, 1990) and pseudorabies, parvoviridae, such as the gastroenteritis virus (Brown, 1981), rotavirus (Berman & Hoff, 1984; Keswick *et al.*, 1985; Springthorpe *et al.*, 1986) and picornaviridae (Peterson *et al.*, 1983; Keswick *et al.*, 1985; Mbithi *et al.*, 1990; Tyler *et al.*, 1990; Best *et al.*, 1994).

Finally, Rodgers *et al.* (1985) found that sodium hypochlorite rapidly removed the outer coat of rotavirus. A study of HBV also showed that sodium hypochlorite (0.525% v/v) severely altered HbsAg and HBcAg (Alder-Storthz *et al.*, 1983).

3.2.2 Viricidal mechanisms of action of iodine

Taylor & Butler (1982) showed that iodine caused severe morphological changes to the poliovirus structure. This observation might be explained by the larger atomic radius of iodine, which might prevent its diffusion through the capsid to the target site inside the virion. Therefore, the mechanism of action of iodine appeared largely to affect the viral capsid rather than viral nucleic acid. Similarly, Olivieri *et al.* (1975) showed that the target site of iodine on f2 coliphage was the amino acid tyrosine of the capsid moiety, with almost no effect on f2 viral RNA.

3.2.3 Viricidal mechanisms of action of bromine

Sharp *et al.* (1975) suggested that bromine (0.2–0.4 mg/l) damaged the capsid proteins of reovirus type 3 and possibly induced a loss of RNA. Olivieri *et al.* (1975) proposed that the primary site of bromine inactivation was more likely to be the protein moiety of the f2 coliphage. Similarly, Keswick *et al.* (1981) showed that high concentrations of bromine chloride (10–20 mg/l) produced a structural degradation of the poliovirus. It was also found that poliovirus RNA remained infectious after treatment with bromine chloride (0.3 mg/l). However, it was suggested that structural degradation and loss of infectivity were not necessarily correlated, since lower concentrations of bromine chloride (0.3–5 mg/l) inactivated the poliovirus without causing structural alterations.

3.3 Biguanides

Chlorhexidine is the most important member of the biguanide family. Chlorhexidine is a membrane-active agent which has been shown to affect the cytoplasmic membrane of bacteria, inducing leakage of intracellular components (Russell & Chopra, 1996). Therefore, it is possible that chlorhexidine interacts with the viral envelope, inducing a rupture of the membrane and consequently liberating a non-infectious viral capsid. This might explain, partially, why chlorhexidine shows a viricidal activity against enveloped viruses, such as the herpes simplex virus (Park & Park, 1989) and HIV (Montefiori *et al.*, 1990), but not against picornaviruses (Mbithi *et al.*, 1990; Best *et al.*, 1994) or larger non-enveloped viruses (Springthorpe *et al.*, 1986).

Furthermore, lack of activity of chlorhexidine against non-enveloped viruses might be caused by a reversible adsorption of the molecule to the viral capsid. A structural study with the phage F116 showed that chlorhexidine diacetate (1%) caused little structural damage to the phage (Maillard *et al.*, 1995a). Similarly, phage proteins (Maillard *et al.*, 1996a) and nucleic acid (Maillard *et al.*, 1996b) were not affected when phage particles were challenged with the bisbiguanide. An energy-dispersive analysis of X-rays (EDAX) study showed that the chlorhexidine molecules did not bind strongly and did not penetrate inside phage particles (Maillard *et al.*, 1995b). However, low concentrations of chlorhexidine were shown to inhibit the transduction ability of F116 (Maillard *et al.*, 1995c).

3.4 Quaternary ammonium compounds

Quaternary ammonium compounds are surface-active agents, benzalkonium chloride being one of the most widely used. They are more active against lipophilic viruses (Resnick *et al.*, 1986; Springthorpe *et al.*, 1986). Since they are surface-active agents, QACs may primarily interact with the viral envelope. It was suggested that QACs might act on the bacterial cytoplasmic membrane by dissociating conjugated proteins (Russell & Chopra, 1996). The activity of QACs against enveloped viruses could possibly be explained by an effect of the agents on the viral proteins of the envelopes, inducing a rupture of the envelope and hence the inactivation of the virus. Cetylpyridinium chloride (CPC) produced a severe alteration of the capsid of F116 bacteriophage (Maillard *et al.*, 1995a), as well as alteration of the phage-protein band pattern (Maillard *et al.*, 1996a) and the transduction ability of the phage (Maillard *et al.*, 1995c). However, CPC had no effect on the phage genome (Maillard *et al.*, 1996b). Similarly, another QAC, cetrimide was shown to alter the structure of rotavirus (Rodgers *et al.*, 1985).

3.5 Alcohols

The presence of water is essential to the antimicrobial activity of alcohols, their optimum activity being shown between 60 and 90% v/v. Ethanol (90%) and isopropanol were shown to be inactive against small non-enveloped viruses, such as picornaviruses (Tyler *et al.*, 1990; Davies *et al.*, 1993) and MS2 coliphage, a leviviridae (Maillard *et al.*, 1994). Ethanol (70%) was found to be highly effective against HIV (Resnick *et al.*, 1986) and the human rotavirus (Rodgers *et al.*, 1985; Springthorpe *et al.*, 1986). The activity of 70% ethanol against small naked viruses varies (Mbithi *et al.*, 1990; Tyler *et al.*, 1990; Maillard *et al.*, 1994) and might be influenced by the testing methodology (Best *et al.*, 1994). Isopropanol inactivated adenoviruses, but not picornaviruses and echovirus II. Parvoviruses, rhinoviruses and vesicular stomatitis virus were little affected when challenged with alcohols (Springthorpe & Sattar, 1990). However, other alcohol solutions were found to be viricidal against the human rotavirus, astrovirus and echovirus II (Kurtz *et al.*, 1980). There is little information on the viricidal mechanisms of action of alcohols. Their activity against enveloped viruses suggests that this could be at the site of the viral envelope. Indeed, several alcohols have been shown to react with the bacterial cytoplasmic membrane (Russell & Chopra, 1996). Their activity against non-enveloped viruses might be partially due to an alteration of viral substructure. Ethanol was shown to remove rapidly the outer coat of the rotavirus (Rodgers *et al.*, 1985) and, with isopropanol, structurally altered the capsid of the phage F116 in a similar manner, producing a high number of folded and fractured capsids (Maillard *et al.*, 1995a). However, it did not affect the substructures of HBV (Thraenhart *et al.*, 1978). An alcohol-based disinfectant (Sterillium) was also found to reduce the activity of HBV DNA polymerase and, to a lesser extent possibly, to denature HBcAg (Howard *et al.*, 1983). Finally, ethanol and isopropanol were shown to be ineffective against the F116 nucleic acid (Maillard *et al.*, 1996b).

3.6 Phenolics

The viricidal activity of phenolic compounds has not been widely investigated, and reports of their antiviral activity sometimes seem controversial (Springthorpe & Sattar, 1990). Phenols might interact with the envelope of viruses in a similar way to their interaction with the prokaryotic membrane (Russell & Chopra, 1996), since they are generally active against lipid-enveloped viruses (Springthorpe *et al.*, 1986; Rubin, 1991). Maillard *et al.* (1996b) showed that phenol did not alter the nucleic acid of F116 bacteriophage or the transduction property of the bacteriophage (Maillard *et al.*, 1995c). However, it might have an effect on capsid proteins, since an electron-microscopic investigation showed that phenol produced a wide range of structural damage to the capsid and tails of the bacteriophage (Maillard *et al.*, 1995a).

3.7 Oxidizing agents

3.7.1 Peroxygens

Peracetic acid is the most widely used peracid and is a powerful oxidizing agent. Its decomposition produces hydrogen peroxide and acetic acid. Not surprisingly, peracetic acid has a wide spectrum of activity among viruses, including picornaviruses (Harakeh, 1984; Springthorpe & Sattar, 1990; Baldry *et al.*, 1991), with the exception of HAV (Mbithi *et al.*, 1990). Peracetic acid was shown to produce several alterations of the F116 phage structure (both capsid and tail) (Maillard *et al.*, 1995a), proteins (Maillard *et al.*, 1996a) and nucleic acid (Maillard *et al.*, 1996b).

The viricidal activity and mechanisms of action of hydrogen peroxide have not been widely studied. As with the peracids, it is an oxidizing agent, reacting with any oxidizable target sites. Unlike peracetic acid, poliovirus has been found to be resistant to hydrogen peroxide (Best *et al.*, 1994).

3.7.2 Ozone

Riesser *et al.* (1976) reported that the capsid protein of the poliovirus type 2 was damaged following ozonation, subsequently inhibiting virus–host-cell specificity and virus uptake. DeMik & DeGroot (1977) also demonstrated damage to the coliphage ØX174 protein coat following treatment with ozone. Breaks in the bacteriophage DNA were also reported. It was suggested that ozone had damaging effects on purine and pyrimidine bases and reacted more strongly with DNA than with RNA (Christensen & Giese, 1954). Similarly, studies investigating the effect of ozone against the bacteriophage T4 showed that ozone attacked the protein capsid, releasing the viral nucleic acid, which was subsequently inactivated (Sproul *et al.*, 1982). Kim *et al.* (1980) showed that treatment of the f2 coliphage with an ozone concentration of 0.8 mg/l for 30 s resulted in broken capsids in many small subunits. They also found that f2 RNA was attacked by ozone. However, it was demonstrated that RNA extracted from the phage prior to ozone treatment was less susceptible than RNA within ozonated bacteriophages. They concluded that capsid proteins were somehow involved in the inactivation of the phage genome. The mechanism of action probably involved a secondary shearing reaction of the RNA with altered capsid proteins. Furthermore, Kim *et al.* (1980) demonstrated that the extent of damage to the phage capsid was proportional to the concentration of ozone and the contact time. Mudd *et al.* (1969) reported that alteration of proteins challenged with ozone was caused by a reaction with cysteine, trytophan and methionine. Damage to the f2 capsid was proposed as a consequence of the alteration of these amino acids contained in the coat proteins (Kim *et al.*, 1980).

Therefore, the primary mechanism of action of ozone appears to be structural damage to the viral capsid, which subsequently loses its virus–host-cell specificity (and therefore its infectivity), followed by an inactivation of the viral nucleic acid within the damaged capsid and/or release of viral nucleic acid from the capsid, which is later attacked by ozone. It was suggested that RNA was possibly inactivated more readily within the viral capsid. Furthermore, within the viral capsid, DNA might be more susceptible to ozonation than is RNA.

3.8 Metallic salts

3.8.1 Silver salts

The viricidal properties of silver might be explained by the oxidation and denaturation (with higher residual concentrations) of complexed sulfhydryl groups (Thurman & Gerba, 1989). Silver has also been shown to bind phage DNA (Rahn & Landry, 1973; Rahn *et al.*, 1973), and phage inactivation by silver nitrate might be explained by its cross-linking with the DNA helix (Fox & Modak, 1974). Viricidal activity of silver has been demonstrated not only against several enveloped viruses, such as the herpes virus (silver sulphadiazine and silver nitrate), vaccinia virus, influenza A virus and pseudorabies virus (Cortisil and Micropur) but also against bovine enteroviruses (Thurman & Gerba, 1989). However, the mechanism by which these viruses were inactivated by silver remains unknown. Since these viruses contain a different genome (i.e. DNA and RNA), the viricidal mechanism of action of silver appears to be more complex than just an effect on viral nucleic acid. Furthermore, it should be noted that the metallic salt has to penetrate within the capsid to affect the viral genome.

3.8.2 Copper salts

The viricidal action of copper might be the binding of copper to thiol or other groups of protein molecules, leading to an alteration of the protein complex (Thurman & Gerba, 1989). Copper has also been reported to have a strong affinity with DNA and to denature DNA reversibly in low-ionic-strength solutions. There are several reports showing that the combination of copper(II) with other compounds produced cleavage of viral nucleic acid in R17 (i.e. via RNA degradation), ØX174 (i.e. via ssDNA scission) and λ DNA bacteriophages (i.e. via cleavage) and the poliovirus RNA (i.e. via scission) (Thurman & Gerba, 1989). Samuni *et al.* (1983) also reported that the action of both copper(II) and ascorbate resulted in impairing phage adsorption and DNA injection. Again, it should be noted that the ability of heavy metal ions to react with viral nucleic acid depends strongly upon the accessibility of viral nucleic acid to these ions.

3.9 Other compounds

3.9.1 Acids

Viruses are usually sensitive to low pH. Virus sensitivity varies when challenged with different mineral acids. Because the viral capsid is composed mainly of proteins, it is not surprising that a variation of pH will produce a conformational change of the viral capsid, which can sometimes increase viral resistance to biocidal compounds (see below). A drastic change in the conformational state might ultimately alter capsid integrity. Citric and phosphoric acids have been shown to inactivate foot-and-mouth disease virus (Russell, 1998) and hydrochloric acid (HCl) human rotavirus and vesicular stomatitis virus (Springthorpe & Sattar, 1990). However, no information on structural changes of these viruses during disinfection is available and the viricidal mechanism of action of acids remains, therefore, theoretical.

3.9.2 Ethylene oxide

Ethylene oxide has been shown to interact with amino, carboxyl, sulfhydryl and hydroxyl groups in bacterial proteins and with nucleic acid (Russell & Chopra, 1996). Although the viricidal mechanisms of action of ethylene oxide have not been studied, the biocide might interact with both protein and nucleic acid components of viruses, inducing a complete inactivation of viral particles. Such broad target sites might then explain its viricidal activity against various lipid-enveloped viruses (Sykes, 1965).

4 Viral resistance to biocide inactivation

4.1 Viral aggregation

Keswick *et al.* (1985) showed that resistance to chlorination by the Norwalk virus was likely to be caused by the presence of viral aggregates (Fig. 6.7). In a previous study with the poliovirus, clumps of virions were associated with the persistence of infectivity after challenge with formaldehyde (Salk & Gori, 1960). Similarly, with the vaccinia virus, the number and frequency of aggregates were correlated with the slope and shape of the survival curve (Sharp, 1968). The size of the viral aggregates is certainly important in the development of resistance to disinfection, as found by Sharp *et al.* (1975) with reovirus challenged with bromine. With poliovirus, persistent infection

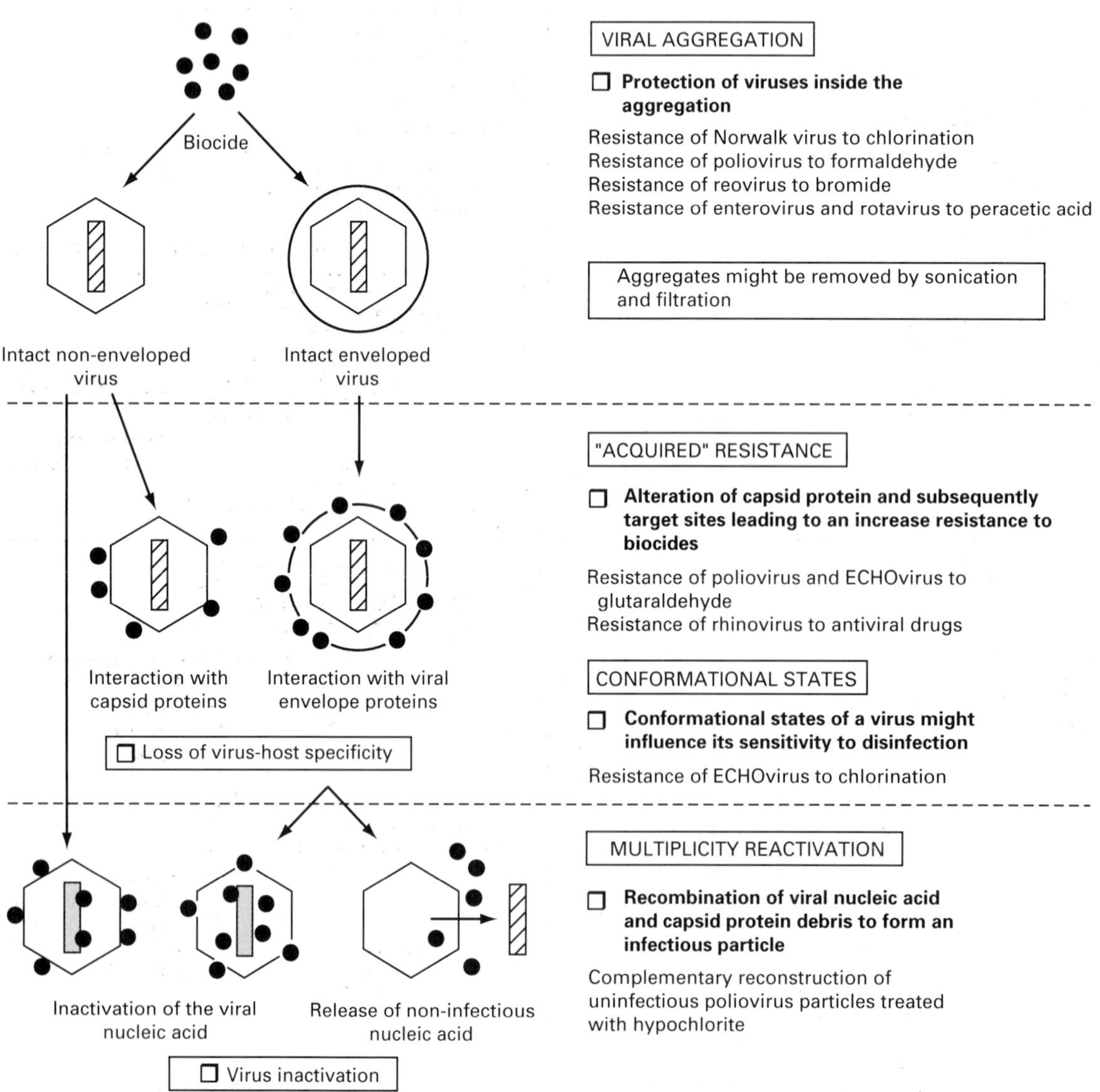

Fig. 6.7 Resistance of viruses to biocidal activity.

could be removed by filtration of the viral aggregates (Salk & Gori, 1960), whereas sonic waves produced the same effect with the vaccinia virus (Sharp, 1968). Harakeh (1984) reported that the effect of peracetic acid against enteroviruses and rotaviruses produced a typical biphasic survival curve, probably due to the presence of viral aggregates.

4.2 Adaptation of viruses to biocides

Viruses might adapt to new environmental conditions and become genetically stable. Thus, residual concentrations of a biocide after disinfection can act as a selective force for the adaptation of viruses (Fig. 6.7). Poliovirus with an increased resistance to chlorine inactivation has been described (Bates

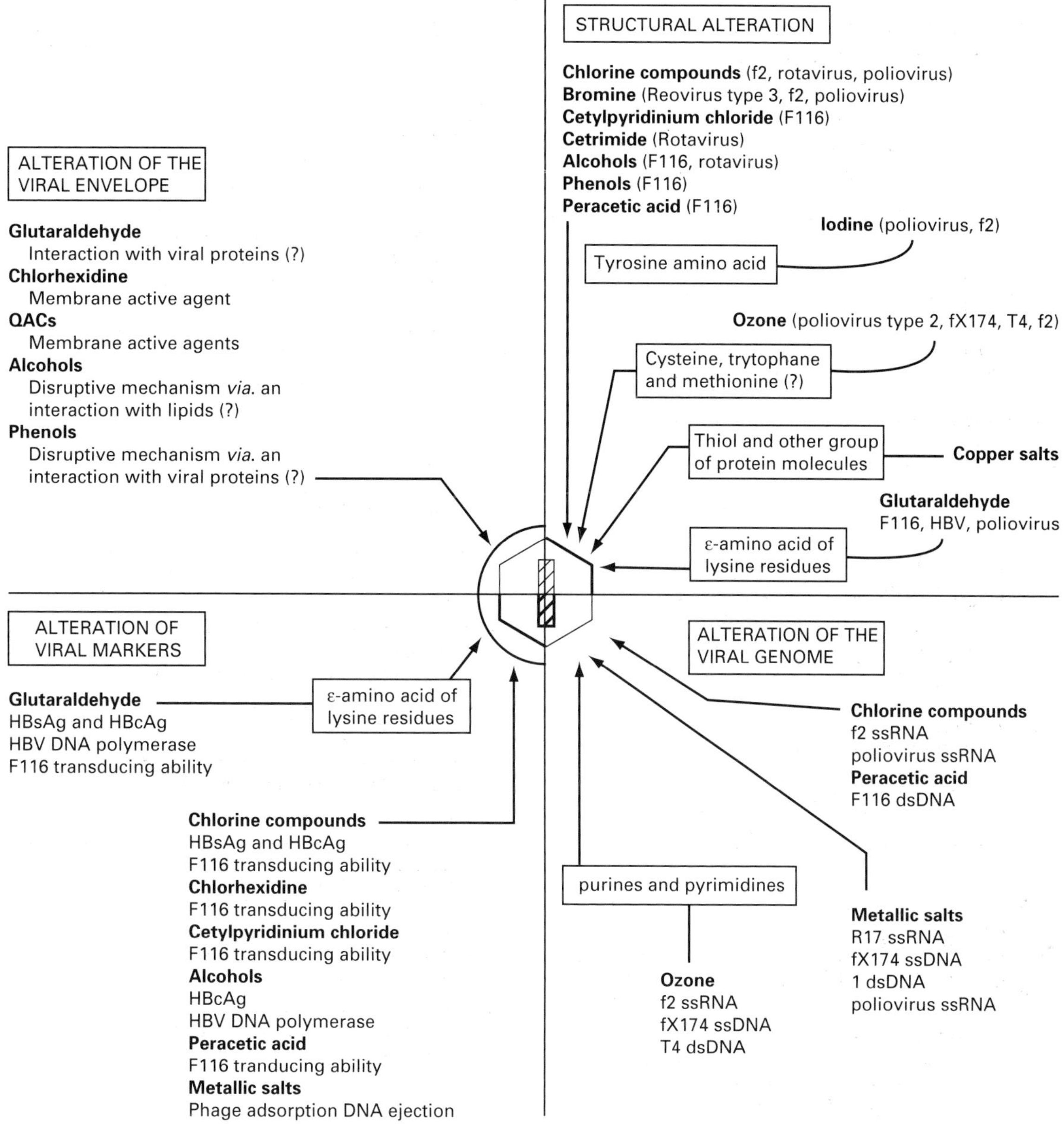

Fig. 6.8 Viral target sites for disinfection.

et al., 1977). Chambon *et al.* (1994) suggested that the resistance to GTA (0.1%) of two echovirus-25 isolates was due to the difference in cross-linking formation of the capsid polypeptides. Heinz *et al.* (1989) showed that mutations in the capsid proteins of rhinovirus 14 conferred viral resistance to antiviral drugs.

Viruses also exist under different forms, depending on the pH. Young & Sharp (1985) reported that echovirus had three conformational states, the efficiency of chlorine disinfection depending on the viral structural state (Fig. 6.7). Vrisjen *et al.* (1983) suggested that some viruses have several isoelectric points and there is evidence of correlation between one of the isoelectric points and the sensitivity to disinfection (Butler *et al.*, 1985). Poliovirus type 1 possesses two isoelectric points associated with two conformational states, A and B, the latter being related to virus inactivation (Mandel, 1971). A change of the isoelectric point is likely to affect the availability of target sites, thus affecting biocide activity (Thurman & Gerba, 1988).

4.3 Multiplicity reactivation

Young & Sharp (1985) noticed that clumping of poliovirus after partial viral inactivation by hypochlorite significantly increased the viral titre. The clumping of non-infectious virions, producing random damage to their capsid proteins or their nucleic acid, can result in complementary reconstruction of an infectious particle by hybridization of the gene pool of the inactivated virions. This phenomenon, first described by Luria in 1947, is the basis of multiplicity reactivation (Thurman & Gerba, 1989) (Fig. 6.7) and underlines the necessity of rendering the viral nucleic acid non-infectious (Thurman & Gerba, 1988).

5 Conclusions

The understanding of the viricidal mechanisms of action of biocides suffers unfortunately from a lack of information and has to rely, when possible, on investigations performed with other microorganisms. Mechanisms of action of biocides against viruses are summarized in Fig. 6.8. It emerges that, although most biocides alter the capsid structure of viruses, only a few alter viral nucleic acid. This is a serious issue, since some viral genomes are known to remain infectious when released from the capsid. Biocides generally have several target sites within the viral structure, unlike chemotherapeutic agents such as antibiotics and antiviral drugs. However, it is conceivable that most biocidal agents will react with primary target sites, which may or may not lead to viral inactivation. The study of viral target sites that are correlated with viral inactivation is important. The alteration of markers, such as antigenic structure and DNA polymerase, is not always related to viral inactivation. Likewise, structural damage to the capsid might not always reflect a loss of infectivity.

Furthermore, studies of the mechanisms of action of biocides against viruses have highlighted the difficulty in selecting an adequate viral model. Likewise, viricidal effects of biocides vary greatly, not only between virus families but also sometimes within a family. The use of bacteriophages, however, offers many advantages and they constitute excellent tools for studying the efficacy and the mechanisms of action of viricides.

Despite the complexity of the task, the study of mechanisms of action of biocides against viruses remains important, if the overall viricidal activity of such agents and our understanding of viral resistance to disinfection are to improve.

6 References

Adler-Storthz, K., Sehulster, L.M., Dreesman, G.R., Hollinger, F.B. & Melnick, J.L. (1983) Effect of alkaline glutaraldehyde on hepatitis B virus antigens. *European Journal of Clinical Microbiology*, **2**, 316–320.

Alvarez, M.E. & O'Brien, R.T. (1982) Effects of chlorine concentration on the structure of poliovirus. *Applied and Environmental Microbiology*, **43**, 237–239.

Bailly, J-L., Chambon, M., Peigue-Lafeuille, H., Laveran, H., De Champs, C. & Beytout, D. (1991) Activity of glutaraldehyde at low concentrations (<2%) against poliovirus and its relevance to gastrointestinal endoscope disinfection procedures. *Applied and Environmental Microbiology*, **57**, 1156–1160.

Baldry, M.G.C., French, M.S. & Slater, D. (1991) The activity of peracetic acid on sewage indicator bacteria and viruses. *Water Science Technology*, **24**, 353–357.

Baltimore, D. & Huang, A.S. (1968) Isopycnic separation of subcellular components from poliovirus-infected and normal HeLa cells. *Science* (New York) **162**, 572–574.

Bates, R.C., Shaffer, P.T.B. & Sutherland, S.M. (1977) Development of poliovirus having increased resistance to chlorine inactivation. *Applied and Environmental Microbiology*, **3**, 849–853.

Berman, D. & Hoff, J.C. (1984) Inactivation of simian rotavirus SA11 by chlorine, chlorine dioxide and monochloramine. *Applied and Environmental Microbiology*, **48**, 317–323.

Best, M., Springthorpe, V.S. & Sattar, S.A. (1994) Feasibility of a combined carrier test for disinfectants: studies with a mixture of five types of microorganisms. *American Journal of Infection Control*, **22**, 152–162.

Bloomfield, S.F., Smith-Burchnell, C.A. & Dalgleish, A.G. (1990) Evaluation of hypochlorite-releasing disinfectants against the human immunodeficiency virus (HIV). *Journal of Hospital Infection*, **15**, 273– 278.

Bond, W.W., Favero, M.S., Petersen, N.J. & Ebert, J.W. (1983) Inactivation of hepatitis B virus by intermediate to high level disinfectant chemicals. *Journal of Clinical Microbiology*, **18**, 535–538.

Brown, T.T. (1981) Laboratory evaluation of selected disinfectants as virucidal agents against porcine parvovirus, pseudorabiesvirus, and transmissible gastroenteritis virus. *American Journal of Veterinary Research*, **42**, 1033–1036.

Bruch, C.W. (1991) Role of glutaraldehyde and other chemical sterilants in the processing of new medical devices. In: *Sterilization of Medical Products*, Vol. 5. (eds Morrissey, R.F. & Prokopenko, Y.I.) pp. 377–396. Morin Heights, Canada: Polyscience Publications Inc.

Butler, M., Medlen, A.R. & Taylor, G.R. (1985) Electrofocusing of viruses and sensitivity to disinfection. *Water Science Technology*, **17**, 201–210.

Chambon, M., Bailly, J-L. & Peigue-Lafeuille, H. (1992) Activity of glutaraldehyde at low concentrations against capsid proteins of poliovirus type 1 and echovirus type 25. *Applied and Environmental Microbiology*, **58**, 3517–3521.

Chambon, M., Bailly, J-L. & Peigue-Lafeuille, H. (1994) Comparative sensitivity of the echovirus type 25 JV-4 prototype strain and two recent isolates to glutaraldehyde at low concentrations. *Applied and Environmental Microbiology*, **60**, 387–392.

Christensen, E. & Giese, A. (1954) Changes in adsorption spectra of nucleic acids and their derivatives following exposure to ozone and ultraviolet radiations. *Archives of Biochemistry and Biophysics*, **51**, 208–216.

Davies, J.G., Babb, J.R., Bradley, C.R. & Ayliffe, G.A. (1993) Preliminary study of test methods to assess the virucidal activity of skin disinfectants using poliovirus and bacteriophages. *Journal of Hospital Infection*, **25**, 125–131.

DeMik, G. & DeGroot, I. (1977) Mechanism of inactivation of bacteriophage ØX174 and its DNA in aerosols by ozone and ozomised cyclohexene. *Journal of Hygiene, Cambridge*, **78**, 191–211.

Eagar, R.G., Leder, J. & Theis, A.B. (1986) Glutaraldehyde: Factors important for microbiocidal efficacy. *Proceedings of the 3rd Conference on Progress in Chemical Disinfection*, pp. 32–49. Binghamton, New York, USA.

Floyd, R.D., Sharp, G. & Johnson, J.D. (1979) Inactivation by chlorine of single poliovirus particles in water. *Environmental Sciences and Technology*, **13**, 438–442.

Fox, C.L. & Modak, S.M. (1974) Mechanisms of silver sulphadiazine action on burn wound infections. *Antimicrobial Agents and Chemotherapy*, **5**, 582– 588.

Frôsner, G., Jentsch, G. & Uthemann, H. (1982) Destroying of antigenicity and influencing the immunochemical reactivity of hepatitis B virus antigens (HBsAg, HBcAg, HBeAg) through disinfectants—a proposed method for testing. *Zentralblatt für Bakteriologie, Parasitenkunde, Infektionskrankheinten und Hygiene. I. Abteilung Originale, Reike*, **176**, 1–14.

Gorman, S.P., Scott, E.M. & Russell, A.D. (1980) Antimicrobial activity, uses and mechanism of action of glutaraldehyde. *Journal of Applied Bacteriology*, **48**, 161–190.

Habeeb, A.F.S.A. & Hiramoto, R. (1968) Reaction of proteins with glutaraldehyde. *Archives of Biochemistry and Biophysics*, **126**, 16–26.

Harakeh, M.S. (1984) Inactivation of enteroviruses, rotaviruses and bacteriophages by peracetic acid in a municipal sewage effluent. *FEMS Microbiology Letters*, **23**, 27–30.

Harakeh, M.S. (1987) The behaviour of viruses on disinfection by chlorine dioxide and other disinfectants in effluent. *FEMS Microbiology Letters*, **44**, 335–341.

Heinz, B.A., Rueckert, R.R., Shepard, D.A. *et al.* (1989) Genetics and molecular analysis of spontaneous mutants of human rhinovirus 14 that are resistant to an antiviral compound. *Journal of Virology*, **63**, 2476–2485.

Hogle, J.M., Chow, M. & Filman, D.J. (1985) Three-dimensional structure of poliovirus at 2.9Å resolution. *Science*, **229**, 1358–1365.

Howard, C.R., Dixon, J.L., Young, P., Van Eerd, P. & Schellekens, H. (1983) Chemical inactivation of hepatitis B virus: the effect of disinfectants on virus-associated DNA polymerase activity, morphology and infectivity. *Journal of Virological Methods*, **7**, 135–148.

Kim, C.H., Gentile, D.M. & Sproul, O.J. (1980) Mechanism of ozone inactivation of bacteriophage f2. *Journal of Environmental Microbiology*, **39**, 210–218.

Keswick, B.H., Fujioka, R.S. & Loh, P.C. (1981) Mechanism of poliovirus inactivation by bromine chloride. *Applied and Environmental Microbiology*, **42**, 824–829.

Keswick, B.H., Satterwhite, T.K., Johnson, P.C. *et al.* (1985) Inactivation of Norwalk virus in drinking water by chlorine. *Applied and Environmental Microbiology*, **50**, 261–264.

Klein, M. & Deforest, A. (1983) Principles of viral inactivity. In *Disinfection, Sterilization and Preservation*, 3rd edn (ed. Block, S.S.), pp. 422–434. Philadelphia: Lea & Febiger.

Kobayashi, H. & Tsuzuki, M. (1984) The effects of disinfectants and heat on hepatitis B virus. *Journal of Hospital Infection*, **5**, 93–94.

Kobayashi, H., Tsuzuki, M., Koshimizu, K. *et al.* (1984) Susceptibility of hepatitis B virus to disinfectants or heat. *Journal of Clinical Microbiology*, **20**, 214–216.

Korn, A.H., Feairheller, S.H. & Filachione, E.M. (1972) Glutaraldehyde: nature of the reagent. *Journal of Molecular Biology*, **65**, 525–529.

Kurtz, J.B., Lee, T.W. & Parsons, A.J. (1980) The action of alcohols on rotavirus, astrovirus and enterovirus. *Journal of Hospital Infection*, **1**, 321–325.

Linemeyer, D.L., Menke, J.G., Martin-Gallardo, A., Hughes, J.V., Young, A. & Mitra, S.W. (1985) Molecular cloning and partial sequencing of hepatitis A viral cDNA. *Journal of Virology*, **54**, 247–255.

McKenna, R., Xia, D., Willingmann, P. *et al.* (1992) Atomic structure of single-stranded DNA bacteriophage Phi X174 and its functional implications. *Nature*, **355**, 137–143.

Maillard, J.-Y. (1996) Bacteriophages: a model system for human viruses. *Letters in Applied Bacteriology*, **23**, 1.

Maillard, J.-Y., Beggs, T.S., Day, M.J., Hudson, R.A. & Russell, A.D. (1994) Effect of biocides on MS2 and K coliphages. *Applied and Environmental Microbiology*, **60**, 2205–2206.

Maillard, J.-Y., Hann, A.C., Beggs, T.S., Day, M.J., Hudson, R.A. & Russell, A.D. (1995a) Electron-microscopic investigation of the effect of biocides on *Pseudomonas aeruginosa* PAO bacteriophage F116. *Journal of Medical Microbiology*, **42**, 415–420.

Maillard, J.-Y., Hann, A.C., Beggs, T.S., Day, M.J., Hudson, R.A. & Russell, A.D. (1995b) Analysis of X-rays: study of the distribution of chlorhexidine and cetylpyridinium chloride on the *Pseudomonas aeruginosa* bacteriophage F116. *Letters in Applied Microbiology*, **20**, 357–360.

Maillard, J.-Y., Beggs, T.S., Day, M.J., Hudson, R.A. & Russell, A.D. (1995c) The effects of biocides on the transduction of *Pseudomonas aeruginosa* PAO by F116 bacteriophage. *Letters in Applied Microbiology*, **21**, 215–218.

Maillard, J.-Y., Beggs, T.S., Day, M.J., Hudson, R.A. & Russell, A.D. (1996a) The effects of biocides on proteins of *Pseudomonas aeruginosa* PAO bacteriophage F116. *Journal of Applied Bacteriology*, **80**, 291–295.

Maillard, J.-Y., Beggs, T.S., Day, M.J., Hudson, R.A. & Russell, A.D. (1996b) Damage to *Pseudomonas aeruginosa* PAO1 bacteriophage F116 DNA by biocides. *Journal of Applied Bacteriology*, **80**, 540–544.

Mandel, B. (1971) Characterization of type 1 poliovirus by electrophoretic analysis. *Virology*, **44**, 554–568.

Mbithi, J.N., Springthorpe, V.S. & Sattar, S.A. (1990) Chemical disinfection of hepatitis A virus on environmental surfaces. *Applied and Environmental Microbiology*, **56**, 3601–3604.

Montefiori, D.C., Robinson, W.E., Jr, Modliszewski, A. & Mitchell, W.M. (1990) Effective inactivation of human immunodeficiency virus with chlorhexidine antiseptics containing detergents and alcohol. *Journal of Hospital Infection*, **15**, 279–282.

Mudd, J.B., Reavitt, R., Ongun, A. & McManus, T.T. (1969) Reaction of ozone with amino acids and proteins. *Atmospheric Environment*, **3**, 669–681.

O'Brien, R.T. & Newman, J. (1979) Structural and compositional changes associated with chlorine inactivation of polioviruses. *Applied and Environmental Microbiology*, **38**, 1034–1039.

Olivieri, V.P., Kruse, C.W., Hsu, Y.C., Griffiths, A.C. & Kawata, K. (1975) The comparative mode of action of chlorine, bromine, and iodine on f2 bacterial virus. In *Disinfection—Water and Wastewater* (ed. Johnson, J.D.), pp. 145–162. Ann Arbor, Michigan: Ann Arbor Science.

Park, J.B. & Park N.-H. (1989) Effect of chlorhexidine on the *in vitro* and *in vivo* herpes simplex virus infection. *Oral Surgery*, **67**, 149–153.

Passagot, J., Crance J.M., Biziagos, E., Laveran, H., Agbalika, F. & Deloince, R. (1987) Effect of glutaraldehyde on the antigenicity and infectivity of hepatitis A virus. *Journal of Virological Methods*, **16**, 21–28.

Peterson, D.A. Hurley, T.R., Hoff, J.C. & Wolfe, L.G. (1983) Effect of chlorine treatment on infectivity of hepatitis A virus. *Applied and Environmental Microbiology*, **45**, 223–227.

Prince, H.N., Prince, D.L. & Prince, R.N. (1991) Principles of viral control and transmission. In *Disinfection, Sterilization and Preservation*, 4th edn (ed. Block, S.S.), pp. 411–444. Philadelphia: Lea & Febiger.

Quinn, L.Y. (1978) Polyconfiguration-model for the A-protein of coliphage MS2. *Biochemical and Biophysical Research Communications*, **83**, 863–868.

Racaniello, V.R. & Baltimore, D. (1981) Molecular cloning of poliovirus cDNA and determination of the complete nucleotide sequence of the viral genome. *Biochemistry*, **78**, 4887–4891.

Rahn, R.O. & Landry, L.C. (1973) Ultraviolet irradiation of nucleic acid complexed with heavy atoms. II. Phosphorescence and photodimerization of DNA complexed with Ag. *Photochemistry and Photobiology*, **18**, 29–38.

Rahn, R.O., Setlow, J.K. & Landry, L.C. (1973)

Ultraviolet irradiation of nucleic acid complexed with heavy atoms. III. Influence of Ag^{+} and Hg^{2+} on the sensitivity of phage and of transforming DNA to ultraviolet radiation. *Photochemistry and Photobiology*, **18**, 39–41.

Resnick, L., Veren, K., Zaki Salahuddin, S., Tondreau, S. & Markham, P.D. (1986) Stability and inactivation of HTLV-III/LAV under clinical and laboratory environments. *Journal of the American Medical Association*, **255**, 1887–1891.

Richards, F.M. & Knowles, J.R. (1968) Glutaraldehyde as a protein cross-linking reagent. *Journal of Molecular Biology*, **37**, 231–233.

Riesser, V.W., Perrich, J.R., Silver, B.B. & McCammon, J.R. (1976) Possible mechanism of poliovirus inactivation by ozone. In *Forum on Ozone Disinfection* (eds Fochtman, E.G., Rice, R.G. & Browning, M.E.), pp. 186–192. Syracuse, New York: International Ozone Institute.

Rodgers, F.G., Hufton, P., Kurzawska, E., Molloy, C. & Morgan, S. (1985) Morphological response of human rotavirus to ultra-violet radiation, heat and disinfectants. *Journal of Medical Microbiology*, **20**, 123–130.

Rubin, J. (1991) Human immunodeficiency virus (HIV) disinfection and control. In *Disinfection, Sterilization and Preservation*, 4th edn (ed. Block, S.S.), pp. 472–481. Philadelphia: Lea & Febiger.

Russell, A.D. (1998) Microbial sensitivity and resistance to chemical and physical agents. In *Topley & Wilson's Microbiology and Microbial Infections*, 9th edn, (eds Balows, A. & Duerden, B.I.), Vol. 2, pp. 149–184. London: Edward Arnold.

Russell, A.D. & Chopra, I. (1996) *Understanding Antibacterial Action and Resistance*, 2nd edn. London: Ellis Horwood.

Salk, J.E. & Gori, J.B. (1960) A review of theoretical, experimental and practical considerations in the use of formaldehyde for inactivation of poliovirus. *Annals of New York Academy of Sciences*, **83**, 609–637.

Samuni, A., Aronovitch, J., Godinger, D., Chevion, M. & Czapski, G. (1983) On the cytotoxicity of vitamin C and metal ions. *European Journal of Biochemistry*, **137**, 119–124.

Sangar, D.V., Rowlands, D.J., Smale, C.J. & Brown, F. (1973) Reaction of glutaraldehyde with foot and mouth disease virus. *Journal of Genetic Virology*, **21**, 399–406.

Sharp, D.G. (1968) Multiplicity reaction of animal viruses. *Progress in Medical Virology*, **10**, 64–109.

Sharp, D.G., Floyd, R. & Johnson, J.D. (1975) Nature of the surviving plaque-forming unit of reovirus in water containing bromine. *Applied Microbiology*, **29**, 94–101.

Springthorpe, V.S. & Sattar, A.S. (1990) Chemical disinfection of virus-contaminated surfaces. *Critical Reviews in Environmental Control*, **20**, 169–229.

Springthorpe, V.S., Grenier, J.L., Lloyd-Evans, N. & Sattar, S.A. (1986) Chemical disinfection of human rotaviruses: efficacy of commercially-available products in suspension tests. *Journal of Hygiene, Cambridge*, **97**, 139–161.

Sproul, O.J., Pfister, R.M. & Kim, C.K. (1982) The mechanism of ozone inactivation of water borne viruses. *Water Science Technology*, **14**, 303–314.

Sykes, G. (1965) *Disinfection and Sterilization*, 24th edn. London: F. & N. Spon.

Taylor, G.R. & Butler, M. (1982) A comparison of the virucidal properties of chlorine, chlorine dioxide, bromine chloride and iodine. *Journal of Hygiene, Cambridge*, **89**, 321–328.

Tenno, K.M., Fujioka, R. & Loh, P.C. (1979) The mechanisms of poliovirus inactivation by hypochlorous acid. In *Proceedings of the 3rd Conference on Water Chlorination: Environmental Impact and Health Effects* (eds Jolley, R., Brungs, W.A. & Cumming, R.B.), pp. 665–675. Ann Arbor, Michigan: Ann Arbor Science Publishers.

Thraenhart, O., Dermietzel, R., Kuwert, E. & Scheiermann, N. (1977) Morphological alteration and disintegration of Dane particles after exposure with 'Gigasept': a first methodological attempt for the evaluation of the virucidal efficacy of a chemical disinfectant against hepatitis virus B. *Zentralblatt für Bakteriologie, Parasitenkunde, Infektionskrankheinten und Hygiene. I. Abteilung Originale, Reike*, **164**, 1–21.

Thraenhart, O., Kuwert, E.K., Dermietzel, R., Kuwert, E., Scheiermann, N. & Wendt, F. (1978) Influence of different disinfection conditions on the structure of the hepatitis B virus (Dane particle) as evaluated in the morphological alteration and disintegration test (MADT). *Zentralblatt für Bakteriologie, Parasitenkunde, Infektionskrankheinten und Hygiene. I. Abteilung Originale, Reike*, **242**, 299–314.

Thurman, R.B. & Gerba, C.P. (1988) Molecular mechanisms of viral inactivation by water disinfectants. *Advances in Applied Microbiology*, **33**, 75–105.

Thurman, R.B. & Gerba, C.P. (1989) The molecular mechanisms of copper and silver ion disinfection of bacteria and viruses. *Critical Reviews of Environmental Control*, **18**, 295–315.

Tyler, R., Ayliffe, G.A.J. & Bradley, C. (1990) Virucidal activity of disinfectants: studies with the poliovirus. *Journal of Hospital Infection*, **15**, 339–345.

Vrisjen, R., Rombaut, B. & Boeye, A. (1983) pH dependent aggregation and electrofocusing of poliovirus. *Journal of Genetic Virology*, **64**, 2339–2342.

Wouters, M., Miller, A.O.A. & Fenwick, M.L. (1973) Distortion of poliovirus particles by fixation with formaldehyde. *Journal of General Virology*, **18**, 211–214.

Young, D.C. & Sharp, D.G. (1985) Virion conformational forms and the complex inactivation kinetics of echovirus by chlorine in water. *Applied and Environmental Microbiology*, **49**, 359–364.

CHAPTER 7

Transmissible Degenerative Encephalopathies:

INACTIVATION OF THE UNCONVENTIONAL CAUSAL AGENTS

1 Introduction

1.1 Disease characteristics

The transmissible degenerative encephalopathies (TDE) form a group of fatal neurological diseases of mammals (Table 7.1) which share many unusual features (Table 7.2). Creutzfeldt–Jakob disease (CJD), Gerstmann–Straussler–Scheinker syndrome (GSS) and fatal familial insomnia (FFI) affect humans worldwide at a collective frequency of only around 1 in 1 000 000 each year. In contrast, scrapie affects sheep in many but not all areas of the world, inflicting losses of up to 30% in affected flocks (Palsson, 1979). Transmissible mink encephalopathy (TME) has occurred sporadically among ranch-bred mink in North America and Europe (Eckroade *et al.*, 1979). Kuru was confined to the Fore tribal population of Papua New Guinea (Alpers, 1987) but has now almost completely disappeared as a result of the abandonment of ritualistic practices which involved contact with

Table 7.1 The transmissible degenerative encephalopathies (TDE).

Disease	Recognized hosts
Scrapie	Sheep, goats, moufflons
Transmissible mink encephalopathy (TME)	Mink
Chronic wasting disease (CWD)	Elk, mule-deer
Bovine spongiform encephalopathy (BSE)	Cattle, exotic ruminants
Feline spongiform encephalopathy (FSE)	Domestic cats, exotic felids
Creutzfeldt–Jakob disease (CJD)	Humans
Gerstmann–Straussler–Scheinker syndrome (GSS)	Humans
Kuru	Humans
Fatal familial insomnia (FFI)	Humans

Table 7.2 Characteristics of the TDE.

Long incubation periods	Afebrile
No antibody response	Fatal
Neuronal vacuolation (normally)	No inflammatory response
Accumulation of modified PrP protein	Unconventional causal agents

the brain tissue of the deceased. Chronic wasting disease (CWD) is confined to North America (Williams & Young, 1980). Bovine spongiform encephalopathy (BSE), which first emerged in 1985, had affected more than 165 000 British cattle by the end of 1996 (Ministry of Agriculture, Fisheries and Food (MAFF), personal communication). Although predominantly a British disease, BSE has occurred to a lesser extent in the indigenous cattle populations of Eire, France, Portugal and Switzerland. It also appears to have been transmitted to British domestic cats and to captive exotic felids and ruminants born in Britain. The possibility that BSE may be transmissible to humans has been suggested by the recent occurrence of a new variant form of CJD, which, apart from one case in France, has been confined to Britain (Will *et al.*, 1996). Not only has the new form of the disease affected an unusually young age-group but the clinical and neurohistopathological features are quite distinct from traditional CJD. It has been suggested that these individuals may have acquired their infections from a dietary source in the 1980s, when it was still permissible to use bovine brain in food products.

Scrapie has existed for at least 250 years, whereas other TDE have been recognized for much shorter periods. More is known about scrapie as a natural disease in sheep and as an experimental disease in rodents, and it is the model for the group.

A feature of all TDE is that a normal sialoglycoprotein (PrP^C), which is expressed predominantly in neurons, converts to a protease-resistant form (PrP^{Sc}) as a consequence of infection (Carp *et al.*, 1985) and accumulates in the central nervous system. This is associated topographically with neuronal vacuolation (Bruce *et al.*, 1989), the principal lesion detectable by histological examination, which is thought to cause the fatal neurological dysfunction which is a clinical hallmark for the TDE.

1.2 Agent characteristics

1.2.1 Nature of the agents

Although the unconventional nature of the scrapie agent has long been recognized (Stamp *et al.*, 1959), no agent-specific nucleic acid has been detected for any of the TDE. The molecular nature of the agents that cause TDE has not been determined, but an abnormal protease-resistant form of a normal host protein is implicated in the pathological process. The normal protein, PrP^C, is a glycoprotein that is associated with cell membranes and is expressed in a variety of cell types. The highest level of expression is in neurons, but its normal function is unknown. During TDE infection, PrP^C is converted progressively to an abnormal protease-resistant form (PrP^{Sc}), which accumulates, particularly in the central nervous system. Because PrP^{Sc} copurifies with infectivity, it has been suggested that the transmissible agent is solely a protein and is devoid of nucleic acid (Prusiner, 1982), but the known hydrophobic nature of PrP could encourage adventitious association with an unindentified agent which would copurify.

The 'prion' hypothesis argues that PrP^{Sc} *per se* is the infectious agent, and that its introduction into, or spontaneous generation within, a previously uninfected host causes a post-translational conformational modification of PrP^C to PrP^{Sc} by some unknown mechanism; the amino acid sequences of PrP^C and PrP^{Sc} are the same. The importance of PrP protein in the development of disease is demonstrated by the inability of scrapie infectivity to replicate in mice in which the *PrP* gene has been ablated (Bueler *et al.*, 1993). The 'virino' theory proposes that, although PrP^{Sc} is probably a required component of the infectious agent, there has to be an additional informational molecule (probably a nucleic acid), which carries strain-specific information and which may trigger the change from PrP^C to PrP^{Sc} (Dickinson & Outram, 1979). The 'virino' model invokes the need for only a very small nucleic acid, which would be difficult to detect; the hypothesis argues that nucleic acid is essential in explaining the diversity of strains and the mutations that are known to occur with scrapie agent (Dickinson *et al.*, 1989). To date there are around 20 strains of rodent-passaged scrapie agent, which can be distinguished by their incubation periods, the distribution and severity of lesions in the brain, clinical manifestations, ease of transmission to new species and susceptibility to thermal inactivation (Bruce, 1993).

Proponents of the 'virino' hypothesis argue that such information must be conveyed by an informational molecule that is independent of the host, but none has been identified. On the other hand, for the 'prion' theory to accommodate strain diversity, there would have to be as many distinct post-translational conformation modifications of PrP^{C} to PrP^{Sc} as there are strains of agent, and this seems unlikely. Nevertheless, recent studies with TME, another of the TDE, have shown that two strains of the causal agent can convert hamster PrP^{C} to PrP^{Sc} in a cell-free system and pass on strain-specific information in the form of differing enzyme cleavage sites for the PrP^{Sc} molecules (Bessen *et al.*, 1995). The authors suggest that this confirms that a messenger molecule, such as a nucleic acid, is not required for conveying strain-specific information. However, the design of these interesting experiments did not permit testing to see if the two types of PrP^{Sc} produced *in vitro* are actually infectious *in vivo*, and this remains to be confirmed.

Another theory that has been proposed to explain strain variation within the framework of the 'prion' hypothesis is that PrP^{Sc} glycosylation patterns confer strain specificity (Hecker *et al.*, 1992). This theory is based on the suggestion that different strains of scrapie agent target to different areas of the brain, and that there are diversely glycosylated forms of PrP^{Sc} in scrapie-infected brain (Endo *et al.*, 1989). The hypothesis is that different subsets of neurons express differently glycosylated forms of PrP^{C}, and that when PrP^{Sc} is injected it will interact preferentially with PrP^{C} molecules which have a matching glycosylation pattern, thus perpetuating strain characteristics. However, some strains target the same areas of the brain. Also, strain specificity is preserved in infectivity which is recovered from lymphoreticular tissues, such as spleen. Current evidence indicates that, within the spleen, agent replication occurs in follicular dendritic cells (Fraser *et al.*, 1989; McBride *et al.*, 1992), and one would not expect this single cell type to have the capacity to donate diverse glycosylation patterns to PrP^{Sc}. There is also an opinion that the causal agents may be conventional viruses, albeit unusual, but there are difficulties with this notion, particularly since there is no detectable immune response in the host to the foreign proteins, which would be associated customarily with conventional viruses. There is clearly a need to determine unequivocally how the strain-specific information that produces phenotypic diversity is processed.

1.2.2 Resistance to inactivation

The agents of TDE are remarkably resistant to inactivation. Because they have not been purified, it is difficult to know to what degree their resistance is intrinsic and how much it is influenced by the protective effect of host tissue to which they are intimately bound; the hydrophobic nature of the cell-membrane domains with which infectivity is associated encourages the formation of aggregates in homogenized tissue preparations (Rohwer & Gajdusek, 1980). The protective effect of such aggregates is recognized for conventional viruses (Salk & Gori, 1960) and may at least partly explain the resistance of TDE agents.

Survival of these agents under harsh conditions could explain outbreaks of scrapie in sheep grazed on pastures that had been unoccupied by sheep for several years (Palsson, 1979), and the rare, sporadic cases of CJD of unknown aetiology. Scrapie agent has been shown to maintain a high degree of viability after burial for 3 years (Brown & Gajdusek, 1991). The CJD agent remains highly infectious after 28 months at room temperature (Tateishi *et al.*, 1987), and scrapie agent survives in a desiccated state for at least 30 months (Wilson *et al.*, 1950).

1.2.3 Accidental transmission through failure of inactivation procedures

The difficulty of inactivating TDE agents became

apparent when about 1800 of 18 000 sheep that had been vaccinated against louping-ill developed scrapie. The vaccine had been contaminated unsuspectedly with scrapie agent, which survived the exposure to 0.35% formalin that inactivated the louping-ill virus (Greig, 1950).

There has also been accidental transmission of CJD through using decontamination methods recognized retrospectively as being inappropriate. Brain electrodes disinfected with ethanol and then 'sterilized' with formaldehyde vapour were implicated on one occasion (Bernoulli *et al.*, 1977). A standard hot-air sterilization process was also considered to have failed to decontaminate CJD-infected surgical instruments, which consequently transmitted the disease to a patient undergoing brain surgery (Foncin *et al.*, 1980).

It is considered generally that BSE was caused by the transmission of scrapie agent to bovines via foodstuff (Dickinson & Taylor, 1988; Wilesmith *et al.*, 1988). Prior to the ban in Britain in July 1988, it was common practice to incorporate ruminant-derived meat and bone-meal into the diets of dairy cattle. It is now known that the heating processes in many of the rendering procedures used traditionally to manufacture meat and bone-meal do not completely inactivate BSE or scrapie agents (Taylor *et al.*, 1995, 1996b).

2 Practical considerations in decontamination studies

No standard methods exist. Experiments have involved various tissue preparations, e.g. crude macerates, unspun 20% homogenates, 10% tissue supernates, biochemically processed and ultracentrifuged material. Exposure times have been varied and the temperature for chemical treatment has been generally either 4°C or room temperature, occasionally with mechanical stirring. These variables undoubtedly contribute to the equivocal results sometimes obtained.

The assumption is sometimes made that procedures effective for partially purified infectivity are applicable equally for dealing with crude tissue contamination, but this is unwarranted (Taylor, 1986). Decontamination experiments should mimic the most adverse conditions, thus enhancing the prospect of detecting residual infectivity after exposure to partially inactivating procedures, especially since bioassay is the only available procedure for detection of TDE infectivity.

Unlike other TDE, distinct strains of scrapie agent have been cloned, and these have reproducible biological characteristics (Dickinson *et al.*, 1989). Because high titres of infectivity in brain tissue combined with a short incubation period are a feature of the 263K strain of scrapie agent in hamsters, it has been regarded as the optimal model for decontamination studies (Rosenberg *et al.*, 1986); this is reasonable for chemical studies, where there is little evidence that TDE agent isolates or strains differ in susceptibility. However, the 22A strain of scrapie agent in mice is relatively thermostable (Dickinson & Taylor, 1978; Kimberlin *et al.*, 1983) and appears to be the most appropriate model for studying thermal destruction of the TDE agents, even though infectivity titres in brain are lower than for 263K (Taylor, 1986).

Little has been done to validate chemical procedures for decontaminating the surfaces of equipment, benches, etc., but preliminary evidence suggests that it may be inadvisable to extrapolate from 'test-tube' studies involving tissue homogenates (Asher *et al.*, 1987).

Decontamination studies have usually involved brain tissue. Reticuloendothelial tissues are also infected, although at a lower level, but it is unknown whether there are differences in the degree of protection afforded to the TDE agents by different tissues.

Autoclaving studies have confirmed that the presence of tissue has an impeding effect on inactivation of scrapie agent. Gravity-displacement autoclaving of scrapie-infected mouse-brain macerate (22A strain) at 126°C for 30 min resulted in a loss of $10^{2.1}$ infective dose for 50% (ID_{50})/g (Kimberlin *et al.*, 1983). When autoclaved at 100°C or 105°C as 10% homogenate (i.e. 10-fold less tissue and infectivity per unit volume), the titre losses were 2.5 and 3.5 logs, respectively (D.M. Taylor & A.G. Dickinson, unpublished data).

Under well-defined experimental conditions, specific strains of scrapie in rodents display highly reproducible inverse relationships between the dose of infectivity administered and the subsequent incubation period before the onset of the clinical signs (Outram, 1976). For any given model, the amount of infectivity present in an inoculum can be calculated by comparing the incubation period of the recipients with an 'incubation period assay' graph, without the need for titration. Unfortunately, this procedure cannot be applied to infectivity exposed to chemical or physical treatments, because these can radically extend the dose–response curves for treated, compared with untreated, agent (Taylor & Fernie, 1996). The same conclusions have been arrived at as a result of other studies involving chemical or physical treatment of scrapie agent (Dickinson & Fraser, 1969; Kimberlin, 1977; Lax *et al.*, 1983; Somerville & Carp, 1983). This means that a meaningful assessment of the amount of infectivity remaining after exposure to partially inactivating procedures can only be obtained by full titration and observing the assay animals for extended periods (Outram, 1976).

3 Inactivation methods

Inactivation studies on TDE agents are conducted either to obtain clues regarding their molecular nature or to establish meaningful decontamination standards. The former generally utilize partially purified materials, whereas the latter involve crude preparations and will be considered here.

3.1 Physical methods

3.1.1 Gamma and ultraviolet irradiation

When CJD, kuru and scrapie agents were exposed to γ (150 kGy) or ultraviolet irradiation (254 nm wavelength; 100 kJ/m^{-2}) infectivity was recoverable (Latarjet, 1979); TME agent is equally resistant (Marsh & Hanson, 1969). Such exposures represent what would be a gross degree of overkill for conventional viruses. The resistance of TDE agents may be attributable at least partially to protective mechanisms afforded by the intimate association of these agents with cell membranes (Millson *et al.*, 1976) and the tendency of infected tissue fragments to form aggregates; these would need to receive as many radiation 'single hits' as there are infectious units within such aggregates to achieve inactivation (Rohwer, 1983). Although the interpretation of irradiation data has caused considerable debate (Alper, 1987), these methods have no practical application for inactivating TDE agents.

3.1.2 Microwave irradiation

Although the inactivating effect of microwave irradiation on conventional microorganisms is considered generally to be attributable to the heat generated, a number of investigators have been forced to the conclusion that inactivation results, at least in part, from non-thermal effects (Culkin & Fung, 1975; Latimer & Matsen, 1977; Diprose & Benson, 1984; Rosaspina *et al.*, 1994). Also, it is considered that the extremely rapid rise in temperature during microwave irradiation in just as important as the final temperature attained. Consequently, the effect of microwave irradiation on the 22A strain of scrapie agent was studied. However, no significant degree of inactivation was observed after the exposure of undiluted, infected brain tissue or 10% saline homogenates (Taylor & Diprose, 1996).

3.1.3 Radiant heat

Thermal studies involving the transfer of heat from water to samples in glass containers have shown that, at temperatures up to 100°C, there is only a small effect on CJD (Tateishi *et al.*, 1987) and scrapie agents (Stamp *et al.*, 1959).

A small amount of infectivity was recoverable after a homogenate of hamster brain infected with the 263K strain of scrapie agent was exposed to dry heat at a temperature of 360°C for an hour (Brown *et al.*, 1990a). However, the brain homogenate had been lyophilized before heating; as with conventional microorganisms, drying of scrapie infectivity is known to enhance its thermostability (Asher *et al.*, 1987). In contrast, when 7 mg samples of (non-lyophilized) macerated mouse brain infected with the ME7 strain of scrapie agent were exposed to dry heat, there was no detectable infectivity after an exposure to 200°C for 1 h, even though some infectivity had survived exposure to 160°C for 24 h or 200°C for 20 min (Taylor *et al.*, 1996c). The survival of lyophilized infectivity after exposure to 360°C in the earlier study led to speculation that the effectiveness of incineration for inactivating scrapie-like agents should be questioned (Brown *et al.*, 1990a). Although temperatures of up to 200°C only were used in more recent studies with non-lyophilized material (Taylor *et al.*, 1996c), it has been possible to use these data to extrapolate to higher temperatures, using a specially designed computer program. These extrapolations indicate that infectivity in 7 mg samples of brain would be destroyed in 1 s at a temperature of 280°C (R.Oberthur, personal communication). This suggests that incineration, which is usually carried out at a minimum temperature of 850°C, should be a reliable procedure for inactivating scrapie-like agents.

3.1.4 *Gravity-displacement autoclaving*

Gravity-displacement autoclaving at 126°C for 2 h inactivates the 139A strain of scrapie agent but not the more thermostable 22A strain (Kimberlin *et al.*, 1983), which is inactivated only after 4 h exposure (Dickinson, 1976). Guinea-pig-passaged CJD agent and the hamster-passaged 263K strain of scrapie agent were reported to be inactivated at 132°C for 1h (Brown *et al.*, 1986b). Consequently, this procedure was adopted as a standard for CJD agent decontamination in the USA (Rosenberg *et al.*, 1986), and has been extended widely as a general decontamination procedure for TDE agents. However, subsequent studies with the 263K strain of scrapie agent have shown that, although high levels of inactivation are achieved, the use of this procedure does not guarantee complete inactivation (Ernst & Race, 1993; M. Pocchiari, unpublished data cited in Horaud, 1993).

3.1.5 *Porous-load autoclaving*

Data indicating that porous-load autoclaving at 136°C for ⩾4 min inactivates both the 139A and 22A strains of scrapie agent (Kimberlin *et al.*, 1983) were used to formulate the UK standard for inactivation of CJD agent by porous-load autoclaving, i.e. 134–138°C for 18 min (DHSS, 1984). This has also become an adopted standard for TDE agents generally. However, more recent studies, involving hamster and mouse brain infected with scrapie agent and bovine brain infected with BSE agent, have indicated that this standard may be unreliable (Taylor *et al.*, 1994). In these more recent studies, infectivity was detectable in samples exposed to 134–138°C for up to 1 h. The major difference between the earlier study and the more recent one was that the average weight of the brain macerates used in the former was 50 mg; in the more recent studies, this was increased to 340 mg. The heavier samples were used because they were considered to be more representative of a worst-case situation in practice, although what constitutes a worst-case scenario in the course of animal or human health care has never been defined officially. Also, previous experience with porous-load autoclaving had indicated that inactivation of samples of intact brain in this weight range would be effective (Taylor & McConnell, 1988; D.M. Taylor, unpublished observations). Upon completion of the more recent porous-load autoclaving studies, it was recognized that, because the samples were 340 mg brain macerates, there had been the potential for a significant amount of smearing and drying of infected tissue on glass surfaces prior to autoclaving, and that this would have been greater than in the earlier study, in which 50 mg samples were used. As stated earlier, it is known that the drying of scrapie infectivity on to glass surfaces enhances thermostability (Asher *et al.*, 1987). Since the drying of infectivity on to glass and other surfaces is exactly what would occur in practice, it is considered that the more recent data are the most relevant. These indicate that the current UK standard for inactivation of TDE agents by exposure to porous-load autoclaving at 134–138°C for 18 min is unreliable.

3.1.6 *Rendering procedures*

These procedures are essentially cooking processes that are applied to waste animal tissues derived mainly from abattoirs. Traditionally, the principal end-product had been tallow, but in the 1920s it was recognized that there were valuable proteins contained in the remaining solids. Until recently, it had been customary to pulverize these solids to produce meat and bone-meal, which could then be incorporated as a protein supplement in animal diets. However, the recognition that the BSE epidemic had probably been caused initially by the survival of scrapie infectivity in meat and bone-meal, and then fuelled by the recycling of subclinically BSE-infected bovine carcasses through the rendering system, resulted in the 1988 British ban on the inclusion of ruminant-derived protein in ruminant diets. In addition, experiments were carried out to establish the effectiveness of rendering procedures used throughout the European Union (EU) with regard to inactivation of BSE and scrapie agents. It should be emphasized that the conditions prevailing during rendering bear no relationship to any of the experimental environments within which the thermostability of TDE agents had been tested previously. During rendering, there is generally (apart from systems using hyperbaric steam) a slowly progressive increase in temperature towards 100°C until the water content is driven off. Thereafter, the temperature in the water-free, fat-rich environment is permitted to increase to a maximum of around 140°C, before there is a detrimental effect on the nutritional value of the rendered proteins. The first rendering study used BSE-spiked abattoir waste. Although the level of the spike proved to be low, infectivity was nevertheless detectable in meat and bone-meal produced by two types of process. One was a continuous process, in which cooking took place at atmospheric pressure for a period of 50 min, and which was designed to achieve a temperature of 112°C or 122°C. The other process was conducted under vacuum with added preheated tallow; exposure times were either 10 or 40 min, by which time the temperatures had reached 120°C or 121°C, respectively (Taylor *et al.*, 1995). As a result of these data, the time/temperature conditions for rendering within the EU were revised (Commission Decision, 1994). In the scrapie-spiked experiments, the level of infectivity introduced into the abattoir waste was approximately 40-fold higher than in the BSE-spiked experiments. In this study, infectivity was detectable in all meat and bone-meal samples, except those produced by procedures involving hyperbaric steam. The procedures that did not inactivate the scrapie agent included a process that achieved a temperature of 138°C over a period of 125 min (Taylor *et al.*, 1996b). It was decided therefore that, as from April 1997, any meat and bone-meal produced as animal feed in the EU (within which the feeding of ruminant-derived proteins to ruminants had already been banned in 1994) should be manufactured by a process involving exposure of the raw materials to a temperature of at least 133°C at 3 bar for 20 min (Commission Decision, 1996)

3.2 Chemical methods

3.2.1 Acids and bases

Little inactivation of scrapie infectivity occurs over the pH range 2–10 (Mould *et al.*, 1965), but it has been reported that a 1 h exposure to 1 mol/l sodium hydroxide (pH 14) inactivates guinea-pig-passaged CJD agent and the hamster-passaged 263K strain of scrapie agent (Brown *et al.*, 1986b). However, the sensitivity of these bioassays was reduced, because it proved necessary to dilute the samples to render them non-toxic for the recipient animals. Residual infectivity has been detected following treatment of 263K scrapie agent with 1 mol/l sodium hydroxide (Diringer & Braig, 1989; Ernst & Race, 1993), even after periods of up to 24 h (Prusiner *et al.*, 1984). Similarly, CJD infectivity has been reported to survive exposure to 1 mol/l (Tamai *et al.*, 1988) or 2 mol/l sodium hydroxide (Tateishi *et al.*, 1988). More recent work with sodium hydroxide, involving the mouse-passaged (ME7) and hamster-passaged (263K) strains of scrapie agent and BSE-infected bovine brain (Taylor *et al.*, 1994), has demonstrated that, if the samples are carefully neutralized, they can be injected without further dilution. Under these circumstances, infectivity can be shown to survive exposure to 2 mol/l sodium hydroxide for up to 2 h. With the 263K strain of scrapie agent, although more than 5 logs of infectivity were lost following such treatments, around 4 logs survived (Taylor *et al.*, 1994).

Although autoclaving or exposure to sodium hydroxide are not completely effective *per se* for inactivating TDE agents, inactivation can be achieved by combining these procedures. Taguchi *et al.* (1991) described the successful inactivation of CJD agent by a sequential process involving exposure to 1 mol/l sodium hydroxide, followed by gravity-displacement autoclaving at 121°C for 30 min. More recently, it has been observed that, if the relatively thermostable 22A strain of scrapie agent is autoclaved at 121°C for 30 min in the presence of 2 mol/l sodium hydroxide (without a prior holding period in sodium hydroxide), inactivation can be achieved (D.M. Taylor, unpublished data). There are practical problems relating to this procedure, such as the potential exposure of operators to splashing with sodium hydroxide and the eventual deleterious effect on the autoclave chamber and other components if they are frequently contaminated with sodium hydroxide. However, given the lack of other reliable decontamination strategies for TDE agents, it would seem sensible to attempt to develop this system by eliminating the practical difficulties that are associated with it at present.

It has been reported that there is little inactivation of CJD agent exposed 1 mol/l hydrochloric acid (pH 0.1) for 1 h (Brown *et al.*, 1986b).

3.2.2 Alkylating agents

The viability of scrapie agent after exposure to 0.35% formalin has been mentioned (Section 1.2.3), but it can survive even more rigorous treatments, e.g. immersion of infected brain tissue for 974 days in 20% formol saline (D.M. Taylor & A.G. Dickinson, unpublished data). The agents of CJD and TME are equally resilient, the former surviving at least 1 year in 10% formol saline (Tateishi *et al.*, 1980); the latter survives formol fixation for at least 6 years (Burger & Gorham, 1977). The agent of BSE is also known to be relatively reistant, having survived an exposure to 10% formol saline for 2 years (Fraser *et al.*, 1992). Although the titre of surviving infectivity was not measured in any of these studies, it could be concluded generally from the number of afffected animals and their incubation periods that little inactivation had occurred. In the one study where titre reduction has been measured, only 1.5 logs of infectivity were lost when 263K-infected hamster brain was exposed to 10% formol saline for 48 h (Brown *et al.*, 1990a).

Scrapie infectivity survived an exposure to 12.5% unbuffered glutaraldehyde (pH 4.5) for 16 h (Dickinson & Taylor, 1978); CJD agent was not inactivated by a 14-day exposure to 5% buffered histological glutaraldehyde at pH 7.3 (Amyx *et al.*, 1981). However, 2% glutaraldehyde buffered to pH 8 is recognized as being more active microbiologically, but there are as yet no reports of it having been tested.

Acetylethyleneimine (Stamp *et al.*, 1959) and β-propiolactone (Haig & Clarke, 1968) have little effect on scrapie agent. Ethylene oxide exposure causes very little loss of CJD (Brown *et al.*, 1982a) or scrapie infectivity (Dickinson, 1976).

3.2.3 Detergents

Mild detergents have little effect on TDE agents (Millson *et al.*, 1976), but sodium dodecyl sulphate has some effect on CJD (Walker *et al.*, 1983) and scrapie infectivity (Millson *et al.*, 1976), which is enhanced by heat (Kimberlin *et al.*, 1983).

3.2.4 Halogens

Sodium hypochlorite solutions containing up to 25 000 parts/10^6 available chlorine have been reported to inactivate guinea-pig-passaged CJD agent and the hamster-passaged 263K strain of scrapie agent (Brown *et al.*, 1986b). In an extensive study with two strains of mouse-passaged scrapie agent, it was demonstrated that a solution containing 14 000 parts/10^6 available chlorine is effective in 30 min, leading to the recommendation that 20 000 parts/10^6 for 1 h should be used in practice (Kimberlin *et al.*, 1983). Such strong solutions are corrosive to metals, but the less corrosive chlorine-releasing compound, sodium dichloroisocyanurate (NaDCC) (see Chapter 2), has been reported to be equally effective for bacterial inactivation at equivalent levels of available chlorine (Coates, 1985). Consequently, a study was conducted, using two sources of BSE-infected brain tissue, which were exposed for 30–120 min to solutions of sodium hypochlorite or NaDCC containing comparable levels of available chlorine (ranging from 8250 to 16 500 parts/10^6). No infectivity was detectable in any of the hypochlorite-treated samples, but infectivity was recoverable from samples that had been treated for up to 120 min with NaDCC solutions containing up to 16 500 parts/10^6 available chlorine (Taylor *et al.*, 1994). It was shown that, at the end of the various exposure periods, the NaDCC solutions had released 3.5 times less chlorine than the hypochlorite solutions.

Only a modest reduction in scrapie infectivity was obtained using 2% iodine in sodium iodide for 4 h (Brown *et al.*, 1982b). Similar results were observed with scrapie and CJD agents, using an iodophor containing 0.8% iodine (Asher *et al.*, 1981).

3.2.5 *Organic solvents*

Numerous studies, particularly with scrapie agent, have shown that organic solvents generally have little effect on TDE infectivity. Experimental exposures have included 1 h with acetone (Hunter & Millson, 1964), 2 weeks with 5% chloroform (D.R. Wilson, unpublished work, cited in Dickinson, 1976), 16 h with ether (Gajdusek & Gibbs, 1968), 2 weeks with 4% phenol (D.R. Wilson, unpublished work, cited in Dickinson, 1976) and 2 weeks with ethanol (Dickinson & Taylor, 1978).

3.2.6 *Oxidizing agents*

Exposure of scrapie agents to chlorine dioxide (50 parts/10^6 for 24 h) inactivated only a small proportion of infectivity (Brown *et al.*, 1982b). Treatment of scrapie agent with 3% hydrogen peroxide for 24 h caused little inactivation (Brown *et al.*, 1982a).

Scrapie-infected brain homogenates were not inactivated by concentrations of up to 18% peracetic acid, but 2% inactivated intact brain tissue (Taylor, 1991). These apparently anomalous results are considered to demonstrate the protective effect of aggregation, which occurs in homogenized preparations.

3.2.7 *Salts and urea*

Oxidizing salts and urea have been tested for their effect on TDE agents, with conflicting results. For example, the report that sodium metaperiodate has a considerable effect on scrapie infectivity (Hunter *et al.*, 1969) is contradicted by several other studies (Adams *et al.*, 1972; A.G. Dickinson, private communication, cited in Hunter *et al.*, 1972; Brown *et al.*, 1982a). Similarly, a claim that potassium permanganate inactivates all CJD and scrapie infectivity in homogenates of brain tissue (Asher *et al.*, 1981) is challenged by data from other experiments (Brown *et al.*, 1982a, 1986b; Kimberlin *et al.*, 1983). The claim that urea is an effective scrapiecide (Millson *et al.*, 1976) is not supported by other studies that have been reviewed (Brown *et al.*, 1986b).

4 Laboratory exposure to transmissible degenerative encephalopathy (TDE) agents

Numerous studies have failed to establish any association between human disease and dietary or occupational exposure to scrapie agent (Taylor, 1989b). Consequently, there are no particular restrictions on working with this agent in the laboratory. Because the data for other animal TDE are not so extensive, it has been recommended that they should be handled with some precautions in the laboratory (ACDP, 1994). This seems sensible, given that there is now a postulated link between BSE and the new variant form of CJD in humans (Will *et al.*, 1996).

Until 1993, CJD had been observed in 24 individuals who had been health-care workers of various types, including a pathologist and two technicians who had worked in neurohistopathology laboratories, but there was no evident association between their development of CJD and any occupational exposure to CJD agent (Berger & David, 1993). Furthermore, there was historically an interval of 40 years between the recognition of CJD as a clinical entity and the suspicion that the disease might be infectious. Even though CJD is a rare disease, brain tissue from CJD-infected individuals must have been handled worldwide without significant precautions during this period by pathologists and laboratory personnel, but without any apparent increased incidence of the disease in such individuals. Nevertheless, the accidental transmission of CJD to human recipients of CJD-contaminated human growth hormone by intramuscular injection (Brown *et al.*, 1992) demonstrates that occupationally acquired disease through trauma is a possibility. This is supported by the data from experiments in which mouse-passaged scrapie infectivity was relatively efficiently transmitted to mice through skin scarification (Taylor *et al.*, 1996a).

Survival of TDE infectivity in brain tissue after exposure to formalin has already been described (see Section 3.2.2). When hamster brain containing $10^{10.2}$ ID_{50}/g of the 263K strain of scrapie agent was fixed in formol saline for 48 h, only 1.5 logs of infectivity were lost (Brown *et al.*, 1990a); even after full histological processing, the titre loss was only 2.8 logs (Brown *et al.*, 1982b). Glutaraldehyde treatment is also known to permit survival of TDE infectivity (see Section 3.2.2). Consequently, the handling of fixed CJD-infected tissues in the histopathology laboratory has been viewed as a potentially risky activity, and a number of procedures have been recommended to reduce this risk. One suggestion has been to fix such tissues in formol saline containing sodium hypochlorite (V.M. Armbrustmacher, personal communication, cited in Titford & Bastian, 1989). High concentrations of sodium hypochlorite inactivate TDE agents (see Section 3.2.4) but there has been no validation of its effectiveness when combined with formalin. The addition of phenol to formol saline has also been suggested (Kleinman, 1980; Brumback, 1988; Esiri, 1989), but the basis of this proposal was flawed (Taylor, 1989a), and phenolized formalin was shown subsequently to be not only ineffective (Brown *et al.*, 1990b) but also to produce poor fixation (Brown *et al.*, 1990b; Mackenzie & Fellowes, 1990). Sections, stained with haematoxylin and eosin, prepared from scrapie-infected formol-fixed brain tissue that had been autoclaved at 134°C for 18 min retained sufficient integrity to permit quantitative scoring of spongiform encephalopathy (Taylor & McBride, 1987), and it has been suggested that autoclaving at 126°C for 30 min (Masters *et al.*, 1985a) or 132°C for 6 min (Masters, *et al.*, 1985b) could be used to inactivate CJD infectivity in formol-fixed brain. However, mouse- or hamster-passaged scrapie agent in formol-fixed brain has been shown to survive porous-load autoclaving at 134°C for 18 min (Taylor & McConnell, 1988) or gravity-displacement autoclaving at 134°C for 30 min (Brown *et al.*, 1990a), with titre losses of <2 logs. The only procedure that has been shown to result in significant losses of infectivity titre in formol-fixed tissues, without significant loss of microscopic morphology, is a 1 h exposure to concentrated formic acid (Brown *et al.*, 1990b). In this study, the level of infectivity in hamster brain infected with the 263K strain of scrapie agent was reduced from $10^{10.2}$ ID_{50}/g to $10^{1.3}$ ID_{50}/g. With mouse brain infected with CJD agent, the original titre of $10^{8.5}$ ID_{50}/g was reduced to $10^{2.3}$ ID_{50}/g. However, in another study, where mouse brain infected with the 301V strain of BSE agent was fixed using paraformaldehyde-lysine-periodate, a necessary prerequisite for the subsequent immunocytochemical investigation that is an important aspect of TDE investigation, the degree of inactivation by formic acid was calculated to be 2 logs less than that achieved with formol-fixed 263K-infected hamster brain, despite the equivalent levels of infectivity of the two agents (Taylor, 1994). This suggests that either infected tissues fixed with paraformaldehyde-lysine-periodate are less amenable to the inactivating effect of formic acid than those fixed with formalin, or that there is a fundamental difference in the susceptibility of the 263K agent compared with 301V; alternatively, both factors may contribute to this observation. Although further studies are in progress to clarify this situation, it is evident that there is no known decontamination procedure that can guarantee the complete absence of infectivity in TDE-infected tissues that have been processed by histopathological procedures. Clearly, autoclaving of histological waste is inappropriate for inactivating scrapie-like agents, and reliance must be placed on incineration.

Precautions in the handling of TDE agents in other types of laboratory are somewhat different from those in the histopathology laboratory. For example, the disruption of infected brain tissue by homogenization has the potential to release many more infectious airborne particles than section-cutting in the histopathology laboratory, especially if the latter tissues were treated with formic acid. In the biochemistry laboratory, there is also the capability, through partial purification procedures, of producing samples that contain infectivity titres higher than those found in naturally infected tissues. Apart from general good laboratory practice, the principal recommendation when handling TDE agents under such conditions is to use microbiological safety cabinets. However, what must be borne in mind is the resistance of TDE agents to inactivation by formalin, which is the customary fumigant for routine decontamination of safety cabinets. The main objective, therefore, is to adopt working procedures that minimize the potential for contamination of the cabinet; these include measures such as the use of disposable covering materials on the work surface and the prevention of aerosol dispersion, e.g. by retaining cotton-wool plugs in glass tissue homogenizers during sample disruption (and for some time thereafter, if possible).

Regardless of these types of precautions, it would be naïve to consider that they would guarantee complete freedom from contamination of the internal surfaces of safety cabinets. Although contamination at this sort of level is unlikely to represent any significant risk to the operator, given that such work should always involve the wearing of disposable gloves and laboratory coats, the potential for cross-contamination from different TDE sources in laboratory experiments has to be considered. This can be addressed by adopting a routine of washing the internal surfaces of safety cabinets with a solution of sodium hypochlorite containing 20 000 parts/10^6 available chlorine; however, a compromise has to be struck between the perceived necessary frequency of such a decontamination procedure and its potential progressive degradative effect on the treated surfaces. Class II safety cabinets are suitable for this type of work and are popular generally, because they combine satisfactory degrees of product and personnel protection under conditions that are not too restrictive for the operator. However, the classical design of such cabinets has been such that contamination of the internal plenum and the air-propulsion units is likely. Although this is not problematic for conventional microorganisms, which can be inactivated by formalin fumigation that penetrates these areas, there is obviously a problem with TDE agents. Although this type of contamination with TDE agents does not represent any significant risk to the operator or the work activity, there is the problem of how to achieve decontamination before engineers are permitted to carry out repairs or servicing, because the plenum and the air-propulsion units are inaccessible, as far as manual hypochlorite decontamination is concerned. There is also the problem of the potential corrosive effects of hypochlorite on the air-propulsion units, even if they were able to be treated with hypochlorite. An improvement in this situation has been achieved by the manufacture of class II safety cabinets with filters positioned immediately below the working surface, which means that contamination of the plenum and the air-propulsion units is avoided unless there is damage to these filters. Because the main filters are readily accessible in such cabinets, it is an easy matter to prevent particle dispersion during their removal, by prior treatment of the filter surface, e.g. with latex solution.

5 References

ACDP (1994) *Precautions for Work with Human and Animal Transmissible Spongiform Encephalopathies*. London: HMSO.

Adams, D.H., Field, E.J. & Joyce, G. (1972) Periodate—an inhibitor of the scrapie agent? *Research in Veterinary Science*, **13**, 195–198.

Alper, T. (1987) Radio- and photobiological techniques in the investigation of prions. In *Prions: Novel Infectious Pathogens Causing Scrapie and Creutzfeldt–Jakob Disease* (eds Prusiner, S.B. & McKinlay, M.P.), pp. 113–146. London: Academic Press.

Alpers, M. (1987) Epidemiology and clinical aspects of kuru. In *Prions: Novel Infectious Pathogens Causing Scrapie and Creutzfeldt–Jakob Disease* (eds Prusiner, S.B. & McKinlay, M.P.), pp. 451–465. London: Academic Press.

Amyx, H.L., Gibbs, C.J., Kingsbury, D.T. & Gajdusek, D.C. (1981) Some physical and chemical characteristics of a strain of Creutzfeldt–Jakob disease in mice. In *Abstracts of the Twelfth World Congress of Neurology*, Kyoto, 20–25 September, p. 255.

Asher, D.M., Gibbs, C.J., Diwan, A.R., Kingsbury, D.T., Sulima, M.P. & Gajdusek, D.C. (1981) Effects of several disinfectants and gas sterilisation on the infectivity of scrapie and Creutzfeldt–Jakob disease. In *Abstracts of the Twelfth World Congress of Neurology*, Kyoto, 20–25 September, p. 225.

Asher, D.M., Pomeroy, K.L., Murphy, L., Gibbs, C.J. & Gajdusek, D.C. (1987) Attempts to disinfect surfaces contaminated with etiological agents of the spongiform encephalopathies. In *Abstracts of the VIIth International Congress of Virology*, Edmonton, 9–14 August, p. 147.

Berger, J.R. & David, N.J. (1993) Creutzfeldt–Jakob disease in a physician: a review of the disorder in health care workers. *Neurology*, **43**, 205–206.

Bernoulli, C., Siegfried, J., Baumgartner, G. *et al.* (1977) Danger of accidental person-to-person transmission of Creutzfeldt–Jakob disease by surgery. *Lancet*, **i**, 478–479.

Bessen, R.A., Kocisko, D.A., Raymond, G.J., Nandan,

S., Lansbury, P.T. & Caughey, B. (1995) Non-genetic propagation of strain-specific properties of scrapie prion protein. *Nature*, **375**, 698–700.

Brown P. & Gajdusek, D.C. (1991) Survival of scrapie virus after 3 years' interment. *Lancet*, **337**, 269–270.

Brown, P., Gibbs, C.J., Amyx, H.L. *et al.* (1982a) Chemical disinfection of Creutzfeldt–Jakob disease virus. *New England Journal of Medicine*, **306**, 1279–1282.

Brown, P., Rohwer, R.G., Green, E.M. & Gajdusek, D.C. (1982b) Effects of chemicals, heat and histopathological processing on high-infectivity hamster-adapted scrapie virus. *Journal of Infectious Diseases*, **145**, 683–687.

Brown, P., Gibbs, C.J. & Gajdusek, D.C. (1986a) Transmission of Creutzfeldt–Jakob disease from formalin-fixed, paraffin-embedded human brain tissue. *New England Journal of Medicine*, **315**, 1614–1615.

Brown, P., Rohwer, R.G. & Gajdusek, D.C. (1986b) Newer data on the inactivation of scrapie virus or Creutzfeldt–Jakob disease virus in brain tissue. *Journal of Infectious Diseases*, **153**, 1145–1148.

Brown, P., Liberski, P.P., Wolff, A. & Gajdusek, D.C. (1990a) Resistance of scrapie agent to steam autoclaving after formaldehyde fixation and limited survival after ashing at 360°C: practical and theoretical implications. *Journal of Infectious Diseases*, **161**, 467–472.

Brown, P., Wolff, A. & Gajdusek, D.C. (1990b) a simple and effective method for inactivating virus infectivity in formalin-fixed tissue samples from patients with Creutzfeldt–Jakob disease. *Neurology*, **40**, 887–890.

Brown, P., Preece, M.A. & Will, R.G. (1992) 'Friendly fire' in medicine: hormones, homografts, and Creutzfeldt–Jakob disease. *Lancet*, **ii**, 24–27.

Bruce, M.E. (1993) Scrapie strain variation and mutation. *British Medical Bulletin*, **49**, 822–838.

Bruce, M.E., McBride, P.A. & Farquhar, C.F. (1989) Precise targeting of the pathology of the sialoglycoprotein, PrP, and vacuolar degeneration in mouse scrapie. *Neuroscience Letters*, **102**, 1–6.

Brumback, R.A. (1988) Routine use of phenolised formalin in fixation of autopsy brain tissue to reduce risk of inadvertent transmission of Creutzfeldt–Jakob disease. *New England Journal of Medicine*, **319**, 654.

Bueler, H., Aguzzi, A., Sailer, A. *et al.* (1993) Mice devoid of PrP are resistant to scrapie. *Cell*, **73**, 1339–1347.

Burger, D. & Gorham, J.R. (1977) Observation on the remarkable stability of transmissible mink encephalopathy virus. *Research in Veterinary Science*, **22**, 131–132.

Carp, R.I., Merz, P.A., Kascsak, R.J., Merz, G. & Wisniewski, H.M. (1985) Nature of the scrapie agent: current status of facts and hypotheses. *Journal of General Virology*, **66**, 1357–1368.

Coates, D. (1985) A comparison of sodium hypochlorite and sodium dichloroisocyanurate products. *Journal of Hospital Infection*, **6**, 31–40.

Commission Decision (1994) On the approval of alternative heat treatment systems for processing animal waste of ruminant origin with a view to the inactivation of spongiform encephalopathy agents, Commission Decision 94/382/EC. *Official Journal of the European Communities*, **L172**, 25–27.

Commission Decision (1996) On the approval of alternative heat treatment systems for processing animal waste with a view to the inactivation of spongiform encephalopathy agents, Commission Decision 96/449/EC. *Official Journal of the European Communities*, **L184**, 43–46.

Culkin, F. & Fung, D.Y.C. (1975) Destruction of *Escherichia coli* and *Salmonella typhimurium* in microwave-cooked soups. *Journal of Milk and Food Technology*, **38**, 8–15.

DHSS (1984) *Management of Patients with Spongiform Encephalopathy, Creutzfeldt–Jakob disease (CJD)*. DHSS Circular DA (84) 16. London: HMSO.

Dickinson, A.G. (1976) Scrapie in sheep and goats. In *Slow Virus Diseases of Animals and Man* (ed. Kimberlin, R.H.), pp. 209–241. Amsterdam: North-Holland.

Dickinson, A.G. & Fraser, H. (1969) Modification of the pathogenesis of scrapie in mice by treatment of the agent. *Nature, London*, **222**, 892–893.

Dickinson, A.G. & Outram, G.W. (1979) The scrapie replication-site hypothesis and its implications for pathogenesis. In *Slow Transmissible Diseases of the Nervous System* (eds Prusiner, S.B. & Hadlow, W.J.), Vol. 2, pp. 13–21. London: Academic Press.

Dickinson, A.G. & Taylor, D.M. (1978) Resistance of scrapie agent to decontamination. *New England Journal of Medicine*, **229**, 1413–1414.

Dickinson, A.G. & Taylor, D.M. (1988). Options for the control of scrapie in sheep and its counterpart in cattle. In *Proceedings of the Third World Congress on Sheep and Beef Cattle Breeding*, Vol. 1, 19–23 June, Paris, pp. 553–564.

Dickinson, A.G., Outram, G.W. , Taylor, D.M. & Foster, J.D. (1989) Further evidence that scrapie agent has an independent genome. In *Unconventional Virus Diseases of the Central Nervous System* (eds Court, LA., Dormont, D., Brown, P. & Kingsbury, D.T.), pp. 446–460. Moisdon la Rivière: Abbaye de Melleray.

Diprose, M.F. & Benson, F.A. (1984) The effect of externally applied electrostatic fields, microwave radiation and electric currents on plants, with special reference to weed control. *Botanical Reviews*, **50**, 171–223.

Diringer, H. & Braig, H.R. (1989) Infectivity of unconventional viruses in dura mater. *Lancet*, **i**, 439–440.

Eckroade, R.J., ZuRhein, G.M. & Hanson, R.P. (1979)

Experimental transmissible mink encephalopathy: brain lesions and their sequential development in mink. In *Slow Transmissible Diseases of the Nervous System* (eds Prusiner, S.B. & Hadlow, W.J.), Vol. 1, pp. 409–449. London: Academic Press.

Endo, T., Groth, D., Prusiner, S.B. & Kobata, A. (1989) Diversity of oligosaccharide structures linked to asparagines of the scrapie prion protein. *Biochemistry*, **28**, 8380–8388.

Ernst, D.R. & Race, R.E. (1993) Comparative analysis of scrapie agent inactivation. *Journal of Virological Methods*, **41**, 193–202.

Esiri, M.M. (1989) *Diagnostic Neuropathology*, Oxford: Blackwell.

Foncin, J.F. Gaches, J., Cathala, F., El Sherif, E. & Le Beau (1980) Transmission iatrogène interhumaine possible de maladie de Creutzfeldt–Jakob avec alteinte des grains du cervulet. *Revue Neurologique*, **136**, 280.

Fraser, H., McConnell, I., Wells, G.A.H. & Dawson, M. (1989) Transmission of bovine spongiform encephalopathy to mice. *Veterinary Record*, **123**, 472.

Fraser, H., Bruce, M.E., Chree, A., McConnell, I. & Wells, G.A.H. (1992) Transmission of bovine spongiform encephalopathy and scrapie to mice. *Journal of General Virology*, **173**, 1891–1897.

Gajdusek, D.C. & Gibbs, C.J. (1968) Slow, latent and temperature virus infections of the central nervous system. In *Infections of the Nervous System* (ed. Zimmerman, H.M.), pp. 254–280. Baltimore: Williams & Wilkins.

Greig, J.R. (1950) Scrapie in sheep. *Journal of Comparative Pathology*, **60**, 263–266.

Haig, D.A. & Clarke, M.C. (1968). The effect of β-propiolactone on the scrapie agent. *Journal of General Virology*, **3**, 281–283.

Hecker, R., Taraboulos, A., Scott, M., Pan, K.-M., Yang, S.-L., Torchia, M., Jendroska, K., De Armond, S.J. & Prusiner, S.B. (1992) Replication of distinct scrapie prion isolates is region specific in brains of transgenic mice and hamsters. *Genes and Development*, **6**, 1213–1228.

Horaud, F. (1993) Safety of medicinal products: summary. *Developments in Biological Standardization*, **80**, 207–208.

Hunter, G.D. & Millson, G.C. (1964) Further experiments on the comparative potency of tissue extracts from mice infected with scrapie. *Research in Veterinary Science*, **5**, 149–153.

Hunter, G.D., Gibbons, R.A., Kimberlin, R.H. & Millson, G.C. (1969) Further studies of the infectivity and stability of extracts and homogenates derived from scrapie affected mouse brains. *Journal of Comparative Pathology*, **79**, 101–108.

Hunter, G.D., Millson, G.C. & Heitzman, R.J. (1972) The nature and biochemical properties of the scrapie agent. *Annales de Microbiologie, Institut Pasteur*, **123**, 571–583.

Kimberlin, R.H. (1977) Biochemical approaches to scrapie research. *Trends in Biochemical Sciences*, **2**, 220–223.

Kimberlin, R.H., Walker, C.A., Millson, G.C. *et al.* (1983) Disinfection studies with two strains of mouse-passaged scrapie agent. *Journal of the Neurological Sciences*, **59**, 355–369.

Kleinman, G.M. (1980) Case records of the Massachusetts General Hospital (case 45-1980). *New England Journal of Medicine*, **303**, 1162–1171.

Latarjet, R. (1979) Inactivation of the agents of scrapie, Creutzfeldt–Jakob disease, and kuru by radiations. In *Slow Transmissible Disease of the Nervous System* (eds Prusiner, S.B. & Hadlow, W.J.), Vol. 2, pp. 387–407. London: Academic Press.

Latimer, J.M. & Matsen, J.M. (1977) Microwave oven irradiation as a method for bacterial decontamination in a clinical microbiology laboratory. *Journal of Clinical Microbiology*, **6**, 340–342.

Lax, A.J., Millson, G.C. & Manning, E.J. (1983) Can scrapie titres be calculated accurately from incubation periods? *Journal of General Virology*, **64**, 971–973.

McBride, P.A., Eikelenboom, P., Kraal, G., Fraser, H. & Bruce, M.E. (1992) PrP protein is associated with follicular dendritic cells of spleens and lymph nodes in uninfected and scrapie-infected mice. *Journal of Pathology*, **168**, 413–418.

Mackenzie, J.M. & Fellowes, W. (1990) Phenolized formalin may obscure early histological changes of Creutzfeldt–Jakob disease. *Neuropathology and Applied Neurobiology*, **16**, 255.

Marsh, R.F. & Hanson, R.P. (1969) Physical and chemical properties of the transmissible mink encephalopathy agent. *Journal of Virology*, **3**, 176–180.

Masters, C.L., Jacobsen, P.F. & Kakulas, B.A. (1985a) Letter to the editor. *Neuropathology and Applied Neurobiology*, **44**, 304–307.

Masters, C.L., Jacobsen, P.F. & Kakulas, B.A. (1985b) Letter to the editor. *Neuropathology and Applied Neurobiology*, **45**, 760–761.

Millson, G.C., Hunter, G.D. & Kimberlin, R.H. (1976) The physico-chemical nature of the scrapie agent. In *Slow Virus Diseases of Animals and Man* (ed. Kimberlin, R.H.), pp. 243–266. Amsterdam: North-Holland.

Mould, D.L., Dawson, A.McL. & Smith, W. (1965) Scrapie in mice: the stability of the agent to various suspending media, pH and solvent extraction. *Research in Veterinary Science*, **6**, 151–154.

Outram, G.W. (1976) The pathogenesis of scrapie in mice. In *Slow Virus Diseases of Animals and Man* (ed. Kimberlin, R.H.), pp. 325–357. Amsterdam: North-Holland.

Palsson, P.A. (1979) Rida (scrapie) in Iceland and its

epidemiology. In *Slow Transmissible Disease of the Nervous System* (eds Prusiner, S.B. & Hadlow, W.J.), Vol. 1, pp. 357–366. London: Academic Press.

Prusiner, S.B. (1982) Novel proteinaceous infectious particles cause scrapie. *Science*, **216**, 136–144.

Prusiner, S.B., McKinlay, M.P., Bolton, D.C. *et al.* (1984) Prions: methods for assay, purification, and characterisation. In *Methods in Virology* (eds Maramorosch, K. & Koprowski, H.), Vol. VIII, pp. 293–345 New York: Academic Press.

Rohwer, R.G. (1983) Scrapie inactivation kinetics—an explanation for scrapie's apparent resistance to inactivation—a re-evaluation of estimates of its small size. In *Virus non conventionnels et affections due système nerveux central* (eds Court, L.A. & Cathala, F.), pp. 84–113. Paris: Masson.

Rohwer, R.G. & Gajdusek, D.C. (1980) Scrapie, virus or viroid: the case for a virus. In *Search of the Cause of Multiple Sclerosis and other Chronic Diseases of the CNS* (Proceedings of the 1st International Symposium of the Hertie Foundation in Frankfurt, September 1979), pp. 335–355. Weinheim: Verlag Chemie.

Rosaspina, S., Salvatorelli, G. & Anzane, D. (1994) The bactericidal effect of microwaves on *Mycobacterium bovis* dried on scalpel blades. *Journal of Hospital Infection*, **26**, 45–50.

Rosenberg, R.N., White, C.L., Brown, P. *et al.* (1986) Precautions in handling tissues, fluids, and other contaminated materials from patients with documented or suspected Creutzfeldt–Jakob disease. *Annals of Neurology*, **19**, 75–77.

Salk, J.E. & Gori, J.B. (1960) A review of theoretical, experimental, and practical considerations in the use of formaldehyde for the inactivation of poliovirus. *Annals of the New York Academy of Sciences*, **83**, 609–637.

Somerville, R.A. & Carp, R.I. (1983) Altered scrapie infectivity estimates by titration and incubation period in the presence of detergents. *Journal of General Virology*, **64**, 2045–2050.

Stamp, J.T., Brotherston, J.C., Zlotnik, I., McKay, J.M.K. & Smith, W. (1959) Further studies on scrapie. *Journal of Comparative Pathology*, **69**, 268–280.

Taguchi, F., Tamai, Y., Uchida, K. *et al.* (1991) Proposal for a procedure for complete inactivation of the Creutzfeldt–Jakob disease agent. *Archives of Virology*, **119**, 297–301.

Tamai, Y., Taguchi, F. & Miura, S. (1988) Inactivation of the Creutzfeldt–Jakob disease agent. *Annals of Neurology*, **24**, 466.

Tateishi, J., Koga, M., Sato, Y. & Mori, R. (1980) Properties of the transmissible agent derived from chronic spongiform encephalopathy. *Annals of Neurology*, **7**, 390–391.

Tateishi, J., Hikita, K., Kitamoto, T. & Nagara, H. (1987) Experimental Creutzfeldt–Jakob disease: inducation of amyloid plaques in rodents. In *Prions: Novel Infectious Pathogens Causing Scrapie and Creutzfeldt–Jakob Disease* (eds Prusiner, S.B. & McKinlay, M.P.), pp. 415–426. New York: Academic Press.

Tateishi, J., Tashima, T. & Kitamoto, T. (1988) Inactivation of the Creutzfeldt–Jakob disease agent. *Annals of Neurology*, **24**, 466.

Taylor, D.M. (1986) Decontamination of Creutzfeldt–Jakob disease agent. *Annals of Neurology*, **20**, 749.

Taylor, D.M. (1989a) Phenolized formalin may not inactivate Creutzfeldt–Jakob disease infectivity. *Neuropathology and Applied Neurology*, **15**, 585–586.

Taylor, D.M. (1989b) Bovine spongiform encephalopathy and human health. *Veterinary Record*, **125**, 413–415.

Taylor, D.M. (1991) Resistance of the ME7 scrapie agent to peracetic acid. *Veterinary Microbiology*, **27**, 19–24.

Taylor, D.M. (1994) Survival of mouse-passaged bovine spongiform encephalopathy agent after exposure to paraformaldehyde-lysine-periodate and formic acid. *Veterinary Microbiology*, **44**, 111–112.

Taylor, D.M. & Diprose, M.F. (1996) The response of the 22A strain of scrapie agent to microwave irradiation compared with boiling. *Neuropathology and Applied Neurobiology*, **22**, 256–258.

Taylor, D.M. & Fernie, K. (1996) Exposure to autoclaving or sodium hydroxide extends the dose–response curve of the 263K strain of scrapie agent in hamsters. *Journal of General Virology*, **77**, 811–813.

Taylor, D.M. & McBride, P.A. (1987) Autoclaved, formol-fixed scrapie brain is suitable for histopathological examination but may still be infective. *Acta Neuropathologica*, **74**, 194–196.

Taylor, D.M. & McConnell, I. (1988) Autoclaving does not decontaminate formol-fixed scrapie tissues. *Lancet*, **i**, 1463–1464.

Taylor, D.M., Fraser, H., McConnell, I. *et al.* (1994) Decontamination studies with the agents of bovine spongiform encephalopathy and scrapie. *Archives of Virology*, **139**, 313–326.

Taylor, D.M., Woodgate, S.L. & Atkinson, M.J. (1995) Inactivation of the bovine spongiform encephalopathy agent by rendering procedures. *Veterinary Record*, **137**, 605–610.

Taylor, D.M., McConnell, I. & Fraser, H. (1996a) Scrapie infection can be established readily through skin scarification in immunocompetent but not immunodeficient mice. *Journal of General Virology*, **77**, 1595–1599.

Taylor, D.M., Woodgate, S.L. & Fleetwood, A.J. (1996b) Scrapie agent survives rendering procedures. In *Abstracts of the Jubilee Meeting of the Association of Veterinary Teachers and Research Workers*, Scarborough, p. 33.

Taylor, D.M., McConnell, I. & Fernie, K. (1966c) The effect of dry heat on the ME7 strain of scrapie agent. *Journal of General Virology*, **77**, 3161–3164.

Titford, M. & Bastian, F.L. (1989) Handling Creutzfeldt–Jakob disease tissues in the laboratory. *Journal of Histotechnology*, **12**, 214–217.

Walker, A.S., Inderlied, C.B. & Kingsbury, D.T. (1983) Conditions for the chemical and physical inactivation of the K.Fu. strain of the agent of Creutzfeldt–Jakob disease. *American Journal of Public Health*, **73**, 661–665.

Wilesmith, J.W., Wells, G.A.J., Cranwell, M.P. & Ryan, J.B.M. (1988) Bovine spongiform encephalopathy: epidemiological studies. *Veterinary Record*, **123**, 638–644.

Will, R.G., Ironside, J.W., Zeidler, M. *et al.* (1996) A new variant form of Creutzfeldt–Jakob disease in the UK. *Lancet*, **347**, 921–925.

Williams, E.S. & Young, S. (1980) Chronic wasting disease of captive mule deer: a spongiform encephalopathy. *Journal of Wildlife Diseases*, **16**, 89–98.

Wilson, D.R., Anderson, R.D. & Smith, W. (1950) Studies in scrapie. *Journal of Comparative Pathology*, **60**, 267–282.

CHAPTER 8

Sensitivity of Protozoa to Disinfectants

A. ACANTHAMOEBA AND CONTACT LENS SOLUTIONS

1 Introduction

Acanthamoeba is one of the most common, free-living amoebae found ubiquitously in the environment (Kilvington & White, 1994). It is found in the air, soil, salt, fresh and drinking-water, chlorinated swimming-pools and hot tubs and from the ice in water at 2°C in northern freshwater lakes (Auran *et al.*, 1987). Some species of *Acanthamoeba* are highly pathogenic to humans. These organisms are increasingly present in corneal infections, causing keratitis (Marshall *et al.*, 1997). If untreated this very painful condition can lead to blindness. It has also been associated with fatal meningoencephalitis in the immunocompromised host (Martinez, 1983). The symptoms of *Acanthamoeba* keratitis are described by Hay *et al.* (1994) as pain, photophobia and recurrent epithelial breakdown, with little infiltrate, dendritiform patterns and localized oedema. The first reported case of *Acanthamoeba* keratitis was in 1973 (Jones & Visvervara, 1975). For a decade, up to 1985, there were only 10 published cases around the world (Wilhelmus, 1991). Since 1985, there has been a rapid increase in the number of cases of *Acanthamoeba* keratitis. This rise in incidence is probably not due to an increase in the number of infections, but to the heightened recognition of the state and therefore better diagnosis.

The occurrence of *Acanthamoeba* keratitis has been linked to the wearing of contact lenses, because over 80% of cases occur in contact lens wearers (Stehr-Green *et al.*, 1989). The use of home-made saline solutions, using non-sterile tap water, is one of the major factors in the cause of this condition (McCulley *et al.*, 1995). The reason that this is such a big problem is that acanthamoebae are found in tap water, as they can survive the chlorine levels found in the water (Jonckheere, 1991). The amoebae then come into contact with both the contact lens and the lens case, which are often contaminated with bacteria. These bacteria are an essential source of nutrients for the protozoa to feed upon.

According to Bottone *et al.* (1992), *Acanthamoeba* shows selective bacterial feeding, particularly on non-fermentative Gram-negatives and coliforms. The contact lens is then a vector for *Acanthamoeba* to the cornea of the eye.

Once in the eye, the acanthamoebae will feed on the natural flora present and the keratocytes on the corneal surface. This will eventually cause damage to the eye.

Acanthamoeba spp. can be considered as being opportunistic pathogens. In addition to causing keratitis, they can produce pneumonitis and a multifocal encaphalitis, termed granulomatous amoebic encephalitis (GAE) (Marshall *et al.*, 1997). MCulley *et al.* (1995) reported that the number of cases is now beginning to fall, which they attributed to better education of contact lens users. Stehr-Green *et al.* (1989) described a rate of approximately 1 in 250 000 infections in the USA, although these figures are hard to prove.

Over 20 species of *Acanthamoeba* have been identified, although only five are pathogenic to humans, namely *A. castellanii*, *A. culbertsoni*, *A. hatchetti*, *A. polyphaga* and *A. rhysodes* (Jones, 1986).

2 Cell forms

Acanthamoeba exists in two forms in nature: as a motile trophozoite or as a highly resistant cyst form. It is the formation of the cyst that enables the parasite to survive adverse conditions. Culbertson (1971) reported that the cyst can withstand saline conditions of up to 0.85% w/v and temperatures from –20 to 42°C. The formation of cysts is also a particular problem in the prevention and treatment of *Acanthamoeba* keratitis, as there are few antimicrobial agents that are active against the highly resilient cyst form.

2.1 Structure of trophozoite

The trophozoite has characteristic fine, spine-like, flexible projections, termed acanthopodia, on its surface and broader 'locomotor' pseudopodia. The cells are flat and irregularly shaped in this phase. The cytoplasm contains a large characteristic nucleus and is enclosed by a cytoplasmic membrane. The trophozoite of *A. castellanii* was described by Bowers & Korn (1968) as 'not differing greatly at the ultrastructure level from a mammalian cell'. The acanthopodia and pseudopodia give the highly irregular 'spiky' appearance of the trophozoite under an electron microscope. Lasman (1977) reported that trophozoites of *Acanthamoeba* are difficult to identify because of the absence of distinctive morphological features.

2.2 Structure of cyst

The cyst form, on the other hand, is polyhedral or convex and almost circular in shape, with a smoother appearance than the trophozoite. The cell wall in the cyst is an important diagnostic aid, having an outer exocyst, which is wrinkled in appearance, and a variably shaped inner endocyst, which closely mimics the shape of the protoplast and lies near the cell surface. The exocyst in mature cysts forms layers parallel to the cell surface, each layer resembling a fibrillar network with an ill-defined amorphous substance. The exocyst measures 0.3–0.5 μm in thickness (Bowers & Korn, 1969).

The endocyst can be differentiated from the exocyst in most species by different texture and staining characteristics. *Acanthamoeba castellanii* shows a large variation between the structure of the two walls, whereas *A. palestinensla* has almost the same structures. The endocyst has a fibrous consistency, is finely granular and occasionally is seen to contain fibrils. The endocyst in the mature cyst is found to be approximately 0.1 m from the plasma membrane; this gap contains a less electron-dense amorphous material.

Neff *et al.* (1964) analysed the constituents of the cyst wall, finding a content of 7% lipid, 33% protein, 35% large alkali-insoluble polysaccharide (shown to be cellulose) and 6.25% nitrogen. The wall contains a large anthrone-reactive carbohydrate, which is also though to be cellulose.

2.3 Life cycle

The life cycle of *A. castellanii* has a growth phase and two cellular differentiation processes, called encystment and excystment. Encystment occurs during unfavourable conditions, such as prolonged starvation, desiccation, cold and heat, when trophozoites are transformed into cysts. Excystment is the process of emergence of trophozoites from the cyst wall under suitable environment conditions (Weisman, 1976). Morphological studies of changes during the encystment and excystment of *A. castellanii* have been undertaken (Neff *et al.*, 1964; Bowers & Korn, 1969; Pasternak *et al.*, 1970; Mattar & Byer, 1971; Chamber & Thompson, 1972).

3 Clinical importance of *Acanthamoeba*

The first case of *Acanthamoeba* keratitis was diagnosed in 1973 in the USA (Visvesvara, 1980) and there were also two early cases in the UK (Nagington *et al.*, 1974). The number of cases has increased significantly since 1985, particularly among contact lens wearers. Daily-wear soft lens or extended-wear soft lens wearers were predominantly at risk (Moore *et al.*, 1987); Stehr-Green *et al.*, 1989; Miller, 1996). However, non-contact-lens-associated *Acanthamoeba* keratitis has also been reported. All cases had the history of either ocular trauma or exposure to a contaminated environment (Sharma *et al.*, 1990). Up to 1992, approximately 90 cases were reported in the UK (Kilvington & White, 1994). According to a *Communicable Disease Report* (CDR) weekly report, in 1993, 12 cases were reported to the centre. In 18 cases, *A. castellanii*, *A. polyphaga*, *A. culbertsoni* and *A. hatchetti* were isolated and identified. A review of all cases of *Acanthamoeba* keratitis at the University of Iowa hospitals and clinics from mid-1993 through 1994 showed that the cases dramatically increased from two to 30 cases per year (Mathews *et al.*, 1996). According to Auran *et al.* (1987), *A. castellanii* is most commonly found in corneal infection, followed by *A. polyphaga*, *A. culbertsoni* and *A. rhysodes*, in that order. Recently, *A. hatchetti* has been isolated (CDR weekly report in 1993). *Acanthamoeba* keratitis is one of the most difficult ocular infections to treat successfully. Without treatment, it can cause blindness. This disease is particulary found among contact lens wearers with poor hygiene. Daily soft contact lens and extended-wear wearers are most likely to get infection (Kilvington & White, 1994). Most cases of *Acanthamoeba* keratitis occur during warmer weather, often subsequent to water exposure, e.g. during swimming (Auran *et al.*, 1987).

4 Prevention of contact-lens contamination

Over 80% of *Acanthamoeba* keratitis could be avoided by the use of a lens-disinfection system effective against the organism (Radford *et al.*, 1995). To reduce the likelihood of contamination, contact lenses should be cleaned and disinfected on a regular basis. Several studies have demonstrated that thorough rinsing and cleaning significantly reduced the number of *Acanthamoeba* trophozoites and cysts attached to both worn and unworn contact lenses (Kilvington & Larkin, 1990; Perkovich *et al.*, 1991; Kilvington, 1993; Gorlin *et al.*, 1996). The use of tap water or home-made saline is not recommended. Wearing contact lenses while swimming should be avoided. It is also recommended that lenses be inserted only after cleaning and disinfection (Dart, 1990). Contact lens storage cases, a primary source of contamination, should be thoroughly cleaned regularly with very hot water (> 70°C), and the case allowed to dry between times to prevent multiplication of microorganisms (Hay & Seal, 1995). Periodic replacement of the case is also essential (Gray *et al.*, 1995).

4.1 Types of contact lenses

Contact lenses can be divided into three types according to their properties: hard, gas-permeable and soft.

4.1.1 Hard lenses

Hard lenses are made from polymethylmethacrylate (PMMA), which is inert and durable and gives better visual acuity than the material used in soft lenses. They are resistant to deposits, such as protein, and allow good tear flow. However, hard lenses are impermeable to oxygen; corneal anoxia may arise and cause oedema. Wearers tend to take longer to adapt to hard lenses. Due to the hydrophobicity of the lens, a wetting solution is required to improve initial comfort (Anderson & Nathan, 1992).

4.1.2 Gas-permeable lenses

Gas-permeable lenses are considered to be the lenses of choice. They are made from one of various polymer materials (varying from low to high gas permeability) to allow more oxygen to reach the cornea. These materials are cellulose acetate butyrate, PMMA and silicone, and fluorocarbon/siloxane copolymer. However, gas-permeable lenses tend to be scratched more easily and lipid deposits accumulate more rapidly than on hard lenses (Anderson & Nathan, 1992; Harvey *et al.*, 1992).

4.1.3 Soft lenses

Soft lenses are less durable and have a shorter life than other types of lens. They are made from polyhydroxyethylmethacrylate (poly-HEMA) and have a high water content (30–80%); this makes the lenses more comfortable to wear and increases wearing time. However, these too are more liable to accumulate lipid and protein deposits. Thus, they need a higher standard of care (Anderson & Nathan, 1992; Harvey *et al.*, 1992).

4.2 Contact-lens solutions

The major deposits on contact lenses are mucoproteins and proteins from tears and abraded corneal material. The other deposits observed include oil from the meibomian gland in the eyelids, calciferous materials, insoluble di- and trivalent salts, cosmetics and atmospheric pollutants (Grant, 1988). The effects of deposits on the lenses may result in a reduction of lens quality, comfort of wearers and effectiveness of disinfectants.

Lens solutions are designed to maintain the lenses in a clean condition for the wearer to use them safely. A guide to contact lens care has been described by Grant (1990) and Anderson & Nathan (1992). Each lens solution has a specific function.

4.2.1 Cleaning solutions

Cleaning solutions are used after removing lenses from the eyes. They are formulated to loosen the deposits and other contaminants, such as dust. There are two types of cleaners (Grant, 1990).

1 Daily—these usually contain a non-ionic or amphoteric surfactant and a preservative. They may also contain a chelating agent, such as disodium edetate, to remove calcium deposits. Daily cleaning with a surfactant is an essential requirement for all types of lenses.

2 Periodic—these solutions are recommended to be used at least once every 2 weeks to remove protein deposits. They contain proteolytic enzymes, such as papain and subtilisin A. Some may contain pancreatin (protease, lipase and amylase enzyme activities). Since the cleaning procedure only loosens the deposits, it is advisable to rinse off the lenses with either a disinfecting solution or 0.9% w/v sterile sodium chloride solution before disinfection (Grant, 1990).

4.2.2 Chemical disinfecting solutions

Chemical disinfecting solutions consist of disinfecting agents and a chelating agent in buffered isotonic solution. This aspect is considered in greater detail below (Section 5).

4.2.3 Wetting solutions

Wetting solutions are required for hard and gas-permeable lenses. Due to the hydrophobicity of the lens, these solutions are designed to improve wettability of the lenses with tear film. They are also slightly viscous to cushion the lens on the eye for greater comfort. Thus, the solutions normally contain hydrophilic polymers, such as polyvinyl alcohol or cellulose derivatives, to enhance viscosity, together with a preservative to prevent microbial growth (Healey, 1982; Grant, 1990).

4.2.4 Multipurpose solutions

Multipurpose preparations are also available for hard and gas-permeable lenses. These can function as combined wetting, cleaning and disinfecting agents. This may be convenient in principle but less effective in practice.

5 Contact lens disinfection

Soft lenses can be disinfected either by thermal disinfection at 80°C for 10 min or by soaking in disinfecting solutions. Hard and gas-permeable lenses can only be disinfected by chemical methods.

5.1 Thermal disinfection

Thermal disinfection is the method of choice for wearers who are sensitive to biocides. This method can be used for low-water-content soft lenses. Ludwig *et al.* (1986) reported that commercial moist heat contact lens disinfection units are effective against *Acanthamoeba* cysts. Kilvington (1991) investigated the effect of moist heat in the disinfection of *Acanthamoeba* cysts and found that *A. polyphaga* cysts were resistant to a temperature of 56°C or 60°C, even after a contact time of 60 min, but were inactivated within 15 min at 65°C and 2 min at 70°C. This suggests that the commercial moist heat contact lens disinfection units are suitable for prevention of *Acanthamoeba* keratitis. However, thermal disinfection can only be used for low-water-content soft lenses. This method does not kill bacterial spores; it may coagulate protein deposits and it does not remove contaminating microbes, particularly those present in the lens container (McTaggard, 1980; Grant, 1990).

5.2 Chemical disinfection

Chemical disinfection consists of disinfecting agents and a chelating agent in buffered isotonic solutions. This method is usually carried out by soaking the cleaned lenses in the disinfecting solution overnight. Except for benzalkonium chloride (BZK), the disinfectants for hard lenses, gas-permeable lenses and soft lenses are basically the same. Benzalkonium chloride is permitted only in disinfecting solutions for hard and gas-permeable lenses. This is because soft-lens materials can absorb this agent, which is gradually released on to the cornea, causing irritation (Anderson & Nathan, 1992).

Based on the *International Contact Lens Year Book* (1995), some biocides commonly present in chemical disinfection products for contact lenses, either alone or in combination, are shown in Table 8.1. The minimal action times recommended by the manufacturers are 10 min for 3% hydrogen peroxide (H_2O_2) and 4–7 h for other biocides (Marques *et al.*, 1991).

6 Types of biocides

6.1 Chlorhexidine diacetate

Chlorhexidine is a member of the N^1, N^5-substituted biguanides. Chlorhexidine dichloride, diacetate and gluconate are used commercially. Chlorhexidine diacetate (CHA) is effective against the vegetative forms of Gram-positive and Gram-negative bacteria but ineffective against acid-fast bacteria, bacterial spores and viruses (Russell & Day, 1993; Ranganathan, 1996). Gram-positive bacteria are more susceptible to CHA than Gram-negative. *Pseudomonas* spp. are less susceptible to CHA than other Gram-negatives (Nicoletti *et al.*, 1993; Russell & Day, 1993). It has antifungal activity but shows only low activity towards

Table 8.1 Biocide concentrations in disinfecting contact-lens solution.

Biocide	Concentration (% w/v)
Chlorhexidine diacetate (CHA)	0.002–0.006
Polyhexamethylene biguanide (PHMB)	0.0001–0.0005
Benzalkonium chloride (BZK)	0.004–0.01
Thiomersal	0.001–0.004
Hydrogen peroxide	3
Sodium dichloroisocyanurate (NaDCC)	3–5*
Halazone (0.16 mg/tablet)	8*
Disodium edetate (EDTA)	0.01–0.3†

*Expressed as parts/10^6 available chlorine (AvCl).
†Present as a chelating agent.

fungal spores (Walters *et al.*, 1983; Russell & Furr, 1996).

Ludwig *et al.* (1986) showed that 0.005% chlorhexidine is effective against cysts of *A. castellanii*, but only delays growth of *A. polyphaga*. However, several studies (Hugo *et al.*, 1991; Kilvington *et al.*, 1991; Rutherford *et al.* 1991; Silvany *et al.*, 1991) have demonstrated that 0.004% chlorhexidine is effective against both species. Variation in the efficacy of chlorhexidine was also reported by Brandt *et al.* (1989), who found that cysts of *A. castellanii*, *A. polyphaga* and *A. culbertsoni* can survive for 6 h to 3 days in a disinfecting solution containing 0.005% chlorhexidine. Khunkitti *et al.* (1997a) studied the uptake of CHA and a polymeric biguanide (polyhexamethylene biguanide (PHMB) by cysts and trophozoites of *A. castellanii*, and Rutherford *et al.* (1991) demonstrated that the efficacy of chlorhexidine is dependent on the number of organisms challenged and the exposure time. Cysts of *A. polyphaga* appear to be more resistant than those of *A. castellanii* (Ludwig *et al.*, 1986; Silvany *et al.*, 1988).

Hay *et al.* (1994) have demonstrated that 0.02% chlorhexidine, alone or in conjunction with 0.1% propamidine, is clinically effective for the treatment of proved *Acanthamoeba* keratitis. However, they recommended the use of the combination system, due to the possibility of an additive effect and prevention of resistance.

Chlorhexidine diacetate is available either as a solution or in tablet form for contact lens disinfection systems. In soaking solutions, it is often used in combination with other biocides, such as thiomersal (TM) and sorbic acid. Green *et al.* (1980) stated that chlorhexidine gluconate had no effects on either the epithelium or the endothelium when used as a soft-lens disinfectant. Burstein (1984) also reported that 0.01–0.02% chlorhexidine gluconate is non-toxic to the human eye.

However, soft-lens materials can absorb and release CHA into the eyes, causing irritation; therefore, it is important to rinse the lens thoroughly before lens insertion (Refojo, 1976). The activity of CHA is reduced by complexation with tear proteins. This complex can form a deposit on lens surfaces, increasing hydrophobicity and leading to chronic ocular irritation (Larke, 1985).

6.2 Polyhexamethylene biguanide

Polyhexamethylene biguanide, also known as polyaminopropyl biguanide and polyhexanide, is a mixture of polymeric hexamethylene biguanides. It has a broad spectrum of activity against Gram-positive and Gram-negative bacteria (Broxton *et al.*, 1983a,b) but is less active against fungi. It is used as a swimming-pool bactericide and algicide (Stewart-Jones *et al.*, 1989).

Silvany *et al.* (1991) demonstrated that PHMB (0.0015%) was effective against *A. polyphaga* after 2 h and *A. castellanii* after 4 h, but at 0.00005% was ineffective against trophozoites of both species. Burger *et al.* (1994) found that 0.0045 to 0.009% of PHMB caused extensive killing of *Acanthamoeba* cysts, whereas, at low concentrations, its lethal action was slow. The time required for PHMB 0.0045% to kill *Acanthamoeba* cysts was 18 min, whereas 0.00225% took 3 h. *Acanthamoeba castellanii* cysts were more sensitive than *A. polyphaga* cysts. However, Hugo *et al.* (1991) showed that 0.0015% PHMB failed to destroy *Acanthamoeba* cysts within 8 h. The presence of organic material greatly reduced PHMB activity against *Acanthamoeba* spp. (Dawson *et al.*, 1983).

Acanthamoeba keratitis can be successfully treated with 0.02% PHMB (Larkin *et al.*, 1992; Elder *et al.*, 1994; Illingworth *et al.*, 1995). Like CHA, it has low mammalian toxicity (Broxton *et al.*, 1983b; Berry & Easty, 1993). However, Volgelberg & Boehnke (1994) have studied the *in vitro* toxicity of PHMB. They suggested that PHMB should be used in selected cases of *Acanthamoeba* keratitis; it was not suitable in cases of corneal ulcer or persistent epithelial defects, due to a possibility of prohibiting re-epithelialization of the diseased cornea.

6.3 Benzalkonium chloride

Benzalkonium chloride is a cation-active quaternary ammonium compound (QAC). It is highly soluble in water and the solution can be sterilized by autoclaving, without loss of effectiveness.

Benzalkonium chloride is active against Gram-positive organisms, but some Gram-negatives and some viruses, fungi and protozoa may be resistant.

It is relatively inactive against spores and moulds and also against some *Pseudomonas* strains and *Mycobacterium tuberculosis*. Its activity against *Pseudomonas aeruginosa* is increased when combined with 0.01–0.1% disodium edetate. However, in the presence of citrate and phosphate but not borate buffers, the activity against *Pseudomonas* can be reduced. Its activity increases with increasing pH (*Handbook of Pharmaceutical Excipients*, 1986). Silvany *et al.* (1991) demonstrated that 0.004% BZK was effective against cysts of *A. castellanii* and *A. polyphaga* at 1h.

Nauheim *et al.* (1990) investigated the survival of *A. polyphaga* in various contact-lens rinsing solutions. They found that exposure to a 0.1% BZK solution for longer than 4h was lethal. Zanetti *et al.* (1995) reported that BZK was very effective against *A. castellanii* trophozoites at short exposure times (30min) but less so against cysts. Similar results were reported by Hugo *et al.* (1991).

A major problem with BZK is that it cannot be used to disinfect hydrophilic soft contact lenses (hydrogel), because it binds to the lens surface due to the presence of water in hydrogels. The QAC will then be released into the eye when the lens is in place, possibly causing hypersensitivity problems.

6.4 Hydrogen peroxide

Hydrogen peroxide is one of the most effective agents available for contact lens solutions for killing both *Acanthamoeba* and other contaminants (Hay & Cairns, 1996; Lever & Sutton, 1996) and is now the recommended system of the Irish Opticians Board (Seal & Hay, 1995).

Hydrogen peroxide is bactericidal and sporicidal (Baldry & Fraser, 1988; Block, 1991). Based on the decimal reduction times (D-values) of 3% H_2O_2 on microorganisms, the 10min disinfection time appears to be adequate for disinfection of bacteria, but not less than 45–60min is required for inactivation of *Candida albicans* (Lever & Sutton, 1996). Ludwig *et al.* (1986), Lindquist *et al.* (1988) and Connor *et al.* (1989) indicated that 3% H_2O_2, when used according to the manufacturer's instructions, is ineffective against *Acanthamoeba* spp. Brandt *et al.* (1989) found that 3% H_2O_2 was slightly effective in killing cysts of *A. castellanii*, *A. polyphaga* and *A. culbertsoni*. Davies *et al.* (1988) demonstrated that 3% H_2O_2 required approximately 2h to kill 99.9% *A. polyphaga*. Kilvington *et al.* (1991) found that *Acanthamoeba* cysts coincubated with bacteria required greater than 4h.

Silvany *et al.* (1988, 1990) compared different brands of H_2O_2 solutions and found that the formulation markedly altered the activity against different *Acanthamoeba* spp., even though the products had identical strengths.

Hydrogen peroxide is an oxidizing agent. It generates free hydroxy radicals for the destruction of bacterial cells by reacting with essential cell components, such as membrane lipids and deoxyribonucleic acid (DNA) (Lever & Sutton, 1996).

As a contact lens disinfecting solution, 3% H_2O_2 is commercially available and is used as a disinfectant for daily- and extended-wear hydrogel lenses (Krezanoski & Houlsby, 1988). One adverse effect of H_2O_2 is eye irritation. Therefore, a neutralizer is required for inactivation of its residues on the lenses prior to insertion into the eyes. Neutralizing agents used to inactivate residual H_2O_2 are listed in Table 8.2.

6.5 Chlorine-releasing agents

The organic chlorine-releasing agents are less irritant and toxic than hypochlorites. They release their chlorine less readily and so exert a more prolonged bactericidal effect (Copley, 1989). Sodium dichloroisocyanurate (NaDCC) is commercially available under the name Softabs (Alcon), containing NaDCC 0.65mg per tablet (*International Contact Lens Year Book*, 1995); when dissolved in 10ml of saline, it releases 3–5 parts/10^6 available chlorine (AvCl) (Stewart-Jones *et al.*, 1989). Halazone is marked under the name Aerotab, containing halazone (BPC, 1994) 0.16mg per tablet (*International Contact Lens Year Book*, 1995). It produces 8 parts/10^6 AvCl (Rosenthal *et al.*, 1992). Organic chlorine-releasing agents give hypochlorous acid, a bactericidally active form, when dissolved in water. Its optimum antimicrobial activity is achieved at pH 5 but activity decreases in alkaline pH (Trueman, 1971). Organic matter reduces its activity considerably.

Table 8.2 Neutralization of residual hydrogen peroxide. (Based upon the *International Contact Lens Year Book* (1995); see also Lever & Sutton (1996) and Sutton (1996) for a general review of neutralizers.)

Neutralizer	Effect	Reference
Platinum	Slow, platinum needs frequent replacing	Stewart-Jones *et al.* (1989)
Catalase	Rapid but unstable	Rogan (1985), Lever & Sutton (1996)
Sodium pyruvate	Rapid, relatively stable	Stewart-Jones *et al.* (1989)
Sodium thiosulphate	As for pyruvate	
Sodium sulphite	As for pyruvate	

$$\underset{\text{Organic chlorine compound}}{RNCl + H_2O} \longrightarrow \underset{\text{Hypochlorous acid}}{RNH + HOCl}$$

$$\underset{\text{active form}}{HOCl} \underset{\text{Acid pH}}{\overset{\text{Alkaline pH}}{\rightleftharpoons}} \underset{\text{inactive form (hypochlorite ion)}}{H^+ + OCl^-}$$

Rosenthal *et al.* (1992) investigated the antibacterial activity of two organic chlorine-releasing compounds against bacteria and fungi. They found that the two commercial products had a rapid bactericidal activity. However, NaDCC had more rapid fungicidal activity against both *C. albicans* and *Fusarium solani* than halazone. Kilvington (1990) demonstrated that halazone was ineffective against *Acanthamoeba* cysts. Wright (1983) claimed that 10 parts/10^6 AvCl from NaDCC inactivated encysted protozoa after 30 min at 20°C and neutral pH. However, viable amoeba cysts have been found frequently in contact lens cases disinfected with an NaDCC system (Seal and Hay, 1992). Devonshire *et al.* (1993) found that seven out of 54 contact lens cases that were disinfected with an NaDCC system contained viable amoebal cysts. Larkin *et al.* (1990) found that two out of nine lens cases were contaminated with *Acanthamoeba* when using a chlorine system, compared with no *Acanthamoeba* isolated from 55 cases of users who used chlorhexidine or H_2O_2.

Halazone is available in tablet form designed to be dispersed by the user in tap water to form the disinfecting solution. From the above results, it would seem to be an extremely inadvisable technique, as *Acanthamoeba* is found in tap water and can easily overcome the relatively low levels of chlorine used in potable water supplies.

6.6 Thiomersal

Thiomersal (TM) is commonly found as a disinfecting agent in contact lens solutions, usually at concentrations of 0.001–0.004%, depending on whether it is being used in combination with other disinfecting agents or on its own. At a concentration of 0.01%, it inhibits the growth of *Ps. aeruginosa*, *Acinetobacter* species, *Escherichia coli* and *Staphylococcus* species (Larke, 1985). Inhibitory concentrations of TM against yeasts are 0.0032% w/v and against moulds 0.0128% w/v. At a concentration of 0.002%, it is ineffective against *Acanthamoeba* cysts (Brandt *et al.*, 1989). Seal & Hay (1992) actually called for it to be discontinued as a disinfectant in contact-lens solutions. Silvany *et al.* (1991) demonstrated that TM (0.004% w/v) in combination with ethylenediamine tetraacetic acid (EDTA) (0.1% w/v) was effective against cysts of *A. castellanii* and *A. polyphaga* at 8 h, whereas TM (0.004%) alone was ineffective. This is somewhat surprising, in view of the fact that EDTA is a known and effective chelator and it would thus be expected to reduce the efficacy of an organomercurial. Brandt *et al.* (1989) showed that TM combined with chlorhexidine killed cysts in approximately 24 h. These contact times are not suitable for contact-lens solutions.

7 Mechanisms of biocidal action on *Acanthamoeba*

Although there is now considerable information about the activity of various biocides against acanthamoebae, surprisingly few data are available about the actual effects of these agents against the trophozoite and cyst forms. With this in mind, recent studies have been undertaken in this laboratory to try to obtain a better understanding of the injury sustained by these cell forms on exposure to these inhibitors.

Khunkitti (1996) and Khunkitti *et al.* (1996) found that the lethal effects of CHA and PHMB were time- and concentration-dependent. Subsequently, Khunkitti *et al.* (1997a) studied the uptake of these cationic agents by cysts and trophozoites of *A. castellanii* and also demonstrated that both biocides induced leakage from both forms. Membrane damage is clearly implicated, although there was no relationship between leakage and trophozoicidal or cysticidal activity. Membrane damage was also observed by electron microscopy (Khunkitti *et al.*, 1998b).

Some preliminary work on the effects of CHA and PHMB on pre-encystment trophozoites, mature cysts and pre-excystment cysts has also been described (Khunkitti *et al.*, 1997b; 1998a,b). Mature cysts were always the most resistant cellular form. Further studies along these lines could be revealing, especially if they could be combined with chemical analyses of the walls of cells as they develop into cysts or trophozoites.

8 Biofilm formation

Acanthamoeba are capable of forming biofilms on surfaces such as contact lenses (Gray *et al.*, 1995). Biofilms are formed when organisms colonize surfaces in layers on top of each other; Lambert (1992) reported that biofilms can be up to 100 cells thick. The cells are surrounded by an external exopolymer matrix, which is made up of polysaccharides or proteins; this is called the glycocalyx. The cells within the biofilm have greater resistance to biocide than isolated cells, for two reasons: the penetration of the biocide into the centre of the biofilm will be greatly reduced and the biocide will not reach its cellular target site as readily as if the cell were isolated (Russell & Chopra, 1996). The actual resistance from cell to cell in the biofilm will also vary. There are three main reasons for this variation. Firstly, at the base of the biofilm, i.e. in contact with the lens surface, there will be less oxygen available and so anaerobic conditions will prevail, which in the case of *Acanthamoeba* will inhibit growth. The second reason is the varied levels of nutrients throughout the film. *Acanthamoeba* requires bacterial cells for its nutrition and so the presence or absence of bacteria in the film will affect viability. The final factor is that all the cells will be growing at different rates, which modulates the action of the biocide on the cells.

This variation in resistance to the biocide may have a large effect on the results of the challenge tests carried out with *Acanthamoeba*. The effect of *Acanthamoeba* biofilms on the effectiveness of biocides is under investigation, and in the future all solutions will have to be tested against single cells and against biofilms.

9 Conclusions

It is difficult to draw any hard conclusions as to the most effective agent available for the disinfection of contact lenses. The results reported vary considerably. These variations may be due to the method of preparation of the *Acanthamoeba* cells, the conditions of the challenge test and the interpretation of the results. The strain of *Acanthamoeba* used is critical in the evaluation of biocidal activity.

Brandt *et al.* (1989) compared the effects of various disinfecting solutions against *A. castellanii*, *A. polyphaga* and *A. culbertsoni*. The results showed that *A. culbertsoni* had a significantly higher resistance than the other two species and that this could be due to a difference in the composition of the cyst wall. Testing with non-pathogenic strains of *Acanthamoeba* would also seem unsuitable, as they will be of little significance in practice. It would seem sensible always to use the cyst form, as this has much greater resistance than the trophozoite and so provides a better reflection of the killing capabilities of the biocide. The sample size used to test the efficacy of the biocide should be standardized. Brandt *et al.* (1989) used an inoculum of 10^7 cysts/ml, whereas Silvany *et al.* (1990) used 8×10^3 organisms/ml (with a 9:1 ratio of cysts to trophozoites). This variation in numbers will obviously affect the kill rate of the biocide.

Termination of biocidal action is also a problem, and in some cases it has been reported that neutralization of the agents was insufficient, thereby creating erroneous, enhanced kill times.

Variations were shown between the same disinfecting agents, but in different formulations. Brandt *et al.* (1989) investigated three commercially available solutions all containing TM (0.001%), chlorhexidine (0.005%) and EDTA (0.1%). Some of the solutions were effective with a 6 h contact time, whereas others required 24 h. These results are even more peculiar when it is noted that these tests were undertaken against the same strain of *Acanthamoeba* and under the same conditions. The only explanation that the authors suggested was a variation in the active constituents, due to leakage or poor manufacture. Standardization of test methods is essential; it is thus surprising to note that, in evaluating contact lens solutions, Gavin *et al.* (1995) did not include *Acanthamoeba* as a test organism.

Hydrogen peroxide is often quoted as being the most effective disinfecting agent against a wide range of organisms. There are still limitations to its use, however, as there will be toxicity problems if it is not fully neutralized. However, with manufacturers recommending a minimum contact time of only 10 min in most systems, there is still a high possibility of contamination of the lens. Khunkitti (1996) recommends a minimum contact time of 4 h.

The use of chlorhexidine in disinfecting systems also provides a suitable level of protection against *Acanthamoeba*. It is not as efficient as H_2O_2, but still has a kill time making it suitable for overnight disinfection of lenses.

The remainder of the disinfecting agents examined are all potentially ineffective at destroying *Acanthamoeba* on contact lenses, even with overnight contact. For example, TM solutions were ineffective against *A. castellanii*, even after 14 days' contact (Brandt *et al.*, 1989), and may cause hypersensitivity. Chlorine-releasing agents, for example halazone, are also poor killing agents, and should be replaced by more effective ones.

Combinations of these agents are often employed, with the aim of increasing their effectiveness. This has resulted in a decrease in the contact time needed to kill *Acanthamoeba*, as shown by Silvany *et al.* (1987); when TM (0.004%) was tested on its own against *A. castellanii* and *A. polyphaga*, it did not kill the organisms within 24 h, but, when used in combination with EDTA, it surprisingly achieved amoebacidal effects within 24 h.

There are other ways of disinfecting contact lenses, apart from the cold chemical methods that have been examined in this study. The most effective is the use of moist heat to achieve disinfection. Kilvington (1991) showed that, at 65°C, a 4 log reduction of *A. polyphaga* cysts was obtained in 15 min. Raising the temperature to 70°C only required 2 min to achieve the same response. A major drawback for heat disinfection is that it cannot be used on a number of different lens types, as it will cause damage to the matrix.

Ultraviolet (UV) light is another possible disinfecting system. Dolman & Dobrogowski (1989) reported sterilization of a suspension of 10^4 *Acanthamoeba*/ml in 3 min. This compares with 2.5 min to destroy 2×10^6 *A castellanii*. This system was tested against a wide range of different types of contact lenses, all of which are suitable to be used with UV, giving it an advantage over moist-heat disinfection.

The use of non-sterile tap water for making saline solutions or for dissolving disinfecting tablets has been shown to be a major risk factor in contracting *Acanthamoeba* keratitis. Tap water has only low levels of chlorine present, which are ineffective against *Acanthamoeba* cysts. It is therefore extremely unwise to use tap water in any step of cleaning contact lenses or lens cases, unless at high temperatures (over 70°C). The elimination of tap water from contact-lens care systems has led to a large decrease in the number of reported cases in the USA (McCulley *et al.*, 1995). In the UK, there are still systems that incorporate tap water in one of the stages; until this practice is stopped, the number of cases of *Acanthamoeba* keratitis will not decrease.

The development of an 'all-in-one' solution is another significant advance. Such a solution is all that is needed to treat contact lenses, where previously up to four separate solutions may have been used. The elimination of multiple solutions will decrease the chance of contamination, as each solution used would heighten the possible risk of contamination of the lens.

Other advances that have been made by the industry should lead to a significant decrease in all types of eye infections, including *Acanthamoeba* keratitis, the most important being the introduction of single-use disposable contact lenses. Each day, a new sterile contact lens is used, the lenses being packaged in a sterile blister pack. This completely eliminates the need for any solutions, and represents a major advance. It should virtually eliminate all eye infections caused by contact lens use.

Of all the commercially available disinfecting solutions on the market, H_2O_2 is the most efficient at killing *Acanthamoeba*, but it still needs a lengthy contact time (about 4–6 h). Of the other disinfecting agents, only chlorhexidine has a kill time that makes it suitable for use as an overnight disinfecting solution.

Little information is available about the mechanisms of inactivation of cysts and trophozoites or about the reasons for the greater resistance of the former to chemical agents, although it is likely that the outer cell layers play a major role.

10 References

Anderson, C. & Nathan, A. (1992) Contact lenses and their care (1). *Pharmaceutical Journal*, **249**, 503–506.

Auran, J.D., Starr, M.B. & Jakobiec, F.A. (1987) *Acanthamoeba* keratitis: a review of the literature. *Cornea*, **6**, 2–26.

Baldry, M.G.C. & Fraser, J.A.L. (1988) Disinfection with peroxygens. In *Industrial Biocides*, Critical Reports on Applied Chemistry, Vol. 23 (ed. Payne, K.R.), pp. 99–166. Chichester: John Wiley & Sons.

Berry, M. & Easty, D.L. (1993) Isolated human and rabbit eye: models of corneal toxicity. *Toxicity* in vitro, **7**, 461–464.

Block, S.S. (1991) Peroxygen compounds. In *Disinfection, Sterilization and Preservation* 4th edn (ed. Block, S.S.), pp. 167–181. Philadelphia: Lea & Febiger.

Bottone, E., Madayag, R. & Quresh, M. (1992) *Acanthamoeba* keratitis: synergy between amoebic and bacterial co-contaminants in contact lens care systems as a prelude to infection. *Journal of Clinical Microbiology*, **30**, 2447–2450.

Bowers, B. & Korn, E. (1968) The fine structure of *A. castellanii*—the trophozoite. *Journal of Cell Biology*, **39**, 95–111.

Bowers, B. & Korn, E. (1969) The fine structure of *A. castellanii*—encystment. *Journal of Cell Biology*, **41**, 786–805.

Brandt, F.H., Ware, D.A. & Visvesvara, G.S. (1989) Viability of *Acanthamoeba* cysts in ophthalmic solutions. *Applied and Environmental Microbiology*, **55**, 1144–1146.

Broxton, P., Woodcock, P.M. & Gilbert, P. (1983a) Action of some polyhexamethylene biguanides upon respiration of *Escherichia coli* ATCC 8739. *Journal of Applied Bacteriology*, **54** (Suppl.), 66P.

Broxton, P., Woodcock, P.M., & Gilbert, P. (1983b) A study of the antibacterial activity of some polyhexamethylene biguanides towards *Escherichia coli* ATCC 8739. *Journal of Applied Bacteriology*, **54**, 345–353.

Burger, R.M., Franco, R.J. & Drlica, K. (1994) Killing *Acanthamoeba* with polyaminopropyl biguanide: quantitation and kinetics. *Antimicrobial Agents and Chemotherapy*, **38**, 886–888.

Burstein, N.L. (1984) Preservative alteration of cornea permeability in humans and rabbits. *Investigative Ophthalmology and Visual Science*, **25**, 1453–1457.

Chambers, J.A. & Thompson, J.E. (1972) A scanning electron microscopic study of the encystment of *Acanthamoeba castellanii*. *Experimental Cell Research*, **73**, 415–421.

Connor, C.G., Blocker, Y. & Pitts, D.G. (1989) *Acanthamoeba culbertsoni* and contact lens disinfection systems. *Optometry and Vision Science*, **66**, 690.

Copley, C.A. (1989) Chlorine disinfection of soft contact lenses. *Clinical and Experimental Optometry*, **72**, 3–7.

Culbertson, C. (1971) The pathogenicity of soil amoebas. *Annual Review of Microbiology*, **25**, 231–254.

Dart, J.K.G. (1990) Contact lens and other risk factors in microbial keratitis. *Lancet*, **338**, 650–653.

Davies, D.J.G., Anthony, Y., Meakin, B.J., Kilvington, S. & White, D. (1988) Anti-acanthamoeba activity of chlorhexidine and hydrogen peroxide. In *Transactions of the BCLA International Conference*, pp. 60–62.

Dawson, M.W., Brown, T.J., Biddick, C.J. & Till, D.G. (1983) The effect of Baquacil on pathogenic free-living amoebae (PFLA). 2. In stimulated natural conditions—in presence of bacteria and/or organic matter. *New Zealand Journal of Marine and Freshwater Resources*, **17**, 313–330.

Devonshire, P., Munco, F.A., Abernethy, C. & Clarke, B.J. (1993) Microbial contamination of contact lenses in the West of Scotland. *British Journal of Ophthalmology*, **77**, 41–45.

Dolman, P. & Dobrogowski, M. (1989) Contact lens disinfection by ultraviolet light. *American Journal of Ophthalmology*, **108**, 665–669.

Elder, M.J., Kilvington, S. & Dart, J.K.G. (1994) A clinical pathologic study of *in vitro* sensitivity testing and *Acanthamoeba* keratitis. *Investigative Ophthalmology and Vision Science*, **35**, 1059–1064.

Gavin, J., Button, N.F., Watson-Craik, I.A. & Logan, N.A. (1995) Efficacy of standard disinfectant test methods for contact lens-care solutions. *International Biodeterioration and Biodegradation*, **36**, 431–440.

Gorlin, A.I., Gabriel, M.M., Wilson, L.A. & Ahearn, D.G. (1996) Binding of *Acanthamoeba* to hydrogel contact lenses. *Current Eye Research*, **15**, 151–155.

Grant, E. (1990) Contact lens care. *Pharmaceutical Journal*, **245**, 148–150.

Gray, T.B., Curson, R.T.M., Sherwan, J.F. & Rose, P.R. (1995) Acanthamoeba, bacterial and fungal contamination of contact lens storage cases. *British Journal of Ophthalmology*, **79**, 601–605.

Green, K., Livington, V. & Bowman, K. (1980) Chlorhexidine effects on corneal epithelium and endothelium. *Archives of Ophthalmology*, **98**, 1273–1278.

Handbook of Pharmaceutical Excipients (1986) London: Pharmaceutical Society of Great Britain.

Harvey, W., Nathan, A. & Anderson, C. (1992) Contact lenses and their care (2). *Pharmaceutical Journal*, **249**, 537–539.

Hay, J. and Cairns, D. (1996) *Acanthamoeba* keratitis [letter]. *Pharmaceutical Journal*, **256**, 110.

Hay, J. & Seal, D.V. (1995) Contact lens wear by hospital health care staff: is there cause for concern? *Journal of Hospital Infection*, **30**, 275–281.

Hay, J., Kirkness, C.M., seal, D.V. & Wright, P. (1994) Drug resistance and *Acanthamoeba* keratitis: the quest for alternative antiprotozoal chemotherapy. *Eye*, **8**, 555–563.

Healey, J.N. (1982) A guide to contact lens care. *Pharmaceutical Journal*, **229**, 650–654.

Hugo, E.R., McLoughlin, W.R., Oh, K. & Tuovinen, O.H. (1991) Quantitative enumeration of *Acanthamoeba* for evaluation of cyst inactivation in contact lens care solutions. *Investigative Ophthalmology and Visual Science*, **32**, 655–657.

Illingworth, C.D., Cook, S.D., Karabatsas, C.H. & Easty, D.L. (1995) *Acanthamoeba* keratitis: risk factors and outcome. *British Journal of Ophthalmology*, **79**, 1078–1082.

International Contact Lens Year Book 1995 (1995) pp. 121–130. London: WB Saunders.

Jonckheere, J. (1991) Ecology of *Acanthamoeba*, *Review of Infectious Disease*, **13** (Suppl. 5), S385–S387.

Jones, D. (1986) *Acanthamoeba*—the ultimate opportunist. *American Journal of Ophthalmology*, **4**, 527–530.

Jones, D., and Visvervara, G. (1975) *Acanthamoeba polyphaga* keratitis and *Acanthamoeba uveitis* associated with fatal meningoencephalitis. *Transactions of the Ophthalmology Society UK*, **95**, 221–232.

Khunkitti, W. (1996) *Acanthamoeba*: Resistance to biocides. PhD thesis, University of Wales, Cardiff.

Khunkitti, W., Lloyd, D., Furr, J.R. & Russell, A.D. (1996) The lethal effects of biguanides on cysts and trophozoites of *Acanthamoeba castellanii. Journal of Applied Bacteriology*, **81**, 73–77.

Khunkitti, W., Lloyd, D., Furr, J.R. and Russell, A.D. (1997a) Aspects of the mechanisms of action of biguanides on trophozoites and cysts of *Acanthamoeba castellanii. Journal of Applied Microbiology*, **82**, 107–114.

Khunkitti, W., Avery, S.V., Lloyd, D., Furr, J.R. & Russell, A.D. (1997b) Effects of biocides on *Acanthamoeba castellanii* as measured by flow cytometry and plaque assay. *Journal of Antimicrobial Chemotherapy* **40**, 227–233.

Khunkitti, W., Lloyd, D., Furr, J.R. & Russell, A.D. (1998a) *Acanthamoeba castellanii*: growth, encystment, excystment and biocide susceptibility. *Journal of Infection* **36**, 43–48.

Khunkitti, W., Hann, A.C., Lloyd, D., Furr, J.R. & Russell, A.D. (1998b) Biguanide-induced changes in *Acanthamoeba castellanii*: an electron microscopic study. *Journal of Applied Microbiology* **84**, 53–62.

Kilvington, S. (1990) Activity of water biocide chemicals and contact lens disinfectants on pathologic free living amoeba. *International Biodeterioration*, **26**, 127–138.

Kilvington, S. (1991) Moist heat disinfection of *Acanthamoeba* cysts. *Reviews of Infectious Diseases*, **13**, (Suppl.), S418.

Kilvington, S. (1993) *Acanthamoeba* trophozoite and cyst adherence to four types of soft contact lens and removal by cleaning agents. *Eye*, **7**, 535–538.

Kilvington, S. & Larkin, D.E.P. (1990) *Acanthamoeba*: adherence to contact lenses and removal by cleaning agents. *Eye*, **4**, 589–593.

Kilvington, S. & White, D.G. (1994) *Acanthamoeba*: biology, ecology and human disease. *Reviews in Medical Microbiology*, **5**, 12–20.

Kilvington, S., Anthony, Y., Davies, D.J.G and Meakin, B.J. (1991) Effect of contact lens disinfectants against *Acanthamoeba* cysts. *Reviews of Infectious Diseases*, **13** (Suppl.), S414–S415.

Krezanoski, J.Z. & Houlsby, R.D. (1988) A comparison of new hydrogen peroxide disinfection systems. *Journal of the American Optometric Association*, **59**, 193–197.

Lambert, P. (1992) Resistance to non antibiotic antimicrobial agents. In *Pharmaceutical Microbiology*, 5th edn, (eds Hugo, W.B. & Russell, A.D.) pp. 295–304. Oxford: Blackwell Science.

Larke, J.R. (1985) Preserved soft lens storage solutions. In *The Eye in Contact Lens Wear*, p. 170. London: Butterworths.

Larkin, D.F.P., Kilvington, S. & Dart, J.K.G. (1992) Treatment of *Acanthamoeba* keratitis with polyhexamethylene biguanide. *Ophthalmology*, **99**, 191.

Lasman M. (1977) Light and electron microscopic

observations on encystment of *Acanthamoeba palestinensis*. *Journal of Protozoology*, **24**, 224–248.

Lever, A.M. & Sutton, S.V.W. (1996) Antimicrobial effects of hydrogen peroxide as an antiseptic and disinfectant. In *Handbook of Disinfectants and Antiseptics* (ed. Ascenzi, J.M.), pp. 159–176. New York: Marcel Dekker.

Lindquist, T.D., Doughman, D.J., Rubenstien, J.B., Moore, J.W. & Campbell, R.C. (1988) *Acanthamoeba*-contaminated hydrogel contact lenses. *Cornea*, 7, 300–303.

Ludwig, I.H., Meisler, D.M., Rutherford, I., Bicon, F.E., Langston, R.H.S. & Visvesvara, G.S. (1986) Susceptibility of *Acanthamoeba* to soft contact lens disinfection systems. *Investigative Ophthalmology and Vision Science*, **27**, 626–628.

McCulley, J., Alizadeh, H. & Niederkorn, J. (1995). *Acanthamoeba* keratitis. *CLAO*, **21**, (1), 73–76.

McTaggard, C. (1980) Care of soft contact lenses. *Pharmaceutical Journal*, **224**, 309–313.

Marques, M.S., Lluch, S., Merindano, M.D., Gonzalez, M. & Saona, C. (1991) Effect of different disinfecting contact lens solutions against ocular bacterial strain growth. *Contact Lens Journal*, **19**, 9–12.

Marshall, M.M., Naumovitz, D., Ortega, Y. & Sterling, C.R. (1997) Waterborne protozoan pathogens. *Clinical Microbiology Reviews*, **10**, 67–85.

Martinez, A. (1983) Free living amoebae: pathogenic aspects. *Protozoology Abstracts*, 7, 293–306.

Mathews, W.D., Sutphin, J.E., Folberg, R., Meier, P.A., Wenzel, R.P. & Elgin, R.G. (1996) Outbreak of keratitis presumed to be caused by acanthamoeba. *American Journal of Ophthalmology*, **121**, 129–142.

Mattar, F.E. and Byer, T.J. (1971) Morphological changes and requirements for macromolecule synthesis during encystment of *Acanthamoeba castellanii*. *Journal of Cell Biology*, **49**, 507–519.

Miller, M.J. (1996) Contact lens disinfectants. In *Handbook of Disinfectants and Antiseptics* (ed. Ascenzi, J.M.), pp. 83–110. New York: Marcel Dekker.

Moore, M.B., McCulley, M.P., Newton, C. *et al.* (1987) *Acanthamoeba* keratitis: a growing problem in soft and hard contact lens wearers. *Ophthalmology*, **94**, 1654–1661.

Nagington, J., Watson, P.G., Playfair, T.J., McGill, J., Jones, B.R. & Steel, A.D. (1974) Amoebic infection of the eye. *Lancet*, **2**, 1537–1540.

Nauheim, R.C., Brockman, R.J., Stopak, S.S. *et al.* (1990) Survival of *Acanthamoeba* in contact lens rinse solutions. *Cornea*, **9**, (4) 290–293.

Neff, R., Benton, W. & Neff, N. (1964) The composition of the mature cyst wall of the soil amoeba *Acanthamoeba* species. *Journal of Cell Biology*, **23**, 66A.

Nicoletti, G., Boghossian, V., Gurevitch, F., Borland, R. & Morgenroth, P. (1993) The antimicrobial activity *in vitro* of chlorhexidine, a mixture of isothiazolinone ('Kathon CG') and cetyltrimethylammonium bromide (CTAB). *Journal of Hospital Infection*, **23**, 87–112.

Pasternak, J.J., Thompson, J.E., Scultz, T.M.G. and Zachariah, K. (1970) A scanning electron microscopic study of the encystment of *Acanthamoeba castellanii*. *Experimental Cell Research*, **60**, 290–298.

Perkovich, B.T. Meisler, D.M., McMahon, J.T. & Rutherford, I. (1991) Adherence of *Acanthamoeba* to soft contact lenses. *Reviews of Infectious Diseases*, **13** (Suppl.), S421–S422.

Pharmaceutical Codex (1994) London: Pharmaceutical Press.

Radford, C.F., Bacon, A.S., Dart, J.K.G. & Minassian, D.C. (1995) Risk factors for *Acanthamoeba* keratitis in contact lens users: a case control study. *British Medical Journal*, **310**, 1567–1570.

Ranganathan, N.S. (1996) Chlorhexidine. In *Handbook of Disinfectants and Antiseptics* (ed. Ascenzi, J.M.), pp. 235–264. New York: Marcel Dekker.

Refojo, M. (1976) Reversible binding of chlorhexidine gluconate to hydrogel contact lenses. *Contact Intraocular Lens Journal*, **2**, 47–56.

Rogan, M. (1985) Systems for hydrogen peroxide disinfection of soft contact lenses. In *Transactions of the BCLA Conference*, pp. 40–42.

Rosenthal, R.A., Schlitzer, R.L., McNamee, L.S., Dassanayake, N.L. & Amass, R. (1992) Antimicrobial activity of organic chlorine releasing compounds. *Journal of the British Contact Lens Association*, **15**, 81–84.

Russell, A.D. & Day, M.J. (1993) Antimicrobial activity of chlorhexidine. *Journal of Hospital Infection*, **25**, 229–238.

Russell, A.D. & Furr, J.R. (1996) Biocides: mechanisms of antifungal action and fungal resistance. *Science Progress*, **79**, 27–48.

Rutherford, I., Katanik, M.T. & Meisler, D.M. (1991) Efficacy of a chlorhexidine tablet system for disinfection of soft contact lenses against *Acanthamoeba* species. *Reviews of Infectious Diseases*, **13**, S416.

Seal, D.V. & Hay, J. (1992) Contact lens disinfection and *Acanthamoeba* problems and practicalities. *Pharmaceutical Journal*, **248**, 717–719.

Seal, D. & Hay, J. (1995) An explosive case from Ireland. *Optician*, **209**, 15.

Sharma, S., Srinivasan, M. & Goerge, C. (1990) *Acanthamoeba* keratitis in non-contact wearers. *Archives of Ophthalmology*, **108**, 676–678.

Silvany, R., Wood, T., Bowman, R., Moore, M. & McCulley, J. (1987) The effect of preservatives in contact lens solutions on two species of *Acanthamoeba*. *Investigative Ophthalmology and Visual Science*, **28** (Suppl.), 371.

Silvany, R.E., Wood, T.S., Bowman, R.B., Moore, M.B. & McCully, J.P. (1988) The effect of contact lens solutions on two species of *Acanthamoeba* [abstract].

Investigative Ophthalmology Vision and Science, **29** (Suppl.), 253.

Silvany, R.E., Dougherty, J.M., McCulley, J.P., Wood, T.S., Bowman, R.W. & Moore, M.B. (1990) The effect of currently available contact lens disinfection systems on *Acanthamoeba castellanii* and *Acanthamoeba polyphaga*. *Ophthalmology*, **97**, 286–290.

Silvany, R.E., Dougherty, J.M. & McCulley, J.P. (1991) Effect of contact lens preservatives on *Acanthamoeba*. *Ophthalmology*, **98**, 854–857.

Stehr-Green, J.K., Bailey, T.M. & Visvesvara, G.S. (1989) The epidemiology of *Acanthamoeba* keratitis in the United States. *American Journal of Ophthalmology*, **107**, 331–336.

Stewart-Jones, J.H., Hopkins, G.A. & Phillips, A.J. (1989) Drugs and solutions in contact lens practice and related microbiology. In *Contact Lenses*, 3rd edn (eds Phillips, A.J. & Stone, J.), pp. 125–185. London: Butterworths.

Sutton, S.V.W. (1996) Neutralizer evaluations as control experiments for antimicrobial efficacy tests. In *Handbook of Disinfectants and Antiseptics* (ed. Ascenzi, J.M.), pp. 43–72. New York: Marcel Dekker.

Trueman, J.R. (1971) The halogens. In *Inhibition and Destruction of the Microbial Cell* (ed. Hugo, W.B.), pp. 144–183. London: Academic Press.

Visvesvara, GDS. (1980) Free-living pathogenic amoeba. In *Manual of Clinical Microbiology*, 3rd edn (eds Lennette, E.H., Balows, A. & Hausler, W.J., Jr) pp. 704–708. Washington, DC: American Society for Microbiology.

Volgelberg, K. & Boehnke, M. (1994) *In vitro* toxicity of polyhexamide (PHMB). *ARVO Annual Meeting Abstracts*, **35**, 1337.

Walters, T.H., Furr, J.R. & Russell, A.D. (1983) Antifungal action of chlorhexidine. *Microbios*, **38**, 195–204.

Weisman, R.A. (1976) Differentiation in *Acanthamoeba castellanii*. *Annual Review of Microbiology*, **30**, 189–219.

Wilhelmus, K. (1991) The increasing importance of *Acanthamoeba*. *Review of Infectious Diseases*, **13**, (Suppl. 5), S367–S368.

Wright, S.G. (1983) Walter sterilisation. *British Medical Journal*, **287**, 741.

Zanetti, S., Fiori, P.L., Usai, S., Carta, F. & Fadda, G. (1995) Susceptibility of *Acanthamoeba castellanii* to contact lens disinfecting solutions. *Antimicrobial Agents and Chemotherapy*, **39**, 1596–1598.

B. INTESTINAL PROTOZOA

1 Introduction

Chapter 8B will focus on the effect of disinfectants on intestinal protozoan parasites: *Cryptosporidium*, a coccidian of the intestinal and occasionally respiratory epithelium of vertebrates, can cause cryptosporidiosis (Sterling and Arrowood, 1993; Fayer *et al.*, 1997); *Entamoeba histolytica*, an amoeba inhabiting the human large intestine, is the aetiological agent of amoebiasis (Martinez-Palomo, 1993); and *Giardia intestinalis* (syn. *lamblia*), a flagellate of the human small intestine, causes giardiasis, the most frequently reported waterborne parasitic in the UK and the USA (Craun, 1990; Kulda and Noyhnkova, 1995). These distinctly different protozoa are considered together because all: (i) are potentially pathogenic to humans; (ii) have a resistant, transmissible cyst (oocyst for *Cryptosporidium*) stage; (iii) are acquired faecal–orally from food, water or fomites; and (iv) are controlled environmentally by filtration, sterilization or disinfection.

2 CT values

In recent studies, the results of chemical disinfection experiments are routinely expressed in terms of *CT* products (in mg·min/l), where *C* is the disinfectant concentration in milligrams per litre and *T* is the contact time. These products are derived theoretically from models by Chick (1908) and Watson (1908) and come from a first-order rate law:

$$\ln N - \ln N_0 = -kC^{\eta}T$$

where k is a constant for a given microorganism exposed to a disinfectant under a fixed set of pH and temperature conditions and η is the coefficient of dilution (see Chapter 3). Plotting *C* and *T* values, respectively, on a logarithmic ordinate and abscissa will result in a straight line, whose slope is η. Values of $\eta < 1$ indicate that time is more important than concentration in cyst inactivation; values of $\eta > 1$ indicate the converse. If $\eta = 1$, then disinfectant concentration and contact time are equally important and the *CT* product is independent of the disinfectant concentration used. The major advantage of using *CT* products for establishing disinfectant concentrations and contact times is that they are based on experimental data; the major disadvantage occurs when the data used to calculate *CT* product are limited so that extrapolation is required (Hoff, 1986). Extrapolation can be quite disconcerting—for example, if pH variations in environmental water treated with chlorine are considered, since the pH influence on chlorine is far less predictable than is the temperature influence. Yet another shortcoming of the Chick–Watson model, as well as a model by Hom (1972), is that there is an assumption, often incorrect, that the disinfectant concentration remains constant throughout the contact time. Finch *et al.* (1994) have proposed other models which take decreasing disinfectant concentration into account. Despite their shortcomings, *CT* products are convenient for comparing disinfectant efficacy on protozoan cysts under a given set of conditions. For the purpose of this section, η is taken as 1 if it is impossible to discern it from the older literature, where *CT* products were not calculated.

3 Effect of disinfectants on protozoa

It is impossible to include all of the historical studies on protozoan disinfection in this chapter. However, earlier studies on *Giardia* have been reviewed by Jarroll (1988), and those on *Cryptosporidium* are included in a review by Fayer *et al.* (1997).

The reader is cautioned that controversy continues regarding the most appropriate method for determing cyst (oocyst) inactivation, especially in the case of *Cryptosporidum*. However, it is important to remember that all these methods are, at best, approximations of what could happen in the human host, and none of them takes a possibly weakened host immune system into account. Campbell *et al.* (1992) reported that *in vitro* excystation compared favourably with fluorogenic-dye staining for estimating viability of *Cryptosporidium parvum* oocysts. However, more recent data suggest that, when disinfection efficacy is being evaluated, *in vitro* excystation and fluorogenic-dye staining should not be used for *Cryptosporidium* oocysts (Finch *et al.*, 1994). In the case of *Cryptosporidium*, excystation tends to underestimate inactivation when compare with animal infectivity (Finch *et al.*, 1994; Owens *et al.*, 1994).

With *Giardia muris*, there was no significant difference between fluorogenic-dye staining and *in vitro* excystation, or between *in vitro* excystation and animal infectivity, but fluorogenic-dye staining significantly underestimated inactivation compared with animal infectivity (Labatiuk *et al.* 1991). *In vitro* excystation was intermediate between fluorogenic-dye staining and animal infectivity. Only animal infectivity has the sensitivity to detect >99.9% inactivation for *G. muris* (Labatiuk *et al.*, 1991).

3.1 Chloramines

Chloramines (NH_2Cl, $NHCl_2$ and NCl_3) are generated when chlorine (either free or as hypochlorite) is added to water in the presence of ammonia (usually as ammonium sulphate). This group of water disinfectants is more complex than those commonly used and generally less effective against protozoan cysts than other halogens. If the chlorine and the ammonia are reacted prior to their addition to water, they are referred to as preformed chloramine. In practice, chloramines are formed by the addition of chlorine and ammonia independently to water; thus, there is a time when a detectable, albeit transient, level of free chlorine exists. This transient level of free chlorine probably enhances the cysticidal effect attributed to chloramine.

Preformed monochloramine exhibited a *CT* product of 7200 mg·min/l against *Cryptosporidium* to reduce animal infectivity significantly. That *CT* value was equivalent to the one for free chlorine at 25°C (Korich *et al.*, 1990). Most of the reports dealing with the effect of chloramines on protozoan cysts are based on studies involving *Giardia* cysts and using *in vitro* excystation as a means of assessing viability (Rubin, 1987; Meyer *et al.*, 1989). In experiments aimed at simulating field conditions (Meyer *et al.*, 1989), chlorine and ammonia were added to water in a Cl_2 : N ratio of 7 : 1, which gave *CT* products for a 99% kill of from 185 mg·min/l at 18°C to 650 mg·min/l at 3°C. Decreasing the temperature and, to a lesser degree, increasing the pH adversely affected chloramine efficacy. A single study assessing preformed chloramines with a 1 : 4 Cl_2 : N ratio showed that, at pH 7 and 15°C, the mean *CT* product was approximately 850 mg·min/l (Hoff, 1986). Comparing these studies suggests that chloramines generated under field conditions are somewhat more effective than those that are used preformed and that chloramines, in general, are less effective than free chlorine.

3.2 Chlorine

Information is sparse regarding the effect of chlorine on *Cryptosporidium* oocyst viability. Korich *et al.* (1990) reported, based on animal infectivity and *in vitro* excystation, that the viability of *Cryptosporidium* oocysts dropped from 80% to 0% after 2 h in 80 mg chlorine/l at pH 7 and 25°C, and that at least 99% were inactivated after the first 90 min. This would translate to a *CT* product of approx. 7200 mg·min/l.

Entamoeba histolytica cysts exhibit a *CT* product of 20 mg·min/l at 30°C and pH 7, with 99% of the cysts inactivated, according to the *in vitro* excystation assay (Stringer *et al.*, 1975). Based on these data, *Entamoeba* and *Giardia* (see below) appear roughly equivalent in their sensitivity to chlorine.

The first *CT* values reported for *Giardia* were calculated from data obtained using *G. muris* cysts and *in vitro* excystation. At pH 7 and 25°C, the *CT* products (Rice *et al.*, 1982) for *G. muris* (murine type and a *G. lamblia* surrogate) ranged from *c.* 26 to 45 mg·min/l; at 5°C, the range was from 449 to 1012 mg·min/l (Leahy *et al.*, 1987). Surprisingly, when the *G. muris* data were plotted with respect to hypochlorous acid (HOCl) concentration vs. pH, cyst inactivation was best at pH 9 > pH 7 > pH 5. Leahy *et al.* (1987) speculated that these unexpected results could be due either to pH-induced changes in the surface of the organism affecting cyst sensitivity to HOCl or to an alteration in the mechanism of action of the disinfectant, allowing for greater sensitivity to the hypochlorite ion (ClO^-) than was believed previously. Too little is known of *Giardia* cyst wall biochemistry (Jarroll *et al.*, 1989; Manning *et al.*, 1992) or cyst physiology (Paget *et al.*, 1989, 1993) to determine which, if either, of these speculations is correct. The *CT* products for *G. lamblia* were reported from *in vitro* excystation experiments (Rubin *et al.*, 1989) in which human-type *Giardia* cysts, collected from infected gerbils (Belosevic *et al.*, 1983), were used. The *CT* products ranged from 120 mg·min/l (pH 7, 15°C) to 1500 mg·min/l (pH 9, 15°C). These data suggest that *G. lamblia* cysts are even more resistant to chlorine than previously thought, since an approximation calculated from earlier data (Jarroll *et al.*, 1981) indicates a *CT* product of 120 mg·min/l at 5°C and pH 7. Hibler *et al.* (1987) estimated *CT* products, using gerbil infectivity as cyst viability measure, of between 157 and 425 mg·min/l at 0.5°C and 5°C.

3.3 Chlorine dioxide

The advantages of chlorine dioxide (ClO_2) over free chlorine or chloramines include the facts that: (i) its efficacy increases threefold in the pH range of 6–9; (ii) it does not disproportionate (transform into two or more dissimilar substances by oxidation and reduction simultaneously) in the normal pH range encountered in water treatment, unlike free chlorine; and (iii) it is less reactive with demand substances than free or combined chlorine. Its disadvantages include: (i) volatilization and thus easy loss from solution; and (ii) disproportionation above pH 10 into non-cysticidal chlorate and chlorite ions (Hoff, 1986).

Of the chlorine-based disinfectants used to treat water, clearly ClO_2 is the most effective protozoan cysticide tested to date. In the case of *Cryptosporidium*, oocysts are more resistant to ClO_2 than *Giardia* cysts, but they are more susceptible to ClO_2 than to either free chlorine or monochloramines. At a ClO_2 concentration of 1.3 mg/l and pH 7, oocyst viability dropped from 87% to 5% at 25°C for 1 h (Korich *et al.*, 1990). While this approximates to a *CT* product of 78 mg·min/l, it highlights *Cryptosporidium*'s extreme resistance to halogen disinfectants, even one as generally effective as ClO_2. Comparable results were found by Ransome *et al.* (1993).

With respect to *Giardia*, ClO_2 surpasses both free chlorine and chloramines, with a mean *CT* product at pH 7 and 5°C of 11.9 mg·min/l; at pH 7 and 25°C, the *CT* product dropped to 5.2 mg·min/l. Rubin (1989) reported that the *CT* at pH 9 and 25°C was about half that at pH 7 (2.8 mg·min/l).

3.4 Iodine

Ransome *et al.* (1993) reported that 120 mg iodine/l reduce *C. parvum* excystation by nearly 93% in 60 min at pH 4 (*CT* = 7200 mg·min/l). At pH 4, 10 mg iodine/l reduced excystation to only 84.5%. Neither of these results supports the use of iodine for inactivating *C. parvum* oocysts in drinking-water.

Iodine exhibited a *CT* product of *c.* 70 mg·min/l at pH 7 and 30°C against *E. histolytica* (99% kill).

This value is at least 3.5 times that for chlorine's efficacy against *E. histolytica*. Iodine is apparently a better *E. histolytica* cysticide in sewage than in buffered water, especially below pH 8 (Stringer *et al.*, 1975).

For elemental iodine, *CT* products ranging from a low of 77 mg·min/l at pH 7 and 25°C to a high of 393 mg·min/l at pH 7 and 5°C were reported for *G. muris*, which suggest that iodine is slightly more effective against *G. muris* than is chlorine, especially at cold temperatures (Rubin, 1987). One of the few small-quantity water disinfectants (Jarroll *et al.*, 1980a,b) currently available that shows efficacy against *Giardia lamblia* is a compound known as Pota-Aqua (chemically equivalent to glycine tetrahydroperiodide in Emergency Drinking Water Germicidal Tablets (EDWGT) and Globaline, Wisconsin Pharmacal, Jackson, Wisconsin).

3.5 Ozone

Ozone is superior to any of the halogens studied to date against *Cryptosporidium* oocysts or *E. histolytica* and *Giardia* cysts. For *Cryptosporidium*, a *CT* product of between 5 and 10 mg·min/l exists, based on the reduction of oocyst viability (excystation and infectivity) from 84% to 0% after 5 min in 1 mg ozone/l at 25°C (Korich *et al.*, 1990). For 99.9% inactivation (infectivity and excystation), *CT* products of from 3.7 (at 22°C) to 10.3 mg·min/l (at 7°C) were calculated by Finch *et al.* (1993); Peeters *et al.* (1989) showed comparable results for *C. parvum* inactivation by ozone. Finch *et al.* (1994), using a non-linear model that takes into account ozone decay in solution with time, provided several families of curves for 99% and 99.9% inactivation at 7 and 22°C. Parker *et al.* (1993) showed that lowering the temperature decreases the efficacy of ozone on *C. parvum* oocysts. By vital-dye inclusion/exclusion, these workers found that, with 5 mg ozone/l of water, greater than 15% of the oocysts remained viable after 10 min at 5°C; all oocysts were inactivated by 5 mg ozone/l after 10 min at 20°C.

Greater than 98% of the *E. histolytica* cysts examined were inactivated following a 5 min exposure to from 0.7 to 1.1 mg ozone/l at pH 7.5–8 in tap water at 19°C (Newton & Jones, 1949). There was little observed difference in this cyst destruction over the temperature range of 10–27°C.

Giardia lamblia is at least an order of magnitude more resistant to ozone (*CT* = 0.17 mg·min/l at pH 7 and 25°C; 0.53 mg·min/l at pH 7 and 5°C) than is *Escherichia coli* (the standard coliform bacterium; *CT* = 0.02 mg·min/l at pH 7.2 and 1°C) and nearly twice as resistant as poliovirus 1 (*CT* = 0.22 mg·min/l at pH 7.2 and 5°C) (Katzenelson *et al.*, 1974; Roy *et al.*, 1982; Wickramayanake *et al.*, 1984a). *Giardia muris* exhibits approximately fourfold higher *CT* products than *G. lamblia* under comparable conditions (Wickramayanake *et al.*, 1984b). Ozone's efficacy decreased as the temperature decreased, and the pH effect on ozone was pH 9 > pH 5 > pH 7 in terms of cysticidal activity.

3.6 Ultraviolet radiation

Lorenzo-Lorenzo *et al.* (1993) showed that UV (ultraviolet) irradiation of 15 000 mW/s for at least 150 min rendered *Cryptosporidium* oocysts incapable of infecting neonatal mice. A recent preliminary report shows that, in aqueous medium, pulsed light (rich in UV frequencies from 260 to 280 nm and *c.* 20 000 times brighter than sunlight) (Arrowood *et al.*, 1996) outperforms conventional UV, which reduced viability by only 2 logs (Campbell *et al.*, 1995). Complete oocyst inactivation was accomplished by as little as 1 J/cm^2 of the pulsed light and was assessed by the fact that mice were not infected by oocysts so exposed (Arrowood *et al.*, 1996).

Giardia lamblia cysts are more resistant to UV than bacteria. *Escherichia coli* viability was reduced nearly 3 logs at 3 mW s/cm^2, while *G. lamblia* cyst viability was not reduced by 1 log at 43–63 mW s/cm^2 (Rice & Hoff, 1981). *Giardia muris* cyst viability was reduced 99% in 20 min, using laser-generated UV at 109.7 mW s/cm^2 (Carlson *et al.*, 1985). These finding suggest that UV of sufficient exposure is effective against *Giardia*. Caveats include the facts that: (i) addition of colour with absorbance of 254 nm, regardless of the source, increases cyst survival; (ii) short-circuiting and the collection of air bubbles in commercial UV disinfection units can decrease the effectiveness of UV; and (iii) large particles

(> 5 mm) may provide shielding from UV, while particles < 5 mm do not apparently offer protection to cysts from UV.

3.7 Miscellaneous disinfectants

Many of the aforementioned disinfectants are frequently used to treat drinking-water for public consumption, and thus studies have focused in the main on this point. Interest is increasing to find compounds effective against protozoa on environmental surfaces as well. Testing for the efficacy of these against *Cryptosporidium* has been more extensive than for any of the other parasites discussed here. For a complete review of the effects of a wide variety of disinfectants on *Cryptosporidium*, see a review by Fayer *et al.* (1997).

Campbell *et al.* (1982) used animal infectivity to test the efficacy of cresylic acid, hypochlorite solution, formaldehyde, benzalkonium chloride, ammonia, sodium hydroxide and an iodophor for use in disinfecting veterinary laboratories for *Cryptosporidium* (from a calf). Of these compounds, formal saline (10% formaldehyde in saline) partially reduced oocyst numbers after 2 h of exposure. After 18 h, 10% formal saline, cresylic acid (5%) and 0.33% iodophor reduced oocyst numbers in intestinal homogenates. However, even after 18 h of exposure to these disinfectants, only ammonia (5%) and formal saline (10%) prevented mice from being infected. Fayer *et al.* (1996) reported that methyl bromide, ethylene oxide and gaseous ammonia completely prevented animal infectivity by *C. parvum* oocysts when the oocysts were exposed to these gases at room temperature for 24 h. Ammonia was also reportedly effective against *Cryptosporidium baileyi*, which has been reported from many species of birds, including chickens and turkeys (Sundermann *et al.*, 1987).

Holton and colleagues (1994) evaluated Cidex (2%; alkaline glutaraldehyde from Surgicos, Scotland), 6% Sactimed Sinald (quatenary ammonium compound from Lever Industrial, England), 1% Virkon (peroxygen compound from Antec International Ltd., England), 0.2% Steris 20 (peracetic acid; Steris, Painesville, Ohio, USA), Phoraid (0.034% iodine, Kalon Chemicals, England), 5% Pentapon DC-1 and HDY (organic beta-enes from Trigon Chemic GmbH, Germany) against *C. parvum*, with *in vitro* excystation as the criterion of viability. After incubating oocysts for 60 min in 37°C Roswell Park Memorial Institute (RPMI) medium alone or with added disinfectant, Pentapon DC-1 and Sactimed Sinald were the most effective. Cidex was a close third. One caveat is that these authors report Steris 20 as being comparable in effect to Pentapon DC-1 and Sactimed, but the data to support this were not shown. What is known of the effects of bromine on *Cryptosporidium* oocysts was reported by Ransome *et al.* (1993). A free bromine residual of 1180 mg/l for 60 min at 10°C only reduced excystation of *C. parvum* oocysts by 88.5%. This represents a *CT* product of 70 800 mg·min/l.

Stringer *et al.* (1975) undertook studies in which *E. histolytica* cysts were exposed to 1.5 mg bromine/l of buffered water at pH 4 and 30°C and then excysted *in vitro*. Under these conditions and in 10 min, 99.9% of the cysts were inactivated, which translates into a *CT* product of 15 mg·min/l. This was nearly equal to the *CT* product for chlorine and *E. histolytica*, but was about a third that for iodine and *E. histolytica*. Adjusting the pH to 10 caused the *CT* product for bromine to rise to 40 mg·min/l, while those for chlorine and iodine rose to 120 and 200 mg·min/l. respectively.

4 Summary

Without exception, ozone is the most effective protozoan cysticide examined to date, with ClO_2 running a distant second. The latter is superior to iodine and free chlorine, which approximate to each other in their cysticidal properties. All of the foregoing oxidants are superior to chloramines as cysticides. Another generality here is that all of these oxidants exhibit enhanced cysticidal properties as temperature increases. Reports differ on the efficacy of the halogens with respect to pH; in some cases, decreasing the pH enhances activity, but the opposite may be true in other cases.

Pulsed light offers some promise of being a non-chemical means of killing protozoa in a variety of environments. Debate still exists as to the suitability of using UV irradiation to treat water. A wide variety of substances are being evaluated as disinfectants for environmental surfaces. To date, formal saline, ammonia, ethylene oxide and methyl bromide and some beta-enes offer the most promise. Many of these products are quite hazardous to human and animal health and care must be exercised in their use.

Virtually all protozoa resist chemical disinfection and UV irradiation better than do most bacteria and viruses. A serious implication of this fact is that the absence of indicator coliform bacteria in treated water should not be considered a reliable indicator of the absence of viable protozoan cysts. Furthermore, the extreme resistance of *Cryptosporidium* to disinfectants that worked well against *Entamoeba* and *Giardia* underscores the idea that these organisms, while similar in many aspects of their epidemiology, are vastly different in their sensitivity to disinfectants. Thus, each organism that represents a potential threat to health must be evaluated rigorously with respect to the disinfectants to be used to control it.

5 References

Arrowood, M., Xie, L., Rieger, K. & Dunn, J. (1996) Disinfection of *Cryptosporidium parvum* oocysts by pulsed light treatment evaluated in an *in vitro* cultivation model. *Journal of Eukaryotic Microbiology*, **43**, 88S.

Belosevic, M., Faubert, G., MacLean, J., Law, C. & Croll, N. (1983) *Giardia lamblia* infections in Mongolian gerbils: an animal model. *Journal of Infectious Diseases*, **147**, 222–226.

Campbell, A., Robertson, L. & Smith, H. (1992) Viability of *Cryptosporidium parvum* oocysts: correlation of *in vitro* excystation with inclusion or exclusion of fluorogenic vital dyes. *Applied and Environmental Microbiology*, **58**, 3488–3493.

Campbell, A., Robinson, L., Snowball, M. & Smith, H. (1995) Inactivation of oocysts of *Cryptosporidium parvum* by ultraviolet irradiation. *Water Research*, **29**, 2583–2586.

Campbell, I., Tzipori, S., Hutchison, G. & Angus, K. (1982) Effect of disinfectants on survival of *Cryptosporidium* oocysts. *Veterinary Record* **111**, 414–415.

Carlson, D. Seabloom, R., Dewalle, F. *et al.* (1985) *Ultra-violet Disinfection of Water for Small Water Supplies*. US Environmental Protection Agency Project Summary No. 600/S2-85/092, September.

Chick, H. (1908) An investigation of the laws of disinfection. *Journal of Hygiene*, **8**, 92–158.

Craun, G. (1990) Waterborne giardiasis. In: *Giardiasis* (ed. Meyer, E.A.), Human Parasitic Diseases, Vol. 3, pp. 267–290. Amsterdam and New York: Elsevier.

Fayer, R., Graczyk, T., Cranfield, M. & Trout, J. (1996) Gaseous disinfection of *Cryptosporidium parvum* oocysts. *Applied and Environmental Microbiology*, **62**, 3908–3909.

Fayer, R., Speer, C. & Dubey, J. (1997) The general biology of *Crytposporidium*. In *Cryptosporidium and Cryptosporidosis* (ed. Fayer, R.), pp. 1–41. Boca Raton, Florida: CRC Press.

Finch, G., Black, E., Gyurek, L. & Belosevic, M. (1993) Ozone inactivation of *Cryptosporidium parvum* in demand-free phosphate buffer determined by *in vitro* excystation and animal infectivity. *Applied and Environmental Microbiology*, **59**, 4203–4210.

Finch, G., Black, E.K., & Gyurek, L. (1994) Ozone and chlorine inactivation of *Cryptosporidium*. In *Water Quality Technology Proceedings (AWWA)*, San Francisco, California, November, pp. 1303–1318.

Hibler, C., Hancock, C., Perger, L., Wergryzn, J. & Swabby, K. (1987) *Inactivation of* Giardia *Cysts with Chlorine at 0.5°C to 5.0°C*. American Waterworks Association Research Report. Denver, Colorado: American Waterworks Association.

Hoff, J. (1986) Strengths and weaknesses of using *Ct* values to evaluate disinfection practice. Paper presented to Water Quality Technology Conference (AWWA), Portland, Oregon, November.

Holton, J., Nye, P. & McDonald, V. (1994) Efficacy of selected disinfectants against *Mycobacterium* and crytposporidia. *Journal of Hospital Infection*, **27**, 105–115.

Hom, L. (1972) Kinetics of chlorine disinfection in an ecosystem. *Journal of Sanitary Engineering Division, American Society of Chemical Engineering*, **98**, 183–193.

Jarroll, E. (1998) Effect of disinfection on *Giardia* cysts. *CRC Reviews in Environmental Control*, **18**, 1–28.

Jarroll, E., Bingham, A. & Meyer, E. (1980a) *Giardia* cyst destruction: effectiveness of six small-quantity water disinfection methods. *American Journal of Tropical Medicine and Hygiene*, **29**, 8–11.

Jarroll, E., Bingham, A. & Meyer, E. (1980b) Inability of an iodination methods to destroy completely *Giardia* cysts in cold water. *Western Journal of Medicine*, **132**, 567–569.

Jarroll, E., Bingham, A. & Meyer, E. (1981) Effect of chlorine on *Giardia lamblia* cyst viability. *Applied and Environmental Microbiology*, **41**, 483–487.

Jarroll, E. Manning, P., Lindmark, D., Coggins, J. & Erlandsen, S. (1989) *Giardia* cyst wall specific carbohydrate: evidence for the presence of galactosamine. *Molecular and Biochemical Parasitology*, **32**, 121–132.

Katzenelson, E., Kletter, B. & Shuval, H. (1974) Inactivation kinetics of viruses and bacteria in water by use of ozone. *Journal of the American Waterworks Association*, **66**, 725–729.

Korich, D., Mead, J., Madore, N., Sinclair, N. &

Sterling, C. (1990) Effects of ozone, chlorine dioxide, chlorine, and monochloramine on *Cryptosporidium parvum* oocyst viability. *Applied and Environmental Microbiology*, **56**, 1423–1428.

Kulda, J. & Nohynkova, E. (1995) *Giardia* in human and animals. In *Parasitic Protozoa*, Vol. VI, 2nd edn (ed. Kreier, J.P.), pp. 225–422. San Diego, California: Academic Press.

Labatiuk, C., Schaefer, F., III, Finch, G. & Belosevic, M. (1991) Comparison of animal infectivity, excystation, and fluorogenic dye as measures of *Giardia muris* cyst inactivation by ozone. *Applied and Environmental Microbiology*, **57**, 3187–3192.

Leahy, J., Rubin, A. & Sproul, O. (1987) Inactivation of *Giardia muris* cysts by free chlorine. *Applied and Environmental Microbiology*, **53**, 1448–1453.

Lorenzo-Lorenzo, M., Ares-Mazas, M., Villa Corta, I. & Duran-Oreiro, D. (1993) Effect of ultraviolet disinfection on drinking water on the viability of *Cryptosporidium parvum* oocysts. *Journal of Parasitology*, **79**, 67–70.

Manning, P., Erlandsen, S. & Jarroll, E. (1992) Carbohydrate and amino acid analyses of *Giardia muris* cysts. *Journal of Protozoology*, **39**, 290–296.

Martinez-Palomo, A. (1993) Parasitic amebas of the intestinal tract. In: *Parasitic Protozoa*, Vol. VI, 2nd edn (ed. Kreier, J.P.), pp. 65–141. San Diego, California: Academic Press.

Meyer, E.A., Glicker, J., Bingham, A. & Edwards, R. (1989) Inactivation of *Giardia muris* cysts by chloramines. *Water Resources Bulletin*, **25**, 335–340.

Newton, W. & Jones, M. (1949) Effect of ozone in water on cysts of *Entamoeba histolytica*. *American Journal of Tropical Medicine*, **29**, 669.

Owens, J., Miltner, R. Schaefer, F., III & Rice, E. (1994) Pilot-scale ozone inactivation of *Cryptosporidium* and *Giardia*. In *Water Quality Technology Proceedings (AWWA)*, San Francisco, California, November, pp. 1319–1328.

Paget, T., Jarroll, E., Manning, P., Lindmark, D. & Lloyd, D. (1989) Respiration in the cysts and trophozoites of *Giardia muris*. *Journal of General Microbiology*, **135**, 145–154.

Paget, T., Manning, P. & Jarroll, E. (1993) Oxygen uptake in cysts and trophozoites of *Giardia lamblia*. *Journal of Eukaryotic Microbiology*, **40**, 246–250.

Parker, J., Greaves, G. & Smith, H. (1993) The effect of ozone on the viability of *Cryptosporidium parvum* oocysts and a comparison of experimental methods. *Water Science Technology*, **27**, 93–96.

Peeters, J., Mazas, E., Masschelein, W., Martinez de Maturana, I. & Debacker, E. (1989) Effect of disinfection of drinking water with ozone or chlorine dioxide on survival of *Cryptosporidium parvum* oocysts. *Applied and Environmental Microbiology*, **55**, 1519–1522.

Ransome, M., Whitmore, T. Carrington, E. (1993) Effect of disinfectants on the viability of *Cryptosporidium parvum* oocysts. **Water Supply**, 11, 75–89.

Rice, E. & Hoff, J. (1981) Inactivation of *Giardia lamblia* cysts by ultraviolet irradiation. *Applied and Environmental Microbiology*, **42**, 546–547.

Rice, E., Hoff, J. & Schaefer, F., III (1982) Inactivation of *Giardia* cysts by chlorine. *Applied and Environmental Microbiology*, **43**, 250–251.

Roy, D., Engelbrecht, R. & Chian, E. (1982) Comparative inactivation of six enteroviruses by ozone. *Journal of the American Waterworks Association*, **74**, 660–664.

Rubin, A. (1987) Factors affecting the inactivation of *Giardia* cysts by monochloramines and comparison with other disinfectants. Paper presented to the conference on Current Research in Drinking Water Treatment, sponsored by the US Environmental Protection Agency and American Waterworks Association Research Foundation, Cincinnati, Ohio, March.

Rubin, A. (1989) Control of protozoan cysts with in water by disinfection with chlorine dioxide. In *Environmental Quality and Ecosystem Stability*: Vol. IV-A: *Environmental Quality* (eds Luria, M., Steinberger, Y. & Spanier, E.), pp. 391–400. Jerusalem, Israel: ISEEQS Publications.

Rubin, A., Evers, D., Eyman, C. & Jarroll, E. (1989) Inactivation of qerbil-cultured *Giardia lamblia* cysts by free chlorine. *Applied and Environmental Microbiology*, **55**, 2592–2594.

Sterling, C. & Arrowood, M. (1993) Cryptosporidia. In *Parasitic Protozoa*, Vol. VI, 2nd edn (ed. Kreier, J.P.), pp. 159–225. San Diego, California: Academic Press.

Stringer, R., Cramer, W. & Kruse, C. (1975) Comparison of bromine, chlorine, and iodine as disinfectants for amoebic cysts. In *Disinfection—Water and Wastewater* (ed. Johnson, J.), pp. 193–209. Ann Arbor, Michigan: Ann Arbor.

Sundermann, C., Lindsay, D. & Blagburn, B. (1987) Evaluation of disinfectants for ability to kill avian *Cryptosporidium* oocysts. *Comparison Animal Practice*, **1**, 36–39.

Watson, H. (1908) A note on the variation of the rate of disinfection with change in the concentration of the disinfectant. *Journal of Hygiene*, **8**, 536–592.

Wickramanayake, G., Rubin, A. & Sproul, O. (1984a) Inactivation of *Naegleria* and *Giardia* cysts in water by ozonation. *Journal of the Water Pollution Control Federation*, **56**, 983–988.

Wickramanayake, G., Rubin, A. & Sproul, O. (1984b) Inactivation of *Giardia lamblia* cysts with ozone. *Applied and Environmental Microbiology*, **48**, 671–672.

CHAPTER 9

Disinfection Mechanisms

1 Introduction

Three areas may be recognized in studies of disinfection mechanisms, and resistance and revival of microbes therefrom.

1 Studies of the kinetics of disinfection.

2 Biochemical and biophysical studies of the basic mechanisms of chemical stress and its reversal.

3 Methods of evaluating disinfectants.

Only the kinetic and the biochemical and biophysical studies concerning the effects of chemical stress and their reversal will be dealt with here. Methods of evaluating disinfectants are dealt with in Chapter 4. Interactions of chemicals with whole cells, cell walls, membranes and the cytoplasm will be considered in turn, followed by suggestions on the possible mechanisms of survival of chemical-disinfectant attack (for reviews, see Hugo, 1971, 1976a,b, 1980; Russell & Hugo, 1988; Denyer, 1995; Russell & Russell, 1995; Russell & Chopra, 1996).

A compilation of experimental methods used to elucidate mechanisms of action has been published by Denyer & Hugo (1991). Russell & Furr (1996) have recently reviewed the mechanisms of antifungal action of biocides and fungal resistance.

They conclude that very little is known in both these areas (see also Chapter 5). Food preservation has been the subject of two excellent and comprehensive books, one edited by Gould (1989) and the other by Russell & Gould (1991).

2 The kinetic approach

In an exemplary paper by Kronig & Paul, published in 1897, and reprinted in English in Brock (1961), the foundation was laid for the kinetic approach to chemical sterilization and the fundamental conditions to be observed in chemical studies of the process. Having codified rules, which included the notion that comparative toxicity studies should be carried out at equimolecular proportions, with known numbers of bacteria in pure culture at constant temperature and under similar conditions of culture, Kronig & Paul (Brock, 1961) went on to apply the emerging rules of chemical kinetics to the disinfection process, a procedure they stated was valid because the process must be a chemical one. They were the first to plot the logarithm of the surviving organisms against time, which they found gave a linear response.

The theme of linear log survival/time was developed by Madsen & Nyman (1907) and survival was investigated by many other workers, notably Chick (1908), Knaysi (1930), Knaysi & Morris (1930), Jordan & Jacobs (1944), Rahn (1945), Berry & Michaels (1947), Eddy (1953), Jacobs (1960) and Prokop & Humphrey (1970).

Departures from true linearity were often encountered, and Madsen & Nyman (1907) concluded that the different rates of destruction of bacteria under the influence of lethal agents were determined essentially by variability of resistance among the cells in a population. Rahn & Schoeder (1941) thought that in each bacterial species there was a single vulnerable molecule the destruction of which was lethal. Such a hypotheses is not supported by our present knowledge of the varied mode of action of lethal chemicals.

Eddy & Hinshelwood (Eddy, 1953) investigated the death rate of *Klebsiella aerogenes* under chemical stress induced by 3, 6-diaminoacridine, *m*-cresol and acid. No satisfactory evidence was found that cells in a given culture possessed variable resistance, and indeed Eddy showed that survivors in a disinfection process gave rise to a population no more resistant than the originals. The often-observed lag phase, before decrease in viability proceeded logarithmically, suggests that a number of events must occur before a significant number of cells begin to die; the number of these events may be the variable factor.

Eddy (1953) believed that at first certain essential metabolic capabilities were impaired. This phase was not considered lethal but gave rise to the initial lag phase. In the light of other evidence, it is probable that this represents bacteriostasis, as it is reversible, at least if the contact time is not prolonged. As time proceeds, the cells die according to the logarithmic law. The slowing up of the death rate after a further lapse of time was taken as indicative of an adaptive (?phenotypic) process, enabling the cells that had survived by chance to adjust to the chemical stress. However, these adapted cells show the same death pattern as in the original experiment when they are subcultured and rechallenged.

The significance of the variation in survival curves continues to be the subject of research, and Casolari (1981) has described a mathematical model in which functions derived from it can describe the varying shapes of survival curves, whether concave, convex, sigmoid or linear. It also claims to explain the tailing-off effect.

A factor that can be calculated from survival data is known as the concentration exponent, η, which measures the effect of dilution on the activity of a stressing agent. It may be calculated from the following expression: (log death time at concentration C_2)−(log death time at concentration C_1)/log C_1−log C_2. Typical values of η for phenol are 6, for mercuric chloride and formaldehyde 1 and for ethanol 9 (see also Chapter 3). There is an exponential relationship between loss of activity and dilution. Thus in the case of phenol, where $\eta=6$, a threefold dilution will mean a decrease in activity by a factor of 3^6 or 729. In practical terms, rapid dilution of a solution of a chemical antimicrobial agent with a high value of η will nullify the stress, and the survivor level among the remaining population will stabilize. Can we learn anything from the vast array of such data? Very little, it is feared, about mechanisms of disinfection, for the curves represent interactions of chemicals having differing cellular targets and modes of action with highly complex microorganisms at different stages of growth, and with different structures and chemical compositions. The subject has been reviewed by Hugo and Denyer (1987).

3 Interactions with the whole cell

However organelle- or enzyme-selective a drug may finally turn out to be, its first apparent interaction is with the whole cell, and this may be examined as an adsorption process or by microelectrophoresis.

3.1 Adsorption

As early as 1911, Herzog & Betzel realized the importance of adsorption in the disinfection process, in their studies with baker's yeast, and since then many others have measured the uptake of drugs by cells. The technique consists essentially of adding a suspension of cells to a solution of the drug and at suitable time intervals removing a sample, centrifuging it and determining the residual amount of drug in the cell-free supernatant solution. If the cells have removed drug from solution, the concentration of the drug in the supernatant fluid will have diminished. From these data, adsorption isotherms may be plotted and information concerning rate and total amount of uptake may be computed. Furthermore, by a consideration of the nature of the isotherm, some notion of the adsorptive mechanism may be inferred (Giles *et al.*, 1960, 1974). These authors considered five main patterns of adsorption, which they called S, L, H, C and Z (Fig. 9.1).

3.1.1 S (S-shaped) pattern

The S pattern in found when the solute molecule is monofunctional, has moderate intermolecular attraction, causing it to orientate vertically, and meets strong competition for substrate sites from molecules of the solvent or by another adsorbed species. Monohydric phenols when adsorbed on a polar substrate from water usually give this pattern.

3.1.2 L (Langmuir) pattern

In the L pattern, as more sites are filled it becomes increasingly difficult for a bombarding solute to find a vacant site. Either the adsorbed solute molecule is not oriented vertically or there is strong competition from the solvent. If vertical orientation does occur, there is a strong intramolecular attraction between the adsorbed molecules. Among the phenols, resorcinol shows this type of behaviour.

3.1.3 H (high-affinity) pattern

The H pattern is obtained when the solute is almost completely adsorbed. Sometimes the process is accompanied by ion exchange, as in many bacteriological staining procedures. It is also shown by the uptake of iodine from an iodophor by yeast (Hugo & Newton, 1964).

3.1.4 C (constant partition) pattern

The C pattern is obtained when the solutes penetrate more readily into the adsorbate than does the solvent. It has been shown to occur when aqueous

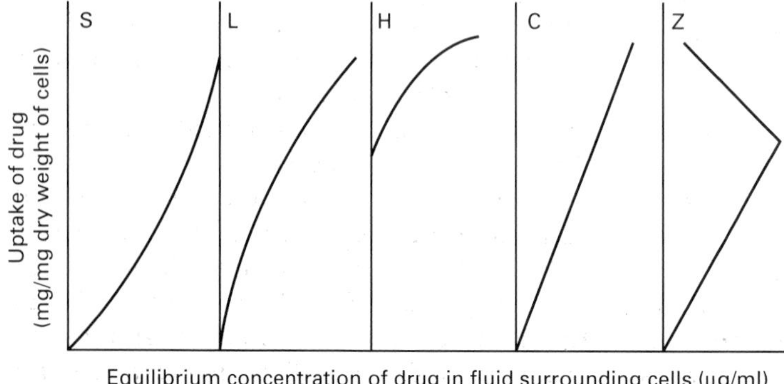

Fig. 9.1 Pattern of adsorption isotherms.

solutions of phenols are adsorbed by synthetic polypeptides, and it might also be expected to occur when phenols are adsorbed from an aqueous solution by bacteria containing a high proportion of lipid in their cell wall.

3.1.5 Z pattern

In the Z pattern, a sharp break in the isotherm is seen, accompanied thereafter by an increased uptake; this is interpreted as being caused by that concentration of adsorbed species which promotes a breakdown in the structure of the adsorbing species and the generation of new adsorbing sites. This was first seen by Giles & Tolia (1974), when studying the uptake of *p*-nitrophenol from organic solvents by cellulose fibres.

3.1.6 Examples of adsorption studies

More recent studies on the adsorption of antibacterial substances by microorganisms include the uptake of cetyltrimethylammonium bromide (CTAB) by bacteria (Salton, 1951), the adsorption of hexylresorcinol by *Escherichia coli* (Beckett *et al.*, 1959), of iodine by *E. coli*, *Staphylococcus aureus* and *Saccharomyces cerevisiae* (Hugo & Newton, 1964), of chlorhexidine by *Staph. aureus*, *E. coli* and *Clostridium perfringens* (Hugo & Longworth, 1964; Hugo & Daltrey, 1974), of basic dyes of fixed yeast cells (Giles & McKay, 1965), of phenols by *E. coli* (Bean & Das, 1966) and *Micrococcus lysodeikticus* (Judis, 1966), of dequalinium by *E. coli* and *Staph. aureus* (Hugo & Frier, 1969), of Fentichlor by *E. coli* and *Staph. aureus* (Hugo & Bloomfield, 1971a), of glutaraldehyde by *E. coli* (Munton & Russell, 1970; Gorman & Scott, 1977), of parabens by *Serratia marcescens* (Furr & Russell, 1972) and of polyhexamethylene biguanides by *E. coli* (Broxton *et al.*, 1984c). Resistant cells may take up less of a biocide, e.g. a benzalkonium chloride-resistant strain of *Pseudomonas aeruginosa* took up less than a pseudomonas-sensitive strain (Sakazami *et al.*, 1989). This is not always true, however.

Gilbert *et al.* (1978) report a most interesting example of the Z pattern referred to above. In studies of the mode of action of 2-phenoxyethanol and some of its analogues on *E. coli*, these workers found very similar isotherms to the cellulose *p*-nitrophenol type.

Extending this work (Gilbert *et al.*, 1978), it was found that a similar pattern was given with the yeast *Candida lipolytica*. When, however, *Ps. aeruginosa* was the test organism, no such inflexion was obtained, a C-type pattern being observed. This is a finding which might well be of significance in explaining, at the cellular level, the greater resistance of *Pseudomonas* to a wide variety of antimicrobial compounds.

Information on the site of adsorption may be obtained by studying the process at different pH values, but it should be borne in mind that the ionization of the disinfectant, as well as receptor sites on the cell surfaces, may be affected by changes in pH.

Adsorption studies of a different nature, involving the uptake of drugs by nucleic acids, have been used extensively to study actions on this molecule, and will be dealt with later.

The action of such substances as serum and organic debris in reducing the stress caused by some chemical bactericides may be due to their ability to compete with the bacterial cell for some of the active agent. In some cases, drugs may be desorbed from the cell after initial adsorption, thereby decreasing the stress.

3.2 Changes in electrophoretic mobility

Bacterial cells are normally negatively charged and, if suspended in water or a suitable electrolyte solution containing electrodes to which a potential has been applied, the cells will migrate to the positively charged electrode. This phenomenon may be placed on a quantitative basis by observing the rate of migration of a single cell to the electrode, by timing over a measured distance using a microscope and calibrated eyepiece micrometer. Once the system has been standardized, the effect of drugs on mobility may be studied, and from the data so obtained some notion of the drug–cell interaction and the effect of drugs on the charged bacterial cell surface may be deduced. The subject of bacterial cell electrophoresis has been reviewed in detail by Lerch (1953), James (1965, 1972) and Richmond & Fisher (1973). In general, it can be said that, while providing an exact tool for studying drug–cell interactions, electrophoresis has not provided much insight into the mechanisms of death.

Electrophoretic studies using antimicrobial compounds include CTAB and *Staph. aureus* (McQuillen, 1950), phenol and *E. coli* (Haydon, 1956), chlorhexidine and *E. coli* and *Staph. aureus* (Hugo & Longworth, 1966) and polyhexamethylene biguanides and *E. coli* (Broxton *et al.*, 1984c).

4 Interactions with the cell wall and other structures external to the cytoplasmic membrane

Antibiotics that have the cell wall as their target include penicillins, cephalosporins, cycloserine, vancomycin and ristocetin. In addition, Pulvertaft & Lumb (1948) showed that *E. coli*, streptococci and staphylococci lysed almost completely when rapidly growing cultures were exposed to low concentrations of antiseptics, such as formalin (0.012%), phenol (0.032%), mercuric chloride (0.0008%), sodium hypochlorite (0.005%) and merthiolate (0.0004%). They presumed that the autolytic enzymes were not inhibited at the low concentrations of antiseptic used, and compared this with the action of penicillin. The involvement of autolytic enzymes in penicillin action has been postulated (Rogers & Forsberg, 1971; Tomasz, 1979). Washed suspensions of *E. coli*, obtained from stationary-phase cultures, are not, however, lysed by low or high phenol concentrations.

Thiomersalate has been shown to increase the susceptibility of *Bacillus anthracis* to lysis, and the observation has been confirmed with *Bacillus cereus*. Low concentrations of some mercury compounds, which include mercuric chloride, phenylmercuric acetate and merthiolate, can lyse growing cultures of *E. coli*.

Sodium lauryl sulphate can lyse non-respiring (cyanide-treated) cells of *E. coli*. The organisms enlarged into globular forms and then lysed rapidly, although actively metabolizing cells were not susceptible. Anionic detergents can cause disaggregation of isolated walls of Gram-negative bacteria, due to their action upon the lipid-containing compounds of the wall, rather than to lytic enzymes (Bolle & Kellenberger, 1958). The lytic effect of anionic detergents on walls of wild-type and envelope mutants of *E. coli* and *Ps. aeruginosa* has been studied by El-Falaha *et al.* (1989). Sodium deoxycholate interferes with the flagellation and mobility of *E. coli* and *Proteus vulgaris* (D'Mello & Yotis, 1987).

Phenol (0.5%) caused lysis of cell pairs of *E. coli* only at the time of separation, i.e. when the cytoplasmic membrane was weak and exposed and its phospholipid content minimal.

Evidence of cell wall damage may be inferred from the phenomenon of drug-induced long forms of bacteria (Hughes, 1956). Thus, long forms may be induced in *Pr. vulgaris* by treatment with 1–2% phenol; a similar effect has been observed with *m*-cresol acting on *K. aerogenes*. Methyl violet, methyl green, fuchsin and methylene blue can induce long forms in *Salmonella typhi*. The involvement of lytic enzymes in long-form induction cannot be excluded.

Other chemicals that have an effect on outer cellular components include glutaraldehyde (Gorman *et al.*, 1980), which combines strongly with amino groups in amino acids and proteins, and permeabilizing agents, e.g. ethylenediamine tetraacetic acid (EDTA), polycations, such as poly-L-lysine, and the iron-binding proteins lactoferrin and transferrin (Vaara & Vaara, 1983a,b; Ellison *et al.*, 1988; Russell & Chopra, 1996; see also Section 4.1 and Chapter 3). Glutaraldehyde also acts elsewhere in the cell, e.g. at the site of the cytoplasmic membrane (Section 5.1) and at cytoplasmic sites (Russell & Chopra, 1996), and EDTA can affect ribosomal stability (Section 6.4).

4.1 Permeabilization

Methods of increasing the penetration of antimicrobial agents into Gram-negative cells have been investigated, in order to overcome the intrinsic resistance of this group of organisms due to the barrier effect of the outer membrane. As stated above, a variety of substances have been used, but EDTA has been extensively investigated as an adjuvant in disinfectant formulations and antibiotic activity (Brown & Richards, 1965; Smith, 1970; Haque & Russell, 1974a,b, 1976; Dankert & Schut, 1976; Russell & Furr, 1977). For general reviews on the subject, see Russell (1971) and Vaara (1992).

Broadley *et al.* (1995) have shown an interesting

potentiation of the effects of chlorhexidine and cetylpyridinium chloride towards mycobacteria by ethambutol; this compound inhibits the synthesis of cell wall components in the mycobacteria and hence may aid the penetration of the antimicrobial agents into the target cells.

5 Interactions with the cytoplasmic membrane

Early work in this area was concerned with drug-induced leakage of material, and there is little doubt that this contributes to stasis or death, according to the time and intensity of exposure to the chemical stress concerned. More recently, reactions at the molecular level have been revealed, and it is these reactions which are currently the most exciting. They include uncoupling of oxidative phosphorylation and inhibition of energy-dependent transport.

5.1 Leakage of cell constituents and modification of cell permeability

Kuhn & Bielig (1940) made the suggestion that cationic detergents of the quaternary ammonium compound (QAC) class might act on the bacterial cell membrane by dissociating conjugated proteins and, in a manner analogous to haemolysis, damage it so much that death would ensue. Hotchkiss (1944) proved that membrane damage was occurring by demonstrating that nitrogen- and phosphorus-containing compounds leaked from staphylococci treated with a QAC or the polypeptide antibiotic, tyrocidin.

Phenol, *p*-chloro-*m*-xylenol, *p*-chloro-*m*-cresol, *p*-chloro-*o*-cresol, 2,4-dichlorophenol, 2,4,6-trichlorophenol, 2,4,-dichloro-*m*-xylenol, CTAB and chlorhexidine all promote a concentration-dependent leakage of cell contents from microbial cells.

In the case of chlorhexidine-induced leakage of intracellular material from *E. coli* and *Staph. aureus*, a diphasic leakage/concentration pattern is found. The first part of the curve represents increasing leakage with increasing concentration of antiseptic, but at high concentrations the protoplasmic contents or cytoplasmic membrane became gradually coagulated, so that the leakage became progressively less. Electron micrographs of thin sections of bacteria taken after suitable dose treatments confirmed this view (Fig. 9.2). A similar pattern is found with hexachlorophene and *Bacillus megaterium*. However, Hugo & Bloomfield (1971a,b,c) in their studies on the mode of action of 2,2′-thiobis-(4-chlorophenol), Fentichlor, found a close correlation between bactericidal action on *E. coli* and *Staph. aureus* and ability to promote leakage of material absorbing at 260 nm. Bacteriostatic concentrations of the drug did not cause leakage.

Many solvents, including butanol, ethanol, toluene and phenylethanol, cause the release of intracellular constituents. The phenylethanol/*E. coli* interaction is reversible, suggesting that the structural integrity of the membrane is not seriously impaired.

Anionic detergents, such as sodium dodecyl sulphate (SDS), are generally less toxic to bacteria, although their target is also the cytoplasmic membrane. This may be due to the fact that in SDS and other anionic detergents the active ion is negatively charged and may be repelled by the negatively charged bacterial surface.

Non-ionic, surface-active agents are practically non-toxic to bacteria; indeed some, e.g. nonidet, are useful biochemical tools for preparing enzymically active bacterial membranes. Non-ionic agents have been shown to act synergistically when combined with various antibacterial compounds, but they also protect cells from phenols (see Chapter 3).

Ion-specific electrodes have allowed very accurate determinations of ion efflux from bacterial cells treated with membrane-active antimicrobial agents. Lambert & Hammond (1973) have concluded that the order of release of cell constituents from *E. coli* treated with 0.2 mmol/l cetrimide was K^+ and then PO_4^{3-}, followed by material absorbing at 260 nm. The release of K^+ was complete in 30 min.

It is clear that solvents and certain antibacterial agents promote leakage of ions and of labile nucleic acids and their component purines, pyrimidines, pentoses and inorganic phosphorus, and detection of all these substances is used to determine membrane damage. It is unlikely that this is a rapidly fatal process, and it is probably associated with bacteriostasis. As might be expected, this type of damage is often reparable.

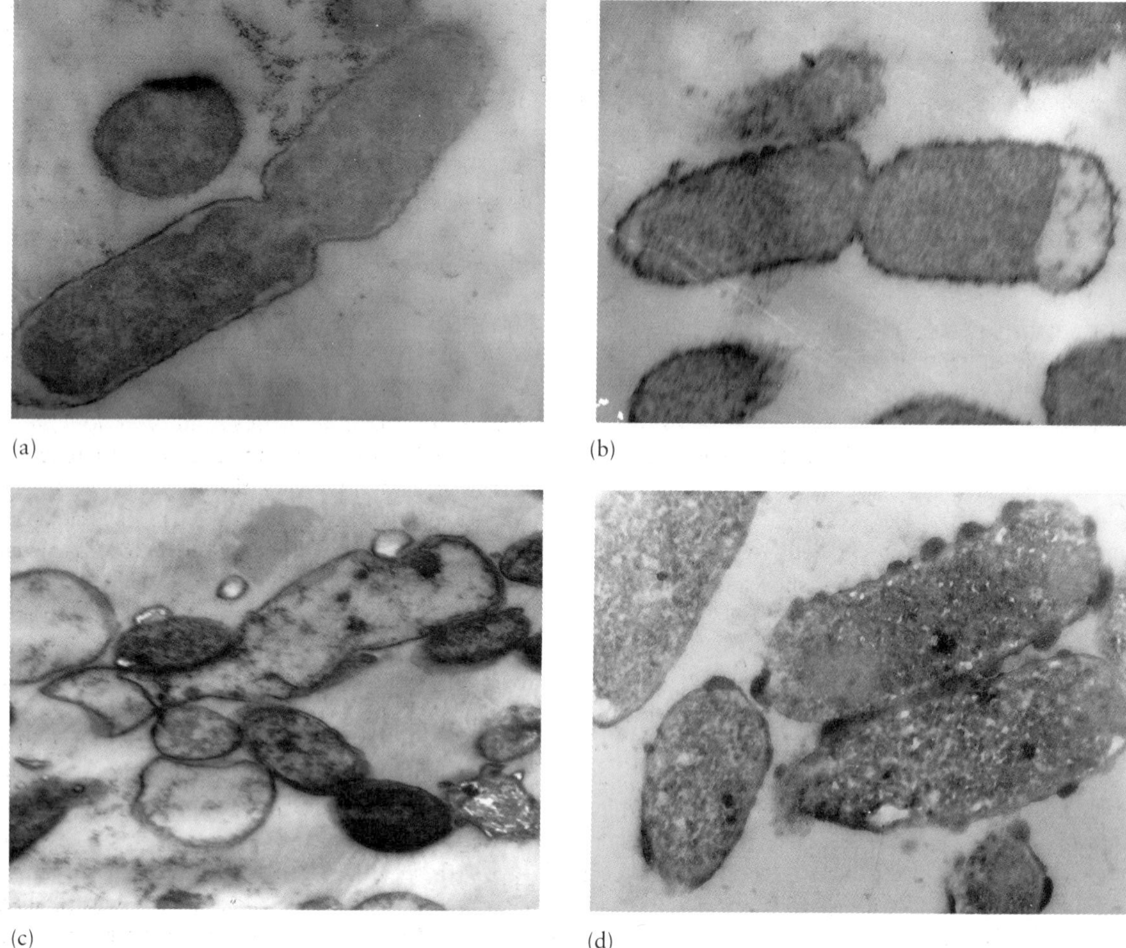

Fig. 9.2 Electron micrographs of thin sections of *Escherichia coli* in phosphate buffer (0.013 mol/l, pH 7.3) after treatment for 6 h with chlorhexidine diacetate at concentrations of: (a) 0 μg/ml; (b) 20 μg/ml; (c) 90 μg/ml; (d) 500 μg/ml (from Hugo & Longworth, 1965).

Salton (1968) has reviewed the mode of action of detergents on bacteria, and he concluded that the sequence of events following exposure of microbes was as follows.

1 Adsorption on to the cell, followed by a penetration into the largely porous cell wall.

2 Reactions with lipid/protein complexes of the cyto-plasmic membrane, leading to its disorganization.

3 Leakage of low molecular weight components from the cytoplasm.

4 Degradation of proteins and nucleic acids.

5 Wall lysis caused by autolytic enzymes.

It is very important, when considering these propositions and any other interaction of drugs with microorganisms, to bear in mind the difference in structure of walls of Gram-positive and Gram-negative bacteria, and especially the role of the outer layers of the walls of the latter group (see Section 9: Chapter 10A).

Glutaraldehyde (pentanedial), $CHO{\cdot}(CH_2)_3{\cdot}CHO$, which first found use as a tanning agent for leather and later as a fixative for tissue prior to embedding and sectioning for electron microscopy, was introduced as an antibacterial agent in 1962 and has been extensively studied (for comprehensive reviews, see Russell & Hopwood, 1976: Gorman *et al.*, 1980).

As might be imagined from a molecule containing two reactive groups, glutaraldehyde has widespread chemical reactivity, combining with $-NH_2$, $-COOH$ and thiol ($-SH$) groups and with many components of the cell which contain these groups. Wall, wall lipopolysaccharide, protein, nucleic acid and lipid have all been implicated and it is hard to decide, to date, which is the reaction (if there is only one) that causes the fatal lesion.

The fact that glutaraldehyde reacts with the ε-amino group of lysine, thus forming an internal protein cross-link, might mean that the function of membrane transport proteins and porins could be impaired. Larger concentrations must kill by a generalized reaction with the many reactive groups of structural and functional components of the cell. *o*-Phthalaldehyde (OPA) has been examined as an endoscope disinfectant (Alfa & Sitter, 1994) and may have a similar mode of action. This disinfectant was considered briefly in Chapter 2.

Other examples of work showing disinfectant-induced leakage of cell constituents include CTAB (Salton, 1951), tetrachlorosalicylanilide and *Staph. aureus* (Woodroffe & Wilkinson, 1966), chlorhexidine and *E. coli* and *Staph. aureus* (Hugo & Longworth, 1965; Russell, 1986; Chawner & Gilbert, 1989a,b; Fitzgerald *et al.*, 1989), phenol and *S. marcescens* (Kroll & Anagnostopoulos, 1981), polyhexamethylene biguanides and *E. coli* (Broxton *et al.*, 1983, 1984a,b) and phenoxyethanol and *E. coli* and *Ps. aeruginosa* (Fitzgerald *et al.*, 1992a,b).

5.2 Inhibition of energy processes

Any discussion on this topic must be linked with both uncoupling of oxidative phosphorylation and the chemiosmotic theory of membrane transport (Mitchell, 1968, 1970, 1972; Harold, 1972; Hamilton, 1975). Mitchell proposed that oxidative phosphorylation, adenosine triphosphate (ATP) synthesis, active transport and the maintenance of intracellular solute levels are powered by a proton-motive force, generated by metabolic oxidoreductions, which are apparent as chemical and electrical gradients or potential differences across the cytoplasmic membrane. It may be expressed in mathematical terms thus:

$$\Delta p = \Delta\psi - Z\Delta\text{pH}$$

where Δp is the proton-motive force, $\Delta\psi$ is the membrane electrical potential in mV, ΔpH is the transmembrane pH gradient and Z is a factor converting pH values to mV, having a value of 62 at 37°C. The expression $-Z\Delta\text{pH}$, therefore, is a pH difference expressed in mV. Typical reported experimental values of these potentials in bacteria at 37°C are 120mV for $\Delta\psi$ and −62mV for $Z\Delta\text{pH}$. Thus

$$\Delta p = 182\text{mV}$$

The proton-motive force may be measured by a pH meter or by measuring the distribution of a weak acid, such as dimethyloxazolidinedione, aspirin or benzoic acid, across the membrane; $\Delta\psi$ may be measured by the distribution of ions, such as K^+, dibenzyldimethylammonium or triphenylmethylphosphonium, by the application of the Nernst equation; ion distribution is measured spectroscopically or with ion-specific electrodes (Niven & Hamilton, 1974).

It will be recalled that the proton-motive force ($\Delta\psi - Z\Delta\text{pH}$) is said to be responsible for the synthesis of ATP as part of the process of oxidative phosphorylation.

It has been known almost from the beginning of this century that nitrophenols, especially 2,4-dinitrophenol (DNP), interfere with oxidative phosphorylation without inhibiting other metabolic processes (Simon, 1953). The name 'uncoupling agent' was coined for DNP, and later was applied to other compounds of similar activity, because they, like DNP, uncoupled oxidation from phosphorylation (Williamson & Metcalf, 1967).

Mitchell (1968, 1970, 1972) showed that DNP caused a backflow of protons across the bacterial and mitochondrial membrane, which resulted in a partial or total collapse of Δp. It was thought that the molecular properties associated with the ability to promote uncoupling were those of a weak acid with lipid solubility. The molecule dissolved in the lipid bilayer of the membrane and acted as a proton conductor by virtue of its ionizability. Since the discovery of this special property, other substances, some of them used as antibacterial agents, have been found to act in a similar manner; examples include Fentichlor and tetrachlorosalicylanilide.

Reviewing the above data, it is possible to see a general pattern of behaviour. The nitrophenols short-circuit the membrane, as it were, causing a rapid backflow of protons into the cell and hence the collapse of Δp: they do not cause leakage of cellular constituents and are active at concentrations of 10^{-6} mol/l. Such compounds are now also called proton ionophores.

Certain other phenolic compounds cause both leakage and collapse of Δp; it is often found that concentrations of 10^{-5} mol/l cause Δp collapse, whereas leakage is promoted by concentrations of the order of 10^{-4} mol/l.

It seemed worthwhile to examine the effect of a membrane-active, non-phenolic substance, such as a cationic detergent, which possesses antibacterial activity and promotes leakage of cytoplasmic constituents. Such a compound is CTAB, and Denyer & Hugo (1977) examined the effect of this extensively investigated compound on its ability to modify Δp.

Using *Staph. aureus*, it was shown that 18 μg/ml (5.3×10^{-5} mol/l) cetrimide caused the discharge of the pH component of Δp; 18 μg/ml was also the bacteriostatic concentration and the concentration that caused the maximum leakage of material absorbing at 260 nm. The results indicated that discharge of all or part of Δp was not the sole prerogative of uncoupling agents, and it became clear that this biochemical effect might be part of the general action of detergents.

From this, it followed that studies on the mode of action of those antibacterial agents which show evidence of membrane activity by traditional techniques, i.e. leakage of cell constituents, must be extended to investigate whether components of Δp are modified. These experimental systems are more difficult to set up; but to omit them and the results they may produce must always leave a doubt in the mind that the fundamental biochemical lesion has been missed (Hugo, 1978). Organic acids, such as sorbic acid, affect Δp and inhibit transport across the membrane, but they might also possess an additional, as yet unidentified, mechanism of action (Eklund, 1985; Sofos *et al.*, 1986; Russell & Hugo, 1988; Cherrington *et al.*, 1990; Russell & Chopra (1996).

5.2.1 Interference with membrane enzymes

Chlorhexidine has been claimed to be an inhibitor of both membrane-bound and soluble adenosine triphosphatase (ATPase) and also of net K^+ uptake in *Streptococcus faecalis*, while hexachlorophane inhibits part of the membrane-bound electron transport chain in *B. megaterium*. However, it is now believed that inhibition of membrane-bound ATPase is not a primary target of chlorhexidine action, since activity is inhibited only at high biguanide concentrations (Chopra *et al.*, 1987; Kuyyakanond & Quesnel, 1992). One explanation of the phenomenon is that chlorhexidine phosphate is very insoluble and may have acted as an ATPase inhibitor by precipitating its substrate!

6 Interactions with the cytoplasm

There are four targets for antibacterial drugs: the cytoplasm itself, cytoplasmic enzymes, the nucleic acids and the ribosomes. Hugo (1965a, 1967) has reviewed the first two of these aspects in considerable detail, but a few of the main points are given below.

6.1 Irreversible coagulation of cytoplasmic constituents

This drastic lesion is usually seen at drug concentrations far higher than those causing general lysis or leakage. It was the first cytological effect to be reported and so most antiseptics were classified as general protoplasmic poisons or as protein precipitants. Indeed, at concentrations used in many practical disinfection procedures, this is undoubtedly the mechanism of rapid killing, the more subtle and more slowly fatal effects being completely masked.

The cytoplasmic components most likely to be coagulated or denatured are proteins and nucleic acids; most studies have been made on the former. Functionally, proteins are of two main kinds in living cells: structural and enzymic. The high specificity of enzymes is due to their unique surface contours and to the distribution of charges on this surface. The latter arise from residual charges, on the carboxylic acid or amino groups of the constituent amino acids, that are left after peptide-bond formation. It is not difficult to imagine that a derangement of this uniquely contoured and electrically charged unit can upset its function.

As early as 1901, Meyer showed that the degree of antibacterial action of phenols was proportional to their distribution between water and protein, thus suggesting that protein was a prime target.

Cooper (1912) came to a similar conclusion and decided that phenols destroy the protein structure within the cell. Bancroft & Richter (1931) actually observed a coagulation of cell protein in *B. megaterium* and *K. aerogenes*, using ultraviolet microscopy.

Three main methods are available for studying protoplasmic coagulation—light and electron microscopy, light-scattering and direct observation of cytoplasm obtained from smashed cells. Examples of studies by electron microscopy include those of Salton *et al.* (1951) and Dawson *et al.* (1953) (with CTAB) on whole cells treated with antibacterial compounds, and those of Hugo & Longworth (1966) (with chlorhexidine) and Bringmann (1953) (with chlorine, bromine, iodine, Cu^{2+}, Ag^{+} and hydrogen peroxide) on thin sections. Hugo & Longworth (1966) found a correlation between the appearance of thin sections and cytoplasmic leakage. Thus, at the concentration which caused maximum leakage, electron micrographs of thin sections showed a significant loss of electron-dense material; at higher concentrations, which promoted no leakage, due to a general coagulation and sealing in of labile protoplasmic constituents, the electron micrographs showed a dense granular cytoplasm, differing markedly in appearance from that seen in untreated cells (Fig. 9.2).

An interesting technique for studying protoplasmic coagulation is based upon protoplast formation and the fact that rod-shaped cells yield globular protoplasts in isotonic media. If this operation is carried out on cells that have been treated with a coagulant or fixative, a rod-shaped protoplast is produced, which, if coagulation is severe, does not undergo lysis or osmotic explosion on subsequent dilution of the medium (Tomcsik, 1955; Hugo & Longworth, 1964; Daltrey & Hugo, 1974). Coagulation of protein may affect the light-scattering properties of cells, and this is a sensitive method of assessing changes in treated bacteria.

Yet another method consists of disrupting the cells and investigating the action of antiseptics on cell-free extracts. Although this system is an artificial one, and the relative concentrations of the protoplasmic constituents change and suffer enzymatic degradation, it gives some indication of the order of concentration required to produce coagulation. Thus, Hugo & Longworth (1966) found that protein and nucleic acid were precipitated from cell-free preparations of *E. coli* at concentrations of chlorhexidine far higher than those causing leakage.

6.2 Effects on metabolism and enzymes

There was a general feeling among early workers that there existed in bacteria a biocide-sensitive enzyme. The reviews of Rahn & Schroeder (1941) and Roberts & Rahn (1946) deal with this notion. Other early work in the field was reviewed by Hugo (1957). Some vindication of these early views has emerged with the identification of –SH enzymes as targets for a variety of biocides. Examples are silver salts (Russell & Hugo, 1994), Cu^{2+}, arsenical compounds, bronopol (Stretton & Manson, 1973), hypochlorous acid (Knox *et al.*, 1948) and the isothiazolones (Fuller *et al.*, 1985; Collier *et al.*, 1990).

6.3 Effects on nucleic acids

There are a number of antibiotics that affect the biosynthesis and functioning of nucleic acids. Among the non-antibiotic antibacterial drugs, the main compounds affecting these targets have been identified; these are the acridine dyes, formaldehyde, phenylethanol, hypochlorites and halamines (Worley & Williams, 1988).

6.3.1 *Acridine dyes*

Acridine dyes, first introduced into medicine as trypanocidal agents, have been used extensively as antibacterial agents and a large amount of work has been carried out on their mode on action. As with the triphenylmethane (TPM) dyes, it was realized early that the cation was the active ion. McIlwain (1941) showed that nucleic acids antagonized the antibacterial action of acridine dyes, and Ferguson & Thorne (1946), after studying the effect of a series of acridine compounds on growth and respiration of *E. coli*, concluded that they inhibited reactions closely connected with synthetic processes. It emerged that, if acridine dyes were only 33% ionized as a cation, there was very little antibacterial action, and for really high activity 98–100% of the molecules should exist in the cationic form. Other studies showed that the flat area of the molecule should be from 0.38 to 0.48 nm^2. Albert (1966) has reviewed acridine chemistry comprehensively.

Studies of deoxyribonucleic acid (DNA) binding with proflavine showed a first-order reaction, which equilibrated with one molecule of proflavine binding to every four or five nucleotides. There was also a slower reaction of higher order, in which a 1:1 binding occurred (Peacocke & Skerrett, 1956; Waring, 1965; Blake & Peacocke, 1968). These interactions also involved marked spectral, viscosity and melting-temperature changes.

From a review of available binding data, Lerman proposed (1961) and later elaborated (1964a,b) an intercalation model, in which it was suggested that proflavine was bound by DNA, through the two primary amino groups being held by ionic links to two phosphoric acid residues and the flat acridine ring system being linked on the purine and pyrimidine residues by van der Waals forces. Pritchard *et al.* (1966) and Blake & Peacocke (1968) have suggested an alternative mechanism, in which the acridine ring lies between two adjacent bases on the same polynucleotide, with the primary amino groups now lying close to the phosphoric acid residues of the DNA. The intercalation theory is compatible with the finding of McIlwain (1941) that nucleic acids antagonize the action of acridines, and with the observation, summarized in Albert (1966), that molecular size and shape are of importance in determining the relative potency of acridines. Pritchard *et al.* (1966) and Blake & Peacocke (1968) made the observation that acridines inhibit synthetic processes (Ferguson & Thorne, 1946).

Ribonucleic acid (RNA) polymerase has also been identified as a target for acridines in cell-free preparations from *E. coli*. Nicholson & Peacocke (1965) suggested that inhibitory acridine molecules, which included proflavine and 9-aminoacridine, occupy sites on the polymerase which normally bind nucleoside triphosphates or the bases in the DNA molecule during copying. Waring (1965) discussed the ability of 23 drugs, including proflavine, to inhibit incorporation of adenosine monophosphate into RNA.

Although the main site of activity of acridines is DNA and RNA polymerase, it is possible that other, possibly secondary, lesions may be induced in bacterial cells under the influence of these compounds. Such secondary sites are discussed by Foster & Russell (1971).

6.3.2 *Formaldehyde and formaldehyde condensates*

Grossman *et al.* (1961) have shown that a reasonably specific reaction occurs between nucleotides and formaldehyde. The amino groups of the purine and pyrimidine rings have been cited as likely sites for the interaction. Collins & Guild (1968) have shown that formaldehyde binding to DNA at 100°C and pH 8 is irreversible. However, Staehelin (1958) found that binding with RNA was reversible if it had not proceeded for longer than 2 h; after 2 h the reaction was slowly reversible only after dialysis. The first reaction was thought to be due to formation of stable methylene bridges, $-NH{\cdot}CH_2NH-$, between bases containing amino groups. Clearly, reactions of this type could occur with cellular amino groups other than those in the nucleic acid molecule.

Formaldehyde condensates have been reviewed by Rossmore & Sondossi (1988).

6.3.3 *Phenylethanol*

Phenylethanol has already been referred to as a membrane-active compound (Woldringh, 1973), but it has also been shown to inhibit initiation of replication at high concentrations (Lark & Lark, 1966). Richardson & Leach (1969) and Richardson *et al.* (1969) re-examined the action of phenylethanol on *Bacillus subtilis*. They concluded that any effects of the drug on DNA function were secondary to its effects on membrane integrity and transport of RNA and DNA precursors into the cells.

6.3.4 *The halogens*

Hypochlorites have been in use as disinfectants since 1774. Chlorine and hypochlorous acid chlorinate and oxidize cell components and, at high concentrations, this indiscriminate chemical onslaught is the general mode of action.

By working with smaller doses, it is possible to dissect out modes of action more precisely. Thus Knox *et al.* (1948) showed that the aldolase of *E. coli* was inhibited by hypochlorite, halazone and succinchloramide. McKenna & Davies (1988) found that, at 50 µmol/l HOCl (≡2.6 parts/10^6), growth was completely inhibited in 5min. Synthesis of DNA decreased by 96%, whereas protein synthesis decreased by only 10–30%. Bacterial membrane disruption and extensive protein degradation were not observed at concentrations below 5 mmol/l (≡2.60 parts/10^6), DNA synthesis appearing to be the sensitive target.

Iodine was introduced as a disinfectant in 1839. Its mode of action differs from that of chlorine in that the hypoiodites are not active and its action is due to direct iodination or oxidation of essential molecules in the microbial cell. Bringmann (1953) has presented electron-microscopic evidence that the mode of action of chlorine is different from that of iodine. Halamines have been reviewed in depth by Worley & Williams (1988).

6.4 Ribosomes

Ribosomes are associated with the formation of peptides from amino acids, ordered by messenger RNA and assembled by transfer RNA. This process is a singular target for many antibiotics and there are some non-antibiotic antibacterial agents whose target lies here.

Treatment of cells with toluene releases ribosomes (Jackson & De Moss, 1965), but this may be taken as a manifestation of the extent of membrane damage by this compound such that a unit the size of a ribosome could be released.

Ethylenediamine tetraacetic acid is a specific chelator of certain metals, including Mg^{2+}, necessary for the integrity of the 50S and 30S ribosome units in prokaryotes. It is not regarded as a primary antibacterial agent, although it is used in conjunction with certain antiseptics to enhance their activity, especially against Gram-negative organisms (Russell, 1971; Leive, 1974). Its possible action on ribosome structure must be borne in mind when it is present in antibacterial systems.

Hydrogen peroxide dissociates the 30S and 50S subunits of the 70S ribosome in *E. coli* (Nakamura & Tamaoki, 1968). This process is 80% reversible upon adding to 10 mmol/l Mg^{2+}, providing the concentration of hydrogen peroxide has not exceeded 0.1%. *p*-Chloromercuribenzoate (0.5 mmol/l) dissociates the 100S ribosomes of *E. coli* into 70S monomers (Wang & Matheson, 1967). This reaction can be reversed by 2-mercaptoethanol but not by Mg^{2+}.

The ribosome cannot be considered a prime target for the specific selective action of any known non-antibiotic antibacterial agent, although it may be destroyed by some chemical agents.

7 Genotypic resistance to disinfectants

Resistance to certain metal ions has been discovered in the penicillinase plasmid of *Staph. aureus* by Novick & Roth (1968), who found that the resistance markers conferred an increase in resistance, ranging from three to 100-fold, depending on the ion involved. Separate genetic loci for resistance to arsenate, arsenite, lead, cadmium, mercuric and bismuth ions were demonstrated. These workers did not attempt to identify the biochemical mechanisms associated with this resistance, but it is interesting to note that a common target for all the resistant ions listed is the –SH group.

A most interesting mechanism for mercury-resistant, plasmid-bearing (P^+) strains of *E. coli*, *Staph. aureus* and *Ps. aeruginosa* involves the biochemical conversion of Hg^{2+} into a volatile organomercury compound (Summers & Lewis, 1973). These workers and Vaituzis *et al.* (1975) have summarized other examples of microorganisms that can produce volatile mercury compounds from Hg^{2+}. Further investigation might reveal that other volatile compounds are produced by strains of microbes resistant to metal ions. Reviews have been published by Foster (1983), Russell (1985), Lyon & Skurray (1987), Chopra (1988), Russell & Gould (1988), Silver & Misra (1988) and Russell & Chopra (1996).

Thornley & Yudkin (1959a,b) and Sinai & Yudkin (1959a,b,c) studied the origin of bacterial resistance to proflavine. They concluded that no single factor determines drug resistance for a single species/single drug combination.

Russell (1972) showed that strains of *Ps. aeruginosa*, with or without R-factors 1822 and 3425, were equally resistant to glutaraldehyde, chloroxylenol solution, Lysol, chlorhexidine, CTAB and phenylmercuric nitrate, suggesting that transferable drug resistance was not occurring with these non-antibiotic antimicrobial agents. Plasmid-bearing strains of *Ps. aeruginosa* have shown transferable drug resistance to antibiotics (Roe *et al.*, 1971). This aspect is discussed in more detail in Chapter 10B.

8 Conversion of a toxic substance to a non-toxic derivative

Many organisms are able to decompose aromatic compounds, many of which are used as disinfectants (Rogoff, 1961; Evans, 1963; Hugo, 1965b; Ribbons, 1965; Gibson, 1968; Beveridge, 1975; Sleat & Robinson, 1984). Beveridge & Hugo (1964) examined the ability of some Gram-negative, non-sporing rods, mainly pseudomonads, to use aromatic compounds, many of them disinfectants, as a sole carbon source. *p*-Cresol, phenol, benzoic acid, *p*-hydroxybenzoic acid and salicylic acid were readily attacked. The metabolic versatility of *Vibrio* 01, an organism now thought to be *Acinetobacter calcoaceticus*, in decomposing many compounds, including some traditional disinfectants, is amply demonstrated in the papers of Fewson (1967) and Beveridge & Tall (1969). Hugo & Foster (1964) found a strain of *Ps. aeruginosa* able to utilize methyl- and propyl-*p*-hydroxybenzoates as sole sources of carbon. Grant (1967) showed a similar capability with *K. aerogenes*. It is clear that this pattern of resistance can be of practical significance, for the hydroxybenzoates were once used as preservatives in eye-drops (Hugo, 1991).

9 Changes in access to the vulnerable site: a possible involvement of lipid

The role of cellular lipid in resistance has attracted considerable interest in recent years. The first hint that bacterial lipid was involved in determining the relative resistance of bacteria to detergents was provided by an experiment of Dyar & Ordal (1946). A strain of *Staph. aureus* with a high lipid content showed exceptional sensitivity to changes in electrophoretic mobility, induced by cetylpyridinium chloride, and acquired a greater apparent negative charge in the presence of SDS.

Following serial subculture, Chaplin (1951) obtained a 43-fold increase in the resistance of a strain of *E. coli* and a 200-fold increase in the resistance of *Serr. marcescens* to a series of QACs. He was unable to demonstrate resistance in *Staph. aureus*. Fischer & Larose (1952) found the adaptive process to be dependent on pH. Thus greater resistance was acquired more rapidly if the serial subcultures were performed at pH 6.8 rather than at pH 7.7. The effect of pH was thought to be on ionization of QAC and hence on drug uptake. In a further paper, Chaplin (1952) stained cells with Sudan Black B, carried out electrophoretic-mobility studies and showed an increase in the lipid content of the resistant cells of *Serr. marcescens*. Strong support for the existence of this lipid and its involvement in resistance came when lipase-treated cells lost their resistance.

Lowick & James (1957) trained *K. aerogenes* to grow in the presence of crystal violet and demonstrated by electrophoretic techniques that the surface of the resistant cells was predominantly lipid, whereas in the case of untrained cells the surface was predominantly polysaccharide. Hugo & Stretton (1966) grew microorganisms in nutrient broth containing glycerol and increased their lipid content. These organisms showed an increased resistance to penicillins. Hugo & Franklin (1968) studied the effect of this lipid enhancement on the resistance to phenols of the Oxford strain of *Staph. aureus*. They used a series of 4-*n*-alkylphenols from phenol to hexylphenol. Enhanced cellular lipid protected the cells from the inhibitory action of only pentylphenol and *n*-hexylphenol. This protection conferred a non-specific blanketing mechanism in which the amyl- and hexylphenols are locked at the interface between the cellular lipid and the aqueous environment. In a similar study, Hamilton (1968) found no significant increase in resistance to tetrachlorosalicylanilide, tribromosalicylanilide, trichloroacetanilide, monochlorophenoxysalicylanilide or hexachlorophene in a glycerol-grown culture of the same organism.

Lipid depletion in *Staph. aureus* and *E. coli* was achieved by Hugo *et al.* (1971) and Hugo & Davidson (1973) by growing biotin-deficient organisms. Only a slight decrease in resistance to a series of phenols and alkyltrimethylammonium bromides was found in both organisms.

Vaczi has published a monograph on the biological role of bacterial lipids, which includes a comprehensive review on lipid content and resistance to both antibiotic and non-antibiotic antimicrobial agents (Vaczi, 1973); see also Chapter 10A.

9.1 Special role of the Gram-negative cell wall in resistance

Gram-negative, rod-shaped bacteria possess lipoprotein and lipopolysaccharide layers outside the peptidoglycan layer, which afford protection from antimicrobial agents. The lipopolysaccharide may be partly removed by EDTA, which results in an increased susceptibility to both antibiotic and non-antibiotic drugs (Russell, 1971; Haque & Russell, 1974a,b; Leive, 1974).

Sanderson *et al.* (1974) and Nikaido (1976) have produced evidence, using mutants of *Salmonella typhimurium* deficient in the carbohydrate

Table 9.1 Cellular targets for non-antibiotic antibacterial drugs.

	Non-antibiotic antimicrobial agents																			
Target or reaction attacked	Acridine dyes	Alcohols	Anilides (TCS, TCC)	Bronopol	Chlorhexidine	Copper(II) salts	Ethylene oxide	Formaldehyde	Glutaraldehyde	Hexachlorophane	Hydrogen peroxide	Hypochlorites, chlorine releasers	Iodine	Mercury(II) salts, organic mercurials	Phenols	β-Propiolactone	Quaternary ammonium compounds	Silver(I) salts	Sulphur dioxide, sulphites	*iso*-Thiazolones
Cell wall								+				+		+	−					
Cytoplasmic membrane																				
Action on membrane potentials			+							+					−					
Action on membrane enzymes																				
Electron-transport chain										+										
Adenosine triphosphate					+	+	+													
Enzymes with thiol groups				+			+		+		+	+	+	+		+		+	−	+
Action on general membranes permeability		+	+		+										−−		+			
Cytoplasm																				
General coagulation					+++	+++			++	+++				+++	−−		+++	+++		
Ribosomes											+			+						
Nucleic acids	+											+								
Thiol groups				+		+	+		+		+	+	+	+		+		+		
Amino groups							+	++	+			+				+			−	+
Highly reactive compounds							+		+			+				+				+

Pluses indicating activity, which appear in several columns for a given compound, demonstrate the multiple actions of the compound concerned. This activity is nearly always concentration-dependent, and the number of pluses indicate the order of concentration at which the effect is elicited, i.e. +, elicited at low concentrations; +++, elicited at high concentrations.
When a plus appears in only one target column, this is the only known site of action of the drug.

components of the lipopolysaccharide, that carbohydrate may play a role in selective exclusions; see also Chapter 10A.

For further reviews, see Hancock (1984), Nikaido & Vaara (1985) and Russell & Chopra (1996).

10 Summary

A summary of the data presented in this chapter is provided as a table (Table 9.1) and diagrammatically (Fig. 9.3).

11 Appendix

The treatment in this chapter has been to examine the action of drugs on each defined structure in the cell and also to examine the role of the structures in resistance. When the mode of action of a new antimicrobial drug is to be elucidated, the approaches as outlined in the chapter are followed systematically to seek the prime target or targets. In this appendix, selected examples of such studies on individual compounds or families of compounds are given to illustrate the experimental approaches used. The references are given in an abbreviated form and may duplicate some given in the main reference section, but are included for completion for those interested in individual compounds.

Mechanisms of antibacterial action are the subject of Technical Series Monograph No. 27, published by the Society of Applied Bacteriology (Denyer & Hugo, 1991), and a theoretical discussion is provided in Russell & Chopra (1996).

Acids

Acids: liphophilic, acetic, benzoic, propionate, sor-

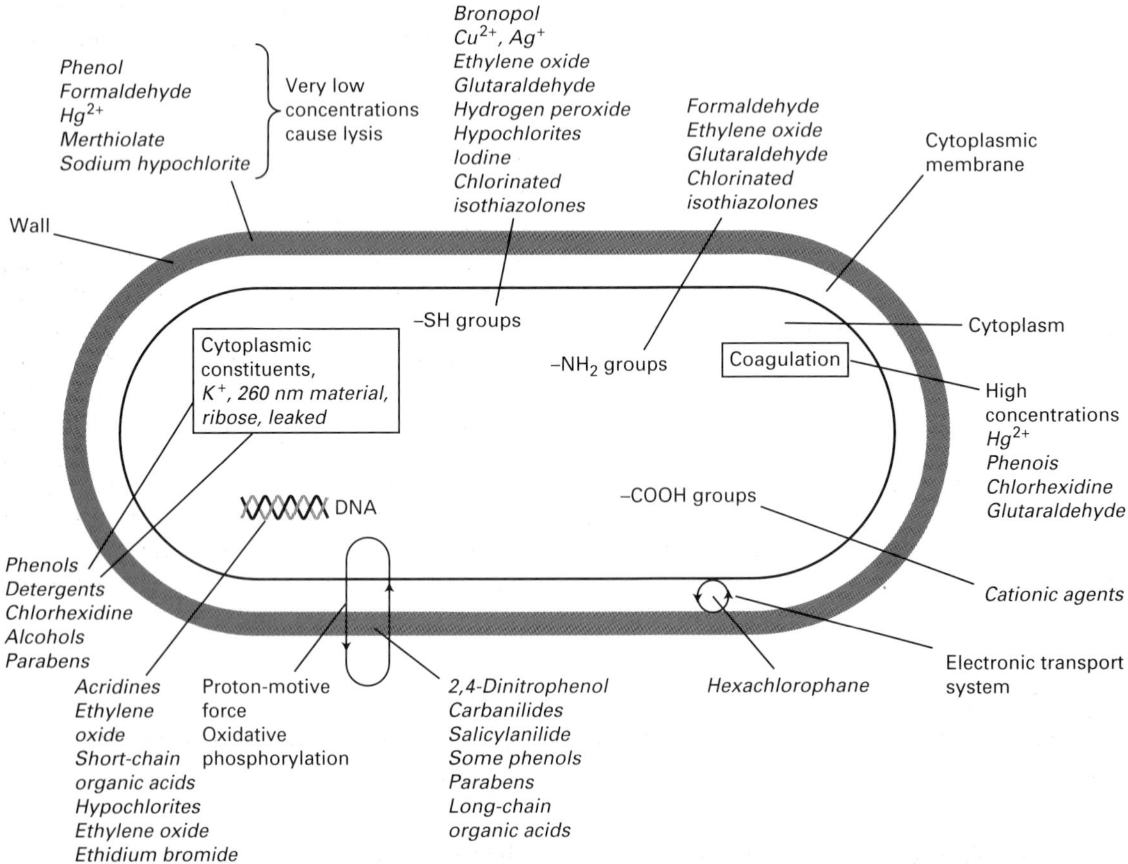

Fig. 9.3 Diagram showing main targets for non-antibiotic antibacterial agents.

bate, caprylic: a review. Freese, E., Sheu, C.W. & Galliers, E. (1973) *Nature, London*, **241**, 321–325; Cherrington, C.A., Hinton, M., Mead, G.C. & Chopra, I. (1991) *Advances in Microbial Physiology*, **32**, 87–108; Eklund, T. (1985) *Journal of General Microbiology*, **131**, 73–76; Russell, J.B. (1992) *Journal of Applied Bacteriology*, **73**, 363–370; Sofos, J.N. *et al.* (1986) *International Journal of Food Microbiology*, **3**, 1–17.

Acridines

Albert, A. (1966) *The Acridines: Their Preparation, Physical, Chemical and Biological Properties and Uses*, 2nd edn. London: Edward Arnold; Waring, M.J. (1966) Cross linking and intercalation in nucleic acids. In *Biochemical Studies of Antimicrobial Drugs*, 16th Symposium of the Society for General Microbiology, p. 235. Cambridge: Cambridge University Press; Albert, A. (1973) *Selective Toxicity*, 5th edn, pp. 282. London: Chapman & Hall.

Alcohols

Ingram, L.O. & Buttke, T.M. (1984) *Advances in Microbial Physiology*, **25**, 253.

Alexidine

Chawner, J.A. & Gilbert, P. (1989) *Journal of Applied Bacteriology*, **66**, 243, 253.

Benzalkonium chloride

Brown, M.R.W. & Tomlinson, E. (1979) *Journal of Pharmaceutical Sciences*, **68**, 146; Lang, M. & Rye, R.M. (1972) *Journal of Pharmacy and Pharmacology*, **24**, 219.

Benzoic acid

Bosund, I. (1962) *Advances in Food Research*, **11**, 331–353 (a review); Krebs, H.A. *et al.* (1983) *Biochemical Journal*, 214, 657.

Bronopol (2-bromo-2-nitropropan-1,3-diol)

Stretton, R.J. & Manson, T.W. (1973) *Journal of Applied Bacteriology*, **36**, 61; Bowman, W.H. & Stretton, R.J. (1972) *Antimicrobial Agents and Chemotherapy*, **2**, 504; Shepherd, J.A., Waigh, R.D. & Gilbert, P. (1988) *Antimicrobial Agents and Chemotherapy*, **32**, 1693–1698.

Cetrimide, cetavlon

Salton, M.R.J. (1950) *Australian Journal of Scientific Research*, **3**, 45; (1951) *Journal of General Microbiology*, **5**; 391; Salton, M.R.J. *et al.* (1981) *Journal of General Microbiology*, **5**, 405; Hugo, W.B. & Denyer, S.P. (1977) *Journal of Pharmacy and Pharmacology*, **29**, 66P; McQuillen, K. (1950) *Biochimica et Biophysica Acta*, **5**, 463; Lambert, P.A. & Hammond, S.M. (1973) *Biochemical and Biochemical Research Communications*, **54**, 796; Smith, A.R. *et al.* (1975) *Journal of Applied Bacteriology*, **38**, 143; Salt, W.G. & Wiseman, D. (1968) *Journal of Pharmacy and Pharmacology*, **20**, 145; (1970) **22**, 261, 767; Dawson *et al.* (1953) *Journal of Pathology and Bacteriology*, **66**, 513.

Chlorhexidine (Hibitane)

Hugo, W.B. & Longworth, A.R. (1964) *Journal of Pharmacy and Pharmacology*, **16**, 62, 751; (1965) **17**, 28; (1966) **18**, 569; Hugo, W.B. & Daltrey, D.C. (1974) *Microbios*, **11**, 119, 131; Elferinck, J.G.R. & Booij, H.L. (1974) *Biochemical Pharmacology*, **23**, 1413; Davies, A. *et al.* (1968) *Journal of Applied Bacteriology*, **31**, 448; Harold, F.M. *et al.* (1969) *Biochemical et Biophysica Acta*, **183**, 129; Rye, R.M. & Wiseman, D. (1964/5) *Journal of Pharmacy and Pharmacology*, **16**, 516; **17**, 295; Kuyyakanond, T. & Quesnel, L.B. (1992) *FEMS Microbiology Letters*, **100**, 211; Barrett-Bee, K. *et al.* (1994) *FEMS Microbiology Letters*, **119**, 249; Chopra, I. *et al.* (1987) *Journal of Antimicrobial Chemotherapy*, **19**, 743.

Dequalinium, dequadin

Hugo, W.B. & Frier, M. (1969) *Applied Microbiology*, **17**, 18.

Dipropalmidine

Woodside, W. (1973) *Microbios*, **8**, 23; Richards,

R.M.E. *et al. Journal of Pharmaceutical Sciences*, **82**, 975.

Dodecyldiethanolamine

Lambert, P.A. & Smith, A.R.W. (1974) *Proceedings of the Society of General Microbiology*, **1**, 49; (1976) *Microbios*, **15**, 191; **17**, 35.

Ethylenediaminetetra-acetic acid

Smith, G. (1970) *Journal of Medical Laboratory Technology*, **27**, 203; Haque, H. & Russell, A.D. (1974) *Antibiotic Agents and Chemotherapy*, **6**, 200; Dankert, J. & Schut, I.K. (1976) *Journal of Hygiene, Cambridge*, **76**, 11.

Fatty acids

Galbraith, H. & Miller, T.B. (1973) *Journal of Applied Bacteriology*, **36**, 635, 647, 659; Cherington, C.A. *et al.* (1991) *Advances in Microbial Physiology*, **32**, 87.

Fentichlor

Hugo, W.B. & Bloomfield, S.F. (1971) *Journal of Applied Bacteriology*, **34**, 557, 569, 579; Bloomfield, S.F. (1974) *Journal of Applied Bacteriology*, **37**, 117.

Formaldehyde

Neely, W.B. (1963) *Journal of Bacteriology*, **85**, 1028, 1420; **86**, 445; (1966) *Journal of General Microbiology*, **45**, 187; Muller, A. (1900) *Archives of Hygiene*, **89**, 363; Rossmore, H.W. & Sondossi, M. (1988) *Advances in Applied Microbiology*, **33**, 223 (includes condensates).

Formaldehyde condensates

Rossmore, H.W. & Sondrossi, I. (1988) *Advances in Applied Microbiology*, **33**, 223.

Glutaraldehyde

Russell, A.D. & Hopwood, D. (1976) *Progress in Medicinal Chemistry*, **13**, 271 (a review); Gorman, S.P., Scott, E.M. & Russell, A.D. (1980) *Journal of Applied Bacteriology*, **48**, 161–190 (a review).

Halamines

Worley, S.D. & Williams, D.E. (1988) *CRC Critical Review of Environmental Control*, **18**, 133.

Halogens

Chlorine

Venkobachar, C. *et al.* (1975, 1977), *Water Research*, **9**, 119; **11**, 727; Khan, A.U. & Kash, M. (1994) *Proceedings of the National Academy of Sciences US*, **91**, 12362; Shih, K.L. & Lederburg, J. (1976) *Journal of Bacteriology*, **125**, 934.

Iodine

Nyiri, W. & DuBois, L. (1931) *Journal of the American Pharmaceutical Association*, **20**, 546; Wyss, D. & Strandskox, F.S. (1945) *Archives of Biochemistry*, **6**, 261.

Hexachlorophane

Gerhart, P. *et al.* (1971) *Journal of Bacteriology*, **108**, 482, 492, 501; (1974) *Antimicrobial Agents and Chemotherapy*, **6**, 712; Lee, C.R. & Garner, T.R. (1975) *Journal of Pharmacy and Pharmacology*, **27**, 694.

8-Hydroxyquinoline, oxine

Rubbo, S.D. *et al.* (1950) *British Journal of Experimental Pathology*, **31**, 425; Albert, A. *et al.* (1953) *British Journal of Experimental Pathology*, **34**, 119; (1954), **34**; Albert, A. (1959) Metal binding agents in chemotherapy: the activation of metals by chelation. In *The Strategy of Chemotherapy*, 8th Symposium of the Society for General Microbiology, p. 112. Cambridge: Cambridge University Press, (a review).

Parabens

Furr, J.R. & Russell, A.D. (1972) *Microbios*, **5**, 189, 237; **6**, 47; Freese, E. *et al.* (1973) *Nature*,

London, **241**, 321; Freese, E. & Levin, B.C. *Developments in Industrial Microbiology*, **19**, 207; Eklund, T. (1985) *Journal of General Microbiology*, **131**, 73; Ness, I.F. & Eklund, T. (1983) *Journal of Applied Bacteriology*, **54**, 237; Russell, A.D. *et al.* (1985) *International Journal of Pharmaceutics*, **27**, 263.

Peroxygens (hydrogen peroxide, peracetic acid)

Baldry, M.G.C. (1983) *Journal of Applied Bacteriology*, **54**, 417; (1984), **57**, 499; (1985), **58**, 315; Davis, B.D. *et al.* (1990) *Microbiology*, 4th edn. London: Harper & Row.

Phenols

Hugo, W.B. (1956) *Journal of General Microbiology*, **15**, 315; Judis, J. *et al.* (1962) *Journal of Pharmaceutical Sciences*, **51**, 261; (1963) **52**, 126; (1964) **53**, 196; (1965) **54**, 417, 1436; James, A.T. *et al.* (1964) *Biochimica et Biophysica Acta*, **79**, 351; Bean, H.S. & Das, A. (1966) *Journal of Pharmacy and Pharmacology*, **18**, 1075: Pullman, J.E. & Reynolds, B.L. (1965) *Australasian Journal of Pharmacy*, **46**, 580; Hugo, W.B. & Bowen, J.G. (1973) *Microbios*, **8**, 139; Beckett, A.H. *et al.* (1959) *Journal of Pharmacy and Pharmacology*, **11**, 360; Gilbert, P. & Brown, M.R.W. (1978) *Journal of Bacteriology*, **133**, 1066; Suter, C.M. (1941) *Chemical Reviews*, **28**, 269; Kroll, R.G. & Anagnostopoulos, G.D. (1981) *Journal of General Microbiology*, **50**, 139.

2-Phenoxyethanol, phenoxetol

Hugo, W.B. (1956) *Journal of General Microbiology*, **15**, 315; Gilbert, P., Beveridge, E.G. & Crone, P.B. (1977) *Microbios*, **19**, 17, 125; **20**, 29.

Phenylethanol

Silver, S. & Wendt, L. (1976) *Journal of Bacteriology*, **93**, 560; Richardson, A.G. & Leach, F.R. (1969) *Biochimica et Biophysica Acta*, **174**, 264, 276; Lang, M. & Rye, R.M. (1972) *Journal of Pharmacy and Pharmacology*, **24**, 219.

Polyethoxyalkyl phenols, tritons

Allwood, M.C. & Lamikanra, A. (1976) *Microbios Letters*, **3**, 131; (1997) *Journal of Applied Bacteriology*, **42**, 379, 387.

Polyhexamethylene biguanides

Davies, A. *et al.* (1968) *Journal of Applied Bacteriology*, **31**, 448; Ikeda, T. *et al.* (1983) *Biochimica et Biophysica Acta*, **735**, 380; Broxton, P. *et al.* (1983) *Journal of Applied Bacteriology*, **54**, 345; (1984), **54**, 115; *Microbios*, **40**, 187; **41**, 15; Gilbert, P. *et al.* (1990) *Journal of Applied Bacteriology*, **69**, 585, 593.

Silver

Russell, A.D. & Hugo, W.B. (1994) Antimicrobial activity of silver. *Progress in Medicinal Chemistry*, **39**, 351–370.

Sorbic acid

Bell, T.A. *et al.* (1959) *Journal of Bacteriology*, **77**, 573; Gooding, C.M. *et al.* (1955) *Food Research*, **20**, 639; Palleroni, N.J. & de Prinz, M.R.J. (1960) *Nature, London*, **185**, 688; York, G.K. & Vaughn, R.H. (1955) *Bacteriological Proceedings*, **55**, 20; Eklund T. (1985) *Journal of General Microbiology*, **131**, 73; Salmond, C.Y. *et al.* (1984) *Journal of General Microbiology*, **130**, 2845.

Sulphur dioxide, sulphites and bisuphites

Hammond, S.M. & Carr, J.G. (1976) The antimicrobial activity of SO_2. In *Inhibition and Inactivation of Vegetative Micro-organisms* (eds Skinner, F.A. & Hugo, W.B.) Society for Applied Bacteriology Symposium Series No. 5, pp. 89–110. London: Academic Press. (A review.)

iso-Thiazolones

Fuller, S.J. (1986) PhD thesis, University of Nottingham; Fuller, S.J. *et al.* (1985) *Letters in Applied Microbiology*, **1**, 13; Collier, P.J. *et al.* (1990) *Journal of Applied Bacteriology*, **69**, 569, 578; Collier, P.J. *et al.* (1991) *International Journal* *of Pharmaceutics*, **66**, 201–220; Chapman, J.S. & Diehl, M.A. (1995) *Journal of Applied Bacteriology*, **78**, 134–141.

Tetrachlorosalicylanilide (TCS)

Hamilton, W.A. (1968) *Journal of General Microbiology*, **50**, 441.

Triclosan

Regos, J. & Hitz, H.R. (1974) *Zeitschrift für Bakteriologie, A*, **226**, 390.

12 References

Albert, A. (1966) *The Acridines*, 2nd edn. London: Edward Arnold.

Alfa, M.J. & Sitter, D.L. (1994) In-hospital evaluation of orthophthalaldehyde as a high level disinfectant for flexible endoscopes. *Journal of Hospital Infection*, **26**, 15–26.

Ayres, H., Furr, J.R. & Russell, A.D. (1993) A rapid method of evaluating permeabilization activity against *Pseudomonas aeruginosa. Letters in Applied Microbiology*, **17**, 149–151.

Bancroft, W.D. & Richter, G.H. (1931) The chemistry of disinfection. *Journal of Physical Chemistry*, **35**, 511–530.

Bean, H.S. & Das, A. (1966) The adsorption by *Escherichia coli* of phenols and their bactericidal activity. *Journal of Pharmacy and Pharmacology*, **18**, 107S–113S.

Beckett, A.H., Patki, S.J. & Robinson, A. (1959b) The interaction of phenolic compounds with bacteria. I. Hexyl-resorcinol and *Escherichia coli. Journal of Pharmacy and Pharmacology*, **11**, 360–366.

Berry, H. & Michaels, I. (1947) The evaluation of the bactericidal activity of ethylene glycol and some of its monoalkylethers against *Bacterium coli. Quarterly Journal of Pharmacy and Pharmacology*, **20**, 331–347.

Beveridge, E.G. (1975) The microbial spoilage of pharmaceutical products. In *Microbial Aspects of the Deterioration of Materials* (eds Lovelock, D.W. & Gilbert, R.J.) pp. 213–235. London: Academic Press.

Beveridge, E.G. & Hugo, W.B. (1964) The resistance of gallic acid and its alkyl esters to attack by bacteria able to degrade aromatic ring structures. *Journal of Applied Bacteriology*, **27**, 304–311.

Beveridge, E.G. & Tall, D. (1969) The metabolic availability of phenol analogues to bacterium NCIB 8250. *Journal of Applied Bacteriology*, **32**, 304–311.

Blake, A. & Peacocke, A.R. (1968) The interaction of amino acridines with nucleic acids. *Biopolymers*, **6**, 1225–1253.

Bolle, A. & Kellenberger, E. (1958) The action of sodium lauryl sulphate on *E. coli. Schweizerische Zeitschrift für Pathologie und Bakteriologie*, **21**, 714–740.

Bringmann, G. (1953) Electron microscope findings on the action of chlorine, bromine, iodine, copper, silver and hydrogen peroxide on *Escherichia coli. Zeitschrift für Hygiene und Infectionskrankheiten*, **138**, 155–166.

Broadley, S.J., Jenkins, P.A. Furr, J.R. & Russell, A.D. (1995) Potentiation of the effects of chlorhexidine diacetate and cetylpyridinium chloride on mycobacteria by ethambutol. *Journal of Medical Microbiology*, **43**, 458–460.

Brown, M.R.W. & Richards, R.M.E. (1965) Effect of ethyline diaminetetra-acetic acid on the resistance of *Pseudomonas aeruginosa* to antibacterial agents. *Nature (Lond.)*, **207**, 1391–1393.

Broxton, P., Woodcock, P.M. & Gilbert, P. (1983) A study of the antibacterial activity of some polyhexamethylene biguanides towards *Escherichia coli* ATCC 8739. *Journal of Applied Bacteriology*, **54**, 345–353.

Broxton, P., Woodcock, P.M. & Gilbert, P. (1984a) Interaction of some polyhexamethylene biguanides and membrane phospholipids in *Escherichia coli. Journal of Applied Bacteriology*, **57**, 115–124.

Broxton, P., Woodcock, P.M. & Gilbert, P. (1984b) Injury and recovery of *Escherichia coli* ATCC 8739 from treatment with some polyhexamethylene biguanides. *Microbios*, **40**, 187–193.

Broxton, P., Woodcock, P.M. & Gilbert, P. (1984c) Binding of some polyhexamethylene biguanides to the cell envelope of *Escherichia coli* ATCC 8739. *Microbios*, **41**, 15–22.

Casolari, A. (1981) A model describing microbial inactivation and growth kinetics. *Journal of Theoretical Biology*, **88**, 1–34.

Chaplin, C.E. (1951) Observations on quaternary ammonium disinfectants. *Canadian Journal of Botany*, **29**, 373–382.

Chaplin, C.E. (1952) Bacterial resistance to quaternary ammonium disinfectants. *Journal of Bacteriology*, **63**, 453–458.

Chawner, J.A. & Gilbert, P. (1989a) A comparative study of the bactericidal and growth inhibitory activities of the bisguanides alexidine and chlorhexidine. *Journal of Applied Bacteriology*, **66**, 243–252.

Chawner, J.A. & Gilbert, P. (1989b) Interaction of the bisbiguanides chlorhexidine and alexidine with phospholipid vesicles: evidence for separative modes of action. *Journal of Applied Bacteriology*, **66**, 253–258.

Cherrington, C.A., Hinton, M.H. & Chopra, I. (1990)

Effects of short-chain organic acids on macromolecular synthesis in *Escherichia coli*. *Journal of Applied Bacteriology*, **68**, 69–71.

Chick, H. (1908) An investigation of the laws of disinfection. *Journal of Hygiene, Cambridge*, **8**, 92–99.

Chopra, I. (1988) Mechanisms of resistance to antibiotics and other chemo-therapeutic agents. *Journal of Applied Bacteriology*, Symposium Supplement, **65**, 149S–166S.

Chopra, I., Johnson, S.C. & Bennett, P.M. (1987) Inhibition of *Providencia stuartii* cell envelope enzymes by chlorhexidine. *Journal of Antimicrobial Chemotherapy*, **19**, 743–751.

Collier, P.J., Ramsey, A., Waigh, R.D., Douglas, K.T., Austin, P. & Gilbert, P. (1990) Chemical reactivity of some *iso*thiazolone biocides. *Journal of Applied Bacteriology*, **69**, 578–584.

Collins, C.A. & Guild, W.R. (1968) Irreversible effects of formaldehyde on DNA. *Biochimica et Biophysica Acta*, **157**, 107–113.

Cooper, E.A. (1912) On the relationship of phenol and *m*-cresol to proteins: a contribution to our knowledge of the mechanism of disinfection. *Biochemical Journal*, **6**, 362–387.

Daltrey, D.L. & Hugo, W.B. (1974) Studies on the mode of action and the antibacterial agent chlorhexidine on *Clostridium perfringens* 2. Effect of chlorhexidine on metabolism and the cell membrane. *Microbios*, **11**, 131–146.

Dankert, J. & Schut, I.K. (1976) The antibacterial activity of chloroxylenol in combination with ethylene diamine tetraacetic acid. *Journal of Hygiene Cambridge*, **76**, 11–22.

Dawson, I.A., Lominski, I. & Stern, H. (1953) An electron microscope study of the action of cetyltrimethylammonium bromide (CTAB) on *Staphylococcus aureus*. *Journal of Pathology and Bacteriology*, **66**, 513–526.

Denyer, S.P. (1995) Mechanism of action of antibacterial biocides. *International Biodeterioration & Biodegradation*, **36**, 227–245.

Denyer, S.P. & Hugo, W.B. (1977) The mode of action of cetyltrimethylammonium bromide (CTAB) on *Staphylococcus aureus*. *Journal of Pharmacy and Pharmacology*, **29**, 66P.

Denyer , S.P. & Hugo, W.B. (1991) eds. *Mechanisms of Action of Chemical Biocides, Their Study and Exploitation*. Society for Applied Bacteriology Technical Series No. 27. Oxford: Blackwell Scientific Publications.

D'Mello, A. & Yotis, W.W. (1987) The action of sodium deoxycholate on *Escherichia coli*. *Applied and Environmental Microbiology*, **53**, 1944–1946.

Dobrogosz, W.J. & De Moss, R.D. (1963) Induction and repression of L-arabinose isomerase in *Pedicoccus pentosaceus*. *Journal of Bacteriology*, **85**, 1350–1364.

Dyar, M.T. & Ordal, E.J. (1946) Electrokinetic studies of bacterial surfaces. I. The effects of surface-active agents on the electrophoretic mobilities of bacteria. *Journal of Bacteriology*, **51**, 149–167.

Eddy, A.A. (1953) Death rate of populations of *Bact. lactis aerogenes*. III. Interpretation of survival curves. *Proceedings of the Royal Society of London, Series B*, **141**, 137–145.

Eklund, P. (1985) The effect of sorbic acid and esters of *p*-hydroxybenzoic acid on the protonmotive force in *Escherichia coli*. *Journal of General Microbiology*, **313**, 73–76.

El-Falaha, B.M.A., Furr, J.R. & Russell, A.D. (1989) Effect of anionic detergents on wild-type and envelope mutants of *Escherichia coli* and *Pseudomonas aeruginosa*. *Letters in Applied Microbiology*, **8**, 15–19.

Ellison, R.T., Giehl, T.J. & La Force, F.M. (1988) Damage of the outer membrane of entire Gram-negative bacteria by lactoferrin and transferrin. *Infection and Immunity*, **56**, 2774–2781.

Evans, W.C. (1963) The microbiological degradation of aromatic compounds. *Journal of General Microbiology*, **32**, 177–184.

Ferguson, T.B. & Thorne, S. (1946) The effects of some acridine compounds on the growth and respiration of *Escherichia coli*. *Journal of Pharmacology and Experimental Therapeutics*, **86**, 258–263.

Fewson, C.A. (1967) The growth and metabolic versatility of the Gram-negative bacterium NC1B 8250 ('*Vibrio 01*'). *Journal of General Microbiology*, **46**, 255–266.

Fischer, R. & Larose, P. (1952) Factors governing the adaptation of bacteria against quaternaries. *Nature, London*, **170**, 715–716.

Fitzgerald, K.A., Davies, A. & Russell, A.D. (1989) Uptake of ^{14}C-chlorhexidine diacetate to *Escherichia coli* and *Pseudomonas aeruginosa* and its reversal by azolectin. *FEMS Micobiology Letters*, **60**, 327–332.

Fitzgerald, K.A., Davies, A. & Russell, A.D. (1992a) Backerial uptake of ^{14}C-chlorhexidine diacetate and the influence of phenoxyethanol. Studies with Gram-positive bacteria. *Biomedical Letters*, **47**, 191–199.

Fitzgerald, K.A., Davies, A. & Russell, A.D. (1992b) Bacterial uptake of ^{14}C-chlorhexidine diacetate and the influence of phenoxyethanol. Studies with Gram-negative bacteria. *Microbios*, **70**, 77–91.

Foster, J.H.S. & Russell, A.D. (1971) Antibacterial dyes and nitrofurans. In *Inhibition and Destruction of the Microbial Cell* (ed. Hugo, W.B.) London: Academic Press.

Foster, T.J. (1983) Plasmid-determined resistance to

antimicrobial drugs and toxic metals in bacteria. *Microbiology Reviews*, **47**, 361–409.

Fuller, S.J., Denyer, S.P., Hugo, W.B., Pemberton, D., Woodcock, P.M. & Buckley, A.J. (1985) The mode of action of 1,2-benzisothiazolone on *Staphylococcus aureus*. *Letters in Applied Microbiology*, **1**, 13–15.

Furr, J.R. & Russell, A.D. (1972) Uptake of esters of *p*-hydroxybenzoic acid by *Serratia marcescens* and by fattened and non-fattened cells of *Bacillus subtilis*. *Microbios*, **5**, 237–246.

Ghuysen, J.M. (1968) Use of bacteriolytic enzymes in determining of wall structure and their role in cell metabolism. *Bacteriological Reviews*, **32**, 425–464.

Gibson, D.T. (1968) Microbial degradation of aromatic compounds. *Science, Washington*, **161**, 1093–1097.

Gilbert, P., Beveridge, E.G. & Crone, B.P. (1977) The lethal action of 2-phenoxyethanol and its analogues upon *Escherichia coli* NCTC 5933, *Microbios*, **19**, 125–141.

Gilbert, P., Beveridge, E.G. & Sissons, I. (1978) The uptake of some membrane-active drugs by bacteria and yeast: possible microbiological examples of Z-curve adsorption. *Journal of Colloid and Interfacial Science*, **64**, 377–379.

Giles, C.H. & McKay, R.B. (1965) The adsorption of cationic (basic) dyes by fixed yeast cells. *Journal of Bacteriology*, **89**, 390–397.

Giles, C.H. & Tolia, A.H. (1974) Studies in adsorption. XIX. Measurement of external specific surface of fibres by solution adsorption. *Journal of Applied Chemistry*, **14**, 186–195.

Giles, C.H., MacEwan, T.H., Nakhwa, S.N. & Smith, D. (1960) Studies in adsorption. XI. A system of classification of solution adsorption mechanisms and measurement of specific surface areas of solids. *Journal of the Chemical Society*, 3973–3993.

Giles, C.H., Smith, D. & Huitson, A. (1974) A general treatment and classification of the solute adsorption isotherm 1. Theoretical. *Journal of Colloid and Interfacial Science*, **47**, 755–765.

Gorman, S.P. & Scott, E.M. (1977) Uptake and media reactivity of glutaraldehyde solutions related to structure and biocidal activity. *Microbios Letters*, **5**, 163–169.

Gorman, S.P., Scott, E.M. & Russell, A.D. (1980) Antimicrobial activity, uses and mechanism of action of glutaraldehyde. *Journal of Applied Bacteriology*, **48**, 161–190.

Gould, G.W. (1989) ed. *Mechanisms of Action of Food Preservation Procedures*. London: Elsevier Applied Science.

Grant, D.J.W. (1967) Kinetic aspects of the growth of *Klebsiella aerogenes* with some benzenoid carbon sources. *Journal of General Microbiology*, **46**, 213–224.

Grossman, L., Levine, S.S. & Allison, W.S. (1961) The reaction of formaldehyde with nucleotides and T2 bacteriophage DNA. *Journal of Molecular Biology*, **3**, 47–60.

Hamilton, W.A. (1968) The mechanism of the bacteriostatic action of tetrachlorosalicyanilide. *Journal of General Microbiology*, **50**, 441–458.

Hamilton, W.A. (1975) Energy coupling in microbial transport. *Advances in Microbial Physiology*, **12**, 1–53.

Hancock, R.E.W. (1984) Alterations in membrane permeability. *Annual Review of Microbiology*, **38**, 237–264.

Haque, H. & Russell, A.D. (1974a) Effect of chelating agents on the susceptibility of some strains of Gram-negative bacteria to some antibacterial agents. *Antimicrobial Agents and Chemotherapy*, **6**, 200–206.

Haque, H. & Russell, A.D. (1974b) Effect of ethylenediamine tetraacetic acid and related chelating agents on whole cells of Gram-negative bacteria. *Antimicrobial Agents and Chemotherapy*, **6**, 447–452.

Haque, H. & Russell, A.D. (1976) Cell envelopes of Gram negative bacteria: composition, response to chelating agents and susceptibility of whole cells to antibacterial agents. *Journal of Applied Bacteriology*, **40**, 89–99.

Harold, F.M. (1972) Conservation and transportation of energy by bacterial membranes. *Bacteriological Reviews*, **36**, 172–230.

Harold, F.M., Favlasova, E. & Baarda, J.R. (1970) A transmembrane pH gradient in *Streptococcus faecalis*: origin and dissipation by proton conductors and *N,N'*-dicyclohexylcarbodiimide. *Biochimica et Biophysica Acta*, **196**, 235–244.

Haydon, D.A. (1956) Surface behaviour of *Bacterium coli*. II. The interaction with phenol. *Proceedings of the Royal Society*, **145B**, 383–391.

Herzog, R.A. & Betzel, R. (1911) Zür Theorie der Dissinfektion. *Physiologische Chemie*, **74**, 221–226.

Hotchkiss, R.D. (1944) Greamicidin, tyrocidin and tyrothricin. *Advances in Enzymology*, **4**, 153–199.

Hughes, W.H. (1956) The structure and development of the induced long forms of bacteria. *Symposia of the Society for General Microbiology*, **6** (eds Spooner, E.T.C. & Stocker, B.A.D.) pp. 341–360. Cambridge: Cambridge University Press.

Hugo, W.B. (1957) The mode of action of antiseptics. *Journal of Pharmacy and Pharmacology*, **9**, 145–161.

Hugo, W.B. (1965a) Some aspects of the action of cationic surface active agents in microbial cells with special reference to their action on enzymes. In *Surface, Activity and the Microbial Cell: SCI Monograph*, **19**, pp. 67–82. London: Society of Chemical Industry.

Hugo, W.B. (1965b) The degradation of preservatives by

micro-organisms. In *Scientific and Technical Symposium. 112th Annual Meeting, American Pharmaceutical Association*, Detroit, CIII. pp. 1–7.

Hugo, W.B. (1967) The mode of action of antibacterial agents. *Journal of Applied Bacteriology*, **30**, 17–50.

Hugo, W.B., ed. (1971) *Inhibition and Destruction of the Microbial Cell*. London: Academic Press.

Hugo, W.B. (1976a) Survival of microbes exposed to chemical stress. In *The Survival of Vegetative Microbes*. (eds Gray, T.G.R. & Postgate, J.R.) 26th Symposium, Society for General Microbiology, Cambridge: Cambridge University Press.

Hugo, W.B. (1976b) The inactivation of vegetative bacteria by chemicals. In *Inhibition and Inactivation of Vegetative Microbes* (eds Skinner, F.A. & Hugo, W.B.) Society for Applied Bacteriology Symposium Series No. 5. London: Academic Press.

Hugo, W.B. (1978) Membrane-active antimicrobial compounds – a reappraisal of their mode of action in the light of the chemi-osmotic theory. *International Journal of Pharmaceutics*, **1**, 127–131.

Hugo, W.B. (1980) The mode of action of antiseptics. In *Handbuch der Antiseptik* (eds Wigert H. und Weifen W.) pp. 39–77. Berlin: VEB Verlag.

Hugo, W.B. (1991) The degradation of preservatives by microorganisms. *International Biodeterioration*, **27**, 185–194.

Hugo, W.B. & Bloomfield, S.F. (1971a) Studies on the mode of action of the phenolic antibacterial agent Fentichlor against *Staphylococcus aureus* and *Escherichia coli*. I. The adsorption of Fentichlor by the bacterial cell and its antibacterial activity. *Journal of Applied Bacteriology*, **34**, 557–567.

Hugo, W.B. & Bloomfield, S.F. (1971b) Studies on the mode of action of the phenolic antibacterial agent Fentichlor against *Staphylococcus aureus* and *Escherichia coli*. II. The effects of Fentichlor on the bacterial membrane and the cytoplasmic constituents of the cell. *Journal of Applied Bacteriology*, **34**, 569–578.

Hugo, W.B. & Bloomfield, S.F. (1971c) Studies on the mode of action of the phenolic antibacterial agent Fentichlor against *Staphylococcus aureus* and *Escherichia coli*. III. The effect of Fentichlor on the metabolic activities of *Staphyloccus aureus* and *Escherichia coli*. *Journal of Applied Bacteriology*, **34**, 579–591.

Hugo, W.B. & Daltrey, D.C. (1974) Studies on the mode of action of the antibacterial agent chlorhexidine on *Clostridium perfringens*. I. Adsorption of chlorhexidine on the cell, its antibacterial activity and physical effects. *Microbios*, **11**, 119–129.

Hugo, W.B. & Davidson, J.R. (1973) Effect of cell lipid depletion in *Staphylococcus aureus* upon its resistance to antimicrobial agents. II. A composition of the response of normal and lipid depleted cells of *S. aureus* to antibacterial drugs. *Microbios*, **8**, 63–72.

Hugo, W.B. & Denyer, S.P. (1987) The concentration exponent of disinfectants and preservatives (Biocides). In *Preservatives in the Food, Pharmaceutical and Environmental Industries*. (eds Board, R.G., Allwood, M.C. & Banks, J.G.) Society for Applied Bacteriology Technical Series No. 22, pp. 281–291. Oxford: Blackwell Scientific Publications.

Hugo, W.B. & Foster, J.H.S. (1964) Growth of *Pseudomonas aeruginosa* in solutions of esters of *p*-hydrobenzoic acid. *Journal of Pharmacy and Pharmacology*, **16**, 209.

Hugo, W.B. & Franklin, I. (1968) Cellular lipid and the antistaphylococcal action of phenols. *Journal of General Microbiology*, **52**, 365–373.

Hugo, W.B. & Frier, M. (1969) Mode of action of the antibacterial compound dequalinium acetate. *Applied Microbiology*, **17**, 118–127.

Hugo, W.B. & Longworth, A.R. (1964) Some aspects of the mode of action of chlorhexidine. *Journal of Pharmacy and Pharmacology*, **16**, 655–662.

Hugo, W.B. & Longworth, A.R. (1965) Cytological aspects of the mode of action of chlorhexidine. *Journal of Pharmacy and Pharmacology*, **17**, 28–32.

Hugo, W.B. & Longworth, A.R. (1966) The effect of chlorhexidine on the electrophoretic mobility, cytoplasmic content, dehydrogenase activity and cell walls of *Escherichia coli* and *Staphylococcus aureus*. *Journal of Pharmacy and Pharmacology*, **18**, 569–578.

Hugo, W.B. & Newton, J.M. (1964) The adsorption of iodine from solution by microorganisms and by serum. *Journal of Pharmacy and Pharmacology*, **16**, 48–55.

Hugo, W.B. & Stretton, R.J. (1966) The role of cellular lipid in the resistance of Gram-positive bacteria to penicillins. *Journal of General Microbiology*, **42**, 133–138.

Hugo, W.B., Bowen, J.G. & Davidson, J.R. (1971) Lipid depletion in bacteria induced by biotin deficiency and its relation to resistance to antibacterial agents. *Journal of Pharmacy and Pharmacology*, **23**, 69–70.

Jackson, R.W. & De Moss, J.A. (1965) Effect of toluene on *Escherichia coli*. *Journal of Bacteriology*, **90**, 1420–1425.

Jacobs, S.E. (1960) Some aspects of the dynamics of disinfection. *Journal of Pharmacy and Pharmacology*, **12**, 9T–18T.

James, A.M. (1965) The modification of the bacterial surface by chemical and enzymatic treatment. In *Cell Electrophoresis* (ed. Ambrose, E.J.) pp. 154–170. London: J. & A. Churchill.

James, A.M. (1972) *The Electrochemistry of Bacterial Surfaces*. Inaugural Lecture. University of London: Bedford College.

Jordan, R.C. & Jacobs, S.E. (1944) Studies on the

dynamics of disinfection. I. New data on the reaction between phenol and *Bact. coli* using an improved technique, together with an analysis of the distribution of resistance amongst the cells of the bacterial population studied. *Journal of Hygiene, Cambridge*, **43**, 275–289.

Judis, J. (1966) Factors affecting binding of phenol derivatives to *Micrococcus lysodeikticus* cells. *Journal of Pharmaceutical Sciences*, **53**, 803–817.

Knaysi, G. (1930) Disinfection I. The development of our knowledge of disinfection. *Journal of Infectious Diseases*, **47**, 293–302.

Knaysi, G. & Morris, G. (1930) The manner of death of certain bacteria and yeast when subjected to mild chemical and physical agents. *Journal of Infectious Diseases*, **47**, 303–317.

Knox, W.E., Stumph, P.K., Green, D.E. & Auerbach, V.H. (1948) The inhibition of sulphydryl enzymes as the basis of the bacterial action of chlorine. *Journal of Bacteriology*, **55**, 451–458.

Kroll, R.G. & Anagnostopoulos, G.D. (1981) Potassium leakage as a lethality index of phenol and the effect of solute and water activity. *Journal of General Microbiology*, **50**, 139–147.

Kuhn, R. & Bielig, H.J. (1940) Uber Invertseifen. I. Die Einwirkung von Invertseifen auf Eiweiss-Stoffe. *Berichte der Deutschen Chemischen Gesellschaft*, **73**, 1080–1091.

Kuyyakanond, T. & Quesnel, L.B. (1992) The mechanism of action of chlorhexidine. *FEMS Microbiology Letters*, **100**, 211–216.

Lambert, P.A. & Hammond, S.M. (1973) Potassium fluxes. First indications of membrane damage in microorganisms. *Biochemical and Biophysical Research Communications*, **54**, 796–799.

Lark, K.G. & Lark, C. (1966) Regulation of chromosome replication in *Escherichia coli* a comparison of the effects of phenylethyl alcohol treatment with those of amino acid starvation. *Journal of Molecular Biology*, **20**, 9–19.

Leive, L. (1974) The barrier function of the Gram-negative envelope. *Annals of the New York Academy of Sciences*, **235**, 109–127.

Lerch, C. (1953) Electrophoresis of *Micrococcus pyogenes* var. *aureus*. *Acta Pathologica et Microbiologica Scandinavica*, **98** (Suppl.), 1–94.

Lerman, L.S. (1961) Structural considerations in the interaction of DNA and acridines. *Journal of Molecular Biology*, **3**, 18–30.

Lerman, L.S. (1964a) Acridine mutagens and DNA structure. *Journal of Cellular and Comparative Physiology*, **64** (Suppl.), 1–18.

Lerman, L.S. (1964b) Amino acid group reactivity in DNA-aminoacridine complexes. *Journal of Molecular Biology*, **10**, 367–380.

Lowick, J.H.B. & James, A.M. (1957) The electrokinetic properties of *Aerobacter aerogenes*. A comparison of the properties of normal and crystal violet-trained cells. *Biochemical Journal*, **65**, 431–438.

Lyon, B.R. & Skurray, R.A. (1987) Antimicrobial resistance of *Staphylococcus aureus*: genetic basis. *Microbiological Reviews*, **51**, 88–137.

McIlwain, H. (1941) A nutritional investigation of the antibacterial action of acriflavine. *Biochemical Journal*, **35**, 1311–1319.

McKenna, S.M. & Davies, K.J.A. (1988) The inhibition of bacterial growth by hypochlorous acid. *Biochemical Journal* **254**, 685–692.

McQuillen, K. (1950) The bacterial surface I. The effect of cetyltrimethylammonium bromide on the electrophoretic mobility of certain Gram-positive bacteria. *Biochimica et Biophysica Acta*, **5**, 463–471.

Madsen, T. & Nyman, M. (1907) Zur Theorie der Desinfektion. I. *Zeitschrift für Hygiene und Infektionskrankheiten*, **57**, 388–395.

Meyer, H. (1901) Zur Theorie der Alkoholnarkose, III. Der Einfluss Wechselnder Temperatur auf Wirkungstark und Narcotics. *Archiv für Experimentielle Pathologie und Pharmakologie*, **46**, 388–342.

Mickelson, M.N. (1974) Effect of uncoupling agents and respiratory inhibitors on the growth of *Streptococcus agalactiae*. *Journal of Bacteriology*, **120**, 733–740.

Mitchell, P. (1961) Coupling of phosphorylation to electron and hydrogen transfer by a chemiosmotic type of mechanism. *Nature, London*, **191**, 144–148.

Mitchell, P. (1968) *Chemiosmotic Coupling and Energy Transduction*. Bodmin: Glyn Research Ltd.

Mitchell, P. (1970) Membranes of cells and organelles. In *Symposia of the Society for General Microbiology*, **20**, (eds Charles, H.P. & Knight, B.C.J.G.) pp. 121–166. Cambridge: Cambridge University Press.

Mitchell, P. (1972) Chemiosmotic coupling in energy transduction: a logical development of biochemical knowledge. *Journal of Bioenergetics*, **3**, 5–24.

Mitchell, P. & Moyle, J. (1967) Acid-base titration across the membrane system of rat-liver mitochondria: catalysis by uncouplers. *Biochemical Journal*, **104**, 588–600.

Munton, T.J. & Russell, A.D. (1970) Aspects of the action of glutaraldehyde on *Escherichia coli*. *Journal of Applied Bacteriology*, **33**, 410–419.

Nakamura, K. & Tamaoki, T. (1968) Reversible dissociation of *Escherichia coli* ribosomes by hydrogen peroxide. *Biochimica et Biophysica Acta*, **161**, 368–376.

Nicholson, B.H. & Peacocke, A.R. (1965) The inhibition of ribonucleic acid polymerase by acridines. *Biochemical Journal*, **100**, 50–58.

Nikaido, H. (1976) Outer membrane of *Salmonella typhimurium*: transmembrane diffusion of some hydrophobic substances. *Biochimica et Biophysica Acta*, **433**, 118–132.

Nikaido, H. & Vaara, M. (1985) Molecular basis of bacterial outer membrane permeability. *Microbiological Reviews*, **49**, 1–32.

Niven, D.F. & Hamilton, W.A. (1974) Mechanisms of energy coupling to the transport of amino acids in *Staphylococcus aureus. European Journal of Biochemistry*, **37**, 244–248.

Novick, R.P. & Roth, C. (1968) Plasmid-linked resistance to inorganic salts in *Staphylococcus. Journal of Bacteriology*, **95**, 1335–1342.

Peacocke, A.R. & Skerrett, J.N.H. (1956) The interaction of aminoacridines with nucleic acids. *Transactions of the Faraday Society*, **52**, 261–279.

Pritchard, N.J., Blake, A. & Peacocke, A.R. (1966) Modified intercalation model for the interaction of amino acridines and DNA. *Nature, London*, **272**, 1360–1361.

Prokop, A. & Humphrey, A.E. (1970) Kinetics of disinfection. In *Disinfection* (ed. Bernarde, M.A.) pp. 61–83. New York: Marcel Dekker.

Pulvertaft, R.J.V. & Lumb, G.D. (1948) Bacterial lysis and antiseptics. *Journal of Hygiene, Cambridge*, **46**, 62–64.

Rahn, O. (1945) Factors affecting the rate of disinfection. *Bacteriological Reviews*, **9**, 1–47.

Rahn, O. & Schroeder, W.R. (1941) Inactivation of enzymes as the cause of death in bacteria. *Byodynamica*, **3**, 199–208.

Ribbons, D.W. (1965) The microbial degradation of aromatic compounds. *Annual Reports on the Progress of Chemistry*, **62**, 455–468.

Richardson, A.G. & Leach, F.R. (1969) The effect of phenylethyl alcohol on *Bacillus subtilis* transformation. I. Characterisation of the effect. *Biochimica et Biophysica Acta*, **174**, 264–275.

Richardson, A.G., Pierson, D.L. & Leach, F.R. (1969) The effect of phenylethanol on *Bacillus subtilis* transformation. II. Transport of DNA and precursors. *Biochimica et Biophysica Acta*, **174**, 276–281.

Richmond, D.V. & Fisher, D.J. (1973) The electrophoretic mobility of microorganisms. *Advances in Microbial Physiology*, **9**, 1–29.

Roberts, M.H. & Rahn, O. (1946) The amount of enzyme inactivation at bacteriostatic and bactericidal concentrations of disinfectants. *Journal of Bacteriology*, **52**, 639–644.

Roe, E., Jones, R.J. & Lowbury, E.J.L. (1971) Transfer of antibiotic resistance between *Pseudomonas aeruginosa* and other Gram-negative bacilli in burns. *Lancet*, **6**, 149–152.

Rogers, H.J. & Forsberg, C.W. (1971) Role of autolysins in killing of bacteria by some bactericidal antibiotics. *Journal of Bacteriology*, **108**, 1235–1243.

Rogoff, M.H. (1961) The oxidation of aromatic compounds by bacteria. *Advances in Applied Microbiology*, **3**, 193–221.

Rossmore, H.W. & Sondossi, I. (1988) Application and mode of action of formaldehyde condensate biocides. *Advances in Applied Microbiology*, **33**, 223–277.

Russell, A.D. (1971) Ethylenediamine tetraacetic acid. In *Inhibition and Destruction of the Microbial Cell* (ed. Hugo, W.B.) pp. 209–224. London: Academic Press.

Russell, A.D. (1972) Comparative resistance of R^+ and other strains of *Pseudomonas aeruginosa* to non-antibiotic antibacterials. *Lancet*, **ii**, 332.

Russell, A.D. (1985) The role of plasmids in bacterial resistance to antiseptics, disinfectants and preservatives. *Journal of Hospital Infection*, **6**, 9–19.

Russell, A.D. (1986) Chlorhexidine: antibacterial action and bacterial resistance. *Infection*, **14**, 212–215.

Russell, A.D. & Chopra, I. (1996) *Understanding Antibacterial Action and Resistance*, 2nd edn. Chichester: Ellis Horwood.

Russell, A.D. & Furr, J.R. (1977) The antibacterial activity of a new chloroxylenol preparation containing ethylenediamineteta-acetic acid. *Journal of Applied Bacteriology*, **43**, 253–260.

Russell, A.D. & Furr, J.R. (1996) Mechanisms of antifungal action and fungal resistance. *Science Progress*, **79**, 27–48.

Russell, A.D. & Gould, G.W. (1988) Resistance of Enterobacteriaceae to preservatives and disinfectants. *Journal of Applied Bacteriology, Symposium Supplement*, **65**, 167S–195S.

Russell, A.D. & Hopwood, D. (1976) The biological uses and importance of glutaraldehyde. *Progress in Medicinal Chemistry*, **13**, 271–301.

Russell, A.D. & Hugo, W.B. (1988) Perturbation of homeostatic mechanisms in bacteria by pharmaceuticals. In *Homeostatic Mechanisms in Microorganisms*: FEMS Symposium no 44 (eds Whittenbury, R., Gould, G.W. & Board, R.G.) pp. 206–219. Bath University.

Russell, A.D. & Hugo, W.B. (1994) Antimicrobial activity of silver. In *Progress in Medicinal Chemistry* (eds Ellis, G.P. & Luscombe, D.K.) **39**, 351–370.

Russell, A.D. & Russell, N.J. (1995) Biocides: activity, action and resistance. In *Fifty years of antimicrobials: past perspectives and future trends* (eds Hunter, P.A., Darby, G.K. & Russell, N.J.) 53rd Symposium of the Society for General Microbiology. Cambridge: Cambridge University Press.

Russell, N.J. & Gould, G.W. (1991) *Food Preservatives*. Glasgow and London, Blackie.

Sakagami, Y., Yokagama, H., Nishimura, H., Ose, Y. & Tashima, T. (1989) Mechanism of resistance to benzalkonium chloride by *Pseudomonas aeruginosa. Applied and Environmental Microbiology*, 55, 2036–2040.

Salton, M.R.J. (1951) The adsorption of cetyltrimethylammonium bromide by bacteria, its action in releasing cellular constituents and its bacterial effect. *Journal of General Microbiology*, 5, 391–404.

Salton, M.R.J. (1968) Lytic agents, cell permeability and monolayer penetratability. *Journal of General Physiology*, **52**, 277S–252S.

Salton, M.R.J., Horne, R.W. & Coslett, V.E. (1951) Electron microscopy of bacteria treated with cetyltrimethylammonium bromide. *Journal of General Microbiology*, **5**, 405–407.

Sanderson, K.E., MacAlistair, T., Costerton, J.W. & Cheng, K.-J. (1974) Permeability of lipopolysaccharide-deficient (rough) mutants of *Salmonella typhinurium* to antibiotics, lysozyme and other agents. *Canadian Journal of Microbiology*, **20**, 1135–1145.

Silver, S. & Misra, S. (1988) Plasmid-mediated heavy metal resistances. *Annual Review of Microbiology*, **42**, 717–743.

Simon, E.W. (1953) Mechanism of dinitrophenol toxicity. *Biological Review*, **28**, 453–479.

Sinai, J. & Yudkin, J. (1959a) The origin of bacterial resistance to proflavine. III. The alleged rapid adaptation to proflavine resistance in *Bacterium lactis aerogenes* (syn. *Aerobacter aerogenes, Klebsiella pneumoniae*). *Journal of General Microbiology*, **20**, 373–383.

Sinai, J. & Yudkin, J. (1959b) The origin of bacterial resistance to proflavine. IV. Cycles of resistance in *Escherichia coli* and their bearing on variations in resistance in cultures. *Journal of General Microbiology*, **20**, 384–399.

Sinai, J. Yudkin, J. (1959c) The origin of bacterial resistance to proflavine. V. Transformation of proflavine resistance in *Escherichia coli. Journal of General Microbiology*, **20**, 400-413.

Sleat, R. & Robinson, J.P. (1984) The bacteriology of anaerobic degradation of aromatic compounds. *Journal of Applied Bacteriology*, **57**, 381–394.

Smith, A.R.W., Lambert, P.A., Hammond, S.M. & Jessup, C. (1975) The differing effects of cetyltrimethylammonium bromide and cetrimide B.P. upon growing cultures of *Escherichia coli*. NCIB 8277. *Journal of Applied Bacteriology*, **38**, 143–149.

Smith, G. (1970) Ethylenediamine tetraacetic acid and the bactericidal efficiency of some phenolic disinfectants against *Pseudomonas aeruginosa. Journal of Medical Laboratory Technology*, **27**, 203–206.

Sofos, J.N., Pierson, M.D., Blocher, J.C. & Busta, F.F. (1986) Mode of action of sorbic acid on bacterial cells and spores. *International Journal of Food Microbiology*, **3**, 1–17.

Staehelin, M. (1958) Reactions of tobacco mosaic virus nucleic acid with formaldehyde. *Biochimica et Biophysica Acta*, **29**, 410–417.

Stretton, R.J. & Manson, T.W. (1973) Some aspects of the mode of action of the antibacterial compound Bronopol (2-bromo-2-nitropropan-1,3-diol). *Journal of Applied Bacteriology*, **36**, 61–76.

Summers, A.O. & Lewis, E. (1973) Volatilization of mercuric chloride by mercury-resistant plasmid-bearing strains of *Escherichia coli. Staphylococcus aureus* and *Pseudomonas aeruginosa. Journal of Bacteriology*, **113**, 1070–1072.

Thornley, M.J. & Yudkin, J. (1959a) The origin of bacterial resistance to proflavine. I. Training and reversion in *Echerichia coli. Journal of General Microbiology*, **20**, 355–364.

Thornley, M.J. & Yudkin, J. (1959b) The origin of bacterial resistance in *Escherichia coli. Journal of General Microbiology*, **20**, 365–372.

Tomasz, A. (1979) The mechanism of the irreversible antimicrobial effects of penicillins: how the β-lactum antibiotics kill and lyse bacteria. *Annual Review of Microbiology*, **33**, 113–137.

Tomcsik, J. (1955) Effects of disinfectants and of surface active agents on bacterial protoplasts. *Proceedings of the Society of Experimental Biology and Medicine*, **89**, 459–463.

Vaara, M. (1992) Agents that increase the permeability of the outer membrane. *Microbiology Reviews*, **56**, 395–411.

Vaara, M. & Vaara, T. (1983a) Polycations sensitise enteric bacteria to antibiotics. *Antimicrobial Agents and Chemotherapy*, **24**, 107–113.

Vaara, M. & Vaara, T. (1983b) Polycations as outer membrane-disorganizing agents. *Antimicrobial Agents and Chemotherapy*, **24**, 114–122.

Vaczi, L. (1973) *The Biological Role of Bacterial Lipids*. Budapest: Akademiai Kiado.

Vaituzis, Z., Nelson, J.D. Jr., Wan, L.W. & Colwell, R.R. (1975) Effects of mercuric chloride on growth and morphology of selected strains of mercury-resistant bacteria. *Applied Microbiology*, **29**, 275–286.

Walsh, C.T. & Kaback, H.R. (1973) Vinylglycolic acid. An inactivator of the phosphoenolpyruvate-phosphate transferase system in *Escherichia coli. Journal of Biological Chemistry*, **248**, 5456–5462.

Wang, J.H. & Matheson, A.T. (1967) The possible role of sulphydryl groups in the dimerization of 70S ribosomes from *Escherichia coli. Biochemical and Biophysical Research Communications*, **23**, 740–744.

Waring, M.J. (1965) The effects of antimicrobial agents on ribonucleic acid polymerase. *Molecular Pharmacology*, **1**, 1–13.

Williamson, R.L. & Metcalfe, R.L. (1967) Salicylanilides: a new group of active uncouplers of oxidative phosphorylation. *Science, Washington*, **158**, 1694–1695.

Woldringh, C.L. (1973) Effects of toluene and phenylethyl alcohol on the ultrastructure of *Escherichia coli. Journal of Bacteriology*, **114**, 1359–1361.

Woodroffe, R.C.S. & Wilkinson, B.E. (1966) The antibacterial activity of tetrachlorosalicylanilide. *Journal of General Microbiology*, **44**, 343–352.

Worley, S.D. & Williams, D.E. (1988) Halamimine water disinfectants. *Critical Review of Environmental Control*, **18**, 133–175.

CHAPTER 10

Bacterial Sensitivity and Resistance

A. INTRINSIC RESISTANCE

1 Introduction

The response of a natural community of microbes to a challenge from a non-antibiotic antibacterial agent will depend on a variety of factors. The pH, temperature, presence of organic debris and other chemical inactivators, and mode and rate of growth of the organisms can all profoundly influence the outcome. In addition, there is considerable variation in the innate sensitivity of the vegetative cells of different groups of bacteria to antiseptics, disinfectants and preservatives (Table 10.1). Generally, Gram-negative organisms are more resistant than Gram-positive species. Special problems of resistance are also posed by *Pseudomonas aeruginosa* and *Mycobacterium tuberculosis*. This resistance phenomenon is consistently demonstrated by natural isolates of these groups of organisms, and it has been described as intrinsic, implying that it is due to some inherent feature of the cells and to distinguish it from acquired resistance, which occurs when resistant strains emerge from previously sensitive species after exposure to antibacterial agents.

Predictably, it has been proposed that the basic features of the Gram-negative cell, which prevent the penetration of crystal violet and result in its accessibility to extraction with alcohol or acetone in the classical Gram-staining procedure, also tend to exclude many antibacterials and prevent them reaching their biochemical or structural targets within the cell. Before examining this in more detail, it is important to point out that Gram-negativity is not always associated with greater resistance to antibacterials. Chlorine, for example, is more active against *Ps. aeruginosa* and *Proteus mirabilis* than against *Staphylococcus aureus* (Trueman, 1971), and similar findings have been reported for phenoxyethanol (Berry, 1944) and silver salts (Sykes, 1958).

2 The Enterobacteriaceae

Many of the antibacterial agents that are less active against Gram-negative cells are believed to exert their effect by inducing metabolic or structural lesions in the cytoplasmic membrane (Hugo, 1967). Hamilton (1971) proposed that the actual cytoplasmic membranes of Gram-positive and Gram-negative cells are equally sensitive to the action of these agents, and that layers of the Gram-negative cell envelope external to the membrane may either constitute a non-absorbing barrier or may absorb and retain the agent, thus protecting the underlying sensitive membrane.

Transmission electron micrographs of Gram-positive cell envelopes show the cytoplasmic membranes to be bounded by cell walls, which typically appear as amorphous structures some 20–30 nm thick. The main macromolecules present in these walls are the peptidoglycans, which provide a rigid framework for the cell, and the teichoic acids,

Table 10.1 Comparative responses of *Staphylococcus aureus*, *Pseudomonas aeruginosa* and some Enterobacteriaceae to antiseptics, disinfectants and preservatives* (based on Wallhäusser, 1984).

	MIC (μg/ml) versus			
Antimicrobial agent	*Staphylococcus aureus*	*Pseudomonas aeruginosa*	*Escherichia coli*	*Klebsiella pneumoniae*
Bronopol	62.5	31.25	31.25	62.5
Phenylethanol	1 250	2 500–5000	2 500	
Propionic acid	2 000	3 000	2 000	1 250
Sorbic acid (pH 6)	50–100	100–300	50–100	50–100
Benzoic acid (pH 6)	50–100	200–500	100–200	100–200
Methyl paraben	800	1 000	800	800
Ethyl paraben	500	800	600	600
Propyl paraben	150	400	300	300
Butyl paraben	120	175	150	100
Chlorocresol	625	1 250	1 250	625
Chloroxylenol	250	1 000	1 000	500
o-Phenylphenol	100	1 000	500	500
Hexachlorophane	0.5	250	12.5	12.5
Triclosan	0.1	> 300	5	5
Propamidine isethionate	2	256	64	256
Dibromopropamidine isethionate	1	32	4	
Hexetidine	5	> 10 000	1 250	> 10 000
8-Hydroxyquinoline	4	128	64	64
Chlorhexidine	0.5–1	5–60	1	5–10
Benzethonium chloride	0.5	250	32	
Cetrimide	4	64–128	16	16
Thiomersal	0.2	8	4	4
Phenylmercuric nitrate	0.1	1–5	0.5	0.5

*Inoculum size *c.* 10^6 cfu/ml.
cfu, colony-forming units; MIC, minimal inhibitory concentration.

which are highly negatively charged and thought to have an important role in the sequestration of divalent cations from the medium (Poxton, 1993). Although mechanically strong, the Gram-positive wall has an open network structure and does not seem to offer any substantial resistance to the diffusion of small molecules, such as antibiotics and other antibacterials, into the cell.

The envelopes of Gram-negative bacteria are more complex, multilayered structures. An important feature is an additional membrane on the external surface of the cell. Sandwiched between this outer membrane and the inner cytoplasmic membrane is the periplasm, which contains the peptidoglycan layer and enzymes, such as β-lactamases, ribonucleases and phophatases, suspended in a highly hydrated polysaccharide gel. The peptidoglycan is less substantial than in Gram-positive cells, typically 3–5 nm thick, and the periplasm is some 10–25 nm in depth (Graham *et al.*, 1991).

Although the outer membrane appears in electron micrographs to be similar in structure to the cytoplasmic membrane, the biochemical composition of the two membranes is quite different. The outer membrane contains less phospholipid, fewer proteins and a unique component, lipopolysaccharide (LPS). There is also an asymmetric organization of these lipid components, with the phospholipids on the inner surface and the LPS molecules confined to the outer leaflet of the membrane. Lipopolysaccharides are large complex structures, with three distinct regions. The lipid A portion, which forms the outer leaflet of the outer membrane, is composed of two glucosamine molecules, each linked to three long-chain fatty acids and phosphate. Extending outwards from the lipid A is the core section of the polysaccharide chain, composed of about 10 sugar residues. Joined to this common core is the O-side-chain, composed of repeating units of four to five sugars. The composition of the O-side-chain is highly variable between strains and species and is responsible for their antigenic specificity.

The influx of essential hydrophilic nutrients from the external medium and the efflux of waste products across the outer membrane take place through channels (porins) in the lipid bilayer, formed by proteins. These outer membrane proteins (OMPs) have been shown to form three types of channels: (i) those which allow non-specific diffusion of solutes; (ii) specific channels, which contain specific binding sites and facilitate the diffusion of special classes of molecules; and (iii) high-affinity receptors, which are involved in the energy-requiring translocation of special large nutrient molecules, such as vitamin B_{12} and iron-chelator complexes (Nikaido, 1994a).

The porin proteins of channels, such as OMP F and OMP C of *Escherichia coli*, which allow the non-specific passage of hydrophilic molecules, form trimers, which fold in such a way as to produce barrel-shaped, water-filled channels traversing the outer membrane (Nikaido, 1994a). The channels have wide entrances and exits, but infolding of parts of the polypeptide chains form short central constrictions, which are only 7 Å x 11 Å in cross-section and which exclude molecules >600 Da in molecular weight. In addition, the constrictions in the porins are lined with negatively charged amino acid residues on one side and positively charged residues on the other. The polar nature of these constricted regions of the porin thus also impedes the entrance of lipophilic molecules.

The Gram-negative cell thus confronts the challenge of an antibacterial agent with an exposed outer surface composed essentially of the LPS and the protein-lined diffusion pores. This layer provides a barrier to the penetration of many chemically unrelated types of antibacterial agents (Russell & Gould, 1988). A number of different approaches have been taken in an attempt to clarify the precise nature of the protection afforded by the outer membrane. These have involved the modification of the membrane by genetic or chemical means and observing the effect of these manipulations on sensitivity to various antibacterial agents.

The availability of a comprehensive collection of mutants of *Salmonella typhimurium* having well-defined alterations in their LPS polysaccharide chains has facilitated an examination of how variations in these structures affect the sensitivity to antibacterials. The results of this approach (Roantree *et al.*, 1969, 1977; Schlecht & Westphal, 1970) indicate that shortening the sugar chains of the LPS has little effect on the antibacterial sensitivity until 80–90% of the chain is deleted. Loss of the next few sugar residues, however, produced cells with greatly increased sensitivity towards some antibiotics and to crystal violet, malachite green and phenol. The sensitivity of these 'deep rough' mutants to a number of other antibiotics was, however, unaffected.

Nikaido (1976) put forward an explanation of these changes. He showed that those agents whose activity was increased in deep rough mutants, as against the wild strain, were generally hydrophobic. Those agents whose activity was unaffected by LPS alteration were mainly small hydrophilic molecules (mol.wt <600). He then proposed that these changes were not a direct result of the alterations in the LPS structure but were due to an extensive reorganization of the outer membrane. The loss of a crucial glucose residue from the LPS blocks the incorporation of many protein molecules into the outer membrane (Ames *et al.*, 1974) and this results in a compensatory reorientation of phospholipid molecules at the outer surface (Smit *et al.*, 1975). These exposed phospholipid-bilayer regions then allow the rapid penetration of hydrophobic molecules such as phenol, by dissolution and diffusion in the lipid (Nikaido & Nakae, 1979).

The so-called *omp* mutants of *Sal. typhimurium*, which have a normal wild-type LPS composition but reduced levels of OMPs, are sensitive to crystal violet and deoxycholate (Ames *et al.*, 1974) and also allow the rapid penetration of a number of hydrophobic antibiotics (Nikaido, 1976). These observations emphasize the integrated nature of the components of the outer membrane and confirm that membrane reorganization, with phospholipid replacing protein at the outer surface, rather than alteration of the LPS structure itself, is the cause of increased hydrophobic permeability in the rough mutants (Nikaido & Vaara, 1985).

In *E. coli*, Tamaki & Matsuhashi (1973) showed that rough mutants with extensive LPS effects were unusually sensitive to the hydrophobic antibiotic novobiocin and hypersensitive to the enzyme lysozyme. Gustafsson *et al.* (1973) studied the uptake of gentian violet into a wild type and a collection of envelope mutants of *E. coli*. They found that all strains they tested bound the dye instantaneously to the outer envelope. The mutants then, however, continued to absorb the dye and permitted its penetration through to the ribosomal fraction of the cytoplasm. The rate of uptake of this second phase increased with increasing deficiency of LPS.

However, it was again clear that LPS is not the only important factor, as *env*A mutants, with some unknown envelope defect but with normal LPS composition, took up the dye extremely rapidly, at a rate equivalent to that observed with spheroplasts.

The observations of Russell *et al.* (1985, 1987) and Russell & Furr (1986a,b, 1987) on rough and deep rough mutants of *E. coli* and *Sal. typhimurium* also suggest that extensive loss of the LPS chain has to occur before sensitivity increases to esters of *p*-(4)-hydroxybenzoic acid, benzalkonium chloride and cetylpyridinium chloride. Deep rough mutants of *E. coli*, however, showed no increase in sensitivity to chlorhexidine, an observation which suggests that this antiseptic has a different cell-entry mechanism from the quaternary ammonium compounds (QACs).

The exposure of *E. coli* cells to 0.2 mmol/l ethylene diaminetetra-acetic acid (EDTA) in 0.12 mol/l tris buffer (pH 8.0) for just 2 min at 37°C results in their sensitization to a wide range of antibacterial agents, including many that are active against the cytoplasmic membrane (Leive, 1968). The cells also release periplasmic enzymes (Neu & Chou, 1967) and become sensitive to lysozyme (Repaske, 1956). These observations indicate that EDTA exerts an effect on a permeability barrier in the cell which is external to the peptidoglycan. The evidence on the precise mode of action has been reviewed by Russell (1971) and Wilkinson (1975). The first stage of the EDTA sensitization process involves the chelation of metal cations, which are bound to the polyanionic polysaccharide chains of LPS. These cations are believed to have a structural function in forming stabilizing cross-bridges between the LPS chains. Dissociation of the outer membrane follows, with the loss of LPS, protein and lipid. The layer is not totally disrupted, however, the amount of LPS released not exceeding 50% of the total present. The remaining LPS fraction, which is still located at the outer surface of the membrane, cannot be removed by raising the EDTA concentration or by re-treating the cells with EDTA (Leive, 1974). These observations have led Nikaido (1976) to suggest that the EDTA-induced loss of protein and LPS results in a reorganization of the outer membrane, similar to that which occurs in the deep rough mutants; phospholipid molecules replace the lost components, thus producing exposed phospholipid-bilayer regions, with all the consequences that this has for permeability.

Lipid bilayers, such as normal cytoplasmic membranes, are highly permeable to lipophilic molecules, the permeability being a function of their fluidity. In the outer membrane of the Gram-negative cell wall, each of the LPS head groups is attached to six covalently linked fatty-acid chains, rather than the two per glycerophospholipid molecule of the cytoplasmic membrane. The fatty acids of the LPS are also devoid of *cis* double bonds. Both these factors produce membranes with lipid interiors tightly packed with hydrocarbon chains and of unusually low fluidity (Nikaido, 1994b). Hydrophobic molecules have been shown to penetrate these LPS-containing membrane bilayers at one-fiftieth to one-hundreth of the rates through the usual phospholipid bilayers (Plesiat and Nikaido, 1992).

Recently, it has been recognized that some species of Gram-negative bacteria also possess active, broad-spectrum, efflux systems, which are capable of pumping out of the cell a diverse range of lipophilic biocidal agents, including dyes, detergents and antibiotics. An example of such an efflux pump is the Acr sytem of *E. coli*. For many years it has been known that acridine-sensitive mutants of *E. coli* also had increased susceptibility to other basic dyes, detergents and hydrophobic antibiotics (Nakamura, 1966). In view of the structural diversity of these antibacterial agents, it was thought that these mutants were likely to have an outer membrane defect of some sort. However, no changes to the LPS or the major OMPs were found and it is now clear that the *acr* genes code for a series of large inner-membrane proteins, which are involved in the pumping of a broad range of antibacterials out of the cell. These efflux pumps span the inner membrane and are thought to be associated with a membrane-fusion protein in the periplasm connecting the pump to a third protein, which forms an outer-membrane channel (Ma *et al.*, 1994).

In summary, then, the protein-lined pores in the outer membrane of *E. coli* restrict the access of hydrophobic and large hydrophilic molecules (> 650 Da) to the vulnerable cytoplasmic membrane. The rigid lipid bed of the outer membrane slows down the penetration of hydrophobic molecules, and powerful efflux systems ensure that lipophilic biocides that do penetrate the envelope are pumped out of the cell. These innate resistance mechanisms are important to enteric bacteria, as their natural habitat of the lower intestinal tract is rich in hydrophobic antibacterials, such as bile salts and fatty acids.

Some members of the Enterobacteriaciae, such as *Pr. mirabilis* and *Providencia stuartii*, exhibit greater degrees of intrinsic resistance to antibacterial agents than typical species, such as *E. coli* (Russell and Gould, 1988). Little is known about the nature of the enhanced resistance in these organisms (Russell, 1996).

3 *Pseudomonas aeruginosa*

Pseudomonas aeruginosa is a Gram-negative bacillus that is particularly resistant to biocides, exhibiting enhanced resistance to a range of agents including QACs, chlorhexidine, triclosan and propamidine (Table 10.1). Evidence that it is the special structure of the cell envelope of this organism that endows it with these characteristics comes from observations on its response to the chelating agent EDTA. *Pseudomonas aeruginosa* is, in fact, extremely sensitive to EDTA; concentrations of the agent that have little effect on other Gram-negative bacilli produce rapid lysis of the pseudomonal cells (Gray and Wilkinson, 1965). At low temperature or in low concentrations of EDTA, the cells will survive exposure, but the chelation of the Mg^{2+}, which is present in high concentrations in the outer membrane and believed to produce strong interlinkage with the LPS chains (Brown, 1975), produces disruption and loss of LPS, protein and lipid. These changes are associated with reduction in the resistance of the cells to agents such as QACs, phenolics and chlorhexidine (Wilkinson, 1975).

Phenotypic variation in the cell envelope composition of *Ps. aeruginosa* has been produced by manipulation of the growth conditions (Robinson *et al.*, 1974), and attempts have been made to correlate these changes with sensitivity to antibacterials. For example, Gilbert & Brown (1978) investigated the effect of nutrient limitation and growth rate on the sensitivity of *Ps. aeruginosa* to 3- and 4-chlorophenol. These substituted phenols increase the permeability of the cytoplasmic membranes to protons and thus uncouple oxidative phosphorylation from respiration. To assess sensitivity to these agents, the rates of drug-induced proton translocation into cells were measured by following the rate of change of pH of the extracellular phase. Variation in the proton permeability is related to the concentration of the agent at the cytoplasmic membrane, so changes in sensitivity were interpreted as variations in the penetration of the agents through the outer membrane. Using these methods, Gilbert & Brown (1978) concluded that rapidly growing cells were generally more sensitive than slower-growing ones and that glucose-limited cells were more sensitive than magnesium-limited ones. It was also shown that uptake of the phenols by cell suspensions varied, sensitive bacteria absorbing more than resistant ones. Using 2-keto-3-deoxyoctonic acid (KDO) as a marker, they concluded that the LPS content was higher in the magnesium-limited cells and that it decreased with increasing growth rates. Lipopolysaccharide content therefore correlated with sensitivity: the less LPS present in the cells, the greater their sensitivity to chlorophenols. The uptake of the agents also correlated with cell LPS content. The LPS content thus appeared to determine the degree of penetration of the cell envelope by these chlorinated phenols.

Kropinski *et al.* (1978) used a genetic approach

to study the effect of LPS on the resistance of *Ps. aeruginosa* to a variety of antibacterials, including dyes, detergents, antiseptics and antibiotics. Of a collection of LPS-deficient mutants, only the roughest strain, which had apparently lost all of the O-specific LPS side-chains and was also deficient in core constituents such as glucose and rhamnose, showed any increased sensitivity to sodium deoxycholate, hexadecylpyridinium chloride and benzalkonium chloride. By analogy with the deep rough mutants of *Sal. typhimurium,* it is possible that the loss of LPS in these strains could result in the relocation of more phospholipid at the outer-membrane surface.

The outer membrane of *Ps. aeruginosa* has a particularly low permeability to hydrophilic molecules. The porin channels are small and inhibit the diffusion of water-soluble agents with molecular weights greater than 400, including many types of antibacterial agents (Nakae, 1995). A multidrug efflux system has also been identified in *Ps. aeruginosa* (Poole, 1994). This MexAB-OprM system is similar in structure to the Acr pump of *E. coli* and has a normal physiological function of exporting the siderophore pyoverdine into the surrounding medium. It has been shown to be able to pump out a wide range of structurally unrelated antibiotics, including tetracyclines, chloramphenicol, fluoroquinolones, novobiocin, erythromycin, fusidic acid and rifampicin (Nikaido, 1996). It may well be that, as in the case of the *E. coli* system, such a pump could also export non-antibiotic biocides. It seems, therefore, that the poor permeability of the outer membrane to hydrophobic and large hydrophilic molecules, together with the effective export of any of these molecules that manage to penetrate to the periplasm or cytoplasm, results in the extraordinary resistance of this species to antibacterial agents.

4 Mycobacteria

The sensitivity of *Mycobacterium* spp. to chemical agents has been reviewed by Croshaw (1971) and Russell (1996). In summary, mycobacteria, including the human tubercle bacillus, are considerably more resistant to acids, alkalis, QACs, chlorhexidine, dyes, halogens and heavy metals than are other vegetative bacterial cells. In addition to their intrinsic resistance, mycobacteria in clinical specimens are notoriously coated in mucous or necrotic caseous materials, which inactivate disinfectants. Viable mycobacterial cells have thus been recovered from, for example, fibre-optic bronchoscopes after disinfection with an alcoholic iodophor (Nelson *et al.*, 1983) or glutaraldehyde (Wheeler *et al.*, 1989). Heat treatment should thus be used whenever possible for the disinfection of objects that may be contaminated with discharges from tuberculous patients (Bergan & Lystad, 1971). Only in circumstances where heat sterilization is not feasible should a chemical disinfectant be used. A clear soluble phenolic (1–2%) or alkaline glutaraldehyde (2%) is suitable for heavily contaminated objects (Ayliffe *et al.*, 1993).

Mycobacteria, of course, fail to take up many of the normal bacteriological dyes. Staining procedures like that of Ziehl–Nielsen, where the arylmethane dye fuchsin, in phenolic solution as carbol fuchsin, is driven into the cells with heat, have to be used to stain these organisms. Once stained, the cells resist decolorization with acid-alcohol. This acid-fastness is a function of their cell-wall structure. The cell wall structure of mycobacteria has been reviewed in considerable detail by Brennan & Nikaido (1995).

External to the cytoplasmic membrane of mycobacterial cells is a peptidoglycan layer, which contains *N*-glycomuramic acid, instead of the usual *N*-acetylmuramic acid. A unique polysaccharide, arabinogalactan is covalently linked to the peptidoglycan, and about 10% of the arabinose residues in this polymer are substituted by mycolic acids. These long-chair (C_{60}–C_{90})fatty acids are tightly packed in parallel arrays perpendicular to the cell surface. They have few double bonds in their hydrocarbon chains and, together with the arabinose head groups, they constitute an almost crystalline inner leaflet of an exceptionally thick lipid bilayer. The lipids of the outer leaflets of these membranes differ from species to species; some have short-chain fatty acids (C_{16}–C_{18}), such as glycerophospholipids and glycopeptolipids, while others have intermediate hydrocarbon chain-length (C_{30}–C_{40}) compounds, such as phenolic glycolipids. These external membranes of mycobacterial cells are thus assymetrical bilayers, with an outer layer of high fluidity overlying one of extremely low fluidity and permeability (Jarlier and Nikaido, 1994). This gradient of fluidity in the mycobacterial cell is analogous to that found in the Gram-negative outer membrane, except that it is in the reverse direction.

Hydrophilic nutrient molecules diffuse into mycobacterial cells through protein-lined porins in the outer membrane. There seem to be relatively few of these proteins per cell, however, and they form narrow channels with diameters of about 2 nm (Jarlier and Nikaido, 1994). As a result, they only permit slow diffusion by small hydrophilic molecules. The permeability of the *Mycobacterium-chelonae* cell walls to hydrophilic cephalosporins, for example, was found to be 10 times lower than that of the outer membrane of *Ps. aeruginosa* and three orders of magnitude lower than that of *E. coli* (Trias *et al*., 1992).

In summary, the influx of lipophilic agents into mycobacterial cells is impeded by a lipid bilayer of extremely low fluidity and exceptional thickness. Hydrophilic agents can gain access only slowly through the small inefficient porins. The unusual structure of these walls is thus a major factor in the intrinsic resistance of mycobacteria to antibacterial agents (Jarlier and Nikaido, 1994). The response of mycobacteria to biocides is considered in more detail in Chapter 10D.

5 Bacterial biofilms and resistance

In many natural habitats bacteria are able to adhere to and colonize available surfaces. The films of microbial growth that develop from these adhered cells are commonly mixed communities containing several different species. It is becoming increasingly clear that, in this mode of growth, bacteria exhibit characteristics that can be quite different from those of the same cells grown in suspension (Costerton *et al.*, 1995). These differences have important environmental, industrial and medical implications. Several groups have reported that bacteria growing in biofilms exhibit reduced sensitivities to antimicrobial agents, when compared with cells of the same organism growing in the dispersed planktonic mode. Gwynne *et al.* (1981) showed that *Ps. aeruginosa*, *E. coli.* and *Staph. aureus* adhering to glass culture vessels could survive in concentrations of β-lactam antibiotics that were bactericidal for the same cells growing in suspension. Marrie & Costerton (1981) demonstrated that *Serratia marcescens* growing on the walls of glass bottles could survive high concentrations (20 000 mg/l) of chlorhexidine. *Pseudomonas cepacia* growing on glass slides has also been shown to be protected against this antiseptic (Pallent *et al.*, 1983; Hugo *et al.*, 1986). The latter refers to early papers on surface colonization.

In an investigation of bladder instillations of antiseptics as a means of controlling urinary-tract infections in patients with indwelling catheters, Stickler *et al.* (1987) used a physical model of the catheterized bladder to examine the effect of chlorhexidine (200 mg/l) on urinary pathogens. *Providencia stuartii*, *Ps. aeruginosa*, *Pr. mirabilis*, *E. coli*, *Klebsiella pneumoniae* and *Streptococcus faecalis* growing in urine in the bladder model rapidly recovered from the initial bactericidal effect of the antiseptic. During these experiments, it was noticed that films of bacterial growth developed on the walls of the model, and cells in these biofilms appeared to be particularly resistant to the antiseptics and initiated the recovery of the cultures after the instillation. More recently, biofilms of *E. coli* and other urinary-tract pathogens established on silicon discs have also been shown to survive well in chlorhexidine (200 mg/l) for up to 2 h, whereas in urine suspension the cells were rapidly killed by this concentration of the antiseptic (Stickler & Hewett, 1991; Stickler *et al.*, 1991).

In many industrial processes, the surfaces of storage tanks, pipelines, water-circulating systems, filtration units and machinery become colonized by biofilms. This biofouling can lead to product contamination and process inefficiency (Bott, 1992; Flemming *et al.*, 1992; Hamilton, 1994; Mittleman, 1995). There are also dangers to public health when biofilms containing *Legionella pneumophila* and other pathogens form in water-supply systems (Walker *et al.*, 1995). Several laboratory investigations have demonstrated the resistance of biofilm cells to chemical agents that are used in attempts to control these problems. Sharma *et al.* (1987), for example, have shown that a QAC, a biguanide and an isothiazolone were less active against sessile than suspended cells of *Desulphovibrio desulfuricans*. *Escherichia coli*, *Sal. typhimurium*, *Yersinia enterocolitica*, *Shigella sonnei* and *K. pneumoniae* showed substantially reduced sensitivities to chlorination when adsorbed to carbon granules (Le Chevalier *et al*., 1988). Similarly, *Enterobacter cloacae* growing on particles sloughed off from a cast-iron pipe was more resistant to disinfection than its planktonic sister cells (Herson *et al*., 1987).

Wright *et al*. (1991) reported that, while 2-bromo-4-nitropropane-1,3-diol (bronopol) and a preparation containing a mixture of isothiazolins (Kathon) were effectively bactericidal against planktonic populations of *L. pneumophila* within 9–12 h, they took up to 48 h to produce similar activity against cells adhering to materials used in water-cooling towers. Green (1994) demonstrated that the resistance of *Legionella bozermanii* to glutaraldehyde and a preparation containing glutaraldehyde and a QAC increased by several orders of magnitude when it was grown as a biofilm on surfaces such as red rubber. Brown *et al*. (1995) reported that biofilms of *Ps. aeruginosa* on polycarbonate membranes exhibited enhanced resistance to povidone iodine.

Gilbert and Brown (1995) reviewed the hypotheses that have been proposed to explain the enhanced resistance of biofilm cells to anfibacterials. Costerton (1984) observed that populations of bacteria growing in biofilms are embedded in an anionic polysaccharide matrix, and suggested that this glycocalyx affords considerable protection to the cells against antimicrobial agents. Nichols *et al*. (1988) examined the hypothesis that the glycocalyx hindered the penetration of bactericidal molecules in the film. In this investigation, they measured the ability of the antibiotic tobramycin to penetrate alginate gels, which chemically resemble the exopolysaccharide of *Ps. aeruginosa* cells, and found that there was an initial inhibition of tobramycin diffusion, until all the gel binding sites were saturated. The antibiotic then diffused freely through the gel. It was calculated that the time required for the concentration of tobramycin at the base of a biofilm 100 μm thick to rise to 90% of the external concentration would increase from 27 s in the absence of any restriction to 77 s in the presence of 1% w/v extracellular polysaccharide. Such an effect is unlikely to be a major contribution to the 1000-fold reduction of sensitivity to tobramycin exhibited by mucoid biofilms of *Ps. aeruginosa*. In this case, at least, it would seem that restriction of penetration of the bactericide is not the sole cause of resistance. If the extracellular polysaccharide glycocalyx of the biofilm matrix reacts in some way with an antibacterial agent, however, it is much more likely to constitute a physical barrier to the penetration of that agent. The activities of biocides such as chlorine and iodine, for example, are substantially reduced by these exopolymers (Characklis and Dydek, 1976; Brown *et al*., 1995) and in these cases the biofilm matrix may well play a direct role in cell protection.

Growth rates of bacteria can have profound effects on their sensitivity to antibacterial agents, slow-growing cells generally being more resistant (Gilbert *et al*., 1987). Brown *et al*. (1988) proposed that the limited availability of nutrients to cells in the depths of biofilms produces populations of metabolically dormant cells and that this reduced growth rate is a major contributing factor to their resistance to antibacterials.

Recent work on effects on cells of attachment to surfaces and cell-to-cell communication in dense communities has produced yet another possible explanation. The accumulation of cell communication signals, such as homoserine lactones, in these circumstances induces the cells to produce sigma factors—proteins capable of switching on or off whole sets of genes (Davies *et al*, 1993; Salmon *et al*., 1995). As a result, attached cells within a biofilm can be phenotypically very different from their corresponding planktonic forms. It has been proposed that such profound changes to the phenotype could well affect the target sites of antibacterials and thus coincidentally produce resistance to these agents (Costerton *et al*., 1995). Exactly how bacteria in biofilms manage to resist the activity of many biocides is thus still uncertain. As biofilm resistance to antibacterial agents has been recorded in so many bacterial species and against such a range of chemically unrelated biocidal molecules, it would be surprising if any single mechanism were responsible for the phenomenon. It may well be, therefore, that a variety of different strategies will have to be employed to control the problem in different circumstances.

6 Disinfection policies and intrinsic resistance

The recognition of the role of the outer membrane of Gram-negative bacteria in inhibiting the passage of so many antibacterial agents provides an opportunity for a rational approach to the design of new antiseptic and disinfectant preparations. The combination of an agent which opens up the outer membrane with compounds which attack, for example, the cytoplasmic membrane could produce a range of new formulations with improved activity against these refractile organisms. In this connection, Dankert & Schut (1976) and Russell & Furr (1977) have shown that the combination of EDTA with chloroxylenol potentiates the activity of this phenolic compound against *Ps. aeruginosa.* Russell & Furr (1977), for example, showed that the EDTA—chloroxylenol mixture withstood a repeated challenge from daily doses of 10^6 viable cells/ml of *Ps. aeruginosa.* Even on day 48, no viable cells could be reisolated from the disinfectant. Chloroxylenol alone, however, at an equivalent concentration, failed the test, cells being recovered from the disinfectant on day 2, and by day 12 the number of viable cells contaminating the solution was $>5\times10^6$ ml. Ayliffe *et al.* (1993) called for hospitals to review their disinfection policies and to reduce the use of disinfectants in circumstances where heating or thorough cleaning will suffice. This makes good economic sense and is also to be approved of on the general grounds that the more extensively an antibacterial agent is used, the more likely it will become that a resistant microbial flora will emerge. In our opinion, hospital committees for control of infection should also think carefully about their antiseptic or disinfectant policies in situations where intrinsically resistant bacteria are producing infections.

This view is based on observations on the mode of development of urinary tract infections in paraplegic patients enduring long-term intermittent bladder catheterization (Stickler *et al.,* 1971; O'Flynn & Stickler, 1972). Catheterization, which was performed three or four times daily, involved the washing of the periurethal area with chlorhexidine (600 mg/l) prior to insertion of the catheter. The effect of this repeated application of antiseptic on the bacterial flora of the urethral meatus was examined in a prospective study of patients from the date of injury and admission to the spinal unit up to the time they developed urinary-tract infection. The urethral flora was examined daily before and after the application of the antiseptic, and the general pattern that emerged was that for the first few days after trauma the meatal skin carried a Gram-positive flora, which was greatly reduced by the application of the antiseptic. A Gram-negative flora usually developed by about day 4 and proved to be more refractory to chlorhexidine. In particular, *Pr. mirabilis, Ps. aeruginosa, Prov. stuartii* and *Klebsiella* spp. frequently survived the meatal cleansing and proceeded to infect the bladder. Many of these strains demonstrated an ability to grow in media containing 200 mg/l of chlorhexidine and some of the *Pr. mirabilis* and *Prov. stuartii* isolates from this source were shown to have minimal inhibitory concentrations (MICs) of up to 800 mg/l, well above the level of 10–50 mg/l originally reported to inhibit the growth of these Gram-negative species (Davies *et al.*, 1954).

In order to ascertain whether this resistance to chlorhexidine was a general phenomenon or was limited to special circumstances, Stickler & Thomas (1980) examined a large collection of isolates of Gram-negative bacilli causing urinary-tract infections in patients from general practice, antenatal clinics and six hospitals. It was observed that chlorhexidine resistance was not a widespread phenomenon. It was limited to *Pr. mirabilis*, *Ps. aeruginosa*, *Prov. stuartii* and *Serr. marcescens*, and the only major source of these resistant strains was another spinal unit, where chlorhexidine was being used extensively in management of patients by long-term indwelling catheterization.

Analysis of the antibiotic sensitivities of the collection revealed a significant correlation between resistance to chlorhexidine and multiplicity of drug resistance, the chlorhexidine-resistant strains generally being resistant to five to seven of the antibiotics tested. These results led us to examine whether the correlation between antibiotic and antiseptic resistance had a basis in an association of the resistance genes. While a transferable resistance factor carrying the genetic information for resistance to commonly used antiseptics and antibiotics would constitute a formidable genetic package for nosocomial organisms, an investigation with strains of *Prov. stuartii* showed no evidence for the existence of such a genetic linkage, and it was suggested that chlorhexidine resistance was an intrinsic property of the cell walls of these organisms, which denies the antiseptic access to its target site of the cytoplasmic membrane, or alternatively that chlorhexidine-resistant strains happen to be efficient recipients for R-factors for some reason (Stickler *et al.*, 1983).

These observations suggest that an antiseptic policy involving the long-term and extensive use of chlorhexidine in clinical situations, such as the catheterized urinary tract, could well be counterproductive and lead to the selection of notoriously drug-resistant nosocomial pathogens (Stickler & Thomas, 1980). Some support for our contention was provided by the report (Walker & Lowes, 1985) of an outbreak of urinary infections in patients at a Southampton hospital. Here, urinary-catheter management involved the use of chlorhexidine for perineal cleaning prior to catheterization. A gel containing chlorhexidine was used as a lubricant for the passage of the catheter, and chlorhexidine was included in the urine drainage bags and instilled into the bags every time they were emptied. The catheter–meatal junction was cleansed daily with chlorhexidine, after which a cream containing the antiseptic was applied to the periurethal area (Southampton Control of Infection Team, 1982). In the outbreak, 90 patients became infected with a chlorhexidine-resistant strain of *Pr. mirabilis,* which was also resistant to sulphafurazole, trimethoprim, ampicillin, mezlocillin, azlocillin, carbenicillin, gentamicin and tobramycin (Dance *et al.*, 1987). The epidemic strain was shown to survive the 'in-use' concentrations of chlorhexidine achieved in the urine reservoir bags (Walker & Lowes, 1985), and these authors considered that the epidemic strain may have been selected by the antiseptic policy, and recommended that the routine addition of chlorhexidine to the catheter bags be abandoned.

In the context of the use of antiseptics in preventing and controlling urinary tract infection, evidence is accumulating that the normal Gram-positive flora of the urethra has a role in protecting the urinary tract from enteric organisms (Kunin & Steele, 1985; Reid *et al.*, 1987). The antiseptics currently used in urethral disinfection are more active against the normal flora, and this may facilitate the colonization of the urethra by the Gram-negative pathogens. It would be most interesting to examine the long-term effects of antiseptic formulations that are selectively active on the urinary pathogens. It is our belief that the careful consideration of which antiseptic to use in special circumstances and the implementation of the general disinfection policies formulated in the guidelines laid down by Ayliffe *et al.* (1993) will help to reduce the accumulation of intrinsically resistant species in the hospital environment.

7 References

Ames, G.F.L., Spudich, E.N. & Nikaido, H. (1974) Protein composition of the outer membrane of *Salmonella typhimurium*: effect of lipopolysaccharide mutations. *Journal of Bacteriology*, **117**, 406–416.

Ayliffe, G.A.J., Coates, D. & Hoffman, P.N. (1993) *Chemical Disinfection in Hospitals*. London: Public Health Laboratory Service.

Bergan, T. & Lystad, A. (1971) Anti-tubercular action of disinfectants. *Journal of Applied Bacteriology*, **34**, 751–756.

Berry, H. (1944) Antibacterial values of ethylene glycol mono-phenyl ether. *Lancet*, **ii**, 175–176.

Bott, T.R. (1992) Introduction to the problem of biofouling in industrial equipment. In *Biofilms—Science and Technology* (eds Melo, L.F., Bott, T.R., Fletcher, M. & Capdeville, B.), pp. 3–12. Dordrecht: Kluwer.

Brennan, P.J. & Nikaido, H. (1995) The envelope of mycobacteria. *Annual Reviews of Biochemistry*, **64**, 29–63.

Brown, M.L., Aldrich, H.C. & Gauthier, J.J. (1995) Relationship between glycocalyx and povidone-iodine resistance in *Pseudomonas aeruginosa* (ATCC 27853) biofilms. *Applied and Environmental Microbiology*, **61**, 187–193.

Brown, M.R.W. (1975) The role of the cell envelop in resistance. In *Resistance of* Pseudomonas aeruginosa (ed. Brown, M.R.W.), pp. 71–105. London: Wiley.

Brown, M.R.W., Allison, D.G. & Gilbert, P. (1988) Resistance of bacterial biofilms to antibiotics: a growth related effect? *Journal of Antimicrobial Chemotherapy*, **22**, 777–780.

Characklis, W.G. & Dydek, S.T. (1976) The influence of carbon-nitrogen ratio on the chlorination of microbial aggregates. *Water Research*, **10**, 512–522.

Costerton, J.W. (1984) The aetiology and persistence of

cryptic bacterial infections: a hypothesis. *Review of Infectious Diseases*, **6** (Suppl. 3), S608–S612.

Costerton, J.W., Lewandowski, Z., Caldwell, D.E., Korber, D.R. & Lappin-Scott, H.M. (1995) Microbial biofilms. *Annual Reviews of Microbiology*, **49**, 711–745.

Croshaw, B. (1971) The destruction of mycobacteria. In *Inhibition and Destruction of the Microbial Cell* (ed. Hugo, W.B.), pp. 420–450. London: Academic Press.

Dance, D.A.B., Pearson, A.D., Seal, D.V. & Lowes, J.A. (1987) A hospital outbreak caused by a chlorhexidine and antibiotic resistant *Proteus mirabilis. Journal of Hospital Infection*, **10**, 10–16.

Dankert, J. & Schut, I.K. (1976) The antibacterial action of chloroxylenol in combination with ethylenediamine tetraacetic acid. *Journal of Hygiene*, **76**, 11–22.

Davies, D.G., Chakrabarty, A.M. & Geesey, G.G. (1993) Exopolysaccharide production in biofilms: substratum activation of alginate gene expression by *Pseudomonas aeruginosa. Applied and Environmental Microbiology*, **59**, 1181–1186.

Davies, G.E., Francis, J., Margin, A.R., Rose, F.L. & Swain, G. (1954) 1:6-di-4-Chlorophenyldiguanidohexane (Hibitane): laboratory investigation of a new antibacterial agent of high potency. *British Journal of Pharmacology and Chemotherapy*, **9**, 192–196.

Flemming, H.C., Schaule, G. & McDonogh, R. (1992) Biofouling on membranes—a short review. In *Biofilms—Science and Technology* (eds Melo, L.F., Bott, T.R., Fletcher, M. & Capdeville, B.), pp. 487–498. Dordrecht: Kluwer.

Gilbert, P. & Brown, M.R.W. (1978) Influence of growth rate and nutrient limitation on the gross cellular composition of *Pseudomonas aeruginosa* and its resistance to 3- and 4-chlorophenol. *Journal of Bacteriology*, **133**, 1066–1072.

Gilbert, P. & Brown, M.R.W. (1995) Mechanisms of the protection of bacterial biofilms from antimicrobial agents. In *Microbial Biofilms* (eds Lappin-Scott, H. & Costerton, J.W.), pp. 118–132. Cambridge: Cambridge University Press.

Gilbert, P., Brown, M.R.W. & Costerton, J.W. (1987) Inocula for antimicrobial sensitivity testing: a critical review. *Journal of Antimicrobial Chemotherapy*, **20**, 147–154.

Graham, L.L., Beveridge, T.J. & Nanninga, N. (1991) Periplasmic space and the concept of periplasm. *Trends in Biochemical Sciences*, **16**, 328–329.

Gray, G.W. & Wilkinson, S.G. (1965) The action of ethylenediamine tetraacetic acid on *Pseudomonas aeruginosa. Journal of Applied Bacteriology*, **28**, 153–164.

Green, P.N. (1994) Biocide efficacy testing against legionella biofilms. In *Bacterial Biofilms and Their Control in Medicine and Industry* (eds Wimpenny, J., Nichols, W., Stickler, D.J. & Lappin-Scott, H.), pp. 105–107. Cardiff: Bioline.

Gustafsson, P., Nordstrom, K. & Normark, S. (1973) Outer penetration barrier of *Escherichia coli* K12: kinetics of the uptake of gentian violet by wild type and envelope mutants. *Journal of Bacteriology*, **116**, 893–900.

Gwynne, M.N., Webb, L.T. & Rolinson G.N. (1981) Regrowth of *Pseudomonas aeruginosa* and other bacteria after the bactericidal action of carbenicillin and other β-lactam antibiotics. *Journal of Infectious Diseases*, **144**, 263–269.

Hamilton, W.A. (1971) Membrane-active antibacterial compounds. In *Inhibition and Destruction of the Microbial Cell* (ed. Hugo, W.B.), pp. 77–93. London: Academic Press.

Hamilton, W.A. (1994) Industrial problems due to biolfilms. In *Bacterial Biofilms and their Control in Medicine and Industry* (ed. Wimpenny, J., Nichols, W., Stickler, D.J. & Lappin-Scott, H.), pp. 109–112. Cardiff: Bioline.

Herson, D.D., McGonigle, B., Payer, M.A. & Baker, K.H. (1987) Attachment as a factor in the protection of *Enterobacter* from chlorination. *Applied and Environmental Microbiology*, **53**, 1178–1180.

Hugo, W.B. (1967) The mode of action of antiseptics. *Journal of Applied Bacteriology*, **30**, 17–50.

Hugo, W.B., Pallent, L.J., Grant, D.J.W., Denyer, S.P. & Davies, A. (1986) Factors contributing to the survival of a strain of *Pseudomonas cepacia* in chlorhexidine solutions. *Letters in Applied Microbiology*, **2**, 37–42.

Jarlier, V. Nikaido, H. (1994) Mycobacterial cell wall: structure and role in natural resistance to antibiotics. *FEMS Microbiology Letters*, **123**, 11–18.

Kropinski, A.M.B., Chan, L. & Milazzo, F.H. (1978) Susceptibility of lipopolysaccharide defective mutants of *Pseudomonas aeruginosa* strain PAO to dyes, detergents and antibiotics. *Antimicrobial Agents and Chemotherapy*, **13**, 494–499.

Kunin, C.M. & Steele, C. (1985) Culture of the surfaces of urinary catheters to sample urethral flora and study of the effect of antimicrobial therapy. *Journal of Clinical Microbiology*, **21**, 902–908.

Le Chevalier, M.W., Cawthon, C.D. & Lee, R.G. (1988) Inactivation of biofilm bacteria. *Applied and Environmental Microbiology*, **54**, 2492–2494.

Leive, L. (1968) Studies on the permeability change produced in coliform bacteria by ethylenediaminetetraacetate. *Journal of Biological Chemistry*, **243**, 2373–2380.

Leive, L. (1974) The barrier of function of the Gram-negative envelope. *Annals of the New York Academy of Sciences*, **235**, 109–129.

Ma, D., Cook, D.N., Hearst, J.E. & Nikaido, H. (1994) Efflux pumps and drug resistance in Gram-negative bacteria. *Trends in Microbiology*, **2**, 489–493.

Marrie, T.J. & Costerton, J.W. (1981) Prolonged survival of *Serratia marcescens* in chlorhexidine. *Applied and Environmental Microbiology*, **42**, 1093–1102.

Mittleman, M.W. (1995) Biofilm development in purifed water systems. In *Microbial Biofilms* (eds Lappin-Scott, H. & Costerton, J.W.), pp. 133–147. Cambridge: Cambridge University Press.

Nakae, T. (1995) Role of membrane permeability in determining antibiotic resistance in *Pseudomonas aeruginosa*. *Microbiology and Immunology*, **39**, 221–229.

Nakamura, H. (1966) Acriflavine-binding capacity of *Escherichia coli* in relation to acriflavine sensitivity and metabolic activity. *Journal of Bacteriology*, **92**, 1447–1452.

Nelson, K.E., Larson, P.A., Schraufnaugel, D.E. & Jackson, J. (1983) Transmission of tuberculosis by flexible fibre bronchoscopes. *American Reviews of Respiratory Diseases*, **127**, 97–100.

Neu, H.C. & Chou, J. (1967) Release of surface enzymes in Enterobacteriaceae by osmotic shock. *Journal of Bacteriology*, **94**, 1934–1945.

Nichols, W.W., Evans, M.J., Slack, M.P.E. & Walmsley, H.L. (1988) The penetration of antibiotics into aggregates of mucoid and non-mucoid *Pseudomonas aeruginosa*. *Jornal of General Microbiology*, **135**, 1291–1303.

Nikaido, H. (1976) Outer membrane of *Salmonella typhimurium*: transmembrane diffusion of some hydrophobic substances. *Biochimica et Biophysica Acta*, **433**, 118–132.

Nikaido, H. (1994a) Porins and specific diffusion channels in bacterial outer membranes. *Journal of Biological Chemistry*, **269**, 3905–3908.

Nikaido, H. (1994b) Prevention of drug access to bacterial targets: permeability barriers and active efflux. *Science*, **264**, 382–387.

Nikaido, H. (1996) Multidrug efflux pumps of Gram-negative bacteria. *Journal of Bacteriology*, **178**, 5853–5859.

Nikaido, H. & Nakae, T. (1979) The outer membrane of Gram-negative bacteria. *Advances in Microbial Physiology*, **20**, 163–250.

Nikaido, H. & Vaara, M. (1985) Molecular basis of the permeability of the bacterial outer membrane. *Microbiological Reviews*, **49**, 1–32.

O'Flynn, J.D. & Stickler, D.J. (1972) Disinfectants and Gram-negative bacteria. *Lancet*, **i**, 489–490.

Pallent, L.J., Hugo, W.B., Grant, D.J.W. & Davies, A. (1983) *Pseudomonas cepacia* and infections. *Journal of Hospital Infection*, **4**, 9–13.

Plesiat, P. & Nikaido, H. (1992) Outer membranes of Gram-negative bacteria are permeable to steroid probes. *Molecular Microbiology*, **6**, 1323–1333.

Poole, K. (1994) Bacterial multidrug resistance–emphasis on efflux mechanisms and *Pseudomonas aeruginosa*. *Journal of Antimicrobial Chemotherapy*, **34**, 453–456.

Poxton, I.R. (1993) Procaryote envelope diversity. *Journal of Applied Bacteriology, Symposium Supplement*, **74**, 1S–11S.

Reid, G., Cook, R.L. & Bruce, A.W. (1987) Examination of strains of lactobacilli for properties that may influence bacterial interference in the urinary tract. *Journal of Urology*, **138**, 330–335.

Repaske, R. (1956) Lysis of Gram-negative bacteria by lysozyme. *Biochimica et Biophysica Acta*, **22**, 189–191.

Roantree, R.J., Kuo, T.T., MacPhee, D.G. & Stocker, B.A.D. (1969) The effect of various rough lesions in *Salmonella typhimurium* upon sensitivity to penicillins. *Clinical Research*, **17**, 157.

Roantree, R.J., Kuo, T.T. & MacPhee, D.G. (1977) The effect of defined lipopolysaccharide core defects upon antibiotic resistances of *Salmonella typhimurium*. *Journal of General Microbiology*, **103**, 223–234.

Robinson, A., Melling, J. & Ellwood, D.C. (1974) Effect of growth environment on the envelope composition of *Pseudomonas aeruginosa*. *Proceedings of the Society for General Microbiology*, **1**, 61–62.

Russell, A.D. (1971) Ethylenediamine tetraacetic acid. In *Inhibition and Destruction of the Microbial Cell* (ed. Hugo, W.B.), pp. 209–224. London: Academic Press.

Russell, A.D. (1996) Mechanisms of bacterial resistance to biocides. *International Biodeterioration and Biodegradation*, **36**, 247–265.

Russell, A.D. & Furr, J.R. (1977) The antibacterial activity of a new chloroxylenol preparation containing ethylenediamine tetraacetic acid. *Journal of Applied Bacteriology*, **43**, 253–260.

Russell, A.D. & Furr, J.R. (1986a) The effects of antiseptics, disinfectants and preservatives on smooth, rough and deep rough strains of *Salmonella typhimurium*. *International Journal of Pharmaceutics*, **34**, 115–123.

Russell, A.D. & Furr, J.R. (1986b) Susceptibility of porin and lipopolysaccharide deficient strains of *Escherichia coli* to some antiseptics and disinfectants. *Journal of Hospital Infection*, **8**, 47–56.

Russell, A.D. & Furr, J.R. (1987) Comparative sensitivity of smooth, rough and deep rough strains of *Escherichia coli* to chlorhexidine, quarternary ammonium compounds and dibromopropamidine isothionate. *International Journal of Pharmaceutics*, **36**, 191–197.

Russell, A.D. & Gould, G.W. (1988) Resistance of Enterobacteriaceae to preservatives and disinfectants. *Journal of Applied Bacteriology Symposium Supplement*, **65**, 167s–195s.

Russell, A.D., Furr, J.R. & Pugh, W.J. (1985) Susceptibility of porin and lipopolysaccharide deficient mutants of *Escherichia coli* to a homologous series of esters of *p*-hydroxybenzoic acid. *International Journal of Pharmaceutics*, **27**, 163–173.

Russell, A.D., Furr, J.R. & Pugh, W.J. (1987) Sequential loss of outer membrane lipopolysaccharides and sensitivity of *Escherichia coli* to antibacterial agents. *International Journal of Pharmaceutics*, **35**, 227–232.

Salmon, G.P.C., Bycroft, B.W., Stewart, G.S.A.B. & Williams, P. (1995) The bacterial 'enigma': cracking the code of cell–cell communication. *Molecular Microbiology*, **16**, 615–624.

Schlecht, S. & Westphal, O. (1970) Untersuchungen zur Typisierung von *Salmonella* R-formen, 4 mitteilung: Typisierung von *S. minnesota* R-mutananen mittels Antibiotica. *Zentralblatt fur Bakteriologie, Parasitenkunde Infectionskrankheiten und Hygiene (Abteilung I)*, **213**, 356–381.

Sharma, A.P., Battersby, N.S. & Stewart, D.J. (1987) Techniques for the evaluation of biocide activity against sulphate-reducing bacteria. In *Preservatives in the Food, Pharmaceutical and Environmental Industries* (eds Board, R.G., Allwood, M.C. & Banks, J.G.), pp. 165–175. Oxford: Blackwell Scientific Publications.

Smit, J., Kamio, Y. & Nikaido, H. (1975) Outer membrane of *Salmonella typhimurium*: chemical analysis and free fracture studies with lipopolysaccharide mutants. *Journal of Bacteriology*, **124**, 942–958.

Southampton Control of Infection Team (1982) Evaluation of aseptic techniques and chlorhexidine on the rate of catheter-associated urinary tract infection. *Lancet*, **i**, 89–91.

Stickler, D.J. & Hewett, P. (1991) Activity of antiseptics against biofilms of mixed bacterial species growing on silicone surfaces. *European Journal of Clinical Microbiology and Infectious Disease*, **10**, 416–421.

Stickler, D.J. & Thomas, B. (1980) Antiseptic and antibiotic resistance in Gram-negative bacteria causing urinary tract infection. *Journal of Clinical Pathology*, **33**, 288–296.

Stickler, D.J., Wilmot, C.B. & O'Flynn, J.D. (1971) The mode of development of urinary tract infection in intermittently catheterised male paraplegics. *Paraplegia*, **8**, 243–252.

Stickler, D.J., Thomas, B., Clayton, C.L. & Chawla, J. (1983) Studies on the genetic basis of chlorhexidine resistance. *British Journal of Clinical Practice, Symposium Supplement*, **25**, 23–30.

Stickler, D.J., Clayton, C.L. & Chawla, J.C. (1987) The resistance of urinary tract pathogens to chlorhexidine bladder washouts. *Journal of Hospital Infection*, **10**, 28–39.

Stickler, D., Dolman, J., Rolfe, S. & Chawla, J. (1991) Activity of some antiseptics against urinary tract pathogens growing as biofilms on silicone surfaces. *European Journal of Clinical Microbiology and Infectious Diseases*, **10**, 410–415.

Sykes, G. (1958) *Disinfection and Sterilisation*, 344 pp. London: E. & F.N. Spon.

Tamaki, S. & Matsuhashi, M. (1973) Increase in sensitivity to antibiotics and lysozyme on deletion of lipopolysaccharides in *E. coli* strains. *Journal of Bacteriology*, **114**, 453–454.

Trias, J., Jarlier, V. & Benz, R. (1992) Porins in the cell wall of *Mycobacteria*. *Science*, **258**, 1479–1481.

Trueman, J.R. (1971) The halogens. In: *Inhibition and Destruction of the Microbial Cell* (ed. Hugo, W.B.), pp. 137–183. London: Academic Press.

Walker, E.M. & Lowes, J.A. (1985) An investigation into *in vitro* methods for the detection of chlorhexidine resistance. *Journal of Hospital Infection*, **6**, 389–397.

Walker, J.T., Mackerness, C.W. Rogers, J. & Keevil, C.W. (1995) In *Microbial Biofilms* (ed. Lappin-Scott, H. & Costerton, J.W.), pp. 196–206. Cambridge: Cambridge University Press.

Wallhäusser, K.H. (1984) Antimicrobial preservatives used by the cosmetic industry. In *Cosmetic and Drug Preservation: Principles and Practice* (ed. Kabara, J.J.), pp. 605–745. New York: Marcel Dekker.

Wheeler, P.W., Lancaster, D. & Kaiser, A.B. (1989) Bronchopulmonary cross-colonization and infection related to mycobacterial contamination of suction valves of bronchioscopes. *Journal of Infectious Diseases*, **159**, 954–958.

Wilkinson, S.G. (1975) Sensitivity to ethylaminediamine tetraacetic acid. In *Resistance of* Pseudomonas aeruginosa (ed. Brown, M.R.W.), pp. 145–188. London: J. Wiley & Sons.

Wright, J.B., Ruseska, I. & Costerton, J.W. (1991) Decreased biocide susceptibility of adherent *Legionella pneumophila*. *Journal of Applied Bacteriology*, **71**, 531–538.

B. PLASMIDS AND BACTERIAL RESISTANCE

1 Introduction

Bacterial resistance to biocides is essentially of two types: (i) intrinsic, a natural (innate), chromosomally controlled property of an organism; (ii) acquired, resulting from genetic changes in a bacterial cell and arising either by mutation or by the acquisition of genetic material, e.g. via plasmids, from another cell (Russell, 1994; Russell, & Russell, 1995; George, 1996; Russell & Chopra, 1996).

Intrinsic resistance has already been considered and this chapter will discuss acquired resistance associated with plasmids. Papers that have described this in detail are those by Russell (1985, 1990), Russell *et al.* (1986). Russell & Gould (1988), Heinzel (1988) and Russell & Chopra (1996). In addition, Chapter 10F, dealing with antibiotic-resistant cocci, should be consulted, together with Russell & Day (1996).

2 Plasmid-mediated resistance

Plasmid-mediated resistance to non-chemotherapeutic agents has been most extensively studied with metals, especially mercury (Nies & Silver, 1995). Although non-mercury metals will form part of the discussion, it must be emphasized that, despite their biocidal activities, they do not have major practical applications as antibacterial agents (Russell & Chopra, 1996). Unlike the situation with antibiotics, the role of plasmids in bacterial resistance to non-metallic biocides has not been widely investigated (Joly, 1995; Russell, 1995; Russell & Day, 1996).

2.1 Heavy-metal resistance

Genetic determinants of resistance to heavy metals are often found on plasmids and transposons, and this resistance may occur with high frequency. Additionally, there is sometimes, but not invariably, an association with antibiotic resistance.

2.1.1 Resistance to mercury

Mercuric chloride is a toxic agent and consequently is no longer widely used as a disinfectant. Organomercury compounds, such as phenylmercuric nitrate (PMN) and acetate (PMA), are, however, widely used as preservatives in pharmaceutical products, and thiomersal in immunological preparations. Merbromin (mercurochrome) is a weak disinfectant.

Mercury resistance is plasmid-borne and not chromosomally mediated. It is transferred from donor cells to recipients by conjugation or transduction. Inorganic mercury and phenylmercury resistance is a common property of clinical isolates of *Staphylococcus aureus* containing penicillinase plasmids (Novick & Roth, 1968; Novick & Bouanchaud, 1971). Plasmids in Gram-negative bacteria may also carry genes specifying resistance to antibiotics and, in some instances, cobalt (Co^{2+}), nickel (Ni^{+}), cadmium (Cd^{+}) and arsenate (As O_3^-) (Foster, 1983; Chopra, 1988; Silver & Misra, 1988). Mercury resistance is always inducible and is not the result of training or tolerance.

Plasmids conferring resistance to mercurials are of two types.

1 'Narrow-spectrum', which encode resistance to inorganic mercury (Hg^{2+}); Fig. 10.1) and to the organomercurials merbromin and fluorescein mercuric acetate in *Escherichia coli*. Othe organomercury compounds are unaffected.

2 'Broad-spectrum', which specify resistance to Hg^{2+}, merbromin and fluorescein mercuric acetate and also to PMN, PMA, thiomersal, *p*-hydroxymercuribenzoate (PHMB), methylmercury and ethylmercury in *E. coli*.

Similar classes of plasmids occur with mercury-resistant strains of *Pseudomonas aeruginosa*, although the 'narrow-spectrum' subclass confers slight resistance to PHMB also (Clark *et al.*, 1977). In *Staph. aureus*, only the 'broad-spectrum' subclass is found (Table 10.2). The mechanism of resistance is shown in Fig. 10.2; see also Ghosh *et al.* (1996).

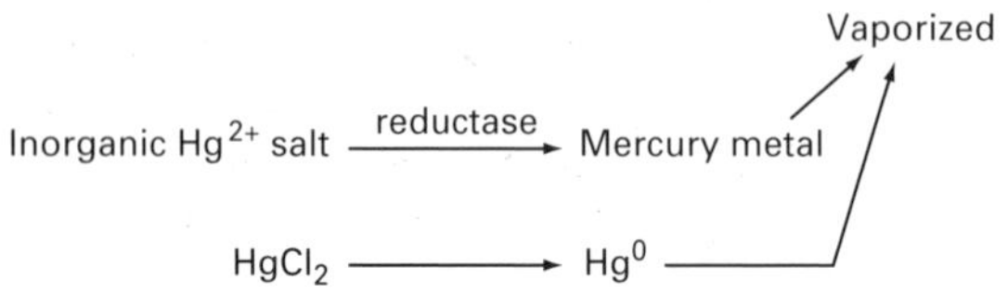

Fig. 10.1 Biochemical mechanism of resistance to inorganic mercury compounds.

Considerable progress has been made in examining the genes responsible for various functions. The most widely studied plasmid is R-100, which confers Hg^{2+} but not organomercury resistance.The genetic map of the mercury resistance determinant, transposon Tn501, consists of the following genes: *mer*R (regulatory gene), *mer*T (Hg^{2+} transport), *mer*P (the product is a periplasmic Hg^{2+}-binding protein), *mer*C (uncertain function), *mer*A (gene product is a subunit of mercuric reductase), *mer*B (if present, the determinant of organomercury lyase) and *mer*D (uncertain function) (Silver & Misra, 1988).

2.1.2 *Resistance to silver*

Of particular interest in the possible context of hospital infection is plasmid-mediated resistance to silver salts, since silver nitrate and silver sulphadiazine (AgSu) have been used topically for preventing infections in severe burns (Russell & Hugo, 1994). In an early study, attempts to transfer silver resistance from silver-resistant (Ag^R) strains of *E. coli* and *Klebsiella* to silver-sensitive (Ag^S) strains of *E. coli* were unsuccessful (Gravens *et al.*, 1969). McHugh *et al.* (1975) isolated a strain of *Salmonella typhimurium* from a burns unit that was resistant to silver nitrate, mercuric chloride and various antibiotics; this resistance could be transferred to *E. coli* in *in vitro* mating

Table 10.2 Plasmid-encoded resistance to mercury compounds.*

Organism	Plasmid-encoded resistance to: Hg^{2+}	Organomercurials	Comment
Escherichia coli	+	+	Narrow- or broad-spectrum plasmids
Salmonella typhimurium	+	–	
Proteus spp.	+	–	
Providencia spp.	+	–	
Pseudomonas aeruginosa	+	+	Narrow- or broad-spectrum plasmids
Staphylococcus aureus	+	+	Broad-spectrum plasmids

* (1) Host cell background might affect pattern of resistance. (2) Although Hg^0 may be formed by volatilization from a number of organomercury substrates, this does not cecessarily indicate that resistance is conferred. Seemingly, a threshold level of Hg^0 must be formed which, if exceeded, confers resistance. (3) Resistance to an organomercury compound does not necessarily involve volatilization of Hg^0; bacterial impermeability might be an alternative mechanism.

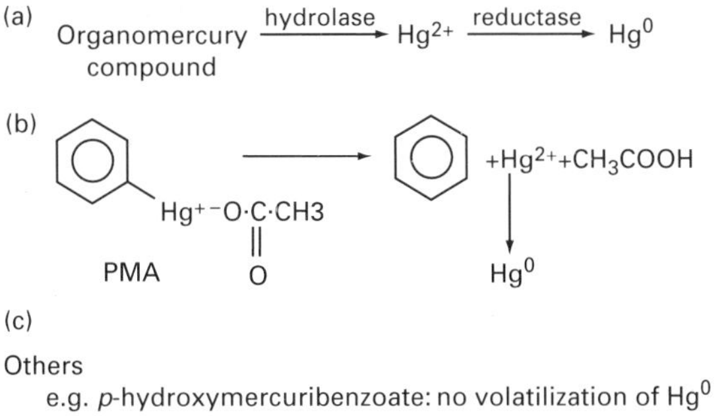

(a) Organomercury compound $\xrightarrow{\text{hydrolase}}$ Hg^{2+} $\xrightarrow{\text{reductase}}$ Hg^0

(b) PMA (C_6H_5–Hg^+–O·C(=O)·CH3) ⟶ C_6H_6 + Hg^{2+} + CH_3COOH; Hg^{2+} ⟶ Hg^0

(c)

Others
e.g. *p*-hydroxymercuribenzoate: no volatilization of Hg^0

Fig. 10.2 Biochemical mechanisms of resistance to organic mercury compounds. (a) General pattern. (b) *Pseudomonas aeruginosa* (broad-spectrum plasmid). (c) Other organomercury derivatives. Permeability barriers may play a role in the resistance of Gram-negative bacteria, and Hg^0 formation does not necessarily confer resistance. PMN, phenylmercuric nitrate.

Table 10.3 Plasmid-encoded resistance to cations and anions

Anion or cation	Plasmid-encoded resistance in
Ag^+	*E. coli, Sal. typhimurium*
Cd^{2+}	*Staph. aureus*
Co^{2+}	*E. coli*
Ni^+	*E. coli*
Zn^{2+}	*Staph. aureus*
Pb^{2+}	*Staph. aureus*
Cu^{2+}	*E. coli*
Arsenate, arsenite, antimony(III)	*E. coli, Staph. aureus*
CrO^{2-}	*Pseudomonas* strains, *Streptococcus lactis*
Tellurate, tellurite	*Alcaligenes* strains

Zn^{2+}, zinc; Pb^{2+}, lead; Cu^{2+}, copper.

experiments, although the authors pointed out the difficulty of transferring silver resistance from Ag^R to Ag^S strains. Nevertheless, plasmid-mediated Ag^+ resistance is determined by the very wide ratio (>100:1) of minimal inhibitory concentrations (MICs) for Ag^R and Ag^S cells.

Silver reduction, analogous to inorganic mercury reduction (Fig. 10.1) is not the basis of resistance. The current hypothesis (Silver & Misra, 1988) is that Ag^S cells bind silver so tightly that they extract it from silver chloride, whereas Ag^R cells do not compete successfully with Ag^+-halide complexes for Ag^+.

2.1.3 Resistance to other cations and to anions

Plasmid-encoded resistance to cations other than mercury and to anions has been demonstrated (Table 10.3). Resistances to arsenate (AsO_4^{3-}), arsenite (AsO_3^{3-}) and antimony(III) are encoded by an inducible operon-like system in both *E. coli* and *Staph. aureus*, and any one of the three ions induces resistance to all three. The mechanism of arsenate resistance involves an energy-dependent efflux of the inhibitor, producing a reduced net accumulation (Silver *et al.*, 1989). This efflux system is mediated by an adenosine triphosphatase (ATPase) transport system.

At least four plasmid-determined systems confer cadmium (Cd^{2+}) resistance. The most widely studied are the *cad*A and *cad*B systems unique to staphylococcal plasmids (Smith & Novick, 1972; Silver & Misra, 1988). The *cad*A gene specifies an approximately 100-fold increase in Cd^{2+} resistance involving Cd^{2+} efflux via a specific efflux ATPase. These *cad*A and *cad*B systems also confer resistance to several other heavy metals. The third system has a *cad*A type mechanism but differs in conferring Cd^{2+} resistance only. The fourth system, found in an *Alcaligenes* strain, involves a plasmid locus simultaneously conferring resistance to Cd^{2+}, (Zn^{2+}) and Co^{2+}, but the mechanism is unknown.

2.2 Resistance to other biocides

The majority of the gentamicin R plasmids associated with methicillin-resistant *Staph. aureus* (MRSA) strains also possess determinants encoding resistance to quaternary ammonium compounds (QACs) and other nucleic-acid-binding (NAB) agents (Lyon & Skurray, 1987; Reverdy *et al.*, 1992, 1993; Russell & Chopra, 1996). In laboratory experiments, resistance to some biocides (chlorhexidine, benzalkonium chloride, acriflavine and ethidium bromide) has been transferred from *Staph. aureus* to *E. coli* (Yamamoto *et al.*, 1988); the resistance levels of the *E. coli* strain carrying recombinant plasmids were some 4–16-fold higher than the isogenic plasmid-free strains. The mechanism of resistance expressed in *E. coli* may be the presence of a biocide efflux system (Midgley, 1986, 1987).

The presence of the R TEM plasmid in *E. coli* or of the RP1 plasmid in *E. coli* or *Ps. aeruginosa* did not increase the resistance of cells to QACs, chlorhexidine, phenols or organomercurials (Ahonkhai & Russell, 1979). Indeed, in some instances the plasmid$^+$ strains appeared to be rather more sensitive, although less so than claimed by Klemperer *et al.* (1980) and Michel-Briand *et al.* (1986). Sutton & Jacoby (1978) observed increased resistance to hexachlorophane (hexachlorophene) in *Ps. aeruginosa* harbouring the RP1 plasmid, although the mechanism is unclear. Curtis & Richmond (1974) found that a lysozyme-sensitive mutant of *E. coli* became lysozyme-resistant upon acquisition of RP1, suggesting cell-surface modifications. The plasmid R124 has also been shown to modify cell-surface changes and biocide response in *E. coli* (Roussow & Rowbury, 1984). About 15% of isolates of Gram-negative bacteria causing urinary-tract infections in paraplegic patients show a high degree of resistance to QACs and chlorhexidine, as well as to antibiotics. These resistant species appear to have been selected as a consequence of the extensive use of cationic antiseptics, but the possibility of a plasmid-linked association of antibiotic and antiseptic resistances has not been established (Stickler *et al.*, 1983). Attempts to transfer QAC and chlorhexidine resistance were unsuccessful.

3 Genetic aspects

Plasmid-encoded biocide resistance has been studied most widely in *Staph. aureus*. In resistant strains of this organism, resistance to biocides is encoded by at least three separate multidrug resistance determinants, namely the *qac*A, *qac*B, *qac*C and *qac*D genes (the last two having identical phenotypes and showing restriction-site homology) (Littlejohn *et al.*, 1990, 1992; Heir *et al.*, 1995; Paulsen *et al.*, 1995). The *qac*A/*qac*B family of genes encodes proton-dependent export-proteins, which demonstrate significant homology to other energy-dependent transporters, e.g. the tetracycline exporters found in various strains of tetracycline-resistant bacteria (Rouch *et al.*, 1990). The *qac*A gene has not been found in susceptible strains of *Staph. aureus* but was present in 70% of clinical *Staph. aureus* isolates resistant to chlorhexidine, benzalkonium, hexamidine and acriflavine (Behr *et al.*, 1994).

These aspects are considered further in Chapter 10F.

4 Mechanisms of plasmid-encoded biocide resistance

Some examples were provided above, especially with plasmid-mediated resistance to mercury compounds. Generally (Table 10.4), such resistance mechanisms consist of: (i) biocide inactivation; (ii) decreased uptake; (iii) cell-surface alterations; and (iv) biocide efflux. Of these, the mechanism that has aroused the greatest interest is the last, since this may be similar to that responsible for bacterial resistance to antibiotics. It has been found to occur in strains of staphylococci resistant to carbonic biocides (QACs, acridines, diamidines, triphenylmethane dyes, possibly chlorhexidine, and also ethidium bromide) (Littlejohn *et al.*, 1992; Leelaporn *et al.*, 1994).

Transferable resistance to formaldehyde and formaldehyde-releasing agents has been described in

Table 10.4 Possible mechanisms of plasmid-encoded biocide resistance.

Mechanism	Example(s)	Comment
Biocide inactivation	Inorganic and organic mercury compounds	See Table 10.1 and Figs 10.2 and 10.3
	Formaldehyde	Formaldehyde dehydrogenase responsible
Decreased uptake	Silver compounds	
Cell-surface alterations	Formaldehyde	Outer-membrane proteins involved
Biocide efflux (expulsion)	Cationic biocides	*Staph. aureus*, *Staphylococcus epidermidis*, *E. coli*

Serratia marcescens (Candal & Eagon, 1984; Hall & Eagon, 1985). Some possible mechanisms are listed in Table 10.4.

Further information is provided by Russell (1997).

5 Conclusions

Apart from mercury compounds and other heavy metals, plasmid-mediated resistance of Gram-negative bacteria to biocides does not appear to be an important mechanism of resistance (Nagai & Ogase, 1990). There is, nevertheless, evidence that some plasmids are responsible for producing surface changes in cells, which, in turn, may modify sensitivity or resistance, and that the response depends not only on the plasmid but also on the host cells. In MRSA strains, certain plasmids are responsible for producing a low-level increase in resistance to QACs and other cationic biocides, the mechanism of which involves efflux. A similar mechanism is operative in biocide-resistant *Staph. epidermidis* strains.

For further information, the review by Russell (1997) should be consulted.

6 References

Ahonkhai, I. & Russell, A.D. (1979) Response of RP1$^+$ and RP1$^-$ strains of *Escherichia coli* to antibacterial agents and transfer of resistance to *Pseudomonas aeruginosa*. *Current Microbiology*, **3**, 89–94.

Behr, H., Reverdy, M.E., Mabilat, C., Freney, J. & Fleurette, J. (1994) Relationship between the level of minimal inhibitory concentrations of five antiseptics and the presence of *qac*A gene in *Staphylococcus aureus*. *Pathologie Biologie*, **42**, 438–444.

Candal, E.J. & Eagon, R.G. (1984) Evidence for plasmid-mediated bacterial resistance to industrial biocides. *International Biodeterioration*, **20**, 221–224.

Chopra, I. (1988) Efflux of antibacterial agents from bacteria. In *FEMS Symposium No. 44: Homeostatic Mechanisms of Micro-organisms*, pp. 146–158. Bath: Bath University Press.

Clark, D.L., Weiss, A.A. & Silver, S. (1977) Mercury and organomercurial resistance determined by plasmids in *Pseudomonas*. *Journal of Bacteriology*, **132**, 186–196.

Curtis, N.A.C. & Richmond, M.H. (1974) Effect of R-factor mediated genes on some surface properties of *Escherichia coli*. Antimicrobial *Agents and Chemotherapy*, **6**, 666–671.

Foster, T.J. (1983) Plasmid-determined resistance to antimicrobial drugs and toxic metal ions in bacteria. *Microbiological Reviews*, **47**, 361–409.

George, A.M. (1996) Multidrug resistance in enteric and other Gram-negative bacteria. *FEMS Microbiology Letters*, **139**, 1–10.

Ghosh, S., Sadhukhan, P.C., Ghosh, D.K., Mandal, A.K., Chaudhuri, J. & Mandal, A. (1996) Studies on the effect of mercury and organomercurial on the growth and nitrogen fixation by mercury-resistant *Azotobacter* strains. *Journal of Applied Bacteriology*, **80**, 319–326.

Gravens, M.L., Margraf, H.W., Gravens, C.K., Thomerson, J.E. & Butcher, H.R. (1969) Silver and intestinal flora: roles in bacterial colonization of burn wounds. *Archives of Surgery*, **99**, 453–458.

Hall, E. & Eagon, R.G. (1985) Evidence for plasmid-mediated resistance of *Pseudomonas putida* to hexahydro-1,3,5-triethyl-*s*-triazine. *Current Microbiology*, **12**, 17–22.

Heinzel, M. (1988) The phenomena of resistance to disinfectants and preservatives. In *Industrial Biocides* (ed. Payne, K.R.), pp. 52–67. Chichester: John Wiley & Sons.

Heir, E., Sundheim, G. & Holck, A.L. (1995) Resistance to quaternary ammonium compounds in *Staphylococcus* spp. isolated from the food industry and nucleotide sequence of the resistance plasmid pST827. *Journal of Applied Bacteriology*, **79**, 149–156.

Joly, B. (1995) La résistance microbienne à l'action des antiseptiques et desinfectants. In *Antisepsie et Désinfection* (eds Fleurette, J., Freney, J. & Reverdy, M.-E.), pp. 52–65. Paris: Editions ESKA.

Klemperer, R.M.M., Ismail, N.T.A.J. & Brown, M.R.W. (1980) Effect of R-plasmid RP1 and nutrient depletion on the resistance of *Escherichia coli* to cetrimide, chlorhexidine and phenol. *Journal of Applied Bacteriology*, **48**, 349–357.

Leelaporn, A., Paulsen, I.T., Tennent, J.M., Littlejohn, T.G. & Skurray, R.A. (1994) Multidrug resistance to antiseptics and disinfectants in coagulase-negative staphylococci. *Journal of Medical Microbiology*, **40**, 214–220.

Littlejohn, T.G., DiBerardino, D., Messerotti, L.J., Spiers, S.J. & Skurray, R.A. (1990) Structure and evolution of a family of genes encoding antiseptic and disinfectant resistance in *Staphylococcus aureus*. *Gene*, **101**, 59–66.

Littlejohn, T.G., Paulsen, I.T., Gillespie, M.T. *et al.* (1992) Substrate specificity and energetics of antiseptic and disinfectant resistance in *Staphylococcus aureus*. *FEMS Microbiology Letters*, **95**, 259–266.

Lyon, B.R. & Skurray, R.A. (1987) Antimicrobial resistance of *Staphylococcus aureus*: genetic basis. *Microbiological Reviews*, **51**, 88–134.

McHugh, G.L., Hopkins, C.C., Moellering, R.C. & Swartz, M.N. (1975) *Salmonella typhimurium* resistant to silver nitrate, chloramphenicol and ampicillin. *Lancet*, **i**, 235–239.

Michel-Briand, Y., Laporte, J.M., Bassignot, A. & Plesiat, P. (1986) Antibiotic resistance plasmids and bactericidal effect of chlorhexidine on Enterobacteriaceae. *Letters in Applied Microbiology*, **3**, 65–68.

Midgley M. (1986) The phosphonium ion efflux system of *Escherichia coli*: a relationship to the ethidium efflux system and energetic studies. *Journal of General Microbiology*, **132**, 3187–3193.

Midgley, M. (1987) An efflux system for cationic dyes and related compounds in *Escherichia coli. Microbiological Sciences*, **4**, 125–127.

Nagai I. & Ogase, H. (1990) Absence of role for plasmids in resistance to multiple disinfectants in three strains of bacteria. *Journal of Hospital Infection*, **15**, 149–155.

Nies, D.H. & Silver, S. (1995) Ion efflux systems involved in bacterial metal resistances. *Journal of Industrial Microbiology*, **14**, 186–199.

Novick, R.P. & Bouanchaud, D. (1971) Extrachromosomal nature of drug resistance in *Staphylococcus aureus. Annals of the New York Academy of Sciences,* **182**, 279–294.

Novick, R.P. & Roth, C. (1968) Plasmid-linked resistance to inorganic salts in *Staphylococcus aureus. Journal of Bacteriology*, **95**, 1335–1342.

Paulsen, I.T. Brown, M.H., Dunstan, S.J. & Skurray, R.A. (1995) Molecular characterization of the staphylococcal multidrug resistance export-protein QacC. *Journal of Bacteriology*, **177**, 2827–2833.

Reverdy, M.E., Bes, M., Nervi, C. Mastra, A. & Fleurette, J. (1992) Activity of four antiseptics (acriflavine, benzalkonium chloride, chlorhexidine digluconate and hexamidine di-isethionate) and of ethidium bromide on 392 strains representing 26 *Staphylococcus* species. *Medical Microbiological Letters*, **1**, 56–63.

Reverdy, M.E., Bes, M., Brun, Y. & Fleurette, J. (1993) Evolution de la résistance aux antibiotiques et aux antiseptiques de souches hospitalières de *Staphylococcus aureus* isolées de 1980 à 1991. *Pathologie Biologie*, **41**, 897–904.

Rouch, D.A., Cram, D.S., DiBerardino, D., Littlejohn, T.G. & Skurray, R.A. (1990) Efflux-mediated antiseptic resistance gene *qac*A from *Staphylococcus aureus*: common ancestry with tetracycline and sugar-transported proteins. *Molecular Microbiology*, **4**, 2051–2062.

Roussow, F.T. & Rowbury, R.J. (1984) Effects of the resistance plasmid R124 on the level of OmpF outer membrane protein and on the response of *Escherichia coli* to environmental agents. *Journal of Applied Bacteriology*, **56**, 63–79.

Russell, A.D. (1985) The role of plasmids in bacterial resistance to antiseptics, disinfectants and preservatives. *Journal of Hospital Infection*, **6**, 9–19.

Russell, A.D. (1990) Mechanisms of bacterial resistance to biocides. *International Biodeterioration*, **26**, 101–110.

Russell, A.D. (1994) Glutaraldehyde: its current status and uses. *Infection Control and Hospital Epidemiology*, **15**, 724–733.

Russell, A.D. (1995) Mechanisms of bacterial resistance to biocides. *International Biodeterioration and Biodegradation*, **36**, 247–265.

Russell, A.D. (1997) Plasmids and bacterial resistance to biocides. *Journal of Applied Microbiology*, **82**, 155–165.

Russell, A.D. & Chopra, I. (1996) *Understanding Antibacterial Action and Resistance,* 2nd edn. Chichester: Ellis Horwood.

Russell, A.D. & Day, M.J. (1993) Antibacterial activity of chlorhexidine. *Journal of Hospital Infection*, **25**, 229–238.

Russell, A.D. & Day, M.J. (1996) Antibiotic and biocide resistance in bacteria. *Microbios*, **85**, 45–65.

Russell, A.D. & Gould, G.W. (1988) Resistance of Enterobacteriaceae to preservatives and disinfectants. *Journal of Applied Bacteriology Symposium Series*, **65**, 167S–195S.

Russell, A.D. & Hugo, W.B. (1994) Antibacterial activity and resistance. *Progress in Medicinal Chemistry*, **31**, 351–371.

Russell, A.D. & Russell, N.J. (1995) Biocides: activity, action and resistance. In *Society for General Microbiology Symposium No. 53*, pp. 327–365. Cambridge: Cambridge University Press.

Russell, A.D., Hammond, S.A. & Morgan, J.R. (1986) Bacterial resistance to antiseptics and disinfectants. *Journal of Hospital Infection*, **7**, 213–225.

Silver, S. & Misra, S. (1988) Plasmid-mediated heavy metal resistances. *Annual Review of Microbiology*, **42**, 717–743.

Silver, S., Nucifora, G., Chu, L. & Misra, T.K. (1989) Bacterial ATPases: primary pumps for exporting toxic cations and anions. *Trends in Biochemical Sciences*, **14**, 76–80.

Smith, K. & Novick, R.P. (1972) Genetic studies on plasmid-linked cadmium resistance in *Staphylococcus aureus. Journal of Bacteriology*, **112**, 761–772.

Stickler, D.J., Thomas, B., Clayton, J.C. & Chawla, J.A. (1983) Studies on the genetic basis of chlorhexidine resistance. *British Journal of Clinical Practice, Symposium Supplement*, **25**, 23–28.

Sutton, L. & Jacoby, G.A. (1978) Plasmid-determined resistance to hexachlorophene in *Pseudomonas aeruginosa. Antimicrobial Agents and Chemotherapy*, **13**, 634–636.

Yamamoto, T., Tamura, Y. & Yokota, T. (1988) Antiseptic and antibiotic resistance plasmid in *Staphylococcus aureus* that possesses ability to confer chlorhexidine and acrinol resistance. *Antimicrobial Agents and Chemotherapy*, **32**, 932–935.

C. RESISTANCE OF BACTERIAL SPORES TO CHEMICAL AGENTS

1 Introduction

Bacterial spores are the most resistant life forms known and their complete destruction will result in the destruction of all other life forms. Chemicals that destroy spores are known as sporicides and have the potential to act as sterilizing agents. In practice, chemical sterilization is rarely achievable at ambient temperatures, although, for thermolabile materials, chemical treatment may be the only alternative to heat sterilization.

Compared with vegetative cells, spores may be as much as 100 000 times more resistant to chemicals (Phillips, 1952). Development of resistance to agents such as chlorhexidine occurs early in the sporulation process, compared with glutaraldehyde resistance, which is a late event. During germination and outgrowth of spores, resistance is lost and cells become sensitive to biocides.

In this chapter the resistance of spores to various chemical agents will be discussed. Factors affecting spore resistance and mechanisms of resistance will also be reviewed. Reviews of spore resistance are also given by Roberts & Hitchins (1969), Russell (1982, 1983, 1991), Gould (1983, 1985), Waites (1985), Quinn (1987), Russell *et al.* (1989), Bloomfield & Arthur (1994) and Russell & Chopra (1996).

2 Factors affecting resistance

When spores are exposed to chemical agents they may be inhibited, sublethally injured or irreversibly damaged. The relative resistance of spores grown in the laboratory and those occurring in their natural environments is unknown, but it is recognized that resistance of laboratory-grown spores may vary considerably depending not only on the chemical agent used but also on the bacterial species and strain, on the method of spore production, preparation and storage and on the conditions used to study resistance. Although the factors affecting heat resistance have been extensively studied, fewer investigations have attempted to explain chemical resistance. The same factors appear to determine resistance to both heat and chemicals, but spores which are particularly resistant to heat are not especially resistant to phenol (Briggs, 1966), ethylene oxide (El-Bisi *et al.*, 1963), chlorine (Dye & Mead, 1972) or hydrogen peroxide (Toledo *et al.*, 1973).

2.1 Species and strain

Spores of different species show marked differences in resistance. Spores of *Bacillus stearothermophilus* were 10^3 times more resistant to hydrogen peroxide than those of *Clostridium botulinum* (Ito *et al.*, 1973), while spores of *Bacillus subtilis* were more resistant to chlorine than those of *Bacillus cereus and Clostridium bifermentens* (Cousins & Allan, 1967; Dye & Mead, 1972). Different strains of the same species may differ in their resistance; spore resistance of various strains of *B. subtilis* to hydrogen peroxide was found to vary by a factor of 10^4 (Waites & Bayliss, 1979b).

2.2 Sporulation media

Alterations in the constituents of the media on which spores are grown will alter their resistance to sporicidal agents. A chemically defined medium has been reported to produce spores or *B. subtilis* that are less variable in resistance to glutaraldehyde (Forsyth, 1975; Stark *et al.*, 1975) than those produced in the soil-extract medium used in the sporicidal test of the Association of Official Analytical Chemists (AOAC), while addition of glucose and metal salts to nutrient agar increased the resistance of spores or *B. subtilis* to hydrogen peroxide 10^4-fold (Waites & Bayliss, 1979a). Partly because of the problems of removing vegetative cells, sporulation media are designed to produce a high percentage of free spores and few vegetative cells or germinated spores (Gould, 1971), but it is possible that the conditions which produce sporulation in most of the population will produce spores with low resistance. Furthermore, spores produced on some media may have little resistance to one chemical but may be particularly resistant to others, while spores grown on different batches of the same media may differ in their resistance, suggesting that small changes in media preparation and harvesting times may alter resistance (Bomar, 1962). Knott *et al.* (1997) have shown that the type of water used in preparation of media can influence spore, germination and outgrowth characteristics.

2.3 Method of harvesting

In addition to dormant free spores, growth on most sporulation media produces vegetative cells, sporangial debris and germinated spores. Numerous methods have been devised to remove unwanted material and leave the dormant spore (Murrell, 1969), but all such methods may alter resistance and should be examined critically before routine use. In particular, sonication, which has been used to remove sporangia from spores, may reduce resistance (St Julian *et al.*, 1967), while the two-phase-system of Sacks & Alderton (1961), which separates free spores from germinated spores and vegetative cells, may initiate germination of a fraction of the spore population (Murrell & Warth, 1965). Nevertheless, a reactive chemical will be rapidly neutralized by vegetative cell debris, so that the spores in a suspension may appear more resistant than those in suspensions containing only spores.

2.4 Methods for storage

Spore resistance may change significantly during periods of prolonged storage (Forsyth, 1975; Waites & Bayliss, 1979a). Spores may be stored in glass-distilled water either refrigerated (although some strains of *Bacillus* may germinate during storage over long periods) or frozen. Alternatively, spores may be stored freeze-dried, which may damage spores of some strains (Marshall *et al.*, 1963) or in ethanol (Molin & Östlund, 1976).

2.5 Conditions of test

In the laboratory, several types of tests are used to determine sporistatic and sporicidal activity. Sporistatic tests usually involve determination of minimum inhibitory concentrations, i.e. the minimum concentration required to prevent germination and/or outgrowth. Sporicidal activity is determined by measuring rates of kill or the time taken for complete destruction of a population. These tests are considered in detail in this volume by

Reybrouck (Chapter 4A) and also by Russell *et al.* (1991).

2.6 Recovery conditions

In common with all microbicidal testing, the quantitative evaluation of sporicides is normally assessed by taking a sample of the biocide-treated spore suspension, which is neutralized by appropriate means, and a sample is plated on nutrient agar to assess the number of colony-forming units. In general, the assumption is made that the spores which form colonies on agar are viable, while those which do not are non-viable. Increasingly, however, there are data which demonstrate that, as with all microbicidal processes, there is a subpopulation of cells within the treated population which is sublethally injured but not killed, and that the ability of these spores to recover and multiply depends upon the recovery conditions employed. The practical implication of this is that, according to the method of recovery employed, it may be possible to over- or underestimate the efficacy of sporicidal products, i.e. there is a possibility that the numbers of damaged spores which might recover under laboratory conditions may be greater or less than those which recover under in-use conditions.

For the evaluation of chemical agents, an important factor in determining the extent of recovery is the neutralization of residual agent at the moment of sampling to prevent continued action and possible sporistasis in the subculture medium. Methods for neutralization of antimicrobial agents are further discussed in Chapter 4A and by Bloomfield (1991).

In order to form colonies on agar, spores must subsequently germinate and outgrow to form a vegetative cell, which then multiplies to produce visible growth. As suggested by Gould (1984), the complexity of the spore cell cycle indicates that the opportunities for sublethal injury and expression of this injury in response to the conditions of recovery are potentially much greater than for vegetative cells. Whereas untreated spores usually germinate rapidly within 20–30 min when transferred to nutrient medium under optimum conditions, it has been shown that, for damaged spores, the rate and extent of recovery are very sensitive to the use of recovery conditions that are less than optimal (Futter & Richardson, 1970a,b; Roberts, 1970). In contrast, other investigations have shown that post-treatment heat shock can enhance the revival of bacterial spores following treatment with hydrochloric acid (HCl) (Ortenzio, 1966), formaldehyde (Spicher & Peters, 1976, 1981) and glutaraldehyde (Gorman *et al.*, 1983a; Power *et al.*, 1988). Lysozyme has also been shown to affect spore revival (Wyatt & Waites, 1975; Gorman *et al.*, 1983b; Gould, 1984). Another agent that has been shown to affect spore revival is alkali (Power *et al.*, 1988, 1989, 1990; Dancer *et al.*, 1989). Dancer *et al.* (1989) showed that, for a challenge inoculum of 10^8 cells ml^{-1} of *Bacillus* spp. spore forms treated with 2% glutaraldehyde, the recovery of viable spores was less than 10^1. In contrast, where spores were treated with 1 mol l^{-1} sodium hydroxide (NaOH) following neutralization of the glutaraldehyde, the recovery was increased up to 10^2–10^3. In contrast, Williams & Russell (1993b) showed that NaOH had no effect on revival of spores treated with formaldehyde, iodine and chlorine-releasing agents (CRAs). In further studies (Williams & Russell, 1992a,b, 1993a,b,c,d,e), in which biocide-treated spores were enumerated on agar containing potential revival agents, such as subtilisin, lysozyme, calcium dipicolinate (CaDPA) and calcium lactate, only calcium lactate was found to have any significant effect, and then only with iodine-treated spores.

Revival of injured spores is reviewed in more detail by Gould (1984), Waites & Bayliss (1984), Russell (1990) and Bloomfield & Arthur (1994).

3 Resistance to chemical agents

Chemical agents that destroy vegetative bacteria are described as disinfectants. Many highly active and widely used disinfectants, such as the phenolics, quaternary ammonium compounds (QACS), alcohols, bisbiguanides, organic acids and esters and mercurials have little or no sporicidal activity but are effective sporistatic agents, i.e. they prevent germination and/or outgrowth of spores. Inhibition of spore germination and outgrowth is reviewed in more detail by Russell (1990).

Chemical agents that are sporicidal include glutaraldehyde, formaldehyde, CRAs, iodine, acids, alkali, hydrogen peroxide, the peroxy acids, ethylene oxide, β-propionolactone and ozone. To achieve sporicidal action with these compounds, much higher concentrations and longer contact times are required compared with those used for destruction of vegetative cells. Table 10.5 lists chemicals in order of their sporicidal efficiency, although all these estimations must be considered as an approximation since the data were obtained under widely differing experimental conditions. The properties of these agents are reviewed in this section. The activity of sporicidal agents is also reviewed by Roberts & Hitchins (1969), Sykes (1970), Russell (1971, 1982, 1990), Block (1983) Waites (1985).

3.1 Glutaraldehyde

Glutaraldehyde is an effective sporicidal agent. Its activity depends on pH, alkaline solutions being more effective (although less stable) than acid solutions. A 2% solution of glutaraldehyde will produce a 4 log reduction in spores of *Clostridium tetani* and *Bacillus anthracis* in 15–30 min (Rubbo *et al.*, 1967). Not all species of *Bacillus* are equally resistant to glutaraldehyde; *B. subtilis* and *Bacillus pumilis* appear to be the most resistant (Rubbo *et al.*, 1967). With suspensions of *B. subtilis*, a contact period of 3 h with 2% alkaline glutaraldehyde produces a *c.* 6 log reduction in viable count (Kelsey *et al.*, 1974; Miner *et al.*, 1977; Gardner & Favero, 1985). Sagripanti & Bonifacino (1996) showed that 2% glutaraldehyde produced only about 1 log reduction in viable count of *B. subtilis* within 30 min at 20°C, but activity increased to a 6 log reduction by increasing the temperature to 40°C. These workers also showed that glutaraldehyde was sensitive to pH and ionic strength; results indicated that sporicidal activity was measurable within a narrow range around pH 9 and activity was increased by addition of sodium carbonate up to 1 mol/l ionic strength. Babb *et al.* (1980) demonstrated that a 2–3 h contact period with 2% glutaraldehyde was required to produce sterilization of *B. subtilis* spores dried on to aluminium foil strips. Potentiation of glutaraldehyde by the use of cationic and anionic surfactant–divalent metal ion combinations and by the addition of sodium phenate and phenol has been described by Boucher (1975), Gorman & Scott (1979) and Isenberg (1985). The properties of glutaraldehyde are reviewed in more detail by Gorman *et al.*, (1980), Russell (1994) and Russell & Chopra (1996).

Table 10.5 Resistance of spores to chemicals.

Chemical	Organism	Kill	Time (h)	Concentration (% w/v)	Temperature (°C)	Reference
Peracetic acid vapour	*B. subtilis* var. *niger*	10^5	0.02	0.0001	25	Portner & Hoffman (1986)
HCl vapour	*B. subtilis*	10^3	0.08	31*	20	Tuynenberg Muys *et al.* (1978)
Ethylene oxide	*B. subtilis*	10^2	0.7	0.07	40	Marletta & Stumbo (1970)
Hydrogen peroxide	*B. subtilis* var. *globigii*	10^3	0.17	25.8	24	Toledo *et al.* (1973)
Hypochlorous acid	*B. subtilis*	10^3	2.0	0.0†	10	Dye & Mead (1972)
Glutaraldehyde	*B. pumilus*	10^3	0.5	2.0	37	Thomas & Russell (1974)
Formaldehyde	*B. subtilis* var. *niger*	10^3	1.5	1.0	40	Trujillo & David (1972)
Propylene oxide	*B. subtilis* var. *niger*	10^3	17.0	0.1	37	Bruch & Koesterer (1961)
Sodium hydroxide	*B. subtilis*	10^3	24.5	5.0	40	Whitehouse & Clegg (1963)
Iodine (as an iodophor)	*B. subtilis*	10^2	>4.0	0.08	21	Cousins & Allan (1967)

*0.25 ml in a 300 ml bottle.
†Free chlorine.

3.2 Formaldehyde

Formaldehyde is used in both liquid and gaseous forms. Formalin is an aqueous solution containing 34–38% formaldehyde, with methanol to delay polymerization. Formaldehyde is sporicidal, but at a slower rate than glutaraldehyde (Rubbo *et al.*, 1967; Sagripanti & Bonifacino, 1996). Mixtures of glutaraldehyde and formaldehyde are found to be 10 times more effective than either chemical alone (Waites & Bayliss, 1984). The properties of other aldehydes are examined by Power & Russell (1990).

3.3 Halogens

Under most conditions, the sporicidal activity of halogens increases in the order bromine : iodine : chlorine (Marks & Strandskov, 1950), spores being more resistant to aqueous iodine than to iodophors (Cousins & Allan, 1967). The activity of halogen-releasing agents is strongly affected by pH, being more active at acid pH. Sodium hypochlorite (NaOCl) at 100–200 parts/10^6 pH and 7–7.6 will produce a 4–5 log reduction in *B. subtilis* spores within a 5 min (Death & Coates, 1979; Bloomfield & Arthur, 1989). Babb *et al.* (1980) demonstrated that buffered solutions of NaOCl at 250 parts/10^6 (pH 7.0) and 1800 parts/10^6 (pH 10.0) produced sterilization of *B. subtilis* spores dried on to aluminium spore strips within 2 min and 60 min, respectively. Similar levels of sporicidal activity are reported by Sagripanti & Bonifacino (1996). Bloomfield & Arthur (1989) showed that, as compared with NaOCl, spores are significantly more resistant to *N*-chloro compounds, such as sodium dichloroisocyanurate (NaDCC) and particularly chloramine-T. Sodium hypochlorite may in turn be less rapidly sporicidal than chlorine dioxide (Ridenour *et al.*, 1949; Benarde *et al.*, 1967). Cousins & Allan (1967) demonstrated that *B. subtilis* spores were more resistant to chlorine than *B. cereus*. Generally, spores of *Clostridium* spp. are more resistant to chlorine than *Bacillus* spores. Death & Coates (1979) have shown that buffered methanol/NaOCl is more rapidly sporicidal than buffered hypochlorite alone. The sporicidal activity of both chlorine and iodine formulations is potentiated by the addition of 1–5% sodium hydroxide (Cousins & Allan, 1967; Bloomfield & Arthur, 1992; Bloomfield & Megid, 1994). Heating of spores reduces their resistance to chlorine (Cousins & Allan, 1967).

3.4 Acid and alkali

Spores are resistant to acid pH, although prolonged incubation at pH 1.5 reduces their resistance (Sacks & Alderton, 1961). Some strains are resistant to constant-boiling HCl at 20°C for up to 30 min but this extreme resistance is dependent on predrying of the spores (Ortenzio *et al.*, 1953). Gaseous HCl is rapidly sporicidal, producing sterility in seconds (Tuynenberg Muys *et al.*, 1978; Lelieveld, 1979). Alkalis are slowly sporicidal at elevated temperatures (von Bockelmann, 1974). Sodium hydroxide is found to sensitize spores of *Clostridium perfringens* (Barach *et al.*, 1975; Labbé *et al.*, 1978) and *Cl. bifermentans* (Wyatt & Waites, 1975) to lysozyme and to the action of CRAs and iodine-releasing compounds (Cousins & Allan, 1967; Bloomfield & Arthur, 1989, 1992; Bloomfield & Megid, 1994). Sodium hydroxide also increases the germination rate of *Cl. bifermentans* (Waites *et al.*, 1972) and *Bacillus megaterium* (Vary, 1973).

3.5 Hydrogen peroxide and other peroxygen compounds

The sporicidal properties of hydrogen peroxide have been extensively investigated (Toledo, 1975; Bayliss & Waites, 1976, 1979; Waites *et al.*, 1976, 1979, 1988; Waites & Bayliss, 1979a; Ando & Tsuzuki, 1986a,b; Sagripanti & Bonifacino, 1996). Hydrogen peroxide is only slowly sporicidal at ambient temperatures, but at elevated temperatures activity is markedly increased (Toledo *et al.*, 1973; Sagripanti & Bonifacino, 1996). Toledo *et al.* (1973) demonstrated that, at ambient temperatures, a 25.8% solution produced 99.99% kill of *B. subtilis* spores within 11 min, but at 76°C the kill time was reduced to 30 s. The action of hydrogen peroxide is potentiated not only by heat but also by transitional-metal ions or by ultraviolet (UV) irradiation (King & Gould 1969; Bayliss & Waites, 1976, 1979; Wallen, 1976). This is thought to be associated with the production of highly reactive free hydroxyl radicals, which is catalysed by heat, irradiation and metal cations, such as Cu. Peracetic acid is rapidly sporicidal (Baldry, 1983, 1988; Sagripanti & Bonifacino, 1996), a 0.1% solution producing a 3 or more log kill of *B. subtilis* spores within 15–30 min (Bayliss *et al.*, 1981; Sagripanti & Bonifacino, 1996). Sagripanti & Bonifacino (1996) also demonstrated that the sporicidal activity of peracetic acid was increased with increasing temperature. Breakdown of peracetic acid produces acetic acid, oxygen and water and leaves no residues. Peracetic acid is more active than hydrogen peroxide and is only slightly affected by the presence of organic matter (Baldry, 1983, 1988; Sagripanti & Bonifacino, 1996). The sporicidal activity of tertiary butyl hydroperoxide has been investigated by Shin & Marquis (1994).

3.6 Ethylene oxide

Ethylene oxide is an active sporicidal agent. In contrast with other sporicides, bacterial spores are generally only about two to 10 times more resistant to ethylene oxide than vegetative cells. Ethylene oxide sterilization is usually slow, taking up to 4 h and sometimes up to 18 h (Znamirowski *et al.*, 1960; Ernst, 1974, 1975; Phillips, 1977; Reich, 1980). Activity of ethylene oxide depends on a number of factors,including temperature, contact time and water vapour. The sporicidal properties of ethylene oxide are reviewed in detail by Phillips (1977) and Caputo & Odlaug (1983); see also Chapter 21.

3.7 Other sporicides

β-propionolactone is an active sporicidal agent but is not widely used because of its allegedly carcinogenic effects. Its sporicidal activity is a direct function of time, temperature, concentration and relative humidity (Hoffman, 1971; Caputo & Odlaug). Ozone is also an active sporicidal agent, but its use is limited by its instability (Hoffman, 1971; Foegeding, 1985; Foegeding & Fulp, 1988).

4 Mechanisms of resistance

4.1 Changes in resistance during spore formation and germination

Bacterial spores (as illustrated in Fig. 10.3) consist of an external protective spore coat, an intermediate cortex and an inner protoplast. The outer coat is made up of protein material, rich in cysteine, whereas the cortex is mainly peptidoglycan. The inner core is surrounded by a protoplast membrane and contains deoxyribonucleic acid (DNA), ribonucleic acid (RNA) and spore enzymes, together with a number of unique constituents, such as dipicolinic acid (DPA). During spore formation, the protoplast contracts and loses water, possibly as a result of expansion of the cortex (Gould & Dring, 1975; Warth, 1978). During germination, the cortex is degraded, the protoplast rehydrates and expands and the structure loses chemical and heat resistance.

Evidence suggests that heat and, to a certain extent, chemical resistance is related to the dehydrated nature of the spore protoplast, but the action of chemicals must be different from that of heat because they must penetrate the outer spore layers before they can exert their action. Whereas a considerable amount of information is available about the way in which antibacterial agents affect vegetative bacterial forms (Russell, 1990), mechan-

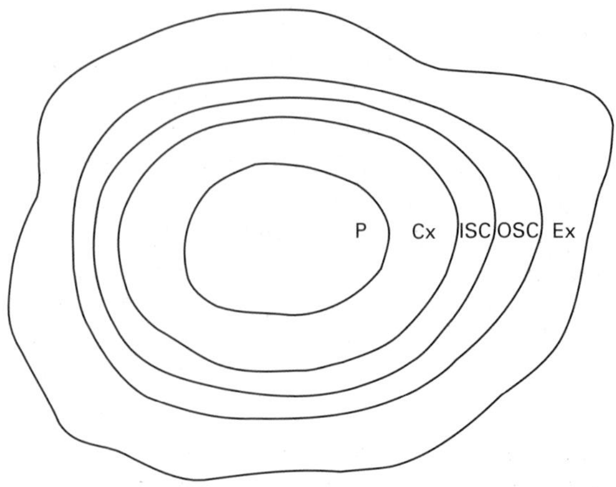

Fig. 10.3 Typical structure of the bacterial spore. Ex, exosporum; OSC, alkali-resistant outer spore coat; ISC, alkali-soluble inner spore coat; Cx, cortex; P, spore protoplast.

isms of sporicidal action are incompletely understood. For the most part, the evidence suggests that the formation of permeability barriers during sporulation, preventing access of the agent to its site of action, plays a significant part in the development of resistance to antimicrobial agents, but changes in cell structure or function at the site of action may also be involved.

Some insight into mechanisms of resistance has been gained by correlating the emergence of resistance to the stage of spore development, using spore mutants blocked at different stages of sporulation. Investigations by Sousa *et al.* (1978), Gorman *et al.*, (1984c) and Shaker *et al.*, (1988) suggest that resistance to toluene and xylene is an early event, while resistance to heat, chlorhexidine, alcohols and halogens occurs at a later stage, which correlates with coat and cortex formation. Resistance to phenols, chloroform lysozyme and finally glutaraldehyde (Power *et al.*, 1988, Knott *et al.*, 1995; Knott & Russell, 1995) appears only late in the sporulation process.

In the following sections, the relationship between spore structure and resistance is reviewed. These aspects are also reviewed by Russell (1983, 1990), Waites (1985) and Bloomfield & Arthur (1994).

4.2 Spore coat and resistance

Experimental evidence suggests that the spore coat is involved in resistance to many antimicrobial agents by preventing penetration of the agent to its site of action. Although, as described above, studies with spore mutants have produced some indications of the importance of the spore coat in antimicrobial resistance, the majority of data have come from studies involving the use of coatless or coat-defective spore forms. These are either coat-deficient mutant strains or, more usually, coat-extracted spores prepared by treatment with NaOH or with combinations of thioglycollic acid (TA), 2-mercaptoethanol (ME) or dithiothreitol, with urea (U) and/or sodium lauryl (dodecyl) sulphate (SLS). Electron microscopy and chemical analysis of extracted spores indicate that the spore coat consists of two layers: an inner coat, which is alkali-soluble, and an outer coat, which is alkali-resistant (Kulikovsky *et al.*, 1975; Labbe *et al.*, 1978; Nishihara *et al.*, 1981). Aronson & Fitz-James (1971), Vary (1973) and Gorman *et al.*, (1983b) have demonstrated that treatment with disulphide-reducing agents produces extraction of both inner and outer spore-coat protein, which can range from 38% of total coat protein for urea–mercaptoethanol (UME) at pH 7.0 to 70% or more for dithiothreitol with urea and SLS (UDS).

Studies by Gould & Hitchins (1963) have shown that spores with intact coats are resistant to the lytic enzyme lysozyme, but spores treated with agents that alter the spore coat will germinate in the presence of lysozyme. Wyatt & Waites (1974) also showed that slow-germination mutants of *Cl. bifermentans*, which were resistant to disulphide-reducing agents, appeared to have reduced permeability to germinants, such as alanine, and altered coats.

Similar studies have been used to indicate the extent to which coat protein protects against the action of chemical agents. Aronson & Fitz-James (1976) found that spores of a *B. cereus* mutant that were lysozyme-sensitive were also more sensitive to octanol than the parent spores. Further work with temperature-sensitive mutants suggested that the outer layers of the coat were responsible for octanol resistance (Stelma *et al.*, 1978). Studies with coat-defective mutants also demonstrated the role of the spore coat in resistance to chloroform (Sousa *et al.*, 1978).

With ethylene oxide, on the other hand, somewhat conflicting results have been obtained. Dadd & Daley (1982) showed that resistance of *B. cereus* spores pre-treated with dithiothreitol remained unchanged, while spores of a coat-defective mutant of *B. subtilis* were actually more resistant to ethylene oxide. In contrast, Marletta & Stumbo (1970) showed that urea–thioglycollic acid (UTA) treatment of *B. subtilis* spores reduced resistance to ethylene oxide, although this resistance was regained on storage. King & Gould (1969) showed that spores treated to allow lysozyme to initiate germination also regained lysozyme resistance during storage, probably as a result of oxidation of reduced disulphide bonds in their coats. Such changes may account for the recovery of resistance to ethylene oxide.

With hydrogen peroxide, NaOH and ethanol Waites & Bayliss (1979b) showed that spores or *B.*

cereus made sensitive to lysosyme by UME treatment were only slightly more sensitive than spores with intact coats, suggesting that the intact coat had little effect in this situation. Experiments with *Cl. bifermentans*, on the other hand, showed that intact spores were 500 times more resistant to hydrogen peroxide than spores pretreated with dithiothreitol (Bayliss & Waites, 1976).

Thomas & Russell (1974) showed that pretreatment with ME or TA had little or no effect on the resistance of *B. pumilis* spores to glutaraldehyde. On the other hand, McErlean *et al.* (1980) and Gorman *et al.* (1984a) indicated that pretreatment of *B. subtilis* spores with UME or UDS (producing 38 and 70% extraction of total coat protein, respectively) caused a progressive increase in sensitivity to glutaraldehyde. Experiments by Munton & Russell (1970) and King *et al.* (1974) showed that, whereas under acid conditions glutaraldehyde resides at the spore surface, treatment of spores with glutaraldehyde under alkaline conditions (in the presence of bicarbonate) facilitated penetration of glutaraldehyde into the spore, with increased activity. This suggests that alkaline but not acid glutaraldehyde causes disruption of spore coats.

Significant increases in sensitivity of *Cl. bifermentans*, *B. cereus* and *B. subtilis* spores to CRAs and iodine-releasing antibacterial agents following treatment with combinations of reagents causing extraction of spore-coat protein has been demonstrated by Cousins & Allan (1967), Wyatt & Waites (1975), Waites & Bayliss (1979), Gorman *et al.* (1983a, 1984b, 1985), Bloomfield & Arthur (1989, 1992) and Bloomfield & Megid (1994). Using agents that produced total coat-protein extraction ranging from 10% (by treatment with 0.2% NaOH or SLS) up to 70% (using UDS), successive increases in sensitivity of *B. subtilis* spores to CRAs, iodine and chlorine/methanol mixtures were found to correlate with the extent of coat protein release (Gorman *et al.*, 1983a; Bloomfield & Arthur, 1989, 1992; Bloomfield & Megid, 1994).

Evidence that the spore coat can play a role in biocide resistance also comes from studies which show that agents such as hydrogen peroxide (Bayliss & Waites, 1976) and NaOCl (Rode & Williams, 1966; Kulikovsky *et al.*, 1975; Wyatt & Waites, 1975; Foegeding & Busta, 1983) themselves cause some disruption and extraction of spore-coat material, thereby facilitating penetration to their site of action. Wyatt & Waites (1975) and Bayliss & Waites (1976) showed that treatment of *Cl. bifermentans*, *B. cereus* and *B. subtilis* spores with chlorine and of *Cl. bifermentans* with hydrogen peroxide produced solubilization of coat protein; gel electrophoresis of protein extracted with chlorine or peroxide produced an identical electrophoretic band to that demonstrated by Vary (1973) from alkali extracts of *Cl. bifermentans*, but other less dense bands, similar to those obtained from urea–dithiothreitol (UD) extracts (corresponding to outer coat-protein material), were absent from chlorine and peroxide extracts. Disruption of spore-coat material by treatment with chlorine is also indicated by studies of Wyatt & Waites (1975) and Foegeding and Busta (1983), which showed that chlorine treatment of *B. subtilis*, *B. cereus*, *Cl. bifermentans* and *Cl. botulinum* spores increased their sensitivity to lysozyme.

Studies with halogen-releasing agents (Bloomfield & Arthur, 1989, 1992; Bloomfield & Megid, 1994) showed that activity against intact *B. subtilis* spores was correlated with the extent of coat protein release. Whereas NaOCl and NaDCC produced substantial coat protein release and were effective at relatively low concentrations, chloramine-T and iodine were only effective at much higher concentrations and produced only limited coat protein extraction under these conditions. With NaOCl, NaDCC and iodine, the addition of up to 1% NaOH potentiated both coat protein extraction and sporicidal activity, while, for chloramine-T, NaOH had little or no effect on either of these properties.

Although these various studies indicate that the intact coat can play an important part in protecting the spore cortex and protoplast against the action of antibacterial agents, interpretation of the data is complicated by the finding that treatment of *B. subtilis* spores with UDS produced substantial extraction, not only of coat protein but also of cortex peptidoglycan, although the effects of other disulphide-reducing agents has not been investigated (Bloomfield & Arthur, 1992; Bloomfield & Megid, 1994). The results of these investigations, as described in more detail below, suggest that, although the coat may play a substantial part in resistance to chemical agents and heat, the cortex may also be involved.

4.3 Spore cortex and resistance

Whereas the role of the spore coat in resistance to biocides is fairly well established, increasingly there is evidence suggesting that the spore cortex may also play a part. Biocidal agents that have been shown to interact with spore cortex material include glutaraldehyde, chlorine, hydrogen peroxide, octanol and butanol, although the nature of this interaction varies considerably from one agent to another. Thus, Hughes & Thurman (1970) and Gorman *et al.* (1984a) report interaction of glutaraldehyde with the cortex of *B. subtilis* spores preventing degradation by lysozyme and nitrite. Waites *et al.* (1976, 1977), Gorman *et al.* (1984b) and Bloomfield & Arthur (1989, 1992), on the other hand, have shown that treatment with hydrogen peroxide or hypochlorite produces degradation of cortex material and, for hypochlorite (Wyatt & Waites, 1975), this treatment increases rather than decreases sensitivity to lysozyme.

For the various oxidizing agents, such as hypochlorites and hydrogen peroxide, it seems unlikely that degradation of spore cortex is responsible for spore death *per se*, since lysozyme treatment alone, under conditions producing cortex degradation, does not result in significant spore death (Fitz-James, 1971; Bloomfield & Arthur, 1989). Rather, it would seem that cortex degradation facilitates penetration of these agents to their site of action on the underlying spore protoplast.

The significance of cortex degradation in sporicidal action is demonstrated by comparative studies of CRAs (Bloomfield & Arthur, 1989, 1992), which showed that, although NaOCl, NaDCC and chloramine-T solutions, buffered to pH 7.4, had similar activity against vegetative cells of *B. subtilis*, there was considerable variation in sporicidal activity. Sodium hypochlorite (100 parts/10^6, 5 min contact) had significantly higher activity than NaDCC at 1000 parts/10^6, while chloramine-T at 5000 parts/10^6 showed little or no activity at 5 min. Pretreatment of spores with NaOH to extract alkali-soluble coat protein increased sensitivity to NaOCl and particularly to NaDCC, but had little effect on chloramine-T, whereas pretreatment of spores with UDS and with UDS followed by lysozyme produced successive increases in sensitivity to all three agents. Chemical analysis of extracted spores confirmed that, while producing significant extraction of coat protein, alkali treatment had no measurable effect on cortex peptidoglycan. In contrast, treatment with UDS and UDS/lysozyme caused progressive extraction of cortex material (50 and 75% of total cortex material, respectively), as well as coat protein. These results suggest that the increasing sensitivity to these CRAs is associated not only with progressive removal of the spore coat but also degradation of cortex peptidoglycan, allowing access to the underlying protoplast. Whereas extraction of alkali-soluble coat protein alone produced substantial increases in sensitivity to NaOCl and NaDCC, degradation of both coat and cortex material was required to achieve significant activity with chloramine-T. Further experiments (Bloomfield and Arthur, 1992, 1994) have shown that NaOCl and NaDCC (in the presence of NaOH) themselves produce degradation of cortex pepti-doglycan) which may be responsible for their rapid sporicidal action under these conditions. Chloramine-T, which produced no degradation of peptidoglycan, was ineffective against normal and alkali-extracted spores. Studies with iodine (Bloomfield & Megid, 1994) were not, however, consistent with those obtained with CRAs; whereas iodine, like chloramine-T, either alone or in the presence of NaOH, showed no evidence of cortex extraction, addition of NaOH produced significant potentiation of the sporicidal action of iodine.

From their experimental observations, Gould and co-workers (Gould, 1977; Gould & Dring, 1974, 1975) have postulated that spore cortex peptidoglycan is responsible not only for mechanical protection of the spore (as with vegetative cells) but is also responsible for maintaining dehydration of the spore protoplast. By maintaining a very low water level and a consequent high viscosity in the protoplast, diffusion of water-soluble antimicrobial agents into the protoplast is reduced. It may be, therefore, that rehydration of the spore protoplast following cortex degradation by the action of CRAs is required to facilitate diffusion of these agents to their site of action on the underlying protoplast.

From their observations of the action of chlorine/methanol mixtures, Death & Coates (1979) suggested that methanol potentiates the action of NaOCl by softening of spore coats, allowing penetration to occur. The results described above suggest rather that the action of chlorine is to produce coat and cortex degradation, thereby facilitating diffusion of methanol to its site of action on the underlying protoplast.

For glutaraldehyde, on the other hand, current evidence suggests that interaction with the cortex may be directly responsible for spore death. Results by Hughes and Thurman (1970) and Thomas & Russell (1974) indicate that low concentrations of glutaraldehyde inhibit spore germination by interacting with and cross-linking amino groups in the cortex peptidoglycan. Further investigations (Thomas, 1977) suggest that, at higher concentrations (10% alkaline glutaraldehyde), extensive irreversible interaction with spore outer layers produces a tough sealed structure, such that germination can no longer occur and spore death results. Gorman *et al.* (1984a) showed that pretreatment with glutaraldehyde protects coatless spores of *B. subtilis* from the lyric action of lysozyme and sodium nitrite and also reduces the solubilization of hexosamines from cortical fragments. If the sporicidal action of glutaraldehyde involves interaction with cortex peptidoglycan, it must follow that glutaraldehyde resistance will be determined by the extent to which this interaction is reversible or irreversible. Studies by Dancer *et al.* (1989) and Power *et al.* (1989, 1990) showed increased recovery of glutaraldehyde-treated spores by treatment with alkali (NaOH or sodium bicarbonate ($NaHCO_3$)) but not with disulphide-reducing agents, lysozyme or protease enzymes.

It is interesting to note that, whereas studies with glutaraldehyde suggest that interaction with spore outer layers produces sealing of spores, thereby preventing germination, the series of changes which occur following treatment with hypochlorite and hydrogen peroxide closely resemble those associated with spore germination, namely decrease in refractility, whereby phase-bright spores become phase-dark (Wyatt & Waites, 1973, 1975; Waites *et al.*, 1976), degradation of cortex peptidoglycan (Gorman *et al.*, 1984c; and Bloomfield & Arthur, 1989, 1992), and decrease in dry weight and optical density (Wyatt & Waites, 1973, 1975; Waites *et al.*, 1976).

There is evidence that other sporicidal agents may also interact with the spore cortex. Imae & Strominger (1976), using mutants of *Bacillus sphaericus* that were defective in the synthesis of *meso*-diaminopimelate (Dap), showed that muramic lactam in the spore cortex increased linearly with an increase in the concentration of Dap in the sporulation medium. When 25% of the maximum cortex concentration was produced, the spores became resistant to both octanol and xylene, but 90% of the maximum cortex development was required for heat resistance. The time at which cortex synthesis occurred during spore formation also coincided with the ordered appearance of resistance to chloroform methanol and octanol (Sousa *et al.*, 1978). Thus, it would seem that a complete cortex is important in conferring resistance to these chemicals. However, an incomplete cortex may affect development of other spore components. Thus, Imae & Strominger (1976) showed that spores without cortices were irregularly shaped, suggesting that coats may also have been defective, thereby reducing resistance.

For both glutaraldehyde and the various oxidizing agents, there is evidence that changes in spore resistance can be achieved by conditions that modify their interaction with spore cortex material. Most particularly, changes that alter the balance of cations and DPA within the spore cortex and protoplast have been investigated. These aspects are discussed in the following section.

4.4 Osmoregulation and resistance

Gould & Dring (1974, 1975) have proposed that the heat resistance of spores probably results from dehydration of the spore protoplast, which is brought about and maintained by the osmotic activity of expanded electronegative peptidoglycan within the spore cortex, the stability of the peptidoglycan being maintained by the presence of mobile, positively charged counterions within the cortex. They found that coat-defective spores treated to allow penetration of multivalent cations showed increased sensitivity to heat and suggested that, in this situation, the multivalent cations interacted with and cross-linked carboxyl groups of the peptidoglycan, causing it to contract, allowing partial rehydration and loss of heat resistance.

It was found that the presence of Cu^{2+} increased the lethal effect of hydrogen peroxide on spores of *Cl. bifermentans* but not of other species, such as *B. subtilis* var. *niger* (Bayliss & Waites, 1976; Wallen, 1976; Waites *et al.*, 1979). Since the protoplasts of *Cl. bifermentans* bound Cu^{2+} but those of *B. subtilis* var. *niger* did not, even when incubated as ultrathin sections with Cu^{2+}, this suggests that the state of the protoplast and cortex may be important in determining the resistance of spores to hydrogen peroxide. Protoplasts of *Cl. bifermentans* bound UO^{2+} and Pb^{2+} more readily than those of other species (Waites *et al.*, 1972), suggesting differences in the availability of groups for binding. Spores of the same *Cl. bifermentans* species were also more sensitive to chlorine (Wyatt & Waites, 1975), to hydrogen peroxide (Bayliss & Waites, 1976) and to a combination of glutaral-dehyde and formaldehyde (W.M. Waites, unpublished) than those of other species, again suggesting that protoplast structure may be important in determining resistance to some chemicals.

Sacks & Alderton (1961) showed that titration with acid to produce H-form spores reduced heat resistances which was recovered by titration with Ca^{2+} to produce Ca-form spores. Gould & Dring (1975) have suggested that, in this situation, acid treatment displaces positively charged cations from the cortex by protonating peptidoglycan carboxyl groups, thus reducing cortex expansion and lowering osmotic pressure. They proposed that re-equilibration at high pH values reimposes expansion and increases the osmotic pressure exerted by the cortex, thereby reinstating heat resistance, as is found experimentally.

Although further investigation is required, it is worth noting the results of Thomas & Russell (1975), McErlean *et al.* (1980) and Gorman *et al.* (1984a). These workers showed that stable Ca^{2+} forms of *B. subtilis* spores were more sensitive to glutaraldehyde, which appears to act by preventing cortical breakdown and spore germination, whereas NaOCl and NaOCl/methanol, which cause cortical breakdown and destabilization of spores, are more effective against unstable H-forms. Tarawatani & Shibaski (1973) have shown that H-form spores were also more sensitive to propylene oxide than normal or Ca-form spores.

At one time, it was thought that DPA played a significant role in the heat resistance of spores, but it has now been shown that mutants of *B. subtilis*, *B. cereus* and B. *megaterium* that contain no DPA and a low level of calcium retain full resistance to heat (Hanson *et al.*, 1972; Zytkovicz & Halvorsen, 1972). It now seems more likely, as stated by Gould (1977), that CaDPA in the spore core plays a role in dormancy as a calcium buffer and a calcium store. It has been calculated (Gould, 1977) that the expanded cortex may exert an osmotic potential of as much as 2 MPa or more, causing water to pass from the core to the cortex until the osmotic pressure is equalized. The water contents of the two compartments at equilibrium will therefore depend on the osmotic activity of the core. As far as is known, the spore protoplast contains mainly macromolecules or insolubilized salts, such as dipicolinate or calcium salts of other weak acids, such as glutamic and phosphoglyceric acids (Nelson *et al.*, 1969), which make only a small osmotic contribution, thereby maintaining an equilibrium position in the direction of a high water-content cortex surrounding a low water-content core.

During germination, as the spore becomes sensitive to heat and other agents and loses its dormancy, calcium previously held by DPA in the core is mobilized in some way to neutralize negative groups in the cortex, so reducing the osmotic pressure and allowing the protoplast to rehydrate. In line with this, it is found that hydrogen peroxide and CRAs produce leakage of Ca^{2+} and/or DPA from spores (Alderton & Halbrook, 1971; Dye & Mead, 1972; Gorman *et al.*, 1984b), while glutaraldehyde, which appears to act by stabilization of the spore cortex, does not (Thomas & Russell, 1974).

Balassa *et al.* (1979) have shown that a mutant of *B. subtilis* that did not synthesize DPA during spore formation and contained less Ca^{2+} than the parent spores was also less resistant to phenol, pyridine and trichloroacetic acid than the parent spores. When DPA was added to the sporulation medium, it was taken up by the spores, which then became more resistant to these three agents. These results suggest that DPA in spore protoplasts may play some role in resistance to heat and chemical agents.

4.5 The spore protoplast and resistance

Although sporicidal agents may interact with spore outer layers, thereby affecting the barrier properties of the coat and the ability of the spore cortex to maintain dehydration of the spore protoplast, there is little evidence to suggest that these effects are responsible *per se* for spore inactivation. With the possible exception of glutaraldehyde, it would seem that the primary lethal action of agents that have a sporicidal action is on the spore protoplast or spore protoplast membrane.

Since the process of sporulation is associated with significant changes in the structure and metabolic function of the cell protoplast and protoplasmic membrane, it is reasonable to assume that these fundamental changes in cell structure must inevitably be associated with significant changes in their interaction with, and therefore their response to, chemical agents, although there has been little investigation of this aspect. Because of the highly reactive nature of bactericides that are also sporicidal, it is likely, as with vegetative cells, that interaction occurs with any number of different structures and/or enzymes within the membrane or protoplasm and that spore inactivation probably results from a number of independent events, such that attempts to elucidate a primary site of action are likely to prove extremely difficult, if not impossible.

Studies by Imlay & Lin (1988), Setlow and Setlow (1993) and Sabli *et al.* (1996) indicate that interaction with cellular DNA contributes to the sporicidal action of peroxygen compounds and CRAs and that changes in DNA structure during sporulation contribute substantially to the development of spore resistance to these agents. A major factor in development of resistance by *B. subtilis* to hydrogen peroxide and hypochlorite appears to be the synthesis of α,β-type small acid-soluble proteins (SASPs) during sporulation, which saturate the spore chromosome and protect the DNA backbone against hydroxyl radical cleavage. This is indicated by the fact that spores of *B. subtilis* deficient in α,β-type SASPs are more sensitive than wild-type spores to both hydrogen peroxide (Setlow & Setlow, 1993) and hypochlorite (Sabli *et al.*, 1996). However, the fact that wild-type spores are largely resistant to DNA damage (Popham *et al.*, 1995) by hydrogen peroxide suggests that the sporicidal action of this compound is not significantly through DNA damage.

In contrast, studies by Bloomfield & Arthur (1989, 1992) and Bloomfield & Megid (1994) indicate that disruption of the protoplast membrane may contribute to both the bactericidal and sporicidal action of halogen-releasing agents and that the increased resistance of spores to iodine and CRAs does not result from alterations in the protoplast membrane during sporulation. This is shown by the fact that concentrations of NaOCl, NaDCC and iodine which are bactericidal to vegetative cells also cause significant damage to isolated *B. subtilis* spore protoplasts, as evidenced by leakage of DPA and phosphate. It is interesting to note that isolated *B. subtilis* spore protoplasts showed sensitivity to the inactivation by halogen-releasing agents similar to that of vegetative forms, which suggests that degradation of the spore cortex must be associated not only with rehydration of the protoplast but also with degradation of the protective SASPs.

5 Conclusions

A review of the literature indicates that the mechanisms which account for the resistance of spores relative to that of vegetative bacterial forms to the action of antimicrobial agents are complex and only partially understood.

Most certainly, it would appear that the spore coat plays an important part in resisting the action of some agents, by limiting penetration to the underlying cortex and protoplast, and that this situation applies even to agents which are known to be actively sporicidal. It is found that sporicidal agents, such as CRAs, peroxide and possibly also glutaraldehyde, applied under conditions in which they cause degradation of outer spore layers, are effective at relatively much lower concentrations, although these are generally in excess of those which kill vegetative cells. In contrast, for agents such as iodine, chloramine-T and NaDCC, under conditions where they produce little or no coat-protein extraction, concentrations and contact times required to achieve adequate penetration required for destruction of spores are very considerably in excess of those which kill vegetative cells. For antimicrobial agents, such as chlorhexidine, which have little or no sporicidal action, it is suggested that these agents may be almost completely excluded from the spore. Shaker *et al.* (1988) have demonstrated that extraction of *B. subtilis* spores decreased resistance to chlorhexidine; whereas 25 μ/ml chlorhexidine produced only a 0.5 log reduction of intact spores within 2 h, the same concentration produce a 2 log reduction with UDS-treated spores.

Increasingly, there is evidence to suggest that the spore cortex also plays a vital role in the resistance of spores to heat and chemical agents. It is suggested that this derives from the stable expanded spore cortex which maintains a stable dehydrated state and a consequent high viscosity within the spore protoplast, thereby limiting diffusion into the protoplast. Experimental studies indicate that resistance imposed by the cortex may be overcome either by interactions within the cortex or by interactions in core which destabilize the cortex, facilitating diffusion of the antimicrobial agent into the sensitive protoplast. Alternatively, the sporicide may interact to prevent cortex degradation, thereby preventing rehydration, germination and outgrowth of the spore. In this situation, treatments that modify these interactions may be used to modify resistance to sporicidal agents.

There is also evidence that, for some agents, changes in the structure of the cell protoplast during spore formation, such as changes in the structure of DNA resulting from the binding of SASPs, can contribute significantly to their resistance to biocides, as compared with that of vegetative cells.

6 Acknowledgement

I would like to acknowledge Professor W.M. Waites, Department of Applied Biochemistry and Food Science, School of Agriculture, Sutton Bonnington, for his significant contribution in writing the original version of this Chapter.

7 References

Alderton, G. & Halbrook, W.V. (1971) Action of chlorine on bacterial spores. *Bacteriological Proceedings*, p. 12.

Ando, Y. & Tsuzuki, T. (1986a) The effect of hydrogen peroxide on spores of *Clostridium perfringens. Letters in Applied Microbiology*, **2**, 65–68.

Ando, Y. & Tsuzuki, T. (1986b) Changes in decoated spores of *Clostridium perfringens* caused by treatment with some enzymatic and non-enzymatic systems. *Letters in Applied Microbiology*, **3**, 61–64.

Aronson, A.I. & Fitz-James, P.C. (1971) Reconstitution of bacterial spore coat layers *in vitro*. *Journal of Bacteriology*, **108**, 571–578.

Aronson, A. & Fitz-James, P.C. (1976) Structure and morphogenesis of the bacterial spore coat. *Bacteriological Reviews*, **40**, 360–402.

Babb, J.R., Bradley, C.R. & Ayliffe, G.A.J. (1980) Sporicidal activity of glutaraldehyde and hypochlorites and other factors influencing their selection for the treatment of medical equipment. *Journal of Hospital Infection*, **1**, 63–75.

Balassa, G., Milhaud, P., Raulet, E., Silva, M.T. & Sousa, J.C.F. (1979) A *Bacillus subtilis* mutant requiring dipicolinic acid for the development of heat-resistant spores. *Journal of General Microbiology*, **110**, 365–379.

Baldry, M.G.C. (1983) The bactericidal, fungicidal and sporicidal properties of hydrogen peroxide and peracetic acid. *Journal of Applied Bacteriology*, **54**, 417–423.

Baldry, M.G.C. (1988) Disinfection with peroxygens. In *Industrial Biocides: Critical Reports on Applied Chemistry* (ed. Payne, K.R.), pp. 91–116. Chichester: John Wiley & Sons.

Barach, J.T., Flowers, R.S. & Adams, D.M. (1975) Repair of heat-injured *Clostridium perfringens* spores during outgrowth. *Applied Microbiology*, **30**, 873–875.

Bayliss, C.E. & Waites, W.M. (1976) The effect of hydrogen peroxide on spores of *Clostridium bifermentans*. *Journal of General Microbiology*, **96**, 401–407.

Bayliss, C.E. & Waites, W.M. (1979) The synergistic killing of spores of *Bacillus subtilis* by hydrogen peroxide and ultra-violet light irradiation. *FEMS Microbiology Letters*, **5**, 331–333.

Bayliss, C.E. & Waites, W.M. & King, N.R. (1981) Resistance and structure of spores of *Bacillus subtilis*. *Journal of Applied Bacteriology*, **50**, 379–390.

Benarde, M.A., Snow, W.B. & Olivieri, V.P. (1967) Chlorine dioxide disinfection temperature effects. *Journal of Applied Bacteriology*, **30**, 159–167.

Block, S.S. (ed.) (1983) *Disinfection, Sterilization and Preservation*, 3rd edn. Philadelphia: Lea & Febiger.

Bloomfield, S.F. (1991) Methods for the assessment of antimicrobial activity. In *Society of Applied Bacteriology Technical Series* No. 27, pp 1–27. London: Academic Press.

Bloomfield, S.F. & Arthur, M. (1989) Effect of chlorine-releasing agents on *Bacillus subtilis* vegetative cells and spores. *Letters in Applied Microbiology*, **8**, 101–104.

Bloomfield, S.F. & Arthur, M. (1992) Interaction of *Bacillus subtilis* spores with sodium hypochlorite, sodium dischloroisocyanurate and chloramine-T. *Journal of Applied Bacteriology*, **72**, 166–172.

Bloomfield, S.F. & Arthur M. (1994) Mechanisms of inactivation and resistance of spores to chemical biocides. *Journal of Applied Bacteriology Symposium Supplement*, **76**, 91s–104s.

Bloomfield, S.F. & Megid, R. (1994) Interaction of iodine with *Bacillus subtilis* spores and spore forms. *Journal of Applied Bacteriology*, **76**, 492–499.

Bomar, M. (1962) The relationship between the age of *Bacillus subtilis* spores and their resistance to ethylene oxide. *Folia Microbiologia Praha*, **7**, 259–261.

Boucher, R.M.G. (1975) On biocidal mechanisms in the aldehyde series. *Canadian Journal of Pharmaceutical Sciences*, **10**, 1–7.

Briggs, A. (1966) The resistance of spores of the genus *Bacillus* to phenol, heat and radiation. *Journal of Applied Bacteriology*, **29**, 490–504.

Bruch, C.W. & Koesterer, M.G. (1961) The microbicidal activity of gaseous propylene oxide and its application to powdered or flaked foods. *Journal of Food Science*, **26**, 428–435.

Caputo, R.A. & Odlaug, T.E. (1983) Sterilization with ethylene oxide and other gases. In *Disinfection, Sterilization and Preservation* (ed. Block, S.S.), pp. 47–64. Philadelphia: Lea & Febiger.

Cousins, C.M. & Allan, C.D. (1967) Sporicidal properties of some halogens. *Journal of Applied Bacteriology*, **30**, 168–174.

Dadd, A.H. & Daley, G.M. (1982) Role of the coat in resistance of bacterial spores to inactivation by ethylene oxide. *Journal of Applied Bacteriology*, **53**, 109–116.

Dancer, B.N., Power, E.G.M. & Russell, A.D. (1989) Alkali-induced revival of *Bacillus* spores after inactivation by glutaraldehyde *FEMS Microbiology Letters*, **57**, 345–348.

Death, J.E. & Coates, D. (1979) Effect of pH on sporicidal and microbicidal activity of buffered mixtures of alcohol and sodium hypochlorite. *Journal of Clinical Pathology*, **32**, 148–153.

Dye, M. & Mead, G.C. (1972) The effect of chlorine on the viability of clostridial spores. *Journal of Food Technology*, **7**, 173–181.

El-Bisi, H.M., Vondell, R.M. & Esselen, W.B. (1963) Studies on the kinetics of the bactericidal action of ethylene oxide in the vapor phase. *Bacteriological Proceedings*, p. 13.

Ernst, R.R. (1974) Ethylene oxide sterilization kinetics. *Biotechnology Bioengineering Symposium*, **4**, 865–878.

Ernst, R.R. (1975) Sterilization by means of ethylene oxide. *Acta Pharmaceutica Suecica*, **12** (Suppl.) 4–64.

Fitz-James, P.C. (1971) Formation of protoplasts from resting spores. *Journal of Applied Bacteriology*, **105**, 1119–1136.

Foegeding, P.M. (1985) Ozone inactivation of *Bacillus* and *Clostridium* spores and the importance of the spore coat to resistance. *Food Microbiology*, **2**, 123–134.

Foegeding, P.M. & Busta, F.F. (1983) Proposed mechanism for sensitization by hypochlorite treatment of *Clostridium botulinum* spores. *Applied and Environmental Microbiology*, **45**, 1374–1379.

Foegeding, P.M. & Fulp, M.L. (1988) Comparison of coats and surface-dependent properties of *Bacillus cereus* T prepared in two sporulation environments. *Journal of Applied Bacteriology*, **65**, 249–259.

Forsyth, M.P. (1975) A rate of kill test for measuring sporicidal properties of liquid sterilizers. *Developments in Industrial Microbiology*, **16**, 37–47.

Futter, B.V. & Richardson, G. (1970a) Viability of clostridial spores and the requirements of damaged organisms. I. Method of colony count, period and temperature of incubation, and pH value of the medium. *Journal and Applied Bacteriology*, **33**, 321–330.

Futter, B.V. & Richardson, G. (1970b) Viability of clostridial spores and the requirements of damaged organisms. II. Gaseous environment and redox potentials. *Journal of Applied Bacteriology*, **33**, 331–340.

Gardner, J.S. & Favero, M.S. (1985) *Guideline for Handwashing and Hospital Infection Control*. HHS Publication No. 99-1117. Atlanta, Georgia: Public Health Service, Centers for Disease Control.

Gorman, S.P. & Scott, E.M. (1979) Potentiation and stabilization of glutaraldehyde biocidal activity utilizing surfactant divalent metal combinations. *International Journal of Pharmaceutics*, **4**, 57–65.

Gorman, S.P., Scott, E.M. & Russell, A.D. (1980) Antimicrobial activity, uses and mechanism of action of glutaraldehyde. *Journal of Applied Bacteriology*, **48**, 161–190.

Gorman, S.P., Hutchinson, E.P., Scott, E.M. & McDermott, L.M. (1983a) Death, injury and revival of chemically-treated *Bacillus subtilis* spores. *Journal of Applied Bacteriology*, **54**, 91–99.

Gorman, S.P., Scott, E.M. & Hutchinson, E.P. (1983b) The effect of sodium hypochlorite-methanol combinations on spores and spore forms of *Bacillus subtilis*. *International Journal of Pharmaceutics*, **17**, 291–298.

Gorman, S.P., Scott, E.M. & Hutchinson, E.P. (1984a) Interaction of *Bacillus subtilis* spore protoplast, cortex, ion-exchange and coatless forms with glutaraldehyde. *Journal of Applied Bacteriology*, **56**, 95–102.

Gorman, S.P., Scott, E.M. & Hutchinson, E.P. (1984b) Hypochlorite effects on spores and spore forms of *Bacillus subtilis* and on a spore lytic enzyme. *Journal of Applied Bacteriology*, **56**, 295–303.

Gorman, S.P., Scott, E.M. & Hutchinson, E.P. (1984c) Emergence and development of resistance to antimicrobial chemicals and heat in spores of *Bacillus subtilis*. *Journal of Applied Bacteriology*, **57**, 153–163.

Gorman, S.P., Scott, E.M. & Hutchinson, E.P. (1985) Effects of aqueous and alocholic providone-iodine on spores of *Bacillus subtilis*. *Journal of Applied Bacteriology*, **59**, 99–105.

Gould, G.W. (1971) Methods for studying bacterial spores. In *Methods in Microbiology* (eds Norris, J.R. & Ribbons, D.W.), Vol. 6A, pp. 326–381. London: Academic Press.

Gould, G.W. (1977) Recent advances in the understanding of resistance and dormancy in bacterial spores. *Journal of Applied Bacteriology*, **42**, 297–309.

Gould, G.W. (1983) Mechanisms of resistance and dormancy. In *The Bacterial Spore* (eds Hurst, A. & Gould, G.W.), Vol. 2, pp. 173–209. London and New York: Academic Press.

Gould, G.W. (1984) Injury and repair mechanisms in bacterial spores. In *The Revival of Injured Microbes* (ed. Andrew, M.H.E. & Russell, A.D.), pp. 199–220. Society for Applied Bacteriology Symposium Series No. 12. London and New York: Academic Press.

Gould, G.W. (1985) Modifications of resistance and dormancy. In *Fundamental and Applied Aspects of Bacterial Spores* (ed. Dring, G.J. Ellar, D.J. & Gould, G.W.), pp. 199–220. Society for Applied Bacteriology Symposium Series No. 12. London and New York: Academic Press.

Gould, G.W. & Dring, G.J. (1974) Mechanisms of spore heat resistance. *Advances in Microbial Physiology*, **11**, 137–164.

Gould, G.W. & Dring, G.J. (1975) Heat resistance of bacterial endospores and concept of an expanded osmoregulatory cortex. *Nature, London*, **258**, 402–405.

Gould, G.W. & Hitchins, A.D. (1963) Sensitization of bacterial spores to lysozyme and to hydrogen peroxide with agents which rupture disulphide bonds. *Journal of General Microbiology*, **33**, 413–423.

Hanson, R.S., Curry, M.V., Gardner, J.V. & Halvorsen, H.O. (1972) Mutants of *Bacillus cereus* strain T that produce thermoresistant spores lacking dipicolinic acid and have low levels of calcium. *Canadian Journal of Microbiology*, **18**, 1139–1143.

Hoffman, R.K. (1971) Toxic gases. In *Inhibition and Destruction of the Microbial Cell* (ed. Hugo, W.B.), pp. 225–258. London and New York: Academic Press.

Hughes, R.C. & Thurman, P.F. (1970). Cross-linking of bacterial cell walls with glutaraldehyde. *Biochemical Journal*, **119**, 925–926.

Imae, Y. & Strominger, J.L. (1976) Relationship between cortex content and properties of spores. *Journal of Bacteriology*, **126**, 907–913.

Imlay, J.A. & Lin, S. (1988) DNA damage and oxygen radical toxicity. *Science*, **240**, 1302–1309.

Isenberg, H.D. (1985) Clinical laboratory studies of disinfection with Sporicidin. *Journal of Clinical Microbiology*, **22**, 735–739.

Ito, K.A., Denny, C.B., Brown, C.K., Yao, M. & Seeger, M.L. (1973) Resistance of bacterial spores to hydrogen peroxide. *Food Technology*, **27**, 58–66.

Kelsey, J.C., MacKinnon, I.H. & Maurer, I.M. (1974) Sporicidal activity of hospital disinfectants. *Journal of Clinical Pathology*, **27**, 632–638.

King, J.A., Woodside, W. & McGucken, P.V. (1974) Relationship between pH and antibacterial activity of glutaraldehyde. *Journal of Pharmaceutical Sciences*, **63**, 804–805.

King, W.L. & Gould, G.W. (1969) Lysis of bacterial spores with hydrogen peroxide. *Journal of Applied Bacteriology*, **32**, 481–490.

Knott, A.G. & Russell, A.D. (1995) Effects of chlorhexidine gluconate on the development of spores of *Bacillus subtilis*. *Letters in Applied Microbiology*, **21**, 117–120.

Knott, A.G., Russell, A.D. & Dancer, B.N. (1995) Development of resistance to biocides during sporulation of *Bacillus subtilis*. *Journal of Applied Bacteriology*, **79**, 492–498.

Knott, A.G., Dancer, B.N., Hann, A.C. & Russell, A.D. (1997) Non-variable sources of pure water and the germination and outgrowth of *Bacillus subtilis* spores. *Journal of Applied Microbiology*, **82**, 267–272.

Kulikovsky, A., Pankratz, H.S. & Sadoff, H.L. (1975) Ultrastructural and chemical changes in spores of *Bacillus cereus* after action of disinfectants. *Journal of Applied Bacteriology*, **38**, 39–46.

Labbé, R.G., Reich, R.R. & Duncan, C.L. (1978) Alteration in ultrastructure and germination of *Clostridium perfringens* type A spores following extraction of spore coats. *Canadian Journal of Microbiology*, **24**, 1526–1536.

Lelieveld, H.L.M. (1979) The effect of pH on microbial growth and destruction. In *Society for Applied Bacteriology Technical Series* No. 15 (eds Gould, G.W. & Corry, J.E.L.), pp. 71–98. London: Academic Press.

McEarlean, E.P., Gorman, S.P. & Scott, E.M. (1980) Physical and chemical resistance of ion-exchange and coat-defective spores of *Bacillus subtilis*. *Journal of Pharmacy and Pharmacology*, **32**, 32P.

Marks, H.C. & Strandskov, F.B. (1950) Halogens and

their mode of action. *Annals of the New York Academy of Sciences*, **53**, 163–171.

Marletta, J. & Stumbo, C.R. (1970) Some effects of ethylene oxide on *Bacillus subtilis*. *Journal of Food Science*, **35** 627–631.

Marshall, B.J., Murrell, W.G. & Scott, W.J. (1963) The effect of water activity, solutes and temperature on the viability and heat resistance of freeze-dried bacterial spores. *Journal of General Microbiology*, **31**, 451–460.

Miner, N.A., McDowell, J.W., Wilcockson, G.W., Bruckner, N.I., Stark, R.C. & Whitmore, J. (1977) Antimicrobial and other properties of a new stabilized alkaline glutaraldehyde disinfectant sterilizer. *American Journal of Hospital Pharmacy*, **34**, 367–382.

Molin, G. & Östlund, K. (1976) Dry heat inactivation of *Bacillus subtilis* var. *niger* spores with special reference to spore density. *Canadian Journal of Microbiology*, **22**, 359–363.

Munton, T.J. & Russell, A.D. (1970) Aspects of the action of glutaraldehyde on *Escherichia coli*. *Journal of Applied Bacteriology*, **33**, 410–419.

Murrell, W.G. (1969) Chemical composition of spores and spore structures. In *The Bacterial Spore* (eds Gould, G.W. & Hurst, A.), pp. 215–273. London: Academic Press.

Murrell, W.G. & Warth, A.D. (1965) Composition and heat resistance of bacterial spores. In *Spores III* (eds Campbell, L.L. & Halvorsen, H.O.), pp. 1–24. Ann Arbor: American Society for Microbiology.

Nelson, D.L., Spudich, J.A., Donsen, P.P.M., Bertsch, L. & Kornberg, A. (1969) Biochemical studies of bacterial sporulation and germination. XVI Small molecules in spores. In *Spores IV* (ed. Campbell, L.L.), Bethesda, Maryland: American Society for Microbiology.

Nishihara, T., Yutsudo, T., Ichikawa, T. & Kondo, M. (1981) Studies on the bacterial spore coat on the SDS-DTT extract from *Bacillus megaterium* spores. *Microbiology, Immunology*, **25**, 327–331.

Ortenzio, L.F. (1966) Collaborative study of improved sporicidal test. *Journal of the Association of Official Analytical Chemists*, **49**, 721–726.

Ortenzio, L.F., Stuart, L.S. & Friedl, J.L. (1953) The resistance of bacterial spores to constant boiling hydrochloric acid. *Journal of the Association of Official Agricultural Chemists*, **36**, 480–484.

Phillips, C.R. (1952) Relative resistance of bacterial spores and vegetative bacteria to disinfectants. *Bacteriological Reviews*, **16**, 135–138.

Phillips, C.R. (1977) Gaseous sterilisation. In *Disinfection, Sterilization and Preservation* (ed. Block, S.S.), pp. 592–610. Philadelphia: Lea & Febiger.

Popham, D.L., Sengupta, S. & Setlow, P. (1995) Heat, hydrogen peroxide, and UV resistance of *Bacillius subtilis* spores with increased core water content and with or without major DNA-binding proteins. *Applied and Environmental Microbiology*, **61**, 3633–3638.

Portner, D.F. & Hoffman, R.K. (1968) Sporicidal effect of peracetic acid vapour. *Applied Microbiology*, **16**, 1782–1785.

Power, E.G.M. & Russell, A.D. (1990) Sporicidal action of alkaline glutaraldehyde: factors influencing activity and a comparison with other aldehydes. *Journal of Applied Bacteriology*, **69**, 261–268.

Power, E.G.M., Dancer, B.N. & Russell, A.D. (1988) Emergence of resistance to glutaraldehyde in spores of *Bacillus subtilis* 168. *FEMS Microbiology Letters*, **50**, 223–226.

Power, E.G.M., Dancer, B.N. & Russell, A.D. (1989) Possible mechanisms for the revival of glutaraldehyde-treated spores of *Bacillus subtilis* NCTC 8236. *Journal of Applied Bacteriology*, **67**, 91–98.

Power, E.G.M., Dancer, B.N. & Russell, A.D. (1990) Effect of sodium hydroxide and two proteases on the revival of aldehyde-treated spores. *Letters in Applied Bacteriology*, **10**, 9–13.

Quinn, P.J. (1987) Evaluation of veterinary disinfectants and disinfection processes. In *Disinfection in Veterinary and Farm Animal Practice* (eds Linton, A.H., W.B. & Russell, A.D.), pp. 66–116. Oxford: Blackwell Scientific Publications.

Reich, R. (1980) Effect of sublethal ethylene oxide exposure on *Bacillus subtilis* spores and biological indicator performance. *Journal of the Parenteral Drug Association*, **34**, 200–211.

Ridenour, G.M., Ingols, R.S. & Armbruster, E.H. (1949) Sporicidal properties of chlorine dioxide. *Water and Sewage Works*, **96**, 279–283.

Roberts, T.A. (1970) Recovering spores damaged by heat, ionizing radiations or ethylene oxide. *Journal of Applied Bacteriology*, **33**, 74–94.

Roberts, T.A. & Hitchins, A.D. (1969) Resistance of spores. In *The Bacterial Spore* (eds Gould, G.W. & Hurst, A.), pp. 611–670. London: Academic Press.

Rode, L.J. & Williams, M.G. (1966) Utility of sodium hypochlorite for ultrastructure study of bacterial spore integuments. *Journal of Bacteriology*, **92**, 1772–1778.

Rubbo, S.D. & Gardner, J.F. (1965) *A Review of Sterilization and Disinfection*. London: Lloyd-Luke.

Rubbo, S.D., Gardner, J.F. & Webb, R.L. (1967) Biocidal activities of glutaraldehyde and related compounds. *Journal of Applied Bacteriology*, **30**, 78–87.

Russell, A.D. (1971) The destruction of bacterial spores. In *Inhibition and Destruction of the Microbial Cell* (ed. Hugo, W.B.), pp. 451–612. London and New York: Academic Press.

Russell, A.D. (1982) *The Destruction of Bacterial Spores*. London: Academic Press.

Russell, A.D. (1983) Mechanisms of action of chemical sporicidal and sporistatic agents. *International Journal of Pharmaceutics*, **10**, 127–140.

Russell, A.D. (1990) The bacterial spore and chemical sporicidal agents. *Clinical Microbiological Reviews*, **3**, 99–119.

Russell, A.D. (1994) Glutaraldehyde: current status and uses. *Infection Control and Hospital Epidemiology*, **15**, 724–733.

Russell, A.D. & Chopra, I. (1996) *Understanding Antibacterial Action and Resistance*, 2nd edn. Chichester: Ellis Horwood.

Russell, A.D., Dancer, B.N., Power, E.G.M. & Shaker, L.A. (1989) Mechanisms of bacterial spore resistance to disinfectants. In *Proceedings of the 4th Conference Programme on Chemical Disinfectants*, Binghamton, New York, pp. 9–29.

Russell, A.D., Dancer, B.N. & Power, E.G.M. (1991) Effects of chemical agents on bacterial sporulation, germination and outgrowth. In *Mechanisms of Action of Chemical Biocides. Their Study and Exploitation. Society of Applied Bacteriology, Technical Series No. 27* (eds Denyer, S.P. and Hugo, W.B.), pp. 23–24. London and New York: Academic Press.

Sabli, Z.H., Setlow, P. & Waites, W.M. (1996) The effect of hypochlorite on spores of *Bacillus subtilis* lacking small acid-soluble proteins. *Letters in Applied Microbiology*, **22**, 405–407.

Sacks, L.E. & Alderton, G. (1961) Behavior of bacterial spores in aqueous polymer two-phase systems. *Journal of Bacteriology*, **82**, 331–341.

Sagripanti, J. & Bonifacino, A. (1996) Comparative sporicidal effects of liquid chemical agents. *Applied and Environmental Microbiology*, **62**, 545–551.

St Julian, G., Pridham, T.G. & Hall, H.H. (1967) Preparation and characterization of intact and free spores of *Bacillus popilliae* Dutky. *Canadian Journal of Microbiology*, **13**, 279–285.

Setlow, B. & Setlow, P. (1993) Binding of small acid-soluble spore proteins plays a significant role in the resistance of *Bacillus subtilis* to hydrogen peroxide. *Applied and Environmental Microbiology*, **59**, 3418–3423.

Shaker, L.A., Dancer, B.N., Russell, A.D. & Furr, J.R. (1988) Emergence and development of chlorhexidine resistance during sporulation of *Bacillus subtilis* 168. *FEMS Microbiology Letters*, **51**, 73–76.

Shin, S.Y. & Marquis, R.E. (1994) Sporicidal activity of tertiary butyl hydroperoxide. *Archives in Microbiology*, **161**, 184–190.

Sousa, J.C.F., Silva, M.T. & Balassa, G. (1978) Ultrastructural effects of chemical agents and moist heat on *Bacillus subtilis*. II Effects on sporulating cells. *Annales de Microbiologie*, **129B**, 377–390.

Spicher, G. & Peters, J. (1976) Microbial resistance to formaldehyde. I. Comparative quantitative studies in some selected species of vegetative bacteria, bacterial spores, fungi, bacteriophages and viruses. *Zentralblatt für Bakteriologie Parasitenkunde, Infektionskrankheiten und Hygiene, I. Abteilung originale, Reihe B*, **163**, 486–503.

Spicher, G. & Peters, J. (1981) Heat activation of bacterial spores after inactivation by formaldehyde: dependence of heat activation on temperature and duration of action. *Zentralblatt für Bakteriologie Parasitenkunde, Infektionskrankheiten und Hygiene, I. Abteilung originale, Reihe B*,**173**, 188–196.

Stark, R.L., Ferguson, P., Garza, & Miner, N.A. (1975) An evaluation of the Association of Offical Analytical Chemists sporicidal test method. *Developments in Industrial Microbiology*, **16**, 31–36.

Stelma, G.N., Aronson, A.I. & Fitz-James, P. (1978) Properties of *Bacillus cereus* temperature-sensitive mutants altered in spore coat formation. *Journal of Bacteriology*, **134**, 1157–1170.

Sykes, G. (1970) The sporicidal properties of chemical disinfectants. *Journal of Applied Bacteriology*, **33**, 147–156.

Tarawatini, T. & Shibasaki, I. (1973) Change in the chemical resistance of heat sensitive and heat resistant bacterial spores against propylene oxide. *Journal of Fermentation Technology*, **51**, 824–891.

Thomas, S. (1977) Effect of high concentrations of glutaraldehyde upon bacterial spores. *Microbios Letters*, **4**, 199–204.

Thomas, S. & Russell, A.D. (1974) Studies on the mechanism of the sporicidal action of glutaraldehyde. *Journal of Applied Bacteriology*, **37**, 83–92.

Thomas, S. & Russell, A.D. (1975) Sensitivity and resistance to glutaraldehyde of the hydrogen and calcium forms of *Bacillus pumilus* spores. *Journal of Applied Bacteriology*, **38**, 315–317.

Toledo, R.T. (1975) Chemical sterilants for aseptic packaging. *Food Technology*, **29**, 102, 104, 105, 108, 110–112.

Toledo, R.T., Escher. F.E. & Ayres, J.C. (1973) Sporicidal properties of hydrogen peroxide against food spoilage organisms. *Applied Microbiology*, **26**, 592–597.

Trujillo, R. & David, T.J. (1972) Sporistatic and sporicidal properties of aqueous formaldehyde. *Applied Microbiology*, **23**, 618–622.

Tuynenberg Muys, G., Van Rhee, R. & Lelieveld, H.L.M. (1978) Sterilization by means of hydrochloric acid vapour. *Journal of Applied Bacteriology*, **45**, 213–217.

Vary, J.C. (1973) Germination of *Bacillus megaterium* spores after various extraction procedures. *Journal of Bacteriology*, **116**, 797–803.

von Bockelmann, I. (1974) The sporicidal action of chemical disinfectants. In *SIK Rapport* No. 359, pp. 86–97.

Waites, W.M. (1985) Inactivation of spores with chemical agents. In *Fundamental and Applied Aspects of Bacterial Spores* (eds Dring, G.J., Ellar, D.J. & Gould, G.W.), pp. 383–396. London: Academic Press.

Waites, W.M. & Bayliss, C.E. (1979a) The preparation of bacterial spores for evaluation of the sporicidal activity of chemicals. In *Society for Applied Bacteriology Technical Series, No. 15* (eds Gould, G.W. & Corry, J.E.L.), pp. 159–172. London: Academic Press.

Waites, W.M. & Bayliss, C.E. (1979b) The effect of changes in spore coat on the destruction of *Bacillus cereus* spores by heat and chemical treatment. *Journal of Applied Biochemistry*, **1**, 71–76.

Waites, W.M. & Bayliss, C.E. (1984) Damage to bacterial spores by combined treatments and possible revival and repair processes. In *The Revival of Injured Microbes* (eds Andrew, M.H.E. & Russell, A.D.), pp. 221–240. Society for Applied Bacteriology Symposium Series, No. 12. London and New York: Academic Press.

Waites, W.M., Wyatt, L.R. & Arthur, B. (1972) Effect of alkali treatment on the germination and morphology of spores of *Clostridium bifermentans*. In *Spores V* (eds Halvorsen, H.O., Hanson, R. & Campbell, L.L.), pp. 430–436. Washington: American Society for Microbiology.

Waites, W.M.,Wyatt, L.R., King, N.R. & Bayliss, C.E. (1976) Changes in spores of *Clostridium bifermentans* caused by treatment with hydrogen peroxide and cations. *Journal of General Microbiology*, **93**, 388–396.

Waites, W.M., King, N.R. & Bayliss, C.E. (1977) The effect of chlorine and heat on spores of *Clostridium bifermentans*. *Journal of General Microbiology*, **102**, 211–213.

Waites, W.M., Bayliss, C.E., King, N.R. & Davies, A.M.C. (1979) The effect of transitional metal ions on the resistance of bacterial spores to hydrogen peroxide and to heat. *Journal of General Microbiology*, **112**, 225–233.

Waites, W.M., Harding, S.E., Fowler, D.R., Jones, S.H., Shaw, D. & Martin, M. (1988) The destruction of spores of *Bacillus subtilis* by the combined effects of hydrogen peroxide and ultraviolet light. *Letters in Applied Microbiology*, **7**, 139–140.

Wallen, S.E. (1976) Sporicidal action of hydrogen peroxide. PhD thesis. University of Nebraska, Lincoln, Nebraska, USA.

Warth, A.D. (1978) Molecular structure of the bacterial spore. In *Advances in Microbial Physiology* (eds Rose, A.H. & Morris, J.G.), Vol. 17, pp. 1–45. London: Academic Press.

Whitehouse, R.L. & Clegg, L.F.L. (1963) Destruction of *Bacillus cereus* spores with solutions of sodium hydroxide. *Journal of Dairy Research*, **30**, 315–322.

Williams, N.D. & Russell, A.D. (1992a) Increased susceptibility of injured spores of *Bacillus subtilis* to cationic and other stressing agents. *Letters in Applied Microbiology*, **15**, 253–255.

Williams, N.D. & Russell, A.D. (1992b) The nature and site of biocide-induced sublethal injury in *Bacillus subtilis* spores. *FEMS Microbiology Letters*, **99**, 277–280.

Williams, N.D. & Russell, A.D. (1993a) Conditions suitable for the recovery of biocide-treated spores of *Bacillus subtilis*. *Journal of Applied Bacteriology*, **74**, 121–129.

Williams, N.D. & Russell, A.D. (1993b) Revival of biocide-treated spores of *Bacillus subtilis*. *Journal of Applied Bacteriology*, **75**, 69–75.

Williams, N.D. & Russell, A.D. (1993c) Revival of *Bacillus subtilis* spores from biocide induced injury in the germination process. *Journal of Applied Bacteriology*, **75**, 76–81.

Williams, N.D. & Russell, A.D. (1993d) Injury and repair in biocide-treated spores of *Bacillus subtilis*. *FEMS Microbiology Letters*, **106**, 183–186.

Williams, N.D. & Russell, A.D. (1993e) Conditions suitable for the recovery of biocide-treated spores of *Bacillus subtilis*. *Microbios*, **74**, 121–129.

Wyatt, L.R. & Waites, W.M. (1973) The effect of hypochlorite on the germination of spores of *Clostridium bifermentans*. *Journal of General Microbiology*, **70**, 383–385.

Wyatt, L.R. & Waites, W.M. (1974) The effect of sodium hydroxide or dithiothreitol–urea on spores of germination mutants of *Clostridium bifermentans*. *Journal of General Microbiology*, **84**, 391–394.

Wyatt, L.R. & Waites, W.M. (1975) The effect of chlorine on spores of *Clostridium bifermentans*, *Bacillus subtilis* and *Bacillus cereus*. *Journal of General Microbiology*, **89**, 337–344.

Znamirowski, R., McDonald, S. & Roy, T.E. (1960) The efficiency of an ethylene oxide steriliser in hospital practice. *Canadian Medical Association Journal*, **83**, 1004–1006.

Zytkovicz, T.H. & Halvorson, H.O. (1972) Some characteristics of dipicolinic acid-less mutant spores of *Bacillus cereus*, *Bacillus megaterium* and *Bacillus subtilis*. In *Spores V* (eds Halvorsen, H.O., Hanson, R. & Campbell, L.L.). Washington, DC: American Society for Microbiology.

D. MYCOBACTERICIDAL AGENTS

1 Introduction

The genus *Mycobacterium* consists of a fairly diverse group of acid-fast bacteria, the best-known and most important members of which are *M. tuberculosis*, the aetiological agent of tuberculosis, and *M. leprae*, the causative agent of leprosy. An organism that is assuming greater clinical importance is *M. avium-intracellulare* (MAI), part of the *M. avium* and *M. intracellulare* (MAIS) complex, which is often associated with respiratory complications in acquired immune deficiency syndrome (AIDS) patients (Collins, 1989; Guthertz *et al.*, 1989; Inderlied *et al.*, 1993; Uttley & Pozniak, 1993; Blessington & O'Sullivan, 1994). Opportunistic pathogenic mycobacteria (Collins *et al.*, 1984) and potentially pathogenic mycobacteria (Goslee & Wolinsky, 1976) may be associated with water supplies.

1.1 Tuberculous and non-tuberculous mycobacteria

Included in the genus *Mycobacterium* are several intracellular bacterial parasites. *Mycobacterium leprae* is an obligate intracellular pathogen, and species that cause progressive lung disease are *M. tuberculosis*, *M. bovis* and *M. avium*, which are facultative intracellular parasites. Species that are rarely pathogenic include *M. gordonae*, *M. fortuitum*, *M. terrae* and *M. smegmatis*, but there are many opportunistic species, such as *M. intracellulare* (Collins, 1989; Grange *et al.*, 1990). The non-tuberculous mycobacteria are often referred to as atypical species.

Contrary to popular feeling, mycobacteria remain a public hazard, with tuberculosis itself still a major killer throughout the world. Added to this are the high isolation rate of mycobacteria from AIDS patients (Hanson, 1988), the prolonged chemotherapeutic treatment of tuberculosis patients and the above-average resistance of mycobacteria to biocides. Readers interested in obtaining further information about the clinical association of mycobacteria with disease should consult Wolinsky (1979), Ratledge & Stanford (1982), Damsker & Bottone (1985), Wayne (1985), Collins (1989), Inderlied *et al.* (1993) and Uttley & Pozniak (1993). Plasmids occur more frequently among clinical isolates of the MAIS complex than among environmental isolates (Jensen *et al.*, 1989).

1.2 Transmission of mycobacterial infection

Mycobacteria do not produce toxins or enzymes that destroy human tissues. They are virulent because they have the ability to survive after macrophage ingestion and they multiply intracellularly. Diseases develop slowly and follow a chronic course, with a granulomatous response. Tuberculosis is more commonly transmitted via inhalation of an aerosol of droplet nuclei from an infected person, with coughing and sneezing being implicated. *Mycobacterium bovis* is usually spread by ingestion of milk from cows with mammary tuberculosis. Atypical (non-tuberculous) mycobacteria have environmental reservoirs, such as soil and water, from which infections may arise, by, for example, ingestion or inhalation of dust particles.

In the context of the present chapter, it is necessary to consider the possible transmission of mycobacteria from medical devices, in particular the nature of these devices and the infection risk following decontamination (Favero, 1991; Medical Devices Directorate, 1993; Russell, 1994). Endoscopes are regarded as being semi-critical items, i.e. they are of intermediate risk to patients. Most are unable to withstand heat, and consequently decontamination is achieved by the use of a chemical agent that produces high-level disinfection. Most episodes of endoscopy-acquired infection arise from inadequate cleaning and disinfection, but transmission of mycobacterial infection is believed to be rare (Axon, 1991; Ayliffe *et al.*, 1993; Babb & Bradley, 1995; Bradley & Babb, 1995; Bradley *et al.*, 1995), although Reeves & Brown (1995) have pointed our that it is, perhaps, an increasing problem. It is, therefore, necessary to have a sound understanding of the effects of biocides on mycobacteria to ensure that these organisms are not transmitted by endoscopy, and especially bronchoscopy. Mycobacteria such as *M. tuberculosis*, MAI and *M. chelonae* (*M. chelonei*) must be considered and further information about these organisms is provided subsequently.

Multidrug-resistant *M. tuberculosis* (MDRTB) is becoming an increasing therapeutic problem (Russell & Chopra, 1996) and consequently ways of inactivating such strains by biocides are important.

1.3 Cell structure

Four closely related genera (*Corynebacterium*, *Mycobacterium*, *Nocardia* and *Rhodococcus*) make up the nocardioform actinomycetes. Most mycobacterial strains occur as unicellular rods, but some develop as mycelial-producing organisms, in which early fragmentation of the mycelium occurs during growth to produce either rods or branched rods. These organisms possess a distinctive cell wall, the composition of which is described below for mycobacteria.

1.4 Cell-wall composition

Mycobacterial cell walls consist of several components. The 'covalent cell-wall skeleton' comprises two covalently linked polymers, namely peptidoglycan and a mycolate (Fig. 10.4) of arabinogalactan. Mycobacterial peptidoglycan contains *N*-glycolmuramic acid, instead of the more widely found *N*-acetylmuramic acid, and differs in other ways also from more typical peptidoglycan. The

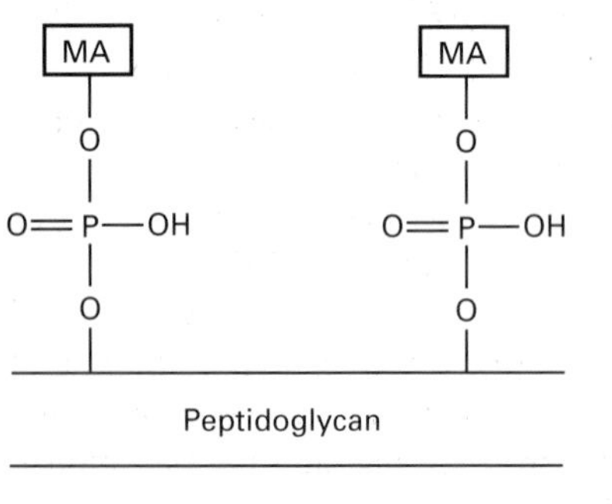

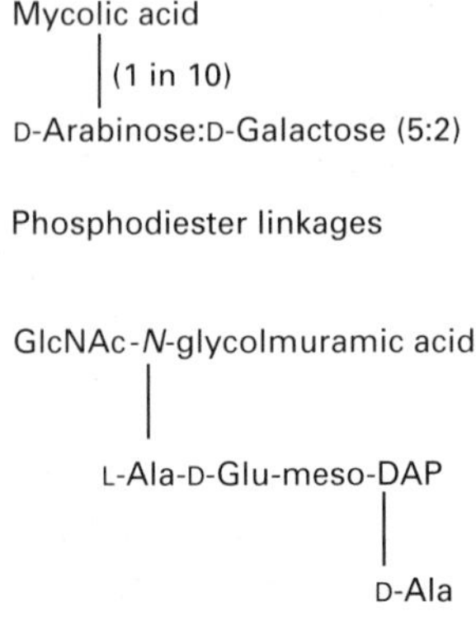

Fig. 10.4 Cell-wall skeleton of mycobacteria. MA, mycolate of arabinogalactan.

arabinogalactan mycolate contains D-arabinose and D-galactose, ratio *c.* 5 : 2, with about 10% of the arabinose residues esterified by a molecule of mycolic acid (Fig. 10.4). The general structure of mycolic acids is depicted in Fig. 10.5.

Other components of mycobacterial cell walls are the lipids and peptides. Lipids occur as free lipids, wax D (considered to be an autolysis product of the cell wall and immunologically identical with cell-wall arabinogalactans) and 6,6'-dimycolates of α_1, α^1-D-trehalose, known as cord factors. The peptides can be removed by proteolytic enzymes. Further details are provided by Draper (1988), Minniken (1991), Russell (1993, 1998), Besa *et al.* (1995) and Russell & Chopra (1996).

2 Response to biocides

2.1 Early findings

Early studies on the response of mycobacteria to biocides were reviewed by Croshaw (1971). This chapter will thus concentrate almost exclusively on subsequent work, with merely an occasional citation to earlier findings. Croshaw's (1971) review can, in essence, be summarized as follows: mycobacteria are resistant to acids, alkalis, chlorhexidine, quaternary ammonium compounds (QACs), non-ionic and anionic surface-active agents, heavy metals and dyes, although many of these agents may inhibit mycobacterial growth without being mycobactericidal. Biocides that were listed by Croshaw (1971) as being mycobactericidal were ampholytic surfactants, e.g. 'Tego' compounds, ethylene oxide gas, iodine (more effective than hypochlorites), alcohols and especially phenolic compounds, notably cresol—soap formulations. Notable omissions from this list are formaldehyde and glutaraldehyde; conflicting results had been noted with the former, although alcoholic solutions were more potent (Rubbo & Gardner, 1965; Rubbo *et al.*, 1967) and glutaraldehyde had been found by Bergan & Lystad (1971) to be surprisingly ineffective against tubercle bacilli. Spaulding (1972) proposed that acid-fast bacteria had a resistance to biocides intermediate between that shown by other non-sporing bacteria on the one hand and bacterial spores on the other. Hirsch (1954) demonstrated that formaldehyde (0.05%), sodium hypochlorite (< 0.05%) and potassium permanganate (0.005%) killed tubercle bacilli, whereas benzalkonium chloride (0.1%) did not. Unfortunately, Tween 80 was present as part of the testing procedure and it is possible that the non-ionic surfactant considerably reduced the effect of benzalkonium. Nevertheless, this compound has been used as a means of isolating *M. tuberculosis* (Patterson *et al.*, 1956).

$$
\begin{array}{lll}
\mathrm{OH} & & \\
| & & \\
\mathrm{CH}- & \mathrm{CH}- & \mathrm{COO^-} \\
| & | & \\
\mathrm{R^2} & \mathrm{R^1} &
\end{array}
$$

Fig. 10.5 General structure of mycolic acids. R^1 and R^2 are alkyl groups that may be saturated or unsaturated.

Croshaw (1971) concluded that comprehensive data on the effects of biocides on mycobacteria were not available, that discrepancies existed (probably because of differences in technique in examining mycobactericidal activity), that many of the (then) newer disinfectants had not been examined and that most of the published work referred only to the tubercle bacillus. The important inference was made that a biocide effective against *M. tuberculosis* was not necessarily lethal to other mycobacteria. For an up-to-date assessment of mycobactericidal activity, see Best *et al.* (1990).

Several of these aspects will be reconsidered in the light of subsequent studies (Section 2.2).

2.2 Recent concepts

The response of mycobacteria to biocides has been reviewed by Rubin (1983) and considered as part of an overall assessment of the sensitivity of microorganisms by Favero (1985), Gardner & Peel (1986) and Russell (1990, 1991, 1998). In addition, Russell (1996) and Russell & Chopra (1996) have provided detailed accounts of the effects of biocides on mycobacteria (Table 10.6).

Spaulding *et al.* (1977), Favero (1985), 1991) and Favero & Bond (1991a,b, 1993) have described three levels of germicidal activity: (i) high-level activity: lethal to vegetative bacteria (including tubercle bacilli), spores, fungi and lipid-enveloped and non-lipid-enveloped viruses; (ii) intermediate activity: lethal to all those listed in (i) except

Table 10.6 Mycobactericidal activity of biocides as described by various authors.

Antibacterial	Mycobacterial susceptibility (S) or resistance (R)	Comment	Reference*
Alcohol	S		1, 2
	S	Reduced in presence of sputum	4
Chlorhexidine	R		1, 3, 4
Ethylene oxide	S		1, 2, 3
Formaldehyde	Moderately S		1
	S?		2
	S	In presence or absence of alcohol	3
	S	Alcoholic solutions	4
Glutaraldehyde†	Moderately S		1
	Generally S		2
	S		3
	S or R	Unproved (1971 ref.)	4
Hypochlorites	Moderately S		1
	S		3
	Moderately R		4
Iodophors†	S		1, 2, 3
	Moderately S	Rather more so than chlorine compounds	4
Peracetic acid	S	Effective vs. glutaraldehyde-resistant *M. chelonae*	5
Phenols	S		1, 2, 3, 4
QACs	R		1, 2, 3
	R	Highly inhibitory	4

* References 1, Gardner & Peel (1986); 2, Rubin (1983); 3, Favero (1985, 1991); 4, Croshaw (1971); 5, Lynam *et al.* (1995)
† See text also

bacterial spores; and (iii) low activity: lethal only to vegetative bacteria (excluding tubercle bacilli), fungi and lipid-enveloped viruses. On the basis of this classification, mycobacteria are clearly more resistant to biocides than other non-sporulating bacteria but less resistant than bacterial spores.

Favero (1991) cites 2% glutaraldehyde, 8%, formaldehyde in 70% alcohol, 6–10% stabilized hydrogen peroxide and gaseous ethylene oxide as being in category (i), with alcohol (70–90%), 0.5% iodine in 70% alcohol, 1% aqueous iodine, chlorine compounds and phenolics in category (ii) and low-level disinfectants, such as QACs and chlorhexidine, in category (iii). It is again noticeable, however, that the only mycobacterial species included in this scheme is the tubercle bacillus. This doubtless reflects its clinical importance in the hospital environment, but other mycobacteria are also important pathogens and their sensitivity or resistance to biocides must also be considered. Depending on its concentration, alcohol is tuberculocidal (Smith, 1947; Rotter, 1996) and might enhance the activity of other agents.

It is not the purpose of this chapter to review the different types of test methods for evaluating mycobactericidal activity. This is the subject of several papers (Sonntag, 1978; Schliesser, 1979; AFNOR, 1981; Borneff *et al.*, 1981; Parkinson, 1981; AOAC, 1984; Ascenzi *et al.*, 1986, 1987; Collins, F.M., 1986a,b; Lind *et al.*, 1986; Quinn, 1987; van

Klingeren & Pullen, 1987, 1993; Eigener, 1988; Isenberg *et al.*, 1988; Cole *et al.*, 1990 Ascenzi, 1991; Broadley *et al*, 1991, 1995; Cutler & Wilson, 1993; Holton *et al.*, 1994; Crémieux, 1995; Sattas *et al.*, 1995; Cole & Robison, 1996; Sutton 1996). Rather, it is the information obtained about mycobactericidal activity allied to the comparative sensitivity or resistance of various types of mycobacteria to a particular biocide that is important. It is also pertinent to point out, however, that conclusions as to efficacy may depend upon the technique employed, and that authors do not always discuss procedural problems (such as cell clumping) and ways of overcoming them.

Recent studies on mycobactericidal activity of various biocides have demonstrated that 2% alkaline glutaraldehyde is effective against *M. tuberculosis*, *M. smegmatis*, *M. fortuitum* and *M. terrae* (Collins & Montalbine, 1976; Collins, F.M., 1986a,b; van Klingeren & Pullen, 1987), although Carson *et al.* (1978) noted a variation in resistance of strains to formaldehyde and glutaraldehyde, and found that strains of *M. fortuitum* and *M. chelonae* in commercial distilled water (CDW) were very resistant to chlorine. The MAIS group undoubtedly presents a higher resistance to glutaraldehyde (Collins, F.M., 1986b; Hanson, 1988; Broadley *et al.*, 1991; Coates & Hutchinson, 1994; Holton *et al.*, 1994) than does *M. tuberculosis*. In accordance with earlier findings (Borick *et al.*, 1964; Borick, 1968; Miner *et al.*, 1977), this important biocide (Russell & Hopwood, 1976; Gorman *et al.*, 1980; Russell & Hugo, 1987) can now be considered as being a mycobactericidal agent (Collins, J., 1986; Cole *et al.*, 1990; Axon, 1991; Babb & Bradley, 1991; Rubin, 1991; Rutala *et al.*, 1991; Ayliffe *et al.*, 1993; Uttley & Pozniak, 1993; Uttley & Simpson, 1994). Ayliffe *et al.* (1993) have, however, pointed out that only small numbers of *M. tuberculosis* were inactivated after a 10 min exposure period. Van Klingeren & Pullen (1993) have isolated *M. chelonae* subspecies *abscessus* from endoscope washes which were not killed by a 60 min exposure to alkaline glutaraldehyde, whereas a reference strain showed an inactivation of 5 $\log_{10}$ after 10 min. The resistant *M. chelonae* strain was also resistant to peracetic acid (Lynam *et al.*, 1995) but not to a phenolic or to sodium dichloroisocyanurate. Other workers (Nye *et al.*, 1990; Uttley & Simpson, 1994) have also noted an above-average resistance of *M. chelonae* to glutaraldehyde. This organism has a particular propensity for adhering to smooth surfaces (Uttley & Simpson, 1994), which might well be a factor contributing to its resistance.

Phenolics are also mycobactericidal (Richards & Thoen, 1979). Chlorhexidine and QACs (see below) inhibit growth of some mycobacterial strains but are not lethal (Fodor & Szabo, 1980; Broadley *et al.*, 1991, 1995).

Nevertheless, it is still apparent that additional studies are necessary, with typical and atypical mycobacterial strains and a wider range of agents. According to Ascenzi *et al.* (1986, 1987), a QAC has a similar tuberculocidal activity to 2% glutaraldehyde, and this claim requires reinvestigation (Merkal & Whipple, 1980). An interesting point made by these authors, however, was the influence of the recovery medium on the apparent numbers of survivors of glutaraldehyde-treated *M. bovis*.

Noteworthy omissions from the list of mycobactericidal agents are hydrogen peroxide and other peroxygens. These important biocides (Baldry & Fraser, 1988) were not mentioned by Rubin (1983) or Baldry & Fraser (1988) in connection with any mycobactericidal activity, although they are sporicidal (Russell, 1990; Bradley *et al.*, 1995). Current opinion suggests an activity of peroxygens well below that level against mycobacteria (Broadley *et al.*, 1993; Cutler & Wilson, 1993; Holton *et al.*, 1994; Taylor *et al.*, 1994). In contrast, peracetic acid has been claimed to be effective against glutaraldehyde-resistant mycobacteria (Lynam *et al.*, 1995).

3 Mechanisms of mycobacterial inactivation

A comprehensive survey of the mechanisms of action of antibacterial agents is provided by Russell & Chopra (1996); see also Chapter 9 in this book. Very few concerted attempts, however, have been made to explain the mechanisms whereby mycobacteria are inactivated or inhibited. Likewise, uptake of biocides into mycobacterial cells is poorly understood, but increasing knowledge about the mycobacterial cell wall (Nikaido *et al.*, 1993) and the demonstration of the presence of porins similar to those found in *Pseudomonas aeruginosa* cell envelopes (Jarlier & Nikaido, 1990) mean that further experimentation could produce useful data.

Potential target sites in the mycobacterial cell are as follows:

1 Cell wall—it is unlikely that this will be a major site for many biocides, although glutaraldehyde could well prove an exception because of its known strong interaction with the surface of bacterial cells (Eager *et al.*, 1986).

2 Cytoplasmic membrane—chlorhexidine and QACs could act here, but their uptake into mycobacterial cells is believed to be greatly reduced by the mycobacterial cell wall (Russell, 1996).

3 Cytosol—proteins, enzymes, (DNA) and ribonucleic acid (RNA) might all be subjected to 'attack' by biocidal agents, but the dearth of current information means that it is impossible to state that mycobactericidal agents have a similar effect on mycobacteria to that on other non-sporulating bacteria (Russell & Chopra, 1996).

4 Mechanisms of biocide resistance

4.1 Intrinsic resistance: the mycobacterial cell wall as a barrier

It is clear from the preceding sections that mycobacteria are much more resistant than other non-sporing bacteria to a variety of biocides, but that differences in sensitivity exist among different mycobacterial species. Evidence was put forward several years ago (Chargaff *et al.*, 1931) that resistance to QACs was related to the lipid content of the cell wall, since *M. phlei* (with low total lipid) was more sensitive than *M. tuberculosis*, which possessed a higher total cell-lipid content. Croshaw (1971) quotes the work of T.H. Shen, who, in 1934, found that the resistance of various species of mycobacteria was related to the content of waxy material in the wall.

Solvent-extractable free lipids account for about 25–30% of the weight of mycobacterial cell walls (Petit & Lederer, 1978) and it is likely that the lipid-rich, hydrophobic layers of the cell wall are responsible for acid-fastness (Fisher & Barksdale, 1973; Barksdale & Kim, 1977) and for resistance to many biocides (Middlebrook, 1965).

As pointed out previously, the mycobacterial cell wall is highly hydrophobic, with a mycoylarabinogalactanpeptidoglycan skeleton. Hydrophilic agents are thus unable to penetrate the cell wall in sufficiently high concentration to produce a lethal effect. Conversely, low concentrations must traverse this permeability barrier, because minimal concentrations inhibiting growth are generally of the same order as those found with other, non-mycobacterial, strains (Russell, 1996), although *M. avium* may be particularly resistant (Broadley *et al.*, 1991).

Chemical agents that inhibit mycobacterial cell-wall synthesis might be of value in elucidating the cell-wall component(s) involved in conferring intrinsic resistance to many antibiotics and biocides. A summary of these findings, presented in Table 10.7 is based on the work of David *et al.* (1988), Sareen & Khuller (1990) Takayama & Kilburn (1988), Rastogi *et al.* (1990), McNeil & Brennan (1991), Wheeler *et al.* (1993) and Broadley *et al.* (1995).

5 Possible methods of potentiating mycobactericidal activity

Very few new biocidal agents are likely to be produced in the foreseeable future. However, one

Table 10.7 Possible cell-wall components involved in mycobacterial resistance to biocides (data from Russell, 1996).

Cell wall component	Inhibitor of synthesis	Relevance to resistance to	
		Antibiotics	Biocides
Mycoside C	*m* -Fl-phe	Yes	Unknown*
Arabinogalactan	Ethambutol	Yes	Yes
Mycolic acid	MOCB	Yes	Unknown*

*Not yet tested.
m-Fl-phe, *m*-fluoro DL-phenylalanine; MOCB, methyl-4-(2-octadecylcyclopropen-1-yl)-butanoate.

such compound is *o*-phthalaldehyde (OPA), which is claimed to be a potent microbicidal agent (Alfa & Sitter, 1994), although its activity against mycobacteria has yet to be assessed. One likely possibility is the use of a combination of two agents to produce an enhanced response, as shown by Gordon *et al.* (1994), who increased the mycobactericidal activity of glutaraldehyde with α,β-unsaturated and aromatic aldehydes.

An improved knowledge of the components of the mycobacterial cell wall responsible for causing intrinsic resistance could also be important. Under specified conditions, L-forms and spheroplasts of mycobacteria can be produced (Willet & Thacore, 1966, 1967), and solutions with a high concentration of soap or other suitable detergent are considered to penetrate the waxy cell wall (Hegna, 1977). The use of specific inhibitors of cell wall synthesis to improve intracellular penetration is likely to be of more significance in chemotherapy than with biocidal compounds (Hoffner *et al.*, 1989; Russell & Russell, 1995; Russell, 1996; Russell & Chopra, 1996). Nevertheless, these approaches could collectively lead to be a better understanding of resistance mechanisms and thence to an improvement of mycobactericidal activity.

6 Clinical and medical uses of mycobactericidal agents

Disinfectants are widely used for various purposes in the hospital environment (Ayliffe *et al.*, 1993, see Chapter 12). In some specific instances, activity against mycobacteria is essential (Favero, 1991). Heat is undoubtedly the most effective method for destroying mycobacteria, which are not especially heat-resistant, and should always be employed if possible. Sterilization or disinfection by heat is not always practicable, however, notably when delicate items of equipment that would be damaged by heat are being used.

A classic example of this occurs with endoscopes. These must be decontaminated effectively and rapidly (Felmingham *et al.*, 1985; Ridgway, 1985; Hanson *et al.*, 1992; Babb & Bradley, 1995; Bradley & Babb, 1995; Reeves & Brown, 1995). Collignon & Graham (1989) have pointed out that even resistant organisms, such as mycobacteria and bacterial spores, are likely to be killed by a disinfectant time for endoscopes of 5min between patients, because of the low number present after effective cleaning. *M. tuberculosis* has been transmitted via a fibre-optic bronchoscope (Leers, 1980) but this has not been reported via gastrointestinal endoscopes (Ridgway, 1985; Ayliffe, 1988). The disinfectant of choice is 2% alkaline glutaraldehyde, although this agent is by no means ideal. Uptake of glutaraldehyde by endoscopes can result (Power & Russell, 1989) and it is possible that—despite a subsequent rinse in sterile saline or water—release of aldehyde inside a patient could occur. Moreover, the disinfection period is often extremely short, to enable rapid turnover of a limited number of endoscopes in an endoscopy unit. Glutaraldehyde is also potentially toxic to personnel. Other biocides are usually unsuitable, because of: (i) corrosive properties, e.g. chlorine disinfectants; or (ii) lack of suitable antibacterial activity, e.g. chlorhexidine and antiseptic-strength iodophors (Favero, 1991). The clear-soluble phenolics show activity against *M. tuberculosis* and are considered to be suitable for the disinfection of rooms occupied by patients with open tuberculosis.

George (1988) has listed the main requirements for preventing hospital-acquired tuberculosis as being: (i) an occupational health scheme; (ii) constant vigilance by staff; and (iii) the implementation of appropriate policies, namely isolation of patients, control of infection and disinfection. Care must be taken in reusing disinfectants (Mbithi *et al.*, 1993; Springthorpe *et al.*, 1995).

7 Conclusions

Several mycobacterial types, especially MDRTB and MAI, are posing serious chemotherapeutic problems. Allied to these has been the recent isolation from endoscope washers of glutaraldehyde-resistant strains of *M. chelonae*. Furthermore, there appears to be a high correlation between virulence of *M. tuberculosis* and resistance to hydrogen peroxide (Gordon & Andrew, 1996).

The mechanism of resistance of mycobacteria to biocides is intrinsic rather than acquired and appears to be involved with the composition of the mycobacterial cell wall. Much remains to be done to enhance biocidal uptake and hence mycobactericidal activity.

8 References

AFNOR (1981) *Recueils de Normes Françaises des Antiseptiques et Désinfectants*, 1st edn. Association Française de Normalisation.

Alfa, M.J. & Sitter, D.L. (1994) In-hospital evaluation of orthophthalaldehyde as a high level disinfectant for flexible endoscopes. *Journal of Hospital Infection*, **26**, 15–26.

AOAC (1984) *Official Methods of AOAC International*, 16th edn, 4th revision. Guthersburg, MD: AOAC.

Ascenzi, J.M. (1991) Standardization of tuberculocidal testing of disinfectants. *Journal of Hospital Infection*, **18**, (Suppl. A), 256–263.

Ascenzi, J.M., Ezzell, R.J. & Wendt, T.M. (1986) Evaluation of carriers used in the test methods of the Association of Official Analytical Chemists. *Applied and Environmental Microbiology*, **51**, 91–94.

Ascenzi, J.M., Ezzell, R.J. & Wendt, R.M. (1987) A more accurate method for measurement of tuberculocidal activity of disinfectants. *Applied and Environmental Microbiology*, **53**, 2189–2192.

Axon, A.T.R. (1991) Disinfection of endoscope equipment. *Baillère's Clinical Gastroenterology*, **4**, 61–77.

Ayliffe, G.A.J. (1988) Equipment-related infection risks. *Journal of Hospital Infection*, **11** (Suppl. A), 279–284.

Ayliffe, G.A.J., Coates, D & Hoffman, P.N. (1993) *Chemical Disinfection in Hospitals*, 2nd edn. London: Public Health Laboratory.

Babb, J.R. & Bradley, C.R. (1991) The mechanics of endoscope disinfection. *Journal of Hospital Infection*, **18** (Suppl. A), 130–135.

Babb, J.R. & Bradley, C.R. (1995) Endoscope decontamination: where do we go from here? *Journal of Hospital Infection*, **30** (Suppl.), 543–551.

Baldry, M.G.C. & Fraser, J.A.L. (1988) Disinfection with peroxygens. In *Industrial Biocides* (ed. Payne, K.R.), Critical Reports on Applied Chemistry, Vol. 23, pp. 91–116. Chichester: John Wiley & Sons.

Barksdale, L. & Kim, K.S. (1977) Mycobacterium. *Bacteriological Reviews*, **41**, 217–372.

Bergan, T. & Lystad, A. (1971) Antitubercular action of disinfectants. *Journal of Applied Bacteriology*, **34**, 751–756.

Besra, G.S. Khoo, W.K., McNeil, M.R., Dell, A., Morris, H.R. & Brennan, P.J. (1995) A new interpretation of the mycolyl-arabinogalactan complex of *Mycobacterium tuberculosis* as revealed through characterization of oligoglycosylalditol fragments by fast-atom bombardment mass spectrometry and ^{1}H nuclear magnetic resonance spectroscopy. *Biochemistry*, **34**, 4257–4266.

Best, M., Sattar, S.A., Springthorpe, V.S. & Kennedy, M.E. (1990) Efficacies of selected disinfectants against *Mycobacterium tuberculosis*. *Journal of Clinical Microbiology*, **28**, 2234–2239.

Blessington, B. & O'Sullivan, J. (1994) Captain of death returns. *Chemistry in Britain*, **30**, 566–569.

Borick, P.M. (1968) Chemical sterilizers (chemosterilizers). *Advances in Applied Microbiology*, **10**, 291–312.

Borick, P.M., Dondershine, F.H. & Chandler, V.L. (1964) Alkalinized glutaraldehyde, a new antimicrobial agent. *Journal of Pharmaceutical Sciences*, **53**, 1273–1275.

Borneff, J., Eggers, H.J., Grün, L. *et al.* (1981) Richtlinien für die Prüfung und Bewertung chemischer Desinfektionsverfahren. *Zentralblatt für Bakteriologie, Mikrobiologie und Hygiene*, **B172**, 534–562.

Bradley, C.R. & Babb, J.R. (1995) Endoscope decontamination; automated vs manual. *Journal of Hospital Infection*, 30 (Suppl.), 537–542.

Bradley, C.R., Babb, J.R. & Ayliffe, G.A.J. (1995) Evaluation of the Steris System 1 peracetic acid endoscope processor. *Journal of Hospital Infection*, **29**, 143–151.

Broadley, S.J., Jenkins, P.A., Furr, J.R. & Russell, A.D. (1991) Antimycobacterial activity of biocides. *Letters in Applied Microbiology*, **13**, 118–22.

Broadley, S.J., Jenkins, P.A., Furr, J.R. & Russell, A.D. (1993) Antimycobacterial activity of Virkon. *Journal of Hospital Infection*, **23**, 189–197.

Broadley, S.J. Jenkins, P.A., Furr, J.R. & Russell, A.D. (1995) Potentiation of the effects of chlorhexidine diacetate and cetylpyridinium chloride on mycobacteria by ethambutol. *Journal of Medical Microbiology*, **43**, 458–460.

Carson, L.A., Petersen, J., Favero, M.S. & Aguero, S.M. (1978) Growth characteristics of atypical mycobacteria in water and their comparative resistance to disinfectants. *Applied and Environmental Microbiology*, **36**, 839–846.

Chargaff, E., Pangborn, M.C. & Anderson, R.J. (1931) The chemistry of the lipoids of tubercle bacilli. XXIII. Separation of the lipoid fractions from the Timothy bacillus. *Journal of Biological Chemistry*, **90**, 45–55.

Coates, D. & Hutchinson, D.N. (1994) How to produce a hospital disinfection policy. *Journal of Hospital Infection*, **26**, 57–68.

Cole, E.C. & Robison, R. (1996) Test methodology for evaluation of germicides. In *Handbook of Disinfectants and Antiseptics* (ed. Ascenzi, J.M.), pp. 1–16. New York: Marcel Dekker.

Cole, E.C., Rutala, W.A., Nessen, L., Wannamaker, N.S. & Weber, D.J. (1990) Effect of methodology, dilution and exposure time on the tuberculocidal activity of glutaraldehyde-based disinfectants. *Applied and Environmental Microbiology*, **56**, 1813–1817.

Collignon, P. & Graham, E. (1989) How well are endoscopes disinfected between patients? *Medical Journal of Australia*, **151**, 269–272.

Collins, C.H., Grange, I.M. & Yates, M.D. (1984) Mycobacteria in water. *Journal of Applied Bacteriology*, **57**, 193–211.

Collins, F.M. (1986a) Kinetics of the tuberculocidal response by alkaline glutaraldehyde in solution and on an inert surface. *Journal of Applied Bacteriology*, **61**, 87–93.

Collins, F.M. (1986b) Bactericidal activity of alkaline glutaraldehyde solution against a number of atypical mycobacterial species. *Journal of Applied Bacteriology*, **61**, 247–251.

Collins, F.M. (1989) Mycobacterial disease, immunosuppression, and acquired immunodeficiency syndrome. *Clinical Microbiology Reviews*, **2**, 360–377.

Collins, F.M. & Montalbine, V. (1976) Mycobactericidal activity of glutaraldehyde solutions. *Journal of Clinical Microbiology*, **4**, 408–412.

Collins, J. (1986) The use of glutaraldehyde in laboratory discard jars. *Letters in Applied Microbiology*, **2**, 103–105.

Crémieux, A. (1995) Méthodes d'étude de l'activité *in vitro* des antiseptiques et des désinfectants sur les bactéries et champignons. In *Antisepsie et Désinfection* (eds Fleurette, J., Freney, J. & Reverdy, M.-E.), pp. 66–83. Paris: Editions ESKA.

Croshaw, B. (1971) The destruction of mycobacteria. In *Inhibition and Destruction of the Microbial Cell* (ed. Hugo, W.B.), pp. 429–449. London: Academic Press.

Cutler, R.R. & Wilson, P. (1993) Disinfectant testing of contaminated endoscopes—a need for standardization. *Journal of Hospital Infection*, **25**, 145–149.

Damsker, B. & Bottone, E.U.J. (1985) *Mycobacterium avium–Mycobacterium intracellulare* from the intestinal tracts of patients with acquired immunodeficiency syndrome: concepts regarding acquisition and pathogenesis. *Journal of Infectious Diseases*, **151**, 179–181.

David, H.L., Rastogi, N., Seres, C.L. & Clement, F. (1988) Alterations in the outer wall architecture caused by the inhibition of mycoside C biosynthesis in *Mycobacterium avium*. *Current Microbiology*, **17**, 61–68.

Draper, P. (1988) Wall biosynthesis: a possible site of action for new antimycobacterial drugs. *International Journal of Leprosy*, **52**, 527–532.

Eager, R.G., Leder, J. & Theis, A.B. (1986) Glutaraldehyde: factors important for microbicidal activity. In *Proceedings of the 3rd Conference on Progress in Chemical Disinfection*, pp. 32–49. New York: SUNY, Binghamton.

Eigener, U. (1988) Disinfectant testing and its relevance in practical application. In *Industrial Biocides* (ed. Payne, K.R.), Critical Reports on Applied Chemistry, Vol. 23, pp. 37–51. Chichester: John Wiley & Sons.

Favero, M.S. (1985) Sterilization, disinfection and antisepsis in the hospital. In *Manual of Clinical Microbiology*, 4th edn (eds Lennette, E.H., Balows, A., Hausler, W.J., Jr & Shadomy, H.J.), pp. 129–137. Washington DC: American Society for Microbiology.

Favero, M.S. (1991) Practical application of liquid sterilants in health care facilities. In *Sterilization of Medical Products* (eds Morrissey, R.F. & Propopenko, Y.I.), Vol. V, pp. 397–405. Morin Heights, Canada: Polyscience Publications.

Favero, M.S. & Bond, W.W. (1991a) Sterilization, disinfection and antisepsis in the hospital. In *Manual of Clinical Microbiology*, 5th edn (eds Balows, A., Hausler, W.J., Jr, Herrman, K.I., Isenber, H.D. & Shadomy, H.J.), pp. 183–200. Washington, DC: American Society for Microbiology.

Favero, M.S. & Bond, W.W. (1991b) Chemical disinfection of medical and surgical materials. In *Disinfection, Sterilization and Preservation*, 4th edn (ed. Block, S.S.), pp. 617–641. Philadelphia, Pennsylvania: Lea & Febiger.)

Favero, M.S. & Bond, W.W. (1993) The use of liquid chemical germicides. In *Sterilization Technology: A Practical Guide for Manufacturers* (eds Morrissey, R.F. & Phillips, G.B.), pp. 309–334. New York: Van Nostrand Reinhold.

Felmingham, D., Mowles, J., Thomas, K. & Ridgway, G.L. (1985) Disinfection of gastro-intestinal fibreoptic endoscopes. *Journal of Hospital Infection*, **6**, 379–388.

Fisher, C.A. & Barksdale, L. (1973) Cytochemical reactions of human leprosy bacilli and mycobacteria: ultrastructural implications *Journal of Bacteriology*, **113**, 1389–1399.

Fodor, T. & Szabo, I. (1980) Effect of chlorhexidine gluconate on the survival of acid-free bacteria. *Acta Microbiologica*, **27**, 343–344.

Gardner, J.F. & Peel, M.M. (1986) *Introduction to Sterilization and Disinfection*. Edinburgh: Churchill Livingstone.

George, R.H. (1988) The prevention and control of mycobacterial infections in hospitals. *Journal of Hospital Infection*, **11** (Suppl. A), 386–392.

Gordon, M.D., Ezzell, R.J., Bruckner, N.I. & Ascenzi, J.M. (1994) Enhancement of mycobactericidal activity of glutaraldehyde with α,β-unsaturated and aromatic aldehydes. *Journal of Industrial Microbiology*, **13**, 77–82.

Gordon, S. & Andrew, P.W. (1996) Mycobacterial virulence factors. *Journal of Applied Bacteriology, Symposium Supplement*, **81**, 10S–22S.

Gorman, S.P., Scott, E.M. & Russell, A.D. (1980) Antimicrobial activity uses and mechanism of action of glutaraldehyde. *Journal of Applied Bacteriology*, **48**, 161–190.

Goslee, S. & Wolinsky, E. (1976) Water as a source of potentially pathogenic mycobacteria. *American Review of Respiratory Diseases*, **113**, 287–292.

Grange, J.M., Yates, M.D. & Broughton, E. (1990) The avian tubercle bacillus and its relatives. *Journal of Applied Bacteriology*, **68**, 411–431.

Griffiths, P.A., Babb, J.R., Bradley, C.R. & Fraise, A.P. (1997) Glutaraldehyde-resistant *Mycobacterium chelonae* from endoscope washer disinfectors. *Journal of Applied Microbiology*, **82**, 519–526.

Guthertz, L.S., Damsker, B., Bottone, E.J., Ford, E.G., Midura, T.F. & Janda, J.M. (1989) *Mycobacterium avium* and *Mycobacterium intracellulare* infections in patients with and without AIDS. *Journal of Infectious Diseases*, **160**, 1037–1041.

Hanson, P.J.V. (1988) Mycobacteria and AIDS. *British Journal of Hospital Medicine*, **40**, 149.

Hanson, P.J.V., Chadwick, M.V., Gaya, H. & Collins, J.V. (1992) A study of glutaraldehyde disinfection of fibreoptic bronchoscopes experimentally contaminated with *Mycobacterium tuberculosis*. *Journal of Hospital Infection*, **22**, 137–142.

Hegna, I.K. (1977) An examination of the effects of three phenolic disinfectants on *Mycobacterium tuberculosis*. *Journal of Applied Bacteriology*, **43**, 183–187.

Hirsch, J.G. (1954) The resistance of tubercle bacilli to the bactericidal action of benzalkonium chloride (Zephiran). *American Review of Tuberculosis*, **70**, 312–319.

Hoffner, S.E., Källenius, G., Breezer, A.E. & Svenson, S.B. (1989) Studies on the mechanisms of synergestic effects of ethambutol and other antibacterial drugs on *Mycobacterium avium* complex. *Acta Leprologia (Geneva)*, **7** (Suppl. 1), 195–199.

Holton, J., Nye, P. & McDonald, V. (1994) Efficacy of selected disinfectants against mycobacteria and cryptosporidia. *Journal of Hospital Infection*, **27**, 105–115.

Inderlied, C.B., Kemper, C.A. & Bermudez, L.E.M. (1993) The *Mycobacterium avium* complex. *Clinical Microbiology Reviews*, **6**, 266–310.

Isenberg, H.D., Giugliano, E.R., France, K. & Alperstein, P. (1988) Evaluation of three disinfectants after in-use stress. *Journal of Hospital Infection*, **11**, 278–285.

Jarlier, V. & Nikaido, H. (1990) Permeability barrier to hydrophilic solutes in *Mycobacterium cheloni*. *Journal of Bacteriology*, **172**, 1418–1423.

Jensen, A.G., Bennedsen, J. & Rosdahl, V.T. (1989) Plasmid profiles of *Mycobacterium avium/intracellulare* isolated from patients with AIDS or cervical lymphadenitis and from environmental samples. *Scandinavian Journal of Infectious Diseases*, **21**, 645–649.

Leers, W.D. (1980) Disinfecting endoscopes: how not to transmit *Mycobacterium tuberculosis* by bronchoscopy. *Canadian Medical Association Journal*, **123**, 275–283.

Lind, A., Lundholm, M, Pedersen, G., Sundaeus, V. & Wahlen, P. (1986) A carrier method for the assessment of the effectiveness of disinfectants against *Mycobacterium tuberculosis*. *Journal of Hospital Infection*, **7**, 60–67.

Lynam, P.A., Babb, J.R. and Fraise, A.P. (1995) Comparison of the mycobactericidal activity of 2% alkaline glutaraldehyde and 'Nu-Cidex' (0.35% peracetic acid). *Journal of Hospital Infection*, **30**, 237–239.

McNeil, M.R. & Brennan, P.J. (1991) Structure, function and biogenesis of the cell envelope of mycobacteria in relation to bacterial physiology, pathogenesis and drug resistance: some thoughts and possibilities arising from recent structural information. *Research in Microbiology*, **142**, 451–463.

Mbithi, J.N., Springthorpe, V.S., Sattar, S.A. & Pacquette, M. (1993) Bactericidal, virucidal and mycobactericidal activities of reused alkaline glutaraldehyde in an endoscopy unit. *Journal of Clinical Microbiology*, **31**, 2933–2995.

Medical Devices Directorate (1993) *Sterilization, Disinfection and Cleaning of Medical Equipment*. London: HMSO.

Merkal, R.S. & Whipple, D.L. (1980) Inactivation of *Mycobacterium bovis* in meat products. *Applied and Environmental Microbiology*, **40**, 282–284.

Middlebrook, G. (1965) The mycobacteria. In *Bacterial and Mycotic Infections of Man*, 4th edn. (eds Dubos, R.J. & Hirsch, J.G.), pp. 490–530. London: Pitman Medical.

Miner, N.A., McDowell, J.W., Willcockson, G.W., Bruckner, I., Stark, R. L. & Whitmore, E.J. (1977) Antimicrobial and other properties of a new stabilized alkaline glutaraldehyde disinfectant/sterilizer. *American Journal of Hospital Pharmacy*, **34**, 376–382.

Minniken, D.E. (1991) Chemical principles in the organization of lipid components in the mycobacterial cell envelope. *Research in Microbiology*, **142**, 423–427.

Nikaido, H., Kim, S.-H. & Rosenberg, E.Y. (1993) Physical organization of lipids in the cell wall of *Mycobacterium chelonae*. *Molecular Microbiology*, **8**, 1025–1030.

Nye, K., Chadha, D.K., Hodgkin, P., Bradley, C., Hancox, J. & Wise, R. (1990) *Mycobacterium chelonae* isolation from broncho-alveolar lavage fluid and its practical implications. *Journal of Hospital Infection*, **16**, 257–261.

Parkinson, E. (1981) Testing of disinfectants for veterinary and agricultural use. In *Disinfectants: Their Use and Evaluation of Effectiveness* (eds Collins, C.H., Allwood, M.C., Bloomfield, S.F. & Fox, A.), pp. 33–36. London: Academic Press.

Patterson, R.A., Thompson, T.L. & Larsen, D.H. (1956) The use of Zephiran in the isolation of *M. tuberculosis*. *American Review of Tuberculosis*, **74**, 284–288.

Petit, J.-F. & Lederer, E. (1978) Structure and immunostimulant properties of mycobacterial cell walls. *Symposium of the Society for General Microbiology*, **28**, 177–199.

Power, E.G.M. & Russell, A.D. (1989) Glutaraldehyde: its uptake by sporing and non-sporing bacteria, rubber, plastic and an endoscope. *Journal of Applied Bacteriology*, **67**, 329–342.

Quinn, P.J. (1987) Evaluation of veterinary disinfectants and disinfection processes. In *Disinfection in Veterinary and Farm Animal Practice* (eds Linton, A.H., Hugo, W.B. & Russell, A.D.), pp. 66–116. Oxford: Blackwell Scientific Publications.

Rastogi, N., Goh, K.S. & David, H.L. (1990) Enhancement of drug susceptibility of *Mycobacterium avium* by inhibitors of cell envelope synthesis. *Antimicrobial Agents and Chemotherapy*, **34**, 759–764.

Ratledge, C. & Standford, J. (eds) (1982) *The Biology of the Mycobacteria*. Vol. 1: *Physiology, Identification and Classification*. London: Academic Press.

Reeves, D.S. & Brown, N.M. (1995) Mycobacterial contamination of fibreoptic bronchoscopes. *Journal of Hospital Infection*, **30** (Suppl.), 531–536.

Richards, W.D. & Thoen, C.O. (1979) Chemical destruction of *Mycobacterium bovis* in milk. *Journal of Food Protection*, **42**, 55–57.

Ridgway, G.L. (1985) Decontamination of fibreoptic endoscopes. *Journal of Hospital Infection*, **6**, 363–368.

Rotter, M.L. (1996) Alcohols for antisepsis of hands and skin. In *Handbook of Disinfectants and Antiseptics* (ed. Ascenzi, J.M.), pp. 177–234. New York: Marcel Dekker.

Rubbo, S.D. & Gardner, J.F. (1965) *A Review of Sterilization and Disinfection*. London: Lloyd-Luke.

Rubbo, S.D., Gardner, J.F. & Webb, R.L. (1967) Biocidal activities of glutaraldehyde and related compounds. *Journal of Applied Bacteriology*, **30**, 78–87.

Rubin, J. (1983) Agents for disinfection and control of tuberculosis. In *Disinfection, Sterilization and Preservation*, 3rd edn (ed. Block, S.S.), pp. 414–421. Philadelphia: Lea & Febiger.

Rubin, J. (1991) Mycobacterial disinfection and control. In *Disinfection, Sterilization and Preservation*, 4th edn (ed. Block, S.S), pp. 375–385. Philadelphia: Lea & Febiger.

Russell, A.D. (1990) The effect of chemical and physical agents on microbes: disinfection and sterilization. In *Topley & Wilson's Principles of Bacteriology and Immunity*, 8th edn (eds Linton, A.H. & Dick, H.M.), pp. 71–103. London: Edward Arnold.

Russell, A.D. (1991) Principles of antimicrobial activity. In *Disinfection, Sterilization and Preservation*, 4th edn (ed. Block, S.S.) pp. 29–34 Philadelphia: Lea & Febiger.

Russell, A.D. (1993) Microbial cell walls and resistance of bacteria and fungi to antibiotics and biocides. *Journal of Infectious Diseases*, **168**, 1339–1340.

Russell, A.D. (1994) Glutaraldehyde: its current status and uses. *Infection Control and Hospital Epidemiology* **15**, 724–733.

Russell, A.D. (1996) Activity of biocides against mycobacteria. *Journal of Applied Bacteriology, Symposium Supplement*, **81**, 87S–101S.

Russell, A.D. (1997) Microbial sensitivity and resistance to chemical and physical agents. In *Topley & Wilson's Microbiology and Microbial Infections. Vol. 2: Systematic Bacteriology* (eds Barlow, A. & Duerden, B.I.) 9th edn, pp. 149–184. London: Arnold.

Russell, A.D. & Chopra, I. (1996) *Understanding Antibacterial Action and Resistance*, 2nd edn. Chichester: Ellis Horwood.

Russell, A.D. & Hopwood, D. (1976) The biological uses and importance of glutaraldehyde. *Progress in Medicinal Chemistry*, **13**, 271–301.

Russell, A.D. & Hugo, W.B. (1987) Chemical disinfectants. In *Disinfection in Veterinary and Farm Animal Practice* (eds Linton, A.H., Hugo, W.B. & Russell, A.D.), pp. 12–42. Oxford: Blackwell Scientific Publications.

Russell, A.D. & Russell, N.J. (1995) Biocides: activity, action and resistance. In *Society for General Microbiology Symposium No. 53*, pp. 327–365. Cambridge: Cambridge University Press.

Rutala, W.A., Cole, E.C., Wannamaker, M.S. & Weber, D.J. (1991) Inactivation of *Mycobacterium tuberculosis* and *Mycobacterium bovis* by 14 hospital disinfectants. *American Journal of Medicine*, **91** (Suppl. B), 267S–271S.

Sareen, M. & Khuller, G.K. (1990) Cell wall composition of ethambutol susceptible and resistant strains of *Mycobacterium smegmatis* ATCC 607. *Letters in Applied Microbiology*, **11**, 7–10.

Sattar, S.A., Best, M., Springthorpe, V.S. & Sanani, G. (1995) Mycobacterial testing of disinfectants: an update. *Journal of Hospital Infection*, **30**, (Suppl.), 372–382.

Schliesser, T. (1979) Testing of chemical disinfectants for veterinary medicine. *Hygiene und Medizin*, **4**, 51–56.

Smith, C.R. (1947) Alcohol as a disinfectant against the tubercle bacillus. *Public Health Reports, Washington*, **62**, 1285–1295.

Sonntag, H.G. (1978) Desinfektionsverfahren bei tuberculose. *Hygiene und Medizin*, **3**, 322–325.

Spaulding, E.H. (1972) Chemical disinfection and antisepsis in the hospital. *Journal of Hospital Research*, **9**, 5–31.

Spaulding, E.H., Cundy, K.R. & Turner, F.J. (1977) Chemical disinfection of medical and surgical materials. In *Disinfection, Sterilization and Preservation*, 2nd edn (ed. Block, S.S.), pp. 654–684. Philadelphia: Lea & Febiger.

Springthorpe, V.S., Mbithi, J.N. & Sattar, S.A. (1995) Microbiocidal activity of chemical sterilants under reuse conditions. In *Chemical Germicides in Health Care* (ed. Rutala, W.), pp. 181–202. Morin Heights: Polyscience Publications.

Sutton, S.V.W. (1996) Neutralizer evaluations as control experiments for antimicrobial efficacy tests. In *Handbook of Disinfectants and Antiseptics* (ed. Ascenzi, J.M.), pp. 43–62. New York: Marcel Dekker.

Takayama, K. & Kilburn, J.O. (1988) Inhibition of synthesis of arabinogalactan by ethambutol in *Mycobacterium smegmatis*. *Antimicrobial Agents and Chemotherapy*, **33**, 1493–1499.

Taylor, E.W., Mehtar, S., Cowan, R.E. & Feneley, R.C.I. (1994) Endoscopy: disinfectants and health. *Journal of Hospital Infection*, **28**, 5–14.

Uttley, A.H.C. & Pozniak, A. (1993) Resurgence of tuberculosis. *Journal of Hospital Infection*, **23**, 249–253.

Uttley, A.H.C. & Simpson, R.A. (1994) Audit of bronchoscope disinfection: a survey of procedures in England and Wales and incidents of mycobacterial contamination. *Journal of Hospital Infection*, **26**, 301–308.

van Klingeren, B. & Pullen, W. (1987) Comparative testing of disinfectants against *Mycobacterium tuberculosis* and *Mycobacterium terrae* in a quantitative suspension test. *Journal of Hospital Infection*, **10**, 292–298.

van Klingeren, B. & Pullen, W. (1993) Glutaraldehyde resistant mycobacteria from endoscope washers. *Journal of Hospital Infection*, **25**, 147–149.

Wayne, L.G. (1985) The 'atypical' mycobacteria: recognition and disease association. *Critical Reviews in Microbiology*, **12**, 185–222.

Wheeler, P.R., Besra, G.S., Minnikin, D.E. and Ratledge, C. (1993) Inhibition of mycolic acid biosynthesis in a cell-wall preparation from *Mycobacterium smegmatis* by methyl 4-(2-octadecylcyclopropen-1-yl) butanoate, a structural analogue of a key precursor. *Letters in Applied Microbiology*, **17**, 33–36.

Willet, H.P. & Thacore, H. (1996) The induction by lysozyme of an L-type growth in *Mycobacterium tuberculosis*. *Canadian Journal of Microbiology*, **12**, 11–16.

Willett, H.P. & Thacore, H. (1967) Formation of spheroplasts of *Mycobacterium tuberculosis* by lysozyme in combination with certain enzymes of rabbit peritoneal monocytes. *Canadian Journal of Microbiology*, **13**, 481–488.

Wolinsky, E. (1979) Nontuberculous mycobacteria and associated diseases. *American Review of Respiratory Diseases*, **119**, 107–159.

E. LEGIONELLA

1 Introduction

Legionella first came to public prominence in 1977, when it was identified as the causative agent of an outbreak of pneumonia that had affected people in the vicinity of a Philadelphia hotel (McDade *et al.*, 1977). The disease had primarily affected delegates at an American Legion's annual convention, and it is after these legionnaires that both the genus and the disease were named. *Legionella pneumophila* is the most notorious of the legionellae. Following the initial identification, retrospective serological studies showed that it had been responsible for disease outbreaks going back to 1965 (Thacker *et al.*, 1978) and the new genus created was shown to contain species isolated as far back as 1947 (McDade *et al.*, 1979).

2 Isolation and cultivation

The organism was originally isolated by guinea-pig inoculation, followed by transfer to the yolk-sac of fertile hens' eggs (McDade *et al.*, 1977). Later, it was shown that the organism could be grown on bacteriological culture media (Feeley *et al.*, 1978). A major breakthrough, however, was the development of charcoal-yeast extract (CYE) agar, supplemented with L-cysteine and ferric pyrophosphate (Feeley *et al.*, 1979). The charcoal probably functions in scavenging toxic oxygen radicals, which are produced when the yeast extract agar is exposed to light. The addition of ACES (N-2-acetamido-2-aminoethane sulfonic acid) buffer increases the buffering capacity of the medium to give buffered CYE (BYCE) agar. The further addition of α-ketoglutarate improved recovery and gave faster initial growth rates. This medium is termed BCYE-α agar (Edelstein, 1981).

The BCYE agars have proved very successful in the routine culturing of legionellae. For the examination of environmental samples, however, selective media have been developed. This has been achieved by including antibiotics in BCYE agar (Wadowski & Yee, 1981) to inhibit the growth of other environmental bacteria.

In addition, several techniques have been developed to increase the selectivity of the isolation procedure. These include an acid pretreatment of the sample, using a pH 2.2 buffer for 5 min (Bopp *et al.*, 1981) and a heat treatment at 50°C for 30 min (Dennis *et al.*, 1984a). These methods have been shown to be successful, but some variation is evident between techniques used (Roberts *et al.*, 1987).

3 Taxonomy

The genus *Legionella* belongs to the family *Legionellaceae* and contains some 30 species, many of which can be subdivided into serogroups and subgroups (Harrison & Taylor, 1988). They are Gram-negative, non-acid-fast, motile, rod-shaped bacteria. Most species are capable of liquefying gelatin and are catalase-positive (Isenberg, 1979). Some species exhibit autofluorescence (Hoffman, 1984), may be weakly oxidase-positive, hydrolyse sodium hippurate and produce a soluble brown pigment on Feeley–Gorman agar (Lattimer & Ormsbee, 1981). Many strains produce β-lactamase, which may explain why β-lactam antibiotics are not clinically effective (Thornsberry & Kirven, 1978). A range of biochemical tests have been utilized in routine identification of the organism (Vesey *et al.*, 1988). Isolates can be identified by their characteristic fatty acid or ubiquinone composition (Wait, 1988) or by the use of specific serological methods, such as indirect or direct immunofluorescence (Harrison & Taylor, 1988). Deoxyribonucleic acid (DNA) hybridization techniques have been developed for the identification of *Legionella*. Grimont *et al.*, (1985) were among the first to report a probe specific for *L-pneumophila*. Subsequently, several polymerase chain reaction (PCR) amplification systems were developed for both environmental and clinical isolates (Bej *et* al., 1993; Nowicki *et al.*, 1993; Tompkins & Loutit, 1993).

4 *Legionella* and disease

There are several clinically distinct diseases caused by *Legionella* species. These include Pontiac fever, Pittsburg pneumonia and, the most serious, legionnaires' disease. Legionnaires' disease is a potentially severe pneumonia-type condition, whereas Pontiac fever is a non-pneumonic, non-fatal illness of short duration. Pittsburg pneumonia appears similar to legionnaires' disease but is caused by *Legionella micdadei* (Rudin *et al.*, 1984). Susceptibility to legionnaires' disease is known to be enhanced by such factors as smoking, use of immunosuppressive drugs and alcoholism, and males are more susceptible than females (Anon., 1981). Once diagnosed, treatment for legionellosis is by erythromycin and rifampicin (Lattimer & Ormsbee, 1981). Infection occurs not by person-to-person spread but by inhalation of infected water droplets. It has been estimated that, taking into account sporadic cases, there have been between 7000 and 8000 cases of legionellosis per year in the USA (Joly, 1993).

4.1 Occurrence

Legionellae are ubiquitous in aquatic habitats and have been regularly isolated from both man-made and natural environments (Fliermans *et al.*, 1979, 1981). The man-made systems include hot and cold water supplies (Hsu *et al.*, 1984), shower heads (Bollin *et al.*, 1985), whirlpool baths (Vogt *et al.*, 1987), specialist medical equipment (Moiraghi *et al.*, 1987), humidifiers (Tobin *et al.*, 1981) and cooling towers (Tobin *et al.*, 1981; Witherall *et al.*, 1984).

Several surveys in the UK have indicated the prevalence of the bacterium in water systems. One survey has reported the isolation of legionellae from 25 of 46 establishments examined. At these 46 sites, 86 discrete cooling water-systems were identified, of which 34 were positive (Bartlett *et al.*, 1985). Other surveys outside the UK have confirmed the ubiquity of the organism in water systems (Ikedo & Yabuuchi, 1986; Tobin *et al.*, 1986).

5 Control of *Legionella*

Legionella can enter both domestic water systems and cooling systems by seeding from low-level contamination in feed-water supplies (Hsu *et al.*, 1984). The primary measures to control the risk of legionellosis therefore involve prevention of the organism growing and multiplying within the systems, and minimizing the possibilities of producing and disseminating aerosols. Several UK government guidance documents have been produced covering this area. These include *The Control of Legionellosis Including Legionnaires' Disease* (Anon., 1993) and *The Prevention and Control of Legionellosis (including Legionnaire's disease): Approved Code of Practice* (Anon., 1995).

5.1 Domestic water systems

In domestic systems, control of *Legionella* growth may be achieved by a combination of good design, construction and maintenance. This includes the use of suitable constructional materials which do not support the growth of legionella (Anon., 1989) and the elimination of 'dead-legs' and stagnant areas.

The water systems should be operated whenever possible at temperatures unfavourable to the growth of legionellae (Dennis *et al.*, 1984b). Cold water supplies should be maintained below 20°C and hot water calorifiers should reach a temperature of 60°C (Anon., 1993). Hot and cold water pipes should not run alongside one another, and hot water should reach the outlet at not below 50°C. Where these conditions cannot be met or where there is a risk of scalding, point-of-use heating should be considered.

Potable water supplies are chlorinated in the UK, but little if any residual chlorine is detectable at the point of use. Chlorine may be used to disinfect contaminated water systems, or pasteurization may be considered in the case of hot-water systems. Reports vary on the efficacy of chlorine against legionellae, some sources stating that they are as sensitive to chlorine as *Escherichia coli* (Hsu *et al.*, 1984), while others report *Legionella* to be more resistant than *E. coli*. (Kuchta *et al.*, 1983; Berg *et al.*, 1984). *Legionella pneumophila* grown in continuous culture exhibits greater chlorine resistance than batch-grown organisms (Berg *et al.*, 1984) and resistant strains have been developed by culturing tap-water-adapted legionellae (Kuchta *et al.*, 1985). Legionellae have been isolated from systems treated with residual chlorine levels of 7.5 parts/10^6 (Tobin *et al.*, 1986), and even hyperchlorination has failed to eradicate *L. pneumophila* (Tobin *et al.*, 1980).

Ultraviolet light has been proposed as an alternative control method in hospital water-distribution systems (Muraca *et al.*, 1987; Liu *et al.*, 1995), as has the use of copper-silver ionization (Liu *et al.*, 1994).

5.2 Recirculating water systems

These systems include cooling water-towers (which may be induced-draught (Fig. 10.6), forced-draught or natural-draught), evaporative condensers and humidification systems, and are all prone to microbial growth.

Generally, humidification systems are operated at temperatures below that required for the growth of legionellae, and biocides are not routinely used

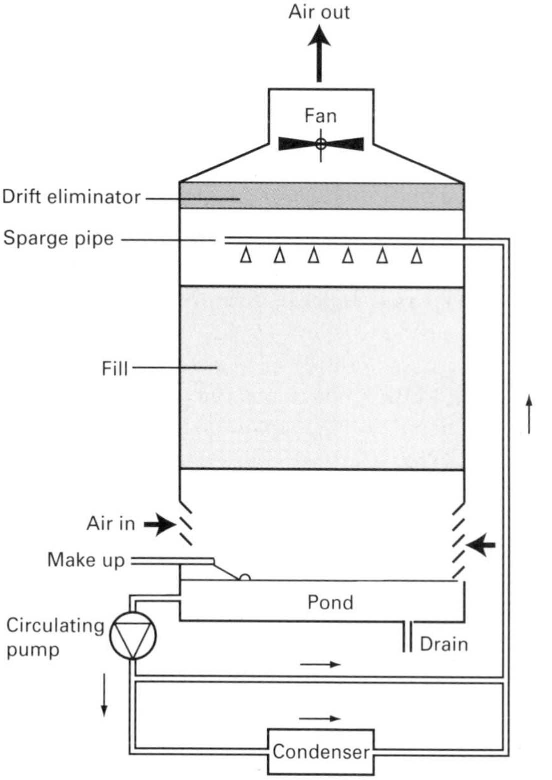

Air out
Fan
Drift eliminator
Sparge pipe
Fill
Air in
Make up
Pond
Circulating pump
Drain
Condenser

Fig. 10.6 Schematic diagram of an induced-draught cooling tower.

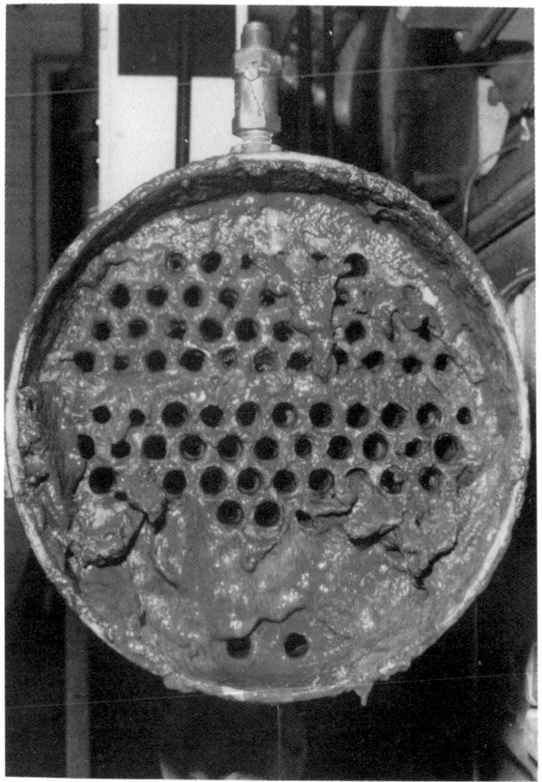

Fig. 10.7 Photograph of tube and shell heat exchanger, showing heavy microbial fouling.

when the systems are in use, as the biocide would be introduced into the conditioned air. Biocides are, however, used in cooling towers and evaporative condensers to control biofouling (Fig. 10.7). This enables the efficient operation of the cooling system, as biological growth and slimes can lead to reduced heat transfer, increased pumping costs, microbially induced corrosion and the degradation of water-treatment chemicals, such as corrosion inhibitors and descalants. Severe microbial growth can even produce structural damage; Fig. 10.8 shows a cooling water tower which has collapsed due to the sheer weight of biofouling.

Many of the industrial biocides used in recirculating water systems have been tested for activity against *L. pneumophila* in laboratory studies (Table 10.8). There is some evidence that *L. pneumophila* is less sensitive than *E. coli* to certain biocides, having a sensitivity similar to *Pseudomonas aeruginosa* (Hollis & Smalley, 1980; Cunliffe, 1990). Biocides tested for activity include chlorine. (Skaliy *et al.*, 1980; Sorraco *et al.*, 1983; Kobayashi & Tsuzuki, 1984; Sawatari *et al.*, 1984), isothiazolinones (Skaliy *et al.*, 1980; Sorraco *et al.*, 1983; Sawatari *et al.*, 1984; Elsmore, 1986; McCoy *et al.*, 1986), quaternary ammonium compounds (Skaliy *et al.*, 1980; Grace *et al.*, 1981; Sorraco *et al.*, 1983; Elsmore, 1986), dibromonitrilopropionamide (Hollis & Smalley, 1980; Skaliy *et al.*, 1980; Sorraco *et al.*, 1983; Elsmore, 1986), dichlorophen (Kobayashi & Tsuzuki, 1984; Elsmore 1986), thiacarbamates (Hollis & Smalley, 1980; Skaliy *et al.*, 1980; Sorraco *et al.*, 1983), sodium pentachlorophenate (Sorraco *et al.*, 1983), methylene bisthiocyanate (Grace *et al.*, 1981), 2-(thiocyanomethylthio)-benzthiazole (Elsmore, 1986), *N*-alkyl-l,3-propanediamine (Grace *et al.*, 1981), bromochlorodimethylhydantoin (McCoy & Wireman, 1989), 2-bromo-2-nitropropane-1,3-diol (BNPD) (Sawatari *et al.*, 1984; Elsmore, 1986; Coughlin & Caplan, 1987) and several others. Non-chemical approaches, such as the use of ultraviolet light, have also been proposed for cooling-water use (Kusnetsov *et al.*, 1994).

The significance of the presence of biofilms in the testing of biocides is becoming more important. It has been shown that biofilms can provide protection for microorganisms (LeChevalier *et al.*, 1988) and also that *L. pneumophila* can grow in biofilms (Colbourne & Dennis, 1988). In addition to suspension tests, the use of biofilm generators and recirculating models has been examined for evaluating biocides against legionellae (Elsmore, 1986; Coughlin & Caplan, 1987). These models can provide a more meaningful testing programme for evaluating biocide efficacy (Walker *et al.*, 1994).

Extrapolation from these laboratory studies to in-use applications may not be realistic because of factors such as possible interaction with other water-treatment chemicals and inactivation by large amounts of slime. This has been indicated by several workers, who have shown that compounds which were deemed to be effective in a laboratory were less than effective in use (Orrison *et al.*, 1981;

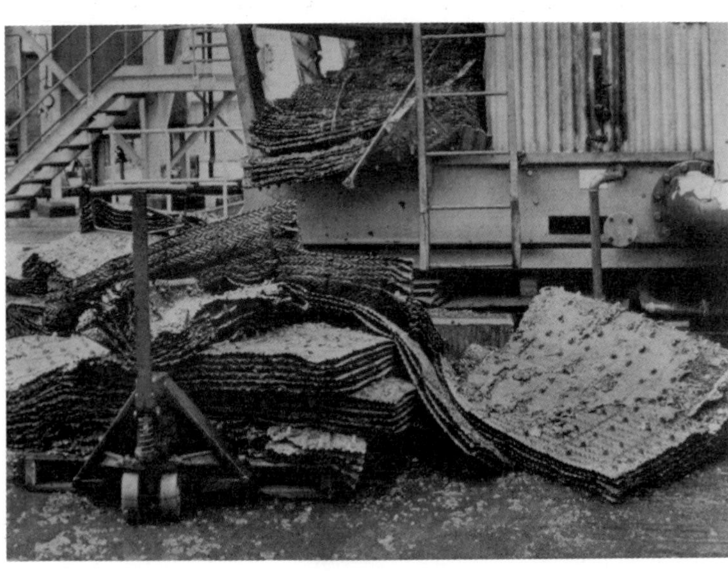

Fig. 10.8 Photograph of part of an open recirculating evaporative cooling tower, showing structural damage due to biofouling.

Table 10.8 Minimum inhibitory concentrations* of several water-treatment biocides against *Legionella* species (Elsmore, 1986). †

Biocide	*L. pneumophila* NCTC 11192	NCTC 11378	NCTC 11405	NCTC 11417	Clinical isolate	Environmental isolate	*L. micdadei* NCTC 11371	*L. oakridgensis* environmental isolate	*L. longbeachae* NCTC 11477	*L. gormanii* NCTC 11401	*L. bozmanii* NCTC 11368	*L. jordanis* NCTC 11533
2-Bromo-2-nitro-propane-1-3-diol (BNPD)	50	50	50	50	50	50	50	50	50	50	50	100
Blend of isothiazolinones	56	56	28	28	28	28	28	56	28	28	28	56
Methylene bisthiocyanate	100	50	100	50	50	50	100	100	50	50	25	100
Chlorinated phenolic thioether	20	20	20	20	20	20	20	20	20	20	20	20
2.2-Dibromo-3-nitrilopropionamide	800	800	400	200	200	200	800	200	100	200	200	400
Sodium dichlorophen	25	25	100	25	25	25	25	25	25	25	25	25
Cationic polyquaternary ammonium compound	800	800	800	800	800	800	400	400	400	400	800	400
Disodium mercaptobenzothiazole	72	72	>576	72	72	72	576	72	72	36	72	576
Dioctyl dimethylammonium chloride	50	50	50	50	50	50	25	50	50	50	25	50
2-(Thiocyanomethylthio) benzothiazole	30	60	240	30	60	30	60	60	30	30	30	60
Paracetic acid	200	200	200	200	200	200	200	200	200	200	200	200
Tetra-alkyl-phosphonium	12.5	12.5	12.5	12.5	6.25	12.5	6.25	12.5	12.5	12.5	12.5	25

* Concentration expressed as parts/10^6 active ingredient.

† Results are from multipoint MIC test carried out in BCYE agar. Note that BCYE may inactivate some of the biocides tested, e.g. BNPD is antagonized by cysteine hydrochloride, a component of the medium.

NCTC, National Collection of Type Cultures; MIC, minimal inhibitory concentration.

England *et al.*, 1982). To date, few extensive field studies have been published on the activity of biocides against *L. pneumophila* in recirculating water applications (Fliermans *et al.*, 1982; Kurtz *et al.*, 1982, 1984; Fliermans & Harvey, 1984; Grow *et al.*, 1984; Elsmore, 1986; Coughlin & Caplan 1987; Elsmore *et al.*, 1987; Muraca *et al.*, 1988; Negron-Alvira *et al.*, 1988; Bentham, 1993; Bentham & Broadbent, 1995).

5.3 Assessment of activity

No standard method exists for the evaluation of biocides against legionellae. The *Report of the Expert Advisory Committee on Biocides* (Wright, 1989) recommends that 'The preparation of a standard procedure should be expedited for the assessment of the efficacy of biocides against legionellae.' This has been partly accomplished in the production of a draft European standard (Anon., 1994). In addition, the Wright report advocates field trials in cooling towers to establish the efficacy of different classes of biocides and the role of continuous or intermittent treatment.

5.4 Factors affecting biocide activity in recirculating water systems

Several factors can affect biocidal activity, including pH, temperature, concentration and the presence of organic matter, e.g. slimes (see also Chapter 3). Figure 10.9 shows the effect of pH on

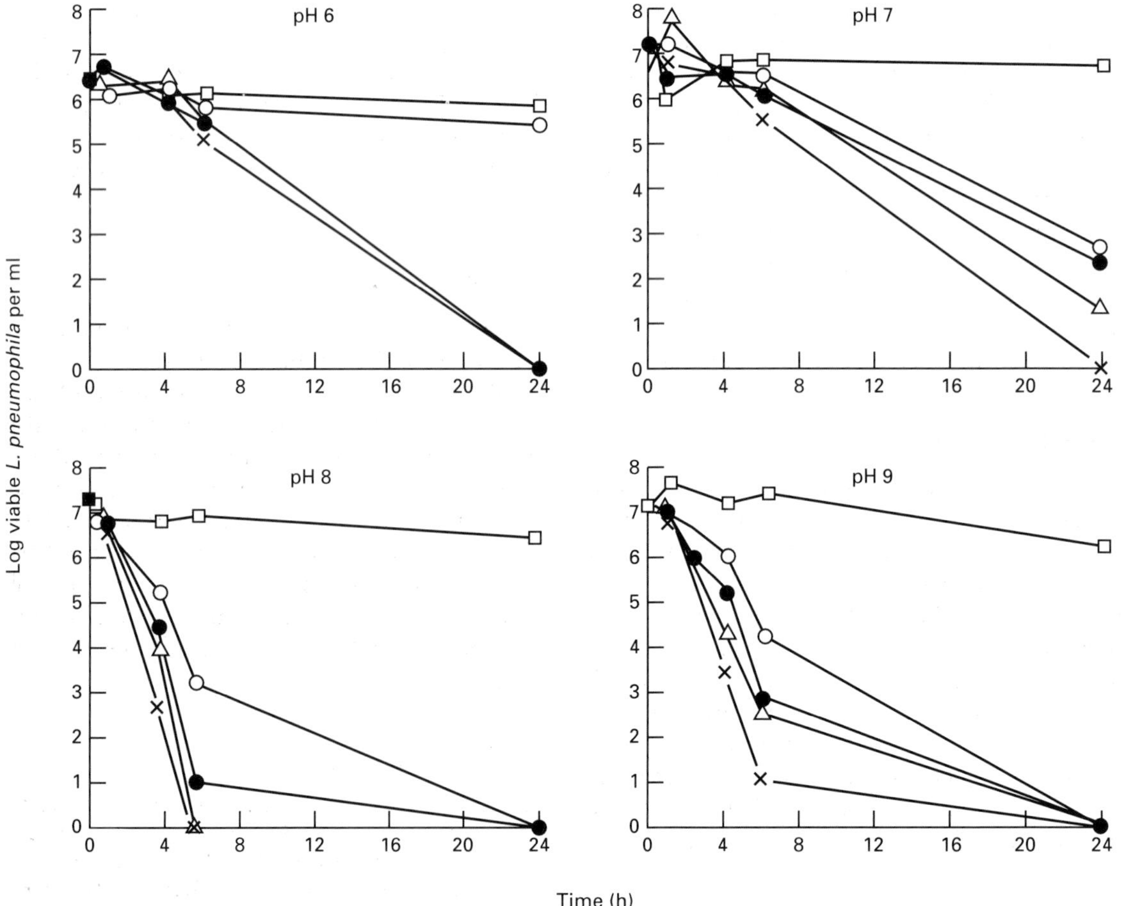

Fig. 10.9 Effects of pH on the activity of BNPD against *L. pneumophila* serogroup 1 (Elsmore 1989). Tested in buffers of pH 6, 7, 8 and 9. □, Control (no BNPD) ○, 15 parts/10^6 BNPD; ●, 25 parts/10^6 BNPD; △, 50 parts/10^6 BNPD; X, 100 parts/10^6 BNDP.

the activity of one biocide (BNPD) against *L. pneumophila* NCTC 11192 in a suspension test. It is known that the stability of the compound is reduced at alkaline pH, with the half-life decreasing from 1.5 years at pH 6 to 2 months at pH 8 (Croshaw & Holland, 1984). The relationship between activity and pH is more complex. Croshaw *et al.*, 1964) reported that the activity of BNPD fell by two to eight times when the pH was increased from 5.3 to 7 or 8. Tuttle *et al.* (1970) indicated that, in certain circumstances, BNPD was more active under alkaline conditions and, in others, it was less active. Moore (1978) stated that the activity of BNPD is not markedly affected by changes in pH over the range 5–8. Moore & Stretton (1981), however, indicated that BNPD was more active at higher pH values, based on extinction-time experiments using *Ps. aeruginosa*. The results obtained may vary, depending on the method used, because, in long contact time tests, the increasing degradation of the BNPD under alkaline conditions may be an important factor. It seems probable that, in the case of *L. pneumophila,* the further the pH varies from the optimum pH for growth (pH 6.9), the more the organism may become stressed and thus more susceptible to any biocide that may be used (States *et al.*, 1987). The majority of recirculating cooling systems are operated at alkaline pH to optimize corrosion-inhibition programmes.

5.5 Resistance to biocides

It is a well-known fact that, under conditions of continuous use, microorganisms can become resistant to certain biocides. The Expert Advisory Committee on Biocides (Wright, 1989) advises the investigation of the possibility of resistance development by *Legionella* spp. to biocides. Furthermore, free-living amoebae have been involved with *L. pneumophila* from cooling water systems; when found within the cysts of *Acanthamoeba polyphaga*, the legionellae are protected and can survive exposure to high concentrations of chlorine (Kilvington & Price, 1990; Kuchta *et al.*,1993).

6 *Legionella* and other microorganisms

It has been suggested that legionellae are more likely to be isolated from systems with high microbial counts (Elsmore *et al.*, 1989) and it would thus be prudent to maintain microbial counts as low as possible, with biocide treatments active against a wide range of common water microorganisms.

It has been postulated that the ability of legionellae to thrive in the natural environment is due to symbiotic-type relationships with other organisms. They have been associated with amoebae (Tyndall & Domingue, 1982; see also Section 5.5), cyanobacteria (Tison *et al.*, 1980), *Tetrahymena* (Fields *et al.*, 1984) and flavobacteria (Wadowski & Yee, 1983). It has therefore been suggested that, if the overall microbial population can be controlled, the growth of legionellae might be minimized (Anon., 1993). It is interesting to note, however, that adaptation of amoebae can occur in the presence of biocides. Srikanth & Berk (1994) indicated that cross-resistance can occur and suggested that exposure to one biocide may boost the amoebae's resistance to a second biocide before the second biocide is used in the cooling-tower. This brings into question the rationale for the usual procedure of alternating biocides on a regular basis.

7 Conclusions

Many biocides have been shown to be active against legionellae in the laboratory.

With the development of standard test methods, more unified results will be obtainable for the assessment of biocide activity. However, direct extrapolation from these laboratory tests to in-use applications may not be valid, due to interactions with water treatment chemicals and biofilms. Biofilm-model systems offer one more meaningful method to evaluate biocide efficacy in the laboratory; however, field trial data still provide the most meaningful results.

8 References

Anon. (1981) *Legionnaires' Disease: Report of a WHO Working Group*. Euro Reports and Studies 72, pp. 1–28. Copenhagen: World Health Organization.

Anon. (1989) *Water Fittings and Materials Directory.* Surrey: Unwin Brothers.

Anon. (1993) *The Control of Legionellosis, Including Legionnaires' Disease*, 2nd edn. HSE: HS (G) 70. London: HMSO.

Anon. (1994) *Chemical Disinfectants and Antiseptics Water Treatment Products Against* Legionella pneumophila *Bacterial Activity: Test Method and Requirements*. CEN/TC 216 N 51, November.

Anon. (1995) *The Prevention and Control of Legionellosis (Including Legionnaires' disease): Approved Code of Practice*. HSE L8. London: HMSO.

Bartlett, C.L.R., Hutchinson, J.G.P., Tillet, H.E., Turner, G.C. & Wright, A.E. (1985) Final Report on a Public Health Laboratory Service collaborative study of *Legionella* species in water systems 1981–1985 (unpublished).

Bej, A.K., Mahbutani, M.H. & Atlas, R.M. (1993) Detection of *Legionella pneumophila* by polymerase chain reaction amplification and restriction enzyme analysis. In Legionella: *Current Status and Emergency Perspectives* (eds Barbaree, J.M., Breiman, R.F. & Dufour, A.P.) pp. 173–174, Washington, DC: American Society for Microbiology.

Bentham, R.H. (1993) Environmental factors affecting the colonisation of cooling towers by *Legionella* spp. in South Australia. *International Biodeterioration and Biodegradation*, **31**, 55–63.

Bentham, R.H. & Broadbent, C.R. (1995) Field trial of biocides for control of *Legionella* in cooling towers. *Current Microbiology*, **30**, 167–172.

Berg, J.D, Hoff, J.C., Roberts, P.V. & Matin, A. (1984) Growth of *Legionella pneumophila* in continuous culture and its sensitivity to inactivation by chlorine dioxide. In Legionella: *Proceedings of the Second International Symposium* (eds Thornsberry, C., Ballows, A., Feeley, J.C. & Jakubowski, W.), pp. 68–70. Washington, DC: American Society for Microbiology.

Bollin, G.E., Plouffe, J.F., Para, M.F. & Hackman, B. (1985) Aerosols containing *Legionella pneumophila* generated by shower heads and hot water faucets. *Applied and Environmental Microbiology*, **50**, 1128–1131.

Bopp, C. A., Sumner, J.W., Morris, G. K. & Wells, J.G. (1981) Isolation of *Legionella* spp. from environmental samples by low-pH treatment and use of selective techniques. *Journal of Clinical Microbiology*, **13**, 714–719.

Colbourne, J.S. & Dennis, P.J. (1988) *Legionella*: a biofilm organism in engineered water systems? In *Biodeterioration* 7 (eds Houghton, D.R., Smith, R.N. & Eggins, H.O.W.), pp. 36–42. London: Elsevier.

Coughlin, M. & Caplan, G. (1987) Microbial efficacy of BNPD against *Legionella pneumophila*. In *Cooling Tower Institute Annual Meeting*, New Orleans. Technical Paper TP 87–18.

Croshaw, B. & Holland, V.R. (1984) Use of Bronopol as a cosmetic preservative. In *Cosmetic and Drug Preservation: Principles and Practice* (ed. Kabara, J.J.), pp. 31–62. New York: Marcel Dekker.

Croshaw, B., Groves, M.J. & Lessel, B. (1964) Some properties of Bronopol, a new antimicrobial agent active against *Pseudomonas aeruginosa*. *Journal of Pharmacy and Pharmacology*, **16**, 127T–130T.

Cunliffe, D.A. (1990) Inactivation of *Legionella pneumophila* by chloramine. *Journal of Applied Bacteriology*, **68**, 453–459.

Dennis, P.J., Bartlett, C.L.R. & Wright, A.E. (1984a) Comparison of isolation methods for *Legionella* spp. In Legionella: *Proceedings of the Second International Symposium* (eds Thornsberry, C., Ballows, A., Feeley, J.C. & Jakubowski, W.), pp. 293–296. Washington, DC: American Society for Microbiology.

Dennis, P.J., Green, D. & Jones, B.P.C. (1984b) A note on the temperature tolerance of *Legionella*. *Journal of Applied Bacteriology*, **56**, 349–350.

Edelstein, P.H. (1981) Improved semi-selective medium for isolation of *Legionella pneumophila* from contaminated clinical and environmental specimens. *Journal of Clinical Microbiology*, **14**, 298–303.

Elsmore, R. (1986) Biocidal control of Legionellae. *Israel Journal of Medical Sciences*, **22**, 647–654.

Elsmore, R. (1989) The activity of BNPD against *Legionella pneumophila* serogroup 1: the influence of pH, inoculum level and test media. *International Biodeterioration*, **25**, 107–113.

Elsmore, R., Guthrie, W.G. & Parr, J.A. (1987) Laboratory and field experience with a bromonitroalkanol biocide in industrial water systems. *Speciality Chemicals*, **7**, 166–176.

Elsmore, R., Corbett, R.J. & Channon, E.J. (1989) Relationship between the common water flora and isolation of *Legionella* species from water systems. In *Airborne Deteriogens and Pathogens* (ed. Flannigan, B.), pp. 83–96. Kew: Biodeterioration Society.

England, A.C., Fraser, D.W., Mallison, G.F., Mackel, D.C., Skaliy, P. & Gorman, G.W. (1982) Failure of *Legionella pneumophila* sensitivities to predict culture results from disinfectant-treated air-conditioning cooling towers. *Applied and Environmental Microbiology*, **43**, 240–244.

Feeley, J.C., Gorman, G.W., Weaver, R.E., Mackel, D.C. & Smith, H.W. (1978) Primary isolation media for the legionnaires' disease bacterium. *Journal of Clinical Microbiology*, **8**, 320–325.

Feeley, J.C., Gibson, K.J., Gorman, G.W. *et al.* (1979) Charcoal–yeast extract agar: primary isolation medium for *Legionella pneumophila*. *Journal of Clinical Microbiology*, **10**, 437–411.

Fields, B.S., Shotts, E.B., Feeley, J.C., Gorman, G.W. & Martin, W.T. (1984) Proliferation of *Legionella pneumophila* as an intracellular parasite of the ciliated protozoan *Tetrahymena pyriformis*. *Applied and Environmental Microbiology*, **47**, 467–471.

Fliermans, C.B. & Harvey, R.S. (1984) Effectiveness of l-bromo-3-chloro-5,5-dimethylhydantoin against *Legio-*

nella pneumophila in a cooling tower. *Applied and Environmental Microbiology*, **47**, 1307–1310.

Fliermans, C.B., Cherry, W.B., Orrison, L.H. & Thacker, L. (1979) Isolation of *Legionella pneumophila* from non-epidemic related aquatic habitats. *Applied and Environmental Microbiology*, **37**, 1239–1242.

Fliermans, C.B., Cherry, W.B., Orrison, L.H., Smith, S.J., Tison, D.L. & Pope, D.H. (1981) Ecological distribution of *Legionella pneumophila. Applied and Environmental Microbiology*, **41**, 9–16.

Fliermans, C.B., Bettinger, G.E. & Fynsk, A.W. (1982) Treatment of cooling systems containing high levels of *Legionella pneumophila. Water Research*, **16**, 903–909.

Grace, R.D., Dewar, N.E., Barnes, W.G. & Hodges, G.R. (1981) Susceptibility *of Legionella pneumophila* to three cooling tower microbiocides. *Applied and Environmental Microbiology*, **41** 233–236.

Grimont, A.D., Grimont, F., Desplaces, N. & Tchen, P. (1985) DNA probe specific for *Legionella pneumophila. Journal of Clinical Microbiology*, **21**, 431–437.

Grow, K.M., Wood, D.O., Coggin, J.H. & Leinbach, E.D. (1984) Environmental factors influencing growth of *Legionella pneumophila* in operating biocide treated cooling towers. In Legionella: *Proceedings of the Second International Symposium* (eds Thornsberry, C., Ballows, A., Feeley, J.C. & Jakubowski, W.), pp. 316–318. Washington, DC: American Society for Microbiology.

Harrison, T.G. & Taylor, A.G. (eds) (1988) *A Laboratory Manual for* Legionella. Chichester: John Wiley and Sons.

Hoffman, P. (1984) Bacterial physiology. In Legionella: *Proceedings of the Second International Symposium* (eds Thornsberry, C., Ballows, A., Feeley, J.C. & Jakubowski, W.), pp. 61–67. Washington, DC: American Society for Microbiology.

Hollis, C.G. & Smalley, D.L. (1980) Resistance of *Legionella pneumophila* to microbiocides. *Developments in Industrial Microbiology*, **21**, 265–271.

Hsu, S.C., Martin, R. & Wentworth, B.B. (1984) Isolation of *Legionella* species from drinking water. *Applied and Environmental Microbiology*, **48**, 830–832.

Ikedo, M. & Yabuuchi, E. (1986) Ecological studies on *Legionella* species. 1. Viable counts of *Legionella pneumophila* in cooling tower water. *Microbiology and Immunology*, **30**, 413–423.

Isenberg, H.D. (1979) Microbiology of legionnaires' disease bacterium. *Annals of Internal Medicine*, **90**, 502–505.

Joly, J.R. (1993) Prevention and control of legionellosis. In Legionella: *Current Status and Emerging Perspective* (eds Barbaree, J.M., Breiman, R.F. & Dufour, A.P.), pp. 291–293. Washington, DC: American Society for Microbiology.

Kilvington, S. & Price, J. (1990) Survival of *Legionella pneumophila* within cysts of *Acanthamoeba polyphaga* following chlorine exposure. *Journal of Applied Bacteriology*, **68**, 519–525.

Kobayashi, H. & Tsuzuki, M. (1984) Susceptibility of *Legionella pneumophila* to cooling tower microbiocides and hospital disinfectants. In Legionella: *Proceedings of the Second International Symposium* (eds Thornsberry, C., Ballows, A., Feeley, J.C. & Jakubowski, W.), pp. 342–343. Washington, DC: American Society for Microbiology.

Kuchta, J.M., States, S.J., McNamara, A.M., Wadowsky, R.M., & Yee, R.B. (1983) Susceptibility of *Legionella pneumophila* to chlorine in tap water. *Applied and Environmental Microbiology*, **46**, 1134–1139.

Kuchta, J.M., States, S.J., McGlaughlin, J.E. *et al.* (1985) Enhanced chlorine resistance of tap water-adapted *Legionella pneumophila* as compared with agar medium-passaged strains. *Applied and Environmental Microbiology*, **50**, 21–26.

Kuchta, J.M., Navratil, J.S., Wadowski, R.M., Dowling, J.N., States, S.J. & Yee, R.B. (1993) Effect of chlorine on the survival and growth of *Legionella pneumophila* and *Hartmannella vermiformis*. In Legionella: *Current Status and Emerging Perspective* (eds Barbaree, J.M., Breiman, R.F. & Dufour, A.P.), pp. 242–245. Washington, DC: American Society for Microbiology.

Kurtz, J.B., Bartlett, C.L.R., Newton, U.A, White, R.A. & Jones, N. (1982) *Legionella pneumophila* in cooling water systems. *Journal of Hygiene, Cambridge*, **88**, 369–381.

Kurtz, J.B., Bartlett, C., Tillett, H. & Newton, U. (1984) Field trial of biocides in control of *Legionella pneumophila* in cooling water systems. In Legionella: *Proceedings of the Second International Symposium* (eds Thornsberry, C., Ballows, A., Feeley, J.C. & Jakubowski, W.), pp. 340–342. Washington, DC: American Society for Microbiology.

Kusnetsov, J.M., Keskitalo, P.J., Ahonen, H.E., Tulkki, A.I., Miettinen, I.T. and Martikainen, P.J. (1994). Growth of *Legionella* and other heterotrophic bateria in a circulating cooling water system exposed to ultraviolet irradiation. *Journal of Applied Bacteriology*, **77**, 461–466.

Lattimer, G.L. & Ormsbee, R.A. (eds) (1981) *Legionnaires' Disease*. New York: Marcel Dekker.

Le Chevalier, M.W., Cawthorn, C.D. & Lee, R.G. (1988) Factors promoting survival of bacteria in chlorinated water supplies. *Applied and Environmental Microbiology*, **54**, 649–654.

Liu, Z., Stout, J.E., Tedesco, L. *et al.* (1994) Controlled evaluation of copper–silver ionisation in eradicating *Legionella pneumophila* from a hospital water distribution system. *Journal of Infectious Disease*, **169**, 919–922.

Liu, Z., Stout, J.E., Tedesco, L., Boldin, M., Hwang, C.

& Yu, V.L. (1995) Efficacy of ultraviolet light in preventing *Legionella* colonization of a hospital water distribution system. *Water Research*, **29**, 2275–2280.

McCoy, W.F. & Wireman, J.W. (1989) Efficacy of bromochlorodimethylhydantoin against *Legionella pneumophila* in industrial cooling water. *Journal of Industrial Microbiology*, **4**, 403–408.

McCoy, W.F., Wireman, J.W. & Lashen, E.S. (1986) Efficiency of methylchloro/methylisothiazolone biocide against *Legionella pneumophila* in cooling tower water. *Journal of Industrial Microbiology*, **1**, 49–56.

McDade, J.E., Shepard, C.C., Fraser, D.W. *et al.* (1977) Legionnaires' disease: isolation of a bacterium and demonstration of its role in other respiratory disease. *New England Journal of Medicine* **297**, 1197–1203.

McDade, J.E., Brenner, D.J. & Bozeman, F.M. (1979) Legionnaires' disease bacterium isolated in 1947. *Annals of Internal Medicine*, **90**, 659–661.

Moiraghi, A., Castellani Pastoris, M., Barral, C. *et al.* (1987) Nosocomial legionellosis associated with use of oxygen bubble humidifiers and underwater chest drains. *Journal of Hospital Infection*, **10**, 47–50.

Moore, K.E. (1978) Evaluating preservative efficacy in pharmaceutical and cosmetic products. PhD thesis, University of Technology, Loughborough, England.

Moore, K.E. & Stretton, J.R. (1981) The effect of pH, temperature and certain media constituents on the stability and activity of the preservative bronopol. *Journal of Applied Bacteriology*, **51**, 483–494.

Muraca, P., Stout, J.E. & Yu, V.L. (1987) Comparative assessment of chlorine, heat, ozone and UV light for killing *Legionella pneumophila* within a model plumbing system. *Applied and Environmental Microbiology*, **53**, 447–453.

Muraca, P.W., Stout, J.E., Yu, V.L. & Lee, Y.C. (1988) Legionnaires' disease in the work environment: implications for environmental health. *American Industrial Hygiene Association Journal*, **49**, 584–590.

Negron-Alvira, A., Perez-Surez, I. & Huzen, T.C. (1988) *Legionella* spp. in Puerto Rico cooling towers. *Applied and Environmental Microbiology*, **54**, 2331–2334.

Nowicki, M., Bornstein, N., Jaulhac, B., Piemont, Y., Monteil, H. and Fleurette, J. (1993) Rapid detection of legionellae in clinical and environmental samples by polymerase chain reaction. In Legionella: *Current status and Emerging Perspectives* (eds Barbaree, J.M., Breiman, R.F. & Dufour A.P.), pp. 178–181. Washington, DC: American Society for Microbiology.

Orrison, L.H., Cherry, W.B. & Milan, D. (1981) Isolation of *Legionella pneumophila* from cooling tower water by filtration. *Applied and Environmental Microbiology*, **41**, 1202–1205.

Roberts, K.P., August, C.M. & Nelson, J.D. (1987) Relative sensitivities of environmental legionellae to selective isolation procedures. *Applied and Environmental Microbiology*, **53**, 2704–2707.

Rudin, J.E., Wing, E.J. & Yee, R.B. (1984) An on-going outbreak of *Legionella micdadii*. In Legionella: *Proceedings of the Second International Symposium* (eds Thornberry, C., Ballows, A., Feeley, J.C. & Jakubowski, W.), pp. 227–229. Washington, DC: American Society for Microbiology.

Sawatari, K., Watanabe, K., Nakasato, H. *et al.* (1984) Bacterial effect of disinfectants against *Legionella pneumophila* and *Legionella bozmanii. Kasenshogaku Zasshi*, **58**, 130–136.

Skaliy, P., Thompson, T.A., Gorman. G.W., Morris, G.K., McEachern, H.V. & Machel, D.C. (1980) Laboratory studies of disinfectants against *Legionella pneumophila. Applied and Environmental Microbiology*, **40**, 697–700.

Sorraco, R.J., Gill, H.K., Fliermans, C.B. & Pope, D.H. (1983) Susceptibilities of algae and *Legionella pneumophila* to cooling tower biocides. *Applied and Environmental Microbiology*, **45**, 1254–1260.

Srikanth, S. & Berk, S.G. (1994) Adaptation of amoebae to cooling tower biocides. *Microbial Ecology*, **27**, 293–301.

States, S.J., Conley, L.F., Towner, S.G. (1987) An alkaline approach to treating cooling towers for control of *Legionella pneumophila. Applied and Environmental Microbiology*, **53**, 1775–1779.

Thacker, S.B., Bennet, J.V., Tsai, T.F. *et al.* (1978) An outbreak in 1965 of severe respiratory illness caused by the Legionnaires' disease bacterium. *Journal of Infectious Diseases*, **138**, 512–519.

Thornsberry, C. & Kirven, L.A. (1978) Beta-lactamase of the Legionnaires' disease bacterium. *Current Microbiology*, **1**, 51–54.

Tison, D.L., Pope, D.H., Cherry, W.B. & Fliermans, C.B. (1980) Growth of *Legionella pneumophila* in association with blue green algae (Cyanobacteria). *Applied and Environmental Microbiology*, **39**, 456–459.

Tobin, J.O'H., Beare, J., Dunnill, M.S. *et al.* (1980) Legionnaires' disease in a transplant unit: isolation of the same causative agent from shower baths. *Lancet*, **ii**, 118–121.

Tobin, J.O'H., Swann, R.A. & Bartlett, C.L.R. (1981) Isolation of *Legionella pneumophila* from water systems: methods and preliminary results. *British Medical Journal*, **282**, 515–517.

Tobin, R.S., Ewan, P., Walsh, K. & Dutka, B. (1986) A survey of *Legionella pneumophila* in water in 12 Canadian cities. *Water Research*, **20**, 495–502.

Tompkins, L.S. & Loutit, J.S. (1993) Detection of *Legionella* by molecular methods. In Legionella: *Current Status and Emerging Perspectives* (eds Barbaree, J.M., Brieman, R.F. & Dufour, A.P.) pp. 163–168. Washington, DC: American Society for Microbiology.

Tuttle, E., Phares, C. & Chiostri, R.F. (1970) Preservation of protein solutions with 2-bromo-2-nitro-l,3-propanediol (bronopol). *American Perfumer and Cosmetics*, **85**, 87–89.

Tyndall, R.L. & Domingue, E.L. (1982) Cocultivation of *Legionella pneumophila* and free-living amoebae. *Applied and Environmental Microbiology*, **44**, 954–959.

Vesey, G., Dennis, P.J., Lee, J.V. & West, A.A. (1988) Further development of simple tests to differentiate the legionellas. *Journal of Applied Bacteriology*, **65**, 339–345.

Vogt, R.L., Hudson, P.J., Orciari, L., Heun, E.M. & Woods, T.C. (1987) Legionnaires' disease and a whirlpool spa. *Annals of Internal Medicine*, **107**, 596.

Wadowski, R.M. & Yee, R.B. (1981) Glycine-containing selective medium for isolation of Legionellaceae from environmental specimens. *Applied and Environmental Microbiology*, **42**, 768–772.

Wadowski, R.M. & Yee, R.B (1983) Satellite growth of *Legionella pneumophila* with an environmental isolate of *Flavobacterium breve*. *Applied and Environmental Microbiology*, **46**, 1447–1449.

Wait, R. (1988) Confirmation of the identity of legionellae by whole cell fatty-acid and isoprenoid quinone profiles. In *A Laboratory Manual for* Legionella (eds Harrison, T.G. & Taylor, A.G.) pp. 69–101. Chichester: John Wiley & Sons.

Walker, J.T., Rogers, J. & Keevil, C.W. (1994) An investigation of the efficacy of a bromine containing biocide on an aquatic consortium of planktonic and biofilm micro-organisms including *Legionella pneumophila*. *Biofouling*, **8**, 47–54.

Witherall, L.E., Novick, L.F., Stone, K.M. *et al.* (1984) *Legionella pneumophila* in Vermont cooling towers. In Legionella: *Proceedings of the Second International Symposium* (eds Thornsberry, C., Ballows, A., Feeley, J.C. & Jakubowski, W.), pp. 315–316. Washington, DC: American Society for Microbiology.

Wright, A.E. (1989) *Report of the Expert Advisory Committee on Biocides*. London: HMSO.

F. ANTIBIOTIC-RESISTANT COCCI

1 Introduction

1.1 Staphylococci

Various species of *Staphylococcus* are known, of which *Staph. aureus* and *Staph. epidermidis* are the most important. These are the only species that will be considered here.

1.1.1 *Staphylococcus aureus*

Staphylococcus aureus is the main pathogen responsible for pyogenic infections. It is a common cause of skin infections, osteomyelitis, wound infections and food poisoning (Shanson, 1989). In a national prevalence survey of hospitals in England and Wales, it was isolated from 3% of urinary-tract, 33% of wound and 6.5% of respiratory-tract infections (Meers *et al.*, 1981). It is carried in the nose of 20–30% of the healthy population and less often, on the skin and mucous membranes. It is thus a ubiquitous organism, which is always present in the hospital environment. For this reason, patients, staff and visitors may all act unknowingly as sources of infection (Wenzel, 1987). Most strains are sensitive to antibiotics and resistant only to penicillin, but some are multiresistant, epidemic in their spread and of high virulence (Crossley *et al.*, 1979; Report, 1986, 1990; Phillips, 1988; Cookson, 1994).

Methicillin-resistant *Staph. aureus* (MRSA) has been recognized as a major cause of sepsis in UK hospitals (Cooke *et al.*, 1986), although not all MRSA strains are of increased virulence. For example, Lacey (1987) often found MRSA in burns in geriatric units without it causing harm. In Ireland, about 30% of all *Staph. aureus* isolated from blood culture were MRSA (Cafferkey *et al.*, 1988). Lyon & Skurray (1987) reported the isolation of strains of *Staph. aureus* resistant to over 20 antimicrobial agents. It has been estimated that the cost of treating infections caused by MRSA strains is about 68% higher than for sensitive strains. One patient in Seattle (Locksley *et al.*, 1982) showed it was possible to act as both a reservoir and a susceptible host. This, together with the mechanisms of gene transfer, presents a major challenge to the formulation of effective clinical control measures. Control includes a reduction in the movement of patients and staff, both within and between hospitals, and screening of patients from 'infected' hospitals.

The term 'epidemic' MRSA (EMRSA) is often used to denote the ease with which these strains can spread (Report, 1986, 1990). Patients particularly at risk are immunocompromised, debilitated ones or those with open sores.

In this chapter, we shall consider the evolution of MRSA strains, the mechanisms of gene transfer, transferable resistance to antibiotics and biocides, and suitable hygienic-control measures. Although antibiotics are outside the scope of this book it is impossible to consider the subject adequately without mention of them in relation to biocides.

The evolution of MRSA has still to be elucidated. However, it is not unreasonable to expect that MRSA strains have evolved by the same mechanisms of mutation and gene transfer that exist in other species. The emergence of gentamicin-resistance plasmids illustrates the evolutionary potential of translocatable elements (Lyon & Skurray, 1987). This evolutionary progression is also believed to have occurred in the formation of the β-lactamase heavy-metal resistance plasmids (Shalita *et al.*, 1980).

Although there are examples of isolates resistant to penicillin via β-lactamase, which predate the use of the compound (Parker, 1983), the spread of the phenotype has most probably resulted from selection due to the widespread use of the antibiotic. This argument can be used to account for the emergence of gentamicin-, antiseptic- and disinfectant-resistant strains. In addition, cadmium has been reported to be selective for R^+ staphylococci (Kondo *et al.*, 1974). Staphylococci do not exist in isolation and appear to share a pool of plasmids with other skin flora, such as the streptococci (Murray, 1987). Similarities between plasmids encoding resistance to tetracycline, chloramphenicol and neomycin in *Staph. aureus* and *Staph. epidermidis* have been reported (Rosendorf & Kayser, 1974), as has identity between plasmids encoding gentamicin (Cohen, *et al.*, 1982), cadmium (Cooksey & Baldwin, 1985) and antiseptic (Lyon & Skurray, 1987) resistance.

Antiseptic resistance is considered in more detail later.

1.1.2 *Staphylococcus epidermidis*

Staphylococcus epidermidis is a coagulase-negative staphylococcus that occurs as a universal skin commensal. It is normally present in the resident skin flora but is also found in the gut and in the upper respiratory tract.

Staphylococcus epidermdis is much less pathogenic than *Staph. aureus*. Infections are rarely caused in healthy people but it may be responsible for infective endocarditis in people with prosthetic heat valves and for wound infection following hip-replacement surgery. Genetic exchange may occur with *Staph. aureus*.

1.2 Streptococci

Pyogenic streptococci consist of the most pathogenic human species, *Streptococcus pyogenes* being the most important. This is Lancefield group A. On blood agar, pyogenic streptococci produce complete (β-type) haemolysis. In contrast, *Streptococcus viridans* produces (α-type) haemolysis, denoted by greenish discoloration.

Streptococcus pyogenes produces several enzymes and toxins and may be present as a commensal in the nasopharynx. It causes tonsillitis and skin infections and, rarely, severe infections, e.g. necrotizing fasciitis.

1.3 Enterococci

Also known as Lancefield Group D streptococci, enterococci do not cause haemolysis on blood agar. The most important *Enterococcus* species are *E. faecium*, *E. faecalis* and *E. durans*, which are found in the human and animal gut.

Enterococci may be responsible for causing urinary and abdominal wound infection. As discussed later (Section 3.1), glycopeptide-resistant enterococci are becoming a matter of increasing clinical concern, as are gentamicin-resistant strains (Simjee & Gill, 1997).

1.4 Other cocci

Pneumococci (*Streptococcus pneumoniae*, *Diplococcus pneumoniae*) are now probably the most important pathogen among the streptococci. They are normal commensals of the upper respiratory tract but can be important pathogens, causing lobar pneumonia, meningitis and acute exacerbation of chronic bronchitis. Antibiotic-resistant pneumococci are now known.

Other important pathogenic cocci are *Neisseria meningitidis* (meningococcus), the main cause of meningitis, and *Neisseria gonorrhoeae*, the cause of the worldwide disease, gonorrhoea.

2 Mechanisms of gene transfer

Each of the traditional processes of transfer (transduction, transformation and conjugation) has been described in *Staph. aureus*. However, gene transfer *in vivo* remains to be demonstrated for all but transduction. For additional information, see Thompson (1986, Townsend *et al.* 1986), Evans & Dyke (1988) and Al-Masaudi *et al.* (1991a,b,c,d).

2.1 Transduction

Many clinical isolates possess more than one phage, as a prophage. This lysogenic state has been reported to influence the ability of the host cell to participate in gene exchange. Transduction was recognized early (Lacey, 1975) and assumed to be a major mechanism in the transfer of resistance genes. Calcium ions were found to promote, and chelating agents to interfere with, the transfer (Lacey, 1980). Both small plasmids and chromosomal genes can be transduced (Novick & Morse, 1968; Stiffler *et al.*, 1974; Kono & Sasatsu, 1976; Iordanescu, 1977). Transduction, via a cell-free lysate, typically occurs at a frequency of 10^{-6} per recipient.

2.2 Transformation

Staphylococcus aureus can be transformed by exogenous deoxyribonucleic acid (DNA), but cells are only competent for a short period, immediately prior to entry into the stationary phase (Rudin *et al.*, 1974; Pattee & Neveln, 1975). This is due to the transient absence of an exonuclease and consequently it is thought that transfer by this route will be low *in vivo*. This conclusion should perhaps be questioned until evidence is presented to demonstrate clearly that cells are not in this physiological state on skin for significant periods.

2.3 Conjugation

Different types of conjugation are known to exist in staphylococci. These are phage-mediated conjugation and plasmid-mediated conjugation. In addition, conjugative transposons have been discovered, which appear mechanistically to fall in the latter class.

2.3.1 Phage-mediated conjugation

Phage-mediated conjugation occurs in mixed cultures of lysogens and recipients (Lacey, 1980). Transfer frequencies per recipient of plasmids can be very high, over 10^{-1}, and Barr *et al.* (1986) have shown that subinhibitory concentrations of β-lactam antibiotics induced a 100–1000-fold increase in plasmid transfer frequency. This process is deoxyribonuclease-insensitive (Schaeffler, 1982).

2.3.2 Plasmid-mediated conjugation

Plasmid-mediated conjugation is a surface preferred system of transfer in *Staph. aureus* (Archer & Johnson, 1983). It is different from phage-mediated transfer, because cell contact is obligatory (Townsend *et al.*, 1986). Plasmids have not been identified in all cases of conjugal transfer. For example, El Solh *et al.* (1986) were unable to detect any plasmid DNA in recipients. This is perhaps indicative of conjugative transposons. Broad host-range plasmids which can transfer resistance between staphylococci and streptococci are known (Buu-Hoi *et al.*, 1984). This and similarities between antibiotic resistances (Schaberg & Zervos, 1986) together suggest that genetic exchange occurs between these genera *in vivo*.

2.3.3 Conjugative transposons

Conjugative transposons (El Solh *et al.*, 1986)

have been identified, although few of these non-plasmid transfer systems have been examined in any detail (Clewell & Gawron-Burke, 1986). These are transferable to and between staphylococci, and their resistances are expressed in a wide variety of Gram-positive bacteria; both properties make their investigation of clinical importance.

3 Transferable resistance to antibiotics and biocides

3.1 Resistance to antibacterial agents

Transfer of penicillin and chloramphenicol resistance plasmids occurs in mixed cultures of *Staph. epidermidis* and *Staph. aureus* (Witte, 1977). Intraspecies transfer of gentamicin resistance plasmids can also occur on skin (Lacey, 1975; Noble & Naidoo, 1978). These plasmids can also mobilize smaller plasmids, encoding resistance to tetracycline, chloramphenicol and erythromycin (Naidoo, 1984). Frequent exchange of natural plasmids between natural bacteria is not unusual (Bale *et al.*, 1988; Courvalin, 1994, 1996). Conjugative plasmids can transfer efficiently among Gram-positive and Gram-negative bacteria of different genera and can conjugate between the two groups; they cannot, however, establish themselves stably by replication into the new host, because their host range for replication is less broad than for transfer (Courvalin, 1996).

Plasmid-mediated resistance to glycopeptide antibiotics has been successfully conjugated from enterococci to *Staph. aureus* in laboratory experiments (Noble *et al.*, 1992), provided that erythromycin and not vancomycin was used as the selective agent. It has also been found, however, that conjugative plasmid transfer in *Staph. aureus* can be enhanced by the exposure of mating cells to subinhibitory concentrations of vancomycin, gentamicin (Al-Masaudi *et al.*, 1991a,b,c,d) or β-lactam antibiotics (Barr *et al.*, 1986).

Inducible resistance to high levels of vancomycin in enterococci is mediated by transposon Tn 1546 or related transposons (Arthur *et al.*, 1996). The transposition of Tn *1546* into plasmids with a broad host range or into conjugative transposons would enable resistance to spread clinically to organisms, such as *Staph. aureus*, which exchange genetic information with enterococci (Arthur *et al.*, 1996).

In intrinsically resistant genera and in *Staph. aureus*, glycopeptide resistance is expressed constitutively, as distinct from the inducible high- and low-level resistance in enterococci (Woodford *et al.*, 1991). High-level resistance to gentamicin in *E. faecium* is well documented (Woodford *et al.*, 1992).

Bacterial drug resistance is an increasing global problem (Parliamentary Office, 1994; Tenover & McGowan 1996). Hospital infections caused by multidrug-resistant (MDR) strains of *Staph. aureus*, enterococci and *Strep. pneumoniae* are of concern and can be difficult to control (Casewell, 1995; McGowan & Metchock, 1995; Wade, 1995).

Tennent *et al.* (1985) reported the finding in a *Staph. aureus* isolate of a plasmid, pSK1, which encoded resistance to ethidium bromide, acriflavine, benzalkonium chloride and other quaternary ammonium compounds (QACs), gentamicin, tobramycin, kanamycin and trimethoprim.

The term 'nucleic-acid-binding (NAB) compound' has been used to describe those compounds that bind strongly to DNA (Townsend *et al.*, 1984a,b; Kigbo *et al.*, 1985). Cetyltrimethylammonium bromide (CTAB), a QAC, has been used (Townsend *et al.*, 1985) for the rapid isolation of plasmid DNA, although it must be pointed out that the concentration (0.5% w/v, 5000 μg/ml) of CTAB used for this purpose is very different, by a factor of 50–100, from those concentrations employed in sensitivity and resistance studies with MRSA strains.

Staphylococcus aureus strains carry a variety of plasmids, many of which encode antibiotic resistance (Bigelow *et al.*, 1989). Resistance to acridines (Ac^R), ethidium bromide (Eb^R), QACs (Qa^R) and propamidine isethionate (PI^R) is mediated by a common determinant on a group of structurally related plasmids (see also below). Many of these plasmids carry the gentamicin, tobramycin and kanamycin resistance transposon Tn *4001* and also encode resistance to the dihydrofolate reductase inhibitor, trimethoprim (Lyon *et al.*, 1984; Gillespie *et al.*, 1986; Skurray *et al.*, 1988). The prototype of this group of plasmids is pSK1; its genes have been cloned into an *Escherichia coli* vector, in which these resistances are then expressed (Tennent *et al.*, 1985). Yamamoto *et al.* (1988) have reported cloning chlorhexidine resistance into *E. coli*.

Townsend *et al.* (1984a) proposed that resistance to CTAB and to the diamidine, propamidine isethionate (PI) was linked, and that these biocides acted as a selective pressure for the retention of plasmids encoding resistance to them. In the laboratory, CTAB could not be employed as a selective genetic marker, because strains with plasmids carrying the R determinant were only about three to four times as resistant as plasmidless strains (Table 10.9). With PI, however, there was up to a 32-fold difference in minimal inhibitory concentration (MIC) values (Table 10.9). Cookson & Phillips (1988) found that resistance to aminoglycoside antibiotics and to PI, cetrimide (equivalent to CTAB) and ethidium bromide always transferred together.

There are at least three genes determining biocide resistance in *Staph. aureus* isolates, (Emslie *et al.*, 1985, 1986; Skurray *et al.*, 1988; Gillespie et *al.*, 1989, 1990). These are *qac*A, located on the pSK1 family of plasmids described above, encoding resistance to acridines, ethidium bromide, QACs and PI; *qac*B, which is similar; and *qac*C, which encodes resistance to QACs and low-level ethidium bromide, but is genetically unrelated to either the *qac*A or *qac*B determinants. The *qac*A determinant also specifies low-level resistance to chlorhexidine (Gillespie *et al.*, 1989). The *qac*C gene is identical to *ebr* and *smr*. Other determinants, *qac*D and *qac*E, have also been described. Properties of the *qac* genes are summarized in Table 10.10, and MICs of cationic biocides

Table 10.9 Effects of biocides on MRSA and MSSA strains.

Biocide	MIC (μg/ml) MSSA	MRSA	References*
Cetrimide/CTAB	1.6	6.25	1
	1.5	2.5–5	2
Chlorhexidine	2	4–8	3
	1.5	2–2.5	2
Benzalkonium chloride	<1	6	1
Acriflavine	30	340	4
Ethidium bromide	4	180	4
Propamidine isethionate (PI)	16	512	1
Parabens			
Methyl	2000	2000	2
Ethyl	1000	1000	2
Propyl	400	400	2
Butyl	125	125	2
Phenols			
Phenol	2000	2000	2
Cresol	750	1250	2
Chlorocresol	200	200	2

*1, Townsend *et al.* (1984a); 2, Al-Masaudi *et al.* (1988); 3, Brumfitt *et al.* (1985); 4, Gillespie *et al.* (1986).
MSSA, methicillin-sensitive *Staph. aureus*.

Table 10.10 The *qac* genes and resistance to quaternary ammonium compounds (QACs) and other biocides.

Multidrug resistance determinant	Gene location	Biocide resistance encoded
*qac*A gene	Predominant: pSK1 family of multiresistance plasmids Other: β-lactamase and heavy-metal resistance plasmids	Intercalating agents, QACs, diamidine, biguanides
*qac*B gene	β-Lactamase and heavy-metal resistance plasmids	Intercalating agents, QACs
*qac*C gene*	Small plasmids (<3 kb) or large conjugative plasmids	Ethidium bromide, some QACs
*qac*D gene*	Large (50 kb), conjugative multiresistance plasmids, e.g. pJE1 and pSK41	Ethidium bromide, some QACs

* Have identical phenotypes and show restriction-site homology.

againts. *Staph. aureus* strains harbouring these genes are presented in Table 10.11.

3.2 Possible genetic linkage between antibiotic and biocide resistance

It was pointed out above (Townsend *et al.*, 1984a) that some cationic biocides acted as a selective pressure for the retention of plasmids encoding resistance to them. Similar conclusions have been reached as a consequence of other studies elsewhere in Australia and in Europe and the USA (Littlejohn *et al.*, 1992; Reverdy *et al.*, 1992, 1993; Behr *et al.*, 1994; Leelaporn *et al.*, 1994; Heir *et al.*, 1995; Paulsen *et al.*, 1996a,b).

Behr *et al.* (1994) detected the *qac*A gene in 85% of clinical isolates of *Staph. aureus* resistant to antiseptics (benzalkonium, hexamidine, chlorhexidine, acriflavine) and ethidium bromide, but not in susceptible strains. Reverdy *et al.* (1992, 1993) postulated that, in the hospital environment, antiseptic usage might select resistant strains. Leelaporn *et al.* (1994) proposed that the prevalence of multidrug export *qac* genes in *Staph. aureus* and in coagulase-negative staphylococci was a consequence of the selective pressure imposed by the use of antiseptics.

Increased resistance, based on MICs, of biocides have been observed in MRSA strains possessing resistance to gentamicin (MGRSA). However, MRSA or MGRSA strains do not always show greater biocide resistance (Almasaudi *et al.*, 1991a,b,d), although this could result from the inherent stability of the GNAB plasmid that encodes resistance to gentamicin and the NAB compounds (Cookson *et al.*, 1991a). Curing of this plasmid reduced the MIC of chlorhexidine. However, MRSA and MGRSA strains were inactivated by the biguanide as readily as methicillin-sensitive (MSSA) ones (Cookson *et al.*, 1991a).

The MRSA strains with low-level resistance to chlorhexidine are sensitive to triclosan, but MRSA strains that express low-level triclosan resistance, but with no resistance to NAB compounds, have been isolated from patients treated with nasal mupirocin and daily triclosan baths (Cookson *et al.*, 1991b). Triclosan resistance could be cotransferred with mupirocin resistance to sensitive *Staph. aureus* strains, but there is no evidence to suggest that the mechanism of triclosan resistance is linked

Table 10.11 MIC values (μg/ml) for strains of *Staph. aureus* carrying various *qac* genes (abstracted from Littlejohn *et al.*, 1992).

		Dyes			Biguanide:	Diamidines		Quaternary ammonium compounds		
qac Gene	Plasmid	Ethidium bromide	Proflavine	Crystal violet	Chlorhexidine	Pentamidine isethionate	Propamidine isethionate	Cetyltrimethylammonium bromide	Benzalkonium chloride	Cetylpyridinium chloride
A	pSK 1	300	>640	2	2	800	>800	4	6	4
B	pSK 21	250	320	2	0.8	800	100	2	6	2
C	pSK 89	100	40	0.25	0.8	<50	50	6	6	6
D	pSK 41	100	40	0.25	0.8	<50	50	6	6	6
–	SK 982 (Host)	<25	40	0.25	0.8	<50	50	1	<2	1

to the efflux mechanism associated with NAB compounds (see Section 4.1). The MIC values of triclosan of 100 μg/ml against sensitive *Staph. aureus* and of > 6400 μg/ml against triclosan-resistant strains (Sasatsu *et al.*, 1993) are highly inaccurate and reflect the use of a triclosan formulation rather than a triclosan solution (Uhl, 1993).

Inorganic (Hg^{2+}) and organomercury resistance is a common property of strains of *Staph. aureus* that carry penicillinase plasmids (Lyon & Skurray, 1987; Silver & Misra, 1998). Inorganic mercury compounds have little if any role to play in antisepsis or disinfection, whereas organomercurials, such as thiomersal, phenylmercuric nitrate and phenylmercuric acetate, are important pharmaceutical preservaties.

4 Mechanisms of biocide resistance in staphylococci

It is always of fundamental importance not only to record bacterial resistance to antibiotics and/or biocides but also to understand the mechanisms of such resistance. For convenience this section is subdivided into two parts, the first of which deals with efflux in MRSA strains and the second, briefly, with other instances of staphylococcal resistance.

4.1 Efflux from methicillin-resistant *Staphylococcus aureus* strains

Resistance of MRSA strains to cationic-type biocides may arise and may be plasmid-associated (Townsend *et al.*, 1983, 1984a,b; Lyon *et al.*, 1984, 1986; Jones & Midgley, 1985; Kigbo *et al.*, 1985; Emslie *et al.*, 1985, 1986; Gillespie *et al.*, 1986, 1989, 1990; Lyon & Skurray, 1987; Skurray *et al.*, 1988; Rouch *et al.*, 1990; Levy 1992; Littlejohn *et al.*, 1992; Leelaporn *et al.*, 1994; Midgley, 1994; Sasatsu *et al.*, 1995; Paulsen *et al.*, 1996a,b). Furthermore, recombinant plasmids have been transferred from *Staph. aureus* to *E. coli* (Tennent *et al.*, 1985; Yamamoto *et al.*, 1988; Table 10.12); these encode resistance to various cationic biocides, although often at fairly low levels.

There are various reasons that could possibly be put forward for biocide resistance in MRSA strains (see Table 10.13 for a summary). First, the surface of these cells could differ from MSSA cells. Al-Masaudi *et al.* (1988a) showed that MSSA strains were typically hydrophobic, a property likely to be determined by a protein or protein-associated molecule located at the celt surface. However, wide differences occurred with MRSA strains, different solvent systems produced different responses and there was little correlation when different methods of assessing hydrophobicity were employed. Secondly, there could be biocide inactivation systems present within MRSA but not MSSA strains—no evidence has been found to support this convention. Finally, reduced uptake of a biocide could result from an efficient efflux mechanism present in MRSA but not in MSSA strains. Evidence to substantiate this hypothesis has been produced by Jones & Midgley (1985) for ethidium bromide, thus explaining the earlier diminished-uptake findings of Johnston & Dyke (1969), and for QACs. Jones & Midgley (1985) cloned a 1.1kb DNA fragment (specifying resistance to ethidium bromide and QACs) from an MRSA strain into a plasmid vector in *E. coli*, but did not examine the Gram-negative cell to determine whether any plasmid-mediated cell envelope changes occurred. These authors reached two interesting conclusions, namely that resistance to QACs and ethidium bromide had the same efflux basis as resistance to Cd^{2+}, tetracyclines, arsenate and arsenite, and that the primary target site of QACs and ethidium bromide must likewise be intracellular.

Active-efflux systems comprise an important mechanism for both intrinsic and acquired resistance (Levy, 1992). Although some of these systems are highly specific, others export a broad

Table 10.12 Plasmid-mediated resistance to cationic biocides in strains of *Staphylococcus aureus* and *Escherichia coli* (based on the data of Yamamoto *et al.*, 1988).

	P^+/P^-:MIC ratio	
Biocide	*Staph. aureus*	*E. coli*
Chlorhexidine gluconate	2	4–8
Benzalkonium chloride	2	4
Acriflavine	128	8
Ethidium bromide	64	16

P^+, Plasmid-bearing strain; P^-, isogenic plasmidless strain; the P^+ *E. coli* strain carries recombinant plasmid from *Staph. aureus*.

Table 10.13 Postulated mechanisms of resistance of MRSA strains to biocides.

Class of biocide	Examples	Resistance mechanism	Comment
QAC	Cetrimide/CTAB Benzalkonium chloride	Efflux	Found in MRSA but not in MSSA strains; low level resistance
Diamidines	Propamidine Dibromopropamidine	Efflux	High-level resistance
DNA-intercalating agents	Acriflavine Acridine orange	Efflux	Reduced uptake; high-level resistance
	Ethidium bromide	Efflux	
Biguanides	Chlorhexidine salts	Efflux	Very low-level resistance only

range of toxic compounds and are termed 'multidrug transporters' (Rouch *et al.*, 1990; Midgley, 1994). In *Staph. aureus*, resistance to intercalating dyes and QACs mediated by the *qac*A gene on the pSK1 plasmid is specified by an energy-dependent mechanism (Rouch *et al.*, 1990). The QacA exporter has a common ancestry with tetracycline-resistance and sugar-uptake proteins. Rouch *et al.* (1990) believe that the *qac*A determinant evolved considerably prior to the widespread use of antiseptics and disinfectants and that, as such, it might aid the survival of *Staph. aureus* in the hospital environment. The *qac*A gene confers resistance via proton-motive force (pmf)-dependent efflux (Paulsen *et al.*, 1996a,b).

The *ebr* gene is identical to the *qac*C/*qac*D gene family (Littlejohn *et al.*, 1991). Sasatsu *et al.* (1994, 1995) detected the *ebr* gene not only in resistant but also in sensitive strains of *Staph. aureus*, as well as in coagulase-negative staphylococci and in enterococcal strains. The authors concluded that, in antiseptic-resistant cells, there was an increase in the copy number of an *ebr* gene on the chro-mosome or on a plasmid, because no mutations were found in the nucleotide sequences of the amplified DNA fragments.

4.2 Other staphylococcal resistance

Other resistance mechanisms of staphylococci to biocides have been described. *Staphylococcus aureus* strains isolated from poultry-processing plants may be resistant to chlorine, either because they grow in macroclumps or because they produce an extracellular slime layer (Bolton *et al.*, 1988). Mucoid-grown *Staph. aureus* cells are less sensitive than non-mucoid ones to several commercial antiseptics and disinfectants; if the mucoid-grown cells are washed in saline or subcultured in brain heart infusion (BHI) broth, they become sensitive to these biocides, demonstrating that the extracellular slime layer, which forms a physical barrier around organisms, is an efficient resistant mechanism (Kolawole, 1984).

The staphylococci referred to by Bolton *et al.* (1988) and Kolawole (1984) are not MRSA strains. It is not known whether MRSA strains *in vivo* produce a slime layer or glycocalyx that could be a contributory factor in conferring resistance to antibiotics and/or biocides.

Little is known about the way in which biocides enter MRSA cells, although presumably this is achieved by passive diffusion across the cell wall. Interestingly, the important topical antiseptic mupirocin is equally effective against MRSA and MSSA strains, whereas deep rough, but not wild-type, strains of Gram-negative bacteria are sensitive, indicating a barrier role in normal Gram-negative bacteria but not in MRSA or MSSA (Al-Masaudi *et al.*, 1988b).

5 Control of methicillin-resistant *Staphylococcus aureus* strains

5.1 Relevance of elevated minimal inhibitory concentrations

It was pointed out above that MRSA strains might

show considerably enhanced resistance to ethidium bromide, crystal violet, acridines and diamidines but only slightly enhanced resistance to QACs and chlorhexidine. Generally, however, the conclusions have been based solely upon MICs and should be put into perspective. Brumfitt *et al.* (1985) found that MRSA strains were only slightly more resistant to chlorhexidine than were MSSA ones. Al-Masaudi *et al.* (1988a) could find no difference in response to chlorhexidine, only a slight difference with QACs but a marked difference with dibromopropamidine isethionate (DBPI). Some of the findings quoted above also demonstrate only a slight increase in resistance to QACs (Lyon *et al.*, 1984; Townsend *et al.*, 1984a) or chlorhexidine (Littlejohn *et al.*, 1992). Lacey *et al.* (1986) confirm much higher resistance of MRSA strains to PI and ethidium bromide, but regard increases in resistance to QACs (2.67–4-fold) and chlorhexidine (twofold) as being 'trivial'. In fact, Lacey & Kruczenyk (1986) are critical of the emphasis placed by the Australian workers on resistance to NAB agents in MRSA strains. This is because they are unlikely to be exposed to agents such as ethidium bromide, whereas gentamicin resistance is considered to be a much more plausible selection pressure. Marples & Cooke (1988) pointed out that resistance to QACs is due to a plasmid-coded efflux system (Section 4.1), but added that resistance at this level probably has no clinical significance.

Furthermore, of the non-antibiotic agents described by the Australian workers, ethidium bromide is not used as an antiseptic or disinfectant, the acridines are used rarely and the diamidines are reserved for specific purposes e.g. PI in the treatment of blepharitis and acute and chronic conjunctivitis, and pentamidine isethionate in the treatment of pneumonia caused by *Pneumocystis carinii*, particularly in acquired immune deficiency syndrome (AIDS) patients, leaving just the QACs and chlorhexidine. Resistance to the former is not particularly marked and to the latter it is slight, if any. The question must be raised, therefore, as to whether antiseptic resistance is of particular significance in terms of the potential for survival in the hospital environment (Gillespie *et al.*, 1986) or whether, as suggested by Lacey (1987), the MRSA strains have been selected by intense antibiotic usage in hospitals. It is particularly interesting to note that antiseptic resistance in clinical MRSA isolates has now been located on the chromosome (Rahman *et al.*, 1988; Gillespie *et al.*, 1989), thereby leading to the acquisition of genes to form a multiresistant chromosome.

It is, perhaps, unfortunate that most studies have expressed resistance in terms of MIC values, because the factor of overriding importance must be the inactivation of MRSA in the clinical situation. Haley *et al.* (1985) have studied the bactericidal activity of antiseptics against MRSA and MSSA. The MSSA strains were more sensitive to Phisohex (containing hexa-chlorophane) and *p*-chloro-*m*-xylenol, but showed the same response as MRSA strains to povidone-iodine and a chlorhexidine-based product.

Cookson *et al.* (1991a) queried whether an elevated MIC of chlorhexidine truly meant a rise in resistance and showed that the biguanide inactivated *Staph. aureus* strains with or without the GNAB plasmid. Likewise, mupirocin- and triclosan-resistant *Staph. aureus* has been found (Cookson *et al.*, 1991b) to be inactivated at a similar rate to that of sensitive strains. Cookson (1994) voiced concern that antiseptice resistance in MRSA strains could be an emerging problem, but, using an *in vivo* rate-of-kill less that mimics a hand-washing procedure, he found no difference in the activity of chlorhexidine on human skin for isolates of MSSA with or without an elevated MIC due to a transferred NAB resistance plasmid.

Further caution is needed when considering some published findings. For example, Sasatsu *et al.* (1994) refer to a high-level resistant strain of *Staph. aureus*; yet MIC values of chlorhexidine, butylparaben and CTAB were identical to those quoted for a low-level resistant strain. Furthermore, the observed MIC (>3200 μg/ml) for methylparaben was well in excess of the known aqueous solubility of this compound.

Attempts to train MSSA (Fitzgerald *et al.*, 1992) or MRSA (Cookson *et al.*, 1991a) to stable chlorhexidine resistance have been unsuccessful. Nicoletti *et al.* (1993) claimed to have trained staphylococci and other bacteria to show stable resistance to chlorhexidine and other biocides, but precipitation of test compounds in their procedure casts considerable doubt on their findings.

5.2 Clinical aspects

Increasing numbers worldwide of nosocomial infections are caused by MRSA strains (Coello *et al.*, 1994). These strains particularly affect patients in intensive-care units (Lejeune *et al.*, 1986). Gentamicin resistance suddenly appeared in the UK in 1976, and MGRSA strains caused severe major hospital outbreaks (Shanson, 1986). The reasons for the re-emergence of MRSA strains are unclear; contributory factors may be the increased use of β-lactam antibiotics especially cephalosporins, and the widespread use of gentamicin, leading to the selection of MGRSA strains. Australian workers have proposed that, since resistance to NAB compounds was prevalent in the staphylococcal population long before the emergence of gentamicin resistance (Emslie *et al.*, 1985, 1986), antiseptic resistance is of particular significance in terms of the potential for their survival in the hospital environment (Gillespie *et al.*, 1986). However, of the NAB compounds, ethidium bromide is not employed as an antiseptic or disinfectant, the acridines and crystal violet find little application in modern medicine, QACs have a limited use in hospitals, because of their narrow spectrum (Ayliffe *et al.*, 1992), and only chlorhexidine is widely used (Russell & Day, 1993, 1996). Furthermore, as pointed out in Section 5.1, MIC tests are unsuitable for assessing clinical usefulness (such as handwashing: Platt & Bucknall, 1988). Diamidines have limited, specific uses.

The studies on antiseptic resistance in staphylococci suggest that antiseptics and disinfectants have little role to play in controlling infections caused by MRSA or EMRSA strains. Doubt has, in fact, been cast on the efficacy of some antiseptic preparations. Shanson (1986), for instance, stated that colonized patient skin sites should be treated with antiseptics, but added that their clinical efficacy for eradicating MRSA had not been established. The uncertainties in the efficacy of topical antibiotic and antiseptic preparations were also pointed out in Report (1986), although mupirocin gave good results and antiseptic detergents for washing and daily bathing appeared to be satisfactory. Tuffnell *et al.* (1987) claimed that antiseptic body washing was of debatable use, but proposed that triclosan, a phenolic that has prolonged surface action, was better for this purpose than hexachlorophane.

Casewell (1995) discussed the evolution of MRSA and, in particular, of EMRSA-16 (the 'Kettering strain'), which has an extraordinary ability for hospital-wide spread and which is impossible to eliminate from some hospitals. Mupirocin was recommended for nasal carriage, although resistance to this antibiotic could emerge. Another strain, EMRSA-15, has spread rapidly in the West Midlands. Ayliffe *et al.* (1992) described appropriate control procedures for EMRSA strains. Nasal treatment with mupirocin was advocated, associated with bathing, washing and shampooing with antiseptic detergents, such as chlorhexidine, povidone-iodine (which has a superior *in vitro* lethal effect to chlorhexidine (McLure & Gordon, 1992)) or triclosan, with similar agents used by staff for hand-washing. A Working party (Report, 1990) had earlier produced revised guidelines for control of MRSA, which were essentially the same. Noticeably, the only QAC recommended was cetrimide, for use as a shampoo (chlorhexidine detergent is drying to the skin), and, although it was observed that some EMRSA strains showed a slightly increased resistance to chlorhexidine, it was concluded that the clinical relevance was doubtful. A similar comment was made by Rutala (1995). Isolation of patients in a purpose-built, dedicated isolation unit, reduction of movement by patients and staff and appropriate screening proceduces all have an important role to play (Coello *et al.*, 1994; Casewell, 1995).

In a review of hospital disinfection policies, Coates & Hutchinson (1994) devoted little attention to the control of MRSA or EMRSA. Baquero *et al.* (1991) quoted work demonstrating that there was no association between the usage of chlorhexidine in a variety of circumstances in the hospital environment and the emergence of chlorhexidine resistance. Nevertheless, they issued a cautionary warning. The presence of specific resistance mechanisms to antibiotics frequently contributes to the long-term selection of resistant variants under *in vivo* conditions, despite large differences in MIC values and the expected drug concentration at the site of the infection. They recommended that antiseptic susceptibility should be tested on a yearly basis. Tenover & McGowan. (1996) discussed the reasons for the emergence of antibiotic-resistant bacteria, including staphylococci, but made no mention of antiseptic resistance as being a possible contributory factor. Of course, adhesion of bacteria to the skin may be an important factor, especially as little is known about local concentrations of antiseptics.

One final observation is worthy of comment here. Millns *et al.* (1994) reported that staphylococci on the hands of dental students and theatre staff retained sensitivity to chlorhexidine and a QAC (cetylpyridinium chloride (CPC)) after exposure to Hibiscrub or CPC-coated gloves.

6 Other cocci

Although other cocci (Sections 1.2–1.4) are important pathogens, there is little published information about their response to biocides although matters are improving (Anderson *et al.*, 1997).

Antibiotic-resistant enterococci have emerged as significant pathogens (Arthur *et al.*, 1996). However, irresponsive of antibiotic susceptibility or resistance, MICs of various strains of *E. faecium* and *E. faecalis* to phenolics and parabens showed a similar pattern, with greater variation when chlorhexidine and two QACs were studied. Variations, but not linked to antibiotic response, were also observed in the lethal effects of chlorhexidine (Alqurashi *et al.*, 1996). Baillie *et al.* (1992) had earlier demonstrated chlorhexidine sensitivity in vancomycin- and gentamicin-resistant *E. faecium*. Bradley & Fraise (1996) observed variation in the tolerance of clinical isolates of enterococci to biocides, but there was no correlation between the effect of a biocide (glutaraldehyde, alcohol or a chlorine-releasing agent) and vancomycin resistance.

An interesting finding was made by Sasatsu *et al.* (1995), who detected the presence of the *ebr* gene (identical to *qac*C/*qac*D) in all strains of enterococci tested. They suggested that its product acted to remove toxic substances.

Baird-Parter & Holbrook (1971) described the sensitivity of various types of cocci to a range of chemical agents. Most of the information provided dealt with staphylococci. However, streptococci were listed as being more sensitive to alcohols and glycols and, in our experience, tend to be rather more sensitive than enterococci to many biocides. The emergence of antibiotic-resistant pneumococci (McGowan & Metchock, 1995) suggests that the effects of different biocides on *Strep. pneumoniae* should be investigated. *Streptococcus mutans*, the main initiating organism of caries, is particularly sensitive to chlorhexidine (Grönroos *et al.*, 1995). *In vitro* development of chlorhexidine resistance in *Streptococcus sanguis* and transmissibility by transformation were claimed by Westergren & Emilson (1980), but this finding remains unsubstantiated.

7 Conclusions

The MRSA/EMRSA strains are capable of causing severe infections, particularly in debilitated patients. They have now spread to many hospitals in most countries of the world, due to selection by widespread use of antibiotics and person-to-person spread. The epidemic strains seem to have a propensity for spreading, but no laboratory test for this factor is available. Lacey & Kruczenyk (1986) considered that too much prominence was given to NAB compounds, such as ethidium bromide, and it is noteworthy that resistance to ethidium bromide was reported to be carried on a penicillinase plasmid as far back as 1969 (Dyke, 1969).

We have seen, and therefore should expect, new disease problems to arise coincidentally with the emergence of new strains with novel gene combinations. These are most likely to arise from gene-transfer processes, as the evolution of novel resistance genes is believed to be a very rare event. If resistance is acquired from coresident strains, it becomes important to understand the process of gene exchange. The key for control is thus to identify ways and means of inhibiting and reducing gene transfer *in vivo*. In a competitive, challenging and changing environment, bacteria have acquired mechanisms for the transfer and receipt of genes from a pool of associated organisms. The adoption of stringent and scientifically planned hygiene practices will no doubt show if infections may be controlled and if past practices and antimicrobial usage have acted to select for MRSA and EMRSA strains, or whether their emergence was due to other factors. Monitoring of clinical isolates of MRSA/EMRSA and of vancomycin-insensitive *Staph aureus* (VISA) for antiseptic resistance on a regular basis should provide useful information.

Studies with other cocci provide little information about biocide suspectibility, and there is a need for additional data in this area.

Effective control measures (Humphreys & Duckworth, 1997) are essential (however, see also Barrett *et al.*, 1998). It is worrying that resistance to mupirocin is now often found in MRSA strains (Eltringham, 1997).

8 References

Al-Masaudi, S.B., Day, M.J. & Russell, A.D. (1988a) Sensitivity of methicillin-resistant *Staphylococcus aureus* strains to some antibiotics, antiseptics and disinfectants. *Journal of Applied Bacteriology,* **65**, 329–337.

Al-Masaudi, S.B., Russell, A.D. & Day, M.J. (1988b) Activity of mupirocin against *Staphylococcus aureus* and outer membrane mutants of Gram-negative bacteria. *Letters in Applied Microbiology*, **7**, 45–47.

Al-Masaudi, S.B., Day, M.J. & Russell, A.D. (1991a) Antimicrobial resistance and gene transfer in *Staphylococcus aureus. Journal of Applied Bacteriology*, **70**, 279–290.

Al-Masaudi, S.B., Day, M.J. & Russell, A.D. (1991b) Effect of some antibiotics and biocides on plasmid transfer in *Staphylococcus aureus. Journal of Applied Bacteriology*, **71**, 239–243.

Al-Masaudi, S.B., Russell, A.D. & Day, M.J. (1991c) Comparative sensitivity to antibiotics and biocides of methicillin-resistant *Staphylococcus aureus* strains isolated from Saudi Arabia and Great Britain. *Journal of Applied Bacteriology*, **71**, 331–338.

Al-Masaudi, S.B., Rusell, A.D. & Day, M.J. (1991d) Factors affecting conjugative transfer of plasmid pWG613, determining gentamicin resistance, in *Staphylococcus aureus. Journal of Medical Microbiology*, **34**, 103–107.

Alqurashi, A.M., Day, M.J. & Russell, A.D. (1996) Susceptibility of some strains of entercocci and streptococci to antibiotics and biocides. *Journal of Antimicrobial Chemotherapy*, **38**, 745.

Anderson, R.L., Carr, J.H., Bond, W.W. & Favero, M.S. (1997) Susceptibility of vancomycin-resistant enterococci to environmental disinfectants. *Infection Control and Hospital Epidemiology*, **18**, 195–199.

Archer, G.L. & Johnson, J.L. (1983) Self transmissible plasmids in staphylococci that encode resistance to aminoglycosides. *Antimicrobial Agents and Chemotherapy*, **24**, 70–77.

Arthur, M., Reynolds, P.E., Depardieu, F. *et al.* (1996) Mechanisms of glycopeptide resistance in enterococci. *Journal of Infection*, **32**, 11–16.

Ayliffe, G.A.J., Babb, J.R. & Bradley, C.R. (1992) 'Sterilization' of arthroscopes and laparoscopes. *Journal of Hospital Infection*, **22**, 265–269.

Ballie, L.W.J., Wade, J.J. & Casewell, M.W. (1992) Chlorhexidine sensitivity of *Enterococcus faecium* resistant to vancomycin, high levels of gentamicin, or both. *Journal of Hospital Infection*, **20**, 127–128.

Baird-Parker, A.C. & Holbrook, R. (1971) The inhibition and destruction of cocci. In *Inhibition and Destruction of the Microbial Cell* (ed. Hugo, W.B.), pp. 369–397. London: Academic Press.

Bale, M.J., Fry, J.C. & Day, M.J. (1988) Transfer and occurrence of large mercury resistance plasmids in river epilithon. *Applied and Environmental Microbiology*, **54**, 972–978.

Baquero, F., Patron, C., Canton, R. & Ferrer, M. (1991) Laboratory and *in-vitro* testing of skin antiseptic: a prediction for *in-vivo* activity? *Journal of Hospital Infection*, **18**, (Suppl. B) 5–11.

Barr, V., Barr, K., Millar, M.R. & Lacey, R.W. (1986) β-Lactam antibiotics increase the frequency of plasmid tranfer in *Staphylococcus aureus. Antimicrobial Agents and Chemotherapy*, **17**, 409–413.

Barrett, S.P., Mummery, S.V. & Chattopadhyay, B. (1998) Trying to control MRSA causes more problems than it solves. *Journal of Hospital Infection*, **39**, 85–93.

Behr, H., Reverdy, M.E., Mabilat, C., Freney, J. & Fleurette, J. (1994) Relationship between the level of minimal inhibitory concentrations of five antiseptics and the presence of *qac*A gene in *Staphylococcus aureus. Pathologie Biologie*, **42**, 438–444.

Bigelow, N., Ng, L.-K., Robson, H.G. & Dillon, J.R. (1989) Strategies for molecular characterisation of methicillin and gentamicin-resistant *Staphylococcus aureus* in a Canadian nosocomial outbreak. *Journal of Medical Microbiology*, **30**, 51–58.

Bolton, K.J., Dodd, C.E.R., Mead, G.C. & Waites, W.M. (1988) Chlorine resistance of strains of *Staphylococcus aureus* isolated from poultry processing plants. *Letters in Applied Microbiology*, **6**, 31–34.

Bradley, C.R. & Fraise, A.P. (1996) Heat and chemical resistance in enterococci. *Journal of Hospital Infection*, **34**, 191–196.

Brumfitt, W., Dixson, S. & Hamilton-Miller, J.M.T. (1985) Resistance to antiseptics in methicillin and gentamicin resistant *Staphylococcus aureus. Lancet*, **i**, 1442–1443.

Buu-Hoi, A., Bieth, G. & Horaud, T. (1984) Broad host range of streptococcal macrolide resistance plasmids. *Antimicrobial Agents and Chemotherapy*, **25**, 289–291.

Cafferkey, M.T., Hone, R. & Keane, C.T. (1988) Sources

and outcome for methicillin-resistant *Staphylococcus aureus* bacteremia. *Journal of Hospital Infection*, **11**, 136–143.

Casewell, M.W. (1995) New threats to the control of methicillin-resistant *Staphylococcus aureus*. *Journal of Hospital Infection*, 30 (Suppl.), 465–471.

Clewell, D.B. & Gawron-Burke, C. (1986) Conjugative transposons and the dissemination of antibiotic resistance in streptococci. *Annual Review of Microbiology*, **40**, 635–659.

Coates, D. & Hutchinson, D.N. (1994) How to produce a hospital disinfection policy. *Journal of Hospital Infection*, **26**, 57–68.

Coello, R., Jiménez, J., Garcia, M. *et al.* (1994) Prospective study of infection, colonization and carriage of methicillin-resistant *Staphylococcus aureus* in an outbreak affecting 990 patients. *European Journal of Clinical Microbiology and Infectious Diseases*, **13**, 74–81.

Cohen, M.L., Wong, E.S. & Falkow, S. (1982) Common R-plasmids in *Staphylococcus aureus* and *Staphylococcus epidermidis* during a nosocomial *Staphylococcus aureus* outbreak. *Antimicrobial Agents and Chemotherapy*, **21**, 210–215.

Cooke, E.M., Casewell, M.W., Emmerson, A.M. *et al.* (1986) Methicillin-resistant *Staphylococcus aureus* in the U K and Ireland: a questionnaire survey. *Journal of Hospital Infection*, **8**, 143–148.

Cooksey, R.C. & Baldwin, J.N. (1985) Program abstract. In *24th Interscience Conference on Antimicrobial Agents and Chemotherapy*, Abstract No. 997.

Cookson, B.D. (1994) Antiseptic resistance in methicillin-resistant *Staphylococcus aureus*: an emerging problem? *Zentralblatt für Bakteriologie*, **26** (Suppl.), 227–234.

Cookson, B.D. & Phillips, I. (1988) Epidemic methicillin-resistant *Staphylococcus aureus*. *Journal of Antimicrobial Chemotherapy*, **21** (Suppl. C), 57–65.

Cookson, B.D., Bolton, M.C. & Platt, J.H. (1991a) Chlorhexidine resistance in methicillin resistant *Staphylococcus aureus* or just an elevated MIC? An *in vitro* and *in vivo* assessment. *Antimicrobial Agents and Chemotherapy*, **35**, 1997–2002.

Cookson, B.D., Farrely, H., Stapleton, P., Garvey, R.R.J. & Price, M.R. (1991b) Transferable resistance to triclosan in MRSA. *Lancet*, **i**, 1548–1549.

Courvalin, P. (1994) Transfer of antibiotic resistance genes between Gram-positive and Gram-negative bacteria. *Antimicrobial Agents and Chemotherapy*, **38**, 1447–1451.

Courvalin, P. (1996) Evasion of antibiotic action by bacteria. *Journal of Antimicrobial Chemotherapy*, **37**, 855–869.

Crossley, K., Leosch, D., Landesman, B., Mead, K., Chern, M. & Strate, R. (1979) An outbreak of infections caused by strains of *Staphylococcus aureus* resistant to methicillin and aminoglycosides: 1. Clinical studies. *Journal of Infectious Diseases*, **139**, 273–279.

Dyke, K.G.H. (1969) Penicillinase production and intrinsic resistance to penicillins in methicillin-resistant cultures of *Staphylococcus aureus*. *Journal of Medical Microbiology*, **2**, 261–278.

El Solh, N., Allignet, J., Bismuth, R., Buset, B. & Fouace, J.M. (1986) Conjugative transfer of antibiotic resistance markers from *Staphylococcus aureus* in the absence of detectable extrachromosomal DNA. *Antimicrobial Agents and Chemotherapy*, **30**, 161–169.

Eltringham, I. (1997) Mupirocin resistance and methicillin-resistant *Staphylococcus aureus* (MRSA). *Journal of Hospital Infection*, **35**, 1–8.

Emslie, K.R., Townsend, D.E., Bolton, S. & Grubb, W.B. (1985) Two distinct resistance determinants to nucleic acid-binding compounds in *Staphylococcus aureus*. *FEMS Microbiology Letters*, **27**, 61–64.

Emslie, K.R., Townsend, D.E. & Grubb, W.B. (1986) Isolation and characterisation of a family of small plasmids encoding resistance to nucleic acid-binding compounds in *Staphylococcus aureus*. *Journal of Medical Microbiology*, **22**, 9–15.

Evans, J. & Dyke, K.G.H. (1988) Characterization of the conjugation system associated with the *Staphylococcus aureus* plasmid pJE1. *Journal of General Microbiology*, **134**, 1–8.

Fitzgerald, K.A., Davies, A. & Russell, A.D. (1992) Sensitivity and resistance of *Escherichia coli* and *Staphylococcus aureus* to chlorhexidine. *Letters in Applied Microbiology*, **14**, 33–36.

Gillespie, M.T., May, J.W. & Skurray, R.A. (1986) Plasmid-encoded resistance to acriflavine and quaternary ammonium compounds in methicillin-resistant *Staphylococcus aureus*. *FEMS Microbiology Letters*, **34**, 47–51.

Gillespie, M.T., Lyon, B.R. & Skurray, R.A. (1989) Gentamicin and antiseptic resistance in epidemic methicillin-resistant *Staphylococcus aureus*. *Lancet*, **i**, 503.

Gillespie, M.T., Lyon, B.R. & Skurray, R.A. (1990) Typing of methicillin-resistant *Staphylococcus aureus* by antibiotic resistance phenotype. *Journal of Medical Microbiology*, **31**, 57–64.

Grönroos, L., Matto, J., Saarela, M. *et al.* (1995) Chlorhexidine sensitivities of mutans streptococcal serotypes and ribotypes. *Antimicrobial Agents and Chemotherapy*, **39**, 894–898.

Haley, C.E., Marling-Cason, M., Smith J.W., Luby, J.P. & Mackowiak, P.A. (1985) Bactericidal activity of antiseptics against methicillin-resistant *Staphylococcus aureus*. *Journal of Clinical Microbiology*, **21**, 9911–992.

Heir, E., Sundhein, G. & Holck, A.L. (1995) Resistance

to quaternary ammonium compounds in *Staphylococcus* spp. isolated from the food industry and nucleotide sequence of the resistance plasmid pST827. *Journal of Applied Bacteriology*, **79**, 149–156.

Humphreys, H. & Duckworth, G. (1997) Methicillin-resistant *Staphylococcus aureus* (MRSA—a re-appraisal of control measures in the light of changing circumstances. *Journal of Hospital Infection*, **36**, 167–170.

Iordanescu, S. (1977) Relationships between contransducible plasmids in *Staphylococcus aureus* NCTC 8325. *Journal of General Microbiology*, **96**, 227–281.

Jaffe, H.M., Sweeney, H.M., Nathan, C., Weinstein, R.A., Kabins, S.A. & Cohen, S. (1980) Identity and interspecific transfer of gentamicin-resistance plasmids in *Staphylococcus aureus* and *Staphylococcus epidermidis*. *Journal of Infectious Diseases*, **141**, 738– 747.

Johnston, L.H. & Dyke, K.G.H. (1969) Ethidium bromide resistance, a new marker on the staphylococcal penicillinase plasmid. *Journal of Bacteriology*, **100**, 1413–1414.

Jones, I.G. & Midgley, M. (1985) Expression of a plasmid borne ethidium resistance determinant from *Staphylococcus* in *Escherichia coli*: evidence for an efflux system. *FEMS Microbiology Letters*, **28**, 355–357.

Kigbo, E.P., Townsend, D.E., Ashdown, N. & Grubb, W.B. (1985) Transposition of penicillinase determinants in methicillin-resistant *Staphylococcus aureus*. *FEMS Microbiology Letters*, **28**, 39–43.

Kolawole, D.O. (1984) Resistance mechanisms of mucoid-grown *Staphylococcus aureus* to the antibacterial action of some disinfectants and antiseptics. *FEMS Microbiology Letters*, **25**, 205–209.

Kondo, I., Ishidawa, T. & Nakahara, H. (1974) Mercury and cadmium resistances mediated by the penicillinase plasmid in *Staphylococcus aureus*. *Journal of Bacteriology*, **117**, 1–7.

Kono, M. & Sasatsu, M. (1976) Association of a penicillin resistance gene with a tetracycline resistance plasmid P_{TP-2} in *Staphylococcus aureus*. *Antimicrobial Agents and Chemotherapy*, **9**, 706–712.

Lacey, R.W. (1975) Antibiotic resistant plasmids of *Staphylococcus aureus* and their clinical importance. *Bacteriological Reviews*, **39**, 1–32.

Lacey, R.W. (1980) Evidence for two mechanisms for plasmid transfer in mixed cultures in *Staphylococcus aureus*. *Journal of General Microbiology*, **119**, 423–435.

Lacey, R.W. (1987) Multi-resistant *Staphylococcus aureus*: a suitable case of inactivity? *Journal of Hospital Infection*, **9**, 103–105.

Lacey, R.W. & Kruezenyk, S.C. (1986) Epidemiology of antibiotic resistance in *Staphylococcus aureus*. *Journal of Antimicrobial Chemotherapy*, **18** (Suppl. C), 207–214.

Lacey, R.W., Barr, K.W., Barr, V.E. & Inglis, T.J. (1986) Properties of methicillin-resistant *Staphylococcus aureus* colonizing patients in a burns unit. *Journal of Hospital Infection*, **7**, 137–148.

Leelaporn, A., Paulsen, I.T., Tennent, J.M., Littlejohn, T.G. & Skurray, R.A. (1994) Multidrug resistance to antiseptics and disinfectants in coagulate-negative staphylococci. *Journal of Medical Microbiology*, **40**, 214–220.

Lejeune, B., Buzit-Losquim, F., Simitzis-Le Flohic, A.M., LeBras, M.P. & Aliz, D. (1986) Outbreak of gentamicin-methicillin-resistant *Staphylococcus aureus* infection in an intensive care unit for children. *Journal of Hospital Infection*, **7**, 21–25.

Levy, S.B. (1992) Active efflux mechanisms for antimicrobial resistance. *Antimicrobial Agents and Chemotherapy*, **36**, 695–703.

Littlejohn, T.G., Diberardino, D., Messerotti, L.J., Spiers, S.J. & Skurray, R.A. (1991) Structure and evolution of a family of genes encoding antiseptic and disinfectant resistance in *Staphylococcus aureus*. *Gene*, **101**, 59–66.

Littlejohn, T.G., Paulsen, I.T., Gillespie, M.T. *et al.* (1992) Substrate specificity and energetics of antiseptic and disinfectant resistance in *Staphylococcus aureus*. *FEMS Microbiology Letters*, **95**, 259–266.

Locksley, R.M., Cohen, M.L., Quinn, T.C. *et al.* (1982) Multiply antibiotic resistant *Staphylococcus aureus*: introduction, transmission and evolution of nosocomial infection. *Annals of Internal Medicine*, **97**, 317–324.

Lyon, B.R. & Skurray, R.A. (1987) Antimicrobial resistance of *Staphylococcus aureus*: genetic basis. *Microbiological Reviews*, **51**, 88–137.

Lyon, B.R., May, J.W. & Skurray, R.A. (1984) Tn *4001*: a gentamicin- and kanamicin-resistance transposon in *Staphylococcus aureus*. *Molecular and General Genetics*, **193**, 554–556.

Lyon, B.R., Tennent, J.M., May, J.W. & Skurray, R.A. (1986) Trimethoprim resistance encoded on a *Staphylococcus aureus* gentamicin resistance plasmid: cloning and transposon mutagensis. *FEMS Microbiology Letters*, **33**, 289–192.

McGowan, J.E., Jr & Metchock, B.J. (1995) Penicillin-resistant pneumococci—an emerging threat to successful therapy. *Journal of Hospital Infection*, **30** (Suppl.), 472–482.

McLure, A.R. & Gordon, J. (1992) *In vitro* evaluation of povidone-iodine and chlorhexidine against methicillin-resistant *Staphylococcus aureus*. *Journal of Hospital Infection*, **21**, 291–299.

Marples, R.R. & Cooke, E.M. (1988) Current problems with methicillin-resistant *Staphylococcus aureus*. *Journal of Hospital Infection*, **11**, 371–392.

Mayon-White, R.T., Ducal, G., Kereselidze, G. & Tikomirov, E. (1988) An international survey of the prevalence of hospital acquired infection. *Journal of Hospital Infection*, **11** (Suppl. A), 43–48.

Meers, P.D., Ayliffe, G.A.J., Emerson, A.M. *et al.* (1981) National survey of infection in hospitals. *Journal of Hospital Infection*, **2** (Suppl.).

Midgley, M. (1994) Characteristics of an ethidium efflux system in *Enterococcus hirae. FEMS Microbiology Letters*, **120**, 119–124.

Millns, B., Martin, M.V. & Field, E.A. (1994) The sensitivity to chlorhexidine and cetylpyridinium chloride of staphylococci on the hands of dental students and theatre staff exposed to these disinfectants. *Journal of Hospital Infection*, **26**, 99–104.

Murray, B.E. (1987) Plasmid-mediated β-lactamase in *Enterococcus faecalis*. In *Streptococcal Genetics* (eds Feretti, J.V. & Curtiss, R., III), pp. 83–86. Washington, DC: American Society for Microbiology.

Naidoo, J. (1984) Interspecific co-transfer of antibiotic resistance in staphylococci *in vivo. Journal of Hygiene, Cambridge*, **95**, 59–66.

Nicoletti, G., Boghossien, V., Gurevitch, Y., Borland, R. & Morgenroth, P. (1993) The antimicrobial activity *in vitro* of chlorhexidine, a mixture of isothiazolinones ('Kathon' CG) and cetyltrimethylammonium bromide (CTAB). *Journal of Hospital Infection*, **23**, 87–111.

Noble, W.C. & Naidoo, J. (1978) Evolution of antibiotic resistance in *Staphylococcus aureus*: the role of the skin. *British Journal of Dermatology*, **98**, 481–489.

Noble, W.C., Virani, Z. & Cree, R.G.A. (1992) Co-transfer of vancomycin and other resistance genes from *Enterococcus faecalis* NCTC 12201 to *Staphylococcus aureus. FEMS Microbiology Letters*, **93**, 195–198.

Novick, R.P. & Morse, S.I. (1968) *In vivo* transmission of drug resistance factors between strains of *Staphylococcus aureus. Journal of Experimental Medicine*, **125**, 45–59.

Parker, M.T. (1983) The significance of phage-typing patterns in *Staphylococcus aureus. Staphylococci and Staphylococcal Infections*, Vol. 1: *Clinical and Epidemiological Aspects* (eds Easmon F.S. & Adlam, C.), pp. 33–62. London: Academic Press.

Parliamentary Office (1994) *Diseases Fighting Back*. London: Parliamentary Office of Science and Technology.

Pattee, P.A. & Neveln, D.E.S. (1975) Transformation analysis of three linkage groups in *Staphylococcus aureus. Journal of Bacteriology*, **124**, 201–211.

Paulsen, I.T., Brown, M.H., Littlejohn, T.G., Mitchell, B.A. & Skurray, R.A. (1996a) Multidrug resistance proteins QacA and QacB from *Staphylococcus aureus*. Membrane topology and identification of residues involved in substrate specificity. *Proceedings of the National Academy of Sciences, USA*, **93**, 3630–3635.

Paulsen, I.T., Skurray, R.A., Tan, R. *et al.* (1996b) The SMR family: a novel family of multidrug efflux proteins involved with the efflux of lipophilic drugs. *Molecular Microbiology*, **19**, 1167–1175.

Phillips, I. (1988) Introduction: hospital infection in the 1990s. *Journal of Hospital Infection*, **11**, (Suppl. A), 3–6.

Platt, J.H. & Bucknall, R.A. (1988) MIC tests are not suitable for assessing antiseptic handwashes. *Journal of Hospital Infection*, **11**, 396–397.

Rahman, M., Nando, J. & George, R.C. (1988) New generic location of gentamicin-resistance in methicillin-resistant *Staphylococcus aureus. Lancet*, **ii**, 1256.

Report (1986) Guidelines for the control of epidemic methicillin resistant *Staphylococcus aureus. Journal of Hospital Infection*, **7**, 193–201.

Report (1990) Revised guidelines for the control of epidemic methicillin-resistant *Staphylococcus aureus. Journal of Hospital Infection*, **16**, 351–377.

Reverdy, M.E., Bes, M., Nervi, C., Mastra, A. & Fleurette, J. (1992) Activity of four antiseptics (acriflavine, benzalkonium chloride, chlorhexidine digluconate and hexamidine di-isethionate) and of ethidium bromide on 392 strains representing 26 *Staphylococcus* species. *Medical Microbiology Letters*, **1**, 56–63.

Reverdy, M.E., Bes, M., Brun, Y. & Fleurette, J. (1993) Évolution de la résistance aux antibiotiques ex aux antiseptiques de souch hospitalières de *Staphylococcus aureus* isolées de 1980 à 1991. *Pathologie Biologie*, **41**, 897–904.

Rosendorf, L.L. & Kayser, F.H. (1974) Transduction and plasmid deoxyribonucleic acid analysis in a multiply antibiotic resistant strain of *Staphylococcus epidermidis. Journal of Bacteriology*, **120**, 677–686.

Rouch, D.A., Cram, D.S., DiBarardino, O., Littlejohn, T.G. & Skurray, R.A. (1990) Efflux-mediated antiseptic resistance gene *qac*A from *Staphylococcus aureus*: common ancestry with tetracycline- and sugar-transport proteins. *Molecular Microbiology*, **4**, 2051–2062.

Rudin, L., Sjostrom, J-E., Lindberg, M. & Phillipson, L. (1974) Factors affecting the competence of transformation in *Staphylococcus aureus. Journal of Bacterioloy*, **118**, 155–164.

Russell, A.D. & Day, M.J. (1993) Antibacterial activity of chlorhexidine. *Journal of Hospital Infection*, **25**, 229–238.

Russell, A.D. & Day, M.J. (1996) Antibiotic and biocide resistance in bacteria. *Microbios*, **85**, 45–65.

Rutala, W.A. (1995) Use of chemical germicides in the United States: 1994 and beyond. In *Chemical Germicides in Health Care* (ed. Rutala, W.A.), pp. 1–22. Morin Heights: Polyscience Publications.

Sasatsu, M., Shimuzu, K., Noguchi, M. & Kono, M. (1993) Triclosan-resistant *Staphylococcus aureus. Lancet*, **341**, 756.

Sasatsu, M., Shidata, Y., Noguchi, N. & Kono, M. (1994) Substrates and inhibitors of antiseptic resistance in *Staphylococcus aureus*. *Biological and Pharmaceutical Bulletin*, **17**, 136 – 138.

Sasatsu, M-, Shirai, Y., Hase, M. *et al.* (1995) The origin of the antiseptic resistance gene *ebr* in *Staphylococcus aureus*. *Microbios*, **84**, 161–169.

Schaberg, D.R. & Zervos, M.J. (1986) Intergeneric and interspecies gene exchange in Gram-positive cocci. *Antimicrobial Agents and Chemotherapy*, **30**, 817–832.

Schaeffler, S. (1982) Bacteriophage-mediated acquisition of antibiotic resistance in *Staphylococcus aureus* type 88. *Antimicrobial Agents and Chemotherapy*, **21**, 460–467.

Shalita, Z., Murphy, E. & Novick, R.P. (1980) Penicillinase plasmids of *Staphylococcus aureus*: structural and evolutionary relationships. *Plasmid*, **3**, 291–311.

Shanson, D.C. (1986) Staphylococcal infection in hospitals. *British Journal of Medicine*, **35**, 312–320.

Shanson, D.C. (1989) *Microbiology in Clinical Practice*, 2nd edn. London: Wright.

Silver, S. & Misra, S. (1988) Plasmid-mediated heavy metal resistances. *Annual Review of Microbiology*, **42**, 711–743.

Simjee, S. & Gill, M.J. (1997) Gene transfer, gentamicin resistance and enterococci. *Journal of Hospital Infection*, **36**, 249–259.

Skurray, R.A., Rouch, D.A., Lyon, B.R. *et al.* (1988) Multiresistant *Staphylococcus aureus*: genetics and evolution of epidemic Australian strains. *Journal of Antimicrobial Chemotherapy*, **21** (Suppl. C), 19–38.

Stiffler, P.W., Sweeney, H.M. & Cohen, S. (1974) Contransduction of plasmids mediating resistance to tetracycline and chloramphenicol in *Staphylococcus aureus*. *Journal of Bacteriology*, **120**, 934–944.

Tennent, J.M., Lyon, B.R., Gillespie, M.T., May, J.W. & Skurray, R.A. (1985) Cloning and expression of *Staphylococcus aureus* plasmid-mediated quaternary ammonium resistance in *Escherichia coli*. *Antimicrobial Agents and Chemotherapy*, **27**, 79–83.

Tenover, F.C. & McGowan, J.E. (1996) Reasons for the emergence of antibiotic resistance. *The American Journal of the Medical Sciences*, **311**, 9–16.

Thompson, R. (1986) R Plasmid transfer. *Journal of Antimicrobial Chemotherapy*, **18** (Suppl. C), 13–23.

Thornsberry, C. (1988) The development of antimicrobial resistance in staphylococci. *Journal of Antimicrobial Chemotherapy*, **21**, (Suppl. C), 9–16.

Townsend, D.E., Ashdown, N., Greed, L.C. & Grubb, W.B. (1983) Plasmid-mediated resistance to quaternary ammonium compounds in methicillin-resistant *Staphylococcus aureus*. *Medical Journal of Australia*, **ii**, 310.

Townsend, D.E., Ashdown, N., Bradley, J.M., Pearman, J.W. & Grubb, W.B. (1984a) 'Australian' methicillin-resistant *Staphylococcus aureus* in a London hospital? *Medical Journal of Australia*, **ii**, 339–340.

Townsend, D.E., Ashdown, N., Greed, L.C. & Grubb, W.B. (1984b) Transposition of gentamicin resistance to staphylococcal plasmids encoding resistance to cationic agents. *Journal of Antimicrobial Chemotherapy*, **14**, 115–134.

Townsend, D.E., Ashdown, N., Bolton, S. & Grubb, W.B. (1985) The use of cetyltrimethylammonium bromide for the rapid isolation from *Staphylococcus aureus* for relaxable and non-relaxable plasmid DNA suitable for *in vitro* manipulation. *Letters in Applied Microbiology*, **1**, 87–94.

Townsend, D.E., Bolton, S., Asdown, N., Taheri, S. & Grubb, W.B. (1986) Comparison of phage mediated and conjugative transfer of staphylococcus plasmid *in vitro* and *in vivo*. *Journal of Medical Microbiology*, **22**, 107–114.

Tuffnell, D.J., Croton, R.S., Hemingway, D.M., Hartley, M.N., Wake, P.N. & Garvey, R.J.P. (1987) Methicillin-resistant *Staphylococcus aureus*: the role of antisepsis in the control of an outbreak. *Journal of Hospital Infection*, **10**, 255–259.

Uhl, S. (1993) Triclosan-resistant *Staphylococcus aureus*. *Lancet*, **342**, 1993.

Wade, J.J. (1995) The emergence of *Enterococcus faecium* resistant to glycopeptides and other standard agents—a preliminary report. *Journal of Hospital Infection*, **30**, (Suppl.), 483–493.

Wenzel, R.P. (1987) Towards a global perspective of nosocomial infections. *European Journal of Clinical Medicine*, **6**, 341–343.

Westergren, G. & Emilson, C.-G. (1980) *In vitro* development of chlorhexidine resistance in *Streptococcus sanguis* and its transmissibility by genetic transformation. *Scandinavian Journal of Dental Research*, **88**, 236–243.

Witte, W. (1977) Transfer of drug resistance-plasmids in mixed cultures of staphylococci. *Zentrablatt für Bakteriologie, Parasitenkunde Infektionskrankheiten Hygiene, I, Abteilung Originale Reihe A*, **237**, 147–159.

Woodford, N., Johnson, A.P. & George, R.C. (1991) Detection of glycopeptide resistance in clinical isolates of Gram-positive bacteria. *Journal of Antimicrobial Chemotherapy*, **28**, 483–486.

Woodford, N., McNamara, E., Smyth, E. & George, R.C. (1992) High-level resistance to gentamicin in *Enterococcus faecium*. *Journal of Antimicrobial Chemotherapy*, **29**, 395–440.

Yamamoto, T., Tamura, Y. & Yokama, T. (1988) Antiseptic and antibiotic resistance plasmid in *Staphylococcus aureus* that possesses ability to confer chlorhexidine and acrinol resistance. *Antimicrobial Agents and Chemotherapy*, **32**, 932–935.

G. LISTERIA

1 Introduction

Listerias are Gram-positive, regular, non-spore-aerobic, microaerophilic or facultatively anaerobic forming, short, rods which exhibit characteristic tumbling motility when cultured at 20–25°C. At the intergeneric level, the genus *Listeria* is most closely related to *Brochothrix* (Collins *et al.*, 1991), while intragenerically *Listeria* contains six species: *L. monocytogenes*, *L. ivanovii* (subspecies *ivanovii* and *londoniensis*), *L. seeligeri*, *L. welshimeri*, *L. innocua*, and *L. grayi* (Rocourt *et al.*, 1987; Boerlin *et al.*, 1992). The former three species have been shown to cause listeriosis, which was recognized primarily as a disease of domestic animals (Seeliger, 1988). However, the recent association of *L. monocytogenes* with several food-borne outbreaks of human listeriosis suggests that contaminated food may be a primary source of the organism in humans.

Numerous animal species are susceptible to listeriosis, with a large proportion of healthy animals shedding *L. monocytogenes* in their faeces. Listeriosis can occur either sporadically or as epidemics, and often leads to fatal forms of encephalitis. Virtually all domestic animals are susceptible to the disease and, unless properly treated, listeriosis in domestic livestock is usually fatal. The disease among these animals is commonly manifested as encephalitis, resulting ultimately in paralysis. However, milder infections in pregnant animals generally give rise to a damaged, dead or aborted fetus (Seeliger, 1961).

Human listeriosis has several different forms and can be divided into five categories: pregnancy infections, neonatal infections, sepsis, meningoencephalitis and focal infections (Bahk & Marth, 1990). Although the highest incidence of infection is usually seen in neonates, followed by those older than 60 years, the proportion of cases not associated with pregnancy appears to be on the increase (McLauchlin, 1990). The disease symptoms may be very severe and can lead to death, where the high mortality rate of around 30% is partly due to the underlying weakened condition of immunocompromised victims (Pearson & Marth, 1990).

2 Characteristics of *Listeria monocytogenes* which make it difficult to eliminate from the environment

Listeria monocytogenes, the species responsible for virtually all cases of human listeriosis, is a highly adaptable bacterium, which survives and grows well over a wide range of environmental parameters.

2.1 Temperature

As a mesophile, the organism has an optimum growth temperature of 30–35°C, at neutral or slightly alkaline pH. However, it also possesses psychrotrophic properties and can grow over a temperature range from 1 to 45°C (Feresu & Jones, 1988). Generation times at 4°C and 10°C of 33.5 and 9.6 h, respectively, have been published (Petran & Zottola, 1989), and growth has been reported below 1°C (Junttila *et al.*, 1988) and down to –0.4°C (Walker *et al.*, 1990). The organism has been described as a rapidly growing mesophile with an unusually low minimal temperature and a growth rate at 10°C characteristic of psychrophiles (Wilkins *et al.*, 1972). It can survive freezing in non-protective media for extended periods, and exhibits a resistance to heat comparable to that of most similar Gram-positive organisms (Farber & Peterkin, 1991).

2.2 pH

The pH range for growth is generally considered to be approximately 4.7–9.2, with some variation between strains, and the optimum is 7.0 (Petran & Zottola, 1989). Growth in laboratory media, however, has been reported at as low as 4.39 (George *et al.*, 1988). Inhibition at low pH is dependent on the nature of the acid, organic acids (acetic > lactic > citric) being more inhibitory than mineral acids, such as hydrochloric acid (Sorrelis *et al.*, 1989). This accounts for the control of the organism in adequately fermented foods or silage. Acid injury has been observed to be greater at optimum growth temperature than under psychrotrophic conditions (Ahamad & Marth, 1989).

2.3 Water activity

The moisture requirement for microbial growth is expressed in terms of water activity (A_w). This is defined as the ratio of the water-vapour pressure of a food substrate to the vapour pressure of pure water at the same temperature. *Listeria monocytogenes* grows optimally at A_w ~0.97 (Petran & Zottola, 1989) but has the ability to multiply in 37.5% (w/v) sucrose solution, with A_w of 0.92 (Petran & Zottola 1989), and in glycerol solution, with A_w of 0.90 (Farber *et al.*, 1992). The organism can grow in 10% sodium chloride (NaCl) (Seeliger & Jones, 1996), which has an A_w ~0.93, and has been recovered from a 25% (w/v) NaCl solution with A_w <9.0, after 18 weeks incubation at 4°C (Shahamat *et al.*, 1980a). This tolerance to high salt concentrations and low A_w values suggests a high resistance to environmental stresses, which is unusual among pathogenic bacteria. These characteristics favour survival, if not growth, in the environment.

2.4 Survival on food and non-food contact surfaces

Since *L. monocytogenes* survives for long periods at low A_w values, it is not surprising that this organism is also remarkably resistant to drying. Palumbo & Williams (1990) suggested that, once the organism has contaminated a food-processing plant, it can persist for long periods in the plant environment if the temperature is low and the organism is protected by various food components. Indeed, Dickgiesser (1980) observed that *L. monocytogenes* survived for 20–30 days on hospital tiles, and attests to the tenacity of this organism on a contact surface similar to that found in the food-processing environment. Scanning electron microscopy has demonstrated that *L. monocytogenes* can attach to various food-contact surfaces (Herald & Zottola, 1988; Mafu *et al.*, 1990; Spurlock & Zottola, 1991). Attached bacteria can be a serious problem in the food-processing industry, where they can form biofilms, within which the bacteria are continually growing, multiplying and being released to the environment. This can be an important source of product contamination. Once a biofilm is firmly established, cleaning and sterilization becomes much more difficult, glycocalyx-protected cells being less susceptible to cleaning/sterilizing agents (Mosteller & Bishop, 1993).

It is due to the organism's ability to survive and grow under a wide range of environmental parameters that control measures which are adequate for other food-borne pathogens may not be sufficient to eliminate the threat posed by *L. monocytogenes*. Hence, a number of preventive measures to reduce numbers and control growth of the organism have been investigated, including preservation of foods by the application of physical processes, sanitization of the food production and processing environment, using disinfectants, and prolonging the shelf-life of food through the use of antimicrobial food additives.

3 Elimination or control of *Listeria monocytogenes* growth in foods by application of food-processing techniques

Food preservation is intended to prevent or delay the growth of microorganisms, a number of methods having been evaluated with respect to the elimination and control of *L. monocytogenes*.

3.1 Thermal inactivation

Thermal processing is the most widely used method of food preservation. Thermal treatment during canning is such that it normally results in sterilization of the product (Stumbo, 1973) and, when carried out under the proper conditions, produces a product that is *Listeria*-free. Pasteurization, which is a milder heat treatment, is applied to foods to eliminate bacterial pathogens without affecting other desirable attributes of the food. The main application of pasteurization has been in milk, where there have been conflicting reports on the thermotolerance of *L. monocytogenes* to the process (Donnelly, 1990). However, it is now generally agreed that the high-temperature short-time (HTST) conditions (71.7°C for 15 s used in commercial pasteurization is a safe process, which reduces the number of *L. monocytogenes* occurring in raw milk to levels that do not pose an appreciable risk to human health (WHO Working Group, 1988). Post-pasteurization contamination by *L. monocytogenes* presents a much greater risk than its survival through pasteurization.

Two recent developments may help to explain some of the discrepancies in the literature regarding the thermotolerance of *L. monocytogenes*. The first is the 'heat-shock' response: several investigators have found that, if *L. monocytogenes* is exposed to sublethal temperatures, ~44–48°C, cells may acquire an enhanced thermotolerance (Fedio & Jackson, 1989; Farber & Brown, 1990; Knabel *et al.*, 1990). Conditions of 'heat shock' may be encountered during minimal processing with products undergoing a mild heat treatment for a long period, e.g. in *sousvide* processing, where heat-stressed survivors may have a greater capacity to recover and grow during storage. This phenomenon must also be considered when heating meats, especially for products heated slowly to a final internal temperature (Mackey & Derrick, 1987; Farber & Brown, 1990). Meat should therefore be kept refrigerated at all times before thermal processing to prevent thermal adaptation by *L. monocytogenes* strains (Kim *et al.*, 1994).

Secondly, different methods for recovering heat-stressed organisms have led to conflicting reports on the thermotolerance of *L. monocytogenes*, since it has been found that the use of anaerobic incubation leads to recovery of significantly more cells than are recovered in the presence of oxygen (Knabel *et al.*, 1990). The oxygen sensitivity of heat-stressed *L. monocytogenes* may be due to inactivation of catalase and superoxide dismutase enzymes during heating (Knabel *et al.*, 1990).

When considering thermal processes with regard to attaining adequate destruction of *L. monocytogenes* in various foods, consideration must be given not only to the organism's inherent thermal resistance but also to the constitution of the food to be processed, e.g. the presence of curing salt has been found to increase resistance of the organism substantially in meats (Farber *et al.*, 1989; Mackey *et al.*, 1990). *Listeria monocytogenes* has been shown to be much more heat-resistant in meat than in milk (Carpenter & Harrison, 1989; Harrison & Carpenter, 1989a,b), survivor curves for meat having a pronounced shoulder (Mackey *et al.*, 1990). Therefore, an equation to achieve a 7D (D = decimal reduction time in minutes) inactivation of *L. monocytogenes* in meat products, allowing for the shoulder, was devised:

$$\log_{10} \text{processing time (min)} = 10.3943 - 0.14618\,t,$$

where t = heating temperature in °C (Mackey *et al.*, 1990) to take account of the effect of meat as a heating menstruum.

3.2 Irradiation

Unlike the conflicting reports on thermal resistance in *L. monocytogenes*, results from several gamma irradiation studies conducted in the USA (Huhtanen *et al.*, 1989), Hungary (Tarjan, 1988) and the UK (Patterson, 1989) have produced similar results. Reported D_{10} values (dose required to inactivate 90% of the population) range from 0.28 to 0.61 kGy for *L. monocytogenes*, depending on the strain, irradiation temperature and substrate. The D_{10} values with poultry meat (Patterson, 1989), which ranged from 0.42 to 0.54 k Gy, were found to be similar to those reported for *Salmonella* spp. irradiated under similar conditions (Idziak & Incze, 1968) and Patterson (1988) suggested that irradiation doses which eliminate salmonellae from poultry carcasses would also be sufficient to remove *L. monocytogenes*. In addition to inactivation studies, Grant *et al.* (1993) compared the growth of *L. monocytogenes* in unirradiated and irradiated cook–chill roast beef and gravy meals at refrigeration temperatures. They concluded that exponential growth of the organism was preceded by an extended lag period of 6–9 days at 5°C and 3–4 days at 10°C, compared with lag periods of 1–2 days and <0.1 day, respectively, in unirradiated beef and gravy stored under the same conditions.

3.3 Packaging

Vacuum packaging is commonly used to extend the shelf-life of perishable food. However, with respect to the growth of *L. monocytogenes*, the composition of the gaseous atmosphere appears to have little effect, similar generation times for the organism having been observed under aerobic, microaerophilic and anaerobic conditions (Ingham *et al.*, 1990). It would appear, however, that multiplication of *L. monocytogenes* can be controlled to some extent using vacuum packaging or modified atmospheric packaging (MAP) in combination with other preservation methods. For example, when compared with gas-permeable packaging, it has been found that vacuum packaging can be effective in suppressing the growth of *L. monocytogenes* on chicken breasts which have been processed using moist heat (Harrison & Carpenter, 1989a) and on cold process smoked salmon preserved with sodium nitrite and NaCl (Pelroy *et al.*, 1994b). The use of nisin spray treatment has also been shown to be effective in reducing the numbers of *L. innocua* and *Brochothrix thermosphacta* on beef when combined with vacuum packaging, hence extending the shelf-life and improving the microbiological safety of fresh refrigerated beef (Cutter & Siragusa, 1996).

It has been shown that MAP is more effective when combined with lactic acid as a preservative in preventing the growth of *L. monocytogenes* in crayfish tail meat at 4°C (Pothuri *et al.*, 1996) and when combined with low-temperature storage to inhibit the growth of *L. monocytogenes* on chicken (Marshall *et al.*, 1991, 1992).

3.4 Freezing

Freezing and subsequent frozen storage extends the shelf-life of foods significantly when compared with preservation by chilling. Temperatures below that for optimum growth reduce metabolic activity and hence have a bacteriostatic effect on microbial-cell growth. The process can also be bactericidal, since death of microorganisms can result as a consequence of the formation of ice crystals, which may grow during extended frozen storage and cause damage to the cell wall. The recall of contaminated ice-cream and other frozen dairy products in the USA between 1986 and 1989 (Ryser & Marth, 1991) and the ability of *Listeria* spp. to survive within a frozen milk product's processing environment and to serve as a source of the organism in finished products (Walker *et al.*, 1991), however, attests to the ability of *L. monocytogenes* to survive the process of freezing and frozen storage. This process is more likely to injure than to kill cells of *L. monocytogenes* (Golden *et al.*, 1988), the type of cell damage and degree of injury having been found to be related to the length of time of frozen storage and strain of *L. monocytogenes* (Hayat, 1986). Studies which have examined the protective effect of foods in the survival of *L. monocytogenes* during freezing and frozen storage have shown that foods offer some degree of protection to *L. monocytogenes* during freezing, sub-lethal injury and cell death being significantly reduced by the presence of various food ingredients (Golden *et al.*, 1988; Palumbo & Williams, 1989; Parish & Higgins, 1989; Lammerding & Doyle, 1990).

3.5 High hydrostatic pressure

The concept of using high hydrostatic pressure as a means of food preservation is not new, with research dating back as far as 1899 on the use of high pressure to improve the keeping quality of milk (Hite, 1899). Recent renewed interest, however, has arisen in high pressure as a means of producing high quality, minimally processed, preservative-free foods which are microbiologically safe. In this context, some recent work has been carried out on evaluating the sensitivity of *L. monocytogenes* to high hydrostatic pressure, where it has been found that a pressure of 37 MPa for 15 min resulted in a 10^5 reduction in numbers of cells in 10 mmol/l phosphate saline at pH 7.0 and 20°C (Patterson *et al.*, 1995). As with all food preservation processes, the nature of the food had an effect on the pressure resistance shown by the organism, with ultrahigh-temperature (UHT) milk providing more protection than poultry meat, which in turn had more protection than buffer. Moreover, there was some evidence of strain variation in pressure sensitivity within *L. monocytogenes* and this, together with the protective effect of the food, must be taken into consideration when making recommendations for improving the safety of pressure-treated foods (Patterson *et al.*, 1995).

It is considered that damage to microorganisms by pressure is similar to that caused by heat (Hoover *et al.*, 1989), although the mechanisms of inactivation remain unknown. Mackey *et al.* (1994) found differences in the ultrastructural changes of *L. monocytogenes* when subjected to a pressure of 25 MPa when compared with that of *Salmonella thompson (Salmonella enterica* subsp. *enterica* serovar Thompson). In this study, pressure-treated cells of *L. monocytogenes* were found to contain vacuolar regions in the cytoplasm, a condition which was not evident in *Sal. thompson*. For both organisms, however, changes in the appearance of nuclear material was evident after pressure treatment.

4 Control of *Listera monocytogenes* through the use of disinfectants

Within the food-processing environment, there is a wide variety of organisms present, including Gram-positive, Gram-negative and spore-forming bacteria, together with other microorganisms, such as yeasts and fungi. Disinfectants that have a broad microbial action against the potential microflora present should therefore be used to ensure that one particular organism, or group of organisms, is not being selected. In this respect, a number of disinfectants and antimicrobial agents employed in the food industry have been tested to evaluate their efficacy against *L. monocytogenes*.

4.1 Chlorine

Chlorine is the most widely used chemical disinfectant in the food industry, where the effect of sodium hypochlorite on free-living, unattached cells of *L. monocytogenes* has been widely studied (Lopes, 1986; Brackett, 1987; El-Kest & Marth, 1988a,b; Tuncan, 1993). Such cells demonstrate no unusual resistance to hypochlorite.

Although the rate of diffusion of chlorine into the microbial cell increases at higher temperatures (El-Kest & Marth, 1988a), it was found that the sterilizing effect remained unchanged when *Listeria* cells were exposed to 25–200 part/10^6 chlorine for 30 s at 2°C, when compared with cells exposed at 25°C (Tuncan, 1993), demonstrating the efficacy of this disinfectant even at low temperatures. The use of chlorine as a disinfectant against *L. monocytogenes*, however, has been found to be influenced by the 'free-chlorine' concentration, exposure time, surface to be cleaned and presence of organic matter (Cordier *et al.*, 1989; Best *et al.*, 1990).

Lee & Frank (1991) have shown that surface-attached cells of *L. monocytogenes* demonstrate an increased resistance to chlorine and, since the organism can attach to various food-contact surfaces (Herald & Zottola, 1988; Mafu *et al.*, 1990; Spurlock & Zottola, 1991), these results have important implications for its inactivation within the food industry. Attached bacteria can be a serious problem in this context, as they can form biofilms, within which the bacteria are continually growing, multiplying and being released into the environment. Mustapha & Liewen (1989) recommended that sodium hypochlorite should be used at a level of 200 parts/10^6 and left on a non-porous surface for approximately 2 min and a solution of 400 parts/10^6 of free chlorine should be left on porous surfaces for about 2 min to allow adequate inactivation of *L. monocytogenes* attached to these surfaces.

Ronner & Wong (1993) compared the activity of chlorine on stainless steel and Buna-n rubber. Biofilm populations were found to be more resistant to chlorine on the latter surface, where a 1–2 $\log_{10}$ reduction in numbers of *L. monocytogenes* occurred, compared with a 3–4 $\log_{10}$ reduction on the former. Mosteller & Bishop (1993) also reported the failure of chlorine to provide an adequate reduction in numbers of *L. monocytogenes* attached to Buna-n rubber and Teflon. The disinfection of other surfaces with chlorine, such as glass (non-porous) and polypropylene (porous), have also been assessed (Mafu *et al.*, 1990), showing that glass surfaces are more easily disinfected with chlorine than is polypropylene. For adequate inactivation of *L. monocytogenes* on polypropylene, > 10 000 parts/10^6 chlorine was required.

With respect to *in situ* inactivation of *L. monocytogenes* in foods, chlorine has not been very effective. For example, total inactivation was not achieved when 100 parts/10^6 of chlorine was applied to shell eggs for 5 min (Bartlett, 1993) or when Brussels sprouts were subjected to 200 parts/10^6 of chlorine for 30 s (Brackett, 1987). When chlorine and chlorine dioxide were applied to fresh-cut vegetables at 200 parts/10^6 and 5 parts/10^6 respectively, for 10 min, they produced only around 1 $\log_{10}$ reduction in numbers of *L. monocytogenes* (Zhang & Farber, 1996).

4.2 Quaternary ammonium compounds

Gram-positive bacteria have been found to be more susceptible to quaternary ammonium compounds (QACs) than Gram-negatives (Lopes, 1986) and many reports verify the efficacy of these compounds in eliminating *L. monocytogenes in vitro* and in the presence of organic matter (Lopes, 1986; Cordier *et al.*, 1989; Mustapha & Liewen, 1989; Best *et al.*, 1990; Mafu *et al.*, 1990; Ren & Frank, 1993). However, when tested against attached *L. monocytogenes* cells, QACs performed poorly (Mosteller & Bishop, 1993). This reduced efficacy towards biofilms may be attributable to the glycocalyx layer, which protects bacterial cells and prevents contact between the QAC and the bacterial cells.

4.3 Iodophors

Iodophors are used in disinfectant solutions within food production and processing, e.g. during and after milking on dairy farms. At their recommended concentrations, iodophors are effective in the elimination of *L. monocytogenes* (Lopes, 1986; Tuncan, 1993). Like other disinfectants, they are less effective in the presence of organic material and when *L. monocytogenes* is dried on to a stainless steel surface (Best *et al.*, 1990). Iodophors were as effective as QACs on Buna-n rubber; however, they were found to be even more effective on Teflon (Mosteller & Bishop, 1993). A reduction in the efficacy of iodophors is observed at low temperatures, i.e. 2°C (Tuncan, 1993) and 4°C (Mafu *et al.*, 1990), where concentrations 5–10 times higher are required to disinfect surfaces at 4°C compared with those at 20°C.

4.4 Combined treatments

Chemical and physical treatments can been combined to control *L. monocytogenes* biofilms effectively within the food industry. For example, adherent cells of *L. monocytogenes* have been shown to be effectively destroyed by the combined application of heat (65°C for 5 min and the monoglyceride, monolaurin, when used at a concentration of 50 µg/ml (Oh & Marshall, 1995). Monolaurin and acetic acid have also been shown to act synergistically as sanitizers for stainless steel surfaces, where, at concentrations of 100 µg/ml and 1%, respectively, applied for 25 min, they completely inactivated a population of 10^5 colony-forming units (cfu)/cm^2 of 1 day-adherent cells on stainless steel. However, like other sanitizers, the effect of this combination diminished when applied to 7 day-adherent cells, demonstrating the increased resistance of *L. monocytogenes* cells with increased culture age (Oh & Marshall, 1996).

4.5 Commercial preparations

On evaluating eight commercial disinfectants, Jacquet & Reynaud (1994) found that only three disinfectants, one containing an amine, one containing QAC and peroxide and a chlorine-based product, were effective in their capacity to cause a 5 $\log_{10}$ reduction in *L. monocytogenes* cell counts. The aldehyde and acid/peroxide-based products examined were inadequate at recommended concentrations in the elimination of *L. monocytogenes*. Cordier *et al.* (1989) and Best *et al.* (1990) also found that, in practice, aldehyde-based preparations were inadequate in eliminating both planktonic cells and those which were surface-attached.

5 Use of food preservatives to inhibit the growth of *Listeria monocytogenes* in foods

Traditionally, foods were preserved by the addition of salt, sugar, vinegar and other acids derived from fermentation, but, more recently, chemically synthesized food additives have been used to prolong the shelf-life of foods and improve safety. Such preservatives include salts, sugars and other solutes which lower A_w, organic acids, esters, sulphites, nitrites, antibiotics, ethanol, carbon dioxide, antioxidants and glycerol esters, all of which have been evaluated, to some extent, for their bacteriostatic or bacteriocidal activity against many food-borne pathogens, including *L. monocytogenes*.

5.1 Organic acids

Organic acids and their salts have been employed for many years as antimicrobial agents. Their effects on the growth and viability of *L. monocytogenes* have been extensively studied (El-Shenawy & Marth, 1988a,b, 1989, 1991; Ahamad & Marth, 1989; Farber *et al.*, 1989; Ita & Hutkins, 1991; Buchanan *et al.*, 1993; Buchanan & Golden, 1994; Pelroy *et al.*, 1994a; Golden *et al.*, 1995; Podolak *et al.*, 1995, 1996) and it has been shown that the organism is more acid-tolerant than most food-borne pathogens, with survival and growth occurring down to pH 4.3. The studies further indicate that the degree of survival varies depending on the acid used, with acetic acid being more listericidal than either lactic, citric or hydrochloric acid (Ahamad & Marth, 1989, 1990; Farber *et al.*, 1989). The listericidal effects of these acids are associated with their dissociation constants (pK_a values) with, in general acids of higher pK_a values being more inhibitory to *L. monocytogenes* at a given pH. It is the undissociated and uncharged weak lipophilic acids, such as acetic acid, which are permeable through the cell membrane and therefore accumulate in cells to higher concentrations than lactic, citric or hydrochloric acid, which are generally unable to passively diffuse into the cell and are thought to be carrier-mediated. Ita & Hutkins (1991) concluded that inhibition of *L. monocytogenes* by acids is caused not by a decrease in the intracellular pH, *per se*, but rather by specific effects of the undissociated acid species on metabolic or other physiological activities.

In addition to the chemical structure of the acid, the antimicrobial activity of organic acids and salts is dependent on the pH, buffering capacity of the system, temperature, acid concentration and strain of bacterium (El-Shenawy & Marth, 1988a,b, 1989; Ahamad & Marth, 1989, 1990). Moreover, O'Driscoll *et al.* (1996) demonstrated that acid tolerance can be induced in *L. monocytogenes* following a 1 h adaptation to mild acid conditions (pH 5.5). This acid-tolerant response has been shown to enhance the survival of the organism in acidic foods and during milk fermentation (Gahan *et al.*, 1996) and therefore should be considered when devising preservation protocols involving the use of acids as antimicrobials. When evaluated as preservatives in food systems, it was found that other food components and/or food additives could also affect their listericidal activity (Pelroy *et al.*, 1994a,b; Golden *et al.*, 1995). These preservatives tend to be more effective at low pH and low temperatures (El-Shenawy & Marth 1988a,b, 1991), but, like most antimicrobials, they are not as effective in destroying bacteria attached to surfaces such as Buna-n rubber or Teflon.

In terms of application within the food industry, lactic, acetic and fumaric acids have been evaluated as decontaminants of beef carcasses (Woolthuis & Smulders, 1985; Podolak *et al.*, 1995, 1996). At concentrations of 1.0% and 1.5%, fumaric acid was found to be more effective than lactic acid, which in turn was more effective than acetic acid, in reducing numbers of *L. monocytogenes* (Dickson & Siragusa, 1994; Podolak *et al.*, 1995, 1996).

5.2 Nitrites

The direct addition of nitrite has been permitted in cured meats in the UK, up to a maximum residual level of 200 μg/g, depending on the food category, where it contributes to the colour, flavour and keeping quality of such products. Sodium nitrite has a bacteriostatic effect against *L. monocytogenes*, and this effect has been shown to be synergistic with other factors, such as salt, pH, availability of oxygen and temperature (Shahamat *et al.*, 1980b; Buchanan *et al.*, 1989). Above pH 6.0, there is little or no inhibitory effect (McClure *et al.*, 1991), with the bacteriostatic effect in meats being maximized by combining with high salt concentrations (3%), vacuum packaging and low-temperature storage.

5.3 Bacteriocins

Bacteriocins are proteins or protein complexes which have bactericidal activity directed against species that are closely related to the producer bacterium (Hof *et al.*, 1997). Their antimicrobial activity against *L. monocytogenes* and other pathogens has been extensively studied, with a view to their use as antimicrobial agents, due to the increasing concern over the safety of food, and consumer resistance to the use of artificial preservatives. In this respect, the bacteriocins from lactic acid bacteria have received most attention, since these organisms have a long history of safe use in fermented foods, e.g. as starter cultures. Of these, nisin, which is produced by *Lactococcus lactis* subsp. *lactis*, has been evaluated and subsequently approved as a food additive in at least 46 countries (Harris *et al.*, 1991).

The primary target of nisin in sensitive vegetative cells is the cytoplasmic membrane, where the protein molecule is incorporated into the membrane to form ion channels or pores, through which efflux of K^+, adenosine triphosphate (ATP) and amino acids results in the destruction of the membrane potential. *Listeria monocytogenes* is sensitive to nisin and, in energized cells, it dissipates the membrane potential and pH gradient, leading to collapse of the proton-motive force (Bruno *et al.*, 1992). However, nisin-resistant strains have also been reported (Harris *et al.*, 1991; Davies & Adams, 1994) and this is clearly an obstacle to the development of food applications. Spontaneous resistance may develop from alteration and/or mutation of the cell surface or cell membrane molecular constituents with which bacteriocins interact. In contrast, true bacteriocin resistance may be observed due to the production of nisinase, to innate or gene-encoded immunity or to inherent resistance, whereby the bacterial cells are naturally not interactive with a bacteriocin (Muriana, 1996).

In terms of application, nisin has been shown to be effective in reducing the level of *L. monocytogenes* in cheese production (Abdalla *et al.*, 1993; Zottola *et al.*, 1994), in meat preservation (Chung *et al.*, 1989; El-Khateib *et al.*, 1993; Fang & Lin, 1994) and in poultry processing (Mahadeo & Tatini, 1994). It has also been used effectively to reduce the levels of *L. monocytogenes* in ice-cream, where the activity of nisin was found to be unaffected by 3 months' storage at −18°C (Dean & Zottola, 1996). However, the latter study, together with that of Jung *et al.* (1992), found that high fat levels reduced the efficiency of nisin.

Although crudely purified nisin has been used directly in foods, many other bacteriocins have been investigated by use of the bacteriocin-producing bacterial strain. These include pediocins (Motlagh *et al.*, 1992), sakacin A (Schillinger *et al.*, 1991), mesentericin Y105 (Héchard *et al.*, 1992), leucocin A (Leistner *et al.*, 1995), piscicocin V1, diverein V41 (Pilet *et al.*, 1995) and bavarcin

(Winkowski & Montville, 1992; Larsen & Nørrung, 1993), produced by *Pediococcus acidilactici*, *Lactobacillus sake*, *Lactobacillus mesenteroides*, *Leuconostoc gelidum*, *Carnobacterium piscicola*, *Carnobacterium divergens* and *Lactobacillus bavaricus*, respectively. Muriana (1996) reviews the use of such bacteriocins for the control of *Listeria* spp. in foods.

5.4 Natural antimicrobial systems

Lysozyme is an antibacterial enzyme which is widely distributed in nature. It lyses certain Gram-positive bacteria by hydrolysing β-1,4 linkages between *N*-acetylmuramic acid and *N*-acetylglucosamine of the peptidoglycan in the cell wall. *Listeria monocytogenes* has been shown to be susceptible to lysozyme at 20–200 mg/l (Hughey & Johnson, 1987), and the addition of the enzyme to certain food products has led to the inhibition or destruction of *Listeria* present in those foods (Hughey *et al.*, 1989).

The listericidal effects of lysozyme are enhanced under alkaline or acidic conditions, and in the presence of ovomucoid and conalbumin, additional antimicrobial agents found together with lysozyme in egg albumen conditions (Wang & Shelef, 1991; Johansen *et al.*, 1994). *Listeria moncytogenes* has been shown to have an increased susceptibility to lysozyme at low temperatures (Smith *et al.*, 1991), but, in terms of its application as a food preservative, it is influenced by other food components. For example, when used in milk, *L. monocytogenes* was highly resistant to egg-white lysozyme, despite being previously sensitive in media and phosphate buffer (Kihm *et al.*, 1994). In raw cod, shrimp homogenates and fresh vegetables, the listericidal activity of lysozyme was dramatically improved when ethylenediamine tetraacetic acid (EDTA) was added (Chander & Lewis, 1980; Hughey *et al.*, 1989; Wang & Shelef, 1992); however, the enzyme appears to be less effective when used in animal-based products, such as cheese, meat and meat products (Hughey *et al.*, 1989).

The lactoperoxidase (LP) antimicrobial system is also a naturally occurring system, found in milk and human saliva. The enzyme LP has been shown to be both bacteriostatic and bactericidal to a variety of Gram-positive and Gram-negative microorganisms, and its antimicrobial activity on *L. monocytogenes*, in broth and sterile milk, has been demonstrated (Siragusa & Johnson, 1989; Bibi & Bachmann, 1990; El-Shenawy *et al.*, 1990). Activation of the LP system prior to pasteurization enhances thermal destruction of the organism (Kamau *et al.*, 1990).

Lactoferricin B, a peptide produced by gastric-pepsin digestion of bovine lactoferrin, has also been found to possess antimicrobial activity against a broad range of Gram-negative and Gram-positive bacteria, including *L. monocytogenes*, where the minimum inhibitory concentration (MIC) was found to be 0.3–0.6 μmol/ml, depending on the strain tested (Bellamy *et al.*, 1992).

5.5 Phenols

Although some food additives are primarily used for their functional properties, they may have an additional antimicrobial role in the foods in which they are used. For example, phenolic antioxidants, including butylated hydroxyanisole (BHA), butylated hydroxytoluene (BHT) and tertiary butylhydroquinone (TBHQ), which are primarily used to prevent the oxidation of fats, have been shown to be active against *L. monocytogenes* (Payne *et al.*, 1989). At MICs of 64 and 128 μg/ml, respectively, TBHQ and BHA effectively inhibited the organism, while BHT was less inhibitory, with an MIC of 512 μg/ml. Subsequently, Yousef *et al.* (1991) examined the growth kinetics of *L. monocytogenes* in the presence of antioxidants and showed that TBHQ was more effective in delaying growth of *L. monocytogenes* than BHA or BHT and could act as a barrier to the growth of *L. monocytogenes* in foods when used at permitted concentrations (up to 200 parts/10^6.

Phenolic compounds are also present in smoke, which contributes to the flavour and safety of meats. Messina *et al.* (1988) studied the efficacy of five liquid-smoke products in reducing numbers of *L. monocytogenes*. At a concentration of 0.5%, three of the five liquid-smoke products were effective in reducing viable cells of *L. monocytogenes* below detection limits within 4 h. Beef frankfurters dipped in the most effective product exhibited >99.9% reduction in numbers of the organism after 72 h at 4°C. Inhibition of *L. monocytogenes* by phenolic compounds found in smoke has been studied by Faith *et al.* (1992). Of the 11 phenolic compounds tested, only isoeugenol demonstrated antilisterial activity. It was also suggested that acetic acid enhanced the antilisterial activity of this compound. Ryser & Marth (1991) reported that the concentrations of liquid smoke required to control the proliferation of listeriae would most probably be organoleptically unacceptable to consumers, and only when it was combined with some other means of preservation could it be used as a means of safeguarding foods from the growth of *Listeria*.

5.6 Herbs and spices

Herbs and spices are primarily added to food to impart desirable flavours and odours. In recent years, a limited number of studies have reported the additional antimicrobial role of spices and their essential oils. Like other antimicrobials, such as salt, the use of spices as growth inhibitors in foods is often limited, since effective antimicrobial doses may be organoleptically unacceptable. Aureli *et al.* (1992) studied the antimicrobial activity of 32 plant essential oils, five of which (cinnamon, clove, origanum, pimento and thyme) showed antibacterial activity to the four strains of *L. monocytogenes* examined. The antilisteric activity of essential oils was shown to be strain-dependent (Aureli *et al.*, 1992; Hefnawy *et al.*, 1993), with increased effect observed with increasing concentration of spice. Ting & Deibel (1992) investigated the antimicrobial activity of 13 spices against *L. monocytogenes* and found that, using a concentration-gradient-plate method, cloves and oregano were the two most effective spices, at MICs ranging from 0.5 to 0.7% (w/v). Sage and rosemary were less inhibitory, with MICs of 0.7–1%, as was nutmeg with an MIC of 1.1–1.4%. When tested in a sterile meat slurry, however, 1% cloves or oregano had little listericidal effect, demonstrating that foods high in protein and fat and with a low water content diminish the antimicrobial ability of spices *in vitro* (Shelef, 1983; Shelef *et al.*, 1984). It is thought that the fat content coats the surface of bacterial cells, hence preventing penetration of the inhibitory substance of spice to the cells.

Pandit & Shelef (1994) screened the antimicrobial activity of 18 spices on brain heart infusion (BHI) agar, with only rosemary (≥0.5% w/v) and cloves (≥1% w/v) revealing listericidal activity. In addition, they tested the various components of rosemary, i.e. oleoresin, encapsulated oil, antioxidant extract of rosemary and the major constituents of rosemary oil, which were cineole, borneole, α-pinene and camphor. The encapsulated oil (5%) and the antioxidant extract (0.3–0.5%) inhibited the growth of *L. monocytogenes*, whereas the oil (1%) was ineffective. Of the major oil constituents only α-pinene delayed listerial growth. More recently, the effect of the essential oil of mint on *L. monocytogenes* was studied in culture medium and in three model food systems, which included pâté (Tassou *et al.*, 1995). No growth was observed over 2 days at 30°C in laboratory media; however, in the model food systems, *L. monocytogenes* survived for about 4 days before numbers declined towards the end of the storage period.

6 Conclusions

Listeria monocytogenes is a robust microorganism in terms of its ability to survive physical processing techniques and to grow in the environmental conditions commonly found in a wide range of foods and in food-processing plants. If it survives the processing techniques or if it reaches food as a postprocessing contaminant, its multiplication is best controlled by a combination of preservatives, whose effects on the growth response of *L. monocytogenes* have been well illustrated (Conner *et al.*, 1986; Buchanan *et al.*, 1989; McClure *et al.*, 1989, 1991; Buchanan & Phillips, 1990; Cole *et al.*, 1990).

7 References

Abdalla, M.O., Davidson, P.M. & Christen, G.L. (1993) Survival of selected pathogenic bacteria in white pickled cheese made with lactic acid bacteria or antimicrobials. *Journal of Food Protection*, **56**, 972–976.

Ahamad, N. & Marth, E.H. (1989) Behaviour of *Listeria monocytogenes* at 7, 13, 21, and 35°C in tryptose broth acidified with acetic, citric, or lactic acid. *Journal of Food Protection*, **52**, 688–695.

Ahamad, N. & Marth, E.H. (1990) Acid injury of

Listeria monocytogenes. *Journal of Food Protection*, **53**, 26–29.

Aureli, P., Costantini, A. & Zolea, S. (1992) Antimicrobial activity of some plant essential oils agains *Listeria monocytogenes*. *Journal of Food Protection*, **55**, 344–348.

Bahk, J. & Marth, E.H. (1990) Listeriosis and *Listeria monocytogenes*. In *Foodborne Diseases* (ed. Cliver, D.), pp. 247–257. Los Angeles: Academic Press.

Bartlett, F.M. (1993) *Listeria monocytogenes* survival on shell eggs and resistance to sodium hypochlorite. *Journal of Food Safety*, **13**, 253–261.

Bellamy, W., Takase, M., Wakabayashi, H., Kawase, K. & Tomita, M. (1992) Antibacterial spectrum of lactoferricin B, a potent bactericidal peptide derived from the *N*-terminal region of bovine lactoferrin. *Journal of Applied Bacteriology*, **73**, 472–479.

Best, M., Kennedy, M.E. & Coates, F. (1990) Efficacy of a variety of disinfectants against *Listeria* spp. *Applied and Environmental Microbiology*, **56**, 377–380.

Bibi, W. & Bachmann, M.R. (1990) Antibacterial effect of the lactoperoxidase–thiocyanate–hydrogen peroxide system on the growth of *Listeria* spp. in skim milk. *Milchwissenschaft*, **45**, 26–28.

Boerlin, P., Rocourt, J., Grimont, F., Grimont, P.A.D., Jacquet, C. & Piffaretti, J. (1992) *Listeria ivanovii* subsp. *londoniensis* subsp. nov. *International Journal of Systematic Bacteriology*, **42**, 69–73.

Brackett, R.E. (1987) Antimicrobial effect of chlorine on *Listeria monocytogenes*. *Journal of Food Protection*, **50**, 999–1003.

Bruno, M.E., Kaiser, A. & Montville, T.J. (1992) Depletion of proton motive force by nisin in *Listeria monocytogenes* cells. *Applied and Environmental Microbiology*, **58**, 2255–2259.

Buchanan, R.L. & Golden, M.H. (1994) Interaction of citric acid concentration and pH on the kinetics of *Listeria monocytogenes* inactivation. *Journal of Food Protection*, **57**, 567–570.

Buchanan, R.L. & Phillips, J.G. (1990) Response surface model for predicting the effects of temperature, pH, sodium chloride content and sodium nitrite concentration and atmosphere on the growth of *Listeria monocytogenes*. *Journal of Food Protection*, **53**, 370–376, 380.

Buchanan, R.L., Stahl, H.G. & Whiting, R.C. (1989) Effects and interactions of temperature, pH, atmosphere, sodium chloride, and sodium nitrite on the growth of *Listeria monocytogenes*. *Journal of Food Protection*, **52**, 844–851.

Buchanan, R.L., Golden, M.H. & Whiting, R.C. (1993) Differentiation of the effects of pH and lactic or acetic acid concentration on the kinetics of *Listeria monocytogenes* inactivation. *Journal of Food Protection*, **56**, 474–478, 484.

Carpenter, S.L. & Harrison, M.A. (1989) Survival of *Listeria monocytogenes* on processed poultry. *Journal of Food Science*, **54**, 556–557.

Chander, R. & Lewis, N.F. (1980) Effect of lysozyme and sodium EDTA on shrimp microflora. *European Journal of Applied Microbiology and Biotechnology*, **10**, 253–258.

Chung, K.-T., Dickson, J.S. & Crouse, J.D. (1989) Effects of nisin on growth of bacteria attached to meat. *Applied and Environmental Microbiology*, **55**, 1329–1333.

Cole, M.B., Jones, M.V. & Holyoak, C. (1990) The effect of pH, salt concentration and temperature on the survival and growth of *Listeria monocytogenes*. *Journal of Applied Bacteriology*. **69**, 63–72.

Collins, M.D., Wallbanks, S., Lane, D.J. *et al.* (1991) Phylogenetic analysis of the genus *Listeria* based on reverse transcriptase sequencing of 16S rRNA. *International Journal of Systematic Bacteriology*, **41**, 240–246.

Conner, D.E., Brackett, R.E. & Beuchat, L.R. (1986) Effect of temperature, sodium chloride and pH on growth of *Listeria monocytogenes* in cabbage juice. *Applied and Environmental Microbiology*, **52**, 59–63.

Cordier, J.L., Putallaz, T. & Cox, L.J. (1989) Impedimetric determination of activity of disinfectants and detergents on *Listeria*: preliminary study. *International Journal of Food Microbiology*, **8**, 293–297.

Cutter, C.N. & Siragusa, G.R. (1996) Reductions of *Listeria innocua* and *Brochothrix thermosphacta* on beef following nisin spray treatments and vacuum packaging. *Food Microbiology*, **13**, 23–33.

Davies, E.A. & Adams, M.R. (1994) Resistance of *Listeria monocytogenes* to the bacteriocin nisin. *International Journal of Food Microbiology*, **21**, 341–347.

Dean, J.P. & Zottola, E.A. (1996) Use of nisin in ice cream and effect on the survival of *Listeria monocytogenes*. *Journal of Food Protection*, **59**, 476–480.

Dickgiesser, N. (1980) *Listeria monocytogenes* als Urasche von krankenhausinfektionen: untersuchungen zum uberleben der Erreger in der Aussenwelt. *Infection*, **8**, 199–201.

Dickson, J.S. & Siragusa, G.R. (1994) Survival of *Salmonella typhimurium, Escherichia coli* 0157:H7 and *Listeria monocytogenes* during storage on beef sanitized with organic acids. *Journal of Food Safety*, **14**, 313–327.

Donnelly, C.W. (1990) Resistance of *Listeria monocytogenes* to heat. In *Foodborne Listeriosis* (eds Millar, A.L., Smith, J.L. & Somkuti, G.A.), pp. 189–194. New York: Elsevier.

El-Kest, S.E. & Marth, E.H. (1988a) Inactivation of *Listeria monocytogenes* by chlorine. *Journal of Food Protection*, **51**, 520–524.

El-Kest, S.E. & Marth, E.H. (1988b) Temperature, pH, and strain of pathogen as factors affecting inactivation of *Listeria monocytogenes* by chlorine. *Journal of Food Protection*, **51**, 622–625.

El-Khateib, T., Yousef, A.E. & Ockerman, H.W. (1993) Inactivation and attachment of *Listeria monocytogenes* on beef muscle treated with lactic acid and selected bacteriocins. *Journal of Food Protection*, **56**, 29–33.

El-Shenawy, M.A. & Marth, E.H. (1988a) Sodium benzoate inhibits growth of or inactivates *Listeria monocytogenes*. *Journal of Food Protection*, **51**, 525–530.

El-Shenawy, M.A. & Marth, E.H. (1988b) Inhibition and inactivation of *Listeria monocytogenes* by sorbic acid. *Journal of Food Protection*, **51**, 842–847.

El-Shenawy, M.A. & Marth, E.H. (1989) Behaviour of *Listeria monocytogenes* in the presence of sodium propionate. *International Journal of Food Microbiology*, **8**, 85–94.

El-Shenawy, M.A. & Marth, E.H. (1991) Organic acids enhance the antilisterial ativity of potassium sorbate. *Journal of Food Protection*, **54**, 593–597.

El-Shenawy, M.A., Garcia, H.S. & Marth, E.H. (1990) Inhibition and inactivation of *Listeria monocytogenes* by the lactoperoxidase system in raw milk, buffer or a semi-synthetic medium. *Milchwissenschaft*, **45**, 638–641.

Faith, N.G., Yousef, A.E. & Luchansky, J.B. (1992) Inhibition of *Listeria monocytogenes* by liquid smoke and isoeugenol, a phenolic component found in smoke. *Journal of Food Safety*, **12**, 303–314.

Fang, T.J. & Lin, L.-W. (1994) Growth of *Listeria monocytogenes* and *Pseudomonas fragi* on cooked pork in a modified atmosphere packaging/nisin combination system. *Journal of Food Protection*, **57**, 479–485.

Farber, J.M. & Brown, B.E. (1990) Effect of prior heat shock on heat resistance of *Listeria monocytogenes* in meat. *Applied and Environmental Microbiology*, **556**, 1584–1587.

Farber, J.M. & Peterkin, P.I. (1991) *Listeria monocytogenes*, a food-borne pathogen. *Microbiological Reviews*, **55**, 476–511.

Farber, J.M., Sanders, G.W., Dunfield, S. & Prescott, R. (1989) The effect of various acidulants on the growth of *Listeria monocytogenes*. *Letters in Applied Microbiology*, **9**, 181–183.

Farber, J.M., Coates, F. & Daley, E. (1992) Minimum water activity requirements for the growth of *Listeria monocytogenes*. *Letters in Applied Microbiology*, **15**, 103–105.

Fedio, W.M. & Jackson, H. (1989) Effect of tempering on the heat resistance of *Listeria monocytogenes*. *Letters in Applied Microbiology*, **9**, 157–160.

Feresu, S.B. & Jones, D. (1988) Taxonomic studies on *Brochothrix, Erysipelothrix, Listeria* and atypical lactobacilli. *Journal of General Microbiology*, **134**, 1165–1183.

Gahan, C.J.M., O'Driscoll, B. & Hill, C. (1996) Acid adaptation of *Listeria monocytogenes* can enhance survival in acidic foods and during milk fermentation. *Applied and Environmental Microbiology*, **62**, 3128–3132.

George, S.M., Lund, B.M. & Brocklehurst, T.F. (1988) The effect of pH and temperature on initiation of growth of *Listeria monocytogenes*. *Letters in Applied Microbiology*, **5**, 153–156.

Golden, D.A., Beuchat, L.R. & Brackett, R.E. (1988) Evaluation of selective direct plating media for their suitability to recover uninjured, heat-injured and freeze-injured *Listeria monocytogenes* from foods. *Applied and Environmental Microbiology*, **54**, 1451–1456.

Golden, M.H., Buchanan, R.L. & Whiting, R.C. (1995) Effect of sodium acetate or sodium propionate with EDTA and ascorbic acid on the inactivation of *Listeria monocytogenes*. *Journal of Food Safety*, **15**, 53–65.

Grant, I.R., Nixon, C.R. & Patterson, M.F. (1993) Comparison of the growth of *Listeria monocytogenes* in unirradiated and irradiated cook-chill roast beef and gravy at refrigeration temperatures. *Letters in Applied Microbiology*, **17**, 55–57.

Harris, L.J., Fleming, H.P. & Klaenhammer, T.R. (1991) Sensitivity and resistance of *Listeria monocytogenes* ATCC 19115, Scott A and UAL500 to nisin. *Journal of Food Protection*, **54**, 836–840.

Harrison, M.A. & Carpenter, S.L. (1989a) Survival of large populations of *Listeria monocytogenes* on chicken breasts processed using moist heat. *Journal of Food Protection*, **52**, 376–378.

Harrison, M.A. & Carpenter, S.L. (1989b) Survival of *Listeria monocytogenes* on microwave cooked poultry. *Food Microbiology*, **6**, 153–157.

Hayat, M. A. (ed.) (1986) *Positive Staining: Transmission Electron Microscopy*. New York: Academic Press.

Héchard, Y., Dérijard, B., Letellier, F. & Cenatiempo, Y. (1992) Characterisation and purification of mesentericin Y105, an anti-*Listeria* bacteriocin from *Leuconstoc mesenteroides*. *Journal of General Microbiology*, **138**, 2725–2731.

Hefnawy, Y.A., Moustafa, S.I. & Marth, E.H. (1993) Sensitivity of *Listeria monocytogenes* to selected spices. *Journal of Food Protection*, **56**, 876–878.

Herald, P.A. & Zottola, E.A. (1988) Attachment of *Listeria monocytogenes* to stainless steel surfaces at various temperatures and pH values. *Journal of Food Science*, **53**, 1549–1562.

Hite, B.H. (1899) The effect of pressure in the preservation of milk. *Bulletin of West Virginia Agricultural Experiment Station*, **58**, 15–35.

Hof, H., Nichterlein, T. & Kretschmar, M. (1997) Management of listeriosis. *Clinical Microbiology Reviews*, **10**, 345–357.

Hoover, D.G., Metrick, C., Papineau, A.M., Farkas, D.F. & Knorr, D. (1989) Biological effects of high hydrostatic pressure on food microorganisms. *Food Technology*, **43**, 99–107.

Hughey, V.L. & Johnson, E.A. (1987) Antimicrobial activity of lysozyme against bacteria involved in food spoilage and food-borne disease. *Applied and Environmental Microbiology*, **53**, 2165–2170.

Hughey, V.L., Wilger, P.A. & Johnson, E.A. (1989) Antibacterial activity of hen egg white lyzozyme against *Listeria monocytogenes* Scott A in foods. *Applied and Environmental Microbiology*, **55**, 631–638.

Huhtanen, C.N., Jenkins, R.K. & Thayer, D.W. (1989) Gamma radiation sensitivity of *Listeria monocytogenes*. *Journal of Food Protection*, **52**, 610–613.

Idziak, E.S. & Incze, K. (1968) Radiation treatment of foods I. Radurization of fresh eviscerated poultry. *Applied Microbiology*, **16**, 1061–1066.

Ingham, S.C., Escude, J.M. & McCown, P. (1990) Comparative growth rates of *Listeria monocytogenes* and *Pseudomonas fragi* on cooked chicken loaf stored under air and two modified atmospheres. *Journal of Food Protection*, **53**, 289–291.

Ita, P.S. & Hutkins, R.W. (1991) Intracellular pH and survival of *Listeria monocytogenes* Scott A in tryptic soy broth containing acetic, lactic, citric and hydrochloric acids. *Journal of Food Protection*, **54**, 15–19.

Jacquet, C. & Reynaud, A. (1994) Differences in the sensitivity to eight disinfectants of *Listeria monocytogenes* strains as related to their origin. *International Journal of Food Microbiology*, **22**, 79–83.

Johansen, C., Gram, L. & Meyer, A.S. (1994) The combined inhibitory effect of lysozyme and low pH on growth of *Listeria monocytogenes*. *Journal of Food Protection*, **57**, 561–566.

Jung, D.S., Bodyfelt, F.W. & Daeschel, M.A. (1992) Influence of fat and emulsifiers on the efficacy of nisin in inhibiting *Listeria monocytogenes* in fluid milk. *Journal of Dairy Science*, **75**, 387–393.

Junttila, J.R., Niemela, S.I. & Hirn, J. (1988) Minimum growth temperatures of *Listeria monocytogenes* and non-haemolytic *Listeria*. *Journal of Applied Bacteriology*, **65**, 321–327.

Kamau, D.N., Doores, S. & Pruitt, K.M. (1990) Enhanced thermal destruction of *Listeria monocytogenes* and *Staphylococcus aureus* by the lactoperoxidase system. *Applied and Environmental Microbiology*, **56**, 2711–2716.

Kihm, D.J., Leyer, G.J., An, G.-H. & Johnson, E.A. (1994) Sensitization of heat-treated *Listeria monocytogenes* to added lysozyme in milk. *Applied and Environmental Microbiology*, **60**, 3854–3861.

Kim, K.-T., Murano, E.A. & Olson, D.G. (1994) Heating and storage conditions affect and recovery of *Listeria monocytogenes* in ground pork. *Journal of Food Science*, **59**, 30–32, 59.

Knabel, S.J., Walker, H.W., Hartman, P.A. & Mendonca, A.F. (1990) Effects of growth temperature and strictly anaerobic recovery on the survival of *Listeria monocytogenes* during pasteurisation. *Applied and Environmental Microbiology*, **56**, 370–376.

Lammerding, A.M. & Doyle, M.P. (1990) Stability of *Listeria monocytogenes* to non-thermal processing conditions. In *Foodborne Listeriosis* (eds Miller, A.J., Smith, J.L.& Somkuti, G.A.), pp. 195–202. Amsterdam: Elsevier.

Larsen, A.G. & Nørrung, B. (1993) Inhibition of *Listeria monocytogenes* by bavarcin A, a bacteriocin produced by *Lactobacillus bavaricus* M1401. *Letters in Applied Microbiology*, **17**, 132–134.

Lee, S.-H. & Frank, J.F. (1991) Effect of growth temperature and media on inactivation of *Listeria monocytogenes* by chlorine. *Journal of Food Safety*, **11**, 65–71.

Leistner, J.J., Greer, G.G., Dilts, B.D. & Stiles, M.E. (1995) Effect of growth of selected lactic acid bacteria on storage life of beef stored under vacuum and in air. *International Journal of Food Microbiology*, **26**, 231–243.

Lopes, J.A. (1986) Evaluation of dairy and plant sanitizers against *Salmonella typhimurium* and *Listeria monocytogenes*. *Journal of Dairy Science*, **69**, 2791–2796.

McClure, P.J., Roberts, T.A. & Otto Oguru, P. (1989) Comparison of the effects of sodium chloride, pH and temperature on the growth of *Listeria monocytogenes* on gradient plates and in liquid medium. *Letters in Applied Microbiology*, **9**, 95–99.

McClure, P.J., Kelly, T.M. & Roberts, T.A. (1991) The effects of temperature, pH, sodium chloride and sodium nitrite on the growth of *Listeria monocytogenes*. *International Journal of Food Microbiology*, **14**, 77–92.

Mackey, B.M. & Derrick, C.M. (1987) Changes in the heat resistance of *Salmonella typhimurium* during heating at rising temperatures. *Letters in Applied Microbiology*, **4**, 13–16.

Mackey, B.M., Pritchet, C., Norris, A. & Mead, G.C. (1990) Heat resistance of *Listeria*: strain differences and effects of meat type and curing salts. *Letters in Applied Microbiology*, **10**, 251–255.

Mackey, B.M., Forestière, K., Isaacs, N.S., Stenning, R. & Brooker, B. (1994) The effect of hydrostatic pressure on *Salmonella thompson* and *Listeria monocytogenes* examined by electron microscopy. *Letters in Applied Microbiology*, **19**, 429–432.

McLauchlin, J. (1990) Human listeriosis in Britain, 1967–85, a summary of 722 cases. 2. Listeriosis in non-pregnant individuals, a changing pattern of infection and seasonal influence. *Epidemiology and Infection*, **104**, 191–201.

Mafu, A.A., Roy, D., Goulet, J., Savoie, J. & Roy, R.

(1990) Efficiency of sanitizing agents for destroying *Listeria monocytogenes* on contaminated surfaces. *Journal of Dairy Science*, **73**, 3428–3432.

Mahadeo, M. & Tatini, S.R. (1994) The potential use of nisin to control *Listeria monocytogenes* in poultry. *Letters in Food Microbiology*, **18**, 323–326.

Marshall, D.L., Wiese-Lehigh, P.L., Wells, J.H. & Farr, A.J. (1991) Comparative growth of *Listeria monocytogenes* and *Pseudomonas fluorescens* on precooked chicken nuggets stored under modified atmospheres. *Journal of Food Protection*, **54**, 841–844.

Marshall, D.L., Andrews, L.S., Wells, J.H. & Farr, A.J. (1992) Influence of modified atmosphere packaging on the competitive growth of *Listeria monocytogenes* and *Pseudomonas fluorescens* on precooked chicken. *Food Microbiology*, **9**, 303–309.

Messina, M.C., Ahmad, H.A., Marchello, J.A., Gerba, C.P. & Paquette, M.W. (1988) The effect of liquid smoke on *Listeria monocytogenes*. *Journal of Food Protection*, **51**, 629–631.

Mosteller, T.M. & Bishop, J.R. (1993) Sanitizer efficacy against attached bacteria in a milk biofilm. *Journal of Food Protection*, **56**, 34–41.

Motlagh, A.M., Holla, S., Johnson, B.R. & Field, R.A. (1992) Inhibition of *Listeria* spp. in sterile food systems by pediocin AcH, a bacteriocin produced by *Pediococcus acidilactici* H. *Journal of Food Protection*, **55**, 337–343.

Muriana, P.M. (1996) Bacteriocins for control of *Listeria* spp. in food. *Journal of Food Protection*, **58** (Suppl.), 54–63.

Mustapha, A. & Liewen, M.B. (1989) Destruction of *Listeria monocytogenes* by sodium hypochlorite and quaternary ammonium sanitizers. *Journal of Food Protection*, **52**, 306–311.

O'Driscoll, B., Gahan, C.G.N. & Hill, C. (1996) Adaptive acid tolerant response in *Listeria monocytogenes*: isolation of an acid-tolerant mutant which demonstrates increased virulence. *Applied and Environmental Microbiology*, **62**, 1693-1698.

Oh, D.-H. & Marshall, D.L. (1995) Destruction of *Listeria monocytogenes* biofilms on stainless steel using monolaurin and heat. *Journal of Food Protection*, **57**, 251–255.

Oh, D.-H. & Marshall, D.L. (1996) Monolaurin and acetic acid inactivation of *Listeria monocytogenes* attached to stainless steel. *Journal of Food Protection*, **59**, 249–252.

Palumbo, S.A. & Williams, A.C. (1989) Freezing and freeze injury in *Listeria monocytogenes*. In *Annual Meeting of the American Society of Microbiology*, 14–18 May, New Orleans, Abstr. P-1.

Palumbo, S.A. & Williams, A.C. (1990) Effect of temperature, relative humidity, and suspending menstrua on the resistance of *Listeria monocytogenes* to drying. *Journal of Food Protection*, **53**, 377–381.

Pandit, V.A. & Shelef, L.A. (1994) Sensitivity of *Listeria monocytogenes* to rosemary (*Rosmarinus officinalis* L.). *Food Microbiology*, **11**, 57–63.

Parish, M.E. & Higgins, D.P. (1989) Survival of *Listeria monocytogenes* in low pH model broth systems. *Journal of Food Protection*, **52**, 144–147.

Patterson, M.F. (1988) Sensitivity of bacteria to irradiation on poultry meat under various atmospheres. *Letters in Applied Microbiology*. **7**, 55–58.

Patterson, M.F. (1989) Sensitivity of *Listeria monocytogenes* to irradiation on poultry meat and in phosphate buffered saline. *Letters in Applied Microbiology*, **8**, 181–184.

Patterson, M.F., Quinn, M., Simpson, R. & Gilmour, A. (1995) Sensitivity of vegetative pathogens to high hydrostatic pressure treatment in phosphate-buffered saline and foods. *Journal of Food Protection*, **58**, 524–529.

Payne, K.D., Rico-Munoz, E. & Davidson, P.M. (1989) The antimicrobial activity of phenolic compounds against *Listeria monocytogenes* and their effectiveness in a model milk system. *Journal of Food Protection*, **52**, 151–153.

Pearson, L.J. & Marth, E.H. (1990) *Listeria monocytogenes*–threat to a safe food supply. *Journal of Dairy Science*, **73**, 912–928.

Pelroy, G.A., Peterson, M.E., Holland, P.J. & Eklund, M.W. (1994a) Inhibition of *Listeria monocytogenes* in cold-process (smoked) salmon by sodium lactate. *Journal of Food Protection*, **57**, 108–113.

Pelroy, G., Peterson, M., Paranjpye, R., Almond, J. & Mel Eklund (1994b) Inhibition of *Listeria monocytogenes* in cold-process (smoked) salmon by sodium nitrite and packaging method. *Journal of Food Protection*, **57**, 114–119.

Petran, R.L. & Zottola, E.A. (1989) A study of factors affecting growth and recovery of *Listeria monocytogenes* Scott A. *Journal of Food Science*, **54**, 458–460.

Pilet, M.-F., Dousset, X., Barré, R., Novel, G., Desmazeaud, M. & Piard, J.-C. (1995) Evidence for two bacteriocins produced by *Carnobacterium piscicola* and *Carnobacterium divergens* isolated from fish and active against *Listeria monocytogenes*. *Journal of Food Protection*, **58**, 256–262.

Podolak, R.K., Zayas, J.E., Kastner, C.L. & Fung, D.Y.C. (1995) Reduction of *Listeria monocytogenes*, *Escherichia coli* O157:H7 and *Salmonella typhimurium* during storage on beef sanitized with fumaric, acetic, and lactic acids. *Journal of Food Safety*, **15**, 283–290.

Podolak, R.K., Zayas, J.E., Kastner, C.L. & Fung, D.Y.C. (1996) Inhibition of *Listeria monocytogenes* and *Escherichia coli* O157:H7 on beef by application of organic acids. *Journal of Food Protection*, **59**, 370–373.

Pothuri, P., Marshall, D.L. & McMillin, K.W. (1996) Combined effects of packaging, atmosphere and lactic acid on growth and survival of *Listeria monocytogenes* in-crayfish tail meat at 4°C. *Journal of Food Protection*, **59**, 253–256.

Ren, T.-J. & Frank, J.F. (1993) Susceptibility of starved planktonic and biofilm *Listeria monocytogenes* to quaternary ammonium sanitizer as determined by direct viable and agar plate counts. *Journal of Food Protection*, **56**, 573–576.

Rocourt, J., Wehmeyer, U. & Stackebrandt, E. (1987) Transfer of *Listeria denitrificans* to a new genus *Jonesia* gen. nov., as *Jonesia denitrificans* comb. nov. *International Journal of Systematic Bacteriology*, **37**, 271–280.

Ronner, A.B. & Wong, A.C.L. (1993) Biofilm development and sanitizer inactivation of *Listeria monocytogenes* and *Salmonella typhimurium* on stainless steel and Bunna-n rubber. *Journal of Food Protection*, **56**, 750–758.

Ryser, E.T. & Marth, E.H. (1991) Incidence and behaviour of *Listeria monocytogenes* in meat products. In *Listeria, Listeriosis and Food Safety* (eds Ryser, E.T. & Marth, E.H.), pp. 405–462. New York: Marcel Dekker.

Schillinger, U., Kaya, M. & Lücke, F.-K. (1991) Behaviour of *Listeria monocytogenes* in meat and its control by a bacteriocin producing strain of *Lactobacillus sake*. *Journal of Applied Bacteriology*, **70**, 473–478.

Seeliger, H.P.R. (ed.) (1961) *Listeriosis*, 2nd edn, p. 37. New York: Hafner.

Seeliger, H.P.R. (1988) Listeriosis–history and actual developments. *Infection*, **16**, S80-S84.

Seeliger, H.P.R. & Jones, D. (1986) Genus *Listeria*. In *Bergey's Manual of Systematic Bacteriology*, Vol. 2 (eds Sneath, P.H.A., Mair, N.S., Sharpe, M.E. & Holt, J.G.), pp. 1235–1245. Baltimore: Williams and Wilkins.

Shahmat, M., Seaman, A. & Woodbine, M. (1980a) Survival of *Listeria monocytogenes* in high salt concentrations. *Zentralblatt für Bakteriologie und Hygiene I. Abt. Org. A*, **246**, 506–511.

Shahamat, M., Seaman, A. & Woodbine, M. (1980b) Influence of sodium chloride, pH and temperature on the inhibitory activity of sodium nitrite on *Listeria monocytogenes*. In *Society for Applied Bacteriology Technical Series No. 14*, pp. 22–37. London: Academic Press.

Shelef, L.A. (1983) Antimicrobial effects of spices. *Journal of Food Safety*, **6**, 29–44.

Shelef, L.A., Jyothi, E.K. & Bulgarelli, M.A. (1984) Growth of enteropathogenic and spoilage bacteria in sage-containing broth and foods. *Journal of Food Science*, **49**, 737–740, 809.

Siragusa, G.R. & Johnson, M. (1989) Inhibition of *Listeria monocytogenes* growth by the lactoperoxidase–thiocyanate–H_2O_2 antimicrobial system. *Applied and Environmental Microbiology*, **55**, 2802–2805.

Smith, J.L., McColgan, C. & Marmer, B.S. (1991) Growth temperature and action of lysozyme on *Listeria monocytogenes*. *Journal of Food Science*, **56**, 1101, 1103.

Sorrells, K.M., Enigl, D.C. & Hatfield, J.R. (1989) Effect of pH, acidulant, time and temperature on the growth and survival of *Listeria monocytogenes*. *Journal of Food Protection*, **52**, 571–573.

Spurlock, A.T. & Zottola, E.A. (1991) Growth and attachment of *Listeria monocytogenes* to cast iron. *Journal of Food Protection*, **54**, 925–929.

Stumbo, C.R. (ed.) (1973) *Thermobacteriology in Food Processing*, 2nd edn. London: Academic Press.

Tarjan, V. (1988) The sensitivity of *Listeria monocytogenes* to gamma radiation. In *Proceedings of the 10th International Symposium: Listeriosis*, Pecs, Hungary, Abstr. P 57.

Tassou, C.C., Drosinos, E.H. & Nychas, G.J.E. (1995) Effects of essential oil from mint (*Mentha piperita*) on *Salmonella enteriditis* and *Listeria monocytogenes* in model food systems at 4°C and 10°C. *Journal of Applied Bacteriology*, **78**, 593-600.

Ting, W.T.E. & Deibel, K.E. (1992) Sensitivity of *Listeria monocytogenes* to spices at two temperatures. *Journal of Food Safety*, **12**, 129–137.

Tuncan, E.U. (1993) Effect of cold temperature on germicidal efficacy of quaternary ammonium compound, iodophor, and chlorine on *Listeria*. *Journal of Food Protection*, **56**, 1029–1033.

Walker, S.J., Archer, P. & Banks, J.G. (1990) Growth of *Listeria monocytogenes* at refrigeration temperatures. *Journal of Applied Bacteriology* **68**, 157–162.

Walker, A.T., Jassim, S.A.A., Holah, J.T., Denyer, S.P. & Stewart, G.S.A.B. (1991) Bioluminescent *Listeria monocytogenes* provide a rapid assay for measuring biocide activity. *FEMS Microbiology Letters*, **91**, 251–256.

Wang, C. & Shelef, L.A. (1991) Factors contributing to antilisterial effects of raw egg albumen. *Journal of Food Science*, **56**, 1251–1254.

Wilkins, P.O., Bourgeois, R. & Murray, R.G.E. (1972) Psychrotrophic properties of *Listeria monocytogenes*. *Canadian Journal of Microbiology*, **18**, 543–551.

Winkowski, K. & Montville, T.J. (1992) Use of meat isolate, *Lactobacillus bavaricus* MN, to inhibit *Listeria monocytogenes* growth in a model meat gravy system. *Journal of Food Safety*, **13**, 19–31.

Woolthuis, C.H.J. & Smulders, F.J.M. (1985) Microbial decontamination of calf carcasses by lactic acid sprays. *Journal of Food Protection*, **48**, 832–837.

World Health Organization (WHO) Working Group (1988) Foodborne listeriosis. *Bulletin of the WHO*, **66**, 421–428.

Yousef, A.E., Gajewski, R.J., II & Marth, E.H. (1991) Kinetics of growth and inhibition of *Listeria monocytogenes* in the presence of antioxidant food additives. *Journal of Food Science*, **56**, 10–13.

Zhang, S. & Farber, J.M. (1996) The effects of various disinfectants against *Listeria monocytogenes* on fresh-cut vegetables. *Food Microbiology*, **13**, 311–321.

Zottola, E.A., Yezzi, T.L., Ajao, D.B. & Roberts, R.F. (1994) Utilisation of cheddar cheese containing nisin as an antimicrobial agent in other foods. *International Journal of Food Microbiology*, **24**, 227–238.

CHAPTER 11

Good Manufacturing Practice

1 Introduction

A good hygienic standard is one of the prime targets in the pharmaceutical, cosmetic and food industries. As well as protecting the consumer, it has an economic basis in the prevention of product loss due to microbial spoilage (Hargreaves, 1990).

Raw materials, including water supplies, are one of the main sources of microorganisms and can result in the contamination of the environment and manufacturing plant. Contamination may also arise from poor hygienic practices by process operators and a failure to follow cleaning and disinfection procedures. Microbial contamination can be controlled by the selection of raw materials and by following the principles of good manufacturing practice (GMP), i.e. providing suitable premises, equipment and environment, with trained personnel to operate approved procedures (Underwood, 1998).

Of equal importance to selecting raw materials with a good microbial quality is the control of the environment to create unfavourable conditions for microbial growth. To achieve this, both cleaning and disinfection must be approached on a technological basis, with trials to evaluate the ability of detergents to remove soil residues, since this will affect the efficiency of the disinfection stage. Cleaning and disinfection should be regarded as a part of the manufacturing process, with written procedures and an adequate time allotted for them to be carried out correctly.

A system which is commonly being introduced is that of hazard analysis of critical control points (HACCP). This is an all-embracing philosophy which examines the risk of microbiological contamination introduced from raw materials, packaging, operatives and the manufacturing environment and methods by which it may be eliminated or controlled by processing or preservation, and identifies critical control points. This procedure, together with any end-point testing, minimizes the risk of product spoilage in a cost-effective manner.

2 Cleaning agents

There is a wide choice of cleaning agents available, including alkalis, both mineral and organic acids, and cationic, anionic or non-ionic surfactants. Careful selection is necessary to ensure that the chosen agent fulfils the following criteria. It must:

1 Suit the surface to be cleaned, and not cause corrosion;

2 Remove the type of soil present without leaving any sort of residue;

3 Be compatible with the water supply.

A suitable detergent must have adequate wetting properties to enable the solvent, usually water, to contact all areas by reducing the surface tension and permitting penetration into all cracks, pinholes and porous materials. In addition, it should disperse any aggregates of soil into small particles and retain any insoluble material in suspension, in order that the soil may be easily flushed from the surface. The detergent itself must be able to be rinsed away without leaving a deposit on the surface.

Ideally, only soft water should be used for cleaning, but, where this is impracticable, it is important that any alkaline detergent used is compatible with the local water-supply or that water-conditioning or sequestering agents are added. If very hard water is used, it may be necessary to incorporate an acid rinse into the cleaning cycle to prevent scale. This is of particular importance in the dairy industry to reduce the problems of 'milkstone'. This use and use as a general cleaner form the main functions of acid detergents.

In selecting an alkaline detergent, the active alkalinity is an important criterion if it is required to deal with fat-containing residues by saponification into a 'soap' or to neutralize acidic constituents. By counterbalancing the active alkalinity against the alkali demand, the optimum pH for soil removal and for protecting the surface from corrosion can be achieved.

Each type of surface-active agent (see also Chapter 2) has different properties: anionics—salts of complex organic acids—are good detergents but poor bactericides; non-ionics—organic compounds but not salts—have good wetting powers; cationics—salts of complex organic bases—are good bactericides but have poorer detergent properties. Cationic and anionic compounds must not be used together, but their two properties are combined in amphoteric compounds.

Cleaning agents are often more effective when used hot, but temperatures of 65°C should not be exceeded when removing fat-containing films, since the emulsion formed with the detergent is destroyed. This temperature restriction also applies to some alkaline detergents when used with hard water. Acid cleaners are normally used cold.

Detergents should be evaluated before their introduction as part of a cleaning cycle. A study of their physical properties, such as solubility in water, active alkalinity reaction, buffering ability, sequestering power and stability in both the dry and liquid forms, will give some guide as to their suitability for a given task, but the final test must be an assessment of the efficiency in removing soil from surfaces. In addition to visual and chemical tests for residues, a fluorescent dye may be introduced with the soil before application of the detergent and the surface examined with ultraviolet (UV) light after cleaning. Many foodstuffs are, however, naturally fluorescent in UV light and it is often standard practice to include the examination of equipment with a specially designed lamp as a postcleaning check.

It is sometimes useful to combine a cleaning and sanitizing stage, but this is only successful where light soiling occurs and a relatively low level of microbial contamination has to be removed. It also has the advantage of providing a bactericide in the wash water, a factor which is often a source of contamination in itself. Not all detergents and disinfectants are compatible, and this must be checked if novel combinations are used. Three main types are commercially available.

1 Alkaline detergents formulated with chlorine-liberating compounds.
2 Alkaline detergents formulated with quaternary ammonium compounds (QACs) or non-ionic surfactants.
3 Acid detergents with iodophors.

Detailed accounts of detergency and cleaning practice in the food (Parker & Litchfield, (1962) and dairy (Anon., 1959a) industries have been published.

2.1 Control of cleaning agents

The effectiveness of in-place cleaning depends upon control of the detergent concentration, and this may be carried out by testing samples at both the start and the end of the circulation period. If the detergent concentration is lower than that established in trials, then all the soil may not be removed; if it is higher, it may require additional rinsing to remove it from the plant, as well as being wasteful. One of the most useful tests is the titratable alkali or acid content.

Regular inspections should be carried out on all equipment, especially behind O-rings, gaskets and rubber diaphragms, where soil may remain. As described previously, inspection with a UV lamp is useful if the soil contains materials that are fluorescent under such conditions.

All cleaning and combined cleaning and disinfection procedures must be validated and controls set with regard to each step, including the strength of the cleaning agent and the temperature and time relationship, for each type of and degree of soiling and for each piece of equipment. Initially, this needs to be carried out in conjunction with microbiological testing, either of the surface which has been cleaned or of the final rinse. Once validated, the procedure may be controlled using set parameters (physical and chemical measurements), with the backup of microbiological testing, to be used on a non-routine basis or when changes are introduced.

3 Disinfection and sterilization

The choice of disinfecting non-disposable equipment and instruments is usually between heat and a chemical agent. Heat is the more reliable and is the first choice for industrial plant used for aseptic preparation and filling operations, but it is usually both too expensive and impracticable for use with large-scale industrial machinery, and chemical agents are employed. Where necessary, buildings, interiors and fittings are treated chemically, but a wider range of techniques are available for the sterilization of water, air and raw materials.

3.1 Chemical disinfectants

The choice of disinfectant is governed by the material or surface to be treated and, in some instances, by the type of contaminating microorganism present. The types of disinfectants and their properties are described in Chapter 2, but Table 11.1 shows some of their industrial applications.

3.1.1 Control and monitoring of chemical disinfectants

With the exception of some halogen-containing preparations, most sterilizing agents are stable chemically in the undiluted state for normal storage periods. Inorganic halogens, such as sodium hypochlorite solution, deteriorate on storage and must be assayed both on receipt and just before use, if stored.

Written instructions should be available for the preparation or dilution of all disinfectants and they should state the source of the water to be used. It is important that water of good microbiological quality is used to dilute disinfectants, particularly those which may support the growth of water-borne organisms, e.g. QACs. Disinfectants prepared for use should be stored for the minimum possible time and be clearly labelled

Table 11.1 The industrial applications for chemical disinfectants.

Disinfectant	Food industry	Pharmaceutical and cosmetic industry
Halogens, e.g. sodium hypochlorite, chlorine gas, iodophors	Water-supplies, equipment, packaging, working surfaces	Water supplies, equipment, packaging, working surfaces
Quaternary ammonium compounds (QACs)	Equipment, building interior fittings, working surfaces	Equipment, building interior fittings, working surfaces
Phenols and related compounds	Not in common use	Building interior fittings, skin disinfectant
Alcohols: ethanol or isopropanol	Working surfaces, equipment. Useful for small-scale treatment after maintenance during a production run	Working surfaces, equipment. Useful for small-scale treatment after maintenance during a production run
Amphoteric compounds	Skin disinfectant, equipment	Skin disinfectant, equipment
Hydrogen peroxide	Used hot for plastic packaging in the dairy industry. Some raw materials	Not in common use
Biguanides	Skin disinfectant	Skin disinfectant
Aldehydes		
Liquid or vaporized formaldehyde, glutaraldehyde	Not in common use	Process water, some equipment
Gaseous	Fumigation of poultry houses	Fumigation of clean or aseptic processing areas, packaging
Ethylene oxide	Some raw materials	Raw materials, finished products, packaging

with the date of preparation and expiry, as well as the contents and the dilution factor. Diluted batches should not be 'topped up' with fresh solutions, but the containers should be emptied and cleaned before refilling. In the case of disinfectants which are vulnerable to colonization by some groups of microorganisms, such as biguanides and QACs, the containers should be washed and either heat-sterilized or treated with an active chemical agent before reuse. This also applies to sprays and other dispensing equipment.

The methods for evaluating chemical disinfectants are given in Chapter 4A,B, and their selection and practical applications are considered in Chapter 2.

Gaseous disinfection is dependent upon both the environmental conditions and the concentration of the agent. When ethylene oxide is used, the temperature and the humidity must both be monitored (Chapter 21) and at least 10 biological indicators, carrying spores of *Bacillus subtilis* (Beeby & Whitehouse, 1965), placed in the load. The spores may be dried on to aluminium or paper strips, which, after the cycle, are tested for viable cells. Some commercial preparations are available in which the spore-bearing strip and medium for bacterial testing are contained in a single, double-walled unit, which is convenient for the process operator to handle. Formaldehyde gas requires a relative humidity of 80–90% to be effective, and monitoring is usually carried out by checking the residual surviving microorganisms on the surface of the treated materials.

In addition to the selection of a disinfectant for a given task, as detailed for cleaning agents, the complete procedure must be validated to ensure efficacy and parameters for disinfectant concentration, temperature and time of exposure set. The validation may take the form of examining the surface disinfected for residual microorganisms, a facet which is considered later in this chapter, or, for liquid disinfectants, it may involve testing a sample of the disinfectant in which instruments or equipment are being treated for the presence of microorganism, or a combination of both. Whichever method is used, it must be in conjunction with the cleaning procedure, and the nature and degree of initial soiling and microbiological load must be taken into consideration. A detailed account of the test devised by Kelsey and Maurer, giving dilution levels and the neutralizing agents required for some disinfectants, is given by Maurer (1985). Records should be kept of all monitoring carried out on chemical disinfection processes; in the pharmaceutical industry, these may be required to be kept with the batch records of the product.

3.2 Disinfection and sterilization by heat

Heat may be used, with or without the aid of moisture, to disinfect or sterilize. The advantage of the pressure of moisture is that lower temperatures are required.

3.2.1 Dry heat

Temperatures in excess of 160°C throughout a hot-air oven are usually recommended for dry heat sterilization. This is used for sterilizing equipment and some dry powders, in both the cosmetic and the pharmaceutical industries. It is usually necessary for sterilizing ovens to be equipped with a fan to distribute heat evenly, and careful packing of the load is important to prevent local cold spots. The temperature should be recorded from a probe sited at the potentially coolest part of the load. An inlet air-sterilizing filter should be fitted to prevent contamination as the load cools. Equipment or instruments sterilized by this method must be wrapped or suitably protected to prevent contamination on removal from the oven.

Containers used for parenteral pharmaceutical preparations are often sterilized at temperatures higher than those required to kill microorganisms, in order to destroy any pyrogenic residues present.

3.2.2 Moist heat

Moist heat may be used in the form of steam under pressure in an autoclave at temperatures which destroy all microorganisms (see Chapter 19A, B) or in the form of hot water or a water-and-steam mixture which kills only a limited range. Additionally, low-temperature steam with formaldehyde has some applications as a sterilizing agent (Chapter 21A). Correctly operated, hot-water pasteurization kills all but the most heat-resistant of bacterial cells in the vegetative phase, but it does not destroy bacterial spores.

The minimum useful temperature for hot-water pasteurization is 65°C, which, with a 10-min holding time, may be used for pasteurizing some small items, such as containers, and for laundering fabric components. The minimum hold period decreases as the temperature increases, and where temperatures in excess of 80°C are possible the time may be reduced to a 1-min hold. It is important that all hot-water pasteurizing equipment is emptied during a standstill to reduce the risk of bacterial colonization (Hambraeus *et al.*, 1968). For large items of equipment, however, steam is more practicable and may be used to treat tanks, pipelines and other equipment whose surface is free from organic residues. If heavy soiling is present, there is the risk of baking it on to the surface and providing a protective layer of insulation around the microorganisms. To monitor the process, the temperature of the steam condensate should be measured. For an efficient process, this should reach 95°C and be maintained for a minimum period of 5 min to destroy vegetative cells. One advantage of this method is that the equipment is rinsed with sterile water.

Moist heat, at temperatures of 121°C and above, is used extensively in the pharmaceutical industry to sterilize equipment, instruments and heat-stable fluids. To ensure sterilization, equipment and instruments must be wrapped in a porous material which allows air to be drawn out and steam to penetrate in, but protects the item from recontamination after sterilization. The temperature must be recorded throughout the cycle by a probe sited in the coolest part of the load or chamber; in practice, this is usually the chamber drain. The pressure may also be recorded, but must not be used to control the process. Precautions must be taken to prevent recontamination of the sterilizer load as it cools; this usually involves the installation of a presterilized filter on the air inlet.

In the food industry, moist heat is used extensively for processing and sterilizing. For the latter, a balance has to be calculated so as to destroy the microbial load with minimal damage to the nutritional and organoleptic properties; the additive value of all heat considered equivalent in minutes to 121.1°C (250°F), i.e. the F or F_0 value, is used. The processing temperature and time thus vary with the type of food, its microbial load and, if being processed in the final container, the size and heat penetration properties of the container. For products that are ultrahigh-temperature (UHT)-processed and aseptically filled, the temperature and time will depend upon the acidity (pH), viscosity and presence of particulate matter; for low-acid foods, the F value is usually in excess of 138°C. There are legal requirements for the conditions of UHT processing of milk and milk-based products.

3.2.3 Monitoring and validation of heat sterilization processes

Five main methods are used to monitor and/or validate both moist and dry heat sterilization processes.

1 Sterility tests, which are tests on the sterilized product or material to detect the presence of microorganisms. For pharmaceutical products, this is usually performed in accordance with the European or United States Pharmacopoeias. The test is, however, destructive and only carried out on relatively few samples and for confidence in microbiological safety should be used as part of a wider quality assurance programme which includes process validation.

2 Challenge tests, using an organism of known heat resistance, which is added to the product before sterilization, samples being examined after sterilization and the level of kill determined. This method, utilizing *Clostridium sporogenes* or another organism of suitable resistance, is often used by the food industry as part of a validation procedure, with the temperature/time relationship of the process being set at optimal, minimum operating conditions and below-minimum operating conditions, as a control, to set the operating parameters. This approach permits a process that will ensure the achievement of commercial sterility with minimum damage to the organoleptic and nutritional properties. Once validated, it is usual to monitor routinely, using a physical test that gives a record of both the temperature and time, and the validation challenge is only repeated if conditions change and/or microbial contamination occurs.

3 Biological indicator tests, which involve determining the viability of microorganisms after processing. These can be of the form of paper strips impregnated with spores of *Bacillus stearothermophilus* (for moist heat) or a specific non-toxic strain of *Clostridium tetani* (for dry heat), which are placed in sealed envelopes or specially designed tubes in the load. An alternative method in use in the food industry is Biorods, in which the microorganism is sealed into a heat-resistant rod, which may be recovered from an individual container after processing and the viability of the microorganism evaluated.

4 Physical tests, which are tests using copper–constantan thermocouples placed in various positions in the load to monitor the temperature. Special fittings are available for determining the temperature inside containers, and for use with rotating moist-heat sterilizers, as well as the stationary type. Used in conjunction with a permanent recording system, they have the advantage of showing both the temperature reached and the duration of hold in the load. They are very important in dry heat sterilizing systems, to ensure that the correct temperature is reached in all areas, and in some steam sterilizers, to ensure that temperature layering, due to the presence of residual air, does not occur.

5 Chemical indicators, of which various types are available, including Browne's tubes, which are both temperature- and time-related; and heat-sensitive tapes, which usually indicate only that a certain temperature was reached, but not the duration of hold, and do not therefore constitute proof of sterilization. Paper sterilization bags printed with a heat-sensitive indicator are, however, a useful visual guide to the operator in industry that the contents have been through a heat process.

The type of monitoring usually reflects the

nature of the finished product and, providing regulatory requirements are met, once the process is validated, it may be practical to routinely use physical tests, together with sterility tests. More detailed accounts of sterilization control are given by Russell (1980) and Denyer (1998), and in Chapter 25.

4 Building and fittings

Ideally, the premises should be purpose-built to a sanitary design, with modern easy-to-clean materials, and sited in surroundings which are free from potential harbourages for rodents, birds and insects. Buildings and sites that do not meet these requirements may be brought up to current standards by rigorous pest-control systems and renovation of interior finishes. Regardless of the age of the building, to maintain a good standard of hygiene a well-planned and adequate waste-disposal system is essential.

4.1 Plant design

The design of a plant, with regard to the separation of different functions and prescribed routes of movement for personnel, raw materials and waste, influences the control of microorganisms. The following are some examples of operations that can influence the microbial quality of the environment, and their siting should be considered at the planning stage.

4.1.1 Large steam usage

Processes that generate or involve large steam usage, which results in high humidity, must be sited away from the production or filling of dry materials preserved by their lack of available water, since moisture in the form of condensate may spoil the product.

4.1.2 Waste-disposal system

This must be designed to prevent the effluent from a potentially contaminated area from flowing through a cleaner one.

4.1.3 Dust generation

Operations that generate dust are usually a potential source of airborne contamination. They include the dispensing of raw materials, in particular flours, sugars and other dried materials from natural sources, packaging involving card- or paper-board, and the soiled linen side of the laundry. These should be physically separated and have different dust-control and air-supply systems from those of functions that require a low microbial count.

4.1.4 Raw materials

Raw materials that have a high microbial count should not pass through areas where clean operations are in process. In areas where a low microbial count is essential, it may be desirable to dedicate fork-lift trucks to serve them and not risk the introduction of contamination from an all-purpose fleet. In addition, unless specified, pallets may not be restricted to use in factories where hygiene is at a premium and may introduce both microorganisms and insects.

4.1.5 Staff

Staff working in a potentially contaminated or dusty area should not have access to cleaner areas without first washing and changing their clothing. In areas where aseptic work is carried out, it is usual to provide a separate changing room—fitted with sanitary washing facilities, such as foot- or elbow-operated taps and hot-air hand-drying machines—through which the staff may pass by a series of airlocks before reaching the work area. The entry into a clean area may be delineated by the use of a contamination-control mat, but this must be selected with care to ensure that it does remove microorganisms, as well as acting as a psychological barrier (Meddick, 1977).

4.2 Floors and drains

To minimize microbial contamination, all floors must be easy to clean, impervious to water and laid on a flat surface. In some areas, it may be necessary for the floor to slope towards a drain, in which case the gradient should be such that no pools of water form. Any joints in the floor, necessary for expansion, should be adequately sealed. The floor-to-wall junction should be coved.

The finish of the floor will often relate to its use or the process being carried out; in areas where little moisture or product is liable to be split, polyvinyl chloride welded sheeting may be satisfactory, but, in wet areas or where frequent washing is necessary, brick tiles or concrete with a hard finish of terrazzo or other ground and polished surfaces are superior. Where concrete is used as a flooring material, it must be adequately sealed with an epoxy resin or substitute to protect it against food acids and alkaline cleaning compounds. Likewise, Portland cement joints cannot be used in food and dairy plants, due to their erosion by food and cleaning acids. Corrosion-resistant resin cements can, however, be used. While easier to clean, excessively smooth finishes must be avoided in wet areas, where they may become very slippery.

In areas where very dirty or heavily contaminated materials are being handled, a high proportion of drains to floor area is necessary, and any such drains should be vented to the outside air and provided with rodent screens. Deep-seal traps (P-, V- or S-shaped but not bell-type) should be fitted to all floor drains and be easily accessible for cleaning. Adequate sealing arrangements must be made in dry- and cold-storage areas where water seals in traps evaporate without replenishment, and a regular inspection is important.

As mentioned earlier, the effluent from a contaminated area must not flow through a cleaner area, and drains should be avoided in locations where aseptic operations are carried out. If drains have to be installed, they must be fitted with effective vented traps, preferably with electrically operated heat-sterilizing devices. Where floor channels are necessary, they should be open, shallow, easy to clean and connected to drains outside the critical area. Routine microbiological checks should be made on all drainage systems in such areas.

4.3 Walls and ceilings

To reduce microbial colonization, the internal surfaces of walls and ceilings must be smooth and impervious to water, and the wall-to-ceiling joint coved to minimize dust collection. The surface should be washable and of a type that will not support mould growth. A modern material which meets this requirement is laminated plastic, but, where a wall is plastered, it can be improved by a coat of hard-gloss paint, which seals the nutrients present in the plaster from microbial attack more effectively than a softer matt finish. The addition of up to 1% of a fungistatic agent, such as pentachlorophenol, 8-hydroxyquinoline or salicylanilide, is also an advantage. In areas of high humidity, painted surfaces are likely to peel, and glazed bricks or tiles adequately sealed are the best finish. Where a considerable volume of steam is used, ventilation at ceiling level is important. Claddings of aluminium or stainless steel have been found to be satisfactory for cold-storage room walls, and thermal cellular-glass insulation blocks are suitable for the construction of partitions or non-load-bearing walls.

To aid cleaning, all electrical cables and other services should be installed either in deep-cavity walls or in a false ceiling, where they are accessible for maintenance but do not collect dust. All pipes that pass through walls or ceilings must be well sealed and flush. Wall and false-ceiling cavities must be included in the rodent and pest control.

Equipment or storage systems should be positioned to allow access to walls and ceilings for cleaning. In warehouse areas, pallets should be stacked away from walls to permit cleaning and adequate rodent control.

4.4 Doors, windows and fittings

Wherever possible, doors and windows should fit flush with the walls, and dust-collecting ledges should be eliminated. Where wood is used in the construction, a hard-gloss finish is the easiest to clean. Doors should be well fitting to reduce the entry of microorganisms, except where a positive air pressure is maintained. Where positive-pressure systems are required, due to the critical nature of the work, they should be fitted with indicator gauges, which must be checked regularly.

Windows in manufacturing areas should serve only to permit light entry and should not be used for ventilation. If, however, they are necessary for ventilation, they must be fitted with insect-proof meshes. An adequate air-control system other than windows must be supplied to all areas where aseptic techniques or operations vulnerable to microbial contamination are being carried out.

Overhead pipes in all manufacturing areas must be sited away from equipment, in order to prevent condensation and possible contaminants from falling into the product. Unless neglected, stainless-steel pipes support little microbial growth, but lagged pipes always present a problem, unless the lagging is well sealed with a waterproof outer membrane and treated regularly with a chemical disinfectant.

Recommendations for the building and standards of interior fittings for the production of pharmaceutical products are given in the *Guide to Good Pharmaceutical Manufacturing Practice* (Anon., 1977).

4.5 Cleaning and disinfection

Walls, ceilings and fittings usually only require a hot water and detergent wash to remove nutrients, which might encourage microbial growth, and dust, which might harbour it. Care must be taken not to scratch plaster surfaces, since this may release additional nutrients to support mould growth. Where chemical disinfection is required, the surface must be cleaned thoroughly, unless a detergent sanitizing agent is used. Suitable disinfectants include QACs and, except in food factories, phenolics.

The cleaning of floors depends upon both their construction and use, but, in all instances, vacuum cleaning, using an industrial sanitary model, which filters the exhaust air to remove microorganisms before discharging it into the atmosphere, is preferable to the use of a broom, which scatters dust and microorganisms. If vacuum cleaning is not possible, damp cleaning may be used. Where brooms are used, they should be made from synthetic materials that can be heat-sterilized.

In processing areas, the floors usually require a hot-water and detergent scrub, which includes all drainage channels and drains. This, followed by a hot-water rinse, is usually sufficient. Where greasy materials are present, drains require regular treatment with an alkali to eliminate residues which may support microbial growth. Where a disinfectant is required, a formulated halogen, a QAC or a phenolic may be used.

Fittings, furnishings and equipment external surfaces should be damp-cleaned with hot water containing a detergent. The detergent acts not only as a cleaning agent but also as a wetting agent for shiny surfaces. Disinfection is usually only necessary where neglect has permitted visible microbial colonization or where aseptic processes are being carried out. Suitable disinfectants include QACs, phenols, alcohols and formaldehyde, but a check on the compatibility with the surface material should be made before use.

With overhead fittings, where regular cleaning is impracticable, a thin smear of liquid paraffin may be used to coat fixtures after cleaning and act as a dust trap. This must, however, be cleaned off and a fresh coat applied on a planned basis.

The techniques for monitoring the microbiological state of building interiors and fittings are similar to those used for equipment, and will be described in Section 6.4.

4.6 Pest control

Pest control, preferably by denying access, is imperative to the maintenance of a good standard of hygiene. Insect control may be by prevention of access, i.e. insect-proof screens on all windows, doors and air-intake fans that are used for ventilation, air currents or plastic strips for fork-lift-truck access, and insectocutors sited at strategic points in the factory. The latter should, ideally, be sited outside manufacturing areas to attract flying insects before they reach the processing plant. Where they are sited inside manufacturing areas, it is important that they are placed to prevent insects attracted by them from flying over open vessels or unprotected food materials. Inspection of raw materials, before acceptance, may reduce infestation in warehouses or manufacturing areas. If insecticides need to be used, either to eliminate infestation or as a prophylactic, only those approved for food use may be used, and all precautions should be taken to ensure they do not gain access to products, raw materials or packaging materials.

Rodents may be successfully controlled by prevention of access and baiting. All door fittings, pipe entry ports, etc. should be checked to ensure that they fit flushly, and rodent-proof strips should be fitted where necessary. Drains should be fitted with rodent-proof traps, and all service ducts baited and inspected regularly for rodent infestation.

Bird access and soiling of the site and roofs are often more difficult to control. Access may be prevented by maintaining the building in good condition and by frequent inspection of the site, in particular warehouse and roof spaces, to ensure that no access points are present. For preference, automatically opening doors should be used for fork-lift-truck access, but, in lieu of this, plastic strips may provide a deterrent. Soiling of roofs, particularly where nutritional powder emissions occur, is very difficult to control, and hygienic measures to ensure they are regularly sanitized, which also controls insect populations, should be carried out. Wherever possible, staff who need access to roofs should not re-enter a building, or, if it is necessary to do so, should change their shoes. Overshoes can be used, or a foot-bath of disinfectant may be used to sanitize the boots or shoes of operatives who have to walk outside the building, where bird-soil contamination may be present.

5 Air

The number of airborne microorganisms is related to the activity in the environment, the amount of dust disturbed and the microbial load of the material being handled. Thus, an area containing working machinery and an active personnel will have a higher microbial count than one with a still atmosphere. Some industrial processes which handle contaminated materials, particularly in the dry form, increase the air count; these include dispensing, blending and the addition to open vessels.

Control of the microflora of the air is desirable in all manufacturing areas and can be improved by air-conditioning (Lidwell & Noble, 1975). Some processes do, however, require a very low microbial air count, and these include the manufacture and packaging of parenteral and ophthalmic preparations in the pharmaceutical and cosmetic industries, and aseptic filling and packaging in the food industry.

5.1 Disinfection

The microbial air count may be reduced by filtration (Chapter 22), chemical disinfection (Chapter 2) and, to a limited extent, by UV light (Chapter 20B). Filtration is the most commonly used method, and filters may be composed of a variety of materials, such as cellulose, glass wool, fibreglass mixtures or polytetrafluoroethylene (PTFE), with resin or acrylic binders. For the most critical aseptic work, it may be necessary to remove all particles in excess of 0.1 μm in size, but for many operations a standard of less than 100 particles/ft^3 (3.5/l) of 0.5 μm or larger (class 100) is adequate. Such fine filtration is usually preceded by a coarser filter stage, or any suspended matter is removed by passing the air through an electrostatic field. To maintain efficiency, all air filters must be kept dry, since microorganisms may be capable of movement along continuous wet films and may be carried through a damp filter.

Filtered air may be used to purge a complete room, or it may be confined to a specific area, incorporating the principle of laminar flow, which permits operations to be carried out in a gentle current of sterile air. The direction of the air flow may be horizontal or vertical, depending upon the type of equipment being used, the type of operation and the material being handled. It is important that there is no obstruction between the air supply and the exposed product, since this may result in the deflection of microorganisms or particulate matter from a non-sterile surface and cause contamination.

Chemical disinfectants are of limited use as sterilants due to their irritant properties, but both atomized propylene glycol, at 0.05–0.5 mg/l, and QACs, at 0.075%, may be used. For areas that can be effectively sealed, formaldehyde gas is useful.

In the food industry, a combination of hydrogen peroxide and filtration is used to sterilize air feeds to aseptic filling machines. Ultraviolet irradiation at wavelengths between 280 and 240 nm may be used to reduce the air count. Additional information is provided in Chapter 2.

5.2 Compressed air

Compressed air has many applications that bring it into direct contact with the product, examples being the conveyance of suspensions or dry powders, fermentations and some products, such as ice-cream and whipped dairy confections, that contain air as an integral part of the structure. Unless the air is presterilized by filtration or a combination of heat and filtration, microorganisms will be introduced into the product.

5.3 Monitoring air for microbial content

Air-flow gauges are essential in all areas where aseptic work is performed. In laminar-flow units, they are necessary for checking that the correct flow rate is obtained and, in complete suites, to ensure that a positive pressure from clean to less-clean areas is always maintained.

The integrity of the air-filtration system must be checked regularly. One method is by counting the particulate matter, both in the working area and across the filter surface. For foodstuffs and some pharmaceuticals that are aseptically filled, it is usual to carry out a count prior to the start of the operation. For systems that have complex ducting or where the surface of the terminal filter is recessed, smoke tests, using a chemical of known particle size, may be introduced just after the main fan and monitored at each outlet. This test has a twofold application, since the integrity of the terminal filter is checked and any leaks in the ducting are detected.

The particulate air count, while rapid and useful, does not replace a count of the viable airborne microorganisms. Common methods for checking this include the following.

1 The exposure of Petri dishes containing a nutrient agar to the atmosphere for a given length of time. This relies upon microorganisms or dust particles bearing them to settle upon the surface.

2 The use of a slit-sampling machine, which is essentially a device for drawing a measured quantity of air from the environment and impinging it upon either a revolving Petri dish containing a nutrient medium or a membrane filter, which may then be incubated with a nutrient medium. This method provides valuable information in areas of low microbial contamination, particularly if the sample is taken close to the working area.

The microbial content of compressed air may be assessed by bubbling a known volume through a nutrient broth, which is then filtered through a membrane. The membrane is incubated on nutrient agar and a total viable count made.

A detailed account of air disinfection and sterilization and methods used for its monitoring was given by Sykes (1965).

6 Equipment

All equipment must be designed and constructed so that all internal contact points and the external surfaces may be cleaned.

While many metals are suitable for the construction of parts that are not in direct contact with the product, copper, lead, iron, zinc, cadmium and antimony must be avoided for contact surfaces. The choice for contact surfaces includes stainless steel, except where corrosive acids are present, titanium, glass and (if excessive heat is not required) plastics. Cloth or canvas belts should not come into contact with the product, since they are absorbent and difficult to clean. Plastics and cloths of synthetic fibres are superior.

Each piece of equipment has its own peculiar area where microorganisms may proliferate, and knowledge of its weak points may be built up by regular tests for contamination. The type and extent of growth will depend upon the source of the contamination, the nutrients available and the environmental conditions, in particular the temperature and pH.

The following points are common to many pieces of equipment, including some used in hospitals, and serve as a general guide to appraising the cleaning programme for the equipment and reducing the risk of microbial colonization.

1 All equipment should be easy to dismantle and clean.

2 All surfaces that are in contact with the product should be smooth, continuous and free from pits. All sharp corners should be eliminated and any junctions welded. Any internal welds should be polished out. There must be no dead ends. All contact surfaces must be inspected on a routine basis for signs of damage; this is very important in

the case of lagged equipment and double-walled and lined vessels, since any cracks or pinholes in the surface may allow the product to seep into an area where it is protected from cleaning and sterilizing agents and where microorganisms may grow and contaminate subsequent batches of product.

3 There should be no inside screw threads, and all outside threads should be accessible for cleaning.

4 Coupling nuts on all pipework and valves should be capable of being taken apart and cleaned.

5 Agitator blades should preferably be of one piece with the shaft and accessible for cleaning. Careful postcleaning checks are usually necessary if the blade shaft is packed into a housing.

6 Rotary seals are superior to packing boxes, since packing material is usually difficult to sterilize and often requires a lubricant, which may gain access to the product.

7 The product must be protected from any lubricant used on moving parts.

8 Valves should be specially selected for the purpose they are to fulfil, and the type of cleaning designed to clean and sterilize all contact parts of the valve. The dairy industry has traditionally used the plug type of valve, incorporated with a cleaning system that will contact all surfaces. With the introduction of aseptic transfer and filling systems, a bellows type of valve, with a steam barrier protection, has been favoured. The pharmaceutical and some food-manufacturing industry processes successfully use a diaphragm type of valve. All valves must be well maintained and have a cleaning system that reaches all contact surfaces. With diaphragm-type valves, it is essential to ensure that the diaphragm is in good condition and the product cannot seep behind it and, in very wet areas, that it is protected so that water from hoses does not enter by the 'dirty' side of the diaphragm.

9 All pipelines should slope away from the product source and all process and storage vessels should be self-draining. Run-off valves should be as near to the tank as possible. Sampling through the run-off valve should be avoided, since any nutrients left in the valve may encourage microbial growth, which could contaminate the complete batch. A separate sampling hatch or cock is preferable.

10 If a vacuum-exhaust system is used to remove air or steam from a preparation vessel, it is necessary to clean and disinfect all fittings regularly. This prevents residues that may be drawn into them from supporting microbial growth, which may later be returned to the vessel with condensate.

11 Multipurpose and mobile equipment requires carefully planned cleaning programmes if used for, or moved into, areas where products of different vulnerability to microbial growth are made.

6.1 Instruments and tools

Any instruments or tools which may be used on product or contact parts of equipment, or for measuring or sampling the product, should be made of hygienic, non-corrosive material and be as simple in design and construction as possible. Tools with hollow handles should be avoided, and one-piece instruments are easier to clean than those with a separate handle. If joints are necessary, their welds should be polished out smooth. For some tasks, such as sampling, presterilized disposable instruments may be preferred.

6.2 Cleaning utensils

These should be as simple in construction as possible, and easy to clean. Stainless-steel bowls and buckets are ideal, since they can be heat-sterilized and their surfaces do not readily scratch or pit. Heat-resistant plastics are also suitable, but types which will not withstand autoclaving and those of galvanized iron are unsuitable. Likewise, brooms and mops should be of the type that can be heat sterilized. For preference, cleaning cloths should be disposable. If this is impracticable, they must withstand boiling. Colquitt & Maurer (1969) found that all cloths and mops used for wet work had to be disinfected by heat, chemical treatment being ineffective. Scrubbing machines with badly designed tanks that cannot be emptied or heat-sterilized have been found to cause contamination in hospitals (Thomas & Maurer, 1972).

6.3 Cleaning and disinfection

Equipment should be cleaned as soon as possible after use and disinfected just before it is used again. If there is a considerable time-lag between uses, the equipment should be washed, disinfected and stored dry. It should then be disinfected again before use. Tanks, pumps, heat-exchange units and other equipment must be drained if standing idle and, if possible, pipelines 'cracked' open at the couplings to remove any moisture. Plant may be cleaned in place or dismantled and cleaned manually; more commonly, a combination of both methods is used. Standard cleaning procedures usually incorporate preflushing, washing, rinsing and disinfecting cycles, and it is important that a written procedure is available which states the concentration of all the agents to be used and the duration of the recycling period.

Sections of pipework are often specially designed for cleaning in place and are welded, where possible, to form continuous lengths; specially designed, crevice-free unions are used where coupling is necessary. An illustrated account of such fittings is given in Anon. (1959b). Cleaning agents are forced through the system at a velocity of not less than 1.5 m (5 ft)/s through the largest pipe diameter of the system. The speed of flow, coupled with the action of a suitable detergent, removes both the soil residues and any microorganisms which may be present, by its scouring action. It is, however, usual to pass a chemical disinfectant through the system after cleaning. Any cross-connections, T-pieces or blank ends must be carefully considered, since they both decrease the efficiency of the system and provide harbours for microorganisms.

In-place cleaning systems are also available for both plate and tubular types of heat-exchange units, pumps, some homogenizers and other equipment. However, valves and T-piece fittings for valves and gauges have to be cleaned manually. Tanks and reaction vessels may be cleaned and sterilized by the use of rotary sprays, which are sited at the point in the vessel where the maximum wall area may be treated. Spray balls, with a hole or jet pattern specifically designed for the individual vessel, are the most efficient. Some fixtures, such as agitators, pipe inlets and outlets and vents, may be blind to the spray pattern and require manual cleaning. Because of the relatively large-capacity storage tanks and pumps required for a totally automatic-cleaning in-place system, it usually has to be fitted when the equipment is installed, but smaller local systems are available and can be accommodated into existing buildings and plant.

The nature of many products or the plant design often renders cleaning in place impracticable, and the plant has to be dismantled for soaking and cleaning, either manually or in an automatic washing-machine.

Some applications for ultrasonic waves of frequencies of 30 000–40 000 Hz converted to mechanical vibrations have been found for the removal of heavy grease and food soils from small pieces of equipment which are difficult to clean, such as valves and parts with small orifices. Combinations of ultrasonics with different disinfectants, such as benzalkonium chloride (Shaner, 1967) and hydrogen peroxide (Ahmed & Russell, 1975), have been found to be suitable for the cold sterilization of instruments.

Equipment may be disinfected using agents such as halogens, QACs, phenolics (except for the food industry), formaldehyde, hot water and steam, or may be sterilized by moist or dry heat or exposure to ethylene oxide. Irradiation by gamma rays (Chapter 20A) is also suitable but is usually applied to disposable equipment only.

6.4 Monitoring the cleaning and disinfection of buildings and equipment

While the efficiency of cleaning procedures can routinely be assessed by visual and chemical tests, the parameters set to control the process must first be established by testing the effectiveness of the cleaning and disinfection system by testing for the presence of residual surviving microorganisms.

There are three main methods for testing surfaces.

1 Collecting a sample of the final rinse water from an automatic cleaning cycle or rinsing the surface with a sterile diluent, and testing for the presence of microorganisms.

2 Using a contact agar surface to replicate the flora present; this has the advantage of being quantitative, but the disadvantage of being suitable for flat planes only of hard surfaces. When this technique is used, residual nutrients may be left on the surface. Where presumptive mould growth is

visible, clear vinyl tape may be used for transferring it from the surface to a microscope slide for detailed examination.

3 Using calcium alginate wool or cotton-wool swabs on the test surface and transferring to a suspending medium, which is then examined for the presence of microorganisms. In the case of calcium alginate wool swabs, quarter-strength Ringer solution containing 1.0% (w/v) sodium hexametaphosphate, which solubilizes the wool of the swab and releases the microorganisms present, is used. Trimarchi (1959) found calcium alginate swabs to be superior to raw-cotton swabs for the examination of cutlery. This technique has the disadvantage that, unless a measuring guide is used, it is not quantitative, but the advantage that it may be used for any surface, including curved pipes and orifices. It does not leave any residue, and for many processes the plant does not have to be recleaned and resterilized.

Modern rapid methods for the detection of microorganisms—for example, changes in impedance, conductivity or bioluminescence, an increase in adenosine triphosphate (ATP) in the growth medium or immunoassays—can prove to be very cost-effective if used for the monitoring of the hygienic quality of the manufacturing environment, as well as for perishable raw materials.

A comparative study of the different methods for sampling surfaces for microbial contamination was made by Favero *et al.* (1968) and Nishannon & Pohja (1977).

7 Water

The microbial quality of water is important, because of its multiple use as a constituent of products, for washing both food and chemicals and for blanching, cooling and cleaning purposes. Microorganisms indigenous to water are usually Gram-negative, saprophytic bacteria, which are nutritionally undemanding and often have a low optimum growth temperature. Other bacteria may be introduced by soil erosion and contamination with decaying plant matter or sewage, which results in a more varied but undesirable flora and frequently includes enterobacteria.

7.1 Raw or mains water

The quality of water from the mains supply varies both with the source and the local authority responsible, and, while it is free from pathogens and faecal contaminants, such as *Escherichia coli*, it may contain other microorganisms, including *Pseudomonas aeruginosa*. While bacteria tend to settle out on prolonged storage and in reservoirs, the reverse is true of industrial storage tanks, where the intermittent throughput ensures that, unless treated, the contents serve as a source of infection. In the summer months, the count may rise rapidly and 10^5–10^6/ml is not unknown. Collins (1964) found 98% of microorganisms in industrial stored waters to be Gram-negative bacteria.

Regular microbiological monitoring is essential for all water supplies, and freedom from enterobacteria is essential for all water used to formulate products or to wash food or chemicals and for all plant-cleaning water. The tolerance of water-borne organisms, such as pseudomonads, will depend upon their ability to grow in and spoil the product.

Water used for cooling heat-processed products in cans or bottles or for spray-cooling fluids in autoclaves must be of a good microbial quality to eliminate the risk of postprocessing contamination due to imperfect seals or seams.

The microbial count of mains water will be reflected in both the softened and deionized water prepared from it.

7.2 Softened water

This is usually prepared either by a base-exchange method, using sodium zeolite, by a lime-soda ash process, or by the addition of sodium hexametaphosphate. Where chemical beds are used, they must be treated regularly to preclude microbial colonization. Where brine is used to regenerate chemical beds, additional flora such as *Bacillus* spp. and *Staphylococcus aureus* may be introduced.

If softened water is used as the cooling agent for a canning or retorting plant, a disinfectant pretreatment to reduce the bacterial count will be necessary. Where it is used as a coolant in a heat-exchange system, the microbial count will rise rapidly unless precautions are taken, and any faults or leaks arising in the heat-exchange plates or the wall of a jacketed vessel may result in the contamination of the product.

Disinfection is also necessary for water used for washing equipment, whether the process is manual or automatic in-place cleaning.

7.3 Deionized or demineralized water

Deionized water is prepared by passing mains water through synthetic anion- or cation-exchange resin beds to remove ions. Thus any bacteria in the mains water will also be present in the deionized water, and beds which are not regenerated frequently with strong acid and alkaline solutions rapidly become contaminated. Deionized water is commonly used for the formulation of pharmaceutical and cosmetic products and for the dilution of disinfectants.

7.4 Distilled water

As it leaves the still, distilled water is free from microorganisms, and any contamination that occurs is the result of either a fault in the cooling system or in storage or distribution. If there is a fault in the cooling system, the water is usually unsatisfactory chemically as well. The flora of distilled water usually consists of Gram-negative bacteria, and, since it is introduced after processing, it is often a pure culture and counts of up to 10^6 organisms/ml have been recorded. Distilled water is used in the pharmaceutical industry for the preparation of oral and parenteral products. For parenteral products, it is usually prepared in a specially designed glass still and a postdistillation sterilization stage is included within 4 h of collecting. Water prepared in this manner is often stored at temperatures in excess of 65°C until required, to prevent both bacterial growth and the production of pyrogenic substances which may accompany it.

7.5 Water treated by reverse osmosis

This plays a similar role to distilled water in the pharmaceutical and cosmetic industry. The process is the reverse of natural osmosis, with the membrane acting as a molecular filter and retaining salts, bacteria and pyrogens. Water may, however, become contaminated in either a storage vessel or the distribution system.

7.6 Storage and distribution systems

If microorganisms colonize a storage vessel, it then acts as a microbial reservoir and contaminates all water passing through it. It is therefore important that the contents of all storage vessels are tested regularly. Reservoirs of microorganisms may also build up in booster pumps, water meters and unused sections of pipeline. Where a high positive pressure is absent or cannot be continuously maintained, outlets such as cocks and taps may permit bacteria to enter the system.

Burman & Colbourne (1977) carried out a survey on the ability of plumbing materials to support growth. They found that both natural and synthetic rubbers used for washers, O-rings and diaphragms were susceptible, but, for jointing, packing and lubricating materials, and silicone-based compounds were superior to those based on natural products, such as vegetable oils or fibres, animal fats and petroleum-based compounds. Some plastics, in particular plasticized polyvinyl chlorides and resins, used in the manufacture of glass-reinforced plastics, are prone to microbial colonization.

7.7 Disinfection of water

The two main methods for treating water are by chemicals (Davis, 1959) or filtration, but UV irradiation has been used successfully, with relatively low flow rates. Sodium hypochlorite or chlorine gas is the most common agent used, and the concentration employed depends both upon the dwell time and the chlorine demand of the water. For most purposes, a free chlorine level of 0.5–5 parts/10^6 with a 20-min dwell time is sufficient, but, for cooling processed cans or bottles, 4–10 parts/10^6 with a similar dwell time is recommended. Pipelines, outlets, pumps and meters may be treated with 50–250 parts/10^6, but it is usually necessary to use a descaling agent first in areas of hard water.

Distilled and deionized water systems may be treated with sodium hypochlorite or formaldehyde solution 1% (v/v). With deionized systems, it is usually necessary to exhaust or flatten the beds with brine before sterilization with formaldehyde, to prevent inactivation to paraformaldehyde.

Membrane filtration is useful where the usage of water is moderate and a continuous circulation of water can be maintained. Thus, with the exception of the water drawn off, the water is continually returned to the storage tank and refiltered. Control of bacteria in non-domestic water-supplies has been reviewed by Chambers & Clarke (1968).

7.8 Monitoring

One of the most useful techniques for checking the microbial quality of water is by membrane filtration, since this permits the concentration of a small number of organisms from a large volume of water. The practical details are described by Windle Taylor & Burman (1964). When chlorinated water supplies are tested, it is necessary to add a neutralizing agent (Russell *et al.*, 1979), such as sodium thiosulphate, to the sample before testing. Although an incubation temperature of 37°C may be necessary to recover some pathogens or faecal contaminants from water, many indigenous species fail to grow at this temperature, and it is usual to incubate at 20–26°C for their detection.

8 Raw materials

Raw materials account for a high proportion of the microorganisms introduced into processing factories and the selection of materials of good microbiological quality aids in controlling the contamination level in the environment. If an HACCP system is in operation, raw materials and their microflora merit special consideration as to any hazard they pose and the necessary control points needed to eliminate them. Together with establishing a realistic but acceptable microbiological standard, the aspects of storage handling and processing must be considered.

8.1 Source

Raw agricultural products support a wide range of microorganisms, including pathogenic types, and can lead to a variety of contamination problems. Treated or refined products may have a higher level of contamination than raw materials, due to handling or the balance of flora may be changed in relation to the refining process. Thus heat-treated materials may have a high bacterial spore load. Semisynthetic and synthetic materials are usually of a good microbial quality, with only casual contaminants present.

8.2 Monitoring

Four main factors must be taken into consideration when monitoring the microbial quality of raw materials.

1 If the material meets the quality demanded by the statutory requirements (if any).
2 If pathogenic organisms are present.
3 If spoilage organisms are present.
4 If the level of microbial contamination is consistent with good hygienic practice and within an agreed specification.

If pathogenic microorganisms or their toxins are present, they must be destroyed by a validated pre- or in-process sterilization stage. Precautions must be taken to prevent cross-contamination of other raw materials or finished products, particularly those which do not receive an in-process sterilization stage, by process operators or the use of common equipment or preparation surfaces.

When spoilage microorganisms are present, they must be eliminated before or during manufacture. If this is not possible, either an alternative source free from such organisms must be sought or a preservative capable of preventing their growth added. The relationship between a product and its spoilage organisms is often quite specific, e.g. the load of spore-forming bacteria is of importance in the canning of low- and medium-acid foods, due to their heat tolerance, but is usually less significant in the manufacture of antacid pharmaceutical preparations with a neutral-to-alkaline reaction, where Gram-negative bacteria pose more serious spoilage problems. The presence of some microorganisms in raw materials presents a threat to the whole factory environment. An example is the fungus *Neurospora sitophila*, which, if present in materials used in a bakery, can spread rapidly throughout the plant.

Changes in the hygienic standard of the supplier can be detected by regular microbiological monitoring, but this is most effective if it is used in conjunction with a supplier-auditing process. Microbiological tests may take the form of a total viable count for bacteria and/or moulds or the specific testing for organisms whose presence indicates an unsatisfactory standard of hygiene. In the water and dairy industry, the presence of *E. coli* is regarded as evidence of faecal contamination and the presence of other coliform bacteria as an index of unsatisfactory hygiene. Studies by Hartman (1960) and Raj *et al.* (1961) indicated that, in the case of frozen foods, enterococci were more relevant than coliform bacteria as an index of hygienic standard. The subject of microbiological standards in foods and the value of indices of sanitary quality was reviewed by Jay (1970).

Staff handling raw materials with pathogens present must have adequate training to prevent both cross-contamination and self-infection.

9 Packaging

Packaging material has a dual role and acts both to contain the product and to prevent the entry of microorganisms or moisture, which may result in spoilage. In addition, it may be an essential barrier against light or oxygen, the entry of which may lead to the deterioration of the product.

For the purpose of sterilization, packaging components may be classified as being of two main types: those which require a presterilization stage before they are used, and those which are sterilized simultaneously with the product, e.g. process cans.

Some packaging materials, such as plastic containers, moulded plastics, cellulose and foil films, have smooth surfaces, free from interstices, and harbour few microorganisms if the standard of hygiene in the production plant and storage area is good. Others, such as paper, cardboard and cork, usually have a higher level of surface flora. Some materials are contaminated by their own packaging or during storage, or by surface-finish treatments, e.g. glass bottles that are sterile when they leave the furnace may be contaminated during packaging and storage or by the use of a surface finish. Tin and aluminium cans often have a protective finish that can support microflora.

When dry materials are being packed, it is often possible to eliminate a presterilization stage for the packaging, but, for dried pharmaceutical products required to pass a test for sterility, the packaging must be presterilized. Unless the product is well preserved, a sterilization stage is usually necessary for liquid and semisolid materials.

Packaging may be treated by both moist and dry heat, irradiation or chemical disinfection. Chemical disinfectants usually selected include sodium hypochlorite, QACs, hydrogen peroxide and, in gaseous form, ethylene oxide or formaldehyde.

In addition to microbiological tests on packaging materials, checks must be made to ensure that the pack is correctly sealed and that screw caps have an adequate torque to prevent both leakage of product and entry of microorganisms.

The product and packaging may be sterilized as a complete assembly by irradiation, ethylene oxide gas and both moist and dry heat. Quality control checks for such operations must include an evaluation of the process, as well as a test for sterility.

Where both the product and container are sterilized by moist heat and the cycle includes a water-cooling stage, checks must be made on the container before processing. In the case of process cans with double-overlap seams, it is usual to measure the percentage overlap of the seam, seam tightness and free space and countersink depth, as well as checking for faults in the seams at both ends of the can. If the balance of the measurements is incorrect and the seam overlap too low or the seam too loose, cooling water and possibly microorganisms may be drawn into the can. If the seams are too tight, damage, such as cut-overs or split droops, may occur and again may permit the entry of postprocessing contaminants. The complete subject of monitoring process cans was reviewed by Put *et al.* (1972). As with glass containers, it is important to check that the container has the correct level of vacuum before processing, since a failure may result in either a 'peaked' or 'panelled' can, the distortion of which weakens the seam and may lead to postprocess contamination.

10 Staff hygiene and protective clothing

All personnel should receive a basic training in hygiene. This should include personal hygiene and an understanding of operator-borne contamination, as well as precautions necessary to prevent cross-infection and the importance of cleaning and disinfection routines.

The type of clothing worn is influenced by the process, but in all instances clean, non-fibre-shedding overalls and hair covering are necessary in all manufacturing areas. Where products are handled, gloves must be worn and, for some processes, face-masks are necessary. For aseptic manufacturing, presterilized clothing, such as single- or two-piece trouser suits, footwear, hair covering (beards included), face-masks and gloves, is necessary. These should be changed on a regular basis, with fresh garments at least once a day.

11 Documentation and records

As mentioned earlier, written procedures should be available for all cleaning and disinfection operations, for both buildings and equipment, and for the monitoring of the efficiency of such processes. In some organizations, it has been found to be advantageous to incorporate these stages into the manufacturing-process sheet, which has to be signed by the operator as each is completed. This not only ensures that the cleaning and disinfection are carried out, but also makes them an integral part of the manufacturing process and provides a permanent record. This system is not applicable to all processes and independent records may be necessary.

All tanks and equipment should bear a label with respect to their current state, e.g. 'in use', 'clean but not sterilized' or 'clean and sterilized'. This is very important in the case of operations carried out by different shifts of operators. The monitoring of disinfection and sterilization processes is often a joint exercise between the production and quality-assurance personnel, but comprehensive records must be maintained by both parties and ideally held at a central location. If an integrated quality-assurance system, such as the ISO 9000 series, and/or an HACCP approach to hygiene is in operation, this will dictate the format of the documentation and assist in maintaining a good system of records.

The concept of good manufacturing practice is embodied in the British Standards Institute Quality Assurance Standard BS5750 and its European equivalent, ISO 9000–9004/EN29000–EN29004, and in the UK Medicines Act and its subsequent code of practice. The European Economic Community (EEC) is currently in the process of preparing regulations on hygienic codes of practice for handling food products and regulations for food-manufacturing areas.

12 References

Ahmed, F.I.K. & Russell, C. (1975) Synergism between ultrasonic waves and hydrogen peroxide in the killing of micro-organisms. *Journal of Applied Bacteriology*, **39**, 31–40.

Anon. (1959a) Cleaning of dairy equipment. In *In-place Cleaning of Dairy Equipment* (ed. Davis, J.G.), pp. 1–8. London: Society of Dairy Technology.

Anon. (1959b) Methods and equipment for in-place cleaning. In *In-place Cleaning of Dairy Equipment* (ed. Davis, J.G.), pp. 16–34. London: Society of Dairy Technology.

Anon. (1977) *Guide to Good Pharmaceutical Manufacturing Practice*. London: HMSO.

Beeby, M.M. & Whitehouse, C.E. (1965) A bacterial spore test piece for the control of ethylene oxide sterilisation. *Journal of Applied Bacteriology*, **28**, 349–360.

Burman, N.P. & Colbourne, J.S. (1977) Techniques for the assessment of growth of micro-organisms on plumbing materials used in contact with potable water supplies. *Journal of Applied Bacteriology*, **43**, 137–144.

Chambers, C.S.W. & Clarke, N.A. (1968) Control of bacteria in non-domestic water supplies. *Advances in Applied Microbiology*, **8**, 105–143.

Collins, V.G. (1964) The freshwater environment and its significance in industry. *Journal of Applied Bacteriology*, **27**, 143–150.

Colquitt, H.R. & Maurer, J.M. (1969) Hygienic mop maintenance in hospitals. *British Hospital Journal and Social Service Review*, **79**, 2177.

Davis, J.G. (1959) The microbiological control of water in dairies and food factories. *Proceedings of the Society for Water Treatment and Examination*, **8**, 31–54.

Denyer, S.P. (1998) Sterilization control and sterility testing. In *Pharmaceutical Microbiology* (eds Hugo, W.B. & Russell, A.D.), 6th edn, pp. 439–452. Oxford: Blackwell Science.

Favero, M.S., McDade, J.J., Robertson, J.A., Hoffman, R.K. & Edward, R.W. (1968) Microbiological sampling of surfaces. *Journal of Applied Bacteriology*, **31**, 336–343.

Hambracus, A., Bengtsson, S. & Laurell, G. (1968)

Bacterial contamination in a modern operating suite. 4. Bacterial contamination of clothes worn in the suite. *Journal of Hygiene, Cambridge*, **80**, 175–181.

Hargreaves, D.P. (1990) Good manufacturing practice in the control of contamination. In *Guide to Microbiological Control in Pharmaceuticals* (eds Denyer, S.P. & Baird, R.M.), pp. 68–86. Chichester: Ellis Horwood.

Hartman, P.A. (1960) Enterococcus: coliform ratio in frozen chicken pies. *Applied Microbiology*, **8**, 114–116.

Jay, J.M. (1970) Indices of food sanitary quality, and microbiological standards. In *Modern Food Microbiology*, pp. 140–193. New York: Van Nostrand Reinhold.

Lidwell, O.M. & Noble, W.C. (1975) Fungi and clostridia in hospital air: the effect of air conditioning. *Journal of Applied Bacteriology*, **39**, 251–261.

Maurer, I.M. (1985) *Hospital Hygiene*, 3rd edn. London: Edward Arnold.

Meddick, H.M. (1977) Bacterial contamination control mats: a comparative study. *Journal of Hygiene, Cambridge*, **79**, 133–140.

Nishannon, A. & Pohja, M.S. (1977) Comparative studies of microbial contamination of surfaces by the contact plate and swab methods. *Journal of Applied Bacteriology*, **42**, 53–63.

Parker, M.E. & Litchfield, J.H. (1962) Effective detergency and cleaning practice. In *Food Plant Sanitation*, pp. 223–263. New York: Reinhold.

Put, H.M.C., Van Doren, H., Warner, W.R. & Kruiswick, J.T.H. (1972) The mechanism of microbiological leaker spoilage of canned foods: a review. *Journal of Applied Bacteriology*, **35**, 7–27.

Raj, H., Weibe, W.J. & Liston, J. (1961) Detection and enumeration of faecal indicator organisms in frozen sea food. *Applied Microbiology*, **9**, 295–308.

Russell, A.D. (1980) Sterilisation control and sterility testing. In *Pharmaceutical Microbiology* (eds Hugo, W.B. & Russell, A.D.), 2nd edn, pp. 317–324. Oxford: Blackwell Scientific Publications.

Russell, A.D., Ahonkhai, I. & Rogers, D.T. (1979) Microbiological applications of the inactivation of antibiotics and other antimicrobial agents. *Journal of Applied Bacteriology*, **46**, 207–245.

Shaner, E.O. (1967) Acoustic–chemical procedures for the ultrasonic sterilization of instruments: a status report. *Journal of Oral Therapy*, **3**, 417–422.

Sykes, G. (1965) Air disinfection and sterilization. In *Disinfection and Sterilization: Theory and Practice*, 2nd edn, pp. 253–288. London: E. & F.N. Spon.

Thomas, M.E.M. & Maurer, I.M. (1972) Bacteriological safeguards in hospital cleaning. *British Hospital Journal and Social Service Review*, **82** (Institutional Cleaning Suppl. 6).

Trimarchi, G. (1959) The bacteriological control of food utensils in public service: methods for the determination of the bacterial content. *Igiene Moderna*, **52**, 95–111.

Underwood, E. (1998) Ecology of microorganisms as it affects the pharmaceutical industry. In *Pharmaceutical Microbiology* (eds Hugo, W.B. & Russell, A.D.), 6th edn, pp. 339–354. Oxford: Blackwell Science.

Windle Taylor, E. & Burman, N.P. (1964) The application of membrane filtration techniques to the bacteriological examination of water. *Journal of Applied Bacteriology*, **27**, 294–303.

CHAPTER 12

Decontamination of the Environment and Medical Equipment in Hospitals

1 Introduction

Infection has always been a problem in hospitals and, before the introduction of antiseptic techniques by Lister (1868), mortality following surgery was often high. John Bell (1801) wrote about the 'hospital sore', describing it as an epidemic ulcer occurring in all hospitals, but particularly in the larger ones. He described how difficult it was for young surgeons in the Hotel Dieu in Paris when they saw many of their patients dying of hospital 'gangrene'. Following Lister's use of antiseptics in surgery (see Chapter 1), a gradual evolution has occurred in aseptic, sterilization and disinfection techniques. Hospitals now have a central sterile supply service for instruments, dressings and many other items, and operating theatres have a mechanical ventilation system providing filtered air. Nevertheless, although mortality has been considerably reduced, morbidity remains and approximately 10% of patients in hospital at any one time have acquired a nosocomial infection (Meers *et al.*, 1981; Mayon-White *et al.*, 1988; Emmerson *et al.*, 1996).

The main hospital-acquired infections are of the urinary tract, surgical operation or traumatic wounds and the respiratory tract. Most of the infections are endogenous in origin (acquired from a patient's own bacterial flora) and may be difficult to prevent (Ayliffe, 1986). The elderly, newborn and the seriously ill are particularly likely to acquire a hospital infection, as are diabetics, leukaemics or patients undergoing radiotherapy or receiving treatment with steroids or immunosuppressive drugs. Infection is also commonly associated with invasive procedures, such as intravenous and urinary tract catheterization and mechanical ventilation of the respiratory tract. Patients are often crowded together in the same environment and some are admitted for the treatment of an existing infection. Hospital staff provide many opportunities for transfer of infection by successive close contact with infected and susceptible patients. The use of antibiotics has been associated not only with more effective treatment of infection, but also with the emergence of antibiotic-resistant organisms and their transmission. In recent years, methicillin-resistant *Staphylococcus aureus* (MRSA) has spread to hospitals in most countries of the world (Wenzel *et al.*, 1991; Ayliffe, 1997) and at least 16 epidemic strains have been described in England and Wales (Report, 1995). These epidemic strains have been difficult to control (Report, 1990; Duckworth, 1993; Cox *et al.*, 1995). However, although usually highly resistant to antibiotics, MRSA do not show significantly increased resistance to disinfectants commonly used in hospitals for environmental and equipment disinfection (see Chapter 10F). Infections caused by coagulase-negative staphylococci have also increased, particularly following intravascular catheterization and implant surgery and in immunocompromised patients. Vancomycin-resistant enterococci are also causing treatment problems in some hospitals (Wade, 1995). Although some strains of enterococci show some increased resistance to heat, they remain sensitive to environmental disinfectants at in-use concentrations (Kearns *et al.*, 1995; Bradley & Fraise, 1996). Outbreaks of diarrhoea in geriatric units caused by *Clostridium difficile* are also being increasingly reported (Cartmill *et al.*, 1994). Antibiotic-resistant strains of Gram-negative bacilli, such as *Pseudomonas aeruginosa, Klebsiella* and *Enterobacter* spp., *Serratia marcescens* and *Acinetobacter* spp., continue to cause infection problems, particularly in high-risk units, such as intensive care and burns. Although they have been exposed to disinfectants for many years, there is little evidence of increased resistance to disinfectants commonly used in US hospitals (Rutala *et al.*, 1997). Despite this, the nature of the hospital population and host susceptibility are more important contributory factors to infection than the inanimate environment, disinfection still has a role in the prevention of the spread of infection.

Disinfectants tend to be used indiscriminately, and a Public Health Laboratory Service Committee (1965) described a wide range of disinfectants in use in hospitals at that time. Although recommendations were made by the committee, the situation had shown little improvement by 1969 (Ayliffe *et al.*, 1969). Disinfectants were often used unnecessarily, and not used at all in situations where they could have been of value. Many of the products were unsuitable for hospital use, but were usually acceptable if they possessed a characteristic 'disinfectant' or 'antiseptic' smell. Dilutions of disinfectants were rarely measured and concentrations were often inadequate and associated with bacterial contamination (Kelsey & Maurer, 1966; Prince & Ayliffe, 1972). Failure to appreciate the effects of concentration and dilution on biocidal activity (Hugo & Denyer, 1987) is common; see concentration exponent (Chapter 3). Although disinfectant policies have been introduced in most hospitals, implementation is still often unsatisfactory (Cadwallader, 1989) and inappropriate disinfectants are still used, particularly in countries where infection-control services are not well developed (e.g. Zaidi *et al.*, 1995). The hospital staff responsible for buying and using disinfectants are often not well trained and have little knowledge of microbiology. They are frequently advised by representatives of disinfectant manufacturers and the advice is usually based on the results of laboratory tests, which do not necessarily mimic hospital conditions (Maurer, 1985). Considerable sums of money are wasted in the unnecessary disinfection of floors and the inanimate environment (Danforth *et al.*, 1987; Daschner, 1991).

The increasing use of complicated medical equipment, often heat-labile, and the presence of potentially hazardous blood-borne infections, such as hepatitis B (HBV), hepatitis C (HCV) and human immunodeficiency virus (HIV), have increased the need for effective and well-defined decontamination procedures (Department of Health Medical Devices Directorate, Parts 1, Principles, 1993, and 2, Protocols, 1996; Part 3, Procedures, to be published). Medical equipment and the hospital environment must be rendered safe to use by a decontamination process, which consists of cleaning and disinfection or sterilization (Ayliffe *et al.*, 1993).

1 Cleaning is a process that removes contaminants, including dust, soil, chemical residues, pyrogens, large numbers of microorganisms and the organic matter protecting them. Cleaning is usually a prerequisite to disinfection or sterilization.

2 Disinfection is a process that reduces the number of organisms, but not necessarily spores; it does not kill or remove all organisms but reduces their number to a level that is not harmful to health. High-level disinfection includes the killing or removal of *Mycobacterium tuberculosis* and enteroviruses, but not necessarily all mycobacteria, spores or prions.

3 Sterilization is a process used to render an object free from all microorganisms, but in practice usually excludes prions.

The decontamination processes vary in their microbiological effect, ranging from cleaning, which is the least effective, to sterilization, which is the most effective. They are not mutually exclusive. Cleaning could remove all organisms. It might be better to redefine these terms on the basis of making an item safe for a specified purpose.

2 A rational approach to disinfection: a disinfectant policy

Every hospital should have a disinfectant policy. The principles of preparing such a policy were described by Kelsey & Maurer (1972) and, more recently, by Ayliffe *et al.* (1993) and Coates & Hutchinson (1994). Policies essentially consist of: listing the purposes for which disinfectants are used; eliminating their use when sterilization rather than disinfection is the object; where heat can be used; where single-use equipment can be economically used; and selecting a limited number of disinfectants for most of the remaining uses. In order to produce a realistic policy, the reason for disinfection should be considered in detail. Risks of infection from equipment or the environment should be categorized, priorities allocated and resources made available on the basis of this assessment.

2.1 Objective

When deciding whether or not disinfection is necessary, it is important to consider the reason for the procedure. The objective is to prevent infection but, in more practical terms, may be defined as the 'reduction of microbiological contamination to such a level that an infective dose is unlikely to reach a susceptible site on a patient'. However, an infective dose cannot easily be determined, due to the variability in virulence of organisms and resistance of the host. In some instances, one virus-containing particle or a single tubercle bacillus will initiate an infection, but for most organisms a much larger number is necessary in a healthy person (Barkley & Wedum, 1977). In experiments with *Staph. aureus* in humans, over 10^6 organisms are required to cause a local infection following intradermal injection, but in the presence of a suture only 10^2 organisms are required (Elek & Conen, 1957). An assessment of the value of disinfection in terms of a reduction in clinical infection would be very useful but is rarely possible. Trials would need to be large and the results could still be inconclusive because of the large number of interrelating factors, although occasional studies have failed to show differences in infection rates between wards using environmental disinfectants and those using detergents only (Danforth *et al.*, 1987). Nevertheless, a rational decision can be made in most situations. For instance, chemical disinfection of an operating-room floor is probably unnecessary, because the bacteria-carrying particles already on the floor are unlikely to reach an open wound in sufficient numbers to cause an infection (Ayliffe *et al.*, 1967; Hambraeus *et al.*, 1978). Cleaning alone, followed by drying, will considerably reduce the bacterial population.

The standards of hygiene expected by patients and staff must also be considered. Even when these standards are illogical, failure to meet them may erode confidence and could cause unnecessary anxiety.

2.2 Categories of risk to patients and treatment of equipment and environment

The objective must be considered carefully in any situation, categories of risk determined (Spaulding, 1977; Rutala, 1996) and the appropriate treatment applied (Ayliffe & Gibson, 1975; Ayliffe *et al.*, 1976). Four categories of risk may be considered: high, intermediate, low and minimal (Ayliffe *et al.*, 1992b).

2.2.1 High risk

These are items of equipment in close contact with a break in the skin or mucous membrane or introduced into a sterile body cavity or into the vascular system. Items in this category should be sterilized by heat, if possible, or, if heat-labile, may be treated with ethylene oxide (EO), low-temperature steam and formaldehyde, gas plasma or commercially by irradiation. In some instances, e.g. a heat-labile laparoscope, high-level disinfection with a chemical agent may be acceptable. The high-risk category includes surgical instruments, implants, surgical dressings, operative endoscopes, urinary and other catheters, parenteral fluids, syringes and needles and other equipment used in surgical operations or aseptic techniques.

2.2.2 Intermediate risk

These are items of equipment in close contact with intact mucous membranes or body fluids or contaminated with particularly virulent or highly transmissible organisms. Items in this category will usually require disinfection. They include respiratory and anaesthetic equipment, fibre-optic gastroscopes and colonoscopes, vaginal speculae, tonometers and thermometers.

2.2.3 Low risk

These are items of equipment in contact with intact skin. Cleaning and drying will usually be sufficient, although some items are usually disinfected, such as stethoscopes, dressing-trolley tops, bedding and baths.

2.2.4 Minimal risk

These are items not in close contact with the patient or his/her immediate surroundings. Items in this category are unlikely either to be contaminated with significant numbers of potential pathogens or to transfer potential pathogens from them to a susceptible site on the patient. Cleaning and drying are usually adequate. Items in this category include floors, walls, ceilings, furniture and sinks. Disinfection may be required for removing contaminated spillage and occasionally for terminal disinfection or surface decontamination during outbreaks caused by organisms that survive well in the inanimate environment, such as MRSA, *Cl. difficile* or enterococci. Pouring disinfectants into sinks and drains is wasteful and of little value in the prevention of hospital infection (Maurer, 1985).

2.3 Requirements of chemical disinfectants

All the requirements or desirable properties of disinfectants are not attainable by any single agent and a choice must be made depending on the particular use, i.e. equipment, environmental surfaces and skin. Requirements are described in more detail in European publications (Reber *et al.*, 1972; Schmidt, 1973; Babb, 1996).

1 The disinfectant should preferably be bactericidal and its spectrum of activity should include all the common non-sporing pathogens, including tubercle bacilli. There is now a greater awareness of the risks of acquiring blood-borne infections, such as HBV, HCV and HIV. Viricidal activity is therefore a requirement for routine disinfection. Narrow-spectrum agents, such as quaternary ammonium compounds (QACs) or pine fluids, may select *Pseudomonas* spp. or other resistant Gram-negative bacilli, which are potentially hazardous to highly susceptible patients.

2 Disinfectants used on surfaces should be rapid in action, since the bactericidal activity ceases when the surface is dry.

3 The disinfectant should not be readily neutralized by organic matter, soaps, hard water or plastics.

4 Toxic effects should be minimal, and in-use dilutions of disinfectants should, if possible, be relatively non-corrosive. Confused or mentally defective patients may accidentally swallow a disinfectant

solution. Many of the environmental disinfectants in routine use are both toxic and corrosive, and care is required in their use and storage. Employers in the UK are now responsible for assessing health risks and measures to protect the health of workers from infection and toxic hazards (*Control of Substances Hazardous to Health Regulations*, 1988).

5 The disinfectant should not damage surfaces or articles treated. This requirement may vary with the particular situation; for example, the criteria for selecting a disinfectant for a toilet are obviously different from those for selecting one for an expensive endoscope.

6 Costs should be acceptable and supplies assured.

2.4 The choice of a method of disinfection

2.4.1 Heat

Heat is the preferred method of disinfection for all medical equipment (Table 12.1). Heat penetrates well, is predictably effective and is readily controlled. Steam at high pressure (for example, 121°C for 15 min, 134°C for 3 min) will sterilize, and, although a sporicidal effect may not necessarily be required, steam is the most reliable method of microbial decontamination. Heat-labile equipment, such as ventilator and anaesthetic tubing and used surgical instruments, may be decontaminated in a washing-machine that reaches an appropriate temperature for disinfection, for example 71°C for 3 min, 80°C for 1 min, 90°C for 1 s (Collins & Phelps, 1985; British Standard BS 2745, 1993).

Low-temperature steam (73°C for 10 min) (see Chapter 19A) or immersion in water at 70-100°C for 5–10 min is effective in killing vegetative organisms and should inactivate most viruses, including HIV.

2.4.2 Chemical

A clear-soluble phenolic and a chlorine-releasing

Table 12.1 Decontamination of equipment.

Method	Temperature (°C)	Time of exposure (min)	Level of decontamination
Heat			
Autoclave	134	3	Sterilization
	121	15	Sterilization
Low-temperature steam	73	10	Disinfection
Low-temperature steam and formaldehyde	73	180	Sterilization
Boilers	100	5–10	Disinfection
Pasteurizers	70–100	Variable	Disinfection
Washing-machines			
Bedpans	80	1	Cleaning and Disinfection
Linen	65	10	Cleaning and Disinfection
	71	3	Cleaning and Disinfection
Others	65–100	Variable	Cleaning and Disinfection
Chemical			
Ethylene oxide	55	60–360	Sterilization
Gas plasma	45	50–70*	Sterilization
Peracetic acid (0.2–0.35%)	RT	5	Disinfection
	RT–45	10	Sterilization
Chlorine dioxide	RT–45	10	Sterilization
(1000–1500 parts/ 10^6 av. ClO_2)	RT	5	Disinfection
2% glutaraldehyde	RT	10–60	Disinfection
		> 180	Sterilization
70% alcohol	RT	5–10	Disinfection

RT, room temperature.
*Total cycle times

agent (Chapter 2) should be sufficient for most environmental disinfection. Clear-soluble phenolics are comparatively cheap, are not readily neutralized and are active against a wide range or organisms, although not usually against viruses. They are suitable for environmental disinfection, but not for skin or for equipment likely to come into contact with skin or mucous membranes, or in food-preparation or storage areas. Their potential toxicity and the poor effect against some viruses have reduced their use in hospitals in recent years. Chlorine-releasing agents are very cheap, are active against a wide range of organisms, including viruses, but are readily neutralized and tend to damage some metals and materials. They are relatively non-toxic when diluted and are useful in food-preparation areas. Powder or tablets containing sodium dichloroisocyanurate (NaDCC) are stable when dry and are useful for environmental decontamination (Bloomfield & Uso, 1985; Coates, 1988). Chlorine-releasing agents at 1000–10 000 parts/10^6 av. Cl are increasingly used for routine disinfection and for removal of spillage, but at these concentrations can cause rapid deterioration of materials. Peroxygen compounds may be useful for the disinfection of some materials, e.g. carpets, which may be damaged by chlorine-releasing compounds (Coates & Wilson, 1992), but some are deficient in activity against mycobacteria (Broadley *et al.*, 1993; Holton *et al.*, 1994). Activated alkaline glutaraldehyde 2% is still the disinfectant of choice for decontaminating flexible endoscopes, but it is likely to be replaced for most purposes within the next few years (see Section 5.10). It is relatively non-corrosive and will kill spores with prolonged exposure (3–10 h) (Babb *et al.*, 1980), but is toxic and irritant. Possible alternatives to glutaraldehyde are peracetic acid, chlorine dioxide (ClO_2) products (such as Tristel) and superoxidized water (sterilox). These agents are rapidly sporicidal, mycobactericidal and viricidal, and some commercial preparations appear to be less irritant to staff than glutaraldehyde (Babb & Bradley, 1995a). However, some are more corrosive, less stable and more expensive. Further tests are required before these products can be accepted for routine use with expensive equipment.

Ethyl or iso propyl alcohol 60–70% is a rapid and effective method for disinfecting skin, trolleys and the surfaces of medical equipment. Compounds of low toxicity, such as chlorhexidine or povidone-iodine (both of which were considered in Chapter 2), may be required for disinfecting skin or mucous membranes and occasionally for inanimate items likely to contact skin or mucous membranes.

2.5 Implementation of the disinfectant policy

Although most hospitals have a policy, implementation is often inefficient. All hospital staff should be aware of the policy and of problems likely to arise if there are any major departures from that policy. Audits of the policy should be carried out at regular intervals in the acute wards and special units.

2.5.1 Organization

The infection-control committee and team have the responsibility for preparing a safe and effective policy and ensuring that the correct disinfectants and methods of application are used. The microbiologist, pharmacist, sterile-services manager and infection-control nurse should be members of the committee. The nursing and domestic staff, who are mainly responsible for the actual practice of disinfection, are also advised through their own organizations, but responsibilities and priorities are often poorly defined. Information is not always passed to those who use the disinfectants (Ayliffe *et al.*, 1992b).

2.5.2 Training

A logical, safe and effective approach to disinfection requires trained staff. They should have some knowledge of microbiology, mechanisms of transfer of infection, health and safety issues and properties of disinfectants. Alternatively, operatives should follow defined schedules and be supervised by trained staff. Decisions are still made too often by staff without adequate training. It is important that external contract cleaners are aware of the policy and are similarly trained to in-house staff. The infection-control team should regularly update the policy.

2.5.3 Distribution and dilution of disinfectants

Since inaccurate dilution is one of the main causes of failure of disinfection, this aspect requires careful consideration. It is preferable to deliver disinfectants to departments at the use dilution, but this is not always possible or convenient. If not possible, suitable dispensers are required and the staff must be trained in their use. As pointed out earlier, the effect of dilution on disinfectant activity should always be borne in mind (Hugo & Denyer, 1987; see also Chapter 3).

2.5.4 Testing of disinfectants

Official tests are available in some countries, e.g. Germany, France, the USA, Switzerland and Holland, but not in the UK (see Chapter 4). The Kelsey–Sykes capacity test has been generally accepted in the UK (Kelsey & Maurer, 1974). However, national tests in Europe will gradually be replaced by agreed standard European suspension, surface and practical tests. These tests will include viricidal, fungicidal, mycobactericidal and sporicidal activity, as well as tests using a range of bacteria (see Chapters 4 and 6). Tests of disinfectants should preferably be carried out by a reliable independent organization and results supplied to hospitals by the manufacturers. The manufacturer should also provide evidence of other properties of the disinfectant, such as the range of susceptible organisms, toxicity, stability and corrosiveness. Manufacturers of reusable medical devices in Europe are required to provide details of acceptable reprocessing methods, including decontamination (Department of Health Medical Devices Directorate, 1996). Surface-disinfection tests on tiles or linen are often used for hospital disinfectants in Europe but not in the UK or USA. In-use tests are useful when a new disinfectant is introduced, and possibly routinely at intervals of 6–12 months (Kelsey & Maurer, 1966; Prince & Ayliffe, 1972). These tests should detect the possible emergence of resistant strains, as well as inadequate dilutions or loss of activity of the disinfectant.

2.5.5 Costs

Excessive costs may be due to unnecessary use, incorrect concentrations or inappropriate disinfectants being used. The cost of the disinfection procedure as well as that of the agent should be considered.

3 Problems with certain microorganisms

3.1 Bacterial spores

A process that kills spores is usually required for articles in the high-risk category (see Section 2.2.1). Liquid preparations, such as glutaraldehyde, peracetic acid, ClO_2, other chlorine-releasing agents or, occasionally, formaldehyde vapour, may be used but are generally less reliable than heat; penetration is often poor, thorough rinsing is required before use, items cannot be packed and recontamination with microorganisms can occur during the rinsing process. Activated alkaline glutaraldehyde 2% requires a minimum exposure time of 3 h for an adequate sporicidal action (Babb *et al.*, 1980) or up to 10 h on the basis of the Association of Official Analytical Chemists (AOAC) test (Spaulding *et al.*, 1977). However, some spores, e.g. *Cl. difficile*, appear to be killed by glutaraldehyde in a much shorter time (Dyas & Das, 1985; Rutala *et al.*, 1993). A number of glutaraldehyde preparations are now available and these show some variation in activity, stability and corrosiveness. Repeated use of a glutaraldehyde solution is common practice, mainly due to expense. The length of time a solution is repeatedly used should depend on the extent of contamination with organic matter or dilution during use and not on stability alone (Babb *et al.*, 1992). Peracetic acid (0.2–0.35%) and ClO_2 (1000–10 000 parts/10^6 av. (ClO_2) are sporicidal in less than 10 min (Babb & Bradley, 1995a). Superoxidized water is also rapidly sporicidal (Selkon *et al.*, in press). Other chlorine-releasing agents are also rapidly sporicidal in high concentrations (Coates, 1996) but have the disadvantage of corroding instruments.

3.2 Blood-borne viruses, hepatitis A and prions

Hepatitis B, HCV and other hepatitis non-A, non-B viruses have not been grown *in vitro*, and reliable laboratory tests for inactivation are not available. Limited studies in chimpanzees have indicated that

HBV is inactivated by a temperature of 98°C for 2 min, but lower temperatures were not investigated. Glutaraldehyde, 70% ethanol, hypochlorite solutions and iodophors also inactivate the virus, e.g. different authors quote 0.1% glutaraldehyde (24°C) in 5 min, 2% glutaraldehyde in 10 min, 70% isopropanol in 10 min, 80% ethanol in 2 min (Bond *et al.*, 1983; Kobayashi *et al.*, 1984). A product containing 3.2% glutaraldehyde reduced HBV surface antigen (HBsAg) activity to low levels in 30 s (Akamatsu *et al.*, 1997). Studies with the duck HBV model showed that the virus was inactivated by 2% glutaraldehyde preparations in 5min (Murray *et al.*, 1991; Deva *et al.*, 1996). The resistance of HCV to disinfectants is unknown, but it can be predicted from its structure that it is not more resistant than HBV. Hepatitis A virus spreads by the faecal–oral route and is one of the most resistant viruses to disinfectants. However, it is rapidly inactivated by 2% glutaraldehyde and high concentrations of chlorine-releasing agents (Mbithi *et al.*, 1990).

Human immunodeficiency virus is an enveloped virus and is readily inactivated by heat and commonly used antiviral disinfectants (Kurth *et* al., 1986; Resnick *et al.*, 1986). It is inactivated by 2% glutaraldehyde in 1 min, but 70% ethanol has shown variable results in surface tests (Hanson *et al.*, 1989; VanBueren *et al.*, 1989). The inconsistent results were probably due to variability of penetration of dried organic material, and it is likely that 70% ethanol is rapidly effective against HIV on precleaned surfaces.

Hepatitis B virus particles are usually present in larger numbers than HIV in blood, and infection is more readily transmissible, but thorough washing of equipment with a detergent to remove blood and body secretions will minimize the risk of infection from these viruses. However, the use of a chorine-releasing solution or powder should be effective in rapidly decontaminating blood spillage before cleaning, and is recommended particularly if the spillage is from an infected or high-risk patient (Coates, 1988; Bloomfield *et al.*, 1990; Ayliffe *et al.*, 1992b; Coates & Hutchinson, 1994). The agents causing viral haemorrhagic fevers, e.g. Lassa, Ebola and Marburg, are transmitted in blood or body fluids. They are inactivated by the same disinfectants as are the other blood-borne viruses, e.g. chlorine-releasing agents and 2% glutaraldehyde (Advisory Committee on Dangerous Pathogens, 1996). The agents causing Creutzfeldt–Jakob disease, kuru, scrapie and bovine spongiform encephalopathy (BSE) are termed prions. They have been transmitted rarely during neurosurgical procedures, from corneal implants and from pituitary growth hormone. They consist of small protein particles, which are highly resistant to heat, EO, glutaraldehyde and formaldehyde. High concentrations of hypochorites (20 000 parts/10^6 av. Cl) for 60 min are effective but are corrosive to most instruments. Moist heat at 134°C for 18 min is sometimes suggested as effective, but even this is uncertain. Thorough cleaning is of great importance, owing to the doubts on the effectiveness of decontamination methods and the probable variation in the resistance of different prions to heat and disinfectants (see Advisory Committee,1998; Chapter 7).

3.3 Mycobacteria

Mycobacterium tuberculosis continues to be a major problem throughout the world, and resistance to useful systemic chemotherapeutic agents is increasing. This and other mycobacteria are often the cause of infections in patients with acquired immune deficiency syndrome (AIDS). Atypical mycobacteria, such as *Mycobacterium chelonae*, have been isolated from the rinsing tank of washer disinfectors and from washings from bronchoscopes. These have been responsible for pseudo-outbreaks and rarely for actual infections of the respiratory tract.

Mycobacterium tuberculosis and some other mycobacteria are more resistant to chemical disinfectants than other non-sporing organisms. Heat is the preferred method of decontamination, but EO is appropriate for heat-labile items. Glutaraldehyde 2% is a less satisfactory alternative, but for practical purposes is still the disinfectant of choice for heat-labile endoscopes. A high-level disinfection process, e.g. immersion for at least 20 min, is required for *M. tuberculosis*. *Mycobacterium avium-intracellulare* is even more resistant to glutaraldehyde and requires immersion for 60–90 min (Collins, 1986; Best *et al.*, 1990; Holton *et al.*, 1994; Lynam *et al.*, 1995; Russell, 1996). Strains of *M. chelonae* resistant to 2% glutaraldehyde have been isolated from washer disinfectors (Van Klingeren and Pullen, 1993; Griffiths *et al.*, 1997). Peracetic acid (0.2–0.35%) and chlorine dioxide (1100 parts/10^6 av. Cl) are effective against most strains of mycobacteria, including *M. avium-intracellulare*, in 5 min. Ethanol 70% and chlorine-releasing compounds in high concentrations (5000–10 000 parts/10^6 av. Cl) are effective against *M. tuberculosis, M. avium-intracellulare* and *M. chelonae* in less than 5 min (Griffiths *et al.*, 1997). The clear-soluble phenolics are active against *M. tuberculosis* and are suitable for disinfection of rooms occupied by patients with open tuberculosis. Quaternary ammonium and peroxygen compounds and chlorhexidine usually show poor activity against tubercle bacilli, although one QAC, Sactimed Sinald, shows useful *in vitro* activity (Holton *et al.*, 1994). The resistance of mycobacteria to disinfectants is also considered in Chapter 10D.

4 Contaminated disinfectant solutions

Solutions contaminated with Gram-negative bacilli are a particular hazard in hospital, and infections originating from them have been reported (Lee & Fialkow, 1961; Bassett *et al.*, 1970; Speller *et al.*, 1971). Contamination is usually due to inappropriate use of disinfectants (Sanford, 1970; Centers for Disease Control, 1974), weak solutions (Prince & Ayliffe, 1972), where there is poor appreciation of the concentration exponent of a particular agent (Hugo & Denyer, 1987), or 'topping up' of containers. The problem can usually be avoided by thorough cleaning and drying of the container before refilling, but an additional biocide is sometimes necessary (Burdon & Whitby, 1967).

5 Treatment of the environment and equipment

In many instances, it is still difficult to decide on the appropriate method of decontamination, even after taking into consideration the nature and risk category of the item concerned. Cleaning alone may be adequate for most routine purposes, but disinfection may be required for the same item during outbreaks of infection. However, it is useful to remember that the risk of transmitting infection on an article that has been thoroughly washed and dried is very small (Nystrom, 1981), Hanson *et al.*, 1990; Babb & Bradley, 1995b). Thorough cleaning also removes potential bacterial nutrients, as well as bacteria themselves. Methods of decontamination of equipment are summarized in Table 12.1. The variable temperatures and exposure times are due to procedural differences and often to practical requirements. Infection risks from equipment have been reviewed by Ayliffe (1988).

Some of the problem areas in hospital are described in this section, but for more information see Maurer (1985), Rutala (1996), Block (1991), Gardner & Peel (1998), Ayliffe *et al.*, (1992b), Bennett & Brachman (1992), Taylor (1992), Wenzel (1993), Philpott-Howard & Casewell (1994) and Mayhall (1996).

5.1 Walls, ceilings and floors

Walls and ceilings are rarely heavily contaminated, provided the surface remains intact and dry (Wypkema & Alder, 1962; Collins, 1988). In our own studies, using contact plates, bacterial counts on walls were in the range of 2–5/25 cm^2 and counts of 10 were unusually high (Table 12.2). The

Table 12.2 Bacterial contamination of walls in an operating theatre.

	Mean counts from 10 contact plates (25 cm^2)	
Time of sampling after washing	Total	*Staph. aureus*
1 day	2.8	0
1 week	5.0	0
3 week	3.4	0.2
5 week	4.6	0.2
12 weeks	1.2	0

Data from Ayliffe *et al.* (1967)

organisms are mainly Gram-positive, coagulase-negative cocci, with occasional aerobic, spore-bearing organisms and, rarely, *Staph. aureus*. The number of bacteria does not appear to increase even if walls are not cleaned, and frequent cleaning has little influence on bacterial counts. Table 12.2 shows bacterial counts from an unwashed operating-theatre wall over a 12-week period (Ayliffe *et al.*, 1967). No increase in contamination occurred over this period. Additional studies showed no further increase over 6 months. Routine disinfection is therefore unnecessary, but walls should be cleaned when dirty.

Floors are more heavily contaminated than walls and a mean count of 380 organisms/25cm^2 was obtained from ward floors in a study by the authors. As on the walls and other surfaces, most of the bacteria are from the skin flora of the occupants of the room. A small proportion—usually less than 1%—are potential pathogens, such as *Staph. aureus*. The number of bacteria in the room environment tends to be related to the number of people in the ward and their activity (Williams *et al.*, 1966; Noble & Sommerville, 1974). Provided these factors remain relatively unchanged, the bacterial population on a surface will usually reach a plateau in a few hours. At this stage, the rates of deposition and death of organisms remain constant (Fig. 12.1); cleaning the floor with a detergent reduces the number of organisms by about 80% and the addition of a disinfectant may increase the reduction to over 95%. In a busy hospital ward, recontamination is rapid and bacterial counts may reach the precleaning or predisinfection level in 1–2 h (Vesley & Michaelson, 1964; Ayliffe *et al.*, 1966). The transient reduction obtained does not appear to justify the routine use of a disinfectant. There is also evidence that skin organisms on the floor are not readily resuspended in the air (Ayliffe *et al.*, 1967; Hambraeus *et al.*, 1978), provided a suitable method of cleaning is used, e.g. a dust-attracting mop, a vacuum cleaner with a filtered exhaust or wet-cleaning techniques.

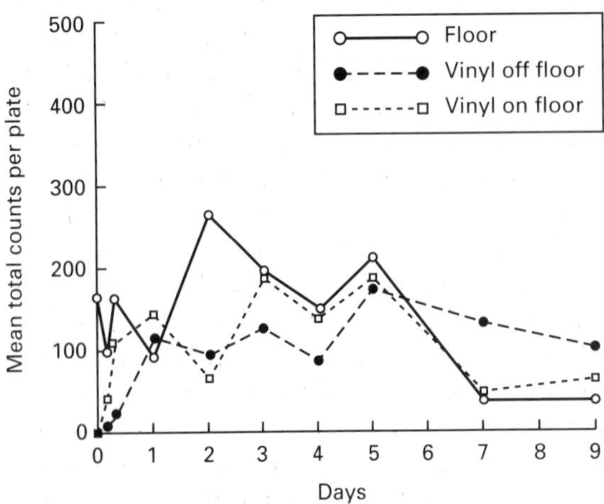

Fig. 12.1 Mean total counts taken on impression plates at intervals after cleaning the floor in a female surgical ward during the course of 9 days.

Disinfection may still be required in areas of high risk or if the number of potential pathogens is thought to be high—for instance, in a room after the discharge of an infected patient—but, even in these circumstances, disinfection of walls and ceilings is rarely necessarily. Carpets are now often found in hospitals and may be exposed to heavy contamination from spillage of food, blood or faeces. The carpets must be able to withstand regular cleaning and should have waterproof backing and the fibres should preferably not absorb water (Ayliffe *et al.*, 1974a; Collins, 1979). There is no evidence that carpets increase the risk of infection in clinical areas (Anderson *et al.*, 1982), and further unpublished studies of the authors over a long period in a surgical ward confirm the original findings of absence of effect on wound infections. Regular routine maintenance is required and many of the failures in the use of carpets have been due to an unpleasant smell associated with inadequate cleaning. This particularly applies to certain wards—for example, the psychogeriatric ward, where spillage is excessive but carpets are preferred for aesthetic reasons. Although the risk of infection is small, careful thought should be given before carpets are fitted in clinical areas or where spillage is likely to be considerable (Collins, 1979).

5.2 Air

Airborne spread of infection in hospitals is less important than previously thought (Brachman, 1971; Ayliffe & Lowbury, 1982), but more recent evidence has demonstrated that airborne spread plays a major role in prosthetic surgery (e.g. Lidwell *et al.*, 1983).

Outbreaks of *Aspergillus* infection have been reported in immunosuppressed patients, probably acquired by the airborne route, mainly during building demolition or structural renovation. This risk may be reduced by nursing susceptible patients in rooms supplied with high efficiency particulate air (HEPA) filtered air (Rogers & Barnes, 1988; Walsh & Dixon, 1989; Rhame, 1991). Legionnaires' disease is caused by the spread of *Legionella* from cooling towers, showers and water-supplies or other aerosol-producing systems (Bartlett *et al.*, 1986; Department of Health, 1994b). It does not spread from person to person. Prevention is possible by regular maintenance of systems, use of biocides and improved design to avoid static water (see Chapter 10E). In the event of an outbreak, chlorination or heating of the hot-water supply to an appropriate temperature for preventing the growth of *Legionella* may be introduced. However, chlorination may corrode the water-storage and supply systems, and excessive heating of water may cause scalding, particularly in children and the elderly.

Disinfection of the air has been reviewed elsewhere (Sykes, 1965), but is now rarely considered necessary in hospital. Good ventilation with filtered air is considered adequate for operating theatres, isolation rooms and safety cabinets (Department of Health, 1994a). Thorough cleaning of surfaces and disinfection are thought to be more reliable than 'fogging', which is the production of a disinfectant aerosol or vapour, usually formaldehyde (Centers for Disease Control, 1972). Methods of air disinfection and air sterilization are considered in Chapters 2 and 11.

5.3 Baths, wash-bowls and toilets

Bath-water contains large numbers of bacteria, including potential pathogens (Ayliffe *et al.*, 1975a). Many bacteria remain on the surface of the bath after emptying and may be transferred to the next patient. Thorough cleaning with a detergent after each use is usually sufficient, but disinfection is necessary in maternity or surgical units when bathing carriers of communicable multiresistant bacteria, such as MRSA, or where patients with open wounds use the same bath. Chlorine-releasing solutions or powders are commonly recommended for disinfection (Boycott, 1956; Alder *et al.*, 1966; Ayliffe *et al.*, 1992b). Abrasive powders may damage certain bath surfaces and non-abrasive chlorine-releasing powders should be used. Wash-bowls are often stacked so that a small amount of residual water remains in each after emptying, and Gram-negative bacilli may grow to large numbers overnight (Joynson, 1978). Routine disinfection is usually unnecessary, but thorough cleaning and drying are always required. Toilets are an obvious infection risk during outbreaks of gastrointestinal infection. Disinfection of the seat of the toilet is probably of some value in these circumstances, but, for routine purposes, cleaning is usually sufficient. Risks of infection from aerosols after flushing are usually small (Newsom, 1972).

5.4 Bedpans and urinals

These are required for patients confined to bed, but are used less often than formerly because of early mobilization of patients after surgical operations. After use, the contents require disposal and the container must be decontaminated, particularly if the patient is suffering from a gastrointestinal or urinary-tract infection. Although bedpan washers without a disinfecting heat cycle are still used without evidence of cross-infection, a thermal disinfection-cycle stage is now recommended on all machines (Ayliffe *et al.*, 1974b; Collins & Phelps, 1985; British Standard BS 2745, part 2 1993). This is the preferred method of decontamination, and chemical methods should be avoided if possible. Immersion of bedpans or urinals in tanks of disinfectant has been associated with the selection and growth of Gram-negative bacilli in the solution (Curie *et al.*, 1978). Macerators are a popular alternative to heat disinfection of metal or polypropylene pans and are satisfactory, if well maintained, but possible disadvantages, particularly drainage requirements, should be considered before installation (Gibson, 1973a,b). They have the advantage of saving nursing time by disposing of several pans in one cycle and avoiding the necessity of handling pans after disinfection. Bedpan supports are, however, reusable and require separate processing.

5.5 Crockery and cutlery

Hand-washed crockery and cutlery are frequently heavily contaminated after processing, but bacterial counts decrease considerably on drying. The addition of a disinfectant to the wash water is unreliable as a disinfection process (Department of Health and Social Security, 1986). Washing in a machine at a minimum temperature of 50–60°C, with a final rinse at 80°C for 1 min or more, followed by a drying cycle, is a satisfactory disinfection process (Maurer, 1985). Table 12.3 shows the difference in contamination of plates after hand- and machine-washing. If a suitable dishwasher is not available, disposable crockery and cutlery may be used for patients with open tuberculosis enteric infections and some other communicable infections, although the risks from washed and dried crockery and cutlery are minimal.

5.6 Cleaning equipment

Floor mops are often heavily contaminated with Gram-negative bacilli. Although the opportunities for these organisms to reach a susceptible site on a patient are small, the presence of a large reservoir of potentially pathogenic Gram-negative bacilli is undesirable. Mops should be periodically disinfected, preferably by heat. Mopheads washed by a machine will usually be adequately disinfected, but soaking overnight in disinfectant is not recommended. Some phenolics may be partially inactivated by plastic floor mops (Leigh & Whittaker, 1967; Maurer, 1985). Moisture retained in mop buckets, trapped in the tanks of scrubbing machines or retained in the reservoir of spray cleaners can also encourage the growth of Gram-negative bacilli (Medcraft *et al.*, 1987). If the fluid used is capable of supporting bacterial growth, the equipment should be dried, cleaned and stored dry. Poorly maintained or badly designed scrubbing machines, carpet cleaners or spray-cleaning equipment can produce contaminated aerosols. Staff should understand the need to decontaminate equipment for use in a certain area, but especially where there is a specific risk of infection.

5.7 Babies' incubators

Surfaces of incubators are rarely heavily contaminated, but there is always a risk of transfer of infection from one baby to the next. Thorough cleaning and drying of surfaces, seals and humidifier are important and are usually sufficient for routine treatment. If disinfection is considered necessary in an addition to cleaning, wiping over with 70% alcohol or a chlorine-releasing solution (125 parts/10^6 av. Cl) is adequate (Ayliffe *et al.*, 1975b).

5.8 Respiratory ventilators and associated equipment

The accumulation of moisture and the warm conditions in ventilators and associated equipment are often associated with the growth of Gram-negative bacilli, particularly *Ps. aeruginosa* and *Klebsiella* spp. There is some experimental evidence that organisms are able to reach the patient from contaminated ventilator tubing (Babington *et al.*, 1971) and that infection can subsequently occur (Phillips & Spencer, 1965). Nebulization of contaminated droplets has caused lung infections (Sanford & Pierce, 1979). Apart from a contaminated nebulizer, the greatest infection risk is from the part of the circuit nearest to the patient. Changing the reservoir bag, tubing and connectors every 48 h is an important measure in the prevention of infection (Craven *et al.*, 1982). Respiratory circuits are preferably decontaminated by heat (see below). Disposable circuits are expensive. Venti-

Table 12.3 Bacterial contamination of crockery (plates) after washing.

		No. of plates in range: bacteria/25 cm²		
Method of washing	No. of plates	0–10	11–1000	>1000
Machine	72	67 (93%)	2	3
Hand	108	40 (37%)	46	22

lators are difficult to clean and disinfect, and most available methods are not entirely satisfactory (Phillips *et al.*, 1974; Ayliffe *et al.*, 1992b).

The use of filters or heat–moisture exchangers for microbiologically isolating the machine from the patient is a better method of preventing contamination of the machine and subsequent cross-infection. The amount of condensate associated with water humidification is minimal if a heat–moisture exchanger is used, and the circuitry can be changed less frequently, e.g. between patients or weekly. Less condensate is also produced with most neonatal ventilating systems, and a change of circuitry every 7 days would often appear to be adequate (Cadwallader *et al.*, 1990). Nevertheless, careful surveillance and monitoring of infection rates are necessary if a reversion to less frequent changing of circuits is introduced. Many ventilators now have reusable circuits, which may be cleaned and disinfected thermally in a dedicated washer-disinfector. Nebulizers should preferably be capable of withstanding disinfection by heat, but, if not, should be chemically disinfected or cleaned and dried every day (La Force, 1992).

5.9 Anaesthetic equipment

Patients are usually connected to anaesthetic machines for a shorter period of time than to respiratory ventilators in intensive-care units, and machines are rarely heavily contaminated, providing that the associated tubing is regularly changed (du Moulin & Saubermann, 1977). It is obviously preferable to provide each patient with a decontaminated circuit, but this could be expensive. Since contamination is usually not great, sessional replacement may be an acceptable compromise, provided decontaminated face-masks, endotracheal tubes and airways are available for each patient during a session of about 9–10 operations (Deverill & Dutt, 1980). The corrugated tubing should be disinfected with low-temperature steam or in a washing-machine that reaches temperatures of 70–80°C (Collins & Phelps, 1985; British Standard BS 2745 Part 3, 1993). Chemical disinfection is less reliable and should be avoided if possible (George, 1975). A single-use circuit may be preferred if a patient with known tuberculosis is anaesthetized. The possible transmission of HCV by anaesthetic equipment has been reported (Ragg, 1994), but this is an unlikely route of spread for a blood-borne virus. Based on this uncertain evidence, it has been suggested that filters should be used and replaced after each patient. Filters can prevent the transfer of bacteria and viruses (Vandenbrouke-Grauls *et al.*, 1995), but there is little evidence from earlier studies that they reduce clinical infection (Feeley *et al.*, 1981; Garibaldi *et al.*, 1981). The cost-effectiveness of using a new filter for each patient requires careful consideration (Snowdon, 1994; Das & Fraise, 1997).

5.10 Endoscopes

Endoscopes are now used for a wide range of diagnostic and therapeutic procedures. Those used for minimal-access surgery, e.g. laparoscopes and arthroscopes, are usually rigid and can be steam-sterilized, whereas the flexible instruments for gastrointestinal endoscopy and bronchoscopy are not. These are often grossly contaminated and difficult to clean and they require chemical sterilization or disinfection processes, which have several disadvantages.

Heat intolerance is not the only problem associated with processing endoscopes. Instrument lumens are often long, narrow, obscure and difficult to clean. The relatively high cost of endoscopes and a substantial increase in demand for endoscopy have resulted in there being too few endoscopes to provide one for each patient during an endoscopy session. Consequently, little time is available for decontamination between patients. Despite this, the incidence of postprocedural infection appears to be low.

Sources of infection during endoscopy are many and varied. If the instrument and accessories are not thoroughly cleaned and disinfected or sterilized between patients, microorganisms may be transferred to patients subsequently undergoing endoscopy. Hepatitis B virus, *M. tuberculosis, Salmonella* and parasitic infections have been transmitted by this route (Spach *et al.*, 1993; Ayliffe, 1996). Fears have also been expressed about the possible transmission of HIV, but this has not yet been reported.

Another source of infection, particularly with immunocompromised patients, is instrument contamination from the processor or the environment. Gram-negative bacilli, particularly *Ps. aeruginosa*, are regularly recovered from poorly processed instruments, automated washer-disinfectors, cleaning solutions and rinse water. These rapidly proliferate in the moist lumens of the instrument and processor between uses, particularly if biofilm is allowed to form (Bradley & Babb, 1995). Instruments and processors should be decontaminated at the start of each session to minimize the risk of infection by this route. Atypical mycobacteria of low virulence, such as *M. chelonae*, have been acquired from rinse water and processors (Reeves & Brown, 1995). These have been deposited in the lumens of bronchoscopes during rinsing and have been transferred to bronchial-lavage samples. This has, on occasion, led to the misdiagnosis of tuberculosis.

The incidence of infection following surgical endoscopy is lower still, presumably because most procedures are clean (Ayliffe *et al.*, 1992a). Endogenous infections have occasionally followed skin or accidental bowel perforation, but instrument-associated infections are rare. Other possible sources of infection are settlement of organisms from air on exposed instruments, the hands and clothing of the surgical team and contaminated dyes, lubricants and irrigation fluids. Sterile or bacteria-free water should be used for rinsing invasive endoscopes and accessories.

Methods of decontamination are shown in Table 12.1. Steam sterilization is the preferred option for rigid endoscopes identified by the manufacturers as autoclavable (Department of Health Medical Devices Agency, 1996a). A porous-load steam sterilizer (134°C $+^{3°C}/_{-0°C}$) with vacuum-assisted air removal, is recommended for packaged lumened endoscopes and accessories. Ethylene oxide at temperatures of 55°C or below may be used for sterilizing flexible and rigid endoscopes, but microbiological validation and aeration considerably lengthen the process and it is rarely practical as a routine. Also, very few hospitals in the UK have an EO-processing facility. In some hospitals, where time permits, EO is used for invasive flexible endoscopes, such as angioscopes, nephroscopes and the duodenoscopes used for endoscopic retrograde cholangiopancreatography (ERCP). Low-temperature steam and formaldehyde (73–80°C) is suitable for sterilizing rigid endoscopes, but cycles are long and immersion in disinfectant or autoclaving is usually preferred (Babb, 1993).

Immersion in a suitable disinfectant is the most widely used option at present (Rutala *et al.*, 1991; Ayliffe, 1993). Aldehyde-based disinfectants, particularly 2% glutaraldehyde, are usually used. These are non-damaging to instrument components and are rapidly effective against viruses and most non-sporing bacteria. Unfortunately, aldehydes, e.g. glutaraldehyde, formaldehyde and succinedialdehyde are irritant and sensitizing to the skin, eyes and respiratory tract (Burge, 1989), and strict precautions must be take to prevent or reduce exposure. If contact with disinfectant is likely, suitable gloves, e.g. nitrile, plastic aprons and eye protection should be worn. Most endoscope washer disinfectors are now equipped with rinsing and vapour containment or extraction facilities (British Society of Gastroenterology Working Party, 1993; Bradley & Babb, 1995).

The manufacturers' glutaraldehyde immersion times vary depending on the nature of microbial contamination anticipated. In the UK and elsewhere, the disinfectant manufacturers and professional societies have produced guidelines for immersion times based on laboratory studies and careful risk assessment (Ayliffe, 1993; Department of Health Medical Devices Agency, 1996a; British Society of Gastroenterology, 1998).

With the introduction of more stringent health and safety legislation in the UK, e.g. Health and Safety at Work Act, *Control of Substances Hazardous to Health Regulations* (COSHH) (1988), and elsewhere, other less toxic disinfectants are being used or investigated (Babb & Bradley, 1995a). These include: alcohol 70% (isopropanol or ethanol); peroxygen products, e.g. Virkon; improved QACs, such as Sactimed Sinald and Dettol ED; peracetic acid, such as Steris and NuCidex; ClO_2, such as Tristel, and superoxidized water, i.e. Sterilox (see Section 3.1). It is important that the disinfectant selected is effective against problematic microorganisms and is non-damaging, user-friendly and affordable. Unfortunately, the most effective agents are usually corrosive and irritant, and it takes a considerable time to establish disinfectant suitability with instrument manufacturers and those responsible for formulating policy.

Alcohol is probably the most widely used alternative instrument disinfectant at present, but it damages lens cements and is flammable and therefore unsafe for use and storage in large volumes, as it would be in automated systems. It is, however, popular for wiping over precleaned surfaces such as fibre-optic cables, cameras and the control box of non-submersible endoscopes. Alcohol is also useful for flushing the lumens of instruments before storage, as it disinfects and evaporates, leaving surfaces dry. Alcohol is not a sporicide but on clean surfaces it is highly effective against non-sporing bacteria, including mycobacteria, and most viruses.

Peracetic acid (0.2–0.35%) is probably the most popular alternative to glutaraldehyde at present. It is rapidly effective and will destroy spores and mycobacteria in under 10 min (Babb & Bradley, 1995a; Bradley *et al.*, 1995). It is, however, more damaging to processing and intrument components, particularly copper-based alloys, and is less stable and more expensive than glutaraldehyde.

Cleaning is an essential prerequisite to disinfection and sterilization (Chapter 3). Thorough cleaning will ensure that microorganisms are largely removed, together with the organic material on which they thrive. Cleaning alone with a neutral or enzymatic detergent will achieve a 3–4 log reduction (99.9–99.99%) in microorganisms (Babb & Bradley, 1995b). In one study, procedure-acquired HIV was totally removed from fibrescopes by thorough cleaning alone (Hanson *et al.*, 1990), and precleaning reduced *M. tuberculosis* to low levels (Hanson *et al.*, 1992). Glutaraldehyde and alcohol are fixatives and, if surfaces are not thoroughly cleaned before disinfection, blockages in lumens may occur and taps and moving parts may stiffen. Ultrasonic cleaning baths are effective on external surfaces but should not be used for rigid telescopes. All lumened devices should be brushed and/or irrigated with detergent before steam sterilization or exposure to disinfectants or chemical sterilants.

Several automated machines are now available which clean, disinfect and rinse the lumens and external surfaces of flexible endoscopes. Studies have shown that these are more reliable in achieving high standards of decontamination than manual processing (Bradley & Babb, 1995). They also protect staff from splashes and skin contact with the disinfectant and are more convenient for endoscopy staff. Before purchasing such equipment, it should be established that it is effective, non-damaging, compatible with the items you intend to process and safe. All channel irrigation with detergent and disinfectant is important, and so is the final water flush. The rinse water must be of good microbiological quality, i.e. sterile or bacteria-free (filtered to $<0.45\,\mu m$), for invasive endoscopes and bronchoscopes; otherwise, infection or specimen contamination, leading to misdiagnosis, could occur. Some machines are capable of flushing endoscope lumens with alcohol to assist drying prior to storage.

The serial processing of endoscopes in automated systems reduces disinfectant potency because of carry-over of water used for cleaning and rinsing. If 2% glutaraldehyde is used, it is recommended that the disinfectant is changed when the postactivation life is reached or when the concentration falls to 1.5% (Babb *et al.*, 1992). Test kits are now available to monitor the fall in concentration.

The more recently introduced automated systems include facilities to contain or remove irritant vapour displaced from immersion and storage reservoirs. If such a facility is not included, machines should be operated in a fume cupboard or under an extraction hood.

In spite of their many advantages, washer-disinfectors may become a source of infection or instrument contamination. Sessional cleaning and disinfection of the machine, particularly the rinsing circuit, is essential if this is to be prevented. Machine disinfection is best done at the beginning of each session if this does not form part of each cycle. Regular cleaning and maintenance will prevent the formation of biofilm and lime scale, which reduce the effectiveness of the disinfection process (Babb, 1993).

Flexible fibre-optic endoscopes are probably the most difficult reusable medical devices to clean, disinfect and sterilize. Improved staff training, the use of validated automated decontamination procedures and the purchase of sufficient, preferably heat-tolerant and cleanable equipment will further reduce the likelihood of infection associated with this equipment.

5.11 Miscellaneous items of medical equipment

5.11.1 Vaginal specula and other vaginal devices

There is little reported evidence of spread of infection from these devices, but there is a potential risk of acquiring HIV, hepatitis viruses, herpes viruses, papillomavirus or other organisms causing sexually transmitted infections. Single-use items are preferred whenever possible, but, if not available or if too expensive, decontamination by thorough cleaning and heat (autoclaving, immersion in boiling water for 5–10 min or processing in a washer-disinfector at 70–100°C) should be effective (Ayliffe *et al.*, 1992b; Working Party Report, 1997). There are no data on the susceptibility of human papillomavirus to disinfectants, but there is no evidence that it is particularly resistant to the usual decontamination processes. If the item is heat-labile, chemical methods after thorough cleaning should be effective, such as immersion in 70% alcohol or a chlorine-releasing agent (1000 parts/10^6 av. Cl_2 for 5–10 min, but these have the disadvantages already described.

5.11.2 Tonometers

Viruses, such as adenovirus 8, herpes virus and HIV, may be transferred from eye to eye by these items if not properly decontaminated after each use. Tonometer heads are usually heat-labile and chemical disinfection is required (Centers for Disease Control, 1985). Thorough rinsing and immersion in a chlorine-releasing agent (500 parts/10^6 av. Cl), 3–6% stabilized hydrogen peroxide or 70% alcohol for 5–10 min is commonly recommended. The manufacturer should state whether the tonometer will be damaged by these processes. Thorough rinsing after disinfection (or allowing alcohol to evaporate) is important to prevent damage to the conjunctiva.

5.11.3 Stethoscopes and sphygmomanometer cuffs

Although these are only in contact with intact skin, transfer of staphylococci can occur (Breathnach *et al.*, 1992; Wright *et al.*, 1995). Thorough cleaning of the stethoscope head with 70% alcohol at regular intervals and after use on patients colonized or infected with MRSA or other organisms transferred by this route should reduce the risks of spread. A sphygmomanometer cuff should be kept for each infected or colonized patient and terminally decontaminated by thorough washing and drying.

5.11.4 Other items

Dressing trolleys, mattress covers, supports, hoists, etc. may require decontamination and similar principles apply. Thorough cleaning is always necessary. Decontamination by heat is preferable to chemical disinfection. Immersion in chlorine-releasing agent may be used if appropriate for the instrument. Wiping with 70% alcohol is less effective than immersion (e.g. 5–10 min) but may be necessary for large items. Glutaraldehyde 2% should be avoided but, if used, appropriate environmental precautions should be taken to contain or extract the irritant vapour.

6 Conclusions

The increased use of invasive techniques in a hospital population consisting of both infected and highly susceptible patients has increased the risk of spread of infection. Disinfection has a role in reducing these risks, but, in the past, too great a reliance has been placed on chemical methods, which are often used in an indiscriminate, illogical and inefficient manner. Heat is the preferred method of microbial decontamination, but the continued use of complex, heat-sensitive equipment means that less satisfactory alternatives are still required. In recent years, there has also been an increase in the use of medical devices labelled 'single-use' (see Chapter 24 for a critical and comprehensive account of the reuse of disposable items). These are often expensive and their use should be discouraged if not cost-effective. Manufacturers should be encouraged to produce equipment that can be readily cleaned and will withstand heat at least to 70–80°C or, preferably, autoclaving at high temperature. A limited range of chemical disinfectants should be available and techniques of application should be standardized according to a well-defined policy. Allocation of resources for disinfection should be related to risks of infction and priorities decided according to the principles already described. Some of the chemical disinfectants, such as glutaraldehyde, are potentially toxic, irritant and allergenic to staff and require special handling and controlled environmental conditions. Alternative agents are required, but prolonged testing under in-use conditions should be undertaken before they are accepted for routine use. All grades of staff should be trained in methods of disinfection and other control-of-infection techniques to an agreed level, depending on their role in the hospital. Decontamination methods should be routinely audited.

7 Acknowledgement

We thank the Editor of the *Journal of Hygiene* for permission to publish Fig. 12.1.

8 References

Advisory Committee on Dangerous Pathogens, Department of Health (1996) *Management and Control of Viral Haemorrhagic Fevers*. London: HMSO.

Advisory Committee on Dangerous Pathogens/ Spongiform Encepholopathy Advisory Committee (1998) *Guidance—"Transmissible Spongiform Encephalopathy agents: Safe Working and the Prevention of Infection"*. London: HMSO.

Akamatsu, T., Tabata, K., Hironaga, M. & Uyeda, M. (1997) Evaluation of the efficacy of a 3.2% glutaraldehyde product for disinfection of fibreoptic endoscopes with an automatic machine. *Journal of Hospital Infection*, **35**, 47–57.

Alder, V.G., Lockyer, J.A. & Clee, P.G. (1966) Disinfection and cleaning of baths in hospital. *Monthly Bulletin of the Ministry of Health and Public Health Laboratories Service*, **25**, 18–20.

Anderson, R.L., Mackel, D.C., Stoler, B.S. & Mallison, D.G.F. (1982) Carpeting in hospital: an epidemiologic evaluation. *Journal of Clinical Microbiology*, **15**, 408–415.

Ayliffe, G.A.J. (1986) Nosocomial infection and the irreducible minimum. *Infection Control*, **7**, 92–95.

Ayliffe, G.A.J. (1988) Equipment-related infection risks. *Journal of Hospital Infection*, **11** (Suppl. A), 279–284.

Ayliffe, G.A.J. (1993) Principles of cleaning and disinfection: which disinfectant? In *Infection in Endoscopy. Gastrointestinal Endoscopy Clinics of North America*, **3**, 411–429.

Ayliffe, G.A.J. (1996) Nosocomial infections associated with endoscopy. In *Hospital Epidemiology and Infection Control* (ed. M.C., Mayhall, C.G.) pp. 680–693. Baltimore: Williams & Wilkins.

Ayliffe, G.A.J. (1997) The progressive intercontinental spread of methicillin-resistant *Staphylococcus aureus*. *Clinical Infectious Diseases*, **24**, (Suppl. 1), S74–S79.

Ayliffe, G.A.J. & Gibson, G.L. (1975) Antimicrobial treatment of equipment in the hospital. *Health and Social Services Journal*, **85**, 598–599.

Ayliffe, G.A.J. & Lowbury, E.J.L. (1982) Airborne infection in hospital. *Journal of Hospital Infection*, **3**, 217–240.

Ayliffe, G.A.J., Collins, B.J. & Lowbury, E.J.L. (1966) Cleaning and disinfection of hospital floors. *British Medical Journal*, **ii**, 442–445.

Ayliffe, G.A.J., Collins, B.J. & Lowbury, E.J.L. (1967) Ward floors and other surfaces as reservoirs of hospital infection. *Journal of Hygiene, Cambridge*, **65**, 515–536.

Ayliffe, G.A.J., Brightwell, K.M., Collins, B.J. & Lowbury, E.J.L. (1969) Varieties of aseptic practice in hospital wards. *Lancet*, **ii**, 1117–1120.

Ayliffe, G.A.J., Babb, J.R. & Collins, B.J. (1974a) Carpets in hospital wards. *Health and Social Services Journal*, 84 (Suppl.), 12–13.

Ayliffe, G.A.J., Collins, B.J. & Deverill, C.E.A. (1974b) Tests of disinfection by heat in a bed-pan washing machine. *Journal of Clinical Pathology*, **27**, 760–763.

Ayliffe, G.A.J., Babb, J.R., Collins, B.J., Deverill, C. & Varney, J. (1975a) Disinfection of baths and bathwater. *Nursing Times, Contact*, 11 September, 22–23.

Ayliffe, G.A.J., Collins, B.J. & Green, S. (1975b) Hygiene of babies' incubators. *Lancet*, **i**, 923.

Ayliffe, G.A.J., Babb, J.R. & Collins, B.J. (1976) Environment hazards—real and imaginary. *Health and Social Services Journal*, **86** (Suppl. 3), 3–4.

Ayliffe, G.A.J., Babb, J.R. & Bradley, C.R. (1992a) 'Sterilization' of arthroscopes and laparoscopes. *Journal of Hospital Infection*, **22**, 265–269.

Ayliffe, G.A.J., Lowbury, E.J.L. Geddes, A.M. & Williams, J.D. (1992b) *The Control of Hospital Infection: A Practical Handbook*, 3rd edn. London: Chapman & Hall.

Ayliffe, G.A.J., Coates, D. & Hoffman, P.N. (1993) *Chemical Disinfection in Hospitals*. London: Public Health Laboratory Service.

Babb, J.R. (1993) Disinfection and sterilization of endoscopes. *Current Opinion in Infectious Diseases*, **6**, 532–537.

Babb, J.R. (1996) Application of disinfectants in hospitals and other health-care establishments. *Infection Control Journal of Southern Africa*, **1**, 4–12.

Babb, J.R. & Bradley, C.R. (1995a) A review of glutaraldehyde alternatives. *British Journal of Theatre Nursing*, **5**, 20–41.

Babb, J.R. & Bradley, C.R. (1995b) Endoscope decontamination: where do we go from here? *Journal of Hospital Infection*, **30** (Suppl.), 543–551.

Babb, J.R., Bradley, C.R. & Ayliffe, G.A.J. (1980) Sporicidal activity of glutaraldehydes and hypochlorites and other factors influencing their selection for the treatment of medical equipment. *Journal of Hospital Infection*, **1**, 63–75.

Babb, J.R., Bradley, C.R. & Barnes, A.R. (1992) Question and answer. *Journal of Hospital Infection*, **20**, 51–54.

Babington, P.C.B., Baker, A.B. & Johnson, H.H. (1971) Retrograde spread of organisms from ventilator to patient via the expiratory limb. *Lancet*, **i**, 61–62.

Barkley, W.E. & Wedum, A.G. (1977) The hazard of infectious agents in microbiological laboratories. In *Disinfection, Sterilization and Preservation* (ed. Block, S.), 2nd edn. Philadelphia: Lea & Febiger.

Bartlett, C.L.R., Macrae, A.D. & Macfarlene, J.D. (1986) *Legionella Infections*. London: Arnold.

Bassett, D.C.J., Stokes, K.J. & Thomas, W.R.G. (1970) Wound infection with *Pseudomonas multivorans*. Lancet, **i**, 1188–1191.

Bell, J. (1801) *The Principles of Surgery*. Edinburgh: Printed for T. Cadell, Jun. & W. Davies (Strand); T.N. Longman & O. Rees (Paternoster Row); W. Creech, P. Hill and Manners & Miller.

Bennett, J.V. & Brachman, P.S. (eds) (1992) *Hospital Infections*, 3rd edn. Boston: Little Brown.

Best, M., Sattar, S.A., Springthorpe, V.S. & Kennedy, M.E. (1990) Efficacies of selected disinfectants against *Mycobacterium tuberculosis*. *Journal of Clinical Microbiology*, **28**, 2234–2239.

Block, S. (ed.) (1991) *Disinfection, Sterilization and Preservation*, 4th edn. Philadelphia: Lea & Febiger.

Bloomfield, S.F. & Uso, E.E. (1985) The antibacterial properties of sodium hypochlorite and sodium dichloroisocyanurate as hospital disinfectants. *Journal of Hospital Infection*, **6**, 20–30.

Bloomfield, S.F., Smith-Burchnell, C.A. & Dalgleish, A.G. (1990) Evaluation of hypochlorite-releasing disinfectants against the human immunodeficiency virus. *Journal of Hospital Infection*, **15**, 273–278.

Bond, W.W., Favero, M.S., Petersen, N.J. & Ebert, J.W. (1983) Inactivation of hepatitis B virus by intermediate to high level disinfectant chemicals. *Journal of Clinical Microbiology*, **18**, 535–538.

Boycott, J.A. (1956) A note on the disinfection of baths and basins. *Lancet*, **ii**, 678–679.

Brachman, P.S. (1971) In *Proceedings of the International Conference on Nosocomial Infections 1970*, pp. 189–192. Chicago: American Hospital Association.

Bradley, C.R. & Babb, J.R. (1995) Endoscope decontamination: automated vs. manual. *Journal of Hospital Infection*, **30** (Suppl.), 537–542.

Bradley, C.R. & Fraise, A.P. (1996) Heat and chemical resistance of enterococci. *Journal of Hospital Infection*, **34**, 191–196.

Bradley, C.R., Babb, J.R. & Ayliffe, G.A.J. (1995) Equipment report: Evaluation of the 'Steris' System 1 peracetic acid endoscope processor. *Journal of Hospital Infection*, **29**, 143–151.

Breathnach, A.S., Jenkins, D.R. & Pedler, S.J. (1992) Stethoscopes as possible vectors of infection by staphylococci. *British Medical Journal*, **305**, 1573–1574.

British Society of Gastroenterology Working Party (1993) Aldehyde disinfectants and health in endoscopy units. *Gut*, **34**, 1641–1645.

British Society of Gastroenterology Working Part (1998) Cleaning and disinfection of equipment for gstrointestinal endoscopy. *Gut*, **42**: 585–593.

British Standard BS 2745 (1993) *Washer Disinfectors for Medical Purposes*, Parts 1–3. London: British Standards Institution.

Broadley, S.J., Furr, J.R., Jenkins, P.A. & Russell, A.D. (1993) Antimicrobial activity of 'Virkon'. *Journal of Hospital Infection*, **23**, 189–197.

Burdon, D.W. & Whitby, J.L. (1967) Contamination of hospital disinfectants with *Pseudomonas* species. *British Medical Journal*, **ii**, 153–155.

Burge, P.S. (1989) Occupational risks of glutaraldehyde. *British Medical Journal*, **299**, 342.

Cadwallader, H. (1989) Setting the seal on standards. *Nursing Times*, **85**, 71–72.

Cadwallader, H.L., Bradley, C.R. & Ayliffe, G.A.J. (1990) Bacterial contamination and frequency of changing ventilator circuitry. *Journal of Hospital Infection*, **15**, 65–72.

Cartmill, T.D.I, Panigrahi, H., Worsley, M.A, McCann, D.C, Nice, C.N. & Keith, E. (1994) Management and control of a large outbreak of diarrhoea due to *Clostridium difficile*. *Journal of Hospital Infection*, **27**, 1–15.

Centers for Disease Control (1972) *Fogging, an Ineffective Measure*. National Nosocomial Infections Study, Third Quarter 1972, pp. 19–22.

Centers for Disease Control (1974) *Disinfectant or Infectant: The Label Doesn't Always Say*. National Nosocomial Infections Study, Fourth Quarter 1973, pp. 18–23.

Centers for Disease Control (1985) Recommendations for preventing possible transmission of human T-lymphotrophic virus type 111/lymphadenopathy-associated virus from tears. *MMWR*, **34**, 533–534.

Coates, D. (1988) Comparison of sodium hypochlorite and sodium dichloroisocyanurate disinfectants: neutralization by serum. *Journal of Hospital Infection*, **11**, 60, 67.

Coates, D. (1996) Sporicidal activity of sodium dichloroisocyanurate, peroxygen and glutaraldehyde disinfectants against *Bacillus subtilis*. *Journal of Hospital Infection*, **32**, 283–294.

Coates, D. & Hutchinson, D.N. (1994) How to produce a hospital disinfection policy. *Journal of Hospital Infection*, **26**, 57–68.

Coates, D. & Wilson, M. (1992) Powders, composed of chlorine-releasing agent acrylic resin mixtures or based on peroxygen compounds, for spills of body fluids. *Journal of Hospital Infection*, **21**, 241–252.

Collins, B.J. (1979) How to have carpeted luxury. *Health and Social Services Journal*, September Suppl.

Collins, B.J. (1988) The hospital environment: how clean should it be? *Journal of Hospital Infection*, **11** (Suppl. A), 53–56.

Collins, B.J. & Phelps, M. (1985) Heat disinfection and disinfector machines. *Journal of Sterile Services Management*, **3**, 7–8.

Collins, F.M. (1986) Bactericidal activity of alkaline glutaraldehyde solution against a number of atypical mycobacterial species. *Journal of Applied Bacteriology*, **61**, 247–251.

Control of Substances Hazardous to Health Regulations (1988) London: HMSO.

Cox, R.A., Conquest, C., Mallaghan, C. & Marples, R.R. (1995) A major outbreak of methicillin-resistant *Staphylococcus aureus* caused by a new phage type (EMRSA 16). *Journal of Hospital Infection*, **29**, 87–106.

Craven, D.I., Connolly, M.G., Lichtenberg, D.A., Primeau, P.J. & McCabe, W.R.(1982) Contamination of mechanical ventilators with tubing changes every 24 or 48 hours. *New England Journal of Medicine*, **306**, 1505–1509.

Curie, K., Speller, D.C.E., Simpson, R., Stephens, M. & Cooke, D.I. (1978) A hospital epidemic caused by a gentamicin-resistant *Klebsiella aerogenes*. *Journal of Hygiene, Cambridge*, **80**, 115–123.

Danforth, D., Nicolle, L.E., Hume, K., Alfierie, N. & Sims, H. (1987) Nosocomial infections on nursing units with floors cleaned with a disinfectant compared with detergent. *Journal of Hospital Infection*, **10**, 229–235.

Das, I. & Fraise, A.P. (1997) How useful are microbial filters in respiratory apparatus? *Journal of Hospital Infection* **37**, 263–272.

Daschner, F. (1991) Unnecessary and ecological cost of hospital infection. *Journal of Hospital Infection*, **18**, (Suppl. A), 73–78.

Department of Health (1994a) *Ventilation in Healthcare Premises*. HTM 2025. London: HMSO.

Department of Health (1994b) *The Control of Legionellae in Healthcare Premises—a Code of Practice*. HTM 2040. London: HMSO.

Department of Health and Social Security (1986) *Health Service Catering Manual: Hygiene*. London: HMSO.

Department of Health Medical Devices Agency (1996) *Decontamination of Endoscopes*. London: Medical Devices Agency.

Department of Health Medical Devices Directorate (1993, 1996) *Sterilization, Disinfection and Cleaning of Medical Devices and Equipment: Guidance on Decontamination from the Microbiological Advisory Committee to Department of Health*, Parts 1 and 2. London: HMSO.

Deva, A.K., Vickery, K., Zou, J., West, R.H., Harris, J.P. & Cossart, Y.E. (1996) Establishment of an in-use method for evaluating disinfection of surgical instruments using the duck hepatitis B model. *Journal of Hospital Infection*, **33**, 119–130.

Deverill, C.E.A. & Dutt, K.K. (1980) Methods of decontamination of anaesthetic equipment: daily sessional exchange of circuits. *Journal of Hospital Infection*, **1**, 165–170.

Duckworth, G.J. (1993) Diagnosis and management of methicillin-resistant *Staphylococcus aureus* infection. *British Medical Journal*, **307**, 1049–1052.

du Moulin, G.C. & Saubermann, A.J. (1977) The anaesthesia machine and circle system are not likely to be sources of bacterial contamination. *Anaesthesiology*, **47**, 353–358.

Dyas, A. & Das, B.C. (1985) The activity of glutaraldehyde against *Clostridium difficile*. *Journal of Hospital Infection*, **6**, 41–45.

Elek, S.D. & Conen, P.E. (1957) The virulence of *Staphylococcus pyogenes* for man. *British Journal of Experimental Pathology*, **38**, 573–586.

Emmerson, A.M., Enstone, J.E., Griffin, M., Kelsey, M.C. & Smyth, E.T.M. (1996) The Second National Prevalence Survey of Infection in Hospitals—overview of the results. *Journal of Hospital Infection*, **32**, 175–190.

Feeley, T.W., Hamilton, W.K., Xavier, B., Moyers, J. & Eger, E.I. (1981) Sterile anesthesia breathing circuits do not prevent post operative pulmonary infection. *Anesthesiology*, **54**, 369–372.

Gardner, J.F. & Peel, M.M (1998). *Introduction to Sterilization, Disinfection and Infection Control*. 3rd edn. London: Harcourt Brace.

Garibaldi, R.A., Britt, M.R., Webster, C. & Pace W.L. (1981) Sterile anesthesia breathing circuits do not prevent pulmonary infection. *Anesthesiology*, **54**, 364–368.

George, R.H. (1975) A critical look at chemical disinfection of anaesthetic apparatus. *British Journal of Anaesthesia*, **47**, 719–721.

Gibson, G.L. (1973a) Bacteriological hazards of disposable bed-pan systems. *Journal of Clinical Pathology*, **26**, 146–153.

Gibson, G.L. (1973b) A disposable bed-pan system using an improved disposal unit and self-supporting bedpans. *Journal of Clinical Pathology*, **26**, 925–928.

Griffiths, P.A., Babb, J.R., & Fraise, A.P. (1998) *Mycobacterium terrae:* a potential surrogate for *Mycobacterium tuberculosis* in a standard disinfectant test. *Journal of Hospital Infection*, **38**, 183–192.

Griffiths, P.A., Babb, J.R., Bradley, C.R. & Fraise, A.P. (1997) Glutaraldehyde-resistant *Mycobacterium chelonae* from endoscope washer disinfectors. *Journal of Applied Microbiology*, **82**, 519–526.

Hambraeus, A., Bengtsson, S. & Laurell, G. (1978) Bacterial contamination in a modern operating suite 3. Importance of floor contamination as a source of airborne contamination. *Journal of Hygiene, Cambridge*, **80**, 169–174.

Hanson, P.J.V., Gor, D., Jeffries, D.J. & Collins, J.V. (1989) Chemical inactivation of HIV on surfaces. *British Medical Journal*, **298**, 862–864.

Hanson, P.J.V., Gor, D., Jeffries, D.J. & Collins, J.V. (1990) Elimination of high titre HIV from fibreoptic endoscopes. *Gut*, **31**, 657–660.

Hanson, P.J.V., Chadwick, M.V., Gaya, H. & Collins, J.V. (1992) A study of glutaraldehyde disinfection of fibreoptic bronchoscopes experimentally contaminated with *Mycobacterium tuberculosis*. *Journal of Hospital Infection*, **22**, 137–142.

Hardie, I.D. (1985) Mycobactericidal efficacy of glutaraldehyde based biocides. *Journal of Hospital Infection*, **6**, 436–438.

Holton, J., Nye, P. & McDonald, V. (1994) Efficacy of selected disinfectants against mycobacteria and cryptosporidia. *Journal of Hospital Infection*, **27**, 105–115.

Hugo, W.B. & Denyer, S.P. (1987) The concentration exponent of disinfectants and preservatives (biocides). In *Preservatives in the Food, Pharmaceutical and Environmental Industries* (eds Board, R.G., Allwood, M.C. & Banks, J.G.), Society for Applied Bacteriology Technical Series No. 22, pp.281–291. Oxford: Blackwell Scientific Publications.

Joynson, D.H.M. (1978) Bowls and bacteria. *Journal of Hygiene, Cambridge*, **80**, 423–425.

Kearns, A.M., Freeman, R. & Lightfoot, N.F. (1995) Nosocomial enterococci: resistance to heat and sodium hypochlorite. *Journal of Hospital Infection*, **30**, 193–199.

Kelsey, J.C. & Maurer, I.M. (1966) An in-use test for hospital disinfectants. *Monthly Bulletin of the Ministry of Health and the Public Health Laboratory Service*, **25**, 180–184.

Kelsey, J.C. & Maurer, I.M. (1972) *The Use of Chemical Disinfectants in Hospitals*. Public Health Laboratory Service, Monograph No. 2. London: HMSO.

Kelsey, J.C. & Maurer, I.M. (1974) An improved Kelsey–Sykes test for disinfectants. *Pharmaceutical Journal*, **213**, 528–530.

Kobayashi, H., Tsuzuki, M., Koshimizu, K. *et al.* (1984) Susceptibility of hepatitis B virus to disinfectants or heat. *Journal of Clinical Microbiology*, **20**, 214–216.

Kurth, R., Werner, A., Barrett, N. & Dorner, F. (1986) Stability and inactivation of the human immunodeficiency virus. *Aids-Forschnung*, **ii**, 601–607.

La Force, F.M. (1992) Lower respiratory tract infections. In *Hospital Infections* (eds Bennett, J.V. & Brachman, P.S.), 3rd edn. Boston: Little Brown, pp. 611–639.

Lee, J.C. & Fialkow, P.J. (1961) Benzalkonium chloride—source of hospital infection with Gram-negative bacteria. *Journal of the American Medical Association*, **177**, 708–710.

Leigh, D.A. & Whittaker, C. (1967) Disinfectants and plastic mop-heads. *British Medical Journal*, **iii**, 435.

Lidwell, O.M., Lowbury, E.J.L., Whyte, W., Blowers, R., Stanley, S. & Lowe, D. (1983) Airborne contamination of wounds in joint replacement operations: the relationship to sepsis rates. *Journal of Hospital Infection*, **4**, 111–131.

Lister, J. (1868) An address on the antiseptic system of treatment in surgery. *British Medical Journal*, **ii**, 53–56, 101–102.

Lynam, P.A., Babb, J.R. & Fraise, A.P. (1995) Comparison of the mycobactericidal activity of 2% alkaline glutaraldehyde and NuCidex (0.35% peracetic acid). *Journal of Hospital Infection*, **30**, 237–239.

Maurer, I. (1985) *Hospital Hygiene*, 3rd edn. London: Edward Arnold.

Mayhall, C.G. (ed.) (1996) *Hospital Epidemiology and Infection Control*. Baltimore: Williams & Wilkins.

Mayon-White, R.T., Ducel, G.I., Kereselidze, T. & Tikomirov, E. (1988) An international survey of the prevalence of hospital-acquired infection. *Journal of Hospital Infection*, **11** (Suppl. A), 43–48.

Mbithi, J.N., Springthorpe, V.S. & Sattar, S.A. (1990) Chemical disinfection of hepatitis A virus on environmental surfaces. *Applied Environmental Microbiology*, **56**, 3601–3604.

Medcraft, J.W., Hawkins, J.M., Fletcher, B.N. & Dadswell, J.V. (1987) Potential hazard from spray cleaning of floors in hospital wards. *Journal of Hospital Infection*, **9**, 151–157.

Meers, P.D., Ayliffe, G.A.J. Emmerson, A.M. *et al.* (1981) Report on the national survey of infection in hospitals, 1980. *Journal of Hospital Infection*, **2** (Suppl.), 1–53.

Murray, S.M., Freiman, J.S., Vickery, K., Lim, D., Cossart, Y.E. & Whiteley, R.K. (1991) Duck hepatitis B virus: a model to assess efficacy of disinfectants against hepadnavirus activity. *Epidemiology and Infection*, **106**, 435–443.

Newsom, S.W.B. (1972) Microbiology of hospital toilets. *Lancet*, **ii**, 700–703.

Noble, W.C. & Somerville, D.A. (1974) *Microbiology of Human Skin*. London: Saunders.

Nÿstrom, B. (1981) Disinfection of surgical instruments. *Journal of Hospital Infection*, **2**, 363–368.

Phillips, I., King, A., Jenkins, S. & Spencer, G. (1974) Control of respirator-associated infection due to *Pseudomonas aeruginosa*. *Lancet*, **ii**, 871–873.

Phillips, I. & Spencer, G. (1965) *Pseudomonas aeruginosa* cross-infection due to contaminated respirators. *Lancet*, **ii**, 1325–1327.

Philpott-Howard, J. & Casewell, M. (1994) *Hospital Infection Control: Policies and Practical Procedures*. London: Saunders.

Prince, J. & Ayliffe, G.A.J. (1972) In-use testing of disinfectants in hospitals. *Journal of Clinical Pathology*, **25**, 586–589.

Public Health Laboratory Service (1965) Committee on the testing and evaluation of disinfectants. *British Medical Journal*, **i**, 408–413.

Ragg, M. (1994) Transmission of hepatitis C via anaesthetic tubings. *Lancet*, **343**, 1419.

Reber, H., Fleury, C., Gaschen, M., Hess, E., Regamey, R., Ritler, P., Tanner, F. & Vischer, W. (1972) Bewertung und Prüfung von Disinfektionsmitteln und Verfahren. Basel: Auftrag der schweizerischen Mikrobiologischen Gesellschaft.

Reeves, D.S. & Brown, N.M. (1995) Mycobacterial contamination of fibreoptic bronchoscopes. *Journal of Hospital Infection*, **30** (Suppl.) 531–536.

Report of a Combined Working Party of the British Society of Antimicrobial Chemotherapy and the

Hospital Infection Society, prepared by G. Duckworth and R. Heathcock (1995) Guidelines on the control of methicillin-resistant *Staphylococcus aureus* in the community. *Journal of Hospital Infection*, **35**, 1–12.

Report of a combined working party of the Hospital Infection Society and the British Society for Antimicrobial Chemotherapy (1990). Revised guidelines for the control of epidemic methicillin-resistant *Staphylococcus aureus Journal of Hospital Infection*, **16**, 351–377.

Resnick, L., Veren. K., Salahuddin, S.Z., Troudeau, S. & Markham, P.D. (1986) Stability and inactivation of HTLV/LAV under clinical and laboratory environments. *Journal of the American Medical Association*, **255**, 1887–1891.

Rhame, F.S. (1991) Prevention of nosocomial aspergillosis. *Journal of Hospital Infection*, **18** (Suppl. A), 466–472.

Rogers, T.R. & Barnes, R.A. (1988) Prevention of airborne fungal infection in immunocompromised patients. *Journal of Hospital Infection*, **11** (Supplement A), 15–20.

Russell, A.D. (1996) Activity of biocides against mycobacteria. *Journal of Applied Bacteriology* **81**, (Symposium Suppl.) 67S–101S.

Rutala, W.A. (1996) APIC guidelines for selection and use of disinfectant. *American Journal of Infection Control*, **24**, 313–342.

Rutala, W.A., Clontz, E.P., Weber, D.J. & Hoffman, K.K. (1991) Disinfection practices for endoscopes and other critical items. *Infection Control Hospital Epidemiology*, **12**, 282–288.

Rutala, W.A., Gergen, M.F. & Weber, D.J. (1993) Inactivation of *Clostridium difficile* spores by disinfectants. *Infection Control and Hospital Epidemiology*, **14**, 36–39.

Rutala, W.A., Stiegel, M.M., Sarubbi, F.A. & Weber, D.J. (1997) Susceptibility of antibiotic-susceptible and antibiotic-resistant hospital bacteria to disinfectants. *Infection Control and Hospital Epidemiology*, **18**, 417–421.

Sanford, J.P. (1970) Disinfectants that don't. *Annals of Internal Medicine*, **72**, 282–283.

Sanford, J.P. & Pierce, A.K. (1979) In *Hospital Infections* (eds Bennett, J.V. & Brachman, P.S.) pp. 255–286. Boston: Little, Brown & Company.

Schmidt, B. (1973) Das 2. Internationale Colloquium uber die Wertbestimmung von Disinfektionsmitteln in Europa. *Zentralblatt für Bakteriologie, Parasitenkunde, Infektions-krankheiten und Hygiene 1. Abteilung Originale Reihe B*, **157**, 411–420.

Snowden, S.L. (1994) Hygiene standards for breathing systems. *British Journal of Anaesthesia*, **72**, 143–144.

Spach, D.H., Silverstein, F.E. & Stamm, W.E. (1993) Transmission of infection by gastrointestinal endoscopy and bronchoscopy. *Annals of Internal Medicine*, **18**, 117–128.

Spaulding, E.H., Cundy, K.R. & Turner, F.J. (1977) Chemical disinfection of medical and surgical materials. In *Disinfection, Sterilization and Preservation*, (ed. Block, S.) 2nd Ed. Philadelphia: Lea & Febiger.

Speller, D.C.E., Stephens, M.E. & Viant, A.C. (1971) Hospital Infection by *Pseudomonas capacia*. *Lancet*, **i**, 798–799.

Sykes, G. (1965) *Disinfection and Sterilization*. 2nd Ed. London: E. & F.N. Spon.

Taylor, E.W. (ed.) (1992) *Infection and Surgical Practice*. Oxford: Oxford Medical Publications.

Van Bueren, J., Cooke, E.M., Mortimer, P.P. and Simpson, R.A. (1989) Inactivation of HIV on surfaces by alcohol. *British Medical Journal*, **299**, 459.

Vandenbrouke-Grauls, C.M.J.E., Teeuw, K.B., Ballemans, K., Lavooij, C., Cornelisse, P.B. & Verhoef, J. (1995) Bacterial and viral removal efficiency, heat and moisture exchange properties of four filtration devices. *Journal of Hospital Infection*, **29**, 45–56.

Van Klingeren, B. & Pullen, W. (1993) Glutaraldehyde resistant mycobacteria from endoscope washers. *Journal of Hospital Infection*, **25**, 147–149.

Vesley, D. & Michaelsen, G.S. (1964) Application of a surface sampling method technique to the evaluation of the bacteriological effectiveness of certain hospital house-keeping procedures. *Health Laboratory Science*, **1**, 107.

Wade, J.J. (1995) Emergence of *Enterococcus faecium* resistant to glycopeptides and other standard agents—a preliminary report. *Journal of Hospital Infection*, **30** (Suppl.), 483–493.

Walsh, T.J. & Dixon, G.M. (1989) Nosocomial aspergillus: environmental microbiology, hospital epidemiology, diagnosis and treatment. *European Journal of Epidemiology*, **5**, 131–142.

Wenzel, R.P. (1997) *Prevention and Control of Nosocomial Infections*. Baltimore and London: Williams & Wilkins.

Wenzel, R.P., Nettleman, M.D., Jones, R.N. & Pfaller, M.A. (1991) Methicillin-resistant *Staphylococcus aureus*: implications for the 1990s and control measures. *American Journal of Medicine*, **91** (Suppl. 3B), 221S–227S.

Williams, R.E.O., Blowers, R., Garrod, L.P. & Shooter, R.A. (1966) *Hospital Infection—Causes and Prevention*. London: Lloyd-Luke.

Working Party Report (1997) *HIV Infection in Maternity Care and Gynaecology*. London: Royal College of Obstetricians and Gynaecologists Press.

Wright, I.M.R., Orr, H. & Porter, C. (1995) Stethoscope contamination in the neonatal intensive care unit. *Journal of Hospital Infection*, **29**, 65–68.

Wypkema, W. & Alder, V.G. (1962) Hospital cross-infection and dirty walls. *Lancet*, **ii**, 1066–1068.

Zaidi, M., Angulo, M. & Sifuentes-Osornio, J. (1995) Disinfection and sterilization practices in Mexico. *Journal of Hospital Infection*, **31**, 25–32.

CHAPTER 13

Special Problems in Hospital Antisepsis

1 Introduction

Long before the discovery of bacteria and the introduction of antiseptic surgery, a variety of substances had been used to prevent putrefaction of meat and to preserve the bodies of the dead. The survival of Egyptian mummies is testimony to their effectiveness. The similarity of wound sepsis and some infections to putrefaction was recognized well before Pasteur's initiation of the science of bacteriology. The word 'antiseptic' seems to have been first used in a book on the plague published in 1721, which contains the following sentence: 'This phenomenon shows the motion of the pestilential poison to be putrefactive it makes use of antiseptics a reasonable way to oppose' (Place, quoted by Thompson, 1934).

The word 'antiseptic' has acquired the special meaning of an antibacterial agent that is bland enough to be applied to body surfaces or wounds without harm, though unsuitable for systemic administration. An antiseptic may be regarded as a special kind of disinfectant, although some would omit its use altogether and say 'disinfection of skin by antiseptics' and others would regard a disinfectant as an antimicrobial agent that is too toxic for application to humans. An antibiotic, strictly speaking, is an antimicrobial agent generated by a living organism. This term is loosely used to cover both naturally and artificially produced chemicals that can be used to treat infections. Some antibiotics are too toxic for systemic use but can be used topically, and so would more properly fall into the role of an antiseptic. However, antibiotics such as neomycin can be absorbed from open wounds or burns, and so their use should be restricted. Other problems with topical antibiotics include generation of resistance (sometimes to unrelated antibiotics) and of skin sensitization.

Although pride of place for considering hands as

vectors for infection must go to Oliver Wendell Holmes (Fischoff, 1982), the scientific foundations of antisepsis were laid down by Ignaz Philip Semmelweis (1818–1865) and Joseph Lister (1827–1912). The two never met, although both were taught by the great Viennese pathologist, Rokitansky (Lister's father was known to Rokitansky as the inventor of the achromatic microscope lens). Semmelweis was one of the first exponents of the scientific method in this sphere: collect data, form a hypothesis and then generate a proof. He was working as a junior member of the obstetrics department in Vienna, where he noted that, although the mothers were admitted at random into the first (medical students) and second (midwives) clinics, the death rate from 'childbed fever' in the former was horrendous, sometimes reaching 18%, while that in the latter averaged around 3%. It could not be the 'atmospheric, cosmic, telluric' theory favoured by the professor, because this would have affected both clinics equally. The sudden death of his friend, the pathologist Kolletschka, after being injured during an autopsy on a deceased woman gave Semmelweis the concept of 'cadaveric particles' carried on the hands of the students and doctors from the mortuary to the wards. The introduction of hand disinfection with 'chlorina liquida', later changed to chlorinated lime (which was cheaper), had a dramatic effect (Fig. 13.1), and mortality dropped to 3%. Semmelweis had great difficulty in gaining acceptance of his work and returned to Budapest, where he also used 'chlorine covers' to protect his hands during surgery. By the time he published his book on prevention of childbed fever in 1861 (Semmelweis, 1861, translated by Frank Murphy, 1981), he was obsessed with the hostile reactions of others, and the result is a mixture of science and diatribe, but still of great interest. Recent work from Vienna (Koller *et al.*, 1995) confirms that his handwashing technique would stand up well to the proposed European Standard for hygienic hand disinfection, and the 'chlorine covers' actually have a persistent action in reducing the number of bacteria on the surgeon's skin (Gottardi & Karl, 1990).

Joseph Lister was an academic surgeon who had the benefit of reading Pasteur's works and learning about bacteria as causes of infection before he ventured into 'antiseptic surgery'. His work came to fruition in the year of Semmelweis's death (1865). He likened the body to the flask in which Pasteur had demonstrated that, by using the barrier of tortuous necks, fermentation was prevented. His solution was to apply some chemical substance" in such a manner that not only would the microbes already present be destroyed, but the germ-killing substance must act as a barrier between the wound and outside sources of infection". Lister hit on the idea of using carbolic acid after learning of its reliable disinfecting activities on the sewage of Carlisle. His first dressings were applied to compound fractures. Later, the method was refined by

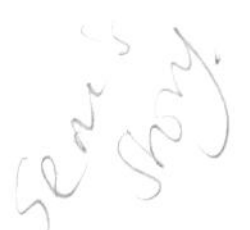

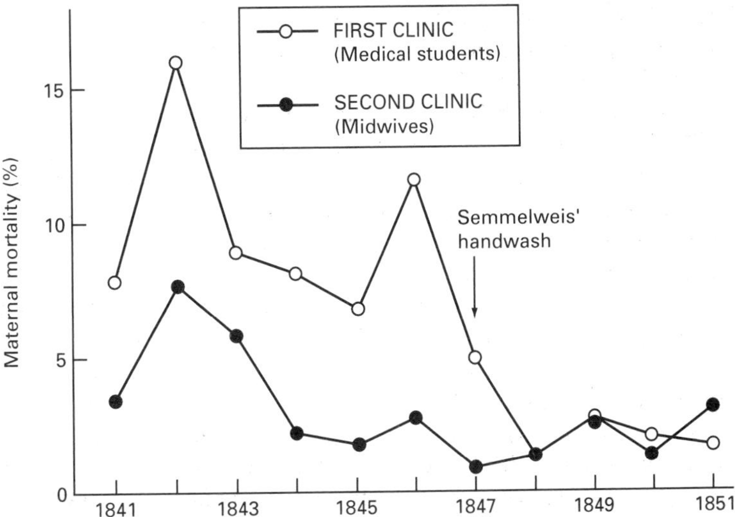

Fig. 13.1 Maternal mortality at the K. K. First and Second obstetric clinics of the University in Vienna.

use of different concentrations of carbolic acid and extended from dressings to use for the surgeon's hands, instruments, ligatures and even the room air (although the latter meant spraying a very irritant substance into the room and was soon abandoned). Lister was already established as a professor in Glasgow at the time of this work, and his results (Lister, 1867, 1909) soon stimulated surgeons in other countries (but not in London) to adopt the antiseptic method. As a result, within a few years hospital gangrene became apparently extinct and more adventurous surgery was possible.

At the start of the twentieth century, Lister's 'antiseptic' barrier was replaced by 'asepsis', i.e. use of heat-sterilized instruments and dressings, plus the use of protective clothing and rubber gloves (by Halstead in 1889) for staff. At first, it seemed that asepsis and antisepsis were antithetical approaches, although it was soon apparent that antiseptics were still required for disinfection of the skin (both of staff and patient) and wounds and for treatment of heat-labile equipment. Recently, the widespread use of antibiotic prophylaxis for surgery has added another dimension. The efficacy of the prophylaxis should not, however, encourage any relaxation of the aseptic methods, especially as antibiotic resistance in bacteria is ever increasing in extent.

In this chapter, the term antisepsis is used in the sense of application of antimicrobial agents to the unbroken skin or mucosae or to burns and open wounds, to prevent sepsis or transfer of infection by removing or excluding microbes. These are essentially hospital practices stemming from the principles laid down by Semmelweis and Lister. Although a century has passed, problems still remain. The epidemic of methicillin-resistant *Staphylococcus aureus* (MRSA) in hospitals worldwide reinforces the need for infection-control policies, but an audit of hospital-acquired infection surveillance (Public Health Laboratory Service, 1997) once again emphasized the lack of proper handwashing policies in hospitals.

2 Skin flora

Price (1938) divided the bacteria found on skin into two types, namely, those normally permanently resident (resident flora) and those picked up by contact with the environment which lodge temporarily on the skin but may remain *in situ* long enough to be transferred, say, from patient to patient (transient flora). This is a good practical approach. However some types of bacteria, for example *Klebsiella* spp., although not normal flora, will survive well on skin (Casewell & Phillips, 1977), and the flora may be increased in both number and spectrum in the presence of certain skin diseases (for example, psoriasis or dermatitis) and systemic illnesses, such as diabetes. Excessive use of wrongly formulated antiseptics or soaps may also be counterproductive, in that the resident flora may multiply on the damaged skin (Ojajarvi, 1991). Finally, the presence of normal pathogens causing skin infection must be remembered; these include *Staph. aureus* and *Streptococcus pyogenes*. One outbreak of infection in the nursery encountered by the author related to a midwife with a whitlow. While not ill enough to prevent her working, the whitlow was the source of 50 infections in the mothers and babies.

2.1 Resident flora

The resident flora consists of species that can resist both the antimicrobial substances excreted on skin and in sweat and also moderate desiccation. In addition, some strains found on skin produce antibacterial agents, for example lysostaphin from *Staphylococcus simulans*, thus helping to maintain a stable ecosystem. Ability to adhere to epithelial cells is also an advantage. The skin flora varies in numbers and spectrum according to location. The count varies, even on closely related areas, such as different parts of the hand, the maximum concentrations being found on the fingertips and under the nails. The predominant flora is composed of coagulase-negative staphylococci, often loosely called *Staphylococcus epidermidis*. There are, in fact, a whole range of species, which can be typed in accordance with the scheme described by Kloos & Schleifer (1975), which is now supported by the API-Staph kit (Bio-Merieux). In moist areas, such as the axillae, or on fingers under a ring, Gram-negative bacteria are commoner, especially *Acinetobacter* spp., and, on occasion, *Klebsiella* and enterobacters, although the latter are more usually transients (Hoffman *et al.*, 1985). *Staphylococcus aureus*, which may be a resident in the nose, is sometimes found as a resident on hands (Larsen *et al.*, 1986), although it is usually present as a transient. Other common resident strains include corynebacteria (both lipophilic and non-lipophilic) and propionibacteria.

The resident flora (Noble, 1981) forms microcolonies on skin and is attached to skin scales, which tend to be shed into the environment at a great rate, the whole superficial layer of the skin being shed every few hours. Counts/cm^2 of skin vary from 10^0 to 10^4 (Noble, 1981). The bacterial flora is normally harmless, if not positively beneficial. However, skin bacteria can create problems when translocated, either into the host or into a patient. Many strains of *Staph. epidermidis* and occasional strains of other coagulase-negative staphylococci produce a slime that allows them to colonize indwelling medical devices, including intravascular catheters, shunts, prosthetic heart valves or joints, peritoneal-dialysis catheters and the total artificial heart (see review, Christensen *et al.*, 1994). Low-grade infections may follow, sometimes with unforeseen results. One of our Cambridge patients unexpectedly developed renal failure, due to immune-complex disease. The immune complexes were shown to contain a staphylococcal antigen and, on investigation, four blood cultures taken at intervals during the previous year were noted to have grown *Staph. epidermidis* and had been assumed to be contaminated. The patient had had a cerebrospinal fluid (CSF) shunt inserted and this was infected.

Use of a detergent hand-wash may loosen the skin scales and also spread out a microcolony, so that the number of bacteria found, say, by making impressions of the hand on a culture plate is increased by washing. Meers and Yeo (1978) showed that the loose skin scales could be released into the air by rubbing the hands after washing and that these could adhere to the plastic used for intravenous-access devices and infusion-fluid containers.

2.2 Transient flora

The transient flora comes from accidental contamination from the environment. That of the hands is of most interest in the hospital situation. The word environment needs some qualification. It can include other parts of the person. For example, a look around a class of 40 students will invariably uncover at least one touching his/her nose. Finger swabs of a class of nurses will often reveal mouth flora as well. This is in addition to the bacteria picked up from the inanimate environment and from patients. Usually, the environment on the hands causes a rapid decline in numbers of transients. Some bacteria (e.g. *Strep. pyogenes*) are rapidly killed by the unsaturated fatty acids, while others—notably the Gram-negative bacilli—are killed by desiccation (Ricketts *et al.*, 1951).

3 Disinfection of staff hands

Correct hand care remains the central pillar of all infection-control procedures, the more so as, with the increasing complexity of medical care, comes more opportunity for infection of patients with normal skin bacteria. The methods used will vary with the circumstances, but by their nature hands can never be rendered 'sterile'. In the operating theatre, methods appropriate for removal of resident flora are required—so-called 'surgical hand disinfection' (Rotter *et al.*, 1980)—and the hands are further protected by use of latex gloves. In the wards, removal of transient organisms is achieved by 'hygienic hand disinfection'. The latter can have various levels. Most transients can be removed by a simple soap-and-water wash. However, in special situations, such as the intensive-care unit (ICU) or haemodialysis unit, where resident organisms could be a problem, or during outbreaks of hospital infection, a more active hand-disinfection procedure is required. The ultimate test of any infection-control measure is the randomized controlled trial, the best example of which was seen in Semmelweis's work. However, in a complex multifactorial situation, this would be hard to achieve. Lidwell (1963) showed that, to demonstrate that a procedure would reduce an infection rate of, say, 3% by a factor of 10% (with an even chance at the 5% level), would require 25 000 observations. None the less, Maki & Hecht (1982) showed that the incidence of infection in an ICU almost halved when unmedicated soap was replaced by antiseptic hand preparations, and another study, in a critical-care unit (Massanari & Hierholzer, 1984), gave similar results. However, it is much easier to test out hand disinfection using laboratory models, and these will be discussed later.

4 Hygienic hand disinfection

4.1 Introduction

The continuing problem of nosocomial transmission of antibiotic-resistant bacteria, such as MRSA and vancomycin-resistant enterococci (VRE), emphasizes the need for efficient methods to remove transient flora, and also for health-care staff sufficiently motivated and trained to use these when necessary. Broughall *et al.* (1984) noted that the rate of hand washing by nurses depended on the acceptability of the products provided, smell and appearance being important factors, in addition to any skin damage produced. They devised an ingenious counter based on a microphone attached to a soap dispenser to record hand washing. Trials on a general medical ward showed an average of 10 hand washes per nurse per shift. The use of washbasins related to their siting. The nurses' perception of hand washes was of 20–24 times per shift, and observations of the time taken showed that, using soap and paper towel, this varied from 2.5 to 24.5 s (mean = 11.6 s). The logistics of hand washing were well described by Gould (1994) from a study in which 360 nurses were 'shadowed' for 2 h by an observer. The nurses were divided equally between two hospitals, using a medical ward, a surgical ward and the ICU in each. The appropriateness and the efficiency (scored by choice of agent, duration of use, number of hand surfaces decontaminated, method of drying and finally disposal) were studied. Overall efficiency correlated well with previous training in hand-washing technique and inversely with workload, except in one ICU, where increased workload resulted in more use of hand rubs instead of hand washes.

The agents used for hygienic hand disinfection include unmedicated soaps, antiseptic soaps and alcoholic hand rubs. The selection of which agents to include in an infection-control policy depends on local attitudes and on the use required. In the UK, use of soap for removal of transient organisms in low-risk clinical areas is recommended, while, in Europe, antiseptic soaps or hand rubs may be used in all areas of the hospital. Washing with soap and water was shown to remove a large proportion of the transient bacteria normally found on hands in early studies by Gardner & Seddon (1946) and Story (1952). However, studies by Lowbury and his colleagues and summarized in the previous edition of this book (Lowbury, 1992) and by Rotter and colleagues (Rotter, 1996) showed that antiseptic-containing preparations were more effective in the removal of heavy concentrations of bacteria either allowed to dry on or actually rubbed into skin. A rub with an alcoholic preparation was the most effective 'degerming' procedure. Ayliffe *et al.* (1988) produced an in-depth report on the topic, including both laboratory and ward aspects, in which these findings were confirmed.

None the less, in areas where the nosocomial infection rate is low, nursing techniques are unlikely to lead to gross hand contamination and the patients are not unduly susceptible to infection, a wash with a bland soap is quite adequate. It has the advantages of being less toxic to staff hands and is cheap. Thus, the author's policy is for use of bland soap throughout the health-care facility unless it is contraindicated. An antiseptic soap or alcoholic hand rub may be preferred in critical-care areas, transplant units, infectious disease wards, haemodialysis units and any clinical area when nosocomial infection is a problem, for example during an outbreak of *Clostridium difficile* infection on a geriatric ward. A hand rub is of particular value when time is at a premium (for example, in the ICU) or if hand-washing facilities are so inconveniently sited as to deter their use. Meers & Yeo (1978) noted that the spread of skin scales into ward air was reduced by use of a rub, which did not loosen them as much as a detergent wash. The increasing use of gloves by ward staff as part of 'universal precautions' can deter them from hand washing; however, it is much easier to remove bacteria from the surface of a glove than from the hand and, if the glove is not damaged, washing is possible. Newsom & Rowland (1989) showed that a single wash with bland soap was 1000 times more effective at removing contaminants from the glove than from the hand.

Whatever agents are employed, it is important that they be user-acceptable and that they are correctly applied. Taylor (1978) showed—by the use of some ingenious experiments with the addition of a dye to the alcoholic preparation—that, when using an alcoholic hand rub, it is easy to miss some parts of the skin. Many surveys have shown that rates of hand disinfection on wards are reduced when an unacceptable preparation is used. Finally, many of these antiseptics have also been widely used in cosmetic formulations to prevent body odour or in mouthwashes, so that systemic toxicity has been an issue, for example with hexachlorophane, and regulatory aspects require consideration (Eirmann, 1981).

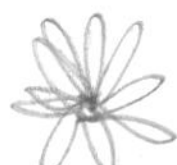

4.2 Laboratory tests

Many tests using artificially contaminated hands have been described. *Staphylococcus aureus* has been favoured as a test strain. This has the advantages of being clinically relevant and being able to survive on skin and is the basis of a reproducible test (Ayliffe *et al.*, 1990). The alternative is *Escherichia coli*, which is also clinically relevant, but has the disadvantage that it dies as it dries. Studies with either strain give similar, but not identical, results. However, in today's ethically aware world, a strain of *E. coli* that has been approved by the Health and Safety Executive as non-toxic to humans seems a reasonable choice (see below). Clearly, other pathogens, such as MRSA or VRE, cannot be tested on staff hands.

The proposed European Standard for hand-degerming agents has therefore taken a stepwise approach. The agent is firstly tested out (phase I) *in vitro* in a suspension test against a single test organism (*E. coli*). If the result is satisfactory, it is tested (phase II, step I) against a range of organisms (*Pseudomonas aeruginosa* ATCC 15442, *Staph. aureus* ATCC 6538, *Enterococcus faecium* ATCC 10541). Finally, when the agent has passed these tests, it is used in the *in vivo* phase 2, step 2 tests.

The proposed standard *in vivo* tests (EN 1499, EN 1500) are based on the Vienna model (Rotter *et al.*, 1977), in which 15 subjects are used. The hands are contaminated by immersion in an overnight culture of the test *E. coli* strain (*E. coli* K12, NCTC 10538 (NCIMB 10083)), allowed to dry and then sampled by kneading the fingertips (Fig. 13.2) in recovery fluid (containing disinfectant neutralizers). The disinfectant neutralizers include polysorbate, lecithin (egg) and histidine, with addition of sodium thiosulphate and bovine serum albumin for halogen-based preparations. For quaternary ammonium compounds, polysorbate is combined with saponin, histidine and cystine, to produce a baseline count (which should be $>10^5$/ml recovery medium). The hands are then treated with the degerming agent according to the manufacturer's instructions, the kneading is repeated and a 'post' value is obtained. The $\log_{10}$ reduction factor is calculated for each of the 15 volunteers and the reduction factors are compared with those produced by a reference degerming procedure. For a hand wash (EN1499), this is use of a bland soap and, for a hand rub (EN1500), it is that produced by propan-2-ol 60% (isopropanol) (v/v). The test agent should be as good as or better than the reference agents.

4.3 In-use monitoring of hand disinfection

Laboratory tests are time-consuming and require a special facility and dedicated trained staff. Otherwise, the test results may be misleading. Newsom & Matthews (1985), for example, showed little difference between *n*-propanol and povidone-iodine using the method described by Rotter *et al.* (1980) for testing hygienic hand disinfection, until taught by the authors to prevent recontamination of the hands from the wrists when doing an alcohol disinfection. The principle of 'on-site' hygienic hand disinfection is to ensure that there is a coherent policy and that staff adhere to it. In

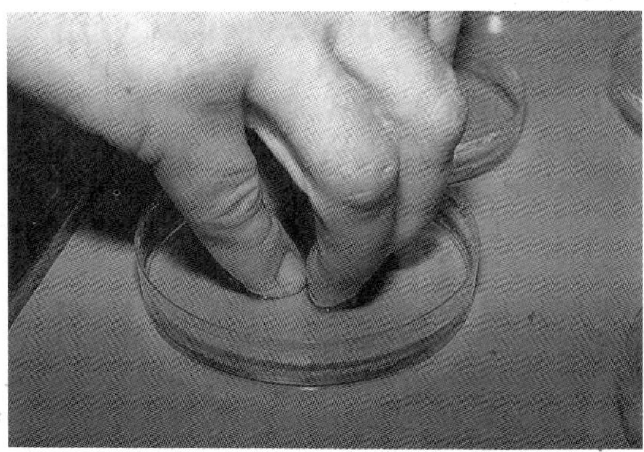

Fig. 13.2 Sampling hands by 'kneading' fingers on the base of a petri-dish containing recovery fluid.

today's budget-conscious health-care facilities, the delegation of budgets to 'end-users' may mean that ward managers may go their own way with regard to choice of hand-degerming agents and not purchase the most relevant or efficient type. The main role of infection-control staff is to check that policies are in place and are used. However, for an occasional simple 'one-off' check, taking a fingerprint impression on a Petri dish after a hand-degerming procedure and then showing the results to the staff may be helpful (Fig. 13.3).

5 Surgical hand disinfection

5.1 Introduction

Systems for surgical hand disinfection have been in place since the days of Semmelweis and Lister but have evolved at different rates in different countries. In Japan, for example, a 5-min scrub is essential, while in the UK a 30-s hand rub may be all that is used after the initial scrub. The value of a surgical scrub is more difficult to demonstrate practically in that the surgeon covers his/her hands with gloves, so providing a barrier. Today's latex gloves in themselves may contain antibacterial substances; for example, the latex accelerator used in some contains zinc and the Biogel coating used in some makes of starch-free gloves has a quaternary ammonium compound (cetylpyridinium chloride) included to provide 'slipperiness' on donning. However, Devenish & Miles (1939), in a classic study, reported a series of staphylococcal infections in a surgical unit that were traced to a single surgeon, who was a heavy nose and skin carrier of the strain. In 54 operations, there was a 25.9% infection rate. In addition, he had a 24% glove-perforation rate and was later shown to shed staphylococci through the damaged gloves.

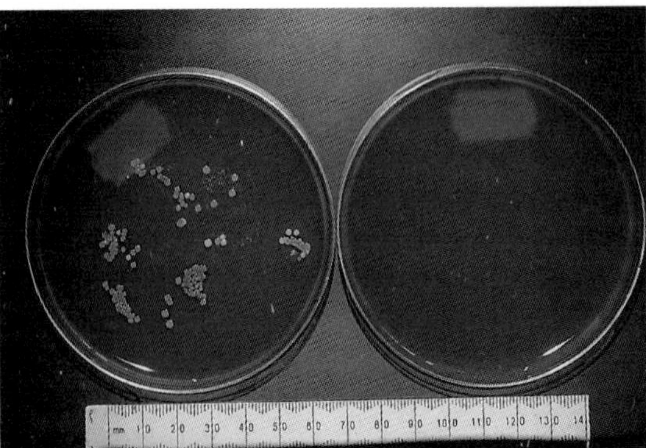

Fig. 13.3 Checking hand-washing technique. Fingerprints from (a) a physiotherapist (b) a cardiac surgeon.

5.2 Laboratory tests

A series of studies from the Birmingham Accident Hospital form the basis of modern surgical hand disinfection. A hand-wash test was used to assess the reduction in yield of bacteria from the skin after cleansing or disinfection. Volunteers moistened their hands in bowls of 100 ml Ringer's solution containing neutralizers and rubbed palm against palm, right palm over left dorsum, left palm over right dorsum and with the fingers interlaced, each procedure three times, followed by thorough rinsing. Pour-plates of nutrient agar with neutralizers were used for viable counts, and tests for carry-over of antiseptic to culture plates were made (Lowbury *et al.*, 1960, 1963, 1964, 1974; Lowbury & Lilly, 1960; Lilly & Lowbury, 1974).

The preparations tested were of two types.

1 Antiseptic detergent solutions, creams or soaps, by the use of which it was envisaged that the combined effects of disinfection and cleansing could be obtained.

2 Alcohol or alcoholic or aqueous solutions of antiseptics.

Antiseptic detergent preparations (see Chapter 2) containing 4% chlorhexidine, 10% povidone iodine (an iodophor), 3% hexachlorophane or 2% Irgasan DP 300 (triclosan) (2,4,4′-trichlor-2′-hydroxydiphenylether) were used, with additions of running water from a tap, in a 2-min vigorous hand wash without a brush, completely covering hands and wrists, allowing the skin to dry while rubbing. Alcoholic preparations studied were ethyl or isopropyl alcohol at 70% or 95%, with 1% added glycerol to prevent excessive drying of the skin. They were used with and without the inclusion of chlorhexidine gluconate (0.5%) or of phenolic compounds. Two aliquots of 5 ml of these fluids were poured into the cupped hand and rubbed vigorously over the entire surface of the hands and wrists, allowing the skin to dry while rubbing. Aqueous solutions were similarly rubbed on the skin, but were rinsed off and the hands were then dried on a sterile towel.

Table 13.1 summarizes some of the findings in these studies; see also Fig. 13.4. Soap and water caused very little reduction in the yield of bacteria from the skin after one standard surgical hand preparation or after six such procedures, three on one day and three on the next. Varying degrees of disinfection were obtained with the antiseptics. Of the detergent antiseptic preparations, the 4% chlorhexidine gave the largest reduction on a single application, but after six applications similar results were obtained with povidone-iodine and Irgasan DP 300. In view of the poor results obtained with soap and water, the benefits of combining detergent action with disinfection are doubtful. The necessity to dilute the antiseptic with water from a tap when this method is used reduces its efficiency. It is therefore not surprising that the best results were obtained with alcohol and with alcoholic solutions rubbed to dryness on the hands. Repeated disinfection brings about a progressive reduction on the skin flora, as judged by the yield of bacteria on sampling, until a low equilibrium level is reached (Fig. 13.4) (Lilly *et al.*, 1979a). If a more effective antiseptic, e.g. alcoholic

Table 13.1 Assessments of alternative methods of surgical hand disinfection and cleansing.

Manner of use	Preparation	Means of percentage reduction in skin sample counts of viable bacteria: After one treatment	After six treatments (2 days)
Detergent used with running water	4% chlorhexidine (Hibiscrub)	86.7 ± 3.0	99.2 ± 0.2
	10% providone-iodine (Disadine)	68.0 ± 6.8	99.7 ± 0.7
	3% hexachlorophane (Disfex)	46.3 ± 9.7	91.9 ± 3.8
	2% Irgasan DP 300 (Zalclense)	11.2 ± 19.9	95.8 ± 1.8
Non-detergent, with no added water during use	0.5% chlorhexidine in 95% ethanol	97.9 ± 1.1	99.7 ± 0.1
	0.1% phenolic in 95% ethanol (Desderman)	91.8 ± 4.6	99.5 ± 0.2
	0.5% chlorhexidine in water	65.1 ± 8.7	91.8 ± 2.4
Soap and water (control)	Experiment 1	3.3 ± 8.3	25.9 ± 5.1
	Experiment 2	12.3 ± 2.2	17.7 ± 3.7

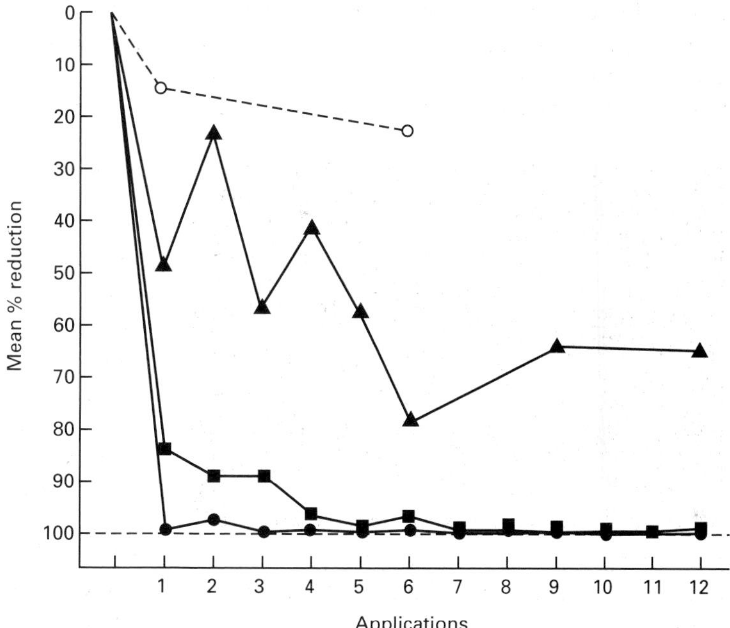

Fig. 13.4 Mean percentage reduction in viable bacteria on hands following disinfection. ▲—▲, 0.3% chlorocresol; ●—●, 95% ethanol; ■—■, Hibiscrub; ○—○, soap and water.

chlorhexidine, is used on skin that has been disinfected to equilibrium level by a detergent antiseptic (e.g. Hibiscrub or Ster-Zac), a further reduction to the equilibrium level of alcoholic chlorhexidine is obtained (two-phase disinfection). There is no further reduction; however, when a less effective antiseptic is used to wash the hands after the low equilibrium level with alcoholic chlorhexidine has been reached, there is a large increase in the yield of bacteria on sampling the skin (Fig. 13.5). These findings agree with the view that the low equilibrium level represents the balance between the killing of the bacteria on the surface by the antiseptic and the emergence of deeper resident organisms to the surface by the friction used in applying the solution. It also illustrates how far we are from being able to sterilize the skin.

5.3 Residual action of antiseptic on the skin

Certain non-volatile antiseptics leave an active residue on the skin after rinsing and drying or

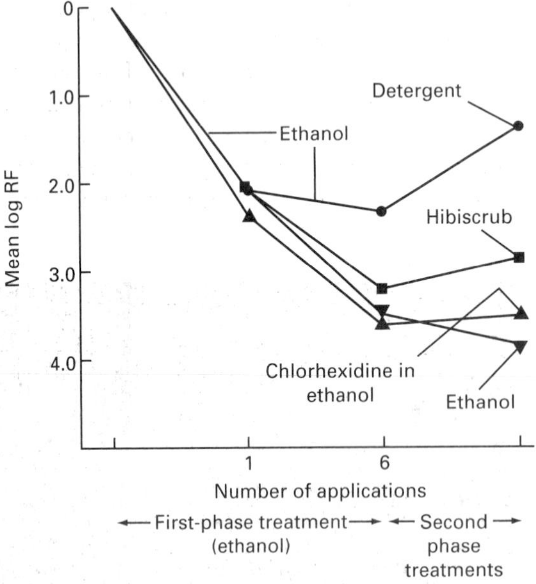

Fig. 13.5 Mean logarithmic reduction factors (RF) of bacteria in samples from hands after one and after six treatments with 95% ethanol, and after an intermediate further treatment with: 95% ethanol, ▼—▼; 0.5% chlorhexidine in 95% ethanol, ▲—▲; Hibiscrub, ■—■; a non-antiseptic detergent (the base of Hibiscrub), ●—●.

deposition from alcoholic solution. This was demonstrated by allowing bacterial suspensions to dry on the skin after it had been cleansed with soap and water or disinfected, and sampling 1 h later for survival of the deposited bacteria in these areas. Large numbers of the deposited bacteria were present in areas that had previously been cleansed with bar soap or disinfected with a volatile antiseptic (alcohol), but very few were present in areas previously disinfected with chlorhexidine, hexachlorophane or povidone iodine (Lowbury *et al.*, 1964; Lowbury & Lilly, 1973).

It is hard to assess the usefulness of residual action by antiseptics deposited on the skin. A study in which volunteers wore gloves for 3 h after having their hands disinfected with various antiseptics showed that the numbers of bacteria present at that time were smaller than those present on the skin immediately before disinfection with the same antiseptics (Lowbury *et al.*, 1974). In other words there was a further fall in the numbers of bacteria on the skin of the surgeon's gloved hands during the course of an operation. This would seem to be due to the continued action by residues of antiseptic, but, surprisingly, a similar effect was obtained with 70% ethyl alcohol, which evaporated completely before the gloves were put on. As a hypothesis to explain this, Lowbury and colleagues suggested that many bacteria damaged by the alcohol would die if left on the skin, but could be resuscitated if they were immediately inoculated on a culture medium. This view was supported by an experiment in which bacteria, exposed briefly to alcohol or water on a membrane filter, were cultured for viable counts immediately and after a 3 h delay (Lilly *et al.*, 1979b). The further reduction in viable counts of bacteria extracted from membrane filters held for 3 h was twice as great when the bacteria had been exposed to alcohol as when they had not been so exposed.

Actual 'in-use' studies have demonstrated the value of persistent activity on the surgeon's hands, especially for prolonged operations, such as open-heart surgery. Glove-rinse studies show a marked increase in bacteria in the glove juice at the end of an operation after a scrub using povidone iodine compared with one using chlorhexidine (Newsom *et al.*, 1988), and, of course, glove-puncture rates increase with time. Cruse & Foord (1973) showed an increase in postoperative infection after clean surgery, in which glove punctures were recorded. In order to compare different surgical hand-disinfection procedures, a reproducible and standard test is required, which must include tests of immediate and persistent activity. Two approaches to testing have been used, depending primarily on the sampling method: either of glove juice or of fingertips. The glove-juice method, described by Peterson (1973), has been adopted by the Food and Drug Administration (FDA) in the USA as the national standard. This method involves donning a rubber glove and sampling by inserting 50 ml of recovery medium into the glove and massaging it over the hand in a standard way. Holloway *et al.* (1990) performed a multicentre comparison between two chlorhexidine preparations using this method, and showed that it gave reproducible results in four centres. The fingertip sampling method is similar to that used in the hygienic hand-disinfection test and has been fully evaluated by Rotter and his colleagues (Rotter *et al.*, 1980, Rotter & Koller, 1990). Both methods have theoretical advantages. The fingertip sampling ensures that the part of the hand with the heaviest contamination is sampled. On the other hand, glove juice might be thought to be more likely to leak through a glove puncture. Thus, the fingertips will be a more stringent test. Whichever test is used, the use of gloves that have no antibacterial coatings or contents is very important. The cetylpyridinium chloride of the Biogel glove, for example, might interfere with the test. A second possible area of contention in testing is selection of a reference agent. The proposed European standard uses 60% *n*-propanol (as in the hygienic hand-rub test). This is one of the most effective agents available and so provides a very stringent standard. Its residual activity lasts at least 3 h; however, to get the best persistent activity, the addition of chlorhexidine is required.

5.4 In-use monitoring of surgical hand disinfection

Surgeons are busy people who do not welcome too much interference with routine. However, some simple monitoring tests can be performed. The easiest test is to ask the surgeon to make a hand impression on a 245 mm × 20 mm plate containing a nutrient medium plus appropriate neutralizers (Fig. 13.6). The comparative numbers of bacteria can then easily be seen. Similarly, the carry-over of residual antibacterial activity can be assessed by using a plate without neutralizers and overlaying it with a nutrient agar preseeded with an overnight culture of *Staph. epidermidis* (Rowland & Newsom, 1985). Analysis of similar cultures can be made more scientific by use of an image analyser (Leyden *et al.*, 1991). An alternative approach is to ask the surgeons to place the gloves in a sterile bag after use, and then to rinse these out with a recovery medium, which is sampled for bacteria.

A recent in-depth study of two surgical teams was reported from Norway (Christensen *et al.*, 1995), using fingerprint impressions before and after surgical hand disinfection, and glove print followed by fingerprint after the operation. The teams used chlorhexidine scrub or occasionally an alcoholic skin preparation. The most important findings of the study, however, related to observation of the hand-washing process. This was extremely variable, despite standard guidelines. Variables included choice of preparation, application time, volumes used and techniques employed, including use of scrubbing brushes. However, only 5.9% of postscrub prints yielded bacteria, on only two occasions were small numbers (1–10) of colonies obtained from postoperative glove prints and 50% of postoperative fingerprints were sterile.

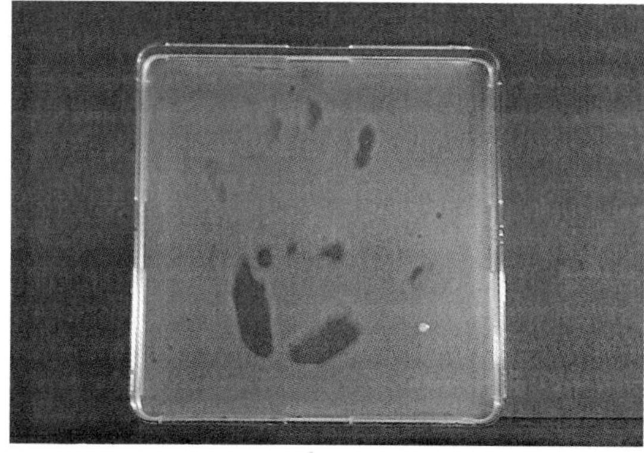

Fig. 13.6 Hand impression to demonstrate persistent activity of surgical hand scrub containing chlorhexidine. Impression made after removing glove following cardiac operation.

5.5 Testing for antiviral activity on hands

In general, hygienic hand disinfection using agents that pass the proposed European Standard will be adequate for removal of viruses from the hands, and at present the European Committee for Standardization (CEN) technical committee has no plans for an 'antiviral' test for hand-degerming agents. However, concerns about human immunodeficiency virus (HIV) infection and occasional epidemics, such as the enterovirus (echo 11) outbreak in a special-care baby unit described by Nagington *et al.* (1983), may mean that users require reassurance about the antiviral activity of their hand-degerming agents.

The choice of model viruses for antiseptic tests presents two major problems: choice of representative strains and, for use on hands, choice of acceptably non-pathogenic viruses. There is general agreement that HIV viruses present no major problem of resistance to antiseptics. The model viruses proposed for the European suspension tests for antiviral activity include an enterovirus (poliovirus type 1, strain LSc-2ab) and an adenovirus (adenovirus type 5, strain ATCC), thus spanning both deoxyribonucleic acid (DNA) and pico-ribonucleic acid (RNA) viruses. However, another picoRNA virus, the hepatitis A virus, has recently been shown to be more resistant to peracetic acid (Thraenhart, personal communication). The topic has been reviewed by (Bellamy (1995), who, with her collaborators (Bellamy *et al.*, 1993), has published a test method for hand-degerming agents, using the challenge of a strain of bovine rotavirus that is not pathogenic for humans. The results confirmed those of Kurtz *et al.* (1981), who showed the effectiveness of alcohols on various viruses.

6 Disinfection of operation sites

Like the surgeon's hands, the patient's operation site requires 'surgical' disinfection, directed against resident as well as transient flora; often, it requires maximum disinfection in a single treatment (i.e. in emergency surgery), without benefit from the progressive effects of repeated application. By the use of a technique similar to that used for assessing disinfection of the surgeon's hands, Lowbury and his colleagues (Lowbury *et al.*, 1960, 1964 compared alternative methods of disinfecting the skin in preparation of the operating site. The greatest reduction in yield of bacteria (about 80%) was obtained with 1% iodine in 70% ethanol and with 0.5% chlorhexidine in 70% ethanol; these were significantly greater than the reductions obtained by application of 70% ethanol, Lugol's iodine solution or aqueous 0.5% chlorhexidine. The antiseptic solution was applied with friction, on gauze swabs, over two hands, in a period of 2 min. The 80% reduction obtained with 0.5% chlorhexidine in 70% alcohol was very poor compared with the reduction of about 99% obtained by use of the same solution for disinfection of the surgeon's hands, as described above. This discrepancy is due to the fact that disinfection on carrying out the surgical hand wash is more effective than that obtained using gauze as an applicator, the usual method for operating-site disinfection. This is shown by a comparison of the two methods of application—by gauze or by the gloved hand—of serial different antiseptics (Lowbury & Lilly, 1975). Table 13.2 shows consistently larger reductions obtained by the gloved hand than by the conventional gauze application of the antiseptics; it also shows a larger reduction when a smaller area—one hand rather than two—was the experimental 'operation site' disinfected in 2 min with a gauze applicator. The role of friction in obtaining good disinfection was further illustrated by the poorer results obtained when an antiseptic solution was sprayed on the skin than when it was rubbed on with gauze (Lowbury *et al.*, 1964).

Davies and her collaborators (Davies *et al.*, 1978) used contact plates as a simple way to sample skin of both volunteers and patients to compare the effectiveness of various preoperative skin preparations. Three plates were used per test—one applied to untreated skin as a control and the others applied 1 and 120 min after treatment. Alcoholic chlorhexidine gave the best results (using 0.5% chlorhexidine), and, interestingly enough, 70% ethanol worked better than 95% ethanol. The best reductions obtained were of the order of 2.8 log; however, the test was constrained by the numbers of bacterial colonies that could be counted on the control plates.

Elimination of bacterial spores from skin is difficult, as most resist the action of alcohols, chlorhe-

Table 13.2 Comparison of gauze applicator and gloved hand for disinfection of operation site (see Lowbury & Lilly, 1975).

	Mean percentage reduction in estimated skin bacteria after disinfection of:			
	One hand			
Antiseptic	With gloved hand	With gauze	*P*	Two hands (with gauze: results of earlier studies)
0.5% chlorhexidine in 70% ethanol	98.8 ± 0.8	90.7 ± 2.1	< 0.01	81.3 ± 2.6 (1960); 84.9 ± 1.4 (1964) 7.9 ± 3.6 (1971); 80.8 ± 4.1 (1973) 81.5 ± 3.4 (1974)
0.5% chlorhexidine in 95% ethanol	99.9 ± 0.02	93.5 ± 2.15	< 0.02	–
0.5% chlorhexidine in distilled water	83.5 ± 5.8	53.7 ± 5.2	< 0.01	60.7 ± 6.0 (1960)
10% povidone-iodine in 70% ethanol	99.7 ± 0.14	86.9 ± 5.9	< 0.1 > 0.05 Not sig.	74.4 ± 5.2 (1971)
Distilled water (control)	25.1 ± 6.5	−4.1 ± 19.1	> 0.1 Not sig.	14.7 ± 5.7 (1960) 8.5 ± 9.8 (1964) 4.7 ± 10.3 (1971)

xidine and the quaternary ammonium compounds. Halogens have some activity but require prolonged contact times. Lowbury *et al.* (1964) showed that a povidone iodine compress laid over skin already contaminated with spores of *Bacillus subtilis* was able to reduce the numbers by 90% in 30 min. The skin of the buttocks and the upper leg often has transient contamination with spores, especially *Clostridium perfringens* from the faeces, and operations involving muscle with poor arterial supply in this area (e.g. amputation of a leg for diabetic gangrene) carry a special risk of endogenous gas gangrene (Ayliffe & Lowbury, 1969). Thus, where possible, this could be considered for before high-risk operations. Iodine in isopropanol has also been recommended by the author for skin preparation before taking blood for culture or performing a lumbar puncture. This approach has recently been justified by Strand *et al.* (1993), who compared the effect of alcoholic iodine with povidone iodine skin preparation on blood-culture contamination. The contamination rate was 6.25% for the iodophor vs. 3.74% for the alcoholic solution ($P < 0.000001$).

Considerable interest has been shown in preoperative measures to reduce skin flora. Use of a chlorhexidine scrub as an adjunct to having a bath was much less effective than its use for hand degerming (Davies *et al.*, 1977). Areas not continuously immersed, such as the chest, showed less reduction in flora, and it is not surprising, given the importantce of friction when applying an antiseptic soap, that this was the case. Brandberg & Anderson (1980) showed that using chlorhexidine scrub in a shower was much more effective at reducing overall skin flora, and Brandberg *et al.* (1980) showed that the showers gave a significant reduction in wound infections among 341 patients undergoing vascular surgery with a groin incision. Hayek *et al.* (1987) compared the use of two preoperative baths or showers in patients undergoing general surgery randomised to use a chlorhexidine scrub or bland soap. They studied a ‘closed’ community and were able to perform a complete follow-up for six weeks. The chlorhexidine scrub reduced wound infections after clean surgery by 30%. However, Ayliffe *et al.* (1983), in a study on 5536 patients in three hospitals, found no difference between bathing with chlorhexidine scrub and with standard soap, and a large multicentre European randomized controlled trial (Rotter *et al.*, 1988) also found no difference. None the less, the subject of preoperative showers continues to be explored (Paulson, 1993). In addition, May *et al.*

(1993) studied the effect of preoperative skin preparation using, 10% aqueous povidone-iodine twice daily for 48 h before elective vascular surgery. Patients had their standard antibiotic prophylaxis, and, in the 64 patients and controls studied, there was no significant difference in postoperative groin-wound infection rates (18.7% in the controls and 17.2% in the test cases).

Thorough decontamination of the skin might have adverse effects. Archer & Armstrong (1983) showed that the skin flora changed after antibiotic prophylaxis for open-heart surgery, with over 50% of patients growing methicillin-resistant strains thereafter. Newsom *et al.* (1990) showed that several preoperative showers using chlorhexidine scrub before open-heart surgery effectively suppressed the skin flora, but that 3 days after operation staphylococci highly resistant to methicillin were obtained. Thirty-two of 59 resistant isolates typed as *Staph. simulans*. This organism was occasionally isolated from patients with deep sternal-wound infections.

The only real test of the efficiency of any technique for preparation of operation sites is by use of a randomized controlled trial, with wound infection as the marker. The number of cases required demands that this be a multicentre trial. However, a clue as to efficacy can be obtained by counting the numbers of bacteria in the wound at the end of the operation. Raahave (1974) described a simple, non-invasive method consisting of making imprints of the wound surfaces, using velvet pads, which were made by gluing pieces of velvet 2.0 cm × 4.5 cm on to larger pieces of aluminium foil. The pads were used to make imprints of the wound cut surface, and then transferred to Petri dishes and an imprint of the pad made on a suitable medium. The author used a variant of this method whereby the pad was immersed in a recovery fluid after use and then processed in a vortex mixer. The bacterial particles were recovered by passing through a membrane filter, which was cultured and the colonies counted. Unpublished results showed a significant lowering in numbers of particles from wounds after comparative operations were performed using standard or 'Goretex' surgical gowns for open-heart surgery. More recently, Taylor *et al.* (1995) assessed wounds by imprints using 47 mm 5 μm mixed cellulose acetate/nitrate membrane filters. The filters were placed on the wound for 10–30 s and then placed on DST agar (Oxoid) containing β-lactamase. Colonies were counted after incubation at 37°C for 48 h and staining with tetrazolium. This method was useful in showing that operating under ultraviolet radiation caused wound disinfection, but could be equally applied to other situations.

7 Antisepsis in burns

7.1 Introduction

Treatment of severe burns has become a highly centralized and specialized affair. In the UK, there are only 39 burns centres, treating an average of 226 patients each. Antiseptics have a major role to play in prevention of infection and, to a much lesser extent, in treatment of established infection. Studies from Birmingham form the basis of current care and are reviewed fully in the previous edition of this book (Lowbury, 1992). Prophylaxis against infection involves the use of first- and second-line defences (i.e. measures used, respectively, to prevent contamination of the burn would and to prevent invasion of the tissues and bloodstream from a colonized wound (Fig. 13.7). Topical application of antimicrobial agents is a component of the first line of defence, and it has been shown to have a valuable role in protecting the patient at a stage when infection presents a special hazard.

Various changes in the incidence, management and key microbial pathogens have been gradually occurring. The current situations in the UK and USA have been reviewed by Papini *et al.* (1995) and Nguyen *et al.* (1996), respectively. In particularly, wound excision and the use of wound growth factors have improved management, so that the problem of sepsis, although still of major concern, is gradually diminishing. *Staphylococcus aureus* is the most common isolate. The prevalence of *Ps. aeruginosa* has lessened and that of *Acinetobacter* has increased (Frame *et al.*, 1992). *Streptococcus pyogenes* is now rarely seen.

Systemic chemotherapy (with erythromycin or a β-lactamase-stable penicillin) is more effective than topical penicillin against *Strep. pyogenes* and (together with oral fucidin) has been shown to have considerable value against *Staph. aureus* (Lowbury

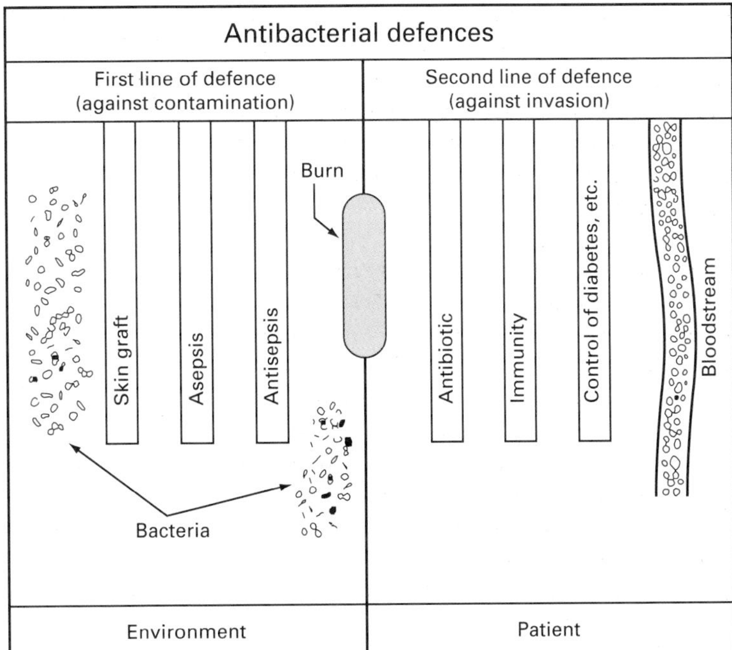

Fig. 13.7 First and second lines of defence against infection in patients with burns.

& Miller, 1962; Lowbury *et al.*, 1962). Gram-negative bacilli are not readily dislodged by systemic chemotherapy, even with antibiotics active against them *in vitro*. Gentamicin, ciprofloxacin and cefotaxime are commonly used, suggesting that there is no consensus (Papini *et al.*, 1995). Topical applications of mafenide (Lindberg *et al.*, 1965) and of silver sulphadiazine cream (Fox, 1968) appear to have some chemotherapeutic effect on *Ps. aeruginosa*, but in most patients systemic therapy is the method of choice.

7.2 Topical chemoprophylaxis

Lister excluded burns from the wounds for which he advocated topical chemoprophylaxis with phenol. Some of his followers tried antisepsis with phenol on burns (Pirrie, 1867), but the method was abandoned because of toxicity. Studies in Birmingham in the 1950s (when *Strep. pyogenes* was the main problem) demonstrated significant prophylaxis with penicillin cream (Jackson *et al.*, 1951). However, penicillin and other antibiotics that have an important role in systemic chemotherapy and a tendency to cause the emergence of resistance in pathogenic bacteria and allergy in patients should not be used for topical application.

This dilemma was largely resolved on the reintroduction of 0.5% silver nitrate solution by Moyer *et al.* (1965). A controlled trial of 0.5% silver nitrate compresses on severely burned patients in Birmingham confirmed Moyer's opinion. *Pseudomonas aeruginosa* was found in about 70% of swabs from burns in the control series, but in only 3% of those kept continuously moist with compresses of 0.5% silver nitrate. This was associated with a large reduction in *Ps. aeruginosa* septicaemia and a reduced mortality (Cason & Lowbury, 1968).

Treatment with silver nitrate compress had some disadvantages—in particular, inadequate prophylaxis against the Gram-negative bacilli that are less sensitive than *Ps. aeruginosa* (notably *Klebsiella* spp.), discomfort and the need for mineral supplements. Alternative chemoprophylatic applications were required. Mafenide 11% (sulfamylon) acetate cream, applied at least once a day and left to dry without dressing cover, proved very effective (Lindberg *et al.*, 1965), but caused severe pain and sometimes a reversible metabolic acidosis. A controlled comparative trial of mafenide cream, silver nitrate compresses and exposure treatment without an antimicrobial application showed that mafenide cream and silver nitrate reduced the incidence and density of bacteria on the burn surface significantly (Lowbury *et al.*, 1971).

A more satisfactory topical prophylactic agent, silver sulphadiazine, was developed by Fox (1968). Controlled trials in Birmingham showed it to be comparable to silver nitrate compresses. Its action against *Klebsiella* spp. and other Gram-negative bacilli was much greater than that of silver nitrate, but it was rather less active than silver nitrate against *Staph. aureus* and slightly less active against *Ps. aeruginosa* and *Proteus* sp. Mortality was lower in the patients treated with silver sulphadiazine (Lowbury *et al.*, 1976). Unfortunately, silver sulphadiazine caused the emergence of plasmid-mediated transferable sulphonamide (Bridges & Lowbury, 1977), so a cream containing 0.5% silver nitrate and 0.2% chlorhexidine gluconate was used. The proportions of sulphonamide-resistant enterobacteria fell, together with resistance to other antibiotics, to which the sulphonamide-resistance plasmid coded a linked resistance. No resistance to silver nitrate or to chlorhexidine occurred. Other antimicrobial agents, including povidone iodine and cerium nitrate (Monafo *et al.*, 1976) have been tried, but have proved less effective in controlled trials (Babb *et al.*, 1977). A cream containing 2% phenoxetol and 0.2% chlorhexidine was comparable to silver nitrate–chlorhexidine cream overall, with significantly greater action against *Staph. aureus*.

7.3 Comment

Though topical antimicrobial propylaxis has proved highly effective and has been shown capable of saving the lives of severely burned patients, there is a disturbingly small number of antimicrobial agents available for this purpose. None is entirely free from potential toxic or sensitizing effects, and none covers the range of potential pathogens and opportunist organisms. The more selectively the agents attack microorganisms, while sparing the host tissues, the greater is the likelihood that strains with intrinsic or acquired resistance will emerge. The topic has changed little since the work done several decades ago, reported by Lowbury (1992) Nguyen *et al.* (1996) note that the development of topical agents, such as silver sulphadiazine, mafenide and silver nitrate, together with the use of perioperative antibiotics and surveillance by wound or blood cultures, has led to a decrease in mortality from infection. The references they quote include nothing new. In the UK survey (Papini *et al.*, 1995), saline or saline with chlorhexidine was used for dressings, while silver suphadiazine was the most popular topical antimicrobial. Other topical dressings included nitrofurazone, silver sulphadiazine plus cerium nitrate, mupirocin, sodium fusidate and povidone-iodine. A review of Medline covering the 1990s revealed only one new potential agent—a zinc compound. So we must assume that the Birmingham work has withstood the test of time, but must be aware of possible future problems from resistant bacterial strains, such as the VRE.

8 Use of antiseptics on skin and mucosae

8.1 Introduction

Topical agents can be used to treat superficial infections of skin and mucosae, to reduce bacterial counts on diseased skin and to try to eliminate carriage of bacteria by staff and patients to prevent nosocomial infection. The use of antibiotics is in general to be discouraged. Some, such as the aminoglycosides, can be absorbed and produce toxic side-effects or may generate antibiotic resistance. β-Lactam antibiotics may cause allergies. However, antibiotics that are not absorbed and may not be associated with the development of resistance, such as sodium fusidate (despite ease of selection of resistant mutants in the laboratory) or peptides (such as ramoplanin or bacitracin), may be used. Pseudomonic acid is another agent that fits the description of an antibiotic *sensu strictu* but is only useful as a local application.

8.2 Laboratory tests of skin disinfection

A simple *in vivo* test for the effectiveness of such agents on skin flora was devised by Williamson & Kligman (1965). This involves occlusion of the skin of the forearm using Occlufol (a type of cling film). Test materials are applied to the skin, and it is then occluded for 24 h. The materials are removed and the bacteria stripped from the skin surface by placing a Perspex cylinder on the skin, adding a harvesting solution (for example, polysorbate in 0.007 mol/l phosphate buffer, pH 7.9, together with appropriate neutralizers) and rubbing vigorously with a glass rod for 2 min (Fig. 13.8) The harvesting solution is removed and the bacterial count measured. Using this technique, a school biology project showed that an occlusive wound dressing was 1000 times better than a plaster in suppression of normal skin flora for 24 h. The reason turned out to be the impregnation of the dressing with domiphen bromide. More recently, the author showed that Ramoplanin was an effective skin antiseptic on skin flora that had been multiplied by pretreatment occlusion for 24 h (Newsom and Webster, 1991, unpublished observations). As an alternative to occlusion, which would allow a broader spectrum of test organisms, Leyden *et al.* (1996) described a 'translocation' method. Swabs moistened with a non-ionic detergent are used to harvest bacteria from the groin or axillae. These are then translocated to the forearm, which is then occluded, as before. The authors suggest that this method is applicable to testing the antimicrobial effectiveness of an agent in a variety of situations. These include use on axillary flora (for deodorants), as a perineal cleanser in the critically ill and for situations where a dense mixed flora exists, e.g. stasis ulcers and infected intertriginous dermatoses.

8.3 Pseudomonic acid (mupirocin) (Bactroban)

This is, strictly speaking, an antibiotic, as it is produced by *Pseudomonas fluorescens*. It is active against staphylococci and certain Gram-negative bacteria. It has a unique action, inhibiting bacterial isoleucyl transfer RNA (tRNA) synthetase, and is structurally unrelated to other antibiotics. It is rapidly metabolized when absorbed, and becomes inactive thereafter. The spectrum includes the MRSA strains and, although mupirocin resistance has been reported in staphylococci, it has not until recently been a problem (see below). Mupirocin shows a good activity against skin flora when tested by the occlusion method, described above (Aly, 1985). Clinical trials have shown a good activity for a 2% ointment against superficial staphylococcal skin and wound infections, and have been reviewed by Lamb (1991).

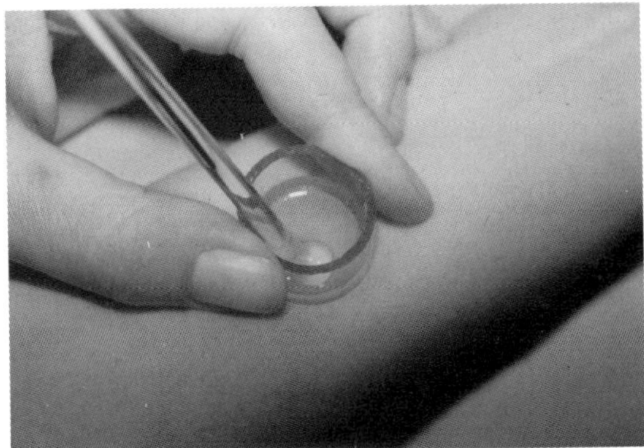

Fig. 13.8 Removal of bacteria from skin by scrubbing with a glass rod.

Casewell *et al.* (1985) showed that 12 volunteers treated four times daily for 5 days with mupirocin ointment had their nasal carriage of *Staph. aureus* eliminated within 48 h. However, the polyethylene glycol used to formulate the ointment was too irritant for intranasal use. A newer formulation, using white soft paraffin and a glycerine ester, has been used instead. Tests on larger numbers of hospital-staff carriers confirmed the results reported by Casewell *et al.* (1985) and have been summarized by Hudson (1994). Unlike the previous regimes for eradication of staphylococci from nasal carriers (such as neomycin with chlorhexidine), mupirocin is swift in action and recurrence of carriage is rare. As a result, use of nasal mupirocin to clear carriage has been enshrined in the UK guidelines for the control of epidemic MRSA (Working Party, 1990).

Although mupirocin–methicillin-resistant strains of *Staph. aureus* (MuMRSA) have been described (Rahman *et al.*, 1987), until recently these have not caused a major problem. However, Irish *et al.* (1998) described an outbreak of an epidemic strain of MuMRSA. The index case had had repeated courses of mupirocin over the previous 9 months. Clearance in patients was attempted, using regimes of 1% chlorhexidine obstetric cream to the nares, plus 2% triclosan (Irgasan) bath concentrate to the skin and hair, or later with the addition of 1% silver sulphadiazine for pressure sores and substitution of 2% triclosan skin cleanser for the bath concentrate. Both regimes failed, as did use of topical bacitracin and fusidic acid in five out of six patients, all of whom turned out to be throat carriers of the organism. The only successful regime for elimination of carriage was the use of systemic antibiotics, namely ciprofloxacin plus rifampicin. Following the use of this regime, the outbreak was controlled. This again brings home the lessons that local antimicrobials do not always work and that repeated courses may generate resistance. Irish *et al.* (1998) also analysed the plasmids coding for resistance and found that these could sometimes occur in coagulase-negative staphylococci. Clearly, the message is: use a short course and only when it is essential, and avoid a blanket treatment, say, of all ward staff, rather than the proved carriers.

9 Practical aspects of disinfectants and antiseptics

9.1 Introduction

Antiseptic formulations and dispensing have created many problems, resulting at best in a product with substandard activity, and at worst in one that is contaminated and positively harmful. Paradoxical as it may seem, the antiseptics are not always sterile. In addition, users may be poorly educated, and they may be subject to financial pressures and makers to commercial constraints.

9.2 Contamination of antiseptics

Contamination of antiseptics has created problems at all levels. Anderson *et al.* (1984) reported on the intrinsic contamination of a commercial iodophor solution with *Ps. aeruginosa*. Laboratory investigations showed that the strain appeared to survive on the polyvinylchloride distribution pipes used in the manufacturing plant, which presumably allowed it to develop resistance to the iodophor solution while protected by a biofilm. Stock solutions of chlorhexidine (Hibitane) contain isopropyl alcohol as a preservative; however, Kahan (1984) reported on septicaemias in six patients with *Burkholderia picketti* from a contaminated 0.05% chlorhexidine wound irrigation. Cardiopulmonary operations were complicated by postoperative infection with *Serratia* from contamination of a quaternary ammonium compound (Ehrenkranz *et al.*, 1980) and with *Burkholderia cepacia* from aqueous chlorhexidine (Speller *et al.*, 1971).

The practice of 'topping up' hand-wash or other containers can lead to trouble. On one occasion, the wall-mounted hand-scrub containers had to be removed from an entire hospital, after it had been supplied with a contaminated batch of scrub solution. A local problem involved a self-dispensing system for the benzalkonium/chlorhexidine mixture (Savlon). The district nurses were issued with marked bottles. The bottle was filled to the first level with concentrate from a stock bottle in the nurses' office and then water was added to a second level. When requiring a refill, the same procedure was used. Samples from all bottles tested grew *Ps. aeruginosa*. Burdon & Whitby (1967) documented a similar incident.

Finally, a more subtle disinfectant contamination was noted in the neurosurgery theatres during an investigation of staphylococcal infections (R.E. Warren, personal communication). Before wound closure, an antiseptic spray was used to coat the wound edges. This came from a pressurized vessel and was administered by a non-scrubbed nurse. Observation showed that she held the canister in such a way as to bounce some spray off her fingertip and into the wound.

Today, hand scrubs tend to come in 800-use disposable cartridges, and should have dispensers that do not intrude on the liquid pathway. Dilutions of antiseptics are best obtained ready-made and in plastic packs that have been presterilized by the manufacturer. The era of refillable containers and ad hoc dilution with hospital tap water is hopefully ending.

9.3 Neutralization of antiseptics

Organic material, such as blood, pus, faeces and oils or fats can inactivate dilute solutions of all antiseptics (Gelinas & Goulet, 1983). The effects are most pronounced with quaternary ammonium compounds, which are adsorbed, and with halogens, which are converted to inactive chlorides or iodides. Chlorhexidine and the quaternary ammonium compounds are electrically charged and can be neutralized by the complementary charge. An episode which shows the effect of a hand wash occurred many years ago in a London hospital.

The scrubbing-brush used was kept in a bowl of a quaternary ammonium compound. It was thickly coated with soap, which neutralized the disinfectant, with the result that the brush was heavily contaminated. The outcome was that, after use of this brush for a hand scrub before performing postoperative eye dressings, three patients developed deep eye infections with *Ps. aeruginosa*.

Bottle closures have been known to inactivate the contents. Linton & George (1966) reported on the inactivation of aqueous chlorhexidine in bottles closed with corks or cork-lined caps. Recently, the Japanese custom of selling swabs soaked in antiseptic has been investigated by Oie & Kamiya (1996). They found that 41/67 samples of gauze swabs impregnated with ethacridine lactate (acrinol) were contaminated with *B. picketti* or *B. cepacia*. When an inoculum of contaminated fluid was put into neat acrinol, no multiplication occurred, but, when placed into a pot containing acrinol and gauze, the contaminant grew well. A further investigation (Oie & Kamiya, 1997) revealed that, while cotton swabs soaked in povidone iodine remained sterile, those soaked in 0.2% benzalkonium chloride were contaminated in a similar way to those in acrinol.

9.4 Toxicity

It may seem surprising that agents aimed at destroying bacterial life by contact are not more toxic; furthermore, the chlorhexidine molecule resembles that of dichlorodiphenyltrichloroethane (DDT). The only real human problem has been with the chronic systemic toxicity of hexachlorophane. This only came to light after 20 years of use, when, in the same year tests on rats (Kimbough 1973) and the occurrence of nervous symptoms in newborn babies both gave warning signs. The rats developed a spongiform encephalopathy after treatment with hexachlorophane, and convulsions and sometimes death occurred in low-birth-weight babies with diseased skin treated with a high-concentration powder (Kopelman, 1973; Powell *et al.*, 1973).

Other serious complications mainly relate to allergy, especially to chlorhexidine or to povidine iodine, which are probably the two most common antiseptics in use. Many health-care staff complain of sore hands when using surgical scrubs or rubs. Usually, this relates more to the formulation than to active ingredients. More serious, however, are the one-off reports of severe reactions, often after exposure to larger concentrations of agent—through broken skin or mucosae. For example, de Groot & Weyland (1994) reported an anaphylactic reaction following use of urethral chlorhexidine gel for bladder catheterization, while Cheung & O'Leary (1985) reported on hypotension in response to use of a dressing containing 0.5% chlorhexidine on a skin-graft donor site. Finally, occupational asthma has been recorded in two nurses, following exposure to a chlorhexidine/alcohol spray (Waclawski *et al.*, 1989). Iodine has separate physiological and pharmacological effects on the body. Thus, in addition to hypersensitivity reactions, there are occasional examples of toxicity from administration of large doses, and regular or prolonged use in patients with thyroid disease should be avoided. Pietsch & Meakins (1978), for example, described metabolic effects, including acidosis, arising in a burned patient after use of topical povidone iodine.

9.5 Financial/commercial aspects

There is no miracle fluid, however much such a one may be advertised. However, antiseptic products have a wide application, both in health care and in the home. Thus, the value of trade names may be important. During an investigation of surgical hand disinfection, the author noted that a particular soap had little effect. The soap in question had contained hexachlorophane, but, on enquiry, although the soap still had the same name, the active ingredient had been changed to triclosan. Another well-known product containing hexachlorophane (Phisohex) had kept the name for a formulation of chlorhexidine, prompting a short report: 'Hexachlorophane, or what's in a name?' (Newsom & Lilly, 1983).

Health-care workers in search of economy may select inadequate products or be misled by terminology. Surgical spirit, alcohol or methylated spirits are time-honoured names, often used to cover all alcohols. On one occasion, the author was trying to repeat studies on a hand rub, using a commercial preparation. The reference procedure failed to give the expected result and, on examination, the hospital pharmacy had changed to a cheaper formulation, based on methylated spirit rather than isopropanol. Hospital staff would have been unaware of the change. The onus is therefore upon the infection-control team to keep a continuous eye on even the most seemingly innocuous parts of the infection-control policy.

10 Conclusions

Since the days of Lister, antiseptic use has been in a state of flux, being supplanted later by asepsis and, more recently, by use of systemic antibiotics for prophylaxis and therapy. However, while some topics, for example the use for hand degerming or for burns, seem to have settled down, new areas are opening up. The increase of antibiotic-resistant Gram-positive bacteria as causes of nosocomial infection provides more of a challenge for the topical antimicrobials. Fortunately, chlorhexidine, suitably applied together with a lotion soft skin conditioner, appears to give a good reduction in numbers of VRE on porcine skin (Frantz *et al.*, 1997). Another challenge is in the increased use of vascular access and urinary catheterization and the insertion of prosthetic materials into the body. Items such as the Silverline controlled-release glass, which allows gradual diffusion of silver ions into a urinary drainage bag, has been shown to reduce biofilms and may reduce catheter-acquired urinary-tract infection (T. Gilchrist, personal communication). This type of technology could well be extended to coatings of other bodily inserts, and the future for antiseptics remains assured.

11 References

Aly, R. (1985) Prophylactic efficacy of Bactroban and other topical antibiotics. Part I: Antimicrobial action of Bactroban ointment applied to normal human skin. In *Bactroban—Proceedings of an International Symposium* (eds Dobson, R.L., Leyden, J.J., Noble, W.C. & Price, J.D.), pp. 47–53. Amsterdam: Excerpta Medica.

Anderson, R.L., Berkelman, R.L., Mackel, D.C., Davies, B.J., Holland, B.W. & Martone, W.J. (1984) Investigation into the survival of *Pseudomonas aeruginosa* in poloxamer-iodine. *Applied and Environmental Microbiology*, **47**, 757–762.

Archer, G.L. & Armstrong, B.C. (1983) Alteration of staphylococcal flora in cardiac surgery patients receiving antibiotic prophylaxis. *Journal of Infectious Diseases*, **147**, 642–649.

Ayliffe, G.A.J. & Lowbury, E.J.L. (1969) Sources of gas gangrene in hospital. *British Medical Journal*, **ii**, 333–337.

Ayliffe, G.A.J., Noy, M.F., Babb, J.R., Davies, J.G. & Jackson, J. (1983) A comparison of pre-operative bathing with chlorhexidine detergent and non-medicated soap in the prevention of wound infection. *Journal of Hospital Infection*, **4**, 237–244.

Ayliffe, G.A.J., Babb, J.R., Davies, J.G. & Lilly, H.A. (1988) Hand disinfection: a comparison of various agents in laboratory and ward studies. *Journal of Hospital Infection*, **11**, 226–243.

Ayliffe, G.A.J., Babb, J.R., Davies, J.G. *et al.* (1990) Hand disinfection tests in three laboratories. *Journal of Hospital Infection*, **16**, 141–149.

Babb, J.R., Bridges, J., Jackson, D.M., Lowbury, E.J.L. & Ricketts, C.R. (1977) Topical chemoprophylaxis: trials of silver phosphate chlorhexidine, silver sulphadiazine and povidone iodine preparations. *Burns*, **3**, 65–71.

Bellamy, K. (1995). A review of test methods used to establish virucidal activity. *Journal of Hospital Infection*, **30**, Suppl, 389–396.

Bellamy, K., Alcock, R., Babb, J.R., Davies, J.G. & Ayliffe, G.A.J. (1993). A test for the assessment of 'hygienic hand disinfection' using rotavirus. *Journal of Hospital Infection*, **24**, 201–210.

Brandberg, A. & Anderson, I. (1980) Whole body disinfection by shower-bath with chlorhexidine soap. In *Problems in the Control of Hospital Infection*, Royal Society of Medicine, International Congress and Symposium Series, 23 (eds Newsom, S.W.B. & Caldwell, A.D.S.), pp. 65–70. London: Academic Press and Royal Society of Medicine.

Brandberg, A., Holm, J., Hammersten, J. & Scherston, T. (1980) Post operative wound infections in vascular surgery: the effect of pre-operative whole body disinfection by shower bath with chlorhexidine soap. In *Problems in the Control of Hospital Infection*. Royal Society of Medicine, International Congress and Symposium Series, 23 (eds Newsom, S.W.B. & Caldwell, A.D.S.), pp. 71–75. London: Academic Press and Royal Society of Medicine.

Bridges, K. & Lowbury, E.J.L. (1977) Drug resistance in relation to use of silver sulphadiazine cream in a burns unit. *Journal of Clinical Pathology*, **31**, 160–164.

Broughall, J.M., Marshman, C., Jackson, B. & Bird, P. (1984) An automatic monitoring system for measuring handwashing frequency in hospital wards. *Journal of Hospital Infection*, **5**, 447–453.

Burdon, D.W. & Whitby, J.L. (1967) Contamination of hospital disinfectants with *Pseudomonas* sp. *British Medical Journal*, **ii**, 153–155.

Casewell, M.W. & Phillips, I. (1977) Hands as a route of

transmission of *Klebsiella* species. *British Medical Journal*, **ii**, 1315–1317.

Casewell, M.W., Hill, R.J.R. & Duckworth, G.J. (1985) The effect of mupirocin (pseudomonic acid) on the nasal carriage of *Staphylococcus aureus*. In *Bactroban—Proceedings of an International Symposium* (eds Dobson, R.L., Leyden, J.J., Noble, W.C. & Price, J.D.), pp. 47–53. Amsterdam: Excerpta Medica.

Cason, J.S. & Lowbury, E.J.L. (1968) Mortality and infection in extensively burned patients treated with silver nitrate compresses. *Lancet*, **i**, 651–654.

Cheung, J. & O'Leary, J.J. (1985) Allergic reaction to chlorhexidine in an anaesthetised patient. *Anaesthetic and Intensive Care,* **13**, 429–439.

Christensen, G.D., Baldassarri, L. & Simpson, W.A. (1994) Colonisation of medical devices by coagulase-negative staphylococci. In *Infections Associated with Indwelling Medical Devices* (eds Bisno, A.L. & Waldvogel, F.). Washington: American Society for Microbiology.

Christensen, J.B., Andersen, B.M., Thomassen, S.M., Johansen, O. & Lie, M. (1995) The effects of 'in-use' surgical handwashing on the pre- and postoperative fingertip flora during cardiothoracic and orthopaedic surgery. *Journal of Hospital Infection*, **30**, 283–293.

Cruse, P.J.E. & Foord, R. (1973) A five-year prospective survey of 23,649 surgical wounds. *Archives of Surgery,* **107**, 206–210.

Davies, J., Babb, J.R., Ayliffe, G.A.J. & Ellis, S.H. (1977) The effect on the skin flora of bathing with antiseptic solutions. *Journal of Antimicrobial Chemotherapy*, **3**, 473–481.

Davies, J., Babb, J.R., Ayliffe, G.A.J. & Wilkins, M.D. (1978) Disinfection of the skin of the abdomen. British Journal of Surgery, **65**, 855–858.

de Groot, A.C. & Weyland, J.W. (1994) Anafylaxie door chloorhexidine na cystoscopie of urethrale catheterisation. *Nederland Tijdschrift Geneeskd*, **138**, 1342–1343.

Devenish, E.A. & Miles, A.A. (1939) Control of *Staphylococcus aureus* in the operating theatre. *Lancet*, **i**, 1088–1094.

Ehrenkranz, N.J., Bolyard, E.A., Wiener, M. & Cleary, T.J. (1980) Antibiotic-sensitive *Serratia marcescens* infections complicating cardio-pulmonary operations: contaminated disinfectant as a reservoir. *Lancet*, **ii**, 1289–1292.

Eirmann, H.J. (1981) Antimicrobials: regulatory aspects. In *Skin Microbiology* (eds Mailbach, A. Aly, R.), pp. 135–147. New York: Springer-Verlag.

Fischoff, E. (1982) *Oliver Wendell Holmes: Physician and Humanist*. Pearson Museum Monographs No. 82/2. Springfield: School of Medicine, Southern Illinois University.

Fox, C.L. (1968) Silver sulphadiazine—a new topical therapy for *Pseudomonas* in burns. *Archives of Surgery*, **96**, 184–188.

Frame, J.D., Kangesu, L. & Malik, W.M. (1992) Changing flora in burn and trauma units: experience in the United Kingdom. *Journal of Burn Care and Rehabilitation*, **13**, 281–286.

Frantz, S.W., Haines, K.A., Azar, C.G., Ward, J.I., Homan, S.M. & Roberts, R.B. (1997) Chlorhexidine gluconate (CHG) activity against clinical isolates of vancomycin-resistant *Enterococcus faecium* (VREF) and the effects of moisturizing agents on CHG residue accumulation on the skin. *Journal of Hospital Infection*, **37**, 157–164.

Gardner, A.D. & Seddon, H.J. (1946) Rapid chemical disinfection of clean, unwashed skin. *Lancet*, **ii**, 683–686.

Gelinas, P. & Goulet, J. (1983) Neutralisation of the activity of eight disinfectants by organic matter. *Journal of Applied Bacteriology*, **54**, 243–247.

Gottardi, W. & Karl, A. (1990) Chloruberzuge auf Hautoberflachen. I. Bestimmung der Belagssstarke mit der DPD-Kuvettenmethode. *Zentralblatt für Bakteriologie und Hygiene*, **190**, 511–522.

Hayek, L.J., Emerson, J.M. & Gardner, A.M.N. (1987) A placebo controlled trial of the effect of two preoperative baths or showers with chlorhexidine detergent on postoperative wound infection rates. *Journal of Hospital Infection*, **10**, 165–172.

Hoffman, P.N., Cooke, E.M., McCarville, M.R. & Emmerson, A.M. (1985) Microorganisms isolated from skin under wedding rings worn by hospital staff. *British Medical Journal*, **290**, 206–207.

Holloway, P.M., Platt, J.H., Reybrouck, G., Lilly, H.A., Mehtar, S. & Drabu, Y. (1990) A multi-centre evaluation of two chlorhexidine containing formulations for surgical hand disinfection. *Journal of Hospital Infection*, **16**, 151–159.

Hudson, I.R.B. (1994) The efficacy of intranasal mupirocin in the prevention of staphylococcal infections: a review of recent experience. *Journal of Hospital Infection*, **27**, 81–98.

Irish, D., Eltringham, I., Teall, A. *et al.* (1998) Control of an outbreak of epidemic methicillin resistant *Staphylococcus aureus* also resistant to mupirocin. *Journal of Hospital Infection,* **39**, 19–26.

Kahan, A. (1984) Is chlorhexidine an essential drug? *Lancet*, **ii**, 759–760.

Kimbough, R.D. (1973) Review of the toxicity of hexachlorophane, including its neurotoxicity. *Journal of Clinical Pharmacology*, **13**, 439–444.

Kloos, W.E. & Schleifer, K.H. (1975) Simplified scheme for routine identification of human staphylococcus species. *Journal of Clinical Microbiology*, **1**, 82–88.

Koller, W., Rotter, M.L. & Gottardi, D. (1995) Do 'chlorine covers' exert a sustained bactericidal effect on the bacterial hand flora? *Journal of Hospital Infection*, **31**, 169–176.

Kopelman, A.E. (1973) Cutaneous absorption of

hexachlorophane in low-birth-weight infants. *Journal of Pediatrics*, **82**, 972–975.

Kurtz, J.B., Lee, T.W. & Parsons, A.J. (1981) The action of alcohols on rotavirus, astrovirus and enterovirus. *Journal of Hospital Infection*, **1**, 321–325.

Lamb, Y.J. (1991) Overview of the role of mupirocin. *Journal of Hospital Infection*, **19** (Suppl. B), 27–30.

Larsen, E., McKinley, K.J. & Grove, G.L. (1986) Physiologic, microbiologic, and seasonal effects of handwashing on the skin of health care personnel. *American Journal of Infection Control*, **14**, 51-59.

Leyden, J.J., McGinley, K.J., Kaminer, M.S. *et al.* & Grover, G.L. (1991) Computerised image analysis of full hand-touch plates: a method for quantification of surface bacteria on hands and the effect of antibacterial agents. *Journal of Hospital Infection*, **18** (Suppl. B), 13–22.

Leyden, J.J., McKinley, K.J., Foglia, A.N., Wharman, J.E., Gropper, C.N. & Vowels, B.R. (1996) A new method for *in vivo* evaluation of antimicrobial agents by translocation of complex dense populations of cutaneous bacteria. *Skin Pharmacology*, **9**, 60–68.

Lidwell, O.M. (1963). Methods of investigation and analysis of results. In *Infection in Hospitals*. (Williams R.E.O. & Shooter R.A.), p. 43 C.I.O.M.S. Oxford: Blackwell Publications.

Lilly, H.A. & Lowbury, E.J.L. (1971) Disinfection of the skin: an assessment of some new preparations. *British Medical Journal*, **iii**, 674–676.

Lilly, H.A., Lowbury, E.J.L. & Wilkins, M.D. (1979a) Limits to progressive reduction of skin bacteria by disinfection. *Journal of Clinical Pathology*, **32**, 382–385.

Lilly, H.A., Lowbury, E.J.L., Wilkins, M.D. & Zaggy, A. (1979b) Delayed antimicrobial effects of skin disinfection by alcohol. *Journal of Hygiene, Cambridge*, **82**, 497–500.

Lindberg, R.B., Moncrief, J.A., Switzer, W.E., Order, S.E. & Mills, W. (1965) The successful control of burn wound sepsis. *Journal of Trauma*, **5**, 601–616.

Linton, K.B. & George, E. (1966) Inactivation of chlorhexidine (hibitane) by bark corks. *Lancet*, **i**, 1353–1355.

Lister, J. (1867) Antiseptic principle in the practice of surgery. *British Medical Journal*, **ii**, 246–248.

Lister, J. (1909) *Collected Papers*. Oxford: Clarendon Press.

Lowbury, E.J.L. (1992) Special problems in hospital antisepsis. In *Principles and Practice of Disinfection, Preservation and Sterilization* (eds Russell, A.D., Hugo, W.B. & Ayliffe, G.A.J.). 2nd edn, pp. 320–329. Oxford: Blackwell.

Lowbury, E.J.L. & Lilly, H.A. (1960) Disinfection of the hands of surgeons and nurses. *British Medical Journal*, **i**, 1445–1450.

Lowbury, E.J.L. & Lilly, H.A. (1973) Use of 4% chlorhexidine detergent solution (Hibiscrub) and other methods of skin disinfection. *British Medical Journal*, **i**, 510–515.

Lowbury, E.J.L. & Lilly, H.A. (1975) Gloved hand as an applicator of antiseptic to operation sites. *Lancet*, **ii**, 153–156.

Lowbury, E.J.L. & Miller, R.W.S. (1962) Treatment of infected burns with BRL 1621 (cloxacillin). *Lancet*, **ii**, 640–641.

Lowbury, E.J.L., Cason, J.S., Jackson, D.M. & Miller, R.W.S. (1962) Fucidin for staphylococcal infection of burns. *Lancet*, **ii**, 478–480.

Lowbury, E.J.L., Lilly, H.A. & Bull, J.P. (1963) Disinfection of the hands: removal of resident bacteria. *British Medical Journal*, **i**, 1251–1256.

Lowbury, E.J.L., Lilly, H.A. & Bull, J.P. (1964) Methods of disinfection of the hands and operation sites. *British Medical Journal*, **ii**, 531–536.

Lowbury, E.J.L., Jackson, D.M., Lilly, H.A. *et al.* (1971) Alternative forms of local treatment for burns. *Lancet*, **ii**, 1105–1111.

Lowbury, E.J.L., Lilly, H.A. & Ayliffe, G.A.J. (1974) Preoperative disinfection of surgeon's hands: use of alcoholic solutions and effects of gloves on the skin flora. *British Medical Journal*, **iv**, 369–374.

Lowbury, E.J.L., Babb, J.R., Bridges, K. & Jackson, D.M. (1976) Topical chemoprophylaxis with silver sulphadiazine and silver nitrate chlorhexidine cream: emergence of sulphonamide-resistant gram-negative bacilli. *British Medical Journal*, **i**, 493–496.

Maki, D. & Hecht, J. (1982) Antiseptic-containing handwashing agents reduce nosocomial infections. In *22nd Interscience Conference on Antimicrobial Agents and Chemotherapy*, p. 303A.

Massanari, R.M. & Hierholzer, W. (1984) A crossover comparison of antiseptic soaps vs. nosocomial infection rates in intensive care units. *American Journal of Infection Control*, **12**, 247–249.

May, J., Brooks, S., Johnstone, D. & Macfie, J. (1993) Does the addition of pre-operative skin preparation with povidone-iodine reduce groin sepsis following arterial surgery. *Journal of Hospital Infection*, **24**, 153–156.

Meers, P.D. & Yeo, G.A. (1978) Shedding of bacteria and skin squames after handwashing. *Journal of Hygiene*, **81**, 99–105.

Monafo, W.W., Tandon, S.N., Ayrzian, W.H., Tuchschmidt, J., Skinner, A.M. & Dietz, F. (1976) Cerium nitrate—a new topical antiseptic for extensive burns. *Surgery*, **80**, 465–473.

Moyer, C.A., Brentano, L., Gravens, D.L., Magraf, H.W. & Monafo, W.W. (1965) Treatment of large burns with 0.5% silver nitrate solution. *Archives of Surgery*, **90**, 812–867.

Nagington, J., Gandy, G., Walker, J., & Gray J.J. (1983) Use of normal immunoglobulin in an echovirus II outbreak in a special care baby unit. *Lancet*, **ii**, 443–446.

Newsom, S.W.B. & Lilly, H.A. (1983) Hexachlorophane, or what's in a name. *Lancet*, **i**, 356–357.

Newsom, S.W.B. & Matthews, J. (1985) Studies on the use of povidone-iodine with the hygienic hand disinfection test. *Journal of Hospital Infection*, **6** (Suppl.), 45–50.

Newsom, S.W.B. & Rowland, C. (1989) Application of the hygienic-hand disinfection test to the gloved hand. *Journal of Hospital Infection*, **14**, 245–247.

Newsom, S.W.B., Rowland, C. & Wells, F.C. (1988) What is in the surgeon's glove. *Journal of Hospital Infection*, **11** (Suppl. A.), 244–259.

Newsom, S.W.B., White, R. & Pascoe, J. (1990) Action of teicoplanin on perioperative skin staphylococci. In *Teicoplanin—Further European Experience* (ed. Gruneberg, R.N.), pp. 1–18. London: Royal Society of Medicine.

Nguyen, T.T., Gilpin, D.A., Meyer, N.A. & Herndon, M.D. (1996) Current treatment of severely burned patients. *Annals of Surgery*, **223**, 14–25.

Noble, W.C. (1981) *In Microbiology of Human Skin* (eds Noble, W.C. and Somerville, D.A.) London: Lloyd-Luke.

Oie, S. & Kamiya, A. (1996) Bacterial contamination of commercial available ethacridine lactate (acrinol) products. *Journal of Hospital Infection*, **34**, 51–58.

Oie, S. & Kamiya, A. (1997) Microbial contamination of antiseptic-soaked cotton balls. *Biology and Pharmacology Bulletin*, **20**, 667–669.

Ojajarvi, J. (1991) Handwashing in Finland. *Journal of Hospital Infection*, **18** (Suppl. B), 35–40.

Papini, R.P.G., Wilson, A.P.R., Steer, J.A., McGrouther, D.A. & Parkhouse, N. (1995) Wound management in burn centres in the UK. *British Journal of Surgery*, **82**, 505–509.

Paulson, D.S. (1993) Efficacy evaluation of a 4% chlorhexidine gluconate as a full-body shower. *American Journal of Infection Control*, **21**, 205–209.

Peterson, A.F. (1973) The microbiology of hands. *Developments in Industrial Microbiology*, **14**, 125–130.

Pietsch, J. & Meakins, J.L. (1978) Complications of povidone-iodine absorption in topically treated burn patients. *Lancet*, **i**, 959.

Pierrie, W. (1867) On the use of carbolic acid in burns. *Lancet*, **ii**, 575.

Powell, H., Swarner, O., Gluck, L. & Lampert, P. (1973) Hexachlorophane myelinopathy in premature infants. *Journal of Pediatrics*, **82**, 976–981.

Price, P.B. (1938) The bacteriology of normal skin: a new quantitative test applied to the study of the bacterial flora and disinfectant action of mechanical cleansing. *Journal of Infectious Disease*, **63**, 301–318.

Public Health Laboratory Service (1997) *Hospital-acquired Infection*. London: Public Health Laboratory Service.

Raahave, D. (1974) Bacterial density in operation wounds. *Acta Chirurgica Scandinavia*, **140**, 585–593.

Rahman, M., Noble, W.C. & Cookson, B.D. (1987) Mupirocin-resistant *Staphylococcus aureus*. *Lancet*, **ii**, 387.

Ricketts, C.R., Squire, J.R., Topley, E. and Lilly, H.A. (1951) Human skin lipids with particular reference to the self-sterilising power of the skin. *Clinical Science*, **10**, 89–111.

Rotter, M.L. (1996) Hand washing and hand disinfection. In *Hospital Epidemiology and Infection Control* (ed. Mayhall, G.). Baltimore: Williams and Wilkins, pp. 691–710.

Rotter, M.L. & Koller, W. (1990) Surgical hand disinfection: effect of sequential use of two chlorhexidine preparations. *Journal of Hospital Infection*, **16**, 161–166.

Rotter, M.L., Koller, W. & Wewalka, G. (1980) Povidone-iodine and chlorhexidine gluconate containing detergents for disinfection of hands. *Journal of Hospital Infection*, **1**, 149–158.

Rotter, M.L., Larson, S.O., Cooke, E.M. (1988) A comparison of the effects of preoperative whole-body bathing with detergent alone and with detergent containing chlorhexidine gluconate on the frequency of wound infections after clean surgery. *Journal of Hospital Infection*, **11**, 310–320.

Semmelweis, I.P. (1861) *Die Aetiologie, der Begriff und die Prophylaxis des Kindbettfiebers*. C.A. Hartleben, Pest, Vienna and Leipzig (translated by F.P. Murphy (1981) Birmingham: Classics of Medicine Library).

Speller, D.C.E., Stephens, M.E. & Viant, A. (1971) Hospital infection by *Pseudomonas cepacia*. *Lancet*, **i**, 798–799.

Story, P. (1952) Testing of skin disinfectants. *British Medical Journal*, **ii**, 1128–1130.

Strand, C.L., Wajsbort, R.R. & Sturmann, K. (1993) Effect of iodophor vs. iodine tincture skin preparation on blood culture contamination rate. *Journal of the American Medical Association*, **269**, 3109–3110.

Taylor, G.J.S., Bannister, G.C. & Leeming, J.P. (1995) Wound disinfection with ultraviolet radiation. *Journal of Hospital Infection*, **30**, 85–94.

Taylor, L.J. (1978) An evaluation of hand washing techniques. *Nursing Times*, **74**, 108–110.

Thompson, C.J.S. (1934) *Lord Lister*, p. 45. London: J Bale and Danielson.

Waclawski, E.R., McAlpine, L.G. & Thomson, N.C. (1989) Occupational asthma in nurses caused by chlorhexidine and alcohol aerosols. *British Medical Journal*, **298**, 929–930.

Williamson, P. & Kligman, A.M. (1965) A new method for the quantitative investigation of cutaneous bacteria. *Journal of Investigative Dermatology*, **45**, 498–503.

Working Party on MRSA Control (1990) Revised guidelines for the control of epidemic methicillin-resistant *Staphylococcus aureus*. *Journal of Hospital Infection*, **16**, 351–357.

CHAPTER 14

Treatment of Laundry and Clinical Waste in Hospitals

1 Laundry

1.1 Hospital linen

Hospital linen may be contaminated with blood, excreta or secretions or may have been used for infected patients and therefore needs to be subjected to a decontamination process. However, although soiled linen can be contaminated with large numbers of microorganisms, the risk of transmission of disease appears to be negligible (McDonald & Pugliese, 1996). After removal from the patient or bed, the linen should be placed in a bag or container which is impervious to bacteria. In the UK, hospital linen is categorized and sorted at source into colour-coded bags/containers (Table 14.1; NHS Executive, 1995). Linen is categorized as used (soiled and foul), infected or heat-labile.

Table 14.1 Categorization of hospital linen (NHS Executive, 1995).

Category	Definition	Colour code (UK)
Used linen (soiled and foul)	All used linen irrespective of state, but on occasion contaminated by body fluids or blood	White or off-white
Infected linen	Linen from patients with or suspected of suffering from enteric fever and other *Salmonella* infections, dysentery (*Shigella* spp.), hepatitis A, hepatitis B, hepatitis C and carriers, open pulmonary tuberculosis, HIV infection, notifiable diseases and other infections in hazard group 3	Red or red on a white or off-white background. Also, carries a bold legend on a prominent yellow label such as: 'INFECTED LINEN'
Heat-labile linen	Fabrics damaged by the normal heat-disinfection process and likely to be damaged at thermal-disinfection temperatures	White with a prominent orange stripe

HIV, human immunodeficiency virus.

Many departments process foul linen (e.g. from incontinent patients in geriatric units) as infected, since manual sorting, which is an unpleasant process, can then be avoided. The sorting of linen is the processing stage most likely to be associated with transmission of infection. However, Weinstein *et al.* (1989) found no difference in bacterial contamination between patients in and those not in isolation. It is recommended that infected linen is double-bagged, with the inner bag being water-soluble or having a water-soluble membrane or seam. The linen is placed within the inner bag into the laundry washing machine and the outer bag is also similarly processed. Used and infected linen is thermally or chemically disinfected. Departments should be encouraged to check for extraneous items (e.g. scissors, needles, surgical instruments, etc.) before bagging the laundry. Their presence means that laundry staff are put at risk of injury and that very often they have to sort the linen, even though in theory it should be unnecessary. Damage may also occur to the washing machines. It has been suggested (Taylor, 1988) that all laundry bags should carry a label stating the ward or department of origin and porters should not accept linen bags that do not carry this identification. It has also been suggested that the linen bags could be passed through metal detectors on arrival in the laundry, but some extraneous items may be plastic or too small to detect.

Staff handling used linen should wear protective clothing, for example gloves and an apron, have adequate access to hand-washing facilities and be trained in basic hygienic techniques, e.g. hand washing.

Special arrangements, such as autoclaving before washing, were recommended for particularly hazardous infections, such as viral haemorrhagic fevers. However, the latest recommendations are that the linen should be placed in an alginate stitched or water-soluble bag and placed directly into the laundry machine. The outer bag should be placed in a clinical-waste bag and sent for incineration (Advisory Committee on Dangerous Pathogens, 1996).

Recently, vancomycin-resistant enterococci (VRE) have been shown to be tolerant to thermal-disinfection temperatures (Bradley & Fraise, 1996). However, Wilcox & Jones (1995) demonstrated that linen test pieces artificially contaminated with a heat-tolerant strain of VRE were free of the test strain after processing in a continuous-batch tunnel washer (CBTW) at 65°C for 10 min. This was thought do be due primarily to the cleansing and dilution effect of the process. Vancomycin-resistant enterococci and their response to biocides are considered in Chapter 10F.

1.1.1 *Disinfection of heat-stable linen*

The UK Department of Health (NHS Executive, 1995) recommends disinfection temperatures of 65°C for 10 min or 71°C for 3 min, after allowing for adequate heat penetration of the load, and the temperature of the load should be recorded. It is preferable to use the higher temperature to ensure correct and thorough disinfection. Heat penetration may not always be adequate, but few organisms remain after the normal drying process (Collins *et al.*, 1987). There is a variation in times and temperatures recommended in other countries (Daschner, 1993; Table 14.2), but the basis for these differences remains uncertain.

1.1.2 *Disinfection of heat-labile linen*

There is an increased use of clothing consisting of man-made fibres, which are damaged or distorted if subjected to the usual hospital laundry-washing temperatures. They are normally laundered at 40°C and dried at 60°C. Chemical

Table 14.2 National recommendations for disinfection of hospital linen (Daschner, 1993).

Country	Methods
Germany	85 °C for 15 min 90 °C for 10 min 60 °C plus phenolic, aldehyde or chloride
USA	71 °C for 25 min < 70 °C plus chemicals (mostly sodium hypochlorite)
Sweden	70 °C for 10 min, no chemicals
UK	71 °C for 3 min 65 °C for 10 min, rarely chemicals
Norway	85 °C for 10 min, no chemicals
Denmark	85 °C for 10 min, no chemicals

disinfection methods are used in the penultimate rinse. Chlorine-releasing agents are the most widely used, at a concentration of 125–150 parts/10^6 available chlorine. However, chlorine can remove colour from fabrics, may damage fire-retardant properties and may damage processing equipment. Other alternative chemicals currently undergoing trials are hydrogen peroxide and quaternary ammonium compounds. It is generally thought that a dilution effect, combined with the terminal drying of the linen, plays a major role in the decontamination process. Triclosan has been shown to have no beneficial effect on the removal of bacteria from patients' dresses compared with ordinary detergent (Tompkins *et al.*, 1988). If decontamination of heat-labile clothing from a patient with a transmissible infection is required, low-temperature steam is a more reliable process. Low-temperature steam and formaldehyde (LTSF) (see Chapter 19A) adequately disinfects woollens and blankets. A residual effect is obtained with the formaldehyde (Alder *et al.*, 1971), but, since most hospital blankets are cotton and can be exposed to an adequate disinfection temperature during the washing process, this method is rarely used routinely.

1.1.3 Dry-cleaning

It is recommended that dry-cleaning should not be used for items potentially contaminated with pathogenic microorganisms. Where there is no alternative method, steam pressing should also be carried out. Bates *et al.* (1993) demonstrated that the dry-cleaning process is not bactericidal and is poorly viricidal for non-enveloped viruses.

1.2 Types of machines

There are two types of washing machines currently used in hospital laundries: washer-extractors and CBTWs (Barrie, 1994).

1.2.1 Washer-extractors

These are similar to domestic washing-machines in that they take in fresh water for each wash and rinse. The risk of recontamination of processed linen from the rinse water is therefore reduced. Washer-extractors can be used to process any type of linen, including bedding and uniforms, most articles of clothing, heat-sensitive fabrics and 'infected' linen, although the processing capacity is relatively low. These machines are recommended by the Department of Health for infected linen, as they are less prone to blockages and therefore maintenance by engineers, who might otherwise be put at risk of infection. Small domestic washing-machines are sometimes found in specialist units, such as special-care baby units, for processing babies clothing, which is very often heat-labile.

1.2.2 Continuous-batch tunnel washers (CBTWs)

Large quantities of linen can be processed in these machines. Linen passes through a number of compartments, where they are prewashed, washed and rinsed. A problem with CBTWs is the reuse of the rinse water. Water from a final rinse may be used for preliminary sluicing of subsequent loads, to avoid wastage of water. When stored overnight or during a weekend, small numbers of residual Gram-negative bacilli and aerobic spore-bearing organisms may multiply to large numbers. These may not be destroyed during the heat cycle and could cause infections in immunocompromised patients. Surviving aerobic spore-bearing organisms on linen have caused infections on rare occasions (Birch *et al.*, 1981; Barrie *et al.*, 1992). Similar problems of overnight growth of organisms can occur in tunnel or batch continuous washers. It is also recommended that these machines should be drained or emptied overnight and linen should be heat-disinfected the following day. Thermal disinfection of the rinse section of the machine prior to production commencing and after the machine has been out of action for 3 h or more is also recommended (NHS Executive, 1995) but may not be possible.

1.3 Microbiological testing of laundry

The routine microbiological testing of laundered items is not recommended, particularly if the time/temperature parameters of a washing cycle can be measured. However, where it is not possible to heat-disinfect linen, testing makes it possible to check that similar standards are being achieved. It may also be of value as an assurance of decontamination during outbreaks and when commissioning and evaluating new washing-machines. Various possible standards have been recommended. Collins *et al.* (1987) suggested that total counts on finished linen should not exceed one organism/10 cm^2 on a regular basis. Walter & Schillinger (1975) proposed that bacterial counts on processed linen of ≤20 colony-forming units (cfu)/100 cm^2 are equivalent to complete pathogen removal, and Christian *et al.* (1983) suggested that a 10^6–10^7 reduction in viable bacteria would be effective in reducing the risk of infection. However, at present, no standards for maximum safe bacterial levels exist (Ayliffe *et al.*, 1990).

Surface/contact sampling of linen yields lower bacterial counts than counting macerated pieces of linen but is easier to perform and does not damage sampled items.

2 Clinical waste

The main problems associated with the disposal of hospital waste are aesthetic and the perception of the public of potential hazards. The overall volume of waste generated in hospitals needs to be reduced. This can be done by decreasing the amount of single-use items used, recycling more items and reducing the amount of packaging. Education of hospital personnel as to the constitution of waste requiring treatment also needs to be addressed. It has been estimated that 50% of clinical waste sent for incineration is actually domestic waste (BMA, 1994). Segregation of waste should preferably take place at the point of production. However, the understanding of the need for waste segregation is low. Correct segregation could save a lot of money, as treatment of clinical waste, i.e. incineration, is approximately 12 times the cost of treatment for domestic waste, i.e. landfill. A study by Mercier & Ellam (1996) demonstrated that the amount of waste inappropriately discarded as clinical waste was substantially reduced by implementing an education programme. The education programme included information on the relative costs associated with disposal, the definitions of clinical waste and the provision of bins clearly labelled and signs explaining the procedures for correct disposal and segregation.

The handling of waste requires a similar policy to that of laundry, but sorting should never be required, so the potential hazard to staff is even less. If sealed in a plastic bag or other appropriate container, waste can safely be transported throughout the hospital and to the site of final disposal. Needles and other sharps should be disposed of in approved leak-proof, puncture-resistant containers (DHSS, 1982).

Hospital waste can be divided into two main categories: 'domestic' and 'clinical'. Clinical waste at present is further categorized into five groups in the UK (Health Services Advisory Committee, 1992; Table 14.3). Similar categorization of waste

Table 14.3 Categories of waste.

Group	Definition
A	All human tissues, including blood (whether infected or not), animal carcasses and tissue from veterinary centres, hospitals or laboratories, and all related swabs and dressings Waste materials where the assessment indicates a risk to staff handling them, e.g. from infectious-disease cases Soiled surgical dressings, swabs and all other soiled waste from treatment areas
B	Discarded syringes, needles, cartridges, broken glass and other sharp instruments
C	Microbiological cultures and potentially infected waste from pathology departments (laboratory and post-mortem rooms) and other clinical or research laboratories
D	Certain pharmaceutical and chemical waste
E	Items used to dispose of urine, faeces and other bodily secretions and excretions assessed as not falling within group A. This includes used disposable bedpan liners, incontinence pads, stoma bags and urine containers

is used in other countries, for example the USA (Rutala & Mayhall, 1992). These categories are based upon a risk assessment of health and safety. Groups A, B, C and D give the highest risk while Group E is the lowest, although this waste may be more visually offensive than the others. Incineration is recommended for all these five groups, although group E cannot be classified as infectious. In the UK, clinical waste is categorized at source into colour-coded bags and containers (Table 14.4).

Hospital-waste disposal is causing problems in many countries. Although incineration is desirable, it is expensive and may be responsible for considerable environmental pollution. There is no epidemiological evidence to suggest that hospital waste is any more infectious than community waste (Hedrick, 1988) and no infections from hospital waste (apart from needle stick injuries) have been reported. However, it seems reasonable to categorize 'sharps', 'microbiological' and 'pathology' waste and waste heavily contaminated with blood and other body fluids as 'infectious' and it should be incinerated. Human tissues are incinerated for aesthetic reasons. Clinical waste from patients with hepatitis B or C, human immunodeficiency virus (HIV), *Salmonella* or *Shigella* infections or with open tuberculosis should be treated as 'infectious' and incinerated. Other clinical waste, i.e. category E, is not hazardous; surgical dressings, which are mainly contaminated with organisms unlikely to harm healthy people, should preferably be incinerated but landfill is adequate. Clinical waste could usefully be divided into two further categories, i.e. 'infected' and 'non-infected', similar to that of laundry. This would reduce the costs without significantly increasing the infection risk to staff.

2.1 Waste-disposal methods

Whatever method is used, the waste should be rendered non-infectious and non-recognizable, it should not pollute the environment and should be safe to handle further if required, i.e. no sharps protruding. There are no microbiological standards for the performance of waste-treatment methods. The waste should be rendered non-infectious, but debate continues as to whether it should be sterilized or disinfected (Ayliffe, 1994). A reasonable standard might require that there are no 'indicator' organisms in 100 g of waste (Collins & Kennedy, 1993). The type of 'indicator' organism to be used needs to be established, but the presence of *Escherichia coli* has been suggested. Tests may need to establish that the operator is not put at risk of infection during processing, for example by the production of aerosols, and that the waste is rendered non-infectious by the process. In the UK, the hospital authorities have a legal responsibility for ensuring the safety of waste handling within the hospital and for the transport procedures of contractors. A waste-disposal/control officer is usually appointed, whose role includes supervision of site staff, contractors, etc., liaison with relevant authorities, education and audit of practices (Blenkharn, 1995).

2.1.1 *Incineration*

This is the most widely used disposal method and is probably one of the few methods that fulfills all the required criteria. However, there are problems with the currently available incinerators in conforming to the requirements of British Standard BS 3316 (1987) for emissions, and careful mainten-

Table 14.4 Colour coding used for clinical waste (UK).

Colour	Type of waste
Black	Normal household waste, not clinical waste
Yellow	Waste destined for incineration
Yellow with a black band	Waste (e.g. from a nursing home) which should preferably be incinerated but which may be landfilled (not widely used)
Light blue or transparent with light blue inscription	Waste for autoclaving (or equivalent treatment) before ultimate disposal

ance is needed to meet environmental standards. Modern incinerators have two chambers. The first chamber heats the waste to 800°C with a limited air supply and the gaseous products of this combustion are moved to a second chamber, where they are further heated to 1000°C or more, with excess air, for at least 2 s to destroy any organic matter that has escaped the first heating and to destroy toxic gases that may otherwise be released into the environment. The effluent gases then pass through scrubbers to remove the gases before release into the environment. Loads with large amounts of fluids should not be incinerated, as they lower the processing temperature. One of the advantages of incinerators is that the energy can be recycled. There are no standards for the microbial content of incinerator emissions, but there are for the emission of smoke, heavy metals, particulate matter, etc. (Collins & Kennedy, 1993). If an incinerator is functioning correctly, it should produce sterile ash (Blenkharn & Oakland 1989). Very few hospitals have functioning incinerators on site, so they have to use safe transport systems to incinerator contractors in the private sector. The waste contract should be reviewed regularly and must include provision of sufficient containers to accommodate the waste, a safe means of transporting the waste to the incinerator and an adequate method for decontamination (thermal or chemical) of the waste containers. The containers should be robust, leak-proof, pest-proof, secure, impact-resistant and easily transportable within the hospital.

2.1.2 Landfill

This method is mainly used for domestic waste and is probably the cheapest method of waste treatment available. It is considered to be unsuitable for untreated clinical waste, mainly for aesthetic, political and practical reasons. However, studies have shown that very few pathogens are present on hospital waste, compared with domestic waste (Rutala & Mayhall, 1992). The availability of landfill sites is gradually disappearing in many countries. Landfill is often used for final disposal after waste has been treated, e.g. after autoclaving.

2.1.3 Autoclaving

This method is mainly used for laboratory waste, such as used culture plates and specimens, etc. The code of practice for the prevention of infection in clinical laboratories (Health Services Advisory Committee, 1991) and the Health and Safety Commission (HSC) (Health Services Advisory Committee, 1992) state that laboratory waste should be autoclaved before it leaves the laboratory. As the capacity of autoclaves is limited, this method is unsuitable for large amounts of clinical waste. The waste is rendered non-infectious but then has to undergo further disposal, such as landfill or incineration, because after autoclaving the waste may still be recognizable and noxious. Provided the waste is safely enclosed, it could be transferred to an incinerator without prior autoclaving.

2.1.4 New methods

The newer methods tend to be smaller, easy-to-use units that treat waste relatively quickly. These units can be placed near the point of waste generation, so that waste can be treated as it is generated, thereby eliminating the need for special handling and storage/transport.

Plastic densification. This method is currently being evaluated in the UK. Plastics—for example, used microbiological culture plates, syringes, specimen pots, etc.—are heated and melted under controlled conditions and densified into briquettes or an unformed mass.

Wet grinding. In this process, the waste is finely ground under running water, similar to the domestic waste-disposal system. The end-product is discharged into the sewer. In agreement with the HSC, this method is used for items in category E, i.e. disposable bedpans, urine containers, incontinence pads and stoma bags. There may be disadvantages to this method, namely that large volumes of water are required, the machinery is noisy and it is prone to blockages if used incorrectly. Wet grinding will not inactivate microorganisms, and aerosols may be generated. Infectious materials should therefore be autoclaved before grinding.

Grinding and chemical disinfection. This method consists of grinding the waste and then mixing it with a chemical disinfectant, usually a chlorine-releasing agent, before it is released into the sewage system. It is reported that this method of waste treatment is used in 14% of US hospitals. A study by Farr & Walton (1993) demonstrated a 4.75 $\log_{10}$ reduction in HIV-1 using mechanical shredding with chlorine dioxide exposure.

Microwave treatment. This method consists of shredding the waste and removing metals before subjecting the waste to microwaves to render it non-infectious. It is still under development.

Other methods. Other methods currently under development include ionizing radiation, radiation, pyrolysis and electrothermal deactivation (Collins & Kennedy, 1993). Further work is required before these methods can be accepted for general use. Most of the newer methods treat waste on a small scale and some may be useful for small health centres. It may therefore be that in the future waste is treated at source as it is generated, rather than in bulk at another location.

The newer treatment methods tend to produce a reduction in bioburdern, with a vast reduction in bulk, but the treatment residues may not be sterile. Blenkharn (1995) suggests that legislative controls governing clinical-waste disposal should be relaxed, as these residues may not present a significant infection risk if suitably contained and handled with care.

3 Conclusions

The risk of infection from laundry and clinical waste is low, provided appropriate precautions are taken. These include segregation into the required categories on the ward into the appropriate coloured bags. All hospital laundry should be disinfected, preferably by heat at 71°C for 3 min, but chemical methods may be required for heat-labile laundry. The important factor is the washing stage of the cycle. Linen requires sorting in the laundry, due to the presence of extraneous items, but linen from infected patients should be placed in a water-soluble bag, which is then placed directly into the washing-machine, thus minimizing the need for further handling.

Clinical waste is less of a risk to the handlers, as no sorting is required. Most hospitals/trusts now appoint a responsible officer/waste-control officer to take responsibility for overseeing the handling and subsequent disposal of clinical waste. Most clinical waste is incinerated, and domestic waste goes to landfill. There are problems with both these methods, as the standards for incinerators are very exacting in order to avoid the possibility of air pollution, and landfill sites will eventually be in short supply. Newer methods are being developed, which may treat smaller volumes of waste and can be installed on site. In an effort to reduce the volume of clinical waste generated, manufacturers should be encouraged to provide reusable items or less packaging.

4 References

Advisory Committee on Dangerous Pathogens (1996) *Management and Control of Viral Haemorrhagic Fevers*. London: HMSO.

Alder, V.G., Boss, E., Gillespie, W.A. & Swarm, A.J. (1971) Residual disinfection of wool blankets treated with formaldehyde. *Journal of Applied Bacteriology*, **34**, 757–763.

Ayliffe, G.A.J. (1994) Clinical waste: how dangerous is it? *Current Opinion in Infectious Diseases*, **7**, 499–502.

Ayliffe, G.A.J., Collins, B.J. & Taylor, L.J. (1990) *Hospital Acquired Infection: Principles and Prevention*. London: Butterworth.

Barrie, D. (1994) Infection control in practice: how hospital linen and laundry services are provided. *Journal of Hospital Infection*, **27**, 219–235.

Barrie, D., Wison, J.A., Hoffman, P.N. & Kramer, J.M. (1992) *Bacillus cereus* meningitis in two neurosurgical patients: an investigation into the source of the organism. *Journal of Infection*, **25**, 291–297.

Bates, C.J., Wilcox, M.H., Smith, T.L. & Spencer, R.C. (1993) The efficacy of a hospital dry cleaning cycle in disinfecting material contaminated with bacteria and viruses. *Journal of Hospital Infection*, **23**, 255–262.

Birch, B.R., Perera, B.S. Hyde, W.A. *et al.* (1981) *Bacillus cereus* cross infection in a maternity unit. *Journal of Hospital Infection*, **2**, 349–354.

Blenkharn, J.I. (1995) The disposal of clinical wastes. *Journal of Hospital Infection*, **30** (Suppl.) 514–520.

Blenkharn, J.I. & Oakland, D. (1989) Emmission of viable bacteria in the exhaust flue gases from a hospital incinerator. *Journal of Hospital Infection* **14**, 73–78.

BMA (1994) *Environmental and Occupational Risks of Health Care*. London: BMA.

Bradley, C.R. & Fraise, A.P. (1996) Heat and chemical resistance of enterococci. *Journal of Hospital Infection*, **34**, 191–196.

British Standard 3316 (1987) *Part 1 Specification for Standard Performance Requirements for Incineration Plant for the Destruction of Hospital Waste*. London: BSI.

Christian, R.R., Manchest, J.T. & Mellor, M.T. (1983) Bacteriological quality of fabrics washed at lower than standard temperatures in a hospital laundry facility. *Applied and Environmental Microbiology*, **45**, 591–597.

Collins, B.J., Cripps, N. & Spooner, A. (1987) Controlling microbial decontamination levels. *Laundry and Cleaning News*, 30–31.

Collins, C.H. & Kennedy, D.A. (1993) *The Treatment and Disposal of Clinical Waste*. HHSC Handbook No. 13. Leeds: H.H. Scientific Consultants Ltd.

Daschner, F. (1993) The hospital and pollution: role of the hospital epidemiologist in protecting the environment. In *Prevention and Control of Nosocomial Infections* (ed. Wenzel, RP) 993–1000. London: Williams and Wilkins.

Department of Health and Social Security (DHSS) (1982) *Specification for Containers for Disposal of Needles and Sharp Instruments*. TSS/S/330.015. London: HMSO.

Farr, R.W. & Walton, C. (1993) Inactivation of human immunodefficiency virus by a medical waste disposal process using chlorine dioxide. *Infection Control and Hospital Epidemiology*, **14**, 527–529.

Health Services Advisory Committee (1991) *Safety in Health Service: Safe Working and the Prevention of Infection in Clinical Laboratories*. London: HMSO.

Health Services Advisory Committee (1992) *Health and Safety Commission: The Safe Disposal of Clinical Waste*. London: HMSO.

Hedrick, E.R. (1988) Infectious waste management—will science prevail? *Infection Control and Hospital Epidemiology*, **9**, 488–490.

McDonald, L.L. & Pugliese, G. (1996) Laundry services. In *Hospital Epidemiology and Infection Control* (ed. Mayhall, C.G.). London: Williams & Wilkins.

Mercier, C. & Ellam, T. (1996) Waste not, want not. *Health Service Journal* **4**, 27.

NHS Executive (1995) *Hospital Laundry Arrangements for Used and Infected Linen*. Health Service Guidelines, HSG(95)18.

Rutala, W.A. & Mayhall, C.G. (1992) SHEA position paper: medical waste. *Infection Control and Hospital Epidemiology*, **13**, 38–48.

Taylor, L.J. (1988) Segregation, collection and disposal of hospital laundry and waste. *Journal of Hospital Infection*, **11** (Suppl. A), 57–63.

Tompkins, D.S., Johnson, P. & Fottall, B.R. (1988) Low-temperature washing of patients' clothing: effects of detergent with disinfectant and a tunnel drier on bacterial survival. *Journal of Hospital Infection*, **12**, 51–58.

Walter, W.G. & Schillinger, J.E. (1975) Bacterial survival in laundered fabrics. *Applied and Environmental Microbiology*, **29**, 368–373.

Weinstein, S.A., Nelson, N.M., Pelletier, C. & Hilbert, D. (1989) Bacterial surface contamination of patient's linen: isolation precautions versus standard care. *American Journal of Infection Control*, **7**, 264–267.

Wilcox, M.H. & Jones, B.L. (1995) Enterococci and hospital laundry. *Lancet*, **344**, 594.

CHAPTER 15

Recreational and Hydrotherapy Pools

1 Introduction

Infections can be transmitted by polluted water and may be acquired from potable or recreational water. The disinfection of drinking water aims to eliminate this infection risk and pool water is also disinfected for the same reason. Disinfecting the pool water also helps to prevent microbial growth, which would otherwise make the water unpleasant for bathing. Such growth may render the water turbid, discoloured or malodorous and may also make it sufficiently aggressive to attack tile grouting and pool fittings. In larger pools, a disinfection system is incorporated and the pool water is also filtered to remove particulate matter, which assists the disinfection process, in addition to maintaining pool-water clarity.

There are many different kinds of pool, including the traditional rectangular 'municipal' pool; competition, diving and learner pools; leisure pools with complex shapes and circulation; splash pools; paddling pools and salt-water pools. Therapeutic pools can take the form of hydrotherapy pools, found in many hospitals and health clinics, and natural thermal pools.

Spa or whirlpools ('jacuzzi') are now quite common; these are usually designed to hold up to six persons at a time. They are fitted with hydrojets and air-induction systems, which agitate the water with the intention of inducing relaxation in the users. Whirlpool baths also have hydrojets and/or air-induction systems but are designed for single-bather use and the bath is drained and refilled between each bather. Other small pools include plunge pools and birthing pools.

2 Pool design

Many aspects of pool design, disinfection and management are detailed in the *Pool Water Guide* (Anon., 1995a).

2.1 The circulation system

Pools designed for multiple-bather use, including hydrotherapy pools, should have a circulation system that is adequate to cope with the anticipated bathing load. In a circulation system, the pool water is pumped through a filter and disinfectant is added before being returned to the pool (Fig. 15.1). Provision is made for the addition of any chemicals required to maintain the pH value of the

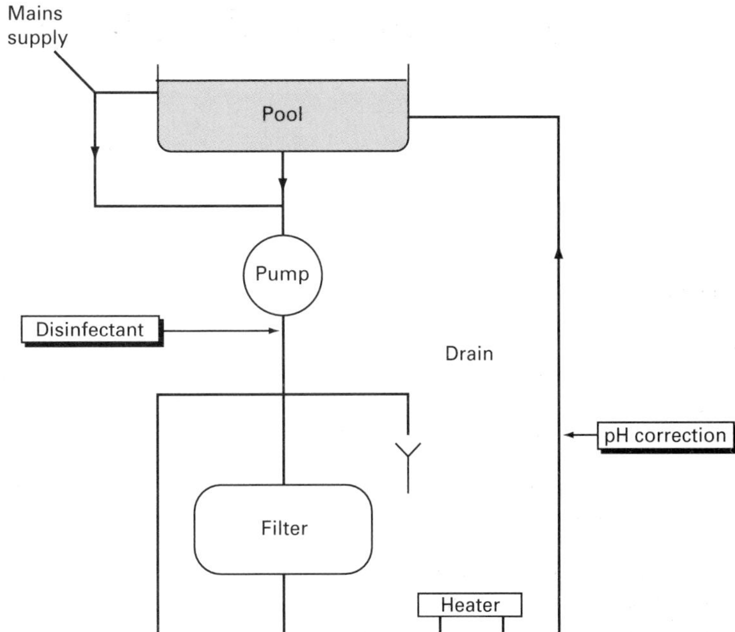

Fig 15.1 Diagrammatic representation of the circulation system.

pool water within the appropriate range, for temperature control, for the addition of fresh water and for the discharge of backwash water to waste. A balance tank may also be incorporated to assist in maintaining the pool water at the correct level; this is essential for so-called 'deck-level' pools, where the water is level with the surrounds. The circulation of the water within the pool itself must ensure that there is a water flow to all parts, with an absence of 'dead spots'. It is an advantage to arrange for a significant proportion of draw-off water from the pool to come from the surface-water layer, where most of the pollutants tend to be concentrated. The water may be withdrawn through overflow channels around the pool sides or skimmers. With deck-level pools, the water overflows into gratings in the surrounds.

The circulation system should be run continuously, even when the pool is not in use, although the turnover time may then be increased. The turnover time is the time taken for a volume of water equal to the total volume of the pool to pass through the treatment plant (including the filters). This time will vary according to the nature of the pool, ranging from around 3–4 h for many swimming-pools, down to $1\text{–}1^1/_2$ h for hydrotherapy pools (and even less for spa pools).

2.2 Filtration

A filtration system will remove particulate matter from the pool water, which assists in maintaining pool clarity and enhances disinfection efficacy. Using a coagulant, such as alum, will precipitate colloidal matter, which can then be removed by the filter. Such systems will be found in pools designed for more than one bather and usually take the form of a pressure sand filter, housed in a steel vessel (more than one in large pools). Filtration efficiency depends on the filtration rate. Medium-rate sand filters have a filtration velocity of between 10 and 25 mh and are suitable for large pools with a high bathing load. High-rate filters (filtration rate > 30 m/h) are less effective at removing particulate matter and should be used only with small, less heavily used pools. Other substances, such as diatomaceous earth or fibre in the form of a pad or cartridge, can be used in filter systems but require more intensive maintenance than sand filters. Ozone systems incorporate an activated carbon filter to remove excess ozone before the water is returned to the pool; this may be housed separately or incorporated within the sand-filter vessel.

In order to be fully effective, filters must be regularly backwashed—at least weekly or whenever the pressure gradient across the filter reaches a figure recommended by the manufacturer. In this process, the flow of pool water is reversed so that the detritus collected in the filter bed is removed. To be fully effective, the back flow should be sufficiently vigorous to fluidize the filter bed; some filters incorporate an air scour to assist this process. The backwash water is discharged to waste and the volume made up with fresh water. This process also removes chemical pollutants and helps to maintain a suitable water balance in the pool. The filtration system is an important means of removing relatively disinfectant-resistant parasites, such as *Giardia* and *Cryptosporidium*.

If not well maintained, filters are readily colonized by microorganisms, *Pseudomonas aeruginosa* being particularly troublesome in this respect. This leads to contamination of the pool water and other parts of the system, and a resistant biofilm may form on the surfaces of the pipework.

2.3 Whirlpool baths and birthing pools

Whirlpool baths and birthing pools are designed for single-bather use. These baths are drained and refilled between each user and so do not have circulation systems, but whirlpool baths do have a means for agitating the water. There is no filtration of the water and any disinfection must be done manually. Colonization of whirlpool baths with *Ps. aeruginosa* has been reported, with evidence of transmission of *Pseudomonas* wound infections by this route (Hollyoak & Freeman, 1995). Birthing pools may also present a possible infection risk, both from mother to infant and to subsequent pool users; microbiological monitoring of the pool water before and after delivery has been advocated (Coombs *et al.*, 1994; Rawal *et al.*, 1994).

Thorough draining and cleaning of these pools with hypochlorite disinfection between each bather use has been recommended. However, some whirlpool baths have plumbing systems that make this difficult to achieve, and this procedure is not always effective at eliminating colonization with *Ps. aeruginosa* in such baths (Hollyoak & Freeman, 1995). The use of chlorine dioxide as an alternative means of disinfection is being evaluated (J.V. Lee, personal communication).

For birthing pools that are plumbed in, it has been suggested that opening the taps for 5 min each day will reduce the risk of contamination from the water which may have been static and tepid in a 'dead leg' if the pool has not been used for several days. For the same reason, the water should be allowed to flow to waste for 2 min before filling the pool (Coombs *et al.*, 1994).

3 Available disinfectants

3.1 Chlorine and its compounds

A variety of pool-water disinfectants are now available, but chlorine in one of its many forms is the most commonly used. Being a powerful oxidizing agent, it will remove pollutants, as well as inactivating microorganisms, including viruses. With most forms of chlorine, the active disinfecting agent is hypochlorous acid (HClO), which, in sufficient concentration, reacts with pollutants until a point ('breakpoint') is reached when no pollutants are left with which to combine. Various compounds are formed, many of which are chloramines (so-called 'combined chlorine'). Depending on the relative concentrations of pollutant and chlorine, monochloramine, dichloramine and nitrogen trichloride are formed. These compounds have little or no disinfecting properties and are largely responsible for the irritant effects of chlorine-disinfected pools. Increasing the hypochlorite concentration beyond this point will lead to the formation of a disinfectant residual ('free chlorine'), which is available to react with any further pollutants or microorganisms that gain entry to the pool. To ensure that this is so, the free chlorine should always be kept at twice the level of the combined; for most pools, a concentration of free chlorine within the range 1–3 mg/l will be found adequate. In practice, free and total chlorine concentrations are regularly monitored; subtracting the concentration of the free chlorine from the total will give the figure for combined chlorine.

Other compounds formed by the action of chlorine on pollutants are termed haloforms; these are stable and their concentration can be reduced only by dilution with fresh water.

For many years, chlorine gas was used as the chlorine source, but handling difficulties have led to a decline in its use. Sodium hypochlorite is the most commonly used substitute, as it is generally easy to control and the dosage can be readily adjusted to cope with increased bather activity. It is considered to be the disinfectant of choice for use in hydrotherapy pools (Anon., 1990). Calcium hypochlorite is a useful alternative for soft-water areas. Sodium hypochlorite can be added by means of a dosing pump, but calcium hypochlorite, being in granular form, must be used in a suitable 'feeder', in which it is slowly dissolved. Sodium hypochlorite can be generated on site by the electrolysis of brine, a system used in some larger pools.

Chlorinated isocyanurates (Chapter 2) have the advantage of stabilizing the free chlorine in the presence of ultraviolet light and are useful for outdoor pools, but the concentration of their dissociation product, cyanuric acid, must not be allowed to exceed 200 mg/l, otherwise the free chlorine will tend to be neutralized. Sodium dichloroisocyanurate (Dichlor) is supplied in the form of rapidly dissolving granules, which can be used for rapid disinfection ('shock chlorination') or for hand-dosing small pools. Trichloroisocyanuric acid (Trichlor) is in the form of sticks, which slowly dissolve. As with calcium hypochlorite, trichloroisocyanurate is used in a feeder. It is important that neither chemical should be used in a feeder designed for, and previously used with, the other, as explosive mixtures may be formed.

Chlorine dioxide is another form of chlorine sometimes used as a pool disinfectant, but it may result in a greenish discoloration of the water and in the formation of chlorates. One system uses tetrachlorodecaoxide, a compound that breaks down to form chlorine dioxide; at present, this is the only chlorine dioxide-based system approved for swimming-pool use by the Department of the Environment's Committee on Chemicals and Materials of Construction for Use in Public Water Supply and Swimming Pools (Anon., 1996).

3.2 Ozone

More recently, ozone systems have become increasingly common, especially in larger pools. Ozone is a very powerful oxidizing agent, with considerable disinfecting properties, but, being toxic, must not be allowed to remain in the pool water. It is therefore used in conjunction with a chlorine disinfectant, which provides a residual disinfectant level in the pool; as most of the pollutants are removed by the ozonation, less combined chlorine is formed, so the free chlorine concentration can be kept below 1 mg/l, with a resulting increase in bather comfort. Ozone is formed on site in a generator, allowed to react with the water and the excess removed by a filter containing activated carbon.

3.3 Bromine and its compounds

Bromine, another powerful oxidizing agent, can also be used for pool disinfection, but elemental liquid bromine, being irritant, requires careful handling and is not often used. A combined form is usually employed, such as bromochlorodimethylhydantoin (BCDMH), supplied in tablet form, which when slowly dissolved in a feeder (brominator), dissociates to form hypobromous acid (see Chapter 2). This acid is similar to HClO in its action, combining with pollutants to form bromamines, but, unlike chloramines, these have useful disinfecting properties. As with the chlorinated isocyanurates, the concentration of the other dissociation product, dimethylhydantoin, must be controlled by dilution with fresh water to avoid impairment of the disinfecting activity and, in this instance, possible toxic effects. Although this system is used successfully in some hydrotherapy pools, it is generally harder to control than those using sodium hypochlorite (Anon., 1990).

Another bromine-based system uses the reaction between sodium bromide and sodium hypochlorite to generate hypobromous acid.

3.4 Other disinfection systems

Other disinfection systems used for pools include ultraviolet radiation, in conjunction with a chlorine residual, and copper/silver ions with chlorine. Both will need further evaluation before gaining general acceptance. Polymeric biguanide (see also Chapter 2) is another compound with disinfecting activity, but it does not combine with pollutants so is not suitable for heavily used pools; it can be used for small domestic pools.

3.5 Laboratory studies

The disinfecting activities of chlorine, bromine, BCDMH, iodine, chlorine dioxide and ozone against *Staphylococcus aureus* have been compared *in vitro* under standard conditions. Of these, ozone was the most effective, with chlorine, bromine, BCDMH and chlorine dioxide next in effectiveness at around the same level; iodine was least effective (Anon., 1984).

4 Pool-water chemistry

The efficiency of a disinfection system greatly depends upon the maintenance of a satisfactory pH value. With a chlorine disinfectant, the value should be kept between 7.2 and 7.8 to ensure the formation of HClO; above pH 7.8, its formation is inhibited. With bromine disinfectants, the formation of hypobromous acid is less affected by a higher pH value. Disinfectants such as sodium and calcium hypochlorite are alkaline and tend to elevate the pH, so that it may be necessary to adjust this by the addition of an acidic chemical, such as sodium bisulphate. The chlorinated isocyanurates and BCDMH have little effect on the pH. The nature of the mains water will also have an effect, soft waters tending to be acidic.

Other important chemical parameters are alkalinity and total dissolved solids (TDS). A sufficient degree of alkalinity of the pool water must be maintained to prevent the water from becoming aggressive and thereby attacking grouting and corroding metallic fixtures, but too high a level may result in scale formation. The TDS should be kept within appropriate limits—too high a concentration will result in a dull appearance to the water and make it unpleasant for bathing. The water will also be corrosive if too high a concentration of sulphates is present; conversely, a minimum level of calcium hardness should be maintained. In practice, regular filter backwashing, with fresh-water replenishment, will usually keep the pool water in a suitable chemical state (with so-called 'balanced water').

5 Health effects

Reported adverse health effects from pool use are relatively infrequent. References are included in the reviews by Galbraith (1980) and Jones & Bartlett (1985), unless otherwise indicated below; see also Kilvington *et al.* (1991).

5.1 Skin irritation and infections

As water is not a natural environment for the human skin, it is not surprising that skin problems are one of the most frequently reported health effects in pool users. An itchy rash covering most of the body exposed to the water is a common presentation of chemical irritation caused by the disinfectant. Chlorine sensitivity is less common than 'bromine rash', which occurs with some BCDMH-disinfected pools; the mechanism for the latter remains unclear, but it may be associated with the dimethylhydantoin element (Penny, 1991; Anon., 1995a). The presence of the rash is usually related to the degree of exposure. Thus, physiotherapists, who may spend much time in a hydrotherapy pool, are particularly at risk, so that immersion periods should be restricted. Such rashes typically appear within 12 h of using the pool and, once sensitized, a person may develop the rash within a few minutes of entering the pool.

In contrast, the itchy rash caused by an infection with *Ps. aeruginosa* develops more than 12 h, and usually more than 24 h, after leaving the pool (Penny, 1991). This rash is the result of infection of the hair follicles and usually resolves within a week in previously healthy persons. It is more particularly associated with spa pools, where the raised temperature and agitation of the water renders the skin more susceptible and, by rendering the disinfection process less effective, enhances the numbers of pseudomonads.

Similarly, otitis externa can be caused by chemical irritation or by infection with *Ps. aeruginosa.* It is more likely to be found in swimming pool users, where head immersion occurs. Frequent diving may assist the process.

Swimming-bath granuloma, caused by *Mycobacterium marinum*, is occasionally reported, usually in association with pools with cracked and roughened surfaces, wherein the organism can proliferate. Fungal infections of the feet and viral warts are often associated with pool use but are more likely to be spread by the pool surrounds than the water.

5.2 Eye irritation and infections

Conjunctivitis is a not uncommon complaint among swimmers but is usually the result of chemical irritation, such as with a low pH value or high combined-chlorine levels. Infective conjunctivitis is more likely to be spread directly from person to person by shared towels than by the water, but adenoviral pharyngoconjunctivitis has been reported in swimmers.

5.3 Respiratory irritation and infections

Some bathers, particularly those with asthma, may experience wheezing as a result of chemical irritation from the pool atmosphere (Anon., 1995b). Otitis media is occasionally associated with swimming, but this appears to be caused by infected mucus being forced up the Eustachian tube as a result of pressure changes while swimming or diving. Other reported infections include legionnaires' disease and Pontiac fever in users of spa pools, where the water agitation can produce aerosol conditions (Bartlett *et al.*, (1986). A Pontiac fever-like illness was associated with a pool contaminated with *Legionella micdadei* (Goldberg *et al.*, 1989). There is one report of *Ps. aeruginosa* pneumonia in a spa-pool user. *Mycobacterium chelonei* infection has been reported in children with cystic fibrosis who used a poorly maintained hydrotherapy pool (Basavaraj *et al.*, 1985).

5.4 Gastrointestinal infections

Outbreaks of giardiasis (Porter *et al.*, 1988) and cryptosporidiosis (Joce *et al.*, 1991) and of infection with Norwalk (Kappus *et al.*, 1989) and hepatitis A viruses (Mahoney *et al.*, 1992) have been associated with using a swimming-pool.

5.5 Other infections

These include a urinary-tract infection with *Ps. aeruginosa* in a spa-pool user and primary amoebic meningoencephalitis in users of warm-water pools. Blood-borne infections, such as hepatitis B and human immunodeficiency virus (HIV) infection, have not been associated with pool use.

6 Pool management

The water in a well-managed pool will appear clear and inviting and be maintained at the appropriate temperature, so enabling the bathers to enjoy a safe and enjoyable experience.

Compliance with the relevant safety standards (e.g. the Control of Substances Hazardous to Health Regulations 1988; Chemicals, Hazard Information and Packaging Regulations 1993; and *Safety in Swimming Pools* (Anon., 1995b)) will require careful management and regular plant maintenance. A record should be kept of the daily bathing load and other events, such as filter backwashing and the results of chemical and bacteriological tests. The pool water will require regular monitoring to ensure that its quality remains satisfactory. Chemical monitoring must be done on a daily basis, which will include, as a minimum, estimations of the residual disinfectant levels and the pH value at frequent intervals throughout the day when the pool is in use. In larger pools, the residual disinfectant and pH values are maintained at the correct levels by an automatic controller. Less frequently, depending on the degree of pool use, estimations of alkalinity, TDS, sulphate and calcium hardness should be done. Other less frequent tests include estimations of cyanuric acid in pools disinfected with a chlorinated isocyanurate and of dimethylhydantoin in pools using a BCDMH system. Table 15.1 gives recommended values for these (Anon., 1990, 1994, 1995a).

Bacteriological monitoring need not to be done often, provided that the chemical parameters are satisfactory. A routine sample should be taken once a month for most pools, but, because of the need for more intensive management, spa and hydrotherapy pools should be tested weekly. A colony count and tests for coliforms (including *Escherichia coli*) should be done routinely and also a test for the presence of *Ps. aeruginosa* in spa and hydrotherapy pools. Tests for other organisms, such as *Staph. aureus* and legionellas, need be done only as part of a special investigation—for example, when health problems have been linked with pool use—following consultation with the relevant public-health officials. Appropriate bacteriological guidelines are given in Table 15.2 (Anon., 1995a).

Table 15.1 Recommended values for chemical parameters.

Disinfectant residual	Value
Free chlorine	1–3 mg/l (less than 1 mg/l for ozone systems, depending on bacteriological-test results) 2.5–5.0 mg/l for chlorinated isocyanurate systems
Combined chlorine	Less than 1 mg/l (always less than half the free chlorine)
Total bromine (BCDMH pools)	4–6 mg/l
pH value	7.2–7.8
Total dissolved solids	Not more than 3000 mg/l
Alkalinity	More than 75 mg/l (as $CaCO_3$)
Sulphate	Not more than 360 mg/l
Calcium hardness	More than 75 mg/l (as $CaCO_3$)
Cyanuric acid	Not more than 200 mg/l
Dimethylhydantoin	Not more than 200 mg/l (a maximum of 100 mg/l advised for spa and hydrotherapy pools)

Table 15.2 Bacteriological guidelines for pool water.*†

Parameter	Guideline
Colony (plate) count	Less than 10 colony-forming units (cfu) after 24 h incubation at 37°C
Coliform count (including *E. coli*)	Not detected in 100 ml
Pseudomonas aeruginosa (spa and hydrotherapy pools)	Not detected in 100 ml

*An occasional colony count between 10 and 100 cfu/ml is acceptable, provided no coliforms or *E. coli* are detected and operating conditions are satisfactory.

†Low numbers of coliforms (less than 10/100 ml, but no *E. coli*) may occasionally be found when the colony count is satisfactory. This may be acceptable provided the residual disinfectant level and pH value are within the normal range and no coliforms are found in consecutive samples.

7 References

Anon. (1984) *The Treatment and Quality of Swimming Pool Water*. Department of the Environment. London: HMSO.

Anon. (1990) *Hygiene for Hydrotherapy Pools*. London: Public Health Laboratory Service Publications.

Anon. (1994) *Hygiene for Spa Pools*. London: Public Health Laboratory Service Publications.

Anon. (1995a) *Pool Water Guide: the Treatment and Quality of Swimming Pool Water*. Diss: Pool Water Treatment Advisory Group.

Anon. (1995b) *Safety in Swimming Pools*. London: Health and Safety Commission and Sports Council.

Anon. (1996) *List of Substances and Products Approved for Use in the Production of Potable Water from Seawater or Brackish Water and for the Treatment of Swimming Pool Water*. London: Drinking Water Inspectorate of the Department of the Environment (updated yearly).

Bartlett, C.L.R., Macrae, A.D. & Macfarlane, J.T. (1986) Legionella *Infections*. London: Edward Arnold.

Basavaraj, D.S., Hooper, W.L., Richardson, E.A., Penny, P., O'Mahony, M. & Begg, N. (1985) *Mycobacterium chelonei* associated with a hydrotherapy pool. *PHLS Communicable Disease Report*, **41**, 3–4.

Coombs, R., Spiby, H., Stewart, P. & Norman P. (1994) Water birth and infection in babies. *British Medical Journal*, **309**, 1089.

Galbraith, N.S. (1980) Infections associated with swimming pools. *Environmental Health*, **88**, 31–33.

Goldberg, D.J., Collier, P.W., Fallon, R.J. *et al.* (1989) Lochgoilhead fever: outbreak of non-pneumonic legionellosis due to *Legionella micdadei*. *Lancet*, **i**, 316–318.

Hollyoak, V.A. & Freeman, R. (1995) *Pseudomonas aeruginosa* and whirlpool baths. *Lancet*, **346**, 644.

Joce, R.E., Bruce, J., Kiely, D. *et al.* (1991) An outbreak of cryptosporidiosis associated with a swimming pool. *Epidemiology and Infection*, **107**, 497–508.

Jones, F. & Bartlett, C.L.R. (1985) Infections associated with whirlpools and spas. *Journal of Applied Bacteriology*, **59** (Suppl.), S61–66.

Kappus, K.D., Marks, J.S., Holman, R.C. *et al.* (1989) An outbreak of Norwalk gastroenteritis associated with swimming in a pool and secondary person-to-person transmission. *American Journal of Epidemiology*, **116**, 834–839.

Kilvington, S., Mann, P.G. & Warhurst, D.C. (1991) Pathogenic *Naegleria* amoebae in the waters of Bath: a fatality and its consequence. In *Hot Springs of Bath* (ed. Kellaway, G.A.), pp. 89–96. Bath: Bath City Council.

Mahoney, F.J., Farley, T.A., Kelso, K.Y., Wilson, S.A., Horan, J.M. & McFarland, L.M. (1992) An outbreak of hepatitis A associated with swimming in a public pool. *Journal of Infectious Diseases*, **165**, 613–618.

Penny, P.T. (1991) Hydrotherapy pools of the future—the avoidance of health problems. *Journal of Hospital Infection*, **18** (Suppl. A), 535–542.

Porter, J.D., Ragazzoni, H.P., Buchanon, J.D., Waskin, H.A., Juranek, D.D. & Parkin, W.E. (1988) *Giardia* transmission in a swimming pool. *American Journal of Public Health*, **78**, 659–662.

Rawal, J., Shah, A., Stirk, F. & Mehtas, S. (1994) Water birth and infection in babies. *British Medical Journal*, **309**, 511.

PART II

Preservation

Many industrial products must be adequately preserved in order to prevent microbial contamination that would be harmful to a patient or other 'consumer' or would render the products themselves unusable. In Part II, therefore, there are chapters on the preservation of pharmaceutical and cosmetic products (Chapter 16), food preservatives (Chapter 17) and preservation in specialized areas (Chapter 18A–F) that have considerable industrial importance.

In many instances, the underlying basis of preservation is similar and all build essentially on the principles laid down in Part I.

CHAPTER 16

Preservation of Medicines and Cosmetics

Dead flies cause the ointment of the apothecary to send forth a stinking savour. (Ecclesiastes 10: 1, The Bible, Authorized Version)

1 The nature of medicines and cosmetics

Medicines are formulated to assist in the administration of drugs to treat or prevent diseases or to alleviate symptoms in patients, making use of a wide variety of routes for administration. Cosmetics, however, are designed to deliver pigments, emollients, perfumes and other agents to enhance personal appearance, modify body odour or assist in body cleaning. Application is largely restricted to the skin, although such products as dentifrices or vaginal deodorants may come into contact with mucous membranes. It must also be anticipated that eye-area cosmetics will come into secondary contact with the cornea and conjunctiva. Although the intended outcomes for medicines and cosmetics are thus fundamentally different, there are many similarities in the nature of the formulations created and the uses (and abuses) to which both can be subjected, as well as fundamentally common microbiological problems which may be encountered. In order to create products that are not only elegant but also efficacious, stable and safe to use throughout their intended life, it is often necessary to include in the formulations a wide variety of other ingredients in addition to those intended to yield the specific therapeutic or cosmetic effect at specific sites in or on the body. While a few formulations may be simple aqueous solutions or dry powders, many are extremely complex, both in the number of ingredients used and in their physicochemical complexity. Some indications of this variation and complexity of medicinal and cosmetic formulations can be obtained from the reviews of Friberg (1984), Eccleston (1990), Frick (1992), Pena *et al.* (1993) and Lund (1994).

One of the problems to be dealt with to ensure the continued stability of the products and safety for the user is the possibility that microorganisms might enter medicines and cosmetics during manufacture, storage or use. The complex chemical and physicochemical nature of many formulations is often found to be conducive to the survival and even multiplication of such contaminants, unless specific precautions are taken to prevent it. Such survival, and even growth, may result in appreciable damage to the product and/or the user. The consequences of this damage will increasingly be reflected in loss of cash and prestige for the manufacturer, as strict product-liability legislation continues to come into operation. Good manufacturing practices should provide adequate control of contamination from raw materials and processing activities (see Chapter 11; Clegg & Perry, 1996). One procedure adopted to limit the establishment of microbial contamination after manufacture is to include one or more specific antimicrobial preservatives in the formulations, although other protective techniques are also available for use independently of, or in combination with, preservatives. Since the behaviour of antimicrobial agents in complex formulations usually differs appreciably from that in simple aqueous solution, it is essential to understand and fully evaluate the preservative needs and problems of individual products before selection of a preservative for any particular system.

2 The consequences of microbial contamination in medicines and cosmetics

The extremely wide diversity of microbial metabolic activity ensures that, if contaminants enter and are allowed to persist in medicines or cosmetics, they may present a variety of hazards, both to the user and to the stability of the products, including the hazards of infection, toxicity and degradation of the formulations, leading to the aggrievement of the user and possible litigation against the manufacturer. Recent reports indicated that UK medicines continue to show the presence of moderate levels of microbial contamination (Baird, 1988; Bloomfield, 1990), although stricter regulatory controls have improved the situation compared with that of the pre-1970 period (Beveridge, 1975). The UK Medicines Control Agency publicly report that, of the medicine recalls issued in recent years, those relating to microbiological defects represent a very small proportion of the total. However, in-use contamination hazards continue to be a particular problem for multidose eye-drops (Geyer *et al.*, 1995) and multidose injections (McHugh & Roper, 1995). In the USA, concern currently centres around the microbial hazards that accumulate during the use of cosmetics (Anon., 1992a; Tran & Hitchins, 1994). Few recent published data have been found for cosmetic contamination in the UK, although anecdotal evidence suggests a similar situation to that in the USA.

The most commonly reported microbial hazards in liquid medicines and cosmetics are pseudomonads and related Gram-negative rods, with bacterial and fungal spores predominating in dry tablets, capsules and cosmetic powders. Shared-use cosmetics accumulate human microflora, such as *Staphylococcus epidermidis, Staphylococcus aureus* and corynebacteria, as well as pathogenic fungi, yeasts and bacterial spores. Those which contain water or become wet during use reveal pseudomonads and related bacteria. The clinical and pharmaceutical significance of such contamination of medicines has been reviewed by Ringertz & Ringertz (1982), Denyer (1988) and Martone *et al.* (1987), and for cosmetics by Sharpell & Manowitz (1991). The implications for product spoilage of both have been discussed by Spooner (1996) and Beveridge (1998).

The risks (likelihood of harm actually occurring) are less clearly determined. These will depend upon the types and quantities of contaminating microorganisms, the route of administration of the product, the degree of tissue damage at the site of application, the immune status and degree of trauma of the patient, the ability of the formulation to encourage microbial survival and the level of preservative protection built into it. Prior to the 1960s, incidents of infection attributed to contaminated products seemed to be regarded as unfortunate but isolated occurrences; these included severe eye infections from contaminated ophthalmic solutions (Theodore & Feinstein, 1952) and tetanus infection of newborn children from contaminated talc dusting powders (Tremewan, 1946). During the 1960s, a number of key investigations demonstrated the existence of a much wider problem. Ayliffe *et al.* (1966) in the UK reported on an extensive outbreak of severe eye infections, traced to traditional but wholly inadequate official guidelines for the preservation and manufacture of ophthalmic solutions. The 'Evans Medical disaster', in which contaminated infusion fluids caused serious injury and probably contributed to some deaths, precipitated public awareness and led to an official inquiry (Clothier, 1972). In Sweden,

Kallings *et al.* (1966) linked an outbreak of salmonellosis to contaminated thyroid tablets and eye and other infections to a range of contaminated pharmaceuticals. Bruch (1972) in the USA similarly reported links between microbial contaminants in medicines and cosmetics and infections, Wilson, in a series of papers leading to Wilson & Ahearn (1977), and Baker (1959) clearly implicated contaminated eye-area cosmetics with severe eye infections. The more general role of opportunistic pathogens, such as the pseudomonads, and their implication in nosocomial infections was also becoming more recognized at this time. These reports stimulated an appreciable tightening of regulatory controls in many countries, and it is generally believed that the present situation is greatly improved. Comprehensive reviews of the earlier work have been made for medicines by Fassihi (1991) and for cosmetics by Sharpell & Manowitz (1991). Appreciable numbers of reports are still, however, being published of causal links between contaminated products and patient damage, of which a limited recent selection is now given.

Although evidence of acute pathogenic infections from medicines has always been rare, a syrup diluted with contaminated water in a West African hospital pharmacy was recently implicated in an outbreak of cholera (1993, personal communication to author).

There are still difficulties in preventing the build-up of pathogenic contaminants in multidose eye-drop containers during use (Geyer *et al.*, 1995), and the limited range of preservatives which are not damaging to the eye is creating problems in controlling microbial proliferation in contact-lens wet-storage cases (Hay *et al.*, 1996). Additionally, there are currently small but serious outbreaks of protozoal infections by *Acanthamoeba*, for which effective and safe preservatives are difficult to find (Seal, 1994). Total parenteral-nutrition infusions, compounded aseptically from sterile components, are conducive to microbial growth but cannot contain preservatives, due to their large volume. Recent cases of fatal infections from contaminated units indicate an urgent need for improved systems for dispensing and protecting them from contamination (Freund & Rimon, 1990; Anon., 1995a). Patients whose resistance has been weakened by trauma, chemotherapy, tissue damage or other disease often succumb to infection by opportunist contaminants, such as in mouthwashes, which are unlikely to cause harm to 'normal' patients Millership *et al.*, 1986). The infection of haemophiliacs with human immunodeficiency virus (HIV) from human-derived factor VIII (Brown *et al.*, 1995) and hepatitis C from blood-derived products (Anon., 1994c) has stimulated action on possible virus contamination of other products derived from human or biotechnology-derived origin, as has the contraction of Creutzfeldt–Jakob disease (CJD) by patients treated with human growth-hormone products from human origin (Anon., 1996a). Despite many well-publicized incidents, infection of patients with burnt or otherwise damaged skin caused by using antiseptic cleaning solutions contaminated with *Pseudomonas* spp. continues (Norman *et al.*, 1986), as does infection from contaminated nebulizer solutions (Hamil *et al.*, 1995).

The liberation of endotoxins by growth of Gram-negative contaminants in large-volume intravenous infusions and peritoneal-dialysis fluids remains a problem (Jarvis & Highsmith, 1984). More recent are incidents of algal toxins, such as mycocystins, surviving in process water and causing damage and even death when used for the dilution of kidney dialysates (Anon., 1996b). The implications of aflatoxin contamination in cosmetics has become of interest (El-Dessouki, 1992), now that there is a suggestion these toxins could penetrate the epidermis (Riley *et al.*, 1985).

With the link between infection and contaminated cosmetics long established (Bruch, 1972; Wilson & Ahearn, 1997), current concerns centre on the practice of in-store cosmetic multiuser 'testers', which have been shown to accumulate appreciable levels of contamination, including a variety of hazardous bacteria, yeasts and fungi, able to initiate severe eye infections (Anon., 1992a; Tran & Hitchins, 1994), and on infections identified with contaminated hand creams and lotions (Anon., 1992a).

Despite major advances in the quality of large-volume parenteral infusions, high numbers of localized and systemic infections occur, directly attributable to the administration devices themselves, such as catheters, for delivering them into the bloodstream (Tebbs *et al.*, 1996).

Papers describing specific incidences of the microbial deterioration of medicines and cosmetics used to be published regularly. However, these have been less frequently disclosed recently, possibly in keeping with the general concerns of both industries about increasingly stringent product-liability legislation. There is good anecdotal and unattributable information to indicate that spoilage problems have not yet disappeared. Recent reviews of the spoilage aspects of microbial contamination of medicines and cosmetics have been made by Parker (1984), Spooner (1996) and Beveridge (1998).

The weight of published evidence, both past and present, on the implications of microbial contamination for medicines and cosmetics demands that a careful and specific microbiological risk assessment is made for each individual product at its design and validation stages, using conventional risk-assessment techniques (Smith, 1984; McIntosh, 1987; Begg, 1990; Rodford, 1996). These must take into account worst-case scenarios, such as the possibility that eye cosmetics may be applied, for example, while driving, where, due to inattention, an applicator might scratch the cornea (Anon., 1991a), or that multidose eye-drop units may well receive varied and appreciable contamination during use by the lay public. Such assessments should take into account the highly critical expectations of the public concerning standards for medicines and other consumer products, which are far greater than those for their food. When a recent survey (Anon., 1996h) showed that 35% of chickens and chicken portions on sale in major UK supermarkets were unfit for human consumption, it generated no more than a few lines in some newspapers on one day.

3 The effect of intrinsic formulation parameters and their manipulation on contamination and spoilage

The overall risk of harm, should microorganisms enter a product during storage or use, will be influenced by their ease of entry into a container, the type and magnitude of the contaminant bioburden, the mode of intended use of the product and the microbiologically conducive, or adverse, chemical and physicochemical characteristics of the formulation. Since the inclusion of antimicrobial preservatives may not always be desirable or possible or offer fully adequate protection, it may be necessary to enhance their action, or replace them, by subtle modification of various intrinsic parameters in order to limit the risks of contamination and spoilage to acceptable levels. Such manipulation forms the basis for the preservation and protection of many foodstuffs, where the ability to add antimicrobial preservatives is strictly limited by law. A wealth of basic and applied food-protection research is available for those who wish to assess these principles for application to medicines and cosmetics, and the reviews of Chirife & Favetto (1992), Dillon & Board (1994a), Gould (1996) and Roberts (1995) are recommended. Their application to pharmaceuticals and cosmetics has been considered briefly by Orth (1993b) and Beveridge (1998).

The ultimate in in-use contamination control would be to provide products as individually packaged, sterile, single-dosage or application units, but this is only cost-effective where there is a high infective risk, such as with eye-drops for hospital use, or where preservatives cannot be used because of overriding toxicity concerns. Possibly the worst-case scenario is that of cosmetic 'tester' kits provided in stores for repeated use by various customers, resulting in appreciable and varied levels of contamination (Tran & Hitchins, 1994). The repeated use and dilution of mascara, eye-liner and eye-shadow with variously moistened applicators also results in a build-up of contamination and attenuation of preservative protection (Orth *et al.*, 1992).

It is generally believed that the replacement of wide-mouthed jars, with ready access for fingers, by flexible tubes for creams and ointments has reduced the degree of contamination of residual product, as has the redesign of bottles to reduce the accumulation of liquid residues around the mouth and neck, and the introduction of plastic 'squeezy' eye-drop bottles is thought to be an improvement over the conventional glass-dropper bottle (Allwood, 1990a). Brannan & Dille (1990) found that slit-top and pump-action closures provided greater protection for a shampoo and skin lotion than a conventional screw-cap closure.

The longer a product is in use, the greater is the

opportunity for contamination to accumulate and the chance of growth and spoilage being initiated, once an adaptive lag period has ensued. Some medicines, extemporaneously prepared or reconstituted in the pharmacy, are dispensed with a short use life of 1–2 weeks, which appears to reduce the risk of contamination and growth acceptably. Oldham & Andrews (1996) found that contamination could be held at reasonable levels in many types of unpreserved eye-drops for up to 7 days, provided they were also stored in a refrigerator.

The response of contaminants to the physicochemically complex environment of many pharmaceutical and cosmetic formulations will differ significantly from that in simple laboratory media (Beveridge, 1998), being markedly influenced by their spatial arrangement (Wimpenny, 1981) and the phase status of the systems (Verrips, 1989). There are many reports of modified behaviour of microorganisms at solid–liquid and liquid–liquid interfaces, but the evidence for increased resistance or longevity compared with freely planktonic situations is far from clear (van Loosdrecht *et al.*, 1990). An increasing understanding of the survival strategies of microorganisms in sparse ecosystems (Roszac & Colwell, 1987) may provide an insight into the longevity of vegetative contaminants in seemingly unlikely products, e.g. *Salmonella* spp. in chocolate (Greenwood & Hooper, 1983) and thyroid tablets (Kallings *et al.*, 1966) or vegetative bacteria in 'dry' ingredients, such as powdered plants, starch powder and powdered hydroxymethylcellulose and aluminium hydroxide gel (Payne, 1990).

The nutritional requirements of most saprophytic non-fastidious spoilage contaminants are likely to be well met in almost all pharmaceuticals and cosmetics, since many ingredients are easily biodegradable, and even the trace residues of non-specific chemical contaminants present in most commercial ingredients are likely to provide ample nutrients to permit growth. For example, even standard distilled and demineralized water contains sufficient trace nutrients to permit ample growth of pseudomonads and related species (Favero *et al.*, 1971). It is usually the physicochemical parameters of the formulation which are the determining factors as to whether growth will or will not take place.

The complex water requirements of microorganisms (Gould, 1989; Wiggins, 1990) necessitate that, if they are to replicate, they must successfully compete for ready access to water against the other ingredients of a formulation that can also interact with it, often in strong and complex manners (e.g. Beveridge & Bendall, 1988). Manipulation of product water activity (A_w, an indicator of the ready availability of water to contaminants) to a level below the minimum essential for growth offers a major potential for protection of some products. It is possible to reduce the A_w of tablets, pastilles, capsules and pharmaceutical and cosmetic powders and powder compacts sufficiently by drying to provide their major mode of spoilage protection, although some contaminants may continue to survive in a senescent state for a considerable time (Sommerville, 1981; Flatau *et al.*, 1996). It is then essential to maintain this low A_w throughout the life of the product, by using water-vapour-resistant bottles or film-strip packing; otherwise protection will be lost. The use of vapour-repellent film coatings (Whiteman, 1995) has been suggested to assist in the control of spoilage of bulk tablets intended for distribution to humid climates (Fassihi *et al.*, 1978). The A_w of some aqueous systems can be lowered sufficiently to give useful protection by the addition of quite large amounts of water-binding low-molecular-weight solutes, such as sucrose (66% w/v, approx. $A_w = 0.86$) in, for example, reconstituted antibiotic syrups, sorbitol (> *c.* 35% w/v) for dentifrice pastes (Morris & Leech, 1996), glycerol (> *c.* 40%) for cosmetic lotions, and urea (10–20%) for some cosmetics (Jackson, 1993). Lintner (1997) described the use of polyacrylamide hydrogels in cosmetic creams to enhance formulation robustness, presumably by very effectively lowering A_w. While even the most osmotolerant bacteria (micrococci) will require A_w levels in excess of *c.* 0.82 for growth and few common fungi or yeast will grow below an A_w of 0.65 (Beuchat, 1983), one needs to be on guard against the rare, rogue, highly osmotolerant mould or yeast, where antimicrobial preservation may also be necessary. Strongly alcoholic formulations, such as perfumes, have a low A_w, as well as being antimicrobial in their own right. Condensed-moisture films can develop with sufficiently high A_w on the surfaces of waxy cosmetics, such as lipsticks, or highly viscous liquids, such as toothpastes, or on compressed cosmetic powders to permit localized fungal growth, when they are persistently exposed to humid environments, such as steamy bathrooms, or if moisture is regularly applied by mouth or applicator during use. Growth of contaminants has occurred in condensed films under the tops of containers formed when hot aqueous products have been packed into cold containers. This effect can also result in appreciable dilution and loss of localized efficiency of any preservative present (Bhadauria & Ahearn, 1980). Should sparse fungal growth be initiated on marginally dried products or those which have become damp during storage, such as tablets packed in bulk, water generated by respiration will create locally raised A_w levels and initiate a cycle of enhanced rates of growth, leading to appreciable levels of spoilage (e.g. Beveridge & Bendall, 1988).

The food industry's wide use of pH reduction or gas environment modification of redox potentials to control spoilage is of limited application to medicines and cosmetics. However, the pH of a product will influence the type of spoilage that might be initiated, although this itself may result in a pH change, allowing other contaminants to take over. Thus, the low pH of fruit juice-flavoured medicines may aid fungal spoilage but suppress bacterial growth, while the slightly alkaline antacid mixtures would favour growth of pseudomonads and related bacteria. It is unlikely that the redox potential of most pharmaceuticals or cosmetics is likely to be low enough to favour anaerobic spoilage, as seen in some foodstuffs. However, Smart & Spooner (1972) reported that initial spoilage and depletion of oxygen tension in a pharmaceutical product by a pseudomonad then permitted establishment of a secondary anaerobic attack, with striking consequences.

Low temperature storage (8–12°C) is used to improve the short-term stability of some unpreserved, or weakly preserved, medicines, such as unpreserved eye-drops (Oldham & Andrews, 1996) and reconstituted antibiotic syrups. Short-term deep freezing (≤ 20°C) is used to further limit the risk of growth of any contaminants introduced during the aseptic dispensing of total parenteral nutrition (TPN) products, prior to use. Where dispensed products are to be 'stored in a cool place' during use, the growth-inhibitory effect of the reduced temperature needs to be balanced against the consequent, and often significant, reduction in efficiency of any preservative present.

Preservative action in most complex formulations usually results in residual, quite low, levels of saprophytic contaminants, which are not considered to be of significant risk. However, in some circumstances, these are able to slowly adapt to their new environment (Orth *et al.* 1985), replicate and initiate gross spoilage, dubbed the Phoenix phenomenon by Orth & Lutes Anderson, (1993c). Additionally, there are an increasing number of reports of inherent and seemingly acquired resistance of contaminants to a wide variety of preservatives. These phenomena and indications of their implications for the formulator have been discussed in detail by Russell & Gould (1988) and Gilbert & Das (1996). Chapman *et al.* (1996) reviewed the phenomenon as it relates to preservative resistance emergence in cosmetic formulations.

4 Attenuation of preservative effectiveness in complex formulations

Replacement in the early 1950s of anionic emulsifiers and relatively simple, slightly alkaline, creams by non-ionic, readily biodegradable, surfactants and more sophisticated formulations of more neutral pH resulted in an increasing number of spoilage problems and a growing realization that preservative molecules were doing appreciably more in these complex systems than merely reacting with microorganisms. Concurrent interest in the physicochemical characteristics of multiphase formulations revealed a variety of interactive possibilities for preservatives (Wedderburn, 1964). Recent reviews by van Doorne (1990), Kostenbauder (1991) and Dempsey (1996) provide detailed and current accounts of these phenomena, and the Cosmetic, Toiletry and Perfumery Association (CTPA) Guidelines place them in a practical context (Anon., 1993b).

It is important to obtain information on the intrinsic properties of any preservative under consideration, from sources such as this book, Wallhaeusser (1984), the *CTPA Guidelines* (Anon., 1993b) and *Martindale: The Extra Pharmaco-*

poeia (Anon., 1996c), in addition to that provided by manufacturers. Detailed monographs for those preservatives commonly used in medicines have been prepared by Wade and Weller (1994). The aqueous solubility of some commonly used preservatives is low and some form salts or complexes with very low-solubility products, which precipitate from solution. Thus, the usefulness of chlorhexidine is restricted by its ability to form insoluble products with chloride, sulphate, phosphate or citrate ions and anionic surfactants. Quaternary ammonium preservatives form insoluble complexes with anionic surfactants and a range of anionic inorganic ions. Benzoates and parabens form insoluble and discolouring complexes with iron salts, chlorocresol precipitates with phosphates, and phenylmercuric nitrate precipitates with chloride ions. Bronopol has formed complexes with unprotected aluminium in flexible tubes. Contrastingly, preservatives with a high vapour pressure, such as chloroform, become appreciably depleted when containers are repeatedly opened during routine use (Lynch *et al.*, 1977).

Preservative stability will be influenced by formulation pH, storage temperature, shelf-life and conditions of processing. Thus, isothiazolinones (Anon., n.d.) and bronopol (McCarthy, 1984) deteriorate significantly if processing temperatures exceed 55°C. Chlorobutanol is unstable around neutral or alkaline pH and suffers appreciable destruction at autoclaving temperatures (Holdsworth *et al.*, 1984). Unless light-proof containers are used, the photocatalysed deterioration of preservatives such as the phenolic, quaternary ammonium and organomercurial agents may become significant. Paraben loss will occur by steam distillation at process temperatures approaching 100°C and have poor stability in slightly alkaline, and above, products (Reiger, 1994). Transesterification between parabens and polyols, such as sorbitol, may occur and result in significant loss of activity (Runesson & Gustavii, 1986) Alternatively, the formaldehyde-releasing agents depend on suitable conditions to provide a slow, steady decomposition and release of formaldehyde to ensure preservative protection over the full life of the product, without too rapid a conversion early on in the product's life leaving little reservoir for the later stages of use; an example is pH 5–6.5 for bronopol (Allwood *et al.*, 1994). It cannot be presumed that preservative degradation products will be inert. Thus, an excessive rate of formaldehyde release might create undue irritancy, and bronopol degradation releases nitrite ions, which might result in the formation of potentially toxic nitrosamines, if ingredients such as amine soaps are present in the formulation or if it comes into contact with dietary amines (Anon., 1992a; Allwood *et al.*, 1994).

Chemical reactions responsible for the inhibition of microorganisms by preservatives are often complex and influenced to a greater extent than for many *in vitro* reactions by variations in preservative concentration, product pH and storage temperature. These are dealt with elsewhere in this book (Chapter 3) and will not be reconsidered here in detail. However, the review of concentration exponents by Hugo & Denyer (1987) is essential reading for formulators. The concurrent influence of these factors on preservative efficiency is believed to be somewhat cumulative. For example, consider that chlorocresol 0.1% w/v (concentration exponent, η, = 6; temperature coefficient, Q_{10}, = 5) was chosen to preserve a multidose injection solution based on experimental data which showed that this would effectively kill an inoculum of contaminant bacteria in 10 min at 30°C. If the injection were actually stored at 10°C in a domestic refrigerator and the final chlorocresol concentration was 20% under strength due to absorptive and evaporative losses during sterilization, then, taking into account the combined influence of η and Q_{10}, one might expect an increase from 10 to 950 min to achieve a similar preservative effect (other factors remaining constant). In practice, such an attenuation in efficiency would probably result in self-sterilizing capability failure.

It is commonly believed that preservatives are usually far less effective at low A_w and virtually inactive at the very low A_w levels expected of powders, tablets or capsules, although there is only limited published work to support this. Low levels of various electrolytes have long been known to influence the activity of phenolic disinfectants, often with enhancement of effect (McCullogh, 1945). Cooper (1947, 1948), Agnostopolous & Kroll (1978) and Kroll & Agnostopolous (1981) generally found marked reductions in the efficiency of phenolic and other disinfectants and preservatives in solutions, with A_w appreciably lowered by addition of higher concentrations of sucrose, glycerol and similar glycols. There is good anecdotal evidence that manufacturers generally find the efficacy of preservatives in syrups and cosmetics such as toothpastes to be appreciably weaker than in simple aqueous solutions with high A_w. This author (E.G. Beveridge, unpublished data) and Boyd (personal communication) also found that the inhibitory properties of a number of phenolic preservatives was generally greatly reduced in liquid media, with A_w appreciably reduced by the addition of low-molecular-weight solutes, such as sucrose, glycerol and polyethylene glycols. Bos *et al.* (1989) found that incorporation of parabens and sorbate into lactose–starch tablets contaminated with *Bacillus brevis* spores did not reduce subsequent spore viability while maintained at a suitably low A_w. Ethylene oxide (Burgess & Reich, 1993) and high temperatures (Wood, 1993) are markedly less effective as sterilizing agents for powders and 'dry' products with very low A_w, when compared with medicines with high A_w. It might be extremely difficult to devise an experiment to evaluate fully the *in situ* efficacy of preservatives under the very low A_w conditions of powders towards vegetative microbial cells, since attempts to assess survivors would generally raise A_w and activate the preservatives during the recovery phase. When the A_w of the external environment is lowered below the osmoregulatory capacity of a microbial cell by non-permeant solutes, growth and other activities cease or are reduced to very low levels, due to the inability of the cell to accumulate sufficient intracellular water for the necessary metabolic reactions to occur (Gould, 1989). Possibly, the apparently minimal efficiency of preservatives at very low A_w indicates a similar critical influence of intracellular water levels upon antimicrobial reactions.

When preservatives are incorporated into multiphase formulations, their efficiency is generally markedly attenuated by a variety of competing interactive possibilities, which have been reviewed by Attwood & Florence (1983), van Doorne (1990) and Dempsey (1996). Partitioning of preservatives between oil and water phases will occur, in line with their partition coefficients, which may be different for commercial-grade systems from those of simple laboratory-devised oil–water mixtures of purified ingredients. Appreciable migration into oil phases of lipophilic preservatives, such as the parabens and phenolic agents, is likely, with less effect on the more hydrophilic preservatives, such as imidazolidinyl urea or the isothiazolinones. The oil : water ratio will also significantly influence the extent of overall migration, and there is the probability that localized preservative concentration will occur at oil–water interfaces. Since microbes also concentrate at interfaces, there are reasonable theoretical grounds for anticipating enhanced activity here (Attwood & Florence, 1983). Some evidence for this was provided by Bean *et al.* (1962), but was discounted by Dempsey (1996).

Preservatives can react with polymeric suspending and thickening agents, such as tragacanth, alginates, starch mucilage and polyethyleneglycols, by displacement of water of hydration, even to the extent of forming insoluble sticky complexes (Wedderburn, 1964; McCarthy, 1984). Cyclodextrins have also been found to interact with a variety of preservatives (Loftsson *et al.*, 1992). However, there are also reports of enhancement of activity for some preservative/polymer combinations (Yousef *et al.*, 1973).

Adsorption on to the surfaces of suspended drug and cosmetic ingredients can also significantly reduce preservative efficiency. Examples include adsorption of parabens on to magnesium trisilicate (Allwood, 1982) and loss of chlorhexidine on to mineral earths, such as kaolin and calamine (Qawas *et al.*, 1986), parabens on to cosmetic pigments (Sakamoto *et al.*, 1987) and benzoic acid on to sulphadimidine particles (Beveridge & Hope, 1967) and various other incidences of adsorption (McCarthy, 1984). In some cases, adsorption is followed by absorption into the solids to form a 'solid' solution. This is a particular problem with preservatives and plastic containers. For example, phenolics and parabens absorb appreciably into nylon and plasticized PVC (Dean, 1992) and chlorobutanol is absorbed appreciably into polyethylene bottles during autoclaving (Holdsworth *et al.*, 1984). Kakemi *et al.* (1971) examined the absorption of parabens and benzalkonium chloride into various container plastics. Aspinall *et al.*

(1983) found that the absorption of phenylmercuric acetate into low-density polythene eye-drop bottles could be inhibited by the presence of phosphate ions, and Miezitis *et al.* (1979) showed that presoaking of polyethylene containers in preservative solutions reduced the amount of subsequent absorption of preservative from the ophthalmic solutions. Appreciable losses of preservative by absorption into 'rubber' sealing wads to injection vials and 'rubber' eye-dropper teats can be reduced by careful selection of elastomer type and by presoaking and autoclaving them in concentrated preservative solution before use. Methods for assessing possible preservative–plastic interactions are provided by Wang & Chien (1984).

When preservatives are added to complex formulations, the above phenomena are likely to interact competitively and the eventual distribution of preservative molecules by the different phenomena between the different ingredients and phases will be determined by the relative affinities of each for the other and the relative proportions of each. In highly viscous and complex systems, full equilibration might never happen within the life of the product. As contaminant microorganisms will represent a minute mass in proportion to the vast amounts of the other components, their 'share' could be expected to be dramatically restricted in many situations. It is generally believed that the proportion of total added preservative responsible ('available') for any inhibition of contaminants is principally that which remains 'free' or unbound to other ingredients in the aqueous phase (Attwood & Florence, 1983; van Doorne, 1990; Dempsey, 1996). Preservative molecules in the oil or micellar phases, or bound to other ingredients, are considered not to contribute directly, except that slow back-migration should occur as preservative concentrations become depleted in the aqueous phase. Experimental evidence for this is limited and might be difficult to obtain. However, there is very good indirect physicochemical evidence to support this contention.

Attempts have been made to develop equations to calculate probable 'free', or 'unbound', preservative concentrations, based on partition coefficients, oil : water ratios, solubilization constants and polymer-binding constants, which have been reviewed by Attwood & Florence (1983). For example, Mitchell & Kamzi (1975) proposed equations such as the following for estimating the 'free' or 'available' preservative in the aqueous phase of an emulsified system:

$$C = C_w\ [1 + nK(M)/(1 + KC_w) + K_w^o\phi](1 + \phi)$$

Where C = gross concentration of preservative in system; C_w = 'unbound' preservative in aqueous phase; n = number of binding sites on surfactant; K = association constant for preservative and surfactant; M = preservative–surfactant ratio for a given surfactant concentration; K_w^o = oil : water partition coefficient; ϕ = oil : water-phase ratio.

They were able to produce some correlation of experimentally determined measurements of bactericidal activity for chlorocresol in cetomacrogol emulsified systems with estimates obtained by their equations (Kamzi & Mitchell, 1978). While these equations have been of value in resolving theoretical concerns and in providing some limited practical information, in general there is difficulty in obtaining adequate values for commercially available ingredients for them to be of general practical application. Another approach has been to estimate the unbound preservative in the aqueous phase by dialysis and measurement of the agent in the dialysate (Attwood & Florence, 1983; McCarthy, 1984), with some formulators believing that useful practical information has been obtained. Kurup *et al.* (1991) compared estimates of 'unbound' preservative in the aqueous phases of emulsified systems as obtained by equilibrium dialysis with direct measurements of antimicrobial activity, and reported that the efficiency of their emulsified systems was greater than that of corresponding simple aqueous solutions containing those concentration of preservatives estimated from the dialysis determinations to be 'available' in the aqueous phase of these systems.

As preservative molecules inactivate microorganisms, they themselves become inactivated and are no longer available to inhibit subsequent additions of contaminants. For those preservatives with high concentration exponents, such as the phenolic agents, this steady depletion of available agent can result in significant attenuation in preservative efficacy during repeated use and in contamination of multidose formulations. The relative non-specificity of preservative reactivity will mean that appreciable preservative depletion will also occur from interaction with the significant amount of non-microbial detritus ('dirt') also introduced during repeated and prolonged use. This must be allowed for, when deciding upon the necessary preservative capacity of a formulation, at the design stage.

It is clear that effective preservation of complex formulations is only likely to be successful if there is a good appreciation of these interactive problems. Even then, it may not be possible to provide highly efficient preservation for many multiphase systems without recourse to more potent preservatives whose enhanced antimicrobial potency is matched by unacceptable levels of irritancy. Provided the problem of preservation is fully explored at the earliest stages of formulation development, it is sometimes possible to reduce the worst interactive effects by knowledgeable selection of ingredients and preservative(s) to maximize the levels of 'free' agent in the aqueous phase.

5 Enhancement of preservative effectiveness

There have been numerous attempts to enhance preservative effectiveness by using preservatives in combination with each other or with various potentiators (Denyer, 1996). For this strategy to be successfully applied, there must be clear evidence of enhancement for any selected combination, rather than the creation of multicomponent preservative systems on the basis of wishful thinking (Parker, 1973).

It is generally believed that, by using combinations of parabens, each approaching its aqueous solubility maximum, greater levels of unbound paraben will remain in the aqueous phase of multiphase systems, with some evidence that this does offer enhanced preservative protection for such formulations (Haag & Loncrini, 1984). It may also be possible to reduce the extent of such migration into the lipophilic regions, by the addition of hydrophilic cosolvents to modify oil : water and micellar distribution coefficients more in favour of preservative retention in the aqueous phase. For example, Darwish & Bloomfield (1995) were able to improve the efficacy of parabens in an emulsion by the incorporation of modest concentrations of ethanol, propylene glycol or glycerol as hydrophilic cosolvents.

Individual preservatives are sometimes less effective against certain microbial species than others, and the careful selection of preservative combinations can offer protection from a wider range of likely contaminants. Thus, it is believed that mixtures of methyl, propyl and butyl parabens have a wider combined antimicrobial spectrum than each individual ester (Haag & Loncrini, 1984). Imidazolidinyl ureas have weak antifungal properties and parabens are less effective against pseudomonads, but combinations of both yield usefully improved protection against both contaminants (Rosen & Berke, 1984). Combinations of parabens with phenoxyethanol are also reported to provide a wider spectrum of activity than either alone (Hall, 1984).

Synergy—activity observed with combinations of agents greater than that anticipated from the sum of their activities when individually applied—is often confused with cases where a widening of antimicrobial spectrum, or simple addition, has been observed. True synergism is often species-specific and most apparent at quite specific ratios of the agents involved. Practically useful examples of preservative synergy include mixtures of parabens (Gilliland *et al.*, 1992), parabens with imidazolidinyl ureas (Rosen & Berke, 1984), parabens with phenoxyethanol (Hall, 1984), chlorocresol with phenoxyethanol (Denyer *et al.*, 1986), parabens with acrylic acid homopolymers and copolymers (Orth *et al.*, 1989) and others (Anon., 1993b). Antagonism between preservatives is uncommon (Pons *et al.*, 1992), but there are reports of antagonism between sorbic acid and parabens (Rehm, 1959) and between benzalkonium chloride and chlorocresol (Pons *et al.*, 1992).

The effectiveness of some preservatives can be enhanced by the presence of a variety of materials which in themselves are not strongly antimicrobial. Thus, the chelating agent ethylenediamine tetraacetic acid (EDTA) usefully potentiates the activity of quaternary ammonium agents, parabens, phenolics, sorbic acid and imidazolidinyl ureas (Hart, 1984) and lauricidin (Kabara, 1980), and is now used to a significant extent in cosmetic formulations. It is also used to potentiate various preservative systems towards pseudomonads and similar microorganisms in medicines, particularly those for use in and around the eyes (Cook & Youssuf, 1994). Essential oils and fragrances may enhance overall preservative protection (Woodruff, 1995). Humectants, such as glycerol and proplylene glycol, in modest concentration can assist in overall protection. The gallate ester antioxidants, butylated hydroxyanisole (BHT) and butylated hydroxytoluene (BHA) also reveal modest antimicrobial activity, which can assist conventional antimicrobial preservatives (Kabara, 1984b).

Biochemical explanations for such enhancements of antimicrobial activity are not always clear. However, in a number of cases, there is good evidence to indicate that enhancement is related to the ability of chaotropic agents, such as EDTA, to disorganize lipopolysaccharides in the outer membranes of Gram-negative bacteria, a well-known barrier to the penetration of many agents (Vaara, 1992). Phenoxyethanol (Gilbert *et al.*, 1977) and benzalkonium chloride (Vaara, 1992) are known to disrupt the barrier properties of the cytoplasmic membrane. In both cases, this would then aid greater penetration of the main preservative to its site of lesion. In other cases, such as the synergy of chlorocresol with phenylethanol (Denyer *et al.*, 1986) and acetates with lactates or propionates (Moon, 1983), there are indications of more specific mechanistic interactions.

Laboratory techniques, such as those described by Pons *et al.* (1992) and Gilliland *et al.* (1992), often demonstrate synergy between combinations of antimicrobial agents, although only a few prove to be of effective value in practical situations. It is therefore essential to confirm any apparent indications of synergy by full testing in complete formulations before placing any commercial reliance upon them.

6 Prediction of preserved-product efficacy

Due to the many interactive possibilities for both microorganisms (Section 3) and preservatives (Section 4) in complex formulations, it is almost impossible to predict, with any reasonable degree of precision, the ultimate effectiveness of a preservative in all but the simplest solutions. It is therefore necessary to obtain some assurance of likely in-use and abuse performance, by conducting a direct, microbiological, preservative-effectiveness test on the complete formulation. Detailed reviews of such test procedures and the problems associated with them have been made recently by Baird (1995) for medicines and by Brannan (1995), Perry (1995) and Leak *et al.* (1996) for cosmetics, while Hopton and Hill (1987) reviewed test methodology for a wider range of commercial materials.

Most conventional preservative-efficacy testing protocols share common features and intentions, although the fine details and interpretation of the results vary significantly. Aliquots of complete formulations should be tested in their final containers, where possible, as these can influence overall efficiency (Akers & Taylor, 1990; Brannan & Dille, 1990). The testing of diluted cosmetic products should also be considered where dilution in use might occur, such as with shampoos in bottles or bars of soap taken into the shower or bath, as well as the addition of an organic load to simulate in-use soiling (Chan & Prince, 1981; Orth, 1993a; Brannan, 1995). Formulations without preservative should be examined for possible inherent inhibitory activity. Samples should be tested within a general-stability test programme to determine whether preservative effectiveness will remain throughout the intended life of the product. A limited range of test microorganisms, representative of likely contaminants, is usually selected from official culture collections, which is often supplemented in individual companies with known problem strains, such as osmophilic yeasts for sugary formulations, 'wild' strains from the factory environment or those isolated from previously spoiled batches (Spooner & Croshaw, 1981). Usually, only elementary methods of cultivation and harvesting of inocula are used, despite much evidence that even minor variations here can dramatically influence the antimicrobial sensitivity of the resultant test suspension (Brown & Gilbert, 1995; Gilbert & Brown, 1995). In general, routine cultivation is well known to attenuate survival and spoilage potential appreciably, and numerous attempts have been made to develop maintenance systems that retain the aggressiveness of wild isolates, often with only limited success. Thus, Spooner and Croshaw (1981) cultivated contaminant isolates in unpreserved product, and Flawn *et al.* (1973) maintained the shampoo-degrading activity of tap-water isolates by routine cultivation in mineralsalt media containing anionic surfactants. The ability of pseudomonads and related environmental isolates to degrade parabens and other phenolic preservatives, as well as a variety of surfactants, could be retained over considerable periods by routine cultivation in minimal liquid media containing the agents as the primary carbon source (E.G. Beveridge, personal observations). There was a formal proposal (Anon., 1992b) that challenge organisms for the *United States Pharmacopoeia* (USP) effectiveness test should be monitored routinely for sensitivity to phenol, but this has not appeared in the final, published, version.

Formulations are usually challenged by intimate mixing with the microbial suspensions and incubation at temperatures relevant to likely use conditions. Where solid formulations, such as powders or cakes, oily or waxy products, such as lipsticks, or viscous creams or gels are to be examined, it may be necessary first to disperse them in an aqueous medium, either directly or with the aid of a dispersant, such as a surfactant; for some solid products, such as soap bars, direct surface inoculation is a more realistic option (Curry *et al.*, 1993; Perry, 1995). Single-species inocula are more commonly used than mixed challenges, although there might be potential advantages to multiple-species inoculation. The latter is not generally used for medicines (Baird, 1995) but is often used for cosmetic testing (Curry *et al.*, 1993; Muscatiello, 1993; Leak *et al.*, 1996). Inocula are commonly added as a single large challenge (single-challenge testing) and monitored for inhibition over a specified period. Multiple challenges (repeat-challenge testing), which repeat the inoculation at set intervals for a specified number of cycles or until the product fails, are also used, particularly for cosmetics (Spooner & Croshaw, 1981; Shaqra & Husari, 1987; Sabourin, 1990).

Preservative efficiency is estimated by cultivating and counting survivors from small aliquots of the inoculated formulation added to culture media, either by conventional colony formation or via membrane filtration or by using most-probable-number schemes with liquid media (Fels, 1995). This presumes an initial uniform distribution of inoculum and any subsequent growth in the product, both assumptions being unlikely to be correct (Brannan, 1995). Not only may it be necessary to ensure the neutralization of residual preservative before recovery is undertaken, but the capability of the recovery media to provide optimal resuscitation conditions for preservative-damaged, but still viable, survivors must also be considered, as many of the standard laboratory media are somewhat stressful to such damaged microorganisms (Baird, 1996). There is a need to confirm that the recovery procedures are not inhibitory to preservative-stressed survivors. One major problem is that of regrowth from very low numbers of survivors after a very long delay—the Phoenix phenomenon (Orth, 1993c). Most official test protocols are not conducted for long enough to provide for this possibility, but some companies include prolonged testing for this reason.

In interpreting the results of challenge tests, most workers would hope to receive an indication of likely performance of their formulation in the market-place. Most official and semiofficial test protocols, however, are guarded in the interpretation of data obtained from their scheme. Thus, the USP preservative-effectiveness test is 'provided to demonstrate, in multiple dose parenteral, otic, nasal and ophthalmic products made with aqueous bases or vehicles, the effectiveness of any added antimicrobial preservative', without clearly indicating effectiveness for what (Anon., 1995c). The *CTPA Guidelines* state that 'the ability to withstand a known microbial insult simply demonstrates the bioavailability of the preservative system in the formulation' (Anon., 1994a).

The *British Pharmacopoeia* (BP) 1998 efficacy of antimicrobial preservation test (Anon., 1998a) covers a wider range of dosage forms and has more stringent compliance criteria than the *European Pharmacopoeia* (EP) Anon., 1996d or the USP (Anon., 1995c; Davison, 1996). It is intended for checking at the development stage that the 'antimicrobial activity of the preparation as such, or with the addition of a suitable preservative or preservative, provides adequate protection from adverse effects that may arise from microbial contamination or proliferation during storage and use of the preparation'. The basic test uses four stock cultures, with no particular record of spoilage or contamination relevance, of *Aspergillus niger,*

Candida albicans, Pseudomonas aeruginosa and *Staph. aureus*, which may be supplemented with other strains or species that may represent likely challenges for that product. A single challenge of 10^5–10^6 microorganisms/g or cm^3 of formulation is used, the product is incubated at 20–25°C and aliquots are tested for survivors at specified intervals by conventional plate count or membrane-filtration techniques. Two levels of criteria, A and B, are given for acceptable performance in the test, level A being the recommended level of efficiency, except where this is not possible for reasons such as toxicity, and then level B applies. The relatively weak compliance criteria for some formulations is indicative of the problems in achieving adequate preservative efficacy in complex products (Table 16.1).

Although preservative-efficacy evaluation with panels of volunteers, using test formulations under controlled conditions, is not generally realistic for medicines, this type of follow-up test is quite common for cosmetics (Lindstrom, 1986; Anon., 1990c). Thus, Farrington *et al.* (1994) developed a panel test whereby volunteers applied the test products for a specified number of times to axillary areas, ensuring that the application fingers came into contact with residual product. Formulations were then examined for any accumulated contamination. There is some agreement that results obtained from in-use panel tests do show a reasonable correlation with estimates obtained from *in vitro* challenge testing and general in-use performance for cosmetics, including the ability to differentiate between products which subsequently perform well during use and those which do not (Anon., 1990c; Farrington *et al.*, 1994; Tran *et al.*, 1994; Brannan, 1995). Spooner & Davison (1993) compared the performance of an extensive array of medicines in the BP efficacy test with levels of contamination detected in used and returned medicines, and concluded that compliance in the official test generally indicated products that would perform adequately in the market-place. However, they considered that the acceptance criteria of the proposed EP and USP tests gave inadequate indications of likely in-use performance, which in some cases might be serious. Fels *et al.* (1987) determined that a wide range of European preserved medicines found to be microbiologically reliable over many years gave predictive indications of failure when submitted retrospectively to the BP efficacy test. Applicants for marketing authorization in the UK for a new medicine must normally demonstrate that, if a preservative is necessary, the product at least satisfies the basic compliance criteria of the BP test, as the licensing authority believes that this gives a reasonable estimate of likely microbial stability in use. Elsewhere in Europe, the EP test is considered to give similar assurance to licensing authorities in a number of member states.

Orth has promoted an alternative to the conventional challenge test, in that, although the methodology is comparable, formal decimal reduction

Table 16.1 Compliance criteria for the BP 1998 preservative-effectiveness test.

Type of product	Type of inoculum	Level criteria	Required $\log_{10}$ reduction of inoculum by time shown					
			6 h	1 day	2 days	7 days	14 days	28 days
Parenteral and ophthalmic medicines	Bacteria	A	2	3	–	–	–	NR
		B	–	1	–	3	–	NI
	Fungi	A	–	–	–	2	–	NI
		B	–	–	–	–	1	NI
Oral medicines	Bacteria	A	–	–	–	–	3	NI
	Fungi	A	–	–	–	–	1	NI
Topical medicines	Bacteria	A	–	–	3	–	NR	NR
	Fungi	A	–	–	–	–	2	NR
Otic medicines	Bacteria	A	2	3	–	–	–	NR
	Fungi	A	–			2	–	NI

NI, no increase in numbers over previous count; NR, no organisms to be recovered.

times (D-values) are determined for the inactivation of inocula, and predictions on the efficiency of formulations are obtained by extrapolation of data to estimate times of contact necessary to yield prescribed log levels of reduction (Orth *et al.*, 1987; Orth, 1993b). Although there is some evidence to show that reliable information can be obtained for preliminary screening purposes, the short time of the test protocol necessitates additional testing to check for possible regrowth phenomena after long delays (Orth, 1993c).

Conventional preservative challenge-test procedures are time-consuming and expensive and, accordingly, attempts have been made to develop alternatives to the conventional tests, using techniques developed for other purposes. Impedance changes during the growth and death of microorganisms can now be readily detected, and Connolly *et al.* (1994) reported on its potential for preservative-efficacy testing. The application of alternative methods to colony counting to estimate cell viability, such as direct epifluorescence (DEF) and adenosine triphosphate (ATP) bioluminescence, have been examined by Connolly *et al.* (1993), who concluded that they were unlikely to prove reliable alternatives in their present state of development.

7 Adverse reactions of users to preservatives

The non-specific and reactive nature of preservatives not only results in interaction with many formulation ingredients (Section 4), but is also reflected in not infrequent incidences of adverse reactions of users to preserved products. Recent large-scale screenings in Europe have recorded significant incidences of sensitization and dermatitis to most of the commonly used preservatives, of the order of 0.5–1.0% of those tested. However, this needs to seen in the context of overall levels of around 5% sensitization to all cosmetic ingredients (de Groot & White, 1995; Jacobs *et al.*, 1995; Berne *et al.*, 1996).

The risk of preservative damage will be related to the frequency and duration of product contact and the route and site of administration, as well as the concentration of preservative used. Thus, preservatives in rinse-off shampoos might be expected to present lower risks of sensitization than those in prolonged-contact products, such as stay-on creams. Direct injection into the central nervous system or ophthalmic tissue is far more likely to be damaging than administration by the oral or topical routes. Concerns over preservative toxicity form an active research area, with over 200 publications appearing in the last 12 years. Regulatory activity exerts appreciable control to limit the risks of adverse reactions, by detailed specification of toxicity-testing requirements, as well as attempting to allay public concerns over the use of animals for the purpose (Loprieno, 1995). The European Union (EU) has agreed to ban the use of animal testing for cosmetic ingredients by 1997, or as soon as reliable alternatives are available. The UK government obtained a voluntary ban on the animal testing of complete cosmetic formulations in November, 1997. This section can only illustrate the problem with selected examples, and interested readers are directed to the reviews of D'Arcy (1990), de Groot & White (1995) and Berne *et al.* (1996) for a detailed treatment of the topic .

Injections preserved with chlorocresol, chlorobutanol, benzyl alcohol and organomercurials have all induced appreciable hypersensitivity and severe adverse reactions (Allwood, 1990b). Benzyl alcohol has been of particular concern with small children, who are unable to metabolize it effectively, and a number of neonatal deaths have been attributed to its use (Anon., 1983). A variety of eye-damaging reactions have been reported due to preservatives in multidose eye-drops, and the particularly distressing condition of 'dry eye' has be related to their use (Burstein, 1985). Benzalkonium chloride and other quaternary ammonium preservatives have been found to be particularly damaging to the cornea, by interfering with tear-film stability and direct toxic effects on the cells (Olsen & White, 1990; Sasaki *et al.*, 1995). Preservatives in nebulizers have induced bronchoconstriction in asthmatic patients (Beasley *et al.*, 1988).

The parabens are by far the most commonly used preservatives in cosmetics (Anon., 1993a), which might reflect a recognition of their low incidence of sensitization, despite possessing only modest preservative efficiency (Anon, 1984). A methylchloroisothiazolone and chloromethylisothiazolone mixture (Kathon CG) has proved to be a most effective preservative, but, with its increasing usage, there has been an increasing number of reports of sensitizing problems (de Groot & White 1995). However, recent formal advice suggests that it is acceptable in rinse-off cosmetics at ≤ 15 parts/10^6 and in leave-on products at ≤ 7.5 parts/10^6, provided they are not used on damaged skin, the periocular area or mucous membranes (Anon., n.d., 1990a). The manufacturers do not recommend its use in medicines, where contact with already damaged skin is more likely. Formaldehyde was regarded as a very effective preservative for rinse-off cosmetics, but fears over its carcinogenicity (still debated; McLaughlin, 1994) and its significant sensitizing record (Imbus, 1985) have limited its use to certain rinse-off care products. The 'formaldehyde-releasing' preservatives, such as diazolidinyl urea (Germal II) and imidazolidinyl urea (Germal 115), which release formaldhyde slowly on storage, do not appear to present major sensitizing problems (Jackson, 1995).

From 14 to 40% of all allergic contact-dermatitis reports implicate the use of topical medicines, the majority of these being related to the therapeutic agents present. From the rather limited range of preservatives used in medicines, parabens are the most commonly reported sensitizers, but they are also the most commonly used. They are more likely to cause problems if applied to damaged skin, particularly on the legs, and are generally well tolerated on healthy skin (Angelini, 1995).

The majority of contact dermatitis reactions recede once the offending product is identified and use ceases. However, re-exposure to the preservative in another formulation will usually provoke further adverse effects (de Groot & White, 1995). Systemic damage from the topical application of preservatives is rare, but there are reports of serious to fatal reactions from skin absorption following the use of cord dusting powders containing hexachlorophene on neonates and its application to burnt and damaged skin or mucous membranes (Anon., 1996c).

8 Regulatory aspects of the preservation of medicines and cosmetics

European Union Directives, commencing with Directive 65/65/EEC (1965), lay down objectives for a common set of standards and procedures for the provision of safe, effective medicines within the European Community. These are reflected in the UK Medicines Act 1968, where permission (marketing authorization) to market a new medicine is only granted, via the Medicines Control Agency, after approval of an extensive submission dossier demonstrating its desirability, safety, efficacy and stability. The new European Medicines Evaluation Agency will play an increasing role in obtaining marketing authorization on a Europe-wide basis. An analogous system operates in the USA for medicines via the Federal Food, Drug, and Cosmetic Act, as Amended (Title 21 USC, 310 *et sqq.*), enforced through the Food and Drug Administration (FDA). Similar control of medicines in Japan is made under the Pharmaceutical Affairs Act of Japan (Law No. 145, 1960), administered through the Pharmaceutical Affairs Bureau.

Specific formal control of cosmetic safety across the EU commenced in 1976 with Council Directive 76/768/EEC, to be followed with a series, of which the most recent is the 6th Amendment, 93/35/EEC, with their objectives to be incorporated into legislation of individual member states. From January 1997, disclosure of cosmetic ingredients, including preservatives, must be made on labels. Cosmetics in the UK are controlled under the the Cosmetic Products (Safety) Regulations 1997 (Anon., 1997), introduced under the Consumer Protection Act 1987 and regulated via the Department of Industry. Although approval prior to sale is not yet required for a new cosmetic, there is an obligation for a suitably qualified person to carry out a safety assessment and for the manufacturers to maintain detailed product and processing information in a product information package (PIP). Formulation content is controlled by prescriptive lists of ingredients. However, regulatory action can only be taken once a product is offered for sale and believed to be defective. In the USA, cosmetics are regulated by the Federal Food, Drug, and Cosmetic Act, as Amended (1990), with the FDA Office of Cosmetics and Colours as the enforcing agency, which can only take action once a product is offered for sale and if it believes that it is unsafe, due to adulteration (which includes microbial problems), or misbranded. While manufacturers must produce cosmetics that are safe, there is no legal obligation to conduct formal assessments and testing prior to sale, although the FDA strongly recommends it. There are only limited lists of banned substances and no formal ingredient recommendations are made. Japanese control of cosmetics is made through the same law as for medicines, via the Pharmaceutical and Cosmetics Division of the Pharmaceutical Affairs Bureau, and prior approval and licensing of cosmetics is required before a cosmetic may be placed on the Japanese market. The following publications provide a wider insight into the legislative arena: Applebe & Wingfield (1993) (EU and UK medicines), Anon. (1997) (UK cosmetics), Anon. (1995b) (US medicines), Anon. (1992a) (US cosmetics), Anon. (1991b) (Japanese medicines and cosmetics) and Schmitt & Murphy (1984) (world overview for cosmetics).

Regulatory bodies generally place the onus on applicants to fully justify the safety, effectiveness and stability of a proposed medicine, including the steps that have been taken to assess and minimize the risks of microbial contamination and spoilage by all relevant means. Where preservatives are deemed necessary, preservative-efficacy tests must demonstrate adequate protection throughout the life of the product, and success in the appropriate national pharmacopoeial efficacy test is usually taken as a minimum requirement. Evidence of the safety of any preservatives used is also required. Lists of approved preservatives are rarely issued, although some official compendia, such as pharmacopoeias may give indications of possible preservatives for various purposes. Acceptance of the suitability of the proposals, including preservatives, usually depends on the panels of experts, who assess the choices in the light of the desirable balanced against the possible. When a preservative system is chosen which has been in common usage for similar medicines, the amount of toxicological data required by licensing authorities is usually considerably less than that for newer and less established preservatives. This tends to encourage applicants to go for the former, despite the possible advantages of the latter. The high cost of extensive toxicological testing for preservatives has minimized the likelihood of novel agents being brought into use.

In both the EU and the UK, there is an obligation on producers of cosmetics to include microbiological-risk assessments in the development process, to take steps to limit such risks and to record this in the PIP. The choice of preservatives is restricted by detailed lists of banned, approved, provisionally approved and restricted-use preservatives. Thus, guaifenesin is banned, mixtures of 4-hydroxybenzoate esters may be used up to a concentration of 0.8% w/v, phenoxyethanol may only be used in rinse-off products and at not more than 1.0% w/v and chlorobutanol may be used at up to 0.5% w/v but not in aerosols. Thiomersal is limited to $\leq$ 0.007% w/v and then only in eye make-up and remover. Confirmation of preservative efficacy is expected, and must form part of the PIP. Although there is no legal obligation to conduct formal risk assessments or carry out preservative-efficacy testing for cosmetics in the USA, it is strongly recommended by the FDA, to prevent subsequent product failure and prosecution should defective products be offered for sale (Anon., 1992a). There are only limited listings of banned or restricted preservatives, such as the banning of bithionol and halogenated salicylanilides or the restriction of mercury-based preservatives to eye-area cosmetics, where greater infective risks balance out toxicity worries. There are no lists of approved preservatives, and public disclosure of ingredients, including preservatives, is required. Applications for cosmetic-product licences in Japan must include full risk assessments for microbiological problems, including details of preservative-efficacy testing and a full toxicity evaluation. Restrictive lists of approved ingredients are published.

Various other regulations will have an impact on preservative usage, such as the banning of chloroform as a preservative, except for medicines, in the UK (SI 1979 No. 382) and in all products in the USA, due to its reported carcinogenicity in animals. Detailed environmental-impact assessments will be required for preservatives (and other ingredients) under environmental-protection legislation being brought into effect in most Western countries, since cosmetic and medicinal components will eventually be disposed of into the biosphere. Increasingly strict direct product-liability laws may offer a clearer route to compensation for users who believe they have suffered damage from a microbiologically inadequate medicine or cosmetic. An international review of the legislation relating to damage from contact dermatitis has recently been made by Frosch & Rycroft (1995).

9 The use of preservatives in medicines and cosmetics

Preceding sections of this chapter have indicated not only that the survival of contaminant microorganisms in medicines and cosmetics may present serious risks for both users and the formulations themselves but also that the use of antimicrobial agents to limit these risks will introduce additional problems, due to the relatively non-specific interactive nature of preservatives, readily combining as they do, with formulation ingredients and users, as well as microbial contaminants. Although the design of sterile single-dose, or application, units would eliminate the need for any preservatives, this option is only economically practical for dosage forms where there is a high risk of serious infection from any contamination present. Additionally, trials with sterile, or very clean, single-application units of cosmetics showed that they were unpopular with consumers, as well as being expensive (Jackson, 1993). There is general acceptance that preservatives should only be included in formulations to deal with possible contamination during storage or use of a product. They should not be required to clean up contamination arising from heavily contaminated raw materials or poor manufacturing processes, which could result in preservative depletion to levels inadequate for postmanufacturing protection. However, the BP still recommends the inclusion of preservatives in aseptically prepared parenteral products, presumably to cater for the risk of erratic failure during processing (Avallone, 1989; Anon., 1993d). Concerns over preservative toxicity by medicine licensing authorities means that applicants for marketing authorizations must fully justify the inclusion or exclusion of any preservative in a formulation, and are expected to adopt alternative strategies for product protection where realistic. With cosmetics, regulatory attitudes often differ, placing the emphasis upon the use of preservatives with acceptable levels of toxicity at specified concentrations, and placing exclusions on others. The formulator in search of an antimicrobial preservative would wish to find one that is highly effective, totally safe, quite stable, and which meets all other criteria of general acceptability. Effectiveness excellence would be judge by a ready ability to inactivate the full range of microbial contaminants likely to be encountered during storage and use, within the intervals between the removal of successive doses. Coupled with this would be a requirement for minimal adverse interaction with the other ingredients of the formulation. This sought-for preservative would be non-toxic, non-irritant and non-sensitizing at the required concentration, duration of product contact and frequency of use. Full stability would be expected throughout the life of the product, including during possibly harsh processing conditions and likely abuse by users. In addition, it should be acceptable to the user and meet any environmental-impact regulations. Naturally, all this should be at minimal cost! Sadly, such expectations are rarely likely to be satisfied, and one is forced to compromise, selecting the least bad preservative for any particular situation.

In general, the more potent antimicrobial agents are usually associated with problems of toxicity. There is only a limited range of materials with both reasonable preservative effectiveness and acceptably low toxicity, and extremely few with sufficient potential to kill bacterial spores. In complex multiphase formulations, attenuating preservative interactions are so appreciable that it can be most difficult to achieve more than weak antimicrobial efficacy, as reflected in the low efficiency criteria set for creams by the BP, and similar, efficacy-test protocols (Table 16.1). The difficulty of adequately balancing efficiency with toxicity considerations has led to an almost complete shift from preserved multidose units to sterile single-dosage forms for parenteral medicines (Anon., 1994b). Occasionally, a higher risk of infection for a product justifies the use of preservatives considered too toxic for general application, such as the FDA's allowance of organomercurial preservatives for cosmetics to be used around the eye, but not for other body-area products (Anon., 1992a).

The instability of agents such as the isothiazolinones and parabens at high temperatures necessitates cautious processing procedures. Chlorobutanol has useful preservative properties but is unstable to autoclaving and has only limited stability on prolonged storage. Parabens have limited shelf-lives in slightly alkaline products, such as antacid suspensions. Formaldehyde-releasers are intended to degrade and release small amounts of formaldehyde during product life, but may degrade too fast in some formulations and create excessive irritancy early on and inadequate protection in the later stages of shelf-life.

Chlorocresol, parabens and other phenolic preservatives impart a distinctively antiseptic odour to formulations, sulphur-containing compounds an 'eggy' smell, and some essential oils give characteristic odours that can be unacceptable to users. Methylparaben in topical formulations can result in unwanted attraction from male dogs, as it is also a major volatile ingredient in the urine of bitches (Person, 1985).

Increasingly, manufacturers are required to assess the environmental impact of formulation ingredients, including preservatives, once they are disposed of into the general biosphere. Halogenated preservatives are somewhat recalcitrant, although the parabens are readily biodegradable, once diluted in effluent (Beveridge, 1975).

While there is little in the manner of official lists of recommended preservatives for medicines, there are bodies of unofficial regulatory beliefs which consider that certain preservatives would or would not be suitable for particular medicines. Thus, the use of bronopol in new applications for oral medicines is most unlikely to be permitted, despite any data submitted to support its by-mouth usage. Since public disclosure of the preservative content of medicines is not generally mandatory, it is difficult to get a detailed pattern of usage. However, examination of partial disclosures in the British National Formulary (Anon., 1996e) and by some manufacturers does provide an indication of UK usage. From published data and anecdotal information received, it would appear that fewer than eight preservatives are in common use in medicines and that parabens are by far the most commonly selected. Detailed monographs on the preservatives commonly used in medicines have been produced by Denyer & Wallhaeusser (1990), Wade & Weller (1994) and Anon. (1996e).

Due to concerns over toxicity and the build-up of contamination in multidose vials (Thompson *et al.*, 1989), preserved multidose containers of injections have been largely replaced by sterile single-dose units without the need for preservatives, leaving only multidose units for parenterals such as campaign vaccines and insulin (Anon., 1996g). Organomercurials seem to be rarely used now, with phenol, chlorocresol, cresol and parabens replacing them. Benzyl alcohol is still used, but not for injections that might be used in children. Preservatives are not permitted in solutions for direct injection into spinal, cranial or ophthalmic tissues, or in doses of greater than $15\,cm^3$, where the risks of toxic damage become greater. As a consequence, these must always be supplied as single-use vials or ampoules. It is possible to achieve reasonable rates of inactivation, except for spores, as the opportunities for attenuating interaction of the preservative with other ingredients is usually limited in these generally simple aqueous solutions. Preservatives are no longer included in oily injections, as they are considered to be ineffective in non-aqueous systems.

Multidose containers of eye-drops are still widely supplied for domestic use, due the perceived high cost of single-dose units, and require good preservative protection to minimize the appreciable risk of *Pseudomonas* and other infection, to which the damaged eye is particularly susceptible. Benzalkonium chloride, often in combination with EDTA, now appears to be the most commonly used preservative, with chlorhexidine and organomercurials occasionally reported (Anon., 1996e). However, concern at the appreciable damaging effect of quaternary ammonium antimicrobial agents on the cornea and their involvement in 'dry-eye' syndrome (see Section 7) has resulted in the widespread use of unpreserved eye-drops and artificial tears, usually in small-dosage units, for people suffering from this and related problems (Anon., 1996f).

The complex distribution of preservatives in creams makes it difficult to obtain rapid inactivation of contamination. However, the major risk is seen as that of spoilage rather than of infection, and the poor levels of inactivation achieved with those preservatives considered to be sufficiently non-irritant for medicinal use is accepted by licensing authorities as the best that is possible. Parabens are again by far the most commonly used preservative, with chlorocresol and benzyl alcohol lagging well behind (Anon., 1996e). Formaldehyde-releasing agents are used, but not widely, and the isothiazolinones are not considered suitable for potentially damaged skin. Most non-aqueous ointments are unpreserved, as the risk of accumulation and replication of contaminants is considered to be low. For high-risk areas, such as the eye, sterile ointments are used. Many UK medicinal creams and ointments which might be used on damaged skin are supplied to microbial specifications approaching those for sterile products.

Parabens are also the most commonly used preservative for oral aqueous medicines, probably due to their long usage with apparent safety and the need to perform expensive oral toxicological evaluation of replacement systems. Weakly alkaline medicines, such as antacid suspensions, are difficult to preserve, as parabens are relatively unstable at these pH levels (Vanhaecke *et al.*, 1987). Chloroform has been an excellent preservative for oral products supplied in well-sealed containers and with a short use life, but is now banned in some countries over fears of toxicity, although it may still be used as a preservative in medicines (only) in the UK. Oral medicines supplied as a dry powder for reconstitution prior to use usually require a preservative to cope with possible in-use contamination once dispensed. Many contain parabens, although the presence of large amounts of sugar or other solutes to provide a low A_w solution for additional protection against spoilage, as well as for taste, often reduces their efficiency.

There are suggestions that the inclusion of preservatives into tablets would give protection should they become damp during storage or use (Fassihi *et al.*, 1978). Bos *et al.*, (1989) suggested that this might be appropriate for tablets for use in tropical and humid environments. These arguments miss the point. If tablets became damp, they would be inherently spoiled, as the low A_w also offers protection against non-biological degradation, which is accelerated in the presence of water, as well as being physically damaged. Whiteman (1995) has recommended the use of water vapour-resistant film coatings to reduce vapour uptake and assist in the maintenance of low A_w for bulk-packed tablets. The main protection must, however, remain adequate A_w reduction during manufacture and the use of water vapour-resistant packaging. It is understood that the UK licensing authorities will not condone the incorporation of preservatives into new tablet formulations.

Some medicinal ingredients have an intrinsic capability to inactivate likely microbial contamination, and no additional preservative is then necessary. Thus, lindane cream, some alkaloid solutions, frusemide injection, some local anaesthetic injections and some broad-spectrum antibiotic creams are able to cope with contaminants adequately without the need for additional preservation. However, the mere presence of an antibiotic should not be presumed automatically to provide an adequate spectrum of preservative cover; there is still the need for a full efficacy-testing programme.

There is some difference of approach to the preservation of cosmetics compared with that for medicines. It is generally accepted that they are for use on a more restricted range of body sites involving healthy skin, and occasionally membranes, or around undamaged eyes, with lower risks of infection from contaminants than for some medicinal routes of administration. Contamination and spoilage possibilities for some cosmetics, however, may be high, due to their physicochemical complexity and the high potential for consumer abuse, such as regular fingering, repeated use of saliva, repeated and communal application and possibilities for in-use dilution of remaining product, such as for shampoos or soap in the shower (Orth *et al.*, 1992). Although some manufacturers do not include preservatives in formulations such as dusting powders, block cosmetics, lipsticks, stick deodorants or alcohol-based perfumes with low A_w many others do so, for added reassurance and to cater for in-use abuse. Considerations of preservative toxicity, irritancy and sensitizing potential take into account the duration of contact and regularity of use on healthy skin for stay-on cosmetics, and the general levels of adverse reactions to other formulation ingredients. Higher levels of potentially more problematic preservatives may be used in rinse-off cosmetics, where the period of contact may be short and /or significant dilution will take place during application. Accordingly, many agents are used which would be considered to be too toxic for medicinal applications. Where the risk of infection by contaminants is deemed to be higher than for most situations, preservatives with greater efficiency may be used, despite their increased toxicity potential, such as the use of organomercurial agents in eye-area cosmetics.

Voluntary disclosure to the FDA revealed the use of over 100 preservatives for cosmetics in the USA (Anon., 1990b, 1993a). Parabens were by far the most commonly used preservatives, followed by imidazolidinyl urea, isothiazolinones, Quaternium 15, formaldehyde, phenoxyethanol and bronopol. The range of preservatives in use in the EU is considerably less, but it is believed that those in most common usage are comparable to those in the USA, with parabens topping the range. Sterile cosmetics are not in common use, except for eye-conditioning, brightening and colouring drops, which should be supplied sterile, and preserved if in multidose containers. The range of preservatives and their applicability to cosmetic protection is indicated in the *CTPA Guidelines* (Anon., 1993b), Orth (1993a) and Anon. (1997).

10 Alternatives to conventional preservatives

In addition to the real technical problems associated with preservatives, adverse public reaction to the use of 'preservatives' in foodstuffs and other domestic products, aroused by various populist publications, ranging from the reasonably sensible *E For Additives* (Hanssen & Marsden, 1988a) to the highly alarmist 'Villejuif List' (Hanssen & Marsden, 1988b), has significantly stimulated manufacturers to investigate alternative strategies to using conventional preservatives for medicines and cosmetics (Morris & Leech, 1996). The manipulation of the intrinsic properties of a formulation for successful preservation, particularly by lowering A_w, as already discussed (see Section 3), as well as the short-term low-temperature storage of preservative-free eye-drops for those patients with dry-eye syndrome and similar problems, has been found to provide satisfactory control over contamination (Anon., 1996f).

In recent years, a variety of 'preservative-free' cosmetics have been promoted to the public. Some indeed appear to contain no commonly recognized preservative, and some do not justify inclusion of a preservative, being of low A_w or having a high alcohol content. In other cases, inhibitory agents not commonly recognized preservatives but providing varying levels of protection have been incorporated, including EDTA alone, antioxidants, such as BHA or BHT, tocopherol, urea, allantoin, propylene glycol, glycerol, lauric acid and citric acid (Jackson, 1993; Orth, 1993b). The term 'hypoallergenic' does not necessarily mean preservative-free, with various of the above agents being used, as well as preservatives regarded as mild, such as phenoxyethanol or bronopol, in lower than usual concentrations. When submitted to the BP preservative-efficacy test, a variety of 'preservative-free' cosmetics on sale in the UK were generally found to fall well below the acceptance criteria for that protocol (unattributable communication to the author).

Naturally occurring ingredients with antimicrobial activity have been found to offer significant protection, alone or in combination with conventional agents, including essential oils (Manon *et al.*, 1998) and perfumery ingredients (Woodruff, 1995), fatty acids, their esters and monoglycerides (Kabara, 1984a). The antibiotic nisin, used in food processing (Delves-Broughton & Gasson, 1994), would be of limited use for cosmetics and medicines, since it has only weak activity against *Pseudomonas* and similar species. Related bacteriocins, currently under examination for food use, might be of greater application (Dillon and Board, 1994b). Lactoferrin binds Fe^{3+} ions so effectively when incorporated into test-food formulations that microbial growth is inhibited (Roller, 1995), and this has been examined for its potential in protecting cosmetics. Lactoperoxidase and glucose oxidase activity liberate traces of hydrogen peroxide and, in combination with almost catalytic levels of anions, such as thiocyanate and iodide, can generate highly antimicrobial chemical species *in situ* (Ekstrand, 1994). A commercial preservative system based on this phenomenon is now in worldwide use for cosmetic creams and toiletry products (Myavert C, Knoll MicroCheck). It performs well in the BP efficacy test, offers shelf-lives of around 2 years and is of low irritancy. However, care must be taken not to use high temperatures during processing (Anon., 1995d). None of these components are classed as preservatives in their own right by regulatory authorities, and users usually refer to products containing it as 'preserved systems'.

11 References

Agnostopoulos, G.D. & Kroll, R.G. (1978) Water activity and solute effect on the bactericidal action of phenol. *Microbios Letters*, **7**, 69–74.

Akers, M.J. & Taylor, C.J. (1990) Official methods of preservative evaluation and testing. In *Guide to Microbiological Control in Pharmaceuticals* (eds Denyer, S.P. & Baird, R.), pp. 292–303. Chichester: Ellis Horwood.

Allwood, M.C. (1982) The adsorption of esters of *p*-hydroxybenzoic acid by magnesium trisilicate. *International Journal of Pharmaceutics*, **11**, 101–107.

Allwood, M.C. (1990a) Package design and product integrity. In *Guide to Microbiological Control in Pharmaceuticals* (eds Denyer, S.P. & Baird, R), pp. 341–355. Chichester: Ellis Horwood.

Allwood, M.C. (1990b) Adverse reactions in parenterals. In *Formulation Factors in Adverse Reactions* (eds Florence, A.T. & Salole, E.G.), pp. 56–74. London: Wright, Butterworth Science.

Allwood, M.C., Denyer, S.P. & Hodges, N. (1994) Bronopol. In *Handbook of Pharmaceutical Excipients*, 2nd edn (eds Wade, A. & Weller, P.J.), pp. 40–42. London: Pharmaceutical Press, and Washington: American Pharmaceutical Association.

Angelini, G. (1995) Topical drugs. In *Texbook of Contact Dermatology*, 2nd edn (eds Rycroft, R.J.G., Menne, T. & Frosch, P.J.), pp. 477–503. Berlin: Springer-Verlag.

Anon. (n.d.) *Kathon CG Microbicide: Cosmetics and Toiletries*. Technical Bulletin. Croydon, UK: Rohm and Haas.

Anon. (1983) Benzyl alcohol: toxic agent in neonatal units. *Pediatrics*, **72**, 356–358.

Anon. (1984) Final report on the safety assessment of methylparaben, ethylparaben, propylparaben, and butylparaben. *Journal of the American College of Toxicology*, **3**, 147–193.

Anon. (1990a) Kathon CG is safe for use in 'leave ons' up to 7.5 ppm. *The Rose Sheet*, 23 April, 2–3.

Anon. (1990b) Frequency of preservative use in cosmetic formulas as disclosed to FDA-1990. *Cosmetics and Toiletries*, **105**, 45–47.

Anon. (1990c) CTFA survey: test methods companies use. *Cosmetics and Toiletries*, **105**, 79–82.

Anon. (1991a) Cosmetic safety: more complex that at first blush. *FDA Consumer*, November, 2.

Anon. (1991b) *Drug Registration in Japan*, 4th edn. Tokyo: Yakuji Nippo.

Anon. (1992a) *Cosmetics Handbook*. Washington: Food and Drugs Administration.

Anon. (1992b) General tests aand assays: microbiological tests. *Pharmacopeial Forum*, **18**, 3047–3052.

Anon. (1993a) Preservative frequency of use: FDA data, June 1993 update. *Cosmetics and Toiletries*, **108**, 47–48.

Anon. (1993b) *CTPA Guidelines for Effective Preservation*. p. 1. London: Cosmetic Toiletry and Perfumery Association.

Anon. (1993d) *British Pharmacopoeia 1993*. General notices, p. xxi. London: HMSO.

Anon. (1994a) *CTPA Guidelines for Preservative Efficacy Testing*, London: Cosmetic Toiletry and Perfumery Association.

Anon. (1994b) Control of microbial contamination and preservation of medicines. In *The Pharmaceutical Codex: Principles and Practice of Pharmaceutics*, 12th edn, pp. 509–529. London: Pharmaceutical Press.

Anon. (1994c) 111 cases of hepatitis C linked to Gamagard. *American Journal of Hospital Pharmacy*, **51**, 2326.

Anon. (1995a) Accidental death verdict on children infected by TPN at a Manchester hospital. *Pharmaceutical Journal*, **254**, 313.

Anon. (1995b) Federal Food, Drug and Cosmetic Act requirements relating to drugs for humans and animals. In *The United States Pharmacopoeia*, 23rd edn, pp. 1888–1907. Rockville: USP Convention.

Anon. (1995c) Microbiological tests: [51] Antimicrobial preservatives—effectiveness. In *United States Pharmacopeia 1995*, 23rd edn, p. 1681. Rockville: United States Pharmacopeial Convention.

Anon. (1995d) *Protection with Myavert: Myavert C*. Knoll MicroCheck Technical Data Sheets. Nottingham: Knoll microcheck.

Anon. (1996a) A case of justice only half done. *New Scientist*, **151**, 3.

Anon. (1996b) Deadly blooms reach Britain's rivers. *New Scientist*, **151**, 5.

Anon. (1996c) *Martindale: The Extra Pharmacopoeia*, 31st edn. London: Pharmaceutical Press.

Anon. (1996d) In *European Pharmacopoeia*, 3rd edn, 5.3.1 General texts: Efficacy of antimicrobial preservation. pp. 286–287. Strasburg: Council of Europe.

Anon. (1996e) *The British National Formulary*, No. 32. London: British Medical Association and Royal Pharmaceutical Society of Great Britain.

Anon. (1996f) Seven day life of unpreserved eye-drops. *Pharmaceutical Journal*, **257**, 206.

Anon. (1996g) Design and use of IV products. *Pharmaceutical Journal*, **257**, 772–773.

Anon. (1996h) How safe is chicken? *Which Magazine*, October, 8–9.

Anon. (1997) *The Cosmetic Products (Safety) Regulations 1997*. London: HMSO.

Anon. (1998a) *British Pharmacopoeia 1998* Appendix XVIC. Efficacy of antimicrobial preservation. 252–253. London: HMSO.

Applebe, G.E. & Wingfield, J. (1993) *Dale and Applebe's Pharmacy Law and Ethics*, 5th edn. London: Pharmaceutical Press.

Aspinall, J.E., Duffy, T.D. & Taylor, C.G. (1983) The effect of low density polyethylene containers on some hospital-manufactured eyedrop formulations II: Inhibition of the sorption of phenylmercuric acetate. *Journal of Clinical and Hospital Pharmacy*, **8**, 233–240.

Attwood, D. & Florence, A.T. (1983) *Surfactant Systems*. London: Chapman & Hall.

Avallone, H.L. (1989) Aseptic processing of non-preserved parenterals. *PDA Journal of Pharmaceutical Science and Technology*, **43**, 113.

Ayliffe, G.A.J., Barry, D.R., Lowbury, E.J.L., Roper-Hall, M.J. & Walker, M. (1966) Postoperative infection with *Pseudomonas aeruginosa*. *Lancet*, **i**, 1113–1117.

Baird, R.M. (1988) Incidence of microbial contamination in medicines in hospitals. In *Biodeterioration 7* (eds Houghton, D.R., Smith, R.N. & Eggins, H.O.W.) pp. 152–156. London: Elsevier Applied Science.

Baird, (1995) Preservative efficacy testing in the pharmaceutical industries. In *Microbiological Quality Assurance: A Guide Towards Relevance and Reproducibility of Inocula* (eds Brown, M.R.W. & Gilbert P.), pp. 149–162. New York: CRC Press.

Baker, J.H. (1959) That unwanted cosmetic ingredient—bacteria. *Journal of the Society of Cosmetic Chemists*, **10**, 133–137.

Bean, H.A., Richards, J.P. & Thomas, J. (1962) The bactericidal activity against *Escherichia coli* of phenol in oil-in-water dispersions. *Boll. Chimica Farmaceutisch*, **101**, 339–346.

Beasley, R., Rafferty, P. & Holgate, S.T. (1988) Adverse reactions to the non-drug constituents of nebuliser solutions. *British Journal of Clinical Pharmacology*, **25**, 283–287.

Begg, D.I.R. (1990) Risk assessment and microbiological auditing. In *Guide to Microbiological Control in Pharmaceuticals* (eds Denyer, S.P. & Baird, R.), pp. 366–379. Chichester: Ellis Horwood.

Berne, B., Bostrom, A., Grahnen, A.F. & Tammela, M. (1996) Adverse effects of cosmetics and toiletries reported to the Swedish Medical Products Agency. *Contact Dermatitis*, **34**, 359–362.

Beuchat, L.R. (1983) Influence of water activity on growth, metabolic activities and survival of yeasts and molds. *Journal of Food Protection*, **46**, 135–141.

Beveridge, E.G. (1975) The microbial spoilage of pharmaceutical products. In *Microbial Aspects of the Deterioration of Materials*, Society for Applied Bacteriology Technical Series No. 9 (eds Lovelock, D.W. & Gilbert, R.J.), pp. 213–235. London: Academic Press.

Beveridge, E.G. (1998) Microbial spoilage and preservation of pharmaceutical products. In *Pharmaceutical Microbiology*, 6th edn. (eds Hugo, W.B. & Russell, A.D.) Oxford: Blackwell Scientific Publications pp. 335–373.

Beveridge, E.G. & Bendall D. (1988) Water relationships and microbial biodeterioration of some pharmaceutical tablets. *International Biodeterioration*, **24**, 197–203.

Beveridge, E.G. & Hope, I.A. (1967) Inactivation of benzoic acid in sulphadimidine mixture for infants BPC. *Pharmaceutical Journal*, **198**, 457–458.

Bhadauria, R. & Ahearn, D.G. (1980) Loss of effectiveness of preservative systems of mascara with age. *Applied and Environmental Microbiology*, **39**, 665–667.

Bloomfield, S.F. (1990) Microbial contamination: spoilage and hazard. In *Guide to Microbiological Control in Pharmaceuticals* (eds. Denyer, S.P. & Baird, R.), pp. 29–52. Chichester: Ellis-Horwood.

Bos, C.E., van Doorne, H. & Lerk, C.F. (1989) Microbiological stability of tablets stored under tropical conditions. *International Journal of Pharmaceutics*, **55**, 175–183.

Brannan, D.K. (1995) Cosmetic preservation. *Journal of the Society of Cosmetic Chemists*, **46**, 199–220.

Brannan, D.K. & Dille, J.C. (1990) Type of closure prevents microbial contamination of cosmetics during consumer use. *Applied and Environmental Microbiology*, **56**, 1476–1479.

Brown, L.K., Schultz, J.R. & Gragg, R.A. (1995) HIV-infected adolescents with hemophilia: adaptation and coping. *Pediatrics*, **96**, 459–463.

Brown, M.R.W. & Gilbert, P. (eds) (1995) *Microbiological Quality Assurance: A Guide to Relevance and Reproducibility of Inocula*. New York: CRC Press.

Bruch, C.W. (1972) Objectionable micro-organisms in non-sterile drugs and cosmetics. *Drug and Cosmetic Industry*, **3**, 51–54, 150–156.

Burgess, D.J. & Reich, R.R. (1993) Industrial ethylene oxide sterilisation. In *Sterilization Technology: A Practical Guide for Manufacturers and Users of Health Care Products* (eds Morrissey, R.F. & Phillips, C.B.), pp. 152–195. New York: Van Nostrand Reinhold.

Burstein, N.L. (1985) The effects of topical drugs and preservatives on the tears and corneal epithelium in dry eye. *Transactions of the Ophthalmological Society of the United Kingdom*, **104**, 402–409.

Chan, M. & Prince, H. (1981) Rapid screeing test for ranking preservative efficacy. *Drug and Cosmetic Industry*, **129**, 34–37, 80–81.

Chapman, J.S., Diehl, M.A. & Fearnside, K.B. (1996)

Preservative tolerance and resistance as a stimulation in perfumery. In *Microbial Contamination, Determination & Eradication*. Proceedings, Society of Cosmetic Chemists Symposium, Daresburg. London: Miller Freeman.

Chirife, J. & Favetto, G.J. (1992) Some physicochemical basis of food preservation by combined methods. *Food Research International*, **25**, 389–396.

Clegg, A. & Perry, B.F. (1996) Control of microbial contamination during manufacture. In *Microbial Quality Assurance in Cosmetics, Toiletries and Non-Sterile Pharmaceuticals*, 2nd edn (eds Baird, R.M. & Bloomfield, S.F.), pp. 49–66. Basingstoke: Taylor & Francis.

Clothier, C.M. (1972) *Roport of the Committee Appointed to Look into the Circumstances, Including the Production, Which Led to the Use of Contaminated Infusion Fluids in the Devenport Section of Plymouth General Hospital*. London: HMSO.

Connolly, P., Bloomfield, S.F. & Denyer, S.P. (1993) A study of the use of rapid methods for preservative efficacy testing of pharmaceuticals and cosmetics. *Journal of Applied Bacteriology*, **75**, 456–462.

Connolly, P., Bloomfield, S. F. & Denyer, S.P. (1994) The use of impedance for preservative efficacy testing of pharmaceuticals and cosmetic products. *Journal of Applied Bacteriology*, **76**, 66–74.

Cook, R.S. & Youssuf, N. (1994) Edetic acid. In *Handbook of Pharmaceutical Excipients*, 2nd edn, pp. 176–179. London: Pharmaceutical Press, and Washington: American Pharmaceutical Association.

Cooper, E.A. (1947) The influence of organic solvents on the bactericidal action of the phenols. Part II. *Journal of the Society of Chemical Industry (London)*, **66**, 48–50.

Cooper, E.A. (1948) The influence of ethylene glycol and glycerol on the germicidal power of aliphatic and aromatic compounds. *Journal of the Society of Chemical Industry (London)*, **67**, 69–70.

Curry, A.S., Graf, J.G. & McEwen, J.D. (1993) *CTFA Microbiology Guidelines*. Washington: Cosmetic, Toiletry and Fragrance Association.

D'Arcy, P.F. (1990) Adverse reactions to excipients in pharmaceutical formulations. In *Formulation Factors in Adverse Reactions* (eds Florence, A.T. & Salole, E.G.), pp. 1–22. London: Wright, Butterworth Science.

Darwish, R.M. & Bloomfield, S.F. (1995) The effect of co-solvents on the antibacterial activity of paraben preservatives. *International Journal of Pharmaceutics*, **119**, 183–192.

Davison, A.L. (1996) Preservative efficacy testing of pharmaceuticals, cosmetics and toiletries and its limitations. In *Microbial Quality Assurance in Cosmetics, Toiletries and Non-Sterile Pharmaceuticals*, 2nd edn (eds Baird, R.M. & Bloomfield, S.F.), pp. 187–216. Basingstoke: Taylor & Francis.

Dean, D.A. (1992) *Packaging of Pharmaceuticals: Packages and Closures*. Practical Packaging Series. Melton Mowbray: Institute of Packaging.

de Groot, A.C. & White, I.R. (1995) Cosmetics and skin care products. In *Textbook of Contact Dermatology*, 2nd edn (eds Rycroft, R.J.G., Menne, T. & Frosch, P.J.), pp. 461–476. Berlin: Springer-Verlag.

Delves-Broughton, J. & Gasson, M.J. (1994) Nisin. In *Natural Antimicrobial Systems and Food Preservation* (eds Dillon, V.M. & Board, R.G.), pp. 99–131. Wallingford: CAB International.

Dempsey, G. (1996) The effect of container materials and multiple-phase formulation components on the activity of antimicrobial agents. In *Microbial Quality Assurance in Cosmetics, Toiletries and Non-Sterile Pharmaceuticals*, 2nd edn (eds Baird, R.M. & Bloomfield, S.F.), pp. 87–97. Basingstoke: Taylor & Francis.

Denyer, S.P. (1988) Clinical consequences of microbial action on medicines. In *Biodeterioration 7* (eds Houghton, D.R., Smith, R.N. & Eggins, H.O.W.), pp. 146–151. London: Elsevier Applied Science.

Denyer, S.P. (1996) Development of preservative systems. In *Microbial Quality Assurance in Cosmetics, Toiletries and Non-Sterile Pharmaceuticals*, 2nd edn (eds Baird, R.M. & Bloomfield, S.F.), pp. 133–147. Basingstoke: Taylor & Francis.

Denyer, S.P. & Wallhaeusser, K.H. (1990) Antimicrobial preservatives and their properties. In *Guide to Microbiological Control in Pharmaceuticals* (eds Denyer), S. & Baird, R.), pp. 274–291. Chichester: Ellis Horwood.

Denyer, S.P., Hugo, W.B. & Harding, V.D. (1986) The biochemical basis of synergy between the antibacterial agents, chlorocresol and 2-phenylethanol. *International Journal of Pharmaceutics*, **29**, 29–36.

Dillon, V.M. & Board, R.G. (1994a) Ecological concepts of food preservation. In *Natural Antimicrobial Systems and Food Preservation* (eds Dillon, V.M. & Board, R.G.), pp. 1–13. Wallingford: CAB International.

Dillon, V.M. & Board, R.G. (1994b) Future prospects for natural antimicrobial food preservation systems. In *Natural Antimicrobial Systems and Food Preservation* (eds Dillon, V.M. & Board, R.G.), pp. 297–305. Wallingford: CAB International.

Eccleston, G. (1990) Multiple-phase oil-in-water emulsions. *Journal of the Society of Cosmetic Chemists*, **41**, 1–22.

Ekstrand, B. (1994) Lactoperoxidase and lactoferroin. In *Natural Antimicrobial Systems and Food Preservation* (eds Dillon, V.M. & Board, R.G.), pp. 15–41. Wallingford: CAB International.

El-Dessouki, S. (1992) Aflatoxins in cosmetics containing substrates for aflatoxin-producing fungi. *Food and Chemical Toxicology*, **30**, 993–994.

Farrington, J.K., Martz, E.L., Wells, S.J. *et al.* (1994) Ability of laboratory methods to predict in-use efficacy of antimicrobial preservatives in an experimental cosmetic. *Applied and Environmental Microbiology*, **60**, 4553–4558.

Fassihi, R.A. (1991) Preservation of medicines against microbial contamination. In *Disinfection, Sterilisation and Preservation* (ed. Block, S.E.), pp. 871–886. Malvern, Pennsylvania: Lea & Febinger.

Fassihi, R.A., Parker, M.S. & Dingwall (1978) The preservation of tablets against microbial spoilage. *Drug Development and Industrial Pharmacy*, **4**, 515–527.

Favero, M.S., Carson, L.A., Bond, W.W. & Peterson, N.J. (1971) *Pseudomonas aeruginosa*: growth in distilled water. *Science*, **173**, 836–838.

Fels, P. (1995) An automated personal computer-enhanced assay for antimicrobial preservative efficacy testing by the most probable number technique using microtiter plates. *Pharmazeutische Industrie*, **57**, 585–590.

Fels, P., Gay, M., Kabay, A. & Uran, S. (1987) Antimicrobial preservation. *Pharmazeutische Industrie*, **49**, 631–637.

Flatau, T.C., Bloomfield, S.F. & Buckton, G. (1996) Preservation of solid oral dosage forms. In *Microbial Quality Assurance in Cosmetics, Toiletries and Non-Sterile Pharmaceuticals*, 2nd edn (eds Baird, R.M. & Bloomfield, S.F.), pp. 113–132. Basingstoke: Taylor & Francis.

Flawn, P.C., Malcolm, S.A. & Woodruffe, R.C.S. (1973). Assessment of the preservative capacity of shampoos. *Journal of the Society of Cosmetic Chemists*, **24**, 229–238.

Freund, H.R. & Rimon, B. (1990) Sepsis during total parenteral nutrition. *Journal of Parenteral and Enteral Nutrition*, **14**, 39–41.

Friberg, S.E. (1984) Microemulsions in relation to cosmetics and their preservation. In *Cosmetic and Drug Preservation: Principles and Practice* (ed. Kabara, J.J.), Cosmetic Science and Technology Series, Vol. 1, pp. 7–20. New York: Marcel Dekker.

Frick, E.W. (1992) *Cosmetic and Toiletry Formulations*, 2nd edn. New Jersey: Noyes Publications.

Frosch, P.J. & Rycroft, R.J.G. (1995) International legal aspects of contact dermatitis. In *Texbook of Contact Dermatology*, 2nd edn (eds Rycroft, R.J.G., Menne, T. & Frosch, P.J.), pp. 752–768. Berlin: Springer-Verlag.

Geyer, O., Bottone, E.J., Podos, S.M., Schumer, R.A. & Asbell, P.A. (1995) Microbial contamination of medicines used to treat glaucoma. *British Journal of Ophthalmology*, **79**, 376–379.

Gilbert, P. & Brown, M.R.W. (1995) Factors affecting the reproducibility and predictivity of performance tests. In *Microbiological Quality Assurance: A Guide to Relevance and Reproducibility of Inocula* (eds Brown, M.R.W. & Gilbert, P. New York: CRC Press pp. 135–147.

Gilbert, P. & Das, J.A. (1996) Microbial resistance to preservative systems. In *Microbial Quality Assurance in Cosmetics, Toiletries and Non-Sterile Pharmaceuticals*, 2nd edn (eds Baird, R.M. & Bloomfield, S.F.), pp. 149–173. Basingstoke: Taylor & Francis.

Gilbert, P., Beveridge, E.G. & Crone, P.B. (1977) The lethal action of 2-phenoxyethanol and its analogues upon *Escherichia coli* NCTC 5933. *Microbios*, **19**, 125–141.

Gilliland, D., Li Wan Po, A. & Scott, E. (1992) Kinetic evaluation of claimed synergistic paraben combinations using a factorial design. *Journal of Applied Bacteriology*, **72**, 258–261.

Greenwood, M.H. & Hooper, W.L. (1983) Chocolate bars contaminated with *Salmonella napoli*: an infectivity study. *British Medical Journal*, **286**, 1394.

Gould, G.W. (1989) Drying, raised osmotic pressure and low water activity. In *Mechanisms of Action of Food Preservation Procedures* (ed. Gould, G.W.), pp. 97–117. London: Elsevier Applied Science.

Gould, G.W. (1996) Methods for preservation and extension of shelf life. *International Journal of Food Microbiology*, **33**, 51–64.

Haag, T.E. & Loncrini, D.F. (1984) Esters of *para*-hydroxybenzoic acid. In *Cosmetic and Drug Preservation: Principles and Practice* (ed. Kabara, J.J.), Cosmetic Science and Technology Series, Vol. 1, pp. 63–77. New York: Marcel Dekker.

Hall, A.L. (1984) Cosmetically acceptable phenoxyethanol. In *Cosmetic and Drug Preservation: Principles and Practice* (ed. Kabara, J.J.), Cosmetic Science and Technology Series, Vol. 1, pp. 79–110. New York: Marcel Dekker.

Hamil, R.J., Houston, E.D., Georghiou, P.R. *et al.* (1995) An outbreak of *Burkholderia* (formerly *Pseudomonas*) *cepacia* respiratory tract colonisation and infection associated with nebulised albuterol therapy. *Annals of Internal Medicine*, **122**, 762–766.

Hanssen, M. & Marsden, J. (1988a) *E For Additives*. London: Thorsons Publishing Group.

Hanssen, M. & Marsden, J. (1988b) Warning: dangerous food additives; the Villjuif List. In *E for Additives* (eds Hanssen, M. & Marsden, J.), pp. 305–307. Appendix II, London: Thorsons Publishing Group.

Hart, J.R. (1984) Chelating agents as preservative potentiators. In *Cosmetic and Drug Preservation: Principles and Practice* (ed. Kabara, J.J.), Cosmetic Science and Technology Series, Vol. 1, pp. 323–337. New York: Marcel Dekker.

Hay, J., Stevenson, R. & Cairns, D. (1996) Single-solution lens care systems. *Pharmaceutical Journal*, **256**, 824–825.

Holdsworth, D.G., Roberts, M.S. & Polack, A.E. (1984) Fate of chlorbutol during storage in polyethylene dropper containers and simulated patient used. *Journal of Clinical and Hospital Pharmacy*, **9**, 29–39.

Hopton, J.W. & Hill, E.C. (eds) (1987) *Industrial Microbiological Testing*. Society for Applied Bacteriology Technical Series No. 23. Oxford: Blackwell Scientific Publications.

Hugo, WB. & Denyer, S.P. (1987) The concentration exponent of disinfectants and preservatives. In *Preservatives in the Food, Pharmaceutical and Environmental Industries*. Society for Applied Bacteriology Technical Series No 22, pp. 281–291. Oxford: Blackwell Scientific Publications.

Imbus, H.R. (1985) Clinical evaluation of patients with complaints related to formaldehyde exposure. *Journal of Allergy and Clinical Immunology*, **76**, 831–840.

Jackson, E.M. (1993) The science of cosmetics. *American Journal of Contact Dermatitis*, **4**, 47–49.

Jackson, E.M. (1995) Diazolidinyl urea: A toxicologic and dermatologic risk assessment as a preservative in consumer products. *Journal of Toxicology—Cutaneous and Ocular Toxicology*, **14**, 3–21.

Jacobs, M.C., White, I.R., Rycroft, J.G. & Taub, N. (1995) Patch testing with preservatives at St John's from 1982 to 1993. *Contact Dermatitis*, **33**, 247–254.

Jarvis, W.R. & Highsmith, A.K. (1984) Bacterial growth and endotoxin production in lipid emulsion. *Journal of Clinical Medicine*, **19**, 17–20.

Kabara, J.J. (1980) GRAS antimicrobial agents for cosmetic products. *Journal of the Society of Cosmetic Chemists*, **31**, 1–10.

Kabara, J.J. (1984a) Medium-chain fatty acids and esters as antimicrobial agents. In *Cosmetic and Drug Preservation: Principles and Practice* (ed. Kabara, J.J.), Cosmetic Science and Technology Series, Vol. 1, pp. 275–304. New York: Marcel Dekker.

Kabara, J.J. (1984b) Food-grade chemicals in a systems approach to cosmetic preservation. In *Cosmetic and Drug Preservation: Principles and Practice* (ed. Kabara, J.J.), Cosmetic Science and Technology Series, Vol. 1, pp. 339–356. New York: Marcel Dekker.

Kakemi, K.K., Sezaki, H., Arakawa, E., Kimura, K. & Ikeda, K. (1971) Interaction of parabens and other pharmaceutical adjuvants with plastic containers. *Chemical and Pharmaceutical Bulletin of Japan*, **19**, 2523–2529.

Kallings, L.O., Ringertz, O. & Silverstolpe, L. (1966) Microbiological contamination of medical preparations. *Acta Pharmaceutica Suecica*, **3**, 219–227.

Kamzi, S.J.A. & Mitchell, A.G. (1978) Preservation of solubilised and emulsified systems II: theoretical development of capacity and its role in antimicrobial activity of chlorocresol in cetomacrogol-stabilised systems. *Journal of Pharmaceutical Sciences*, **67**, 1266–1271.

Kostenbauder, H.B. (1991) Physical factors influencing the activity of antimicrobial agents. In *Disinfection, Sterilization, and Preservation*, 4th edn (ed. Block, S.E.), pp. 59–71. Philadelphia: Lea & Febinger.

Kroll, R.G. & Agnostopoulos, G.D. (1981) Potassium leakage as a lethality index of phenol and the effect of solute and water activity. *Journal of Applied Bacteriology*, **50**, 139–147.

Kurup, T.R.R., Wan, L.S.C. & Chan, L.W. (1991) Availability and activity of preservatives in emulsified systems. *Pharmaceutica Acta Helvetiae*, **66**, 76–83.

Leak, R.F., Morris, C. & Leech, R. (1996) Challenge tests and their predictive ability. In *Microbial Quality Assurance in Cosmetics, Toiletries and Non-Sterile Pharmaceuticals*, 2nd edn (eds Baird, R.M. & Bloomfield, S.F.), pp. 199–216. Basingstoke: Taylor & Francis.

Lindstrom, S.M. (1986) Consumer use testing: assurance of microbiological product safety. *Cosmetics and Toiletries*, **101**, 71–73.

Limtner, K. (1997) Physical methods of preservation. *Inside Cosmetics*, **March**, 1997, 23–29.

Loftsson, T., Stefansdottir, O., Frioriksdottir, H. & Guomundsson, O. (1992) Interactions between preservatives and 2-hydroxypropyl-β-cylcodextrin. *Drug Development and Industrial Pharmacy*, **18**, 1477–1484.

Loprieno, N. (1995) *Alternative Methods for the Safety Evaluation of Chemicals in the Cosmetic Industry*. New York: CRC Press.

Lund, W. (1994) *The Pharmaceutical Codex: Principles and Practice of Pharmaceutics*, 12th edn. London: Pharmaceutical Press.

Lynch, M., Lund, W. & Wilson, D.A. (1977) Chloroform as a preservative in aqueous systems. *Pharmaceutical Journal*, **219**, 507–510.

Manou, I., Bouillard, L., Devleeschouwer, M.J. & Barel, A.O. (1998) Evaluation of the preservative properties of *Thymus vulgaris* essential oil in topically applied formulations under a challenge test. *Journal of Applied Microbiology*, **84**, 368–376.

McCarthy, T.J. (1984) Formulated factors affecting the activity of preservatives. In *Cosmetic and Drug Preservation: Principles and Practice* (ed. Kabara, J.J.), Cosmetic Science and Technology Series, Vol. 1, pp. 359–388. New York: Marcel Dekker.

McCulloch, E.C. (1945) *Disinfection and Sterilisation*, 2nd edn, p. 221. London: Henry Kimpton.

McHugh, G.J. & Roper, G.M. (1995) Propofol emulsion and bacterial contamination. *Canadian Journal of Anesthesia*, **42**, 801–804.

McIntosh, D.A. (1987) Risk assessment and protection against civil and criminal liability in the pharmaceutical industry. In *Proceedings of the 9th BIRA Annual Symposium*, pp. 18–29.

McLaughlin, J.K. (1994) Formaldehyde and cancer: a critical review. *International Archives of Occupational and Environmental Health*, **66**, 295–301.

Martone, W.J., Tablan, O.C. & Jarvis, W.R. (1987) The epidemiology of nosocomial epidemic *Pseudomonas cepacia* infections. *European Journal of Epidemiology*, **3**, 222–232.

Miezitis, E.O., Polack, E.A. & Roberts, M.S. (1979) Concentration changes during autoclaving of aqueous solutions in polyethylene containers: an examination of some methods for reduction of solute loss. *Australian Journal of Pharmacy*, **8**, 72–77.

Millership, S.E., Patel, N. & Chattopadhyay, B. (1986) The colonisation of patients in an intensive treatment unit with Gram-negative flora: the significnce of the oral route. *Journal of Hospital Infection*, **7**, 226–235.

Mitchell, A.G. & Kamzi, J.A. (1975) Preservative availability in emulsified systems. *Canadian Journal of Pharmaceutical Sciences*, **10**, 67–68.

Moon, N.J. (1983) Inhibition of the growth of acid tolerant yeasts by acetate, lactate and propionate and their synergistic mixtures. *Journal of Applied Bacteriology*, **55**, 453–460.

Morris, C. & Leech, R. (1996) Natural and physical preservative systems. In *Microbial Quality Assurance in Cosmetics, Toiletries and Non-Sterile Pharmaceuticals*, 2nd edn (eds Baird, R.M. & Bloomfield, S.F.), pp. 69–97. Basingstoke: Taylor & Francis.

Muscatiello, M.J. (1993) CTFA's preservation guidelines: a historical perspective and review. *Cosmetics and Toiletries*, **108**, 53–59.

Norman, P. & Gosden, P.E. & Platt, J. (1986) Pseudobacteraemia associated with contaminated skin cleaning agent. *Lancet*, **i**, 209.

Oldham, G.B. & Andrews, V. (1996) Control of microbial contamination in unpreserved eyedrops. *British Journal of Ophthalmology*, **80**, 588–591.

Olson, R.J. & White, G.L. (1990) Preservatives in ophthalmic topical medications: a significant cause of disease. *Cornea*, **9**, 362–364.

Orth, D.S. (1993a) Preservation of cosmetic products. In *Handbook of Cosmetic Microbiology* (ed. Orth, D.S.), pp. 75–102. New York: Marcel Dekker.

Orth, D.S. (1993b) Microbiological considerations in product development. In *Handbook of Cosmetic Microbiology* (ed. Orth, D.S.), pp. 103–118. New York: Marcel Dekker.

Orth, D.S. (1993c) Microbial injury and the Phoenix phenomenon. In *Handbook of Cosmetic Microbiology*, (ed. Orth, D.S.), pp. 119–150. New York: Marcel Dekker.

Orth, D.S. & Lutes Anderson, C.M. (1985) Adaptation of bacteria to cosmetic preservatives. *Cosmetics and Toiletries*, **100**, 57–64.

Orth, D.S., Lutes, C.M., Milstein, S.R. & Allinger, J.J. (1987) Determination of shampoo preservative stability and apparent activation energies by the linear regression method of preservative efficacy testing. *Journal of the Society of Cosmetic Chemists*, **38**, 307–319.

Orth, D.S., Lutes Anderson, C.M., Smith, D.K. & Milstein, S.R. (1989) Synergism of preservative system components: use of the survival curve slope method to demonstrate anti-*Pseudomonas* synergy of methyl paraben and acrylic acid homoploymers and copolymers *in vitro*. *Journal of the Society of Cosmetic Chemists*, **40**, 347–365.

Orth, D.S., Barlow, R.F. & Gregory, L.A. (1992) The required D-value: evaluating product preservation in relation to packaging and consumer use/abuse. *Cosmetics and Toiletries*, **107**, 39–43.

Parker, M.S. (1973) Some aspects of the use of preservatives in combination. *Soap, Perfumery and Cosmetics*, **46**, 223–225.

Parker, M.S. (1984) Microbial biodeterioration of pharmaceutical preparations. *International Biodeterioration*, **20**, 151–156.

Payne, D.N. (1990) Microbial ecology of the production process. In *Guide to Microbiological Control in Pharmaceuticals* (eds Denyer, S.P. & Baird, R.), pp. 53–67. Chichester: Ellis Horwood.

Pena, L.E., Lee, B.L. & Stearns, J.F. (1993) Consistency development and destabilisation of a model cream. *Journal of the Society of Cosmetic Chemists*, **44**, 337–345.

Perry, B.F. (1995) Preservation efficacy testing in the cosmetics and toiletries industries. In *Microbiological Quality Assurance: A Guide Towards Relevance and Reproducibility of Inocula* (eds Brown, M.R.W. & Gilbert, P.), pp. 163–187. New York: CRC Press.

Person, J.R. (1985) Mounting evidence of paraben sensitivity in dogs. *Archives of Dermatology*, **121**, 1107.

Pons, J.-L., Bonnaveiro, N., Chevalier, J. & Cremieux, A. (1992) Evaluation of antimicrobial interactions between chlorhexidine quaternary ammonium compounds, preservatives and exipients. *Journal of Applied Bacteriology*, **73**, 395–400.

Qawas, A., Fulayyeh, I.Y.M., Lyall, J., Murray, J.B. & Smith G. (1986) The adsorption of bactericides by solids and the fitting of adsorption data to the Langmuir equation by a non-linear least-squares method. *Pharmaceutical Acta Helvetica*, **61**, 314–319.

Rehm, H.-J. (1959) Untersuchung zur Wirkung von Konservierungsmittelkombinationen. Die Wirkung einfacher Konserviersmittelkombinationen auf *Escherichia coli*. *Z. Lebensm. Unters. Forsch.*, **110**, 356–363.

Reiger, M.M. (1994) Methylparaben. In *Handbook of Pharmaceutical Excipients*, 2nd edn, pp. 310–313. London: Pharmaceutical Press, and Washington: American Pharmaceutical Association.

Riley, R.T., Kemppainen, B.W. & Norred, W.P. (1985) Penetration of aflatoxins through isolated human epidermis. *Journal of Toxicology and Environmental Health*, **15**, 769–777.

Ringertz, O. & Ringertz, S. (1982) The clinical significance of microbial contamination in pharmaceutical and allied products. In *Advances in Pharmaceutical Sciences*, Vol. 5 (eds Bean, H.S., Beckett, A.H. & Careless, J.E.), pp. 201–226. London: Academic Press.

Roberts, T.A. (1995) Microbial growth and survival: developments in predictive modelling. *International Biodeterioration and Biodegradation*, **36**, 297–309.

Rodford, R (1996) Safety of preservatives. In *Microbial Contamination–Determination–Eradication. Proceedings, Society of Cosmetic Chemists Symposium, Daresbury*. London; Miller Freeman Publishers. pp. 1–23.

Roller, S. (1995) The quest of natural antimicrobials as novel means of food preservation: status report on a European research project. *International Biodeterioration and Biodegradation*, **36**, 333–345.

Rosen, W.E. & Berke, P.A. (1984) German 115: a safe and effective preservative. In *Cosmetic and Drug Preservation: Principles and Practice* (ed. Kabara, J.J.), Cosmetic Science and Technology Series, Vol. 1, pp. 191–205. New York: Marcel Dekker.

Roszac, D.B. & Colwell, R.R. (1987) Survival strategies of bacteria in the natural environment. *Microbiological Reviews*, **51**, 365–379.

Runesson, B. & Gustavii, K. (1986) Stability of parabens in the presence of polyols. *Acta Pharmaceutica Suecica*, **23**, 151–162.

Russell, A.D. & Gould, G.W.G. (1988) Resistance of Enterobacteriaceae to preservatives and disinfectants. *Journal of Applied Bacteriology, Symposium Supplement*, 167S–195S.

Sabourin, J.R. (1990) Evaluation of preservatives for cosmetic products. *Drug and Cosmetic Industry*, **147**, 24–27, 64–65.

Sakamoto, T., Yanagi, M., Fukushimi, S. & Mitsui, T. (1987) Effects of some cosmetic pigments on the bactericidal activities of preservatives. *Journal of the Society of Cosmetic Chemists*, **38**, 83–98.

Sasaki, H., Nagano, T., Yamamara, K., Nishida, K. & Nakamara, J. (1995) Ophthalmic preservatives as absorption promoters for ocular drug delivery. *Journal of Pharmacy and Pharmacology*, **47**, 703–707.

Schmitt, W.H. & Murphy, E.G. (1984) An overview of worldwide regulatory programs. In *The Cosmetic Industry: Scientific and Regulatory Foundations* (ed. Estrin, N.F.), pp. 131–161. Cosmetic Science and Technology Series. New York: Marcel Dekker.

Seal, D.V. (1994) *Acanthamoeba* keratitis. *British Medical Journal*, **308**, 1116–1117.

Shaqra, Q.M. & Husari, N. (1987) Preservation of some commercially available antacid suspensions against *Pseudomonas aeruginosa* (ATCC 9027). *International Biodeterioration*, **23**, 47–51.

Sharpell, F. & Manowitz, M. (1991) Preservation of cosmetics. In *Disinfection, Sterilisation and Preservation* (ed. Block, S.E.), pp. 887–900. Malvern, Pennsylvania: Lea & Febinger.

Smart, R. & Spooner, D.F. (1972) Microbiological spoilage in pharmaceuticals and cosmetics. *Journal of the Society of Cosmetic Chemists*, **23**, 721–737.

Smith, J.L. (1984) Evaluating your microbiology programme. In *The Cosmetic Industry: Scientific and Regulatory Foundations*, (ed. Estrin, N.F.), pp. 301–320. Cosmetic Science and Technology Series. New York: Marcel Dekker.

Sommerville, P.C. (1981) A survey into microbial contamination of non-sterile pharmaceutical products. *Farmaceutische Tijdschrift, Belgica*, **58**, 345–450.

Spooner, D.F. (1996) Hazards associated with the microbiological contamination of cosmetics, toiletries, and non-sterile medicines. In *Microbial Quality Assurance in Cosmetics, Toiletries and Non-Sterile Pharmaceuticals*, 2nd edn (eds Baird, R.M. & Bloomfield, S.F.), pp. 9–27. Basingstoke: Taylor & Francis.

Spooner, D.F. & Croshaw, B. (1981) Challenge testing: the laboratory evaluation of the preservation of pharmaceutical preparations. *Antonie van Leeuwenhoek Journal of Serology*, **47**, 168–169.

Spooner, D.F. & Davison, A.L. (1993) The validity of the criteria for pharmacopoeial antimicrobial preservative efficacy tests. *Pharmaceutical Journal*, **251**, 602–605.

Tebbs, S.E., Ghose, S.E. & Elliott, T.S.J. (1996) Microbial contamination of intravenous and arterial catheters. *Intensive Care Medicine*, **22**, 272–273.

Theodore, F.H. & Feinstein, R.R. (1952) *Serratia* keratitis transmitted by contaminated eye droppers. *American Journal of Ophthalmology*, **93**, 723–726.

Thompson, D.F., Letassy, N.A., Gee, M. & Kolar, R. (1989) Contamination risks of multidose medication vials: a review. *Journal of Pharmacy Technology*, **5**, 249–253.

Tran, T.T. & Hitchins, A.D. (1994) Microbial survey of shared-use cosmetic test kits available to the public. *Journal of Industrial Microbiology*, **13**, 389–391.

Tran, T.T., Hurley, F.J., Shurbaji, M. & Koopman, L.P. (1994) Adequacy of cosmetic preservation: chemical analysis, microbiological challenge and in-use testing. *International Journal of Cosmetic Science*, **16**, 61–76.

Tremewan, H.C. (1946) Tetanus neonatorum in New Zealand. *New Zealand Medical Journal*, **45**, 312–313.

Vaara, M. (1992) Agents that increase the permeability of the outer membrane. *Microbiological Reviews*, **56**, 395–411.

van Doorne, H. (1990) Interactions between preservatives and pharmaceutical components. In *Guide to Microbiological Control in Pharmaceuticals* (eds Denyer, S. & Baird, R.), pp. 274–291. Chichester: Ellis Horwood.

Vanhaecke, E., Remon, J.P., Pijck, J., Aerts, R. &

Herman, J. (1987) A comparative study of the effectiveness of preservatives in twelve antacid suspensions. *Drug Developments in Industrial Pharmacy*, **13**, 1429–1446.

van Loosdrecht, M.C.M., Lyklema, J., Norde, W. & Zehnder, A.J.B. (1990) Influence of interfaces on microbial activity. *Microbiological Reviews*, **54**, 75–87.

Verrips, C.T. (1989) Growth of micro-organisms in compartmentalised producs. In *Mechanisms of Action of Food Preservation Procedures* (ed. Gould, G.W.), pp. 363–399. London: Elsevier Applied Science.

Wade, A. & Weller, P.J. (1994) *Handbook of Pharmaceutical Excipients*, 2nd edn. London: Pharmaceutical Press, and Washington: American Pharmaceutical Association.

Wallhaeusser, K.-H. (1984) Antimicrobial preservatives used by the cosmetic industry. In *Cosmetic and Drug Preservation: Principles and Practice* (ed. Kabara, J.J.), Cosmetic Science and Technology Series, Vol. 1, pp. 605–745. New York: Marcel Dekker.

Wang, Y.J. & Chien, Y.W. (1984) *Sterile Pharmaceutical Packaging: Compatibility and Stability.* Parenteral Drug Association Technical Report No. 5. Pennsylvania: Parenteral Drug Association.

Wedderburn, D.L. (1964) Preservation of emulsions against microbial attack. In *Advances in Pharmaceutical Sciences*, Vol. I (eds Bean, H.A., Beckett, A.H. & Carless, J.), pp. 195–268. London: Academic Press.

Whiteman, M. (1995) Evaluating the performance of tablet coatings. *Manufacturing Chemist*, **66**, 24–27.

Wiggins, P.W. (1990) Role of water in some biological processes. *Microbiological Reviews*, **54**, 432–449.

Wilson, L.A. & Ahearn, D.G. (1977) *Pseudomonas*-induced corneal ulcers associated with contaminated eye mascaras. *American Journal of Ophthalmology*, **84**, 114–119.

Wimpenny, J.W.T. (1981) Spatial order in microbial ecosystems. *Biological Reviews*, **56**, 295–342.

Wood, R.T. (1993) Sterilization with dry heat. In *Sterilization Technology: A Practical Guide for Manufacturers and Users of Health Care Products* (eds Morrissey, R.F. & Phillips, C.B.), pp. 81–119. New York: Van Nostrand Reinhold.

Woodruff, J. (1995) Preservatives to fight the growth of mould. *Manufacturing Chemist*, **66**, 34–35.

Yousef, R.T., El-Nakeeb, M.A. & Salama, S. (1973) Effect of some pharmaceutical materials on the bactericidal activities of preservatives. *Canadian Journal of Pharmaceutical Sciences*, **18**, 54–56.

CHAPTER 17

Chemical Food Preservatives

1 Introduction

It is becoming obvious that our global society is experiencing major advances and expansion in the commercial development and manufacturing of processed foods; marketing of more perishable food products; advances in food-processing and distribution procedures; acceptance of, as well as demand for, convenience foods by modern consumers; and reduction in numbers of people involved in food production. These developments are coupled with increases in total world population and changes in lifestyles—especially more foods prepared outside the home, which have resulted in increased demands for more and different foods, as well as a higher potential for the mishandling of foods during various stages of processing, storage, distribution and preparation for consumption (CAST, 1998). In addition, food safety and utilization of chemicals in food processing and preservation have become important concerns of consumers, health professionals and government regulators. Furthermore, recognition of potential public-health problems caused by psychrotrophic pathogenic microorganisms and increases in numbers of immunodeficient persons, who are especially sensitive to microbial food-borne illness, have emphasized the need for appropriate preservation of perishable foods. Consequently, food preservation has attained greater significance in the survival and well-being of the human race (Foegeding & Busta, 1991).

Certain methods of food processing and preservation, such as drying (dehydration), salting, smoking and fermentation, have been used by humans since prehistoric times; preserved foods could have been used during periods of shortages, such as the winter months, when crop production and hunting were limited. As the human population increased, food preservation became more important. Added objectives were to diminish food waste and to maintain the wholesomeness and safety of food, allowing consumption during periods of production failures due to adverse climatic conditions or during migrations (Foegeding & Busta, 1991; CAST, 1998).

Preservation of foods in modern times relies on systems involving handling or decontamination procedures that minimize contamination (e.g. aseptic handling/packaging, washing, filtration, centrifugation); destruction of contamination through application of thermal or radiation energies; or inhibition of microbial proliferation through control of factors that affect growth, and which include addition of chemical food preservatives (Foedgeding & Busta, 1991; Gould, 1995, 1996; CAST, 1998).

Improvements of methods involving food preservation by heat, storage at low temperature, packaging in modified atmosphere environments and drying have resulted in increased application of these processes in recent years. However, there are many foods where such processes cannot be applied or their useful application is limited, due to potentially adverse effects on product quality and acceptability. In these instances, preservation by the application of chemical additives as hurdles to microbial growth increases in significance.

Chemicals exerting antimicrobial activity are present in food products either as natural constituents, introduced by direct incorporation as additives or developed during processing of the food. Some chemical compounds have been used accidentally or intentionally in the preservation of foods for many centuries. These traditional preservatives include common salt, sugars, spices, acids and components of smoke, and are introduced through processes such as fermentation, salting (curing) and smoking. Meat and fish products were widely preserved by such processes in ancient times. Additional natural food components with antimicrobial activity have been recognized through the years (CAST, 1997).

During the past century, some specific and well-identified compounds have been used as chemical food preservatives. In general terms, chemical preservation can include a variety of compounds employed in the processing of foods, and may affect the appearance, colour, texture, flavour, odour, nutrient value, wholesomeness and safety. However, this chapter only deals with chemicals acting as antimicrobial agents in foods. In this text, compounds that are introduced into the food during processing and before consumption with the objective of preventing or delaying microbial spoilage and the development of pathogenic microorganisms are considered in some detail. Certain chemicals reported as having the potential to inhibit microbial growth in food systems are also presented briefly.

2 Need for food preservation

Growth of microorganisms in foods leads to chemical and enzymatic reactions that result in changes in the general appearance, colour, flavour, texture, consistency and nutritive value, as well as safety. Food that has experienced undesirable microbial growth becomes unfit for human consumption and is considered a loss, thus contributing to worldwide food shortages, which are expected to become even more noticeable as the world population increases. Other unwanted consequences of such growth are health problems for individuals consuming the food, loss of life, and adverse effects to private and national economies (Foegeding & Busta, 1991). In addition, increases in urban population densities intensify the need for extension of food-product shelf-life in order for it to remain of acceptable quality and safe during the longer periods of time that are needed for its destination to consumers (CAST, 1998). It is estimated that food losses are extensive and that their impact will be maximized in light of continued increases in world population. Furthermore, proliferation of toxic microorganisms may result in human illness, which sometimes leads to death, costing national economies billions of dollars and precious human lives (Roberts, 1989; Todd, 1989; Bryan, 1992; CAST, 1994, 1998; Mossel *et al.*, 1995; ICMSF, 1996; Ray, 1996). Microbial food-borne-illness concerns have intensified in recent years, due to recognition or emergence of sometimes psychrotrophic pathogenic bacteria and their undesirable health effects on immunodeficient humans, especially the young, elderly and infirm. Recognition of food-borne-disease problems caused by pathogenic bacteria, such as *Listeria monocytogenes* and verotoxigenic *Escherichia coli* (e.g. *E. coli* O157:H7) has increased the need for microbial control in food products (CAST, 1994).

In general, it is a well-accepted fact that there is a need for preservation of our food supply, both in its state as a raw agricultural commodity and as products of modern food-processing techniques. The main objectives of chemical food preservation are to extend the shelf-life, retain wholesomeness and ensure the safety of our food supply, by delaying or preventing microbial decomposition and by inhibiting or suppressing the growth of pathogenic microorganisms (Foegeding & Busta, 1991). As indicated above, food preservation also allows variety in our diet throughout the year and in locations of the globe where climatic and soil conditions do not allow production or processing of certain foods.

Physical control processes such as dehydration (drying), low-temperature storage (refrigeration–freezing) and heat processing (Chapter 19D) constitute commonly used methods of food preservation, but their application is limited to certain types of food products and the degree of such application is also limited by their influence on product characteristics. Even though they are used extensively, changes in product identity and functionality, energy requirements of the processes, available technology, method reliability and consumer acceptance are some major factors limiting the widespread application of the physical control methods. Treatment of foods by irradiation, even though classified as an additive by USA regulation (CFR, 1996), is a physical process of microbial inactivation and control. Even though approved uses in food have increased, the main application of irradiation treatments is still restricted to medical fields (Chapter 20A). In most countries, even approved food uses are not widely applied, due to labelling requirements, undocumented health concerns, equipment availability and potentially economic concerns (Loaharanu, 1995). Newer methods of microbial control through disinfection or inactivation include application of high hydrostatic pressures, pulsed electric fields and light, ultrasonic waves and microwaves. Their application in foods, however, is still at the experimental stage.

Physical (e.g. heating) methods of food preservation are often used in combination with a variety of chemical additives. Such combinations of multiple hurdles or barriers to microbial growth allow these processes or agents to be used at lower intensity or concentration and the food still retains good keeping quality, with only minor changes in characteristics (Leistner, 1978, 1985, 1995; Sofos, 1993; Giese, 1994).

For the purposes of this chapter, the inhibition of undesirable microorganisms by chemical compounds in a food system is characterized as chemical food preservation. Other deteriorative changes in food resulting from chemical or enzymatic reactions may also be retarded or prevented through use of chemical preservatives. Such deterioration may include alterations of flavour, odour, colour, appearance, texture and nutritive value, and is not considered in this chapter.

3 Interactions of multihurdle preservation systems

Preservation of food products is often accomplished through the combined or synergistic activity of several additives, intrinsic product parameters (e.g. composition, acidity, water activity (A_w)) and extrinsic factors (e.g. processing temperature, storage atmosphere and temperature). Use of this multihurdle approach, based on additive or synergistic antimicrobial influences, should continue in the future (Leistner, 1985, 1995; Wagner & Moberg, 1989; Sofos, 1993), because it minimizes undesirable changes in product properties and reduces concentration of additives and extent of processing treatments, while maintaining product quality and safety. The concept of combinations of preservatives and treatments to preserve foods is frequently called the hurdle or barrier concept (Leistner, 1978, 1985, 1995; Sofos, 1993). Combinations of additives and preservative systems provide multiple preservation alternatives for application in food products to meet consumer demands for wholesome, healthy and safe foods (Foegeding & Busta, 1991; CAST, 1998).

The evaluation of the antimicrobial activity of multihurdle preservation systems is feasible through the use of predictive microbiology principles and the application of mathematical models (Farber, 1986; Labuza *et al.*, 1992; Buchanan *et al.*, 1993; McMeekin *et al.*, 1993; Ross & McMeekin, 1994; Haas *et al.*, 1997; Miller *et al.*, 1997; Roberts, 1997; Schaftner & Labuza, 1997; Whiting, 1997). The selected multihurdle preservation systems can also be correlated with quantitative risk-assessment models (Whiting & Buchanan, 1994; Buchanan & Whiting, 1996) to predict accurately the anticipated shelf-life for a product (CAST, 1998). The preservation system can then be validated and, after its application in a commercial product, it can be managed through process control by the hazard-analysis critical control-point (HACCP) system (ICMSF, 1988; Tompkin, 1990; NACMCF, 1992; Pierson & Corlett, 1992; Sofos, 1992a; Mortimer & Wallace, 1994).

4 Selection of chemical food preservatives

No single, currently available, food preservative satisfies all the requirements of the ideal, or is capable of being used in a wide range of food products (Foegeding & Busta, 1991). Factors affecting preservative function should be closely evaluated when a food preservative is to be selected for a specific food (Ingram *et al.*, 1964; Mossel, 1975; Jarvis & Burke, 1976; Lueck, 1992; Davidson & Branen, 1993; Giese, 1994; Welbourn, 1994). Major factors affecting the antimicrobial activity of individual compounds include the types of microorganisms likely to be encountered and the nature of the food to be preserved (Foegeding & Busta, 1991; CAST, 1997). It is highly desirable that the antimicrobial spectrum of a preservative be wide, and that its activity should not inhibit the growth of one kind of microorganism and as a consequence permit the growth of another, possibly pathogenic, type. In many instances, one group of microorganisms suppresses the growth of another. If the first group is inhibited, the second may predominate and cause problems not encountered previously. Therefore, antimicrobials should exhibit inhibitory activity against a wide range of microorganisms (Foegeding & Busta, 1991). A chemical food preservative is preferred when it does not interfere with useful microorganisms, such as lactic acid bacteria in fermented foods, and when it does not lead to development of resistant strains, as is the case for strains of yeasts and moulds, which have developed resistance to benzoate and sorbate (Sofos, 1989a; Foegeding & Busta, 1991).

The antimicrobial activity of chemical food preservatives is influenced by their physical and chemical properties and by their interaction with the food to be preserved (Foegeding & Busta, 1991). Important properties include solubility, dissociation constant (pK_a) and chemical reactivity (Table 17.1). The preferential solubility of parabens (esters of *p*-hydroxybenzoic acid: see Chapter 2) in lipids is considered the main reason for their extensive performance in aqueous culture media and their low performance in lipid-containing food systems. The antimicrobial activity of weak-acid preservatives is attributed mostly to their undissociated form. Thus, the pK_a value of a particular compound will predict its efficacy in a food system with a specified pH level (Sofos, 1989a). Since the potassium salt of sorbic acid is more soluble in water than the acid itself, the salt is preferred in spray or brine applications. However, in applications made directly into the products, the acid form may be used. Since the antimicrobial activity of parabens increases with chain length and water solubility decreases, a mixture of two or more of these compounds can yield the most practical preservative action (Foegeding & Busta, 1991).

The most commonly used chemical food preservatives are weak acids or their salts or esters. Acidity

Table 17.1 Some properties of the most commonly used chemical food preservatives.

Agent	Chemical formula	Water solubility (g/100 ml, 25 °C)	pK_a	Effective against
Lactic acid	$CH_3CHOHCOOH$	High	3.1	Bacteria, yeasts, moulds (Lactic acid to Methylparaben)
Citric acid	$CH_2COOHCOHCOOHCH_2COOH$	High	3.1	
Acetic acid	CH_3COOH	High	4.75	
Sodium diacetate	$CH_3COONa \cdot CH_3COOH \cdot \frac{1}{2}H_2O$	100.0	4.75	
Sodium benzoate	C_6H_3COONa	50.0	4.2	
Sodium propionate	CH_3CH_2COONa	100.0	4.9	
Potassium sorbate	$CH_3CH{=}CHCH{=}CHCOOK$	139.2	4.75	
Methylparaben	HO–⟨benzene ring⟩–$COOCH_3$	0.25	8.5	
Sodium nitrite	$NaNO_2$	66.0		Bacteria
Sulphur dioxide	SO_2	85.0		Bacteria, yeasts, moulds

is the main means of preservation in fermented products, such as sauerkraut, pickles, yoghurt and fermented meats. The method of preserving foods by increasing their acidity, either naturally by fermentation or by addition of acids, has been in use for thousands of years. In certain instances, the effect of acids may be combined with other factors, such as heat processing, dehydration (A_w) or other chemical compounds. Acidity also potentiates the preservative action of the salts of weak mineral acids, such as nitrites and sulphites, which are common preservatives. The preservative action of weak acids is twofold. The concentration of free hydrogen ions (H^+) is increased and the undissociated form of the acid directly affects the microorganisms. The growth and survival of microorganisms during processing and storage are affected by the pH of the product. Low pH not only inhibits microbial growth but also reduces microbial heat resistance during processing. The major effect of organic-acid preservatives is the result of the toxic effect of their undissociated molecule. The pK_a values of most food preservatives, except parabens, are below pH 5.0 (Table 17.1). This is very important, considering that the optimum pH range for the growth of most bacteria is between 5.5 and 7.0, whereas yeasts and moulds can grow at pH values as low as 2.0.

In general, pH not only directly influences the growth and survival of microorganisms, but also the effects of the most commonly used preservatives are dependent on it. A low pH generally favours effective preservation. This is either due to its direct effect on the microorganisms (especially bacteria) or due to the increased effectiveness of most preservatives at lower pH values. It is fortunate or maybe fortuitous that most foods fall toward the acid side of the pH range, where the available preservatives are generally effective. Table 17.2 lists some of the commonly used chemical food preservatives, their levels of incorporation and acceptable daily intake by humans. More details on these aspects are found in the text.

In addition to the properties of the preservatives to be used and the pH of the food, selection of a chemical for food preservation is affected by its interaction with the food and other ingredients or processes involved in the manufacturing of the

Table 17.2 Common uses of chemical food preservatives.

Agent	Acceptable daily intake used levels (mg/kg body weight)	Commonly Food products of (%)	common usage
Lactic acid	No limit	No limit	Olives, salad-dressings, mayonnaise, desserts, bakery goods
Citric acid	No limit	No limit	Carbonated beverages, fruit juices, wines
Acetic acid	No limit	No limit	Salad-dressings, mayonnaise, olives, sauces, pickled meats, vegetables
Sodium diacetate	15	0.3–0.5	Bread and bakery goods
Sodium benzoate	5	0.03–0.2	Pickles, beverages, salads, syrups, fish, preserves, jams, jellies, margarine
Sodium propionate	10	0.1–0.3	Bread and bakery products, cheese products, fruits, vegetables
Potassium sorbate	25	0.05–0.2	Dairy products, baked goods, fruits, vegetables, soft drinks, margarine, pickled products, jams, jellies, meat and fish products
Methylparaben	10	0.05–0.1	Fruit products, pickles, syrups, baked goods, creams, preserves, pastes
Sodium nitrite	0.2	0.01–0.02	Cured meats, cheese, fish
Sulphur dioxide	0.7	0.005–0.2	Wines, fruit juices, syrups, meat and fish products

food (Foegeding & Busta, 1991). Certain ingredients act synergistically or exert additional antimicrobial activity, while processes (e.g. heating, drying) which may cause microbial injury enhance antimicrobial activity of chemical compounds. As indicated above, there is a major contribution of interacting hurdles in food preservation, which should be considered when chemical food preservatives or total food preservation systems are selected.

The stringent considerations needed to be met for approval of a compound as a food preservative, as well as the complexity of foods and the variety of influential and interacting factors, often make selection of the appropriate preservative difficult. Selection of the proper chemical food preservative is also difficult because only a few compounds are currently approved for use as preservatives; all approved chemical food preservatives have certain disadvantages; the demand for food preservation is increasing; and listing of chemical additives on product labels is undesirable from a marketing standpoint (Foegeding & Busta, 1991).

5 Methods of application

Chemical food preservatives may be applied to foods as additives or they develop in the product during processes such as fermentation (Foegeding & Busta, 1991). Addition of chemical food preservatives may be through direct addition in the formulation; by spraying with or immersing in a solution; by dusting with a powder; through application with an organic carrier, such as ethanol, vegetable oil or propylene glycol, applied to the coating or packaging material that comes in contact with the surface of the food; or as an ingredient of multicomponent formulations applied in a single action (Sofos, 1989a; CAST, 1998).

Selection of the method of application is based on the properties of the preservative, processing procedures, convenience in processing and type of food product. Properties of chemical food preservatives, such as solubility and volatility, are major determinants of the method of application. One important consideration in spray or dipping applications is to use adequate concentrations in order to achieve sufficient uptake by the food for its preservation, without exceeding legal limits or sensory thresholds. Often the method of application is selected on the basis of the ease with which the preservative can be added through existing processing and packaging procedures.

6 Mechanisms of chemical food preservation

The objective of chemical food preservation is the prevention or delay of microbiologically induced changes in a food product. In some instances, and under certain circumstances, some physical control methods of food preservation (e.g. heat) or chemical compounds (e.g. alkylating agents) may result in product sterilization by actually killing the indigenous microbial flora. Frequently, however, the microbial population remains viable in the product, but its proliferation is inhibited or retarded by the chemical compounds added to the product as food preservatives or by the total preservation system of the food in instances where chemical food preservatives are applied in combination with physical control processes or other chemical compounds.

The specific effects and the mechanisms through which microbial control is accomplished may vary among compounds and other conditions. The mechanisms of chemical food preservation may differ among compounds used as preservatives, food systems being preserved, microorganisms to be controlled and other constituents of the system, and between culture media and actual foods. The complexity of food systems, the diversity of microbial species and the extensive interactions occurring in multicomponent non-homogeneous systems are major reasons why the mechanisms of food preservation in most instances are not well defined. Several reviews of pertinent information exist in the literature (Wyss, 1948; Bosund, 1962; Oka, 1964; Hugo, 1967, 1976a,b; Vinter, 1970; Skinner & Hugo, 1976; Freese *et al.*, 1973; Warth, 1977; Freese & Levin, 1978; Sofos *et al.*, 1986; Sofos, 1989a; Denyer & Hugo, 1991; Russell, 1991; Russell & Chopra, 1996), but many effects still remain unexplained and, in most instances, definite answers are still lacking.

Determination of specific mechanisms of microbial inhibition will facilitate the search for new preservatives; may explain the development of resistant microbial strains; and may result in selection or development of ideal chemical food preservatives or preservation systems. As indicated above, a very important factor in chemical food preservation is the pH of the system. The growth of most microorganisms reaches an optimum at pH values near neutrality (7.0). The pH range for growth, however, is different among microbial groups, genera, etc. In general, bacteria do not grow well at pH values below 4.5, while yeasts and moulds are more resistant to acidity and some can even grow at pH values below 2.0. A high level of acidity may directly inhibit microbial growth or it may facilitate the action of other preservatives, such as lipophilic acids, by increasing the proportion of their more effective undissociated form. Of the commonly used chemical food preservatives, only the esters of *p*-hydroxybenzoic acid have a high pK_a value (8.5) and are effective at higher pH values (>7.0). The range of pH values in which certain microorganisms can grow is also affected by environmental factors, such as oxygen tension, other microbial species present, storage temperature, A_w, heat processing, gas atmosphere, nutrient availability and means of acidification.

The internal pH of microbial cells may be considerably affected by the pH of their environment. Acidification of the interior of the cell can result in growth inhibition. Such inhibition, however, varies among microbial species, since different species exhibit different tolerances toward internal acidity (Neal *et al.*, 1965; Freese *et al.*, 1973; Hunter & Segel, 1973). In the case of acid preservatives, especially lipophilic acids, a lowering of the pH of the medium can have a dual effect. One is direct acidification, and the second an increase in the effective undissociated form as the pH approaches the pK_a value of the compound. Chemical food preservatives, in general, exert their antimicrobial activity through some type of a reaction with components of the microbial cell (Oka, 1964). This reaction may be interference with the proton-motive force, cell membranes and their permeability; with the genetic apparatus of the cell; or with enzymatic or other chemical activities within the cell (Wyss, 1948; Freese *et al.*, 1973; Eklund, 1985, 1989; Dillon & Cook, 1994; Russell & Chopra, 1996). The antimicrobial effect of food preservatives may depend on their sorption on to the cell surface or on membrane permeability and uptake by the cell (Oka, 1964). Lipophilic acid preservatives have been reported to uncouple substrate transport and oxidative phosphorylation from the electron-transport system by making the cytoplasmic membrane freely permeable to protons, thereby destroying part of the proton-motive force (Chapter 9). As a result, growth inhibition may occur through inhibition of active cellular uptake of compounds such as amino acids, organic acids and phosphate. Several studies have suggested that the microbial inhibition by sorbic acid and similar compounds is the result of inhibition of various dehydrogenase enzymes (Sofos, 1989a), while Warth (1991a,b) indicated that the primary action of benzoic acid against *Zygosaccharomyces bailii* and *Saccharomyces cerevisiae* was through depletion of adenosine triphosphate (ATP).

On the basis of indirect but conclusive evidence, Tompkin (1978, 1993) has suggested that nitrite may react with an iron-containing compound (ferredoxin) within the germinated botulinal cell and consequently could interfere with energy metabolism to prevent outgrowth and toxin production. Woods *et al.* (1981) have suggested that, through nitric oxide, nitrite inhibits the phosphoroclastic system of clostridia.

The above highlight only some of the theories presented to explain the effectiveness of some chemicals used in preventing microbial growth in food systems. Final conclusions are yet to be reached and the subject is still open. It is very likely, however, that more than one mechanism is involved in inhibition of microorganisms by chemical food preservatives. Additional information on mechanisms of antimicrobial activity is presented in the discussion of certain individual food preservatives.

7 Naturally occurring antimicrobials

Chemical ingredients with antimicrobial properties are found in many plants and animal tissues and secretions, as well as in insects and microorganisms (CAST, 1998). These naturally occurring antimicrobial components have probably evolved as natural defence mechanisms against enemy invasion. Natural antimicrobial agents present in plant tissues include essential oils, phenolic compounds, low molecular weight components of herbs and spices, phytoalexins and pigments (Dallyn, 1994; Walker, 1994; Delaquis & Mazza, 1995). Animal tissue-derived antimicrobials include lysozyme, lactoperoxidase, lactotransferrin, ovotransferrin, fatty acids and polyamines. Antimicrobials produced by microorganisms include acids, bacteriocins, alcohol, hydrogen peroxide and diacetyl (CAST, 1998). These latter items will be discussed in another section.

Many spices, herbs, seasonings and their essential oils are classified as generally recognized as safe (GRAS) for use in foods by the Food and Drug Administration (FDA) in the USA, or are approved (CFR, 1996) and used in food processing mainly as flavouring ingredients; in some instances their use covers thousands of years (Conner, 1993; Beuchat, 1994). Furthermore, a long list of synthetic flavouring substances and adjuvants are approved for use in the USA (CFR, 1996). Some of these flavouring components of processed foods contain substances with bacteriostatic or even bactericidal activity. Information on the antimicrobial activity of spices, plant materials and their components and on other naturally occurring antimicrobial systems can be found in several reviews (Habtanen, 1980; Davidson *et al.*, 1983; Shelef, 1984; Banks *et al.*, 1986; Zaika, 1988; Beuchat & Golden, 1989; Wilkins & Board, 1989; Gould, 1992, 1995, 1996; Conner, 1993; Beuchat, 1994; Dillon & Board, 1994; Lattanzio *et al.*, 1994; Walker, 1994; CAST, 1998).

Common plants known for their antimicrobial activity include garlic, onion and leek of the genus *Allium*, which contain the antimicrobial compound allicin, acting on sulph-hydryl-containing enzymes. Some widely known spices with antimicrobial activity include cinnamon, clove and allspice, while common phenolic antimicrobials are eugenol, thymol, cinnamic aldehyde and oleuropein. Natural antimicrobial activity is also present in the flowers of hops, used in beer making, as well as in coffee, tea and cocoa, which contain the antimicrobials caffeine, theobromine and theophylline. The antimicrobial activity of spices and their extracts is well documented against Gram-positive as well as Gram-negative bacteria and fungi (CAST, 1998).

The amounts of spices commonly introduced into the food are generally small and antimicrobial action of their components may be only synergistic with the total preservative system in the product. Future research on the subject, however, may lead to identification and potential manufacturing of new preservatives with regulatory, industrial and consumer acceptance.

Various other naturally occurring compounds have demonstrated antimicrobial activity and may play key roles in preservation of natural foods (Davidson *et al.*, 1983; CAST, 1998). Such compounds are found in various foods, but especially in milk and eggs. They include lysozyme, lactoperoxidase, lactotransferrin, casein, fatty acids, conalbumin and others. However, very little use has been made of these food components as intentional chemical food preservatives (Banks *et al.*, 1986; Beuchat & Golden, 1989; CAST, 1998).

The naturally occurring enzyme lysozyme, or muramidase, which is present in many biological systems, including several foods (e.g. milk and egg-white), has been suggested as a preservative for other foods and beverages. The maximum antimicrobial activity of lysozyme is at pH 7.0 and it degrades the cell wall of bacteria, but it is of high cost (Busta & Foegeding, 1983; Hughey & Johnson, 1987; Tranter, 1994). Lysis of bacteria occurs through hydrolysis of the beta linkage between muramic acid and glycosamine of the glycopolysaccharides in the bacterial cell wall (Beuchat & Golden, 1989). The enzyme is active against pathogens, such as *Clostridium botulinum* and *L. monocytogenes* (Hughey *et al.*, 1989). Gram-negative bacteria need to be sensitized to lysozyme by treatment with chelators, such as ethylenediaminetetra-acetic acid (EDTA), which acts on the protective lipoprotein/lipopolysaccharide layers (El-Kest & Marth, 1992; Erickson & Jenkins, 1992; CAST, 1998). Lysozyme is used to prevent gas formation by clostridia, resulting in 'blowing' of cheeses, and has been evaluated as a preservative in foods such as sausages, seafood, tofu and sake (Tranter, 1994). Other antimicrobials present in milk and eggs include vitamin-binding proteins, such as avidin, casein, aprotinin, protamine and histones (CAST, 1998).

Oxidase enzymes can lead to antimicrobial action by generating hydrogen peroxide and, in the presence of catalase, by depleting oxygen, while peroxidases produce toxic metabolites (Ekstrand, 1994; CAST, 1998). Lactoperoxidase occurs in high amounts in milk and other body fluids, and oxidizes thiocyanate and other halides in the presence of hydrogen peroxide to produce the lactoperoxidase antimicrobial system (LPS) (Reiter & Harnulv, 1984; Beuchat & Golden, 1989; Ekstrand, 1994). The components of the system occur naturally or are formed through microbial action (i.e. hydrogen peroxide) in milk. The system has been used in some developing countries in the preservation of milk (Medina *et al.*, 1989), and has potential in preserving infant formulas (Banks & Board, 1985). The system was also found inhibitory against the pathogenic bacteria *L. monocytogenes* (Denis & Ramet, 1989; Earnshaw & Banks, 1989), *Campylobacter jejuni* (Borch *et al.*, 1989) and *Salmonella typhimurium* (Earnshaw *et al.*, 1990).

It should be noted that the inhibitory activity of the LPS is neutralized by other enzymes (e.g. catalase), heating, reducing agents and with storage time (Davidson *et al.*, 1983). It has been suggested, however, that this and other natural systems should be developed and applied in food preservation (Banks *et al.*, 1986; CAST, 1998). The LPS has been used or tested in various parts of the world as a preservative of raw milk in places of limited refrigeration. Other products than may be preserved with the LPS include infant milk formula, cheese, ice-cream, salad-dressings and toothpaste (Ekstrand, 1994; CAST, 1998).

Another peroxidase with antimicrobial activity is myeloperoxidase, found in mammalian cells. It binds hydrogen peroxide and oxidizes chlorine to hypochlorous acid (CAST, 1998). A system that is related to the LPS, and which is considered safe and highly antimicrobial, is the so-called glucose oxidase/glucose system. Glucose oxidase catalyses the reaction between glucose and oxygen to yield gluconic acid or D-glucon-*S*-lactose and hydrogen. Actually, this system may act as a source of hydrogen peroxide, which can be used in the LPS (Dziezak, 1986; Tiina & Sandholm, 1989; Joeng *et al.*, 1992; Kantt & Torres, 1993). Glucose oxidase and catalase have been used in egg products, meat and potatoes to prevent browning and off-flavour reactions, and can also inhibit growth of oxygen-requiring microorganisms, such as yeasts in beer, wine and other beverages (CAST, 1997).

Polypeptides and peptides with antimicrobial activity are present in many plant and animal tissues (Gabay, 1994; Tranter, 1994; Owen Fields, 1996). In addition to lytic enzymes and oxidases, natural antimicrobial activity is also attributed to iron-binding peptides, such as transferrins (e.g. ovotransferrin or conalbumin and lactoferrin), found in foods such as eggs and milk (Ekstrand, 1994; Tranter, 1994).

Other natural peptides with antimicrobial activity include bacteriocins, defensins, killer toxins and antimicrobials present in insects (Casteels, 1990; Lehrer *et al.*, 1991; Dillon, 1994; CAST, 1998). Bacteriocins are discussed later. Killer toxins are produced by yeasts and attack other yeasts. Various components of insects, including the cuticle, gut, secretions and haemolymph, exhibit antimicrobial activity. At present, the only insect that may contribute antimicrobial activity to a food is the honey-bee, which introduces antimicrobials such as royalicin and hydroxydecenoic acid in honey (Dillon, 1994; CAST, 1998). In addition to organic acids and bacteriocins, certain microorganisms produce additional antimicrobials, such as ethanol, diacetyl, natamycin and hydrogen peroxide, some of which are approved food preservatives (CAST, 1998) and are discussed in other parts of this chapter.

Other natural compounds with antimicrobial activity include lipids, such as monoacylglycerols, fatty acids, lipopeptides and lipid oxidation products (Wang & Johnson, 1992; Kabara, 1993; CAST, 1998). Lipid compounds with antimicrobial activity have been evaluated in various foods and under certain conditions have been found to be bacteriostatic or bactericidal against microorganisms such as *L. monocytogenes* (Unda *et al.*, 1991; Wang & Johnson, 1992; Wang *et al.*, 1993). Their antimicrobial activity depends however, on the type of food, presence of additional antimicrobials and presence of neutralizers of lipid antimicrobial activity, such as sequesterants, starch and serum albumen (CAST, 1998). Certain lipid substances or fatty acids and their derivatives are considered as GRAS or are approved for use in foods in the USA (CFR, 1996). The presence of fats and oils can also influence the thermal properties of foods, leading to cell protection from thermal destruction and a need for longer heating times to achieve uniform heating and desirable microbial inactivation (Ababouch & Busta, 1987; Ababouch *et al.*, 1987, 1992).

8 Traditional chemical food preservatives

8.1 General

Substances that have been added to foods for centuries and have traditionally contributed to their stability and safety include common salt, sugars, wood smoke and spices. Their initial introduction into foods is lost in history, but they still continue to constitute basic adjuncts to our food supply. Their application may have started accidentally; evidently, the first and foremost reason for their use was their effect on flavour. However, with time, their antimicrobial activity was also noticed. Their preservative action is either direct, indirect or through interactions among the preservatives, as well as with other components of the food system or other additives (Prescott & Proctor, 1937; Jensen, 1954; Reddish, 1957; Lueck, 1980; Sofos, 1984; Foegeding & Busta, 1991; Davidson & Branen, 1993).

8.2 Common salt

Sodium chloride (NaCl), or common salt, has been widely used as a flavouring or preservative agent in foods since ancient times (Jensen, 1954; Sofos, 1984). Common foods preserved with salt include meat and fish products, butter, margarine, cheeses and brined vegetables (Shelef & Seiter, 1993). It is the main ingredient of curing mixtures or brines. The use of salt in meat preservation led to the accidental and subsequent intentional use of nitrate and nitrite in meat curing (Binkerd & Kolari, 1975; Sofos *et al.*, 1979c). The preservative system of cured meats consists of salt, nitrite and other factors, including mild heat processing, low-temperature storage, smoking in certain instances and sugar (Sofos *et al.*, 1979c; Sofos & Busta, 1980).

The molecular weight of sodium chloride is 58.44 and it is a very water-soluble, white, cubic crystal. The compound is a dietary constituent which, in excessive amounts, may retard the growth and shorten the lifespan of laboratory animals (Meneely *et al.*, 1953). It should be noted that the acute toxicity dose (LD_{50}) of this traditional, widely and, often, freely used substance is half (5g/kg body weight) that of sorbic acid, i.e. it is twice as toxic (Sofos & Raharjo, 1994b).

As stated, salt has been used for centuries and continues to be an approved substance for use in foods. In recent years, however, there is a trend for reduction or elimination of sodium chloride and other sodium-containing substances in food formulations. This trend has arisen from evidence linking dietary sodium intake with development of hypertension in certain sensitive individuals (Sofos, 1984; Sofos & Raharjo, 1994b). One proposed method for reduction of sodium chloride amounts used in food processing is partial replacement with potassium chloride or phosphates (Sofos, 1984, 1986a,b). Other developments that have allowed reduction in salt levels in foods include the expanded use of mechanical refrigeration and product packaging in food preservation (Sofos, 1993).

Various microorganisms exhibit varying tolerances to sodium chloride, with mesophilic Gram-negative rods and psychrotrophic bacteria being the most sensitive, since they tolerate only 4–10% of the compound. Spore-forming and lactic-acid-producing bacteria tolerate 4–16% sodium chloride, while halophiles (i.e. salt-loving) need relatively high salt concentrations for growth. The resistance to salt of yeasts and moulds varies, with some species being extremely tolerant (Banwart, 1989). Antimicrobial effects of sodium chloride may include dehydration, interference with enzymes and their action, plasmolysis or cellular toxicity of high sodium or chloride concentrations (Sofos, 1984; Shelef & Seiter, 1993). A 10% sodium chloride concentration reduces the A_w of the system to levels below 0.935, a situation which is inhibitory to all types of *Cl. botulinum* (Schmidt, 1964). Lower salt levels act synergistically with other preservatives, including nitrite, sorbate and benzoate (Sofos, 1984; Shelef & Seiter, 1993). Due to the reduced A_w, the effects of salt on microorganisms are related to preservation by drying, in conjunction with which salt is frequently used. Halophilic bacteria and osmophilic microorganisms in general, however, are capable of proliferating in the presence of high salt concentrations and, if present, may result in food spoilage (Tanner,

1944; Walker, 1977). The pathogens *Staphyloccus aureus* and *L. monocytogenes* can tolerate sodium chloride concentrations exceeding 5% (Papageorgiou & Marth, 1989; Sofos, 1993).

8.3 Sugars

Sugars (glucose, fructose, sucrose, syrups and other corn-derived products) are widely used as sweeteners, fermentable materials, flavourings, etc. They are usually highly soluble in water and sweet-tasting (CAST, 1998). In many instances, sugars exhibit antimicrobial activity in food systems directly through increased osmotic pressure; through interactions with other components and processing of the food; or indirectly by serving as substrates in food fermentations.

Sucrose is the most commonly used disaccharide ($C_{12}H_{22}O_{11}$), with a molecular weight of 342.30. In recent years, sucrose is being replaced in food formulations with high-fructose corn-syrup solids or non-nutritive sweeteners, in combination with bulking agents. A 50% sucrose concentration decreases water activity to 0.935, which is inhibitory to growth of *Cl. botulinum*. Increased sugar concentrations result in high osmotic pressures, which prevent growth and multiplication of bacteria, since the moisture of the food is being tied up by the sugar and becomes unavailable to the organism. Direct inhibition of microorganisms, however, requires high concentrations of sugar. Examples of foods preserved by high sugar concentrations include jellies, preserves, syrups, juice concentrates, condensed milk and a variety of sweets. Bacteria are generally less tolerant to increased osmotic pressure (or reduced A_w) than yeasts and moulds. Certain species of yeast, especially those of *Zygosaccharomyces* and *Torulopsis*, and the mould *Aspergillus glaucus* are very osmotolerant or saccharophilic. Such organisms may develop and spoil foods even in the presence of high sugar concentrations (Foegeding & Busta, 1991).

Small concentrations of sugars support growth of many spoilage and pathogenic microorganisms (Hobbs, 1976). In addition, through their osmotic effects, sugars may increase the heat resistance of moulds and other organisms (Doyle & Marth, 1975). Sugar–metal-ion complexes, especially iron, may influence bacterial growth and control (Charley *et al.*, 1963; Sams & Carroll, 1966; Tompkin, 1978). Xylitol is not, or is only slowly, fermented by many food-borne microorganisms, but it may have a unique antimicrobial activity (Makinen & Soderling, 1981; Foegeding & Busta, 1991).

Interactions of sugar with other ingredients or preservatives and processes such as drying and heating are of more practical importance in food preservation than using high concentrations of sugar, which is limited to only certain applications. In products where fermentation is important for preservation and flavour development, native or added sugars constitute the substrate for production of acid, alcohol and other antimicrobial agents, which results in indirect food preservation by sugar (Christiansen *et al.*, 1975; Smith & Palumbo, 1981).

8.4 Smoke

Exposure of certain products, such as meat and fish, to smoke (smoking) is an ancient practice, which is still being used in many places. Smoke from wood, besides contributing to flavour, may have preservative activity, through heating and drying and also through the introduction into the product of certain chemical components of smoke (Maga, 1988). Phenolic compounds, formaldehyde, acetic acid and creosote may lower the pH of the smoked product. They are also likely to be active in other ways in preventing spoilage, since they prevent spore formation and control growth of certain microorganisms (Sink & Hsu, 1977; Maga, 1988). Even though smoking continues to be one of the basic methods of food preservation, its action is mostly a surface phenomenon, since the components do not penetrate deeply into the product (Christiansen *et al.*, 1968; Tatini *et al.*, 1976).

Direct addition of refined liquid-smoke flavourings to food products has been increasing in recent years. In addition to their flavouring properties, these preparations offer some advantages over the use of traditional open-fire wood smoking (Hollenbeck, 1979; Sofos & Maga, 1988). Liquid smoke is easier to apply uniformly and the concentrations used can be controlled for uniformity in flavour, colour and preservative action (Eklund *et al.*, 1982). Furthermore, use of liquid smoke minimizes pollution and crude tar, and polycyclic aromatic hydrocarbon carcinogens have been removed (White *et al.*, 1971). Compositional differences in liquid smokes, however, will result in differences in antimicrobial activity, depending on the type of wood used to produce the preparations (Boyle *et al.*, 1988; Sofos *et al.*, 1988). Liquid-smoke preparations or derivatives were reported to be inhibitory to *L. monocytogenes* (Messina *et al.*, 1988; Lindner, 1991).

9 Antimicrobials produced by microorganisms

9.1 General

Microorganisms present in food may produce antimicrobial agents, other than acids, which include bacteriocins, hydrogen peroxide, alcohols and other compounds. Certain of these compounds are produced commercially in industrial fermentations for use as additives in foods or other applications.

9.2 Ethyl alcohol

Ethyl alcohol (ethanol, CH_3CH_2OH) is a colourless liquid which is miscible in water. To be used as a food, it is obtained from yeast fermentation of sugar-containing liquid substrates, while heterofermentative bacteria may also produce small amounts of the compound (Luecke & Earnshaw, 1991). Use of alcohol for food preservation is not always regulated, because the compound is a natural constituent of several food products. Products containing natural or added alcohol include wines, liquors, beers, other alcoholic beverages, flavour extracts and some intermediate-moisture food products. Consumption of 200–400 ml pure alcohol in a short period of time is hazardous for humans, while levels of 40–80 ml daily over longer periods of time may be tolerable (Foegeding & Busta, 1991). Ethanol is listed as GRAS in the USA (CFR, 1996), but it is not a specified food additive in the UK (Seiler & Russell, 1991). Its main use by the food industry is as a solvent for colourings and flavourings. In the USA, ethyl alcohol may be used as an antimicrobial agent on pizza crusts prior to final baking at levels not to exceed 2% (Foegeding & Busta, 1991; Seiler & Russell, 1991).

Alcohol acts on microorganisms through non-specific denaturation of proteins in the protoplast, when used at concentrations of 60–80%, because the presence of water is needed for disinfectant activity (Seiler & Russell, 1991; Shelef & Seiter, 1993). Concentrations of 5–20% alcohol act as inhibitors of microbial growth (Foegeding & Busta, 1991; Seiler & Russell, 1991). The non-specific protein denaturation of alcohol affects all types of microorganisms, with the exception of bacterial spores, but Gram-negative are more sensitive than Gram-positive bacteria (Foegeding & Busta, 1991). The primary site of action by ethanol is believed to be the cytoplasmic membrane, where it may have a direct effect on the membrane or on membrane enzymes, or it may indirectly impair membrane biosynthesis (Seiler & Russell, 1991). However, ethanol has been found to affect not only enzymes, but also peptidoglycan synthesis, deoxyribonucleic acid, (DNA), ribonucleic acid (RNA), protein and fatty acid synthesis.

Microorganisms resistant to ethanol include *Lactobacillus* spp., *Zymomonas mobilis* and osmophilic yeasts (Seiler & Russell, 1991). The antimicrobial activity of ethanol is increased by decreasing a_w but is reduced in the presence of organic matter (Shelef & Seiter, 1993). Antimicrobial activity is often increased when ethanol is applied in combination with compounds such as acids (Parish & Caroll, 1988; Splittastoesser & Stoyla, 1989).

9.3 Hydrogen peroxide

Hydrogen peroxide or hydrogen dioxide (H_2O_2) is a water-miscible, colourless liquid which is formed through hydrolysis of peroxides, such as peroxidisulphuric acid. Concentrations of more than 30% are caustic, and it decomposes to oxygen and water in the presence of organic matter and metal ions, without being a toxicological hazard (Foegeding & Busta, 1991). The compound is useful as an oxidizing or bleaching agent (Cords & Dychdala, 1993) and is approved for use in several countries, since, when used in adequate amounts, it inactivates microorganisms (Stevenson & Shafer, 1983). In addition, the compound may be produced naturally by lactic acid bacteria in fermented foods (Dillon & Cook, 1994).

Hydrogen peroxide is active against bacteria, including spore-formers, yeasts, moulds and viruses, but its effectiveness varies with type of microorganism and environmental conditions (Toledo *et al.*, 1973; El-Gendy *et al.*, 1980; Stevenson & Shafer, 1983; Cords & Dychdala, 1993; Setlow & Setlow, 1993; CAST, 1998). The antimicrobial activity of hydrogen peroxide depends on concentration, level of contamination, pH, temperature and exposure time (Smith & Brown, 1980). The antimicrobial activity of hydrogen peroxide is due to its intense oxidizing properties, but its effect is brief, since it decomposes rapidly when exposed to organic matter (Cords & Dychdala, 1993). The combination of nitrite and hydrogen peroxide inactivated *E. coli* in the presence of lactate, but not in the presence of acetate or phosphate. The results suggested that nitrogen dioxide, formed from the reaction of peroxynitrous acid with lactate, was responsible for lactate-dependent killing of *E. coli*, induced by the reaction of protonated nitrite and hydrogen peroxide (Kono *et al.*, 1994).

Uses of hydrogen peroxide, which is GRAS in the USA (CFR, 1996), include treatment of milk (0.05%) for manufacture of certain cheeses and addition to whey (0.04%) and starch (0.15%). Excess of the compound after treatment is inactivated by heat or by addition of catalase, which catalyses its conversion to water and oxygen. Other approved uses, as an oxidizing or bleaching agent, in the USA include dried eggs, tripe, beef feet, herring, wine, instant tea, etc. (CFR, 1996). Hydrogen peroxide also inhibits microbial spoilage in fish marinades, and it can be used to decontaminate packaging materials for aseptic processing of juices and other foods (CFR, 1996; CAST, 1998). Care should be taken, however, to avoid oxidized flavours, bleached colours and loss of sensitive nutrients, such as vitamin C.

As indicated, hydrogen peroxide is also produced and accumulates during growth of lactobacilli, which lack catalase, and then inhibits other bacteria (Daeschel, 1989). The intermediary oxidation products formed inhibit microorganisms (Banks *et al.*, 1986). In addition, hydrogen peroxide may react with other components to form microbial inhibitors, such as in the LPS and glucose oxidase system (Banks *et al.*, 1986; Field *et al.*, 1986). Growth of lactobacilli in milk produces hydrogen peroxide, which reacts with thiocyanate, with lactoperoxidase activity as the catalyst (Gaya *et al.*, 1991). Hydrogen peroxide is also produced by oxidation of glucose to gluconic acid, which is catalysed by glucose oxidase (Kantt & Torres, 1993). Hydrogen peroxide solutions have also been evaluated in spraying applications to decontaminate beef carcasses during the slaughtering process (Gorman *et al.*, 1995, 1997).

9.4 Bacteriocins

Bacteriocins are naturally produced small peptides with potent bactericidal activity (Daeschel, 1989; McMullen & Stiles, 1996). They are produced by a large and diverse assortment of Gram-positive and Gram-negative bacteria, including lactic-acid bacteria used in food fermentations (Klaenhammer, 1988, 1993; Daeschel, 1989; Hoover, 1992; Ray & Daeschel, 1992, 1994; Hoover & Steenson, 1993; Nettles & Barefoot, 1993; Stiles, 1994; Sahl *et al.*, 1995; Muriana, 1996). In terms of bacteria that produce them, as well as chemical properties, antibacterial activity and mode of action, bacteriocins are a rather diverse and heterogeneous group of compounds. The most widely studied bacteriocins are the colicins, derived from *E. coli*, while the bacteriocins produced by lactic-acid bacteria have also become the subject of extensive investigations (CAST, 1998).

In general, bacteriocins have become popular subjects of investigation, because they present the opportunity to preserve foods through natural means (Gombas, 1989; Hansen *et al.*, 1989; Montville, 1989; Muriana, 1996; Owen Fields, 1996). They can be present in foods subjected to fermentation or through growth of spoilage microorganisms. Being proteins, they are susceptible to digestive enzymes and thus are considered safe. Their susceptibility to enzymes and, in some instances, to heat, however, may limit their use to applications after thermal processing and denaturation of enzymes in foods. Among the microorganisms inhibited by certain bacteriocins, numerous reports have included the fatal pathogen *L. monocytogenes* (Harris *et al.*, 1989; Spelhaug & Harlander, 1989; Muriana, 1996).

The antimicrobial activity of bacteriocins appears to be exerted on membranes, where they cause leakage and dissipation of the proton-motive force, through pore formation (Montville & Bruno, 1994; Muriana, 1996). For example, the activity of the bacteriocin nisin is on the phospholipid fraction of the cytoplasmic membrane, where it acts as a depolarizing agent, to cause leakage (Abee *et al.*, 1994a,b; Demel *et al.*, 1994; Winkowski *et al.*, 1994, 1996). Bacteria (e.g. *L. monocytogenes*) may develop resistance to nisin, which appears to involve a reduction in the accessibility or presence of suitable absorption sites (Davies & Adams, 1994). As peptides, bacteriocins are of low molecular weight, but larger than antibiotics. This makes them susceptible to biochemical reactions, which may limit their antimicrobial activity (Muriana, 1996). Activity is affected by concentration, microorganisms, pH, temperature and interactions (CAST, 1998). Microorganisms may develop bacteriocin resistance, as a result of mutations or due to the activity of proteolytic enzymes (Ming & Daeschel, 1993, 1995; Rekhif *et al.*, 1994; Muriana, 1996).

The common bacteriocin nisin is used as a food preservative and is the most extensively studied bacteriocin produced by *Lactococcus lactis* subsp. *lactis*. The nisin molecule consists of 34 amino acids, including lanthionine, dehydroalanine and β-methyllanthionine. Nisin is sensitive to α-chymotrypsin, but it is resistant to pronase and trypsin, as well as to 100°C for 10 min in acidic environments. Its stability to heat increases at higher pH values (Foegeding & Busta, 1991; Hurst & Hoover, 1993).

Nisin may be present naturally in milk and fermented dairy products, and its main use is in the preservation of dairy products and especially processed-cheese spreads. Amounts permitted and used in foods, such as processed-cheese products, are in the range of 100–400 iu/g (Hurst & Hoover, 1993). In the USA, the FDA has affirmed a nisin preparation as a GRAS substance for use in pasteurized cheese spreads and various pasteurized processed-cheese spreads for inhibition of outgrowth of *Cl. botulinum* (CFR, 1996). The toxicity of nisin is low (Shtenberg & Ignat'ev, 1970), and it is not used in animal or human medicine. Countries and products in which use of nisin is permitted are listed by Hurst and Hoover (1993).

Nisin is exclusively effective against Gram-positive bacteria; against its activity appears to be greater against bacterial spores than against vegetative cells and it may even inhibit spore germination (Hurst & Hoover, 1993; Delves-Broughton & Gasson, 1994). It is usually used in combination with heat because it enhances bacterial spore sensitivity to heat and inhibition of outgrowth of surviving spores (Hoover, 1992; Thomas *et al.*, 1993; Rao & Mathur, 1996). Bacteria inhibited by nisin include species of *Bacillus* and *Clostridium*, *L. monocytogenes*, *Staph. aureus* and *Mycobacterium* spp. (Daeschel, 1989). The reduction of activity of nisin against *L. monocytogenes* in milk with fat was counteracted by the addition of the emulsifier Tween 80 (Jung *et al.*, 1992a). Nisin is effective in combination with sorbate against *L. monocytogenes*, and it becomes active against Gram-negative bacteria, such as *Salmonella* spp. and *E. coli*, when combined with chelators, such as EDTA, lactate, citrate, phosphate and ethyl maltol (Stevens *et al.*, 1991, 1992; Cutter & Siragusa, 1995a,b; Schved *et al.*, 1995).

In processed cheeses, where nisin finds its major application, it inhibits butyric acid bacteria and clostridia (Somers & Taylor, 1987). Another potential use is in canned products, where, through its sensitizing effect, it may reduce the intensity of heat treatments needed to inactivate bacterial spores. Nisin has also been tested as an alternative to nitrite for inhibition of *Cl. botulinum* in meat products. Its activity, however, was variable and depended on factors such as pH and properties of the substrate (Hurst, 1981; Rayman *et al.*, 1981, 1983; Scott & Taylor, 1981a,b; Taylor *et al.*, 1985; McMullen & Stiles, 1996).

Numerous bacteriocins produced by species and strains of lactic-acid bacteria were identified in the 1980s and 1990s. These include lactocin and helveticin (*Lactobacillus helveticus*), lactacin B and F (*Lactobacillus acidophilus*), curvacins (*Lactobacillus curvatus*), propionicin (*Propionibacterium* spp.), plantaricin A (*Lactobacillus plantarum*), Las 5 and diplococcin (*Streptococcus cremoris*), mesenterosins and leuconosins (*Leuconostoc* spp.) and pediocins (*Pediococcus acidilactici* and *Pediococcus pentosaceous*) (Klaenhammer, 1988; Daeschel, 1989; Hoover & Steenson, 1993; Ray &

Daeschel, 1994; Hill, 1995; McMullen & Stiles, 1996; CAST, 1997). However, commercial uses are slow to gain approval and application. Characteristics of these bacteriocins include: broad-spectrum antimicrobial activity; maintenance of activity in variable environments; no effect on food quality; cost-effectiveness; and adequate information to support approval by regulatory authorities (Ray & Daeschel, 1994).

9.5 Other

Microorganisms play a major role in food preservation throughout the world. In addition to acids, alcohol, hydrogen peroxide and bacteriocins, they also produce small quantities of other compounds that exhibit activity against undesirable microorganisms (Vandenbergh, 1993). Preservation of fermented foods may also be enhanced by changes in A_w, oxygen levels and changes in nutrients brought about by microbial growth (Luecke & Earnshaw, 1991; Dillon & Cook, 1994). Miscellaneous antimicrobial agents produced by bacteria, yeasts or moulds include diacetyl, carbon dioxide, glycerol and acetoin (Dillon & Cook, 1994).

Diacetyl 2,3-butanedione, ($C_4H_6O_2$) is chemically synthesized from methyl ethyl ketone, and is GRAS for use as a food flavouring and adjuvant in the USA (CFR, 1996). The compound is also synthesized biologically by heterofermentative, citrate-fermenting lactic-acid bacteria, providing the buttery odour or flavour in certain fermented dairy products, at levels of 0.0001–0.0007% (Daeschel, 1989; Luecke & Earnshaw, 1991). Diacetyl is also found in wine, brandy and coffee. As an antimicrobial agent, diacetyl (0.2–0.03%) has inhibited yeasts, Gram-negative and non-lactic Gram-positive bacteria, but higher levels (> 0.05%) were needed to inhibit lactics and clostridia (Jay, 1982a,b). The antimicrobial activity increased at pH 5.5 compared with pH 8.0, while acetate, glucose and Tween 80 interfered with inhibition. Addition of (0.04%) diacetyl caused lower aerobic plate counts in ground beef (Jay, 1982b). The compound was not effective against *L. monocytogenes*, but it inhibited *Yersinia enterocolitica* in broth (Motlagh *et al.*, 1991), which confirms that diacetyl is more active against Gram-negative bacteria. It has been suggested that its antimicrobial action involves binding of arginyl residues on proteins, while Gram-positive bacteria may be more resistant, because they lack periplasmic binding proteins and large amino acid pools (Jay *et al.*, 1983; Shelef & Seiter, 1993; CAST, 1997). Although it is a GRAS compound, its usefulness as a food preservative is questionable, because of its flavour at the relatively large (> 0.02%) amounts needed for microbial inhibition (Motlagh *et al.*, 1991). Diacetyl may be effective as a sanitizer of equipment, but its usefulness is also limited by its volatility (Jay *et al.*, 1983).

Another example of a biologically derived antimicrobial was identified in the 1980s and has been named reuterin (3-hydroxyproponaldehyde) . It is a low molecular weight non-protein, which is highly soluble and pH-neutral. Reuterin is produced by the heterofermentative *Lactobacillus reuterii,* and it appears to be a broad-spectrum antimicrobial acting against certain Gram-negative and Gram-positive bacteria, yeasts, moulds and protozoa, including pathogens (Daeschel, 1989; CAST, 1998).

10 Acidulants

10.1 General

Several common and naturally occurring acids are added to or formed in foods during fermentation (Foegeding & Busta, 1991; Dillon & Cook, 1994). In addition to antimicrobial activity, they act as flavouring agents, buffers, synergists to antioxidants, modifiers of certain properties and curing adjuncts (Gardner, 1972). In addition to antimicrobial action, caused by reduced pH, they enhance the antimicrobial activity of other additives or physical methods of food preservation. Moreover, the decrease in pH facilitates destruction of microorganisms by heat, permitting shorter sterilization or processing times, which are less detrimental to the quality of the product (Foegeding & Busta, 1991). Low pH values also prevent or delay spore germination and bacterial growth and most lipophilic, weak-acid preservatives are more effective at lower pH values, where their undissociated portion, the effective form, increases. Inhibition of microbial growth, however, is variable with type of acidulant, among other factors (Sorrels *et al.*, 1989; CAST, 1998).

Acidification is required by law for products such as canned figs, artichokes and several other fruits and vegetables in some countries. A pH value of 4.6 or less is still required for the canning of certain foods in order to prevent growth of, or toxin production by, *Cl. botulinum*, even though botulinum toxin may be formed at pH values below 4.6 under certain conditions (Sugiyama & Sofos, 1988). Acidulants are also very important in cases where the lipophilic, weak-acid preservatives are added as salts for increased solubility. In products of high pH (> 5.5), an acidulant should be included (except for parabens) if no adverse effect on product characteristics and quality is encountered. Prior exposure to acidic conditions, however, may lead to development of microbial resistance, as is the case for *E. coli* 0157:H7 (Doores, 1993; Zhao *et al.*, 1993; Miller & Kaspar, 1994; Leyer *et al.*, 1995). Common acids used as additives or naturally present in foods are lactic, acetic, malic, fumaric, citric, etc.

10.2 Lactic acid

Lactic acid (2-hydroxypropanoic acid, CH_3CHOH COOH) is the main product of many food fermentations. It is formed by microbial degradation of sugars in products such as cheese, sauerkraut, pickles, olives and fermented meat products (Daeschel, 1989). The acid produced in such fermentations decreases the pH to levels unfavourable for growth of spoilage organisms, such as putrefactive anaerobes and butyric acid-producing bacteria. Yeasts and moulds that can grow at such pH levels can be controlled by the inclusion of other preservatives, such as sorbate and benzoate, or by packaging (Lueck, 1980; Sofos, 1989a).

The main species of bacteria that produce lactic acid belong to the genera *Lactobacillus*, *Lactococcus*, *Leuconostoc* and *Pediococcus*, but some mould species and certain other bacteria are also capable of producing lactic acid. Other end-products formed by lactic acid bacteria during food fermentations include acetic acid, ethyl alcohol, carbon dioxide, diacetyl, bacteriocins and mannitol. The lactic acid produced by fermentation of added fermentable sugars (glucose, sucrose) should decrease the pH to levels sufficient to inhibit growth and toxin production by pathogens such as *Cl. botulinum* and *Staph. aureus*. A process was allowed in the USA for the production of bacon, where addition of sugar and lactic acid-producing bacteria promotes faster nitrite depletion and inhibition of *Cl. botulinum* toxin production due to lower pH levels (USDA, 1979).

Lactic acid has a pK_a of 3.83, is highly water-soluble and is usually manufactured commercially by a fermentation process. Being a natural constituent of foods and a product of fermentation, it is one of the oldest food preservatives and is of low toxicity and non-mutagenic. Thus, it is a GRAS substance (CFR, 1996), and the Food and Agriculture Organization of the United Nations (FAO) has set no limit for the acceptable daily intake of the acid and several of its salts (Foegeding & Busta, 1991). Besides being an acidulant and exhibiting preservative action, due to decreased pH, lactic acid may also be used as a flavouring agent in Spanish-type olives and in frozen desserts or as an emulsifier in leavened bakery products (Gardner, 1972) . Some lactic acid derivatives are also employed as direct food acidulants. Glucono-δ-lactone is GRAS in the USA (CFR, 1996) and can be used as a curing and pickling agent. This compound, following ring opening to give gluconic acid, functions in a similar manner to added lactic acid. Sodium, calcium and potassium lactates are also approved for use as flavour enhancers in meat products in the USA.

Lactic acid is also used as a preservative, in combination with carbon dioxide, in certain carbonated beverages (Foegeding & Busta, 1991). Its food-grade DL form is available as an aqueous solution, which is colourless and odourless. It is very soluble in water and its taste is acrid. Lactic acid and lactates (i.e. sodium lactate, potassium lactate) inhibit bacteria, including spore-formers, such as putrefying anaerobes and butyric-acid producers, or vegetative-cell pathogens, such as *L. monocytogenes*, *Cl. botulinum*, *Salmonella*, *Staph. aureus*, *Y. enterocolitica*, etc. (Woolford, 1975; Wong & Chen, 1988; Shelef & Yang, 1991; Bradford *et al.*, 1993; Doores, 1993; Harmayani *et al.*, 1993; Houtsma *et al.*, 1994; Meng & Genigeorgis, 1994; Miller & Acuff, 1994; Pelroy *et al.*,

1994; Shelef, 1994; Buncic *et al.*, 1995). Lactic- and acetic-acid solutions have been recommended as sprays for decontamination of animal carcasses after slaughter (Smulders *et al.*, 1986; Adams & Hall, 1988; Sofos, 1994b; Hardin *et al.*, 1995).

Lactic acid, as well as citric acid, inhibits formation of mycotoxins, such as aflatoxins and sterigmatocystin (Reiss, 1976), although, at certain concentrations, lactic acid stimulated formation of aflatoxin (El-Gazzar *et al.*, 1987). As indicated above, sodium lactate is used in poultry-meat products in the USA, as a flavouring agent and flavour enhancer, at levels of 1–3%. The compound also enhances product shelf-life by inhibiting spoilage and pathogenic bacteria (Debevere, 1989; Maas *et al.*, 1989; Wederquist *et al.*, 1994, 1995). It should be noted that microbial inhibition by lactate may be variable and affected by environmental conditions and properties of the substrate (Harmayani *et al.*, 1991; Maas, 1993). Combinations of lactic acid and potassium sorbate were found effective in extending the shelf-life of fresh, refrigerated, vacuum-packaged poultry meat (Kolsarici & Candogan, 1995).

10.3 Acetic acid

Acetic acid (ethanoic acid, CH_3COOH) is produced through the oxidation of alcohol by bacteria of the genus *Acetobacter* and *Gluconobacter*. In the form of vinegar (i.e. 4% or more acetic acid), it constitutes one of the oldest preservatives and flavouring agents. Substrates for vinegar production include grapes, cider, wine, a variety of sugars and malt. Generally, two successive bioconversions, the first alcoholic (anaerobic fermentation) and the second acetic (aerobic oxidation), are employed in the production of acetic acid (Jacobs, 1958; Foegeding & Busta, 1991; Reed, 1982).

Acetic acid is a general preservative, inhibiting many species (CFR, 1996). It is also a product of lactic acid fermentation (CAST, 1998). Bacteria inhibited by acetic acid include *Bacillus* spp., *Clostridium* spp., *Salmonella* spp., *Staph. aureus* and *L. monocytogenes*, while *E. coli* O157:H7 is reported to survive in acidic environments better than other serotypes of *E. coli* (Doores, 1993; Zhao *et al.*, 1993; Miller & Kaspar, 1994; Leyer *et al.*, 1995). The main applications of vinegar (acetic acid) include products such as mayonnaise, salad-dressings, pickles, olives, sauces and ketchup (catsup).

As a liquid solution of 1.5–2.5%, acetic acid has been applied in sprays to decontaminate meat-animal carcasses and cuts (Dickson, 1992; Dickens & Whittemore, 1994; Dickens *et al.*, 1994; Sofos, 1994b; Gorman *et al.*, 1995, 1997; Hardin *et al.*, 1995). In the vapour form, acetic acid showed promising results for the control of fruit decay by postharvest fungi (Sholberg & Gaunce, 1995). Increased involvement of fruit and vegetable products in the incidence of food-borne illness has increased the need for control of pathogenic bacteria in these products. Acetic acid dipping of fresh parsley reduced total bacteria and *Y. enterocolitica* populations (Karapinar & Gonul, 1992).

Besides acetic acid, several related compounds (acetates) yield acetic acid and are used in food processing. The selection of the compound is dictated by flavour and economic reasons (Chichester & Tanner, 1972; Foegeding & Busta, 1991). Acetates (calcium acetate, sodium diacetate) have been reported to be effective against rope and mould in bread. Sodium diacetate has the advantage of not introducing off-flavours in bread when used as a mould and rope inhibitor. The use of propionates, however, has replaced acetic acid as a rope-inhibiting agent in bread (Chichester & Tanner, 1972; Foegeding & Busta, 1991). Sodium acetate inhibited *L. monocytogenes* in catfish fillets and in sausages (Wederquist *et al.*, 1994, 1995; Kim *et al.*, 1995; Rong-Yu *et al.*, 1996). Combinations of sodium acetate or sodium propionate with EDTA and acetic acid may be useful in inactivating *L. monocytogenes* in mildly acidic, refrigerated foods (Golden *et al.*, 1995). The antimicrobial activity of acetate is reported to increase at lower pH values ($pK_a = 4.76$), where the amount of the undissociated acid is greater. Peracetic acid is an oxidized derivative of acetic acid, and it decomposes to acetic acid and oxygen in the presence of organic substrates. The compound has been recommended as a disinfectant of food-contact surfaces (Foegeding & Busta, 1991; Doores, 1993).

Dehydroacetic acid ($C_8H_8O_4$, pK_a 5.27) inhibits yeasts and moulds more than it does bacteria, and it is effective against secondary fermentations in alcoholic beverages. Sodium dehydroacetate was more effective than sodium benzoate against *Sacch. cerevisiae*, *Penicillium glaucum* and *Aspergillus niger* (Banwart, 1989). In the USA (CFR, 1996), the compound and its sodium salt are GRAS and may be used to treat cut or peeled squash and as a fungistat in cheese wrappers (Doores, 1993).

10.4 Other

Several other acids may be present as natural components in various food products or be produced or added to foods for various reasons. Included in this group are compounds such as adipic, ascorbic, isoascorbic, caprylic, citric, formic, fumaric, malic, succinic and tartaric acid (Foegeding & Busta, 1991; CAST, 1998).

Malic (1-hydroxy-1,2-ethanedicarboxylic, COOH $CH_2CHOHCOOH$) or hydrosuccinic acid is a common natural acid found in apples, peaches, cherries, grapes, apricots, bananas, carrots, broccoli, potatoes, peas, rhubarb, citrus fruits, figs, tomatoes and beans (Gardner, 1972; Foegeding & Busta, 1991; Doores, 1993). In the USA, it is a GRAS substance (CFR, 1996) used to acidify and preserve salad-dressings, including mayonnaise, fruit preserves, sherberts, jams, jellies and beverages. It has pK_a values of 3.4 and 5.1 and it inhibits bacteria and yeasts (Banwart, 1989; Foegeding & Busta, 1991; Doores, 1993).

Citric acid ($COOHCH_2C(OH)(COOH)CH_2$ COOH) is the major acid in citrus fruits and it is widely used as an acidifier in carbonated beverages and other foods (e.g. fruit preserves, jams, jellies, canned vegetables, dairy products, ice-cream and salad-dressing), because of its solubility and its unique and pleasant flavour properties (Foegeding & Busta, 1991). The acid and several of its salts are considered GRAS in the USA. Monoglyceride citrate is approved in the USA for use as a synergist and solubilizer for antioxidants in oils and fats (CFR, 1996). The ability of many microorganisms to metabolize citrate and its low pK_a values (3.1, 4.8 and 6.4) make it a less effective antimicrobial agent than other acids (Foegeding & Busta, 1991; Doores, 1993).

Fumaric acid (*trans*-butenedioic acid, COOH CH:CHCOOH) is non-hygroscopic, is of low solubility and has a strong acidic taste (Doores, 1993). It is used in gelatin desserts, pie fillings, biscuit doughs, wines and fruit drinks. In foods, it can act as an antioxidant and antifungal agent (Gardner, 1972; Conner & Beuchat, 1987). Esters of fumarates may inhibit *Cl. botulinum*, while in wine the acid inhibits the malolactic fermentation (Huhtanen, 1983; Dymicky *et al.*, 1987; Doores, 1993). Fumaric acid solutions inhibited *L. monocytogenes*, *E. coli* O157:H7 and *Sal. typhimurium* during storage of fresh beef to a greater extent than acetic and lactic acids (Podolak *et al.*, 1995).

Formic acid (HCOOH) is a colourless, transparent liquid with a pungent odour and is miscible in water. Its pK_a value is 3.75 and it has an LD_{50} value of 1–2 g/kg body weight (Lueck, 1980). High concentrations may irritate the skin and mucous membranes, but its sodium and potassium salts are of lower acute toxicity. The acid is readily absorbed through the skin and mucous or intestinal membranes and is a normal constituent of human blood and other tissues involved in transfer of one-carbon substrates (Foegeding & Busta, 1991). Its antimicrobial activity is more potent against yeasts and, to a lesser degree, against bacteria. Ethyl formate is considered GRAS in the USA for use as a flavouring agent (CFR, 1996).

Tartaric acid ($COOH(CHOH)_2COOH$) is the common acid of grapes and is manufactured from waste products of the wine industry. The compound is a GRAS substance in the USA (CFR, 1996), and it is used in fruits, jams, jellies, preserves, sherberts and beverages. Cream of tartar (monopotassium tartrate) is used in the baking industry (Foegeding & Busta, 1991). In addition to its antimicrobial properties, it is a synergist of antioxidants (Doores, 1993).

Adipic acid ($COOH(CH_2)_4COOH$) is a low-solubility, non-hygroscopic acid, useful as an acidulant in dry, powdered-food products. Its antimicrobial activity is attributed only to its acidifying capacity. The compound is classified as GRAS in the USA, when used according to good manufacturing practices (GMP) as a buffering or neutralizing agent (Doores, 1993; CFR, 1996). Specific food uses include baking-powders, powdered fruit beverages, sweets biscuits and gelatin desserts. It may also be used in canned vegetables, as a sequestrant in oils and to improve the melting characteristics of processed cheeses (Gardner, 1972).

Succinic acid ($COOH(CH_2)_2COOH$)and its anhydride are used mostly as acidulants in bakery products (Foegeding & Busta, 1991; Doores, 1993). The compound has pK_a values of 4.2 and 5.6 and is considered GRAS in the USA (CFR, 1996). Succinic acid has reduced microbial loads on poultry carcasses, but it impaired the appearance of the product (Cox *et al.*, 1974).

Caprylic (octanoic, $CH_3(CH_2)_6COOH$) acid has a pK_a value of 4.9. The compound, which is a colourless oil of slight solubility in water, is GRAS in the USA and is approved for use as an antimicrobial in cheese wraps (CFR, 1996). It may be used as a flavouring adjuvant in cheese, baked foods, fats, oils, frozen dairy desserts, gelatins, puddings, meat products, snack foods and soft sweets (Doores, 1993).

Glutaric acid ($COOH(CH_2)_3COOH$) occurs naturally in foods and has pK_a values of 4.3 and 5.2. The compound has been suggested for use as a food acidulant (Merten & Bachman, 1976; Foegeding & Busta, 1991).

Salicylic (*o*-hydroxybenzoic) acid is a white crystal of 138.12 molecular weight, with a solubility of 0.2% (w/v) in room-temperature water. The compound reacts with proteins and damages microbial cells (Lueck, 1980), but only a few countries still permit its use in pickled olives, at concentrations of 0.04–0.06% (Foegeding & Busta, 1991).

Boric acid (H_3BO_3) and borax ($Na_2B_4O_7 \cdot 10H_2O$) are white powders or crystals of 5% (w/v) solubility at room temperature. The pK_a value of boric acid is 9.14, which makes it almost completely undissociated in environments of even neutral pH. Because of their high toxicity, the compounds are not permitted for food use in the USA, but they have been employed in food applications in other countries (Foegeding & Busta, 1991).

Monohalogenacetic acids, which include monochloroacetic and monobromoacetic acid, are not permitted for use in foods, but in the past they were used, along with their esters, to stabilize juices and wines (Lueck, 1980). They are effective inhibitors of bacteria, moulds and especially yeasts (Busta & Foegeding, 1983; Foegeding & Busta, 1991).

Ascorbic acid ($C_6H_8O_6$) or vitamin C, its isomer isoascorbic or erythorbic acid and their salts are highly soluble in water and safe to use in foods. The pK_a values are 4.17 and 11.57. At high concentrations (e.g. 0.05%), ascorbate enhances depletion of residual nitrite and reduces nitrosamine formation in cured meats, while, at lower concentrations (e.g. 0.02%), it increases the anticlostridial activity of nitrite (Tompkin, 1984; Sofos & Raharjo,1994a). Ascorbate alone has shown no major antimicrobial activity, although it has inhibited pseudomonads in liquid substrates (Banwart, 1989) and *Cl. botulinum* in cooked potatoes, when used in combination with citric acid (Notermans *et al.*, 1985).

The inorganic acids phosphoric (H_3PO_4) and hydrochloric (HCl) acids are strong acidulants, causing microbial inhibition due to increased hydrogen-ion concentration, and are GRAS in the USA (CFR, 1996). Of these two GRAS inorganic acids, phosphoric is a common acidulant in carbonated beverages.

11 Lipophilic acids

11.1 General

The organic lipophilic acids benzoic, propionic and sorbic acid are among the compounds most commonly used in food preservation. Some of these weak acids are found as natural ingredients in food products, e.g. benzoic acid in cranberries and sorbic acid in rowan-berries (Lueck, 1976, 1980; Sofos, 1989a). Organic acids of chain length greater than C_{10} are also very effective against pathogenic bacteria (Roth & Halvorson, 1952), but their potential use is restricted because of their low solubility.

The antimicrobial efficacy of these acids is optimal in an acidic environment, since their pK_a values are generally between pH 3 and 5 (Sauer, 1977). At lower pH values, the amount of undissociated acid is greater, and this is believed to be the major contributor (Eklund, 1980, 1983) to antimicrobial activity (see also Chapter 2). If feasible, in foods of higher pH, the lipophilic-acid preservatives may be used in combination with an acidulant (CAST, 1998). In general, their usefulness is limited to foods with pH values of less than 5.5–6.0. The esters of *p*-hydroxybenzoic acid (parabens) have a pK_a value of 8.5, permitting their use in foods with pH values around neutrality (Davidson, 1993).

It is believed that the protonated (i.e. undissociated, uncharged) acid diffuses through the cell membranes into the cytoplasm, where it dissociates under the neutral pH of the cell interior. Inhibition of growth is then believed to be due to acidification of the cytoplasm, leading to interference with transport of chemicals across the cell membrane or with enzymatic activity. The dissociated acid, however, has also shown antimicrobial activity (Eklund, 1980, 1983, 1985; Sofos, 1989a; Doores, 1993). In order for constant pH to be maintained in the cytoplasm, the proton must be pumped out of the cell and this leads to disruption of the proton-motive force and interference with metabolic activity (Chang & Piper, 1994; Dillon & Cook, 1994). Prior exposure to subinhibitory levels may increase resistance of yeasts, moulds and bacteria to these preservatives (Warth, 1977, 1985; Goodson & Rowbury, 1989; Sofos, 1989a).

Besides chain length, the antimicrobial activity of lipophilic acids increases with the degree of unsaturation, and the *cis*-isomers are more effective than the *trans*-isomers (Kodicek, 1956). However, as mentioned previously, the better solubility, lower toxicity and more acceptable taste of short-chain lipophilic acids are major reasons contributing to their selection as antimicrobial agents. Antimicrobial activity is also affected by type of acid and food, temperature and other environmental factors.

11.2 Benzoic acid

Benzoic (phenylformic, benzenecarboxylic, C_6H_5COOH) acid, first described in 1875, in the form of its sodium salt constitutes one of the most common chemical food preservatives. Naturally, the compound is present in products such as cranberries, prunes, strawberries, plums, apples and ripe olives. In the pure state, benzoate is a white granular or crystalline powder, with a sweet or somewhat astringent taste. The water solubility of benzoic acid is low (0.35 g in 100 ml) but increases with a rise in temperature (Sofos, 1994a). The widely used sodium salt, sodium benzoate, a white powder or flakes, has an increased solubility in water (50 g in 100 ml) and in alcohol (1.3 g in 100 ml), but is insoluble in ether, in other organic non-polar solvents and in lipids (Sofos, 1994a; Sieber *et al.*, 1995).

Sodium benzoate has a molecular weight of 144.1 and a pK_a of 4.19. The maximum pH for antimicrobial activity is 4.5, while it is most effective in the pH range 2.5–4.0 (Sofos, 1994a). At pH values above 4.5, its antimicrobial activity diminishes (at pH 6.0, its activity is 100 times less than at 4.0) and the introduction of an acidulant or other preservative should be considered. As with other lipophilic acids, the antimicrobial activity of benzoate is due to its undissociated molecule. There is evidence that benzoate in part inhibits nutrient uptake through acidification of the cytoplasm (Eklund, 1980, 1983, 1985, 1988, 1989), and it interferes with enzymatic activity (Bosund, 1962; Chipley, 1993).

Benzoic acid is a GRAS compound in the USA (CFR, 1996), but it is more toxic to rats than is sorbic acid. However, humans are believed to have a high tolerance to benzoate, which does not accumulate in the human body, since it is conjugated with glycine or gluconic acid to produce hippuric acid or benzyl glucuronide, which are excreted (Chipley, 1993; Sofos, 1994a). Benzyl coenzyme A (CoA) is an intermediate in the detoxification process formed at the expense of ATP. Benzoate is not mutagenic in *Salmonella* or *Drosophila*, but it may interact with nucleosides and DNA *in vitro* (Njagi & Gopalan, 1980).

Sodium benzoate is the form used most widely in food preservation, due to its higher solubility in water. It is a common preservative in acid or acidified foods, such as carbonated and still beverages, fruit juices, salads, syrups, sauces, jams, jellies, purées, margarine, sauerkraut, pickles, olives, relishes, pie fillings, syrups, preserves, fish, minced meat and fruit cocktails. It is used at concentrations ranging from 0.03 to 0.30% in the USA, and, as indicated, it is a natural component in many berries, cinnamon, ripe cloves, plums and prunes. Maximum levels permitted in various countries are 0.00075–1.25%, depending on country and type of food (Chipley, 1993). Application as a spray solution (0.7%) on beef carcasses was active against some fungi, but others were able to proliferate (Nassar *et al.*, 1995).

Benzoate is probably the most widely used food

preservative, and its low cost is one of its advantages. In cases where it introduces a noticeable flavour to products, such as beverages, a lower level of benzoate in combination with another preservative (sorbate, parabens) may be considered (Jermini & Schmidt-Lorenz, 1987). To avoid product discoloration due to benzoate, sulphurous acid may be introduced to retard oxidative changes. In such cases, however, sedimentation may increase, since both compounds influence the colloidal balance of juices (Kimble, 1977).

Microorganisms inhibited by benzoate include *Bacillus cereus*, *E. coli*, *E. coli* O157:H7, *Vibrio parahaemolyticus*, *Staph. aureus*, *Lactobacillus* spp., *L. monocytogenes*, *Pseudomonas* spp., *Candida krusei*, *Debaryomyces hansenii*, *Hansenula* spp., *Pichia* spp., *Rhodotorula* spp., *Saccharomyces* spp., *Zygosaccharomyces* spp., *Alternaria solani*, *Aspergillus* spp., *Byssochlamys nivea*, *Cladosporium herbarum*, *Mucor racemosus*, *Penicillium* spp. and *Rhizopus nigrificans* (Chipley, 1993; Zhao *et al*., 1993). Yeasts are inhibited by benzoate to a greater extent than moulds and bacteria. Osmotolerant yeasts, such as *Z. bailii*, however, may be resistant to benzoate and limit the shelf-life of intermediate-moisture foods and fruit drinks (Warth, 1977, 1985, 1988, 1989a,b,c; Jermini & Schmidt-Lorenz, 1987; Wind & Restaino, 1995). Extent of resistance or sensitivity to benzoate may be affected by species sensitivity and by the rate of uptake and capacity of the cells to remove the compound (Warth, 1989c). The most important mechanism, however, may be the inducible energy-requiring system of transport of the compound out of the cell (Warth, 1989a,b). Certain bacteria can metabolize benzoate through a pathway involving β-ketoapidate. These include members of the family Enterobacteriaceae, *Corynebacterium glutamicum* and *Gluconobacter oxydans* (Chipley, 1993; Sofos, 1994a).

11.3 Propionic acid

Propionic acid (CH_3CH_2COOH) is an aliphatic, monocarboxylic acid, having a strong, pungent, rancid odour. Characteristically, as much as 1% of the compound is produced by bacteria of the genus *Propionibacterium* during the ageing of Swiss-type cheeses, where it provides flavour and acts as a mould inhibitor. *Propionibacterium* also forms carbon dioxide gas, which leads to formation of the characteristic cavities ('eyes') in Swiss-type cheeses. Propionic acid is also formed by bacteria in the gastrointestinal tract of ruminants. As indicated, propionic acid has a strong odour, and, since it is also somewhat corrosive, usually the sodium and calcium salts are used as food preservatives. The sodium salt is more water-soluble than the calcium salt, their solubilities at 100°C being 150 and 55.8 g/100 ml water, respectively (Doores, 1993; Sofos, 1994a). Propionates are white, free-flowing powders, with a slightly cheese-like flavour.

The main application of propionates is in the baking industry, where they are used to suppress growth of bacteria (*Bacillus mesentericus*) causing rope in bread and the growth of moulds in bread and cakes (O'Leary & Kralovec, 1941; Seiler, 1964). In addition to *B. mesentericus*, other specific microorganisms inhibited by propionates include *E. coli*, *Salmonella*, *L. monocytogenes*, *Staph. aureus*, *Proteus vulgaris*, *Pseudomonas* spp., *Sarcina lutea*, *Aspergillus* spp., *Torula* spp., *Trichophyton metagrophytes* and *Saccharomyces ellipsoideus* (El-Shenawy and Marth, 1989, 1992; Doores, 1993).

Bakery products in which propionates are used as preservatives include breads, fruit cakes, cheesecake, chocolate cake, devil's food cake, pie fillings and piecrusts. Other applications are to control surface-mould growth on cheese, fruits, vegetables, tobacco and malt extract (Olson & Macy, 1945; Jacobs, 1947; Chichester & Tanner, 1972; Gardner, 1972). Propionate inhibits microbial growth through interference with nutrient-transport functions (Eklund, 1980) and inhibition of enzymes (Sofos, 1994a). Inhibition of *L. monocytogenes* by propionate was associated with reduced lactic-dehydrogenase activity (Buazzi & Marth, 1992). Calcium propionate appears to be more inhibitory to aflatoxin formation than mould growth (Lueck, 1980). Both the calcium and sodium salts mix well with emulsifying agents and the basic dough ingredients. However, calcium propionate is preferred in yeast-raised bread as a means of calcium enrichment, while the sodium salt is better in cakes, since calcium ions may interfere with chemical leavening. As a mould inhibitor, in addition to being directly added to the product, propionate may also be applied to wrappers and packages (Foegeding & Busta, 1991).

The effectiveness of propionates in controlling mould growth is generally greater than that of sodium benzoate, but the propionates have minimal activity against yeasts (Walters & Levin, 1994). Actually, many yeasts metabolize propionate, which makes it useful in the preservation of yeast-leavened bakery products, since it does not interfere with the fermentation. As with other lipophilic acids, the effect of propionates increases at lower pH levels, since their pK_a value is 4.88 (Foegeding & Busta, 1991; CAST, 1998). Their optimum pH level is around 5.0 and in some foods they can be used at pH values up to 6.0. The type and amount of propionate to be employed depends upon the product and its acidity (Chichester & Tanner, 1972; Kimble, 1977). Propionic acid was a more effective antimicrobial than lactic acid in minced pork (Ogden *et al.*, 1995). Inhibition of some bacteria (e.g. *E. coli*) may be reversed by addition of β-alanine, while in other microorganisms (e.g. *Aspergillus clavatus*, *Bacillus subtilis* and *Pseudomonas* spp.) inhibition was not reversed with addition of β-alanine (Doores, 1993).

Propionic acid and its calcium and sodium salts are considered GRAS in the USA (CFR, 1996).The compound is metabolized like any fatty acid, and levels as high as 0.38% may be used in food applications (Chichester & Tanner, 1972). The FAO has set no limits on the acceptable daily intake (ADI) for humans.

11.4 Sorbic acid

Sorbic acid 2,4-hexadienoic acid, CH_3–CH=CH–CH=CH–COOH) is a straight-chain, *trans–trans*, unsaturated, fatty acid. It was discovered in 1859 from the reaction of rowan-berry oil with strong alkali, and it was first synthesized in 1900 (Lueck, 1976, 1980). The first patent for its use as an antimicrobial agent was issued in 1945 (Gooding, 1945). Details on sorbate food preservatives can be found in a book by Sofos (1989a).

The carboxylic group of sorbic acid reacts to yield sorbate salts and esters, which in dry form are remarkably stable to oxidation. Aqueous solutions, however, are relatively unstable and degrade by first-order reaction kinetics (Sofos, 1989a). Derivatives of sorbic acid include its potassium, calcium and sodium salts, as well as aldehydes, alcohols, esters and amides, such as sorboyl palmitate, sorbamide, sorbohydroxanic acid, methyl sorbate, ethyl sorbate and sorbic anhydride (Sofos, 1989a, 1994a). Because of their high aqueous solubility, salts of sorbic acid, especially potassium sorbate, are important food preservatives. The acid, which is more soluble in lipid materials than in water, has a weak acid odour and acid taste. Its solubility is better in alcohol and in anhydrous acetic acid than in water. The water solubility of sorbic acid is only 0.15% w/v at 20°C, but it increases with temperature and in buffered solutions with pH values above 4.4. Solubility, stability, uptake, diffusion and partition of sorbate in foods are important processes which affect its antimicrobial activity (Sofos, 1989a).

Sorbic acid and potassium sorbate are available as granular or fluffy, white powders. The potassium salt is very soluble in water (over 50%) and, when added to acidic foods, it is hydrolysed to the acid form. Sodium and calcium sorbates are also available and have preservative activities, but their application is limited compared with that for the potassium salt, which is employed because of its stability, general ease of preparation and water solubility. The water solubility of the sodium and calcium salts is 32% and 1.2%, respectively. Sorbic acid and its salts are practically tasteless and odourless in foods, when used at reasonable levels (< 0.2%).

Sorbic acid is generally considered non-toxic and is metabolized, as are the longer-chain fatty acids (Deuel *et al.*, 1954a,b), by β- and ω-oxidation. Among other common food preservatives, sorbic acid has the highest ADI (25 mg/kg body weight) (Lueck, 1980). The LD_{50} for sorbic acid is 7–11 g/kg body weight, while that for sodium sorbate is 6–7 g. High levels of sorbic acid (> 1%) may irritate mucous membranes of highly sensitive individuals, but no mutagenic, teratogenic or carcinogenic effects have been observed in laboratory animals when used at reasonable levels (Jung *et al.*, 1992b; Wuergler *et al.*, 1992; Sofos, 1994a). A report on potential allergenic reactions from consumption of sorbate-treated bacon in the USA has not been confirmed (Sofos, 1989a). Reports of mutagenic effects due to possible nitrite–sorbate reactions have not been verified in realistic food systems (Kada, 1974; Hayatsu *et al.*, 1975; Namiki & Kada, 1975; Sofos, 1981, 1989a). In the USA, sorbates are classified as GRAS (CFR, 1996), at maximum permissible levels in various foods of 0.05–0.3%.

Like all other lipophilic acid preservatives, sorbate is more effective in its undissociated form. However, reports exist that even the dissociated sorbate molecule has shown antimicrobial activity, even though it was 10–600-fold less than that of the undissociated acid (Eklund, 1983; Skirdal & Eklund, 1993). Since its value pK_a is 4.76, the activity is higher at lower pH values (Gooding *et al.*, 1955; Bell *et al.*, 1959). The maximum pH for sorbate activity is 6.0–6.5, with measurable activity detected at pH 6.5–7.0. These higher pH levels for sorbate activity, compared with other similar lipophilic-acid preservatives, extend its use to foods with higher pH values. It can sometimes replace benzoate, partially or totally, in order to avoid possible off-odour and to extend the range of microorganisms inhibited. Even at low pH values (2.5–4.0), sorbate has a broader spectrum of activity compared with that of benzoate and propionate (Smith & Rollin, 1954; Gooding *et al.*, 1955; Sofos & Busta, 1981, 1993). The inhibitory activity of potassium sorbate against *Z. bailii* in salsa mayonnaise stored at 23–25°C was greater than that of sodium benzoate (Wind & Restaino, 1995).

At concentrations of 0.05–0.3%, sorbates inhibit growth of yeasts and moulds and many bacteria. Their effect against bacteria, however, is not as comprehensive as that against yeasts and moulds, but it was found to inhibit several pathogens, including *Cl. botulinum* (Sofos, 1989a), *L. monocytogenes* (El-Shenawy & Marth, 1988), and *Y. enterocolitica* (Tsay & Chou, 1989). Yeasts inhibited by sorbates include *Brettanomyces*, *Candida*, *Cryptococcus*, *Debaryomyces*, *Endomycopsis*, *Hansenula*, *Kloeckera*, *Rhodotorula*, *Saccharomyces*, *Sporobolomyces*, *Torulaspora*, *Torulopsis* and *Zygosaccharomyces* (Sofos, 1989a; Sofos & Busta, 1993). Among the genera of moulds inhibited by sorbate are *Acternaria*, *Botrytis*, *Cephalosporium*, *Cladosporium*, *Collectotrichum*, *Cunninghamella*, *Fusarium*, *Geotrichum*, *Gliocladium*, *Helminthosporium*, *Humicola*, *Monilia*, *Mucor*, *Penicillium*, *Phoma*, *Pullalaria*, *Rhizoctonia*, *Rhizopus*, *Sporotrichum* and *Trichoderma* (Sofos, 1989a; Sofos & Busta, 1993). The list of bacteria inhibited by sorbates includes *Acetobacter*, *Achromobacter*, *Acinetobacter*, *Enterobacter*, *Bacillus*, *Campylobacter*, *Clostridium*, *Escherichia*, *Klebsiella*, *Listeria*, *Micrococcus*, *Moraxella*, *Mycobacterium*, *Proteus*, *Pseudomonas*, *Salmonella*, *Serratia*, *Staphylococcus*, *Vibrio* and *Yersinia* (Sofos, 1989a; Sofos & Busta, 1981, 1993).

Sorbic acid has been used to inhibit yeasts in situations such as cucumber fermentations, where it allows growth of catalase-negative, lactic acid-producing bacteria (Phillips & Mundt, 1950; Jones & Harper, 1952; Costilow *et al.*, 1956, 1957). Sorbates are used for mould and yeast inhibition in a variety of foods, including cheese products, baked goods, fruits and vegetables, wines, soft drinks, fruit juices, pickles, sauerkraut, syrups, jellies, jams, preserves, salads, margarine and certain meat and fish products. There are certain exceptions to the application of sorbates. Since they are effective yeast inhibitors, their use may cause problems in yeast-raised bakery products. No such problem exists, however, when sorbate is used to preserve chemically leavened or unleavened items. Alternatives that may be used in yeast-leavened products include employment of reduced sorbate levels; increased level of yeast inoculum; extension of fermentation time; application of sorbate sprays after baking; or use of slow-releasing sorbate preparations (Sofos, 1989a).

Sorbic acid retards bacterial spore germination (loss of heat resistance) in comminuted meat systems and culture media (Sofos *et al.*, 1979b,d, 1986). The action of sorbate on bacterial spore germination appears to occur during the connecting reactions that follow triggering or initiation in the germination process. This inhibitory effect appears to involve spore membranes or protease enzymes involved in germination (Sofos *et al.*, 1986). Inhibition of metabolic function in vegetative cells has been associated with alterations in membranes, the proton-motive force and the morphological structure of the cells and with inhibition of cell-transport processes and enzymatic activity (Sofos, 1989a). It is likely that more than one mechanism of inhibition may be involved under various conditions (Sofos & Busta, 1993).

Evidence exists that some strains of moulds, bacteria and yeasts are resistant or can metabolize sorbic acid through biochemical pathways similar to those of other fatty acids (Melnick *et al.*, 1954; Troller, 1965; Marth *et al.*, 1966; Warth, 1977, 1985; Sofos, 1989a; Splittstoesser & Churney, 1992; Sofos & Busta, 1993; Neves *et al.*, 1994; Thakur *et al.*, 1994). Sorbate has been found to be decomposed in cheese and fruit products by moulds of the genera *Penicillium*, *Aspergillus* and *Mucor*. Decomposition depended on prior exposure of the microorganism to subinhibitory levels of sorbate, high microbial load, low concentration of sorbate and type of product. Degradation of sorbate by mould in cheese has resulted in the accumulation of 1,3-pentadiene and development of a kerosene-like or plastic paint-type odour. Metabolism of sorbate by lactic-acid bacteria in wine and fermented vegetables has resulted in production of ethyl sorbate, 4-hexanoic acid, 1-ethoxyhexa-2,4-diene and 2-ethoxyhexa-3,5-diene (Liewen & Marth, 1985; Sofos, 1989a; Sofos & Busta, 1993). Under certain conditions, mycotoxin formation by certain moulds has been enhanced in the presence of sorbate (Liewen & Marth, 1985; Sofos, 1989a). Since high concentrations of contamination with certain microorganisms may degrade sorbate and result in product defects, it should be expected to preserve products only when manufactured under sanitary conditions. It should not be thought of as a replacement of GMP. This, of course, applies to all chemical food preservatives or other methods of food preservation.

After the extensive research on sorbate in the 1950s, a new wave of investigations was initiated in the 1970s in an effort to expand its applications, and sorbates were found effective against several pathogenic bacteria (Sofos, 1989a, 1992b; Sofos & Busta, 1993). Sorbates were examined extensively as a preservative of meat products after a report showed that potassium sorbate delayed toxin production by *Cl. botulinum* in an uncured sausage product (Tompkin *et al.*, 1974). Earlier reports had indicated not only that was sorbic acid ineffective against clostridia, but also that it could be used as a selective agent for such organisms (Emard & Vaughn, 1952; York & Vaughn, 1954, 1955; Hansen & Appleman, 1955). The above conclusions were probably the result of the low solubility of sorbic acid in aqueous media and the pH levels at which the studies were performed. Consequently, the observation by Tompkin *et al.* (1974) of activity against clostridia stimulated additional research.

The call for elimination or reduction of nitrite in cured meat products, due to concern over potential carcinogenic properties, and the perceived necessity to find a replacement with antibotulinal activity stimulated interest in sorbate as an antibotulinal agent. The lack of new preservatives, the drawbacks of the existing ones and the properties of sorbate contributed to the expansion of the research beyond cured meats to other microbial species and food products. These studies on sorbate as an antibotulinal agent in meat products, either by itself or with low nitrite levels (40–80 parts/10^6), demonstrated effectiveness in meat products, such as frankfurters, bacon and comminuted pork (Ivey & Robach, 1978; Ivey *et al.*, 1978; Sofos *et al.*, 1979a,b,c,d, 1980a,b). However, the use of sorbate as a direct additive to all meat products in the USA was not permitted. The only approved use in meats in the USA to date is the dipping of casings for dry sausages to prevent growth of surface moulds.

Several studies have reported on synergistic antimicrobial effects and interactions of sorbate with salt, sugar and other compounds, as well as processing and storage conditions (Gooding *et al.*, 1955; Robach, 1979; Beuchat, 1981a,b,c, 1982; Restaino *et al.*, 1982; Roland & Beuchat, 1984; Sofos, 1985, 1989a; Robach, 1987). A combination of sodium benzoate (0.1%) and potassium sorbate (0.1%) inactivated *E. coli* O157:H7 in apple cider (Zhao *et al.*, 1993). Taking advantage of such interactions should be useful in minimizing levels of additives and processes in order to enhance product shelf-life, while maintaining sensory quality. Antimicrobial effects of sorbate derivatives have also been described; sorbohydroxamic acid, sorbic aldehyde and other derivatives are more effective than sorbic acid over a wider pH range against several microorganisms (Dudman, 1963; Troller & Olsen,1967; Sofos, 1989a).

12 Esters

12.1 General

In addition to acids and their salts, esters of various acids have been proposed or tested or are in use as chemical preservatives in foods. Esters with antimicrobial activity include those of *p*-hydroxybenzoic acid, dicarbonic acid, fatty acids, fumaric acid and sucrose fatty-acid esters.

12.2 Esters of *p*-hydroxybenzoic acid

The methyl, ethyl, propyl, butyl and heptyl esters of *p*-hydroxybenzoic acid ($C_6H_4(COH)COOH$), also known as parabens, parasepts or PHB esters, find use as preservatives in pharmaceuticals, cosmetics and food products (see Chapters 2 and 3). They are generally white, free-flowing powders, with properties similar to those of benzoic acid, but the modification improves their usefulness. Their water solubility decreases as the number of carbon atoms in the ester group increases, whereas their solubility in ethanol, propylene glycol and oil increases with increasing numbers of carbon atoms in the ester group (Chichester & Tanner, 1972; Davidson,1993). The water solubility of the methyl ester is 0.25% (w/v) at 25°C, but the upper total limit permitted in foods is 0.1%. The toxicity of parabens is low, with an LD_{50} ranging from 180 to over 8000 mg/kg body weight, depending on the form and methods of administration (Matthews *et al*., 1956; Chichester & Tanner, 1972; Lueck, 1980; Sofos, 1994a). The ADI is set at 10 mg/kg body weight (Foegeding & Busta, 1991; Sofos, 1994a). Methyl and propyl parabens are considered as GRAS in the USA (CFR, 1996).

Parabens inhibit or prevent the growth of a variety of yeasts, moulds and bacteria. They are more effective against yeasts and moulds than against bacteria, especially Gram-negative bacteria (Ingram *et al*., 1964; Foegeding & Busta, 1991; Davidson, 1993). They may be used as preservatives in baked goods (except yeast-leavened products), fruit products, jams, jellies, preserves, pickles, olives, syrups, beverages, creams and pastes (von Schelhorn, 1951; Jermini & Schmidt-Lorenz, 1987). Heptyl paraben is approved for use in the USA for the inhibition of spoilage bacteria in fermented malt beverages (≤0.0012%) and in non-carbonated soft drinks and fruit-based beverages (≤0.002%) (CFR, 1996). The ethyl and butyl esters are also approved for certain uses in other countries. Products in which parabens have been tested experimentally include meats, margarine, soy sauce, maple syrup, beer and butter (Frank & Willits, 1961). In meat products in the USA, they may be used as mould inhibitors by dipping the casings of dry sausages in a 3.5% solution. They were also proposed as antibotulinal agents in a five-compound patent suggested as an alternative to nitrite in the USA (Sweet, 1975). Whereas Robach & Pierson (1978) found that the methyl and propyl esters were very effective antibotulinal agents in laboratory media, they appear to be ineffective against *Cl. botulinum* in meat. Their antimicrobial activity has been demonstrated against a variety of species, including *E. coli*, *Pseudomonas* spp., *Aeromonas hydrophila*; *Y. enterecolitica*, *Vibrio* spp., *Staph. aureus*, *B. subtilis*, *Salmonella typhi*, *L. monocytogenes*, *Alternaria* spp., *Aspergillus* spp., *Sacch. cerevisiae*, *R. nigrificans*, etc. (Fung *et al*., 1985; Payne *et al*., 1989; Foegeding & Busta, 1991; Moir & Eyles, 1992; Davidson, 1993; Sofos, 1994a). Propyl paraben, at 0.03–0.05%, inhibited *Sal. typhimurium* and *Staph. aureus* (Pierson *et al*., 1980). Inhibition of nutrient transport appears to be the primary mode of antimicrobial action by parabens (Eklund, 1980), as demonstrated with *E. coli*, *Pseudomonas aeruginosa* and *B. subtilis*. Parabens have also inhibited bacterial spore germination (Parker, 1969), as well as microbial respiration (Shiralkar & Rege, 1978), protease secretion (Venugopal *et al*., 1984) and synthesis of DNA, RNA and protein (Nes & Eklund, 1983).

The high pK_a value (8.5) of parabens allows their use as antimicrobials in foods of higher pH, compared with other common preservatives. Their antimicrobial activity increases with the number of carbon atoms in the ester group, while the activity of branched-chain esters is low (Huppert, 1957; Dymicky & Huhtanen, 1979). Since solubility decreases with chain length, the lower esters are more often used in practice. However, a more common procedure is a combination of the methyl and propyl esters to include both good antimicrobial activity and solubility (Foegeding &

Busta, 1991). In slightly acidic foods and where problems of flavour may arise, parabens can be combined with benzoate, which is also less expensive. In many cases, benzoate is preferred to parabens, since yeasts and moulds can grow at acidic pH values, where benzoate is more effective. Thus, the main application of parabens is at higher pH values (above 6.8 or 7.0), where the other preservatives are ineffective.

12.3 Other

Di- or pyrocarbonic-acid esters (R^1O–CO–O–CO–OR^2) include diethyl and dimethyl esters. The diethyl ester of dicarbonic acid is known as diethyl pyrocarbonate (DEDC or DEPC), while the dimethyl ester is known as dimethyl dicarbonic acid (DMDC). The compounds have been reviewed by Ough (1993b). While DMDC has a molecular weight of 134.1 and its water solubility is 3.65%, DEDC (molecular weight 162.1) is of lower water solubility (0.6%); both are miscible with ethanol. The compounds are colourless liquids, with faint fruity odours. In water solutions, DMDC and DEDC hydrolyse to yield methanol and ethanol, respectively, and carbon dioxide. Hydrolysis is faster for DMDC than for DEDC and proceeds more rapidly in acidic conditions (Foegeding & Busta, 1991).

Both DEDC and DMDC are fungicidal for yeasts, as well as bactericidal. The list of fungi sensitive to DEDC is very long, while DMDC and sorbate/benzoate were very effective against fungi and bacteria in tomato juice at 5 and 20°C, but juice treated with DMDC had lower amounts of glucose, fructose, lycopene, β-carotene, ascorbic acid and amino acids (Bizri & Wahem, 1994). The antimicrobial activity is more potent at higher temperatures and at pH values below 4.0 (Chichester & Tanner, 1972). The antimicrobial activity of these esters is due to their interaction with microbial-enzyme nucleophilic groups (Ough, 1993b). Diethyl pyrocarbonate has been used as a yeast inhibitor in wines, non-carbonated beverages, fruit juices, fermented malt beverages and beer. The compound acts as a sterilant, so the product should be maintained free of subsequent contamination (Foegeding & Busta, 1991).

The dicarbonates are expected to decompose in foods before consumption and therefore the safety of their reaction products may be of more concern than that of the original compounds. However, DEDC and DMDC irritate the skin and mucous membranes, and thus eye contact should be avoided (Foegeding & Busta, 1991). Details on the toxicology and safety of the dicarbonic-acid esters are presented by Ough (1993b). The potential toxicity of the products of their hydrolysis and decomposition, such as methanol and ethyl carbonate, has resulted in banning most of their uses in the USA and other countries. In the USA, DMDC is still permitted as an inhibitor of yeasts in wines at levels of up to 0.02% and in ready-to-drink tea at levels up to 0.025% (CFR, 1996). The FAO World Health Organization (WHO) Expert Committee on Food Additives has recommended that the human daily intake of ethyl carbonate, a carcinogen resulting from reaction of ammonia with DEDC, should not exceed 10 μg/day.

Sucrose fatty acid esters, derived from sucrose esterified with a mixture of palmitic and stearic acids, are approved emulsifiers in the USA. There is evidence that these esters, in combination with sorbate or propionate, may provide added antimycotic activity at pH values higher than the optimum for either inhibitor alone (Sofos, 1989a). The compounds have also inhibited heat-damaged, as well as unheated, bacterial spores (Tsuchido *et al.*, 1983). Also, some aliphatic esters of phenylalanine have been reported as bacterial and mould inhibitors in foods and beverages, at levels as low as 0.005% (Kiritaguchi *et al.*, 1973).

Monoglycerides of lauric acid, known as monolaurin or lauricidin, are classified as GRAS emulsifiers in the USA (CFR, 1996). Monolaurin has shown antimicrobial activity against psychrotrophic as well as spore-forming and pathogenic bacteria (e.g. *Clostridium sporogenes*, *Cl. botulinum*, *Clostridium perfringens*, *B. cereus*, *Staph. aureus* and *L. monocytogenes*), moulds and osmophilic yeasts (Kabara, 1981, 1984, 1993; Schlievert *et al.*, 1992; Wang & Johnson, 1992; Wang *et al.*, 1993; Chaibi *et al.*, 1996a,b, 1997). Monolaurin has been proposed as a component of multicompound antimicrobial systems in foods (Kabara, 1993). In Japan, monocylglycerols have been used as antimicrobials in situations where duration of action and off-flavours do not become problems (CAST, 1997). Sanitation of food-contact surfaces with organic acid/monolaurin combinations has been presented as less effective than that of other commonly used sanitizers (Deog-Hwan & Marshall, 1996).

Esters of fumaric (*trans*-butenedioic) acid, such as monomethyl fumarate (methyl fumarate) and dimethyl fumarate, have exhibited inhibitory activity against fungi and *Cl. botulinum* (Huhtanen *et al.*, 1981). At levels of 0.15–0.2%, these compounds were suggested as alternatives to nitrite in preservation of bacon (Doores,1993). In addition, the *n*-monoalkyl maleates and fumarates esterified with C_{13}, C_{18} to alcohols have exhibited antimicrobial activity (Dymicky *et al.*, 1987).

13 Gases

13.1 General

Several gases or vapours are used in food processing, either as antimicrobial agents or for other purposes exhibiting indirect antimicrobial activity. Gases such as carbon dioxide, sulphur dioxide, epoxides and chlorine have been used commercially as antimicrobial food preservatives, water disinfectants, sterilants or sanitizers. Nitrogen and oxygen, frequently used or their concentrations modified in packaging of food products, have no direct adverse effect on microorganisms and are not considered chemical food preservatives. Lack of oxygen, however, affects growth of aerobic microorganisms. Nitrogen can be used as a cryogenic agent, or inert gas, in controlled-atmosphere storage, and may indirectly affect some microorganisms, especially through elimination of oxygen (Huffman, 1974). Oxygen levels may be reduced in the storage of fruits, vegetables and meat, mainly for physiological reasons (Clark & Lentz, 1973). Other biocidal gases, mostly used in medicine, are not included in the discussion, nor are carbon monoxide and acetaldehyde, also shown to possess potential preservative action (Clark *et al.*, 1976).

13.2 Sulphur dioxide and sulphites

Sulphur dioxide (SO_2) has been used for many centuries as a fumigant and especially as a wine preservative (Amerine & Joslyn, 1951; Joslyn & Braverman, 1954; Hammond & Carr, 1976). It is a colourless, pungent-smelling, non-flammable gas with a suffocating odour and is very soluble in cold water (85 g in 100 ml at 25°C) and in organic solvents. Sulphur dioxide is used as gas or in the form of its sulphite, bisulphite and metabisulphite salts, which are powders. The gaseous form is produced either by burning sulphur or by its release from the compressed, liquefied form. The sulphites, including sodium sulphite, sodium hydrogen sulphite, sodium metabisulphite, potassium metabisulphite and calcium sulphite, are easier to handle and use than the gas or liquid forms of SO_2 (Ough, 1993a; Sofos, 1994a). Sulphur dioxide and the various sulphite salts dissolve in water and, at low pH values, yield sulphurous acid, bisulphite and sulphite ions. The various sulphite salts contain 50–68% active SO_2 (Foegeding & Busta, 1991). A pH-dependent equilibrium is formed in water and the proportion of SO_2 ions increases with decreasing pH values. At pH values less than 4.0, the antimicrobial activity reaches its maximum (Wyss, 1948; Sofos, 1994a). Metabisulphites are more stable to oxidation than bisulphites, which, in turn, show greater stability than sulphites.

Sulphites are GRAS in the USA (CFR, 1996), but levels of application in wines are restricted to 350 mg/l by the Bureau of Alcohol, Tobacco and Firearms. Sulphites are not permitted or recommended for preservation of foods considered as important sources of vitamin B_1 (thiamine), because they destroy this nutrient (Ough, 1993a; Sofos, 1994a). Sulphur dioxide and sulphites do not accumulate in the body, because they are rapidly oxidized to sulphate and excreted in the urine. The LD_{50} values vary from 40 to 2000 mg/kg in equivalent amounts of SO_2, depending on the sulphiting agent and type of animal (Ough, 1993a). Sulphur dioxide has shown mutagenic effects in bacterial tests, but sulphites are not mutagenic (Hayatsu & Miura, 1970; Mukai *et al.*, 1970). Sulphites have also been associated with the triggering of asthma attacks and other acute allergenic responses in a small number of susceptible individuals. This has led to a decreased use of the compounds in foods, special labelling requirements (e.g. salads, wines) and concerns about foods with no ingredient labels, such as vegetable salads treated with sulphites to prevent browning in restaurants (Walker, 1985; IFT, 1986; Sofos, 1994a).

The antimicrobial action of SO_2 is selective, with some species being more resistant than others (Clark & Takacs, 1980). In water, SO_2 forms sulphurous acid (H_2SO_3), with pK_a values of 1.8 and 7.2, which is more inhibitory to microbial growth than sulphite ions. Thus, it is not surprising that the undissociated acid was 1000 times more effective than sulphite and bisulphite ions against *E. coli*, 100–500 times more effective against yeasts (*Sacch. cerevisiae*) and 100 times more effective against moulds (*A. niger*) (Joslyn & Braverman, 1954). Antimicrobial activity is influenced by pH, concentration, SO_2 binding and duration of contact (Foegeding & Busta, 1991; Ough, 1993a).

Due to its high reactivity, SO_2 can interact with thiol groups in proteins, enzymes, vitamins, cofactors, nucleotides, nucleic acids and lipids in microbial cells and cause highly inhibitory or lethal effects (Woodzinski *et al.*, 1978; Clark & Takacs, 1980; Lueck, 1980; Foegeding & Busta, 1991; Ough, 1993a). Sulphur dioxide cleaves disulphide bonds of proteins, resulting in changed enzyme conformation and modification of active sites. In addition, SO_2 causes inhibition of enzymes by binding enzyme intermediates or end-products, which may alter enzyme equilibria. The lipid peroxidation of SO_2 may cause interference with membrane functions.

Sulphur dioxide and sulphites are used in the preservation of a variety of food products (Sofos, 1994a), including wines, as well as dehydrated fruits and vegetables, fruit juices, acid pickles, salads, syrups and meat and fish products in certain countries. In fruits, they control *Botrytis* and *Cladosporium* moulds, in order to extend the processing period of products such as grapes, cherries and other berry fruits. In fruit juices, they prevent undesirable fermentations during processing and storage (Foegeding & Busta, 1991). A combination of 0.01% SO_2 and 0.05% sorbate was recommended for the preservation of intermediate-moisture fruit products as an inhibitor of osmotolerant yeasts (Tapia-de-Daza *et al.*, 1995). Excessive amounts of sulphites may induce off-flavours and product discoloration.

In wine-making, sulphites are added to the expressed grape juice (must) to inactivate the naturally occurring undesirable flora before the desirable fermentative yeasts are added (Amerine & Joslyn, 1951; Joslyn & Braverman, 1954; Rose, 1993). The condition of the grapes, type of wine, pH, sugar concentration and contamination determine the amount (50–100 parts/10^6) of sulphite to be used in wine-making (Amerine & Joslyn, 1951). In wine preservation, sulphite is also important for cleaning the equipment; it prevents undesirable changes and bacterial spoilage during storage; and it may serve as an antioxidant and clarifying agent (Foegeding & Busta, 1991; Ough, 1993a).

Sulphites are not permitted for use in fresh and processed meats in the USA. However, they are used as sausage preservatives in the UK and as dried-fish and shrimp preservatives in France, and they were shown to delay *Cl. botulinum* growth and toxin production in meat (Tompkin *et al.*, 1980). They are also used to prevent 'black spot', a discoloration caused by oxidation, in shrimp in the USA. The reason that they are prohibited from meats in the USA is that they destroy thiamine, and may restore the colour of old meat, which could be misleading to the consumer. Their use in fresh sausage in the UK is to delay the growth of yeasts, moulds and Gram-negative mesophilic bacteria (Foegeding & Busta, 1991). This is associated with the fact that sulphites favour the development of acid-producing bacteria (*Lactobacillus* spp. and *Brochotrix thermosphacta*), especially under refrigerated storage (Dyett & Shelley 1966). The most commonly used form in sausage is sodium metabisulphite, at a maximum concentration of 450 parts/10^6 as SO_2. In addition to its antimicrobial effects, SO_2 added to foods for its antioxidant and reducing properties, and to prevent enzymatic and non-enzymatic browning reactions (IFT, 1986; Foegeding & Busta, 1991; Ough, 1993a).

13.3 Carbon dioxide

Carbon dioxide (CO_2) is a colourless, odourless, acidic in odour and flavour, non-combustible gas, and is considered as GRAS in the USA (CFR, 1996). In commercial practice, it is sold as a liquid under pressure (58 kg/cm^2) or solidified as dry ice. The gas is readily dissolvable in water (171 ml/100 ml at 0°C) and in the liquid phase of foods, where carbonic acid is formed. Amounts of 30–60% (v) CO_2 in the presence of 20% (v) oxygen (O_2) cause rapid death to animals, while lung exposure in humans to atmospheres of more than 10% CO_2 causes unconsciousness (Lueck, 1980). Inhalation of lower concentrations over long periods of time may also be dangerous (Sofos, 1994a). The compound, however, is virtually not subject to food regulations. The antimicrobial activity of CO_2 is dependent on concentration, the microorganisms under consideration, their stage during growth, the water activity of the system and the temperature of storage (Foegeding & Busta, 1991). Depending on these factors, CO_2 may have no effect, have a stimulatory effect, inhibit growth or be lethal to microorganisms (King & Nagel, 1967, 1975; Parekh & Solberg, 1970; Foegeding & Busta, 1983c, 1991). Low concentrations of CO_2 may stimulate microbial growth, but concentrations of 100% have killed species of *Bacillus*, *Aerobacter*, *Flavobacterium* and *Micrococcus*, while strains of *Proteus*, *Lactobacillus* and *Cl. perfringens* were only inhibited (Ogilvy & Ayres, 1951, 1953; Parekh & Solberg, 1970). Carbon dioxide at atmospheric pressure inhibited spore germination of *B. cereus* spores, but enhanced germination of clostridia (Enfors and Molin, 1978). Concentrations of 10 and 25 atm of CO_2, however, inhibited germination of *Cl. sporogenes* and *Cl. perfringens*, respectively. Generally, CO_2 concentrations of 5–50% are inhibitory to most yeasts, moulds and bacteria (Hales, 1962; Smith, 1963), and high CO_2 concentrations increase the lag phase and generation time of microorganisms (Tomkins, 1932). However, increasing concentrations do not increase activity indefinitely. From a concentration of 5 to about 25–50%, inhibitory action increases almost linearly but, at higher concentrations, activity increases only slightly or not at all (Ogilvy & Ayres, 1951, 1953; Clark & Lentz, 1969, 1973). With decreasing temperatures, both CO_2 solubility and antimicrobial activity increase (Golding, 1945). Combinations of CO_2 and nisin were found effective against *L. monocytogenes* in pork (Fang & Lo-Wei, 1994).

Carbon dioxide is used as a solid (dry ice) in many countries as a means of chilling products, for low-temperature storage and in transportation of food products. Besides keeping the temperature low, as it sublimates, the gaseous CO_2 inhibits growth of psychrotrophic microorganisms and prevents spoilage of the food. Foods in which CO_2 controls psychrotrophic spoilage include meats and meat products, poultry, eggs, fish, fruits and vegetables (Foegeding & Busta, 1991). Moulds are generally most sensitive to CO_2, while yeasts (fermentative) are more resistant, and Gram-positive bacteria are more resistant than Gram-negative types (Tomkins, 1932; Ogilvy & Ayres, 1953). Among bacteria, meat-spoilage organisms, such as *Pseudomonas*, micrococci and bacilli, are very sensitive to CO_2, while acid-producing organisms (lactobacilli) are generally resistant (Ogilvy & Ayres, 1953; King & Nagel, 1975; Gill & Tan, 1979; Foegeding & Busta, 1991; Sofos, 1994a).

As a gas, CO_2 is used as a direct additive in the storage of fruits and vegetables, meats and beverages. The use of increased CO_2 levels in modified-atmosphere storage of foods has been increasing, because the appropriate gaseous composition minimizes chemical and biological product decomposition (Finne, 1982; Rowe, 1988; Baker & Genigeorgis, 1990). In vacuum-packaged meats, generated CO_2 inhibits the growth of aerobic spoilage organisms, while the growth of lactobacilli is encouraged. The handling of meat in this fashion has been a very important innovation in meat storage and transportation. A concentration of 10–20% CO_2 is usually common in the controlled/modified-atmosphere storage of fresh meats. Higher concentrations may cause undesirable odours and the increase in antimicrobial activity is only marginal (Clark & Lentz, 1969; Silliker *et al.* 1977). In fruits and vegetables, stored under controlled or modified atmospheres, the correct combination of O_2 and CO_2 delays respiration and ripening, as well as retarding mould and yeast growth. These effects allow for an extended storage of the products for transportation and for consumption during the off-season. The amount of CO_2 (5–10%) is determined by factors such as the nature of the product, variety, climate and extent of storage (von Schelhorn, 1951; Smith, 1963).

One major safety concern with products preserved under modified-atmosphere storage is whether pathogens will outgrow spoilage organisms and render the product unsafe for human consumption before any visible signs of spoilage (Ito & Bee, 1980; Genigeorgis, 1985; Post *et al.*, 1985; Garcia *et al.*, 1987; Hintlian & Hotchkiss, 1987). This concern is especially valid for seafood stored under modified atmospheres, which may allow production of toxin by non-proteolytic, psychrotrophic strains of *Cl. botulinum* (Sofos, 1994a).

A major application of CO_2 is in carbonated soft drinks and mineral waters, where it serves the dual purpose of having both an antimicrobial and an effervescing effect. Levels of 3–5 atm of CO_2 are common, since they strongly inhibit or destroy spoilage and pathogenic microorganisms. The antimicrobial action of CO_2 in carbonated beverages increases with CO_2 reassure and decreases with sugar content (Insalata, 1952). The presence of CO_2, along with exclusion of O_2, prevents oxidative deterioration in beer and ale (Foegeding & Busta, 1991). The inhibitory effect of CO_2 is a direct antimicrobial action, as well as an indirect effect due to a decrease in pH caused by carbonic-acid formation from CO_2 (Koser & Skinner, 1922; Hays *et al.*, 1959). Another application of CO_2 is the preservation of eggs during refrigerated storage with a concentration of 2.5% CO_2.

13.4 Other

The various forms of chlorine constitute the most widely used chemical sanitizer in the food industry. These chlorine forms include chlorine (Cl_2) gas, sodium hypochlorite (NaOCl), calcium hypochlorite ($Ca(OCl)_2$) and chlorine dioxide (ClO_2) gas. These compounds are used as water adjuncts in processes such as product washing, transport and cooling of heat-sterilized cans; in sanitizing solutions for equipment surfaces; and in washing treatments to reduce microbial loads on the surface of meat, poultry and seafood (Foegeding & Busta, 1991; Cords and Dychdala, 1993; CFR, 1996). Elemental chlorine is highly corrosive and causes severe inflammation of the skin and mucous membranes, and inhalation of air with more than 20 parts/10^6 chlorine for 15 min may be fatal (Lueck, 1980; Foegeding & Busta, 1991).

Owing to its strong penetrating ability and oxidizing effect, adequate chlorine concentrations result in rapid inactivation of microorganisms. It has been reported that chlorine disrupts bacterial spore coats, damaging germination mechanisms, preventing outgrowth of germinated spores and causing leakage of spore contents (Foegeding & Busta, 1983a,b, 1991; Foegeding, 1983). Since chlorine is highly reactive, depending on concentration, its antimicrobial activity is reduced or eliminated in the presence of organic matter. The antimicrobial activity of chlorine is higher at neutral or slightly acidic pH values, where the active form (HOCl) is present in higher concentrations. Heat also increases the antimicrobial activity of chlorine, which is active against all types of microorganisms, including *L. monocytogenes* (El-Kest & Marth, 1988a,b,c). Important applications of chlorine include disinfection of drinking-water, sanitation of food-processing equipment and decontamination of water used in meat and poultry processing for chilling and for bacterial reduction by washing or rinsing (Sofos, 1994b). Chlorine dioxide is approved in the USA (CFR, 1996) for use as an antimicrobial agent in water used in poultry processing (up to 3 parts/10^6 residual chlorine).

Ozone (O_3) is a water-soluble, unstable, blue gas, which has a pungent, characteristic odour and occurs freely in nature. Maximum amounts tolerated by humans are 0.04 mg/kg, while concentrations of 0.1 mg/kg are objectionable, because they cause eye, nose, throat and mucous-membrane irritation. Ozone is produced commercially by passing electrical discharges or ionizing radiation through air or oxygen (Nagy, 1959). When exposed to air and water, it decomposes rapidly and forms oxygen. Thus, it is usually generated at the point of its use (Foegeding & Busta, 1991).

Yeasts and moulds are not as sensitive to ozone as bacteria, while bacterial spores are more resistant than vegetative cells (Foegeding, 1985). Of bacteria, Gram-negative species are less sensitive than Gram-positives. Lethality of microorganisms from ozone is due to its strong oxidizing activity, which may affect sulphydryl groups of enzymes and cell wall lipids. This may result in loss of enzymatic activity and leakage of vital cell components. The antimicrobial activity of ozone is affected by pH, stage of microbial growth, temperature, relative humidity and organic matter present in the substrate (Clark and Takacs, 1980).

Applications of ozone in various countries have included sterilization and removal of off-odours, flavours and colours from water. In the USA, ozone is considered as GRAS, approved as an antimicrobial for bottled water and foods (CFR, 1996). In addition, it is used as a maturing agent in wines and ciders and to sterilize beverage containers (Torricelli, 1959). Ozone can also preserve eggs and other foods, and it inactivates mycotoxins (Foegeding & Busta, 1991). In recent years, ozonation treatments have been evaluated for the decontamination of meat-animal carcasses and produce (Gorman *et al.*, 1995, 1997).

Ethylene (C_2H_4O) and propylene (C_3H_6O) oxides are organic epoxides or cyclic ethers possessing antimicrobial and sterilant properties. In their molecule, an oxygen is linked to two adjacent carbon atoms of the same chain. Ethylene oxide (Chapters 2 and 21) is a colourless, non-corrosive gas at ambient temperatures, which liquefies at 10.8°C and freezes at −111.3°C. It is highly reactive and, as a liquid, it is miscible in water and organic solvents. It is inflammable, and at concentrations of more than 700 parts/10^6 the gas form has an ether-like odour. Low concentrations (3%) of ethylene oxide are explosive in air and this constitutes a drawback in its handling and application. Mixtures of 10–20% ethylene oxide with 80–90% carbon dioxide are non-flammable and are recommended for use. Mixtures of ethylene oxide and fluorinated hydrocarbons or methyl formate have also been available for commercial application.

Ethylene oxide does not lose its antimicrobial activity in such mixtures, which are commonly used as sterilizing agents (Mayr & Suhr, 1972). Ethylene oxide at 0.1–0.2 g/l of air may be fatal to humans (Lueck, 1980). Concentrations higher than 100 mg/kg result in lung and eye irritations and may cause nausea and mental disorientation (Foegeding & Busta, 1991). Propylene oxide has similar properties to ethylene oxide but it is less volatile and its antimicrobial activity is lower. It is an inflammable, colourless gas that liquefies at 34.5°C and freezes at −110°C. It is less reactive and less penetrating than ethylene oxide and has a narrower explosive range (2–22%). The toxicity of propylene oxide has been reported to be only one-third that of ethylene oxide (Bruch, 1961).

Ethylene oxide gas penetrates most organic materials without causing any damage. This is advantageous, since it can be used for sterilization of sensitive materials. Its breakdown products include glycol and ethylene chlorohydrin (Bruch, 1972; Wesley *et al.*, 1965). The epoxides are removed from the food by evacuating the chamber, accompanied by agitation and gentle heating, and the remaining glycols are considered generally as non-toxic. The epoxides are antimicrobial in both aqueous and gaseous phases (Marletta & Stumbo, 1970). Through the years, epoxides were used to decontaminate products such as dried fruits, maize starch, potato flour, maize wheat, barley, dried eggs, gelatin, gums and cereals (Whelton *et al.*, 1946; Pappas & Hall, 1952; Mayr & Kaemmerer, 1959; Bruch & Koesterer, 1961). Questions about the safety of ethylene chlorohydrin, a product of ethylene oxide hydrolysis, have limited the application of ethylene oxide in recent years to spices only. The regulatory authorities of the USA have set a gas-residue limit in spices of only 50 parts/10^6 and other countries have similar rules and requirements (Foegeding & Busta, 1991). Approval of irradiation treatments to disinfect spices in the USA were aimed at reducing dependence on epoxides for such applications. Both epoxides, ethylene and propylene, have been widely used for equipment sterilization, and they have both been reported to kill a variety of yeasts, moulds, bacteria and viruses (Whelton *et al.*, 1946; Phillips & Kaye, 1949; Pappas & Hall, 1952; see also Chapters 2 and 21).

14 Nitrite and nitrate

Nitrite (NO_2) and nitrate (NO_3) sodium and potassium salts are approved (CFR, 1996) and used as curing agents in meat, poultry and fish proceeing (Tompkin, 1993; Sofos & Rarharjo, 1994a). Their use started accidentally as impurities of common salt (NaCl), which was used to preserve meats in ancient times (Binkerd & Kolari, 1975; Sofos *et al.*, 1979c). Potassium nitrate is known as saltpetre or nitre, and calcium nitrate from caves (wall saltpetre) was used by ancient people in the curing of meat (Binkerd & Kolari,

1975). Observations that these nitrate impurities caused a reddening effect on meat led to the regular of nitrate in meat curing in order to achieve uniform colour.

At the end of the nineteenth century, it was shown that nitrite, and not nitrate, was responsible for cured-meat colour fixation, through reaction with the haem proteins haemoglobin and myoglobin. At the beginning of the twentieth century, the use of nitrite in meat curing was officially permitted in the USA and other countries and its functions were defined. The curing reaction is accelerated with addition of compounds such as ascorbic acid, isoascorbic or erythorbic acid, their sodium salts, fumaric acid, glucono-δ-lactone, citric acid, sodium citrate and sodium acid pyrophosphate (Sofos & Raharjo, 1994a). Besides meats, nitrite and nitrate are sometimes used in cheese processing.

In addition to reacting with haem proteins to fix the characteristic cured-meat colour, other nitrite functions include a not very well-defined effect on the flavour of cured-meat products; a mild antioxidant effect, which prevents rancidity and 'warmed-over' flavour in such products; and finally an antimicrobial effect, especially against *Cl. botulinum* (Skovgaard, 1992; Freybler *et al.*, 1993; Sofos & Raharjo, 1994a). In general, concentrations of more than 100 parts/10^6 are necessary for botulism control, but lower nitrite concentrations (40–80 parts/10^6) may be sufficient for antimicrobial activity when sorbate (Ivey & Robach, 1978; Ivey *et al.*, 1978; Sofos *et al.*, 1979a,b,c,d, 1980a,b; Robach & Sofos, 1982; Sofos, 1989a) or sugar and a starter culture (Tanaka *et al.*, 1980, 1985) are included in the formulations. Nitrite concentrations lower (15–50 parts/10^6) than those needed for antimicrobial activity are necessary for chemical effects (colour, flavour). Levels of nitrite permitted to be added to muscle foods are generally in the range of 0.001–0.02% and in the USA they should not result in more than 0.02% of nitrite in the finished product (Sofos & Raharjo, 1994a).

Nitrate is not believed to have a direct effect on the above properties; it functions only as a source of nitrite (Christiansen *et al.*, 1973, 1974; Binkerd & Kolari, 1975), and most of its uses have been discontinued. The good safety record against botulism of commercially processed cured-meat products is believed to be related to nitrite addition (Silliker *et al.*, 1958; Ingram, 1974, 1976; Roberts, 1975; Lechowich *et al.*, 1978; Sofos *et al.*, 1979c; Sofos & Busta, 1980; Tompkin, 1993). Other factors (heat processing, product pH and composition, microbial contamination, refrigeration, NaCl concentration), however, are also important.

The antimicrobial effects of nitrite were observed early in its regular use against several bacterial genera (*Achromobacter, Aerobacter, Escherichia, Flavobacterium, Micrococcus* and *Pseudomonas*) (Tarr, 1941a,b, 1942). The most important antimicrobial action of nitrite, however, is against *Cl. botulinum*, which produces highly potent neurotoxins, and its value as an insurance factor contributing to the botulinal safety of cured-meat products that may be temperature-abused has been demonstrated in a number of studies (Sofos *et al.*, 1979c; Sofos & Busta, 1980). The presence of nitrite in a meat system, however, does not inhibit botulinal outgrowth indefinitely. The safety of the product is the result of interactions among a variety of the factors mentioned above. Among these factors, nitrite is a very important one, since it has a direct antibotulinal effect and it also interacts with most of the other factors. The eventual result is an extended botulism-safety of the product (Silliker, 1959; Roberts, 1975; Sofos *et al.*, 1979c; Roberts *et al.*, 1981; Robinson *et al.*, 1982).

The effect of nitrite is not the same against all genera and species of microorganisms. Some bacteria (salmonellae, lactobacilli, bacilli, *Cl. perfringens, L. monocytogenes*) are affected less by nitrite than is *Cl. botulinum* (Castellani & Niven, 1955; Grever, 1974; Buchanan *et al.*, 1989; Junttila *et al.*, 1989). Increased nitrite concentrations, however, may eliminate such resistance. Nitrite was the least inhibitory preservative, compared with benzoate and sorbate, especially against *Staph. aureus*. Antimicrobial activity was influenced, not only by type of microorganisms, but also by temperature, pH and NaCl concentration (Thomas *et al.*, 1993). In combination with low pH, high NaCl and temperature effectively inhibited growth of *Shigella flexneri* (Zaika *et al.*, 1991). The nitrite effects are generally greater under vacuum packaging than in aerobic conditions (Barber & Deibel, 1972; Herring, 1973; Labots,

1977). However, the major application of nitrite as a chemical food preservative is that of an antibotulinal agent in cured-meat products (Tompkin, 1993; Sofos & Raharjo, 1994a).

When added to meat, nitrite is involved in a variety of chemical reactions (Cassens *et al.*, 1979; Walters, 1992). The rate of these reactions is affected by product pH, temperature, composition and microbial contamination, and they result in the depletion of the compound. As the pH of the environment decreases, nitrite depletion is increased through increased production of nitrous acid and nitric oxide, which constitute the reactive forms of nitrite.

Tompkin (1993) presented a chronological review of the research that has contributed to our understanding of the antimicrobial activity of nitrite. No precise mechanism of antimicrobial activity by nitrite has been presented, but several theories have been proposed. Possible explanations of the antimicrobial activity of nitrite include (Sugiyama & Sofos, 1988) reactions of nitrite with food components and the formation of antibotulinal compound(s), such as the Perigo factor(s) (Benedict, 1980; National Research Council, 1981, 1982), which is considered to be unimportant, because it forms at higher temperatures (e.g. >105°C) and loses its activity in the presence of meat particles. The presence of meat with a high iron content or blood fractions interferes with the antibacterial activity of nitrite (Miller & Menichillo, 1991; Brewer *et al.*, 1992; Tompkin, 1993). Other possible mechanisms are based on the premise that nitrite or its derivatives, nitrous acid and nitric oxide, act directly on the organism and/or restrict the availability to the organism of an essential nutrient (Vahabzadeh *et al.*, 1983; Kim *et al.*, 1987; Sugiyama & Sofos, 1988). Woods *et al.* (1981) reported that nitrite and nitric oxide inhibited the phosphoroclastic system in clostridia.

During the 1970s, a series of reports demonstrated the occurrence of carcinogenic *N*-nitroso compounds (nitrosamines) in some cured-meat products (e.g. bacon) when cooked under certain conditions (e.g. >171°C). Numerous nitrosamines were found to be carcinogenic (Magee & Barnes, 1967; Sebranek & Cassens, 1973; Crosby & Sawyer, 1976; Gray & Randall, 1979; Tricker & Kubacki, 1992; Sofos & Raharjo, 1994a). Nitrosamine incidence and levels of occurrence in meat products have decreased through research and product control, and in the US the appropriate authorities have set maximum levels of acceptance, monitored by strict regulations (Cassens, 1995). The levels of residual nitrite in US commercial cured meats have decreased to approximately 20% of those present 25 years ago (Cassens, 1997).

A report published in 1979 indicated nitrite itself as being a direct carcinogen in laboratory animals (Newberne, 1979). The unconfirmed results indicated increased carcinogenicity with nitrite consumption in mice. Ignoring the nitrosamine–nitrite carcinogenicity controversy, nitrite used under existing regulations is not considered a health hazard. The ADI for nitrite is set at 0–0.2 mg/kg. At high concentrations, however, nitrite is toxic. The intravenous lethal dose for a 60–70 kg adult is estimated to be 1.5 to 2.5 g of nitrite. Since it oxidizes haemoglobin to methaemoglobin at these high intakes, the condition of methaemoglobinaemia occurs, which can result in death, due to oxygen shortage (Sofos & Raharjo, 1994a). Additional potential toxic effects of nitrite are discussed by Sofos & Raharjo (1994a). The nitrite issue caused an extensive debate among scientists, consumers, producers and regulatory authorities in several countries, especially in the USA, but the debate finally subsided (Cassens, 1995). The predominant sources of nitrate/nitrite in the diet may be water and vegetables (Hoffman, 1995). The subject of nitrite in foods has been summarized in an overview paper published by the Institute of Food Technologists (IFT, 1987).

Of the various compounds and process modifications tested as alternatives to nitrite in cured-meat products during the 1970s and early 1980s, only the use of a starter culture (e.g. *P. acidilactici*), along with sugar and 80 mg/kg nitrite, was permitted by the US Department of Agriculture for use in bacon. This product is organoleptically acceptable and gives rise to substantially less nitrosamine when fried. Furthermore, if the bacon is temperature-abused, the starter culture grows and produces lactic acid from the added sugar, which reduces the pH and inhibits *Cl. botulinum* (Tanaka *et al.*, 1985). Combinations of starter-culture bacteria and nitrite were also found effective against *Y. enterocolitica* in fermented sausages (Asplund *et al.*, 1993). Nitrite-free meat-curing systems have also been developed (Shahidi & Pegg, 1992).

15 Antibiotics

Antibiotics were frequently tested and used in food preservation in the 1950s and 1960s, but their commercial application as chemical food preservatives has been either restricted or prohibited. However, trace amounts of antibiotics may be present in foods originating from sources treated with the compounds (Katz & Brady, 1993). Such residues are considered food additives in the USA by the FDA. In the USA in 1967, the FDA prohibited the approved use of chlortetracycline and oxytetracycline in foods and introduced specifications to eliminate residues in food products carried over from treated animals. Their main uses included preservation of meat, poultry, fish, milk and its products, fresh fruits and vegetables and canned foods. Reviews on the subject of antibiotics in foods include those by Marth (1966), Fukusumi (1972) and Katz & Brady (1993).

The major reason that the use of antibiotics in food preservation was restricted or prohibited was the development and discovery of antibiotic-resistant strains of microorganisms (Anon., 1969; Levy, 1987; Tomasz, 1994). Microbial resistance to antibiotics is the result of genetic mutation or of selection of existing resistant organisms. If antibiotic-resistant strains of microorganisms colonize the digestive tract of humans and animals and cause disease, the antibiotics used in medicine may then become ineffective. Continuous use of antibiotics as food preservatives meant that microorganisms were exposed to sublethal doses of these drugs, and the development of resistant strains might also result in loss of their value in food preservation (Katz & Brady, 1993; Tomasz, 1994). In the UK the Swann Committee (Anon., 1969) and in the USA and FDA Task Force (Anon., 1972) reported that the use of antibiotics in farm animals may result in the development of antibiotic-resistant bacteria, which could be transferred from animals to humans. In order to avoid such undesirable consequences, the use of antibiotics in farm animals should be restricted to those which do not show cross-resistance with therapeutically important antibiotics.

Following these discoveries, the use of antibiotics came under attack and they were prohibited or restricted in most countries. The only antibiotic still remaining in some use as a food preservative in certain countries is natamycin (pimaracin). The presence of antibiotics in foods today is generally due to their use in animal feeds at subtherapeutic levels to improve efficiency of production and reduce costs (Franco *et al.*, 1990). The presence of antibiotic residues in foods such as milk and meat is not permitted in the USA and other countries. The subject, however, has become controversial and has led to trade restrictions among various countries.

Natamycin or pimaricin, a metabolic product of *Streptomyces natalensis*, is active as an inhibitor of yeasts and mycotoxin-producing moulds. The compound is a polyene macrolide ($C_{33}H_{47}NO_{13}$) antibiotic, which forms white crystalline needles and is of low solubility in water (0.003–0.01%, 25°C) and alcohols (Brik, 1981; CAST, 1997). Macrolides are characterized by a large lactone ring, which is glycosidically linked to rare sugars. Natamycin is highly soluble in acetic acid, glycol and glycerol (Clark *et al.*, 1964; Lueck, 1980). Its LD_{50} is 0.45–4.7 mg/kg body weight, depending on animal species (Levinskas *et al.*, 1966).

Although it is active against yeasts and moulds, natamycin is inactive against bacteria, viruses and actinomycetes (Foegeding & Busta, 1991; Davidson & Doan, 1993; Gould, 1996). In addition, some moulds, such as *Aspergillus flavus*, inactivate the compound with enzymes they produce. This, of course, is a problem only when the antibiotic is applied to foods after mould growth is initiated. Inhibition depends on concentration (Rusul & Marth, 1988b), and it appears to be due to interaction with cell membranes which results in loss of cellular components (Lueck, 1980). Inhibitory concentrations against yeasts and moulds range between 0.0001% and 0.0025% (CAST, 1998). The inhibitory activity of natamycin is affected by pH, oxidants, heavy metals, temperature and light. The pH actually affects the stability of natamycin, but, in the range of most foods (pH 5–7), the compound is stable. Its activity is believed to be through binding of sterol groups in cell membranes of fungi, which results in inhibition of sterol biosynthesis and distortion of and leakage from cell membranes (Davidson & Doan, 1993; CAST, 1997).

Natamycin has been used as a surface treatment in cheese, and such use has also been proposed for sausage products, fruits, juices and poultry, as an antifungal agent (Bullerman, 1977; Holley, 1981; Gourama & Bullerman, 1988; Davidson & Doan, 1993). In the USA (CFR, 1996), natamycin is approved for use as a mould inhibitor on the surface of cuts and slices of cheese. Methods for such applications include dripping or spraying with aqueous solutions of 0.02–0.03%. Since it does not penetrate into the product, it does not affect its flavour (Shibata *et al.*, 1991). The ADI for natamycin is 0.3 mg/kg body weight.

Two tetracycline antibiotics that have been used as food preservatives are oxytetracycline (Terramycin) and chlortetracycline (Aureomycin). Their basic structure consists of a four-membered tetracaine ring, with characteristically distributed polar side-groups. They are weakly basic, poorly soluble in water (Kurytowicz, 1976) and stable to temperatures up to boiling (Foegeding & Busta, 1991). Tetracyclines were used to extend the shelf-life of fresh meat, poultry and fish (Goldberg, 1964). Common applications included immersing fresh poultry or fish in tetracycline solutions of 3–100 mg/kg for 0.6–2 h, followed by refrigerated or ice storage (Kohler *et al.*, 1955; Lee *et al.*, 1967).

16 Indirect chemical food preservatives

Chemical substances added to foods with the objective of inhibiting microbial growth for extension of product shelf-life and assurance of consumer safety from pathogenic microorganisms may be classified as direct chemical food preservatives. In contrast, indirect chemical food preservatives may be called the chemical additives added to foods (CFR, 1996) as processing aids or to improve or preserve chemical and sensory qualities, but which may also contribute to inhibition of microbial growth. Among others, chemicals permitted to be added to foods for various reasons and which have exhibited antimicrobial activity include phenolic antioxidants, phosphates, EDTA, disodium EDTA, fatty acids and sodium bicarbonate (Shelef & Seiter, 1993; CFR, 1996).

Derivatives of phenol have been known as antiseptic agents for a long time (Davidson, 1993). In addition to parabens, which are phenolic compounds approved for use in foods as antimicrobials, additional phenolic compounds occur naturally in foods or are introduced through food processing. Phenolic compounds are also added to foods as antioxidants. Common phenolic antioxidants which may also have antimicrobial activity include butylated hydroxyanisole (BHA), butylated hydroxytoluene (BHT), tertiary butylhydroquinone (TBHQ) and propyl gallate (PG).

Butylated hydroxyanisole ($C_{11}H_{16}O_2$; 2- and 3-isomer of tertiary-butyl-4-hydroxyanisole) has exhibited antimicrobial properties against various microorganisms, including *Aspergillus parasiticus*, *Sacch. cerevisiae*, *Cl. perfringens*, *Sal. typhimurium Staph. aureus*, *E. coli* and *V. parahaemolyticus* (Raccach, 1984; Rusul & Marth, 1988a; Payne *et al.*, 1989; Davidson, 1993). Inhibitory concentrations have varied with substrate, pH and type of microorganism, but they exceed 0.01%. It should be noted, however, that most tests on the antimicrobial activity of this and other phenolic antioxidants have involved aqueous culture media, while in food systems their inhibitory effects may be reduced drastically (Dawson *et al.*, 1975).

Butylated hydroxytoluene ($C_{15}H_{24}O$; 2,6-ditertiary-butyl-*p*-cresol) has also exhibited antimicrobial properties in culture media and at concentrations greater than 0.01%. Among the organisms inhibited are *Cl. botulinum* and *Staph. aureus*, while *Salmonella senftenberg* was not inhibited by 1% BHT (Davidson, 1993). In general, BHT is less effective as an antimicrobial agent than other phenolic antioxidants.

Tertiary butylhydroquinone was shown to be inhibitory against bacteria and yeasts at concentrations of even less than 0.01%. The antimicrobial activity of PG appears to be limited. Other phenolic compounds which may have antimicrobial activity, as well as those microoganisms inhibited by these compounds, are discussed by Davidson (1993). In the USA, BHA, BHT and TBHQ are permitted for use as antioxidants in foods (CFR, 1996).

Several phosphate compounds, such as sodium acid pyrophosphate ($Na_2H_2P_2O_7$), sodium tripolyphosphate ($Na_2P_3O_{10}$), sodium hexametaphosphate ($(NaPO)_{13}$–Na_2O) and tetrasodium pyrophosphate ($Na_5P_2O_7$) are approved for use in processed foods in the USA and other countries. Their contribution to various food products relates to water retention, binding, emulsification, coagulation, texture, colour and flavour (Tompkin, 1984; Sofos, 1986a,b, 1989b; Wagner, 1986). In processed-meat products, especially in formulations with reduced sodium chloride, phosphates improve water and fat retention, meat-particle cohesion, texture, colour and flavour. The influence of phosphates on microbial growth is variable and depends on individual type and concentration, substrate, pH, microbial contamination, heat treatment, chemical additives and storage conditions. It is believed that their antimicrobial activity is due to chelation of metal ions useful in microbial metabolism. It has also been suggested that phosphates inhibit enzymes involved in transport functions, metabolism and activation of microbial toxins (Wagner, 1986; Sofos, 1989b; Shelef & Seiter, 1993). Trisodium phosphate solutions have been approved in the USA as decontaminants of meat and poultry (Gorman *et al.*, 1995, 1997).

Ethylenediamine tetraacetic acid (versene, $(HOOCCH_2)_2$–NCH_2CH_2N–$(CH_2COOH)_2$) and its salts are chelating agents used as synergists of antioxidants in foods (Shelef & Seiter, 1993). The compounds are approved for use in foods in the USA and other countries. Chelation of trace metal ions by EDTA results in inhibition of certain microorganisms, including *Cl. botulinum* (Winarno *et al.*, 1971; Tompkin, 1978). Several studies have reported inhibition of microbial growth and extension of shelf-life in products such as fish (Levin, 1967; Russell, 1971; Kuusi & Loytomaki, 1972; Wilkinson, 1975; Russell & Fuller, 1979; Ward & Ashley, 1980; Bulgarelli & Shelef, 1985). Calcium disodium EDTA and disodium EDTA are permitted for use in various foods in the USA for reasons such as retention of colour or flavour (CFR, 1996).

17 Other antimicrobials

A variety of compounds either have found some limited use as chemical food preservatives but their use has been discontinued, or have been found active against microorganisms and have been suggested for use (Foegeding & Busta, 1991). Low molecular weight glycols, such as propylene ($CH_3CHOHCH_2OH$) and butylene ($CH_3CHOHCHOHCH_3$) glycol, are permitted for use in foods (CFR, 1996) as A_w-reducing humectants, and they also retard microbial growth. They find major application in intermediate-moisture foods for inhibiting fungi (McIver *et al.*, 1978).

Diphenyl, biphenyl or phenyl benzene ($C_6H_5C_6H_5$) is a permitted food additive in the UK and other countries, because it inhibits a large number of microorganisms, especially moulds (e.g. *Penicillium italicum* and *Penicillium digitatum*). The compound is applied to wrapping materials to preserve citrus fruits during storage and transportation (Hopkins & Loucks, 1947; Lueck, 1980).

The compound *N*-trichloromethylmercapto-4-cyclohexene-1,2-dicarboximide (Captan, $C_9H_8Cl_3NO_2S$) has found application as a fungistat for raisin grapes. Glutaraldehyde ($HOC(CH_2)_3CHO$) may inactivate viruses and it is a natural component of various foods (Saitanu & Lund, 1975).

The compound *o*-phenylphenol (*o*-hydroxybiphenyl, orthoxenol, Dowicide 1, SOPP, 2-phenylphenol, $C_6H_5C_6H_4OH$) denatures microbial cell-wall components and inhibits enzymes (Lueck, 1980). Concentrations of 0.001–0.005% inhibit moulds, while higher concentrations are needed for inhibition of bacteria. The compound may preserve citrus fruits when immersed for 0.5–1 min in a 0.5–2% solution (Foegeding & Busta, 1991).

Potassium bromate ($KBrO_3$) increases the oxidation-reduction potential, which causes some antimicrobial activity. One application, which was discontinued due to off-flavours, involved the use of up to 0.04% bromate to inhibit butyrics and anaerobes in processed cheeses (Lueck, 1980). Quaternary ammonium chloride combinations are permitted in the USA to be used as antimicrobial agents in raw sugar-cane juice, added prior to clarification, when further processing of the sugar-cane juice must be delayed. Calcium chloride, potassium chloride, potassium hydroxide, potassium and sodium carbonates, sodium bicarbonate and sodium hypophosphite are also listed as GRAS in the USA and may exhibit antimicrobial activity. Sodium bicarbonate was found to inhibit aflatoxin formation in maize (Montville & Goldstein, 1989), yeasts in apple juice (Curran & Montville,

1989) and bacteria and yeasts in culture media (Corral *et al.*, 1988).

Fluorides (NaF, KF) act on enzymes and inhibit microorganisms, but they are toxic and their use for the preservation of dairy products, meat, beer and wine has been discontinued. Wine has been stabilized with allyl isothiocyanate (CH_2=$CHCH_2$ NCS), but it has an undesirable odour (Foegeding & Busta, 1991). Thiourea (H_2NCSNH_2) has been applied on the surface or on wrappers to protect citrus fruit from mould spoilage, but its use is prohibited in the USA due to toxicity. Tobacco and some foods have been preserved with 8-oxyquinoline (C_9H_7NO), 8-hydroxyquinoline or hydroxybenzopyridine (Lueck, 1980). The amino acid glycine (NH_2CH_2COOH) has inhibited several bacteria (Hammes *et al.*, 1973). Due to adverse effects on experimental animals, the US FDA no longer regards glycine and its salts as GRAS for use in human foods, but they can still be used in animal feeds, since the amino acid is an essential nutrient for certain animals (CFR, 1996).

Nitrofuran derivatives, such as furyl furamide ($C_{11}H_8O_5N_2$; AF-2) and nitrofuryl acrylamide (nitrofuran 2) inhibit electron transfer of aerobic bacteria, but they have been reported as mutagenic and carcinogenic (Sugiyama *et al.*, 1975; Takayama & Kuwabara, 1977). Furyl furamide use to preserve tofu and meat in Japan was disallowed (Foegeding & Busta, 1991). Thiabendazole ($C_{10}H_7N_3S$) is considered safe at concentrations permitted for preservation of citrus fruits, apples and bananas in several countries. The compound is an effective fungistatic agent (Robinson *et al.*, 1964; Rizk & Isshak, 1974). Hexamethylenetetramine ($C_6H_{12}N_4$) was used as a preservative in several countries of Europe, but its use was discontinued because it is mutagenic (Natvig *et al.*, 1971; Hurni & Ohder, 1973). Silver (Ag) has been used to disinfect drinking water, vinegar, fruit juices, drinks and wine. It is active against bacteria and, to a lesser extent, against yeasts and moulds, but it is inactivated by suspended matter, proteins, chlorides and calcium ions (Lueck, 1980).

A variety of other compounds have demonstrated antimicrobial activity in model or food systems, either alone or in combination with other additives or processing factors. Such compounds include hinokitiol (*m*-isopropyltropolon, 2-hydroxy-4-isopropylol, or 2,4,6-cycloheptatriene), idoacetamide, chloroacetamide, lactulose, xylitol, glutamine, glutathione, etc. (Davidson *et al.*, 1983; Foegeding & Busta, 1991; Erfan, 1992). The compound *n*-dodecyldimethylbenzylammonium chloride, in combination with other quaternary ammonium chloride compounds, is permitted in the USA as an antimicrobial agent in raw sugar-cane juice (CFR, 1996).

18 Regulation of chemical food preservatives

The use of additives and preservatives in foods is controlled by legislation in most countries (Jarvis & Burke, 1976; Ahlborg *et al.*, 1977; Young, 1989; Owen Fields, 1996; Post, 1996). A substance or compound is allowed for use as a legal food preservative only when its safety has been demonstrated by its manufacturer. In the USA, the Food Additives Amendment to the Food, Drug and Cosmetic Act of 1938 and its subsequent revisions or amendments specify the conditions and the processes under which any substance may be approved as a chemical additive. The use of chemical compounds in food preservation is regulated by the FDA of the Department of Health and Human Services in the USA, and by the appropriate authorities of other countries. At the international level, the FAO and the WHO are concerned with food preservation and establish ADI doses for food preservatives. Assuming that the safety of the compound is established, the regulations specify applications, amounts to be used and any other necessary conditions to protect the public well-being. Information on food-preservative regulations is useful when preparing products for export markets and may be obtained from individual countries. In the USA, Title 21, parts 170–199 and other parts of the Code of Federal Regulations list chemicals permitted for use as antimicrobials or preservatives in foods and conditions for their use (CFR, 1996).

Certain food additives, including some chemical preservatives (benzoate, propionate, sorbate, parabens) are characterized as GRAS and are exempted from the Food Additive Regulations in the USA. However, the additive's intended use must fall within its spectrum of activity; it must be approved for the food product; and the principles of GMP must be employed when no limits in the use concentration are set in the GRAS list. Every chemical food preservative used in the USA must be stated on the label of the product (Foegeding & Busta, 1991). For specific information about the rules and legislation concerning the use of chemical food preservatives in a certain country, the appropriate domestic authorities should be contacted.

Some common arguments against the use of chemical compounds as food preservatives are that they are harmful to the consumer, they reduce the nutritional quality of foods, they make faulty food appear normal by masking undesirable characteristics and their use could be eliminated if GMP are followed (Foegeding & Busta, 1991; Parke & Lewis, 1992). However, the regulatory authorities of each country are responsible for preventing abuses that may lead to hazards. These authorities will generally approve the use of chemicals as food preservatives only when the following conditions are fulfilled (Foegeding & Busta, 1991).

1 There should be a need for preservation of the food concerned.

2 The chemical must be proved effective at performing the described preservative action under the specific conditions of the described food product.

3 The compound suggested as a food preservative must be non-toxic.

4 It must be proved safe and non-carcinogenic, at concentrations well above the intended use levels.

5 It must not change the identity of the food by altering its flavour, appearance or other properties.

6 Its application to the food must be practicable and its properties (e.g. solubility) should not interfere with such application.

7 Its cost should not be prohibitive.

8 It should be readily available.

9 Its total consumption (including consumption from other uses) should not exceed specified safe levels.

Most of the original preservatives, some of which have been proved to be effective and safe by long customary or empirical accidental use, are still applied, despite well-known limitations. Few new preservatives have been approved in recent years, due to the existence of strict controls and requirements. In some cases, it is even difficult to extend the application of commonly used preservatives to food products other than those currently approved and regulated (Foegeding & Busta, 1991) An example of this is potassium sorbate, which is widely used in foods but was not approved for use in cured-meat products in the USA.

19 Future of chemical food preservatives

Chemical food preservatives will continue to be important and their use may expand in the future. As the world population increases, the demands for a more abundant food supply will increase and chemical additives will play a role in assuring proper shelf-life and safety in our food supply. Furthermore, as consumer demands for minimally processed foods of long shelf-life and convenience in preparation increases, the use of preservative systems, including existing or new preservatives derived from natural sources, will expand. Consumer concerns over the use of chemical additives in food may lead to further exploration of naturally occurring chemical preservatives, but rapid increases in world population will also ensure a continued need for existing chemical food preservatives. Advances in understanding the mechanisms of microbial control will be beneficial in developing preservative systems for newly evolving or emerging microbial concerns.

20 References

Ababouch, L. & Busta, F.F. (1987) Effect of thermal treatments in oils on bacterial spore survival. *Journal of Applied Bacteriology*, **62**, 491–502.

Ababouch, L., Dikra, A.J. & Busta, F.F. (1987) Tailing of survivor curves of clostridial spores heated in edible oils. *Journal of Applied Bacteriology*, **62**, 503–511.

Ababouch, L., Chaibi, A. & Busta, F.F. (1992) Inhibition of bacterial spore growth by fatty acids and their sodium salts. *Journal of Food Protection*, **55**, 980–984.

Abee, T., Klaenhammer, T.R. & Letlellier, L. (1994a) Kinetic studies of the action of lactacin F, a bacteriocin produced by *Lactobacillus johnsonii* that forms poration complexes in the cytoplasmic membrane. *Applied and Environmental Microbiology*, **60**, 1006–1013.

Abee, T., Rombouts, F.M., Hugenholtz, J., Guihard, G. & Letellier, L. (1994b) Mode of action of nisin Z against *Listeria monocytogenes* Scott A grown at high and low temperatures. *Applied and Environmental Microbiology*, **60**, 1962–1968.

Adams, M.R. & Hall, C.J. (1988) Growth inhibition of food-borne pathogens by lactic and acetic acids and their mixtures. *International Journal of Food Science and Technology*, **23**, 287–292.

Ahlborg, U.G., Dich, J. & Eriksson, H.-B. (1977) Data on food preservatives. *Var Foda*, **29**, 41–96.

Amerine, M.A. & Joslyn, M.A. (1951) *Table Wines: The Technology of Their Production*. Berkeley, California: University of California Press.

Anon. (1969) *Swann Report: Report to the Joint Committee on the Use of Antibiotics in Animal Husbandry and Veterinary Medicine*. London: HMSO.

Anon. (1972) *Report to the Commissioner of the Food and Drug Administration by the FDA Task Force on the Use of Antibiotics in Animal Feeds*. Rockville, Maryland, USA: United States Department of Health, Education and Welfare, Food and Drug Administration.

Asplund, K., Nurmi, E., Hirn, J., Hirvi, T. & Hill, P. (1993) Survival of *Yersinia enterocolitica* in fermented sausages manufactured with different levels of nitrite and different starter cultures. *Journal of Food Protection*, **56**, 710–712.

Baker, D.A. & Genigeorgis, C. (1990) Predicting the safe storage of fresh fish under modified atmospheres with respect to *Clostridium botulinum* toxigenesis by modeling length of the lag phase of growth. *Journal of Food Protection*, **53**, 131–140.

Banks, J.G. & Board, R.G. (1985) Preservation by the lactoperoxidase system (LP-S) of a contaminated infant formula. *Letters of Applied Microbiology*, **1** , 81–85.

Banks, J.G., Board, R.G. & Sparks, N.H.C. (1986) Natural antimicrobial systems and their potential in food preservation of the future. *Biotechnology and Applied Biochemistry*, **8**, 103–147.

Banwart, G. (1989) *Basic Food Microbiology*, 2nd edn. Westport, Connecticut, USA: AVI Publishing.

Barber, L.E. & Deibel, R.H. (1972) Effect of pH and oxygen tension on staphylococcal growth and enterotoxin formation in fermented sausage. *Applied Microbiology*, **24**, 891–898.

Bell, T.A., Etchells, J.L. & Borg, A.F. (1959) Influence of sorbic acid on the growth of certain species of bacteria, yeast and filamentous fungi. *Journal of Bacteriology*, **77**, 573–580.

Benedict, R.C. (1980) Biochemical basis for nitrite inhibition of *Clostridium botulinum* in cured meat. *Journal of Food Protection*, **43**, 877–891.

Beuchat, L.R. (1981a) Combined effects of solutes and food preservatives on rates of inactivation of and colony formation by heated spores and vegetative cells of molds. *Applied and Environmental Microbiology*, **41** , 472–477.

Beuchat, L.R. (1981b) Influence of potassium sorbate and sodium benzoate on heat inactivation of *Aspergillus flavus, Penicillium puberulum* and *Geotrichum candidum*. *Journal of Food Protection*, **44**, 450–454.

Beuchat, L.R. (1981c) Effects of potassium sorbate and sodium benzoate on inactivating yeasts heated in broths containing sodium chloride and sucrose. *Journal of Food Protection*, **44**, 765–769.

Beuchat, L.R. (1982) Thermal inactivation of yeasts in fruit juices supplemented with food preservatives and sucrose. *Journal of Food Science*, **47** , 1679–1682.

Beuchat, L.R. (1994) Antimicrobial properties of spices and their essential oils. In *Natural Antimicrobial Systems in Food Preservation* (eds Board, R.G. & Dillon, V.), pp. 167–179. Wallingford, Oxon, UK: CAB International.

Beuchat, L.R. & Golden, D.A. (1989) Antimicrobials occurring naturally in foods. *Food Technology*, **43** (1), 134–142.

Binkerd, E.F. & Kolari, O.E. (1975) The history and use of nitrate and nitrite in the curing of meat. *Food and Cosmetics Toxicology*, **13**, 655–661.

Bizri, J.N. & Wahem, I.A. (1994) Citric acid and antimicrobials affect microbiological stability and quality of tomato juice. *Journal of Food Science*, **59**, 130–134.

Borch, E., Wallentin, C., Rosen, M. & Bjorck, L. (1989) Antibacterial effect of the lactoperoxidase/thiocyanate/hydrogen peroxide system against strains of *Campylobacter* isolated from poultry. *Journal of Food Protection*, **52**, 638–641.

Bosund, I. (1962) The action of benzoic and salicylic acids on the metabolism of microorganisms. *Advances in Food Research*, **11**, 331–353.

Boyle, D.L., Sofos, J.N. & Maga, J.A. (1985) Inhibition of spoilage and pathogenic microorganisms by liquid smoke from various woods. *Lebensmittel Wissenschaft und Technologie*, **21**, 54–58.

Bradford, D.D., Huffman, D.L., Egbert, W.R. & Mikel, W.B. (1993) Potassium lactate effects on low fat fresh pork sausage chubs during simulated retail distribution. *Journal of Food Science*, **58**, 1245–1248.

Brewer, M.S., McKeith, F., Martin, S.E., Dallmier, A. & Meyer, J. (1992) Sodium lactate effects on shelf-life, sensory and physical characteristics of fresh pork sausage. *Journal of Food Science*, **56**, 1176–1178.

Brik, H. (1981) Natamycin. In *Analytical Profiles of Drug Substances* (ed. Flory, K.), p. 513. New York: Academic Press.

Bruch, C.W. (1961) Gaseous sterilization. *Annual Reviews of Microbiology*, **15**, 245–262.

Bruch, C.W. (1972) Sterilization of plastics: toxicity of ethylene oxide residues. In *Industrial Sterilization* (eds Phillips, G.B. & Miller, W.S.), pp. 49–77. Durham, North Carolina, USA: Duke University Press.

Bruch, C.W. & Koesterer, M.G. (1961) The microbiocidal activity of gaseous propylene oxide and its application to powdered or flaked foods. *Journal of Food Science*, **26**, 428–435.

Bryan, F.L. (1992) Public health problems of foodborne diseases and their prevention. In *Handbook of Natural Toxins*, Vol. 7, *Food Poisoning* (eds Tu, A.T. & Maga, J.A.), pp. 3–22. New York: Marcel Dekker.

Buazzi, M.M. & Marth, E.H. (1992) Sites of action by propionate on *Listeria monocytogenes*. *International Journal of Food Microbiology*, **15**, 109–119.

Buchanan, R.L. & Whiting, R.C. (1996) Risk assessment and predictive microbiology. *Journal of Food Protection*, **58**, 1–7.

Buchanan, R.L., Stahl, H.G. & Whiting, R.C. (1989) Effects and interactions of temperature, pH, atmosphere, sodium chloride, and sodium nitrite on the growth of *Listeria monocytogenes*. *Journal of Food Protection*, **52**, 844–851.

Buchanan, R.L., Whiting, R.C. & Palummbo, S.A. (eds) (1993) Proceedings of workshop on the application of predictive microbiology and computer modeling techniques to the food industry. *Journal of Industrial Microbiology*, **12** , 137–359.

Bulgarelli, M.A. & Shelef, L.A. (1985) Effect of ethylenediamine tetraacetic acid (EDTA) on growth from spores of *Bacillus cereus*. *Journal of Food Science*, **50**, 661–664.

Bullerman, L.B. (1977) Incidence and control of mycotoxin producing molds in domestic and imported cheeses. *Annals of Nutritional Alimentation*, **31**, 435–446.

Buncic, S., Fitzgerald, C.M., Bell, R.G. & Hudson, J.A. (1995) Individual and combined listericidal effects of sodium lactate, potassium sorbate, nisin and curing salts at refrigeration temperature. *Journal of Food Safety*, **14**, 247–264.

Busta, F.F. & Foegeding, P.M. (1983) Chemical food preservatives. In *Disinfection, Sterilization and Preservation*, 3rd edn (ed. Block, S.S.), pp. 656–694. Philadelphia, Pennsylvania: Lea & Febiger.

Cassens, R.G. (1995) Use of sodium, nitrite in cured meats today. *Food Technology*, **49** (7), 72–80, 115.

Cassens, R.G. (1997) Residual nitrite in cured meat. *Food Technology*, **51** (2), 53–55.

Cassens, R.G., Greaser, M.L., Ito, T. & Lee, M. (1979) Reactions of nitrite in meat. *Food Technology*, **33** (7), 48–57.

CAST (Council of Agricultural Science and Technology) (1994) *Foodborne Pathogens: Risks and Consequences*. Task Force Report No. 122. Ames, Iowa, USA: Council of Agricultural Science and Technology.

CAST (Council of Agricultural Science and Technology) (1998) *Naturally Occurring Antimicrobials in Food*. Task Force Report No. 132. Ames, Iowa, USA: Council of Agricultural Science and Technology.

Casteels, P. (1990) Possible applications of insect antibacterial peptides. *Research in Immunology*, **141**, 940–942.

Castellani, A.G. & Niven, C.F., Jr (1955) Factors affecting the bacteriostatic action of sodium nitrite. *Applied Microbiology*, **3**, 154–159.

CFR (Code of Federal Regulations) (1996) *Foods and Drugs*, 21 CFR Parts 170–199. Washington, DC: United States National Archives of Records Administration.

Chaibi, A., Ababoush, L.H. & Busta, F.F. (1996a) Inhibition of bacterial spores and vegetative cells by glycerides. *Journal of Food Protection*, **59**, 716–722.

Chaibi, A., Ababoush, L.H. & Busta, F.F. (1996b) Inhibition by monoglycerides and L-alanine-triggered *Bacillus cereus* and *Clostridium botulinum* spore germination and outgrowth. *Journal of Food Protection*, **59**, 832–837.

Chaibi, A., Ababoush, L.H., Belasri, K., Bouretta, S. & Busta, F.F. (1997) Inhibition of germination and vegetative growth of *Bacillus cereus* and *Clostridium botulinum* 62A spores by essential oils. *Food Microbiology*, **14** , 161–174.

Chang, L. & Piper, P.W. (1994). Weak acid preservatives block the heat shock response and heat shock-element-directed lacZ expression of low pH *Saccharomyces cerevisiae* cultures, an inhibitory section partially relieved by respiratory deficiency. *Microbiology*, **140**, 1085–1096.

Charley, P.J., Sarkar, B., Stitt, C.F. & Saltman, P. (1963) Chelation of iron by sugars. *Biochimica et Biophysica Acta*, **69**, 313–321.

Chichester, D.F. & Tanner, F.W. (1972) Antimicrobial food additives. In *Handbook of Food Additives*, 2nd edn (ed. Furia, T.E.), pp. 115–184. Boca Raton, Florida: CRC Press.

Chipley, J.R. (1993) Sodium benzoate and benzoic acid. In *Antimicrobials in Foods*, 2nd edn (eds Davidson, P.M. & Branen, A.L.), pp. 11–48. New York: Marcel Dekker.

Christiansen, L.N., Deffner, J., Foster, E.M. & Sugiyama, H. (1968) Survival and outgrowth of *Clostridium botulinum* type E spores in smoked fish. *Applied Microbiology*, **16**, 133–137.

Christiansen, L.N., Johnston, R.W., Kautter, D.A., Howard, J.W. & Aunan, W.J. (1973) Effect of nitrite and nitrate on toxin production by *Clostridium botulinum* and on nitrosamine formation in perishable canned comminuted cured meat. *Applied Microbiology*, **25**, 357–362.

Christiansen, L.N., Tompkin, R.B., Shaparis, A.B. *et al.* (1974) Effect of sodium nitrite on toxin production by *Clostridium botulinum* in bacon. *Applied Microbiology*, **27**, 733–737.

Christiansen, L.N., Tompkin, R.B., Shaparis, A.B.,

Johnston, R.W. & Kautter, D.A. (1975) Effect of sodium nitrite on *Clostridium botulinum* growth in a summer-style sausage. *Journal of Food Science*, **40**, 488–490.

Clark, D.S. & Lentz, C.P. (1969) Microbiological studies in poultry processing plants in Canada. *Canadian Institute of Food Science and Technology Journal*, **2**, 33–36.

Clark, D.S. & Lentz, C.P. (1973) Use of mixtures of carbon dioxide and oxygen for extending shelf-life of pre-packaged fresh beef. *Canadian Institute of Food Science and Technology Journal*, **6**, 194–196.

Clark, D.S. & Takacs, J. (1980) Gases as preservative. In *Microbial Ecology of Foods*. Vol. I. *Factors Affecting Life and Death of Microorganisms* (ed. International Commission on Microbiological Specifications of Foods), pp. 170–192. New York: Academic Press.

Clark, D.S., Lentz, C.P. & Roth, L.A. (1976) Use of carbon monoxide for extending shelf-life of pre-packaged fresh beef. *Canadian Institute of Food Science and Technology Journal*, **9**, 114–117.

Clark, W.L., Shirk, R.J. & Kline, E.F. (1964) Pimaracin, a new food fungistat. In *Microbial Inhibitors in Food* (ed. Molin, N.), pp. 167–184. Stockholm: Almquist and Wiksell.

Conner, D.E. (1993) Naturally occurring compounds. In *Antimicrobials in Foods* 2nd edn, (eds Davidson, P.M. & Branen, A.L.), pp. 441–468. New York: Marcel Dekker.

Conner, D.E. & Beuchat, L.R. (1987) Heat resistance of ascospores of *Neosartorya fischeri* as affected by sporulation and heating medium. *International Journal of Food Microbiology*, **4**, 303–312.

Cords, B.R. & Dychdala, G.R. (1993) Sanitizers: halogens, surface-active agents and peroxides. In *Antimicrobials in Foods*, 2nd edn (eds Davidson, P.M. & Branen, A.L.), pp. 459–538. New York: Marcel Dekker.

Corral, L.G., Post, L.S. & Montville, T.J. (1988) Antimicrobial activity of sodium bicarbonate. *Journal of Food Science*, **53**, 981–982.

Costilow, R.N., Coughlin, F.M., Robach, D.L. & Ragheb, H.S. (1956) A study of acid-forming bacteria from cucumber fermentations in Michigan. *Food Research*, **21**, 27–33.

Costilow, R.N., Coughlin, F.M., Robbins, E.K. & Hus, W.-T. (1957) Sorbic acid as a selective agent in cucumber fermentations. II. Effect of sorbic acid on the yeast and lactic acid fermentation in brined cucumbers. *Applied Microbiology*, **5**, 373–379.

Cox, N.A., Mercuri, A.J., Juven, B.J., Thompson, J.E. & Chew, V. (1974) Evaluation of succinic acid and heat to improve the microbiological quality of poultry meat. *Journal of Food Science*, **39**, 985–987.

Crosby, N.T. & Sawyer, R. (1976) *N*-nitrosamines: a review of chemical and biological properties and their estimation in foodstuffs. *Advances in Food Research*, **22**, 1–71.

Curran, D.M. & Montville, T.J. (1989) Bicarbonate inhibition of *Saccharomyces cerevisiae* and *Hansenula wingei* growth in apple juice. *International Journal of Food Microbiology*, **8**, 1–9.

Cutter, N.N. & Siragusa, G.R. (1995a) Population reductions of Gram-negative pathogens following treatments with nisin and chelators under various conditions. *Journal of Food Protection*, **58**, 977–983.

Cutter, N.N. & Siragusa, G.R. (1995b) Treatments with nisin and chelators to reduce *Salmonella* and *Escherichia coli* on beef. *Journal of Food Protection*, **58**, 1029–1030.

Daeschel, M.A. (1989) Antimicrobial substances from lactic acid bacteria for use as food preservatives. *Food Technology* **43** (1), 164–167.

Dallyn, H. (1994) Antimicrobial properties of vegetable and fish oils. In *Natural Antimicrobial Systems and Food Preservation* (eds Dillon, V.M. & Board, R.G.), pp. 205–221. Wallingford, Oxon, UK: CAB International.

Davidson, P.M. (1993) Phenolic compounds. In *Antimicrobials in Foods*, 2nd edn (eds Davidson, P.M. & Branen, A.L.), pp. 37–74. New York: Marcel Dekker.

Davidson, P.M. & Branen, A.L. (eds) (1993) *Antimicrobials in Foods*. New York: Marcel Dekker.

Davidson, P.M. & Doan, C.H. (1993) Natamycin. In *Antimicrobials in Foods*, 2nd edn (eds Davidson, P.M. & Branen, A.L.), pp. 395–408. New York: Marcel Dekker.

Davidson, P.M., Post, L.S., Branen, A.L. & McCurdy, A.R. (1983) Naturally occurring and miscellaneous food antimicrobials. In *Antimicrobials in Foods* (eds Branen, A.L. & Davidson, P.M.), pp. 371–419. New York: Marcel Dekker.

Davies, E.A. & Adams, M.R. (1994) Resistance of *Listeria monocytogenes* to the bacteriocin nisin. *International Journal of Food Microbiology*, **21**, 341–347.

Dawson, L.E., Stevenson, K.E. & Gertonson, E. (1975) Flavor, bacterial and TBA changes in ground turkey patties treated with antioxidants. *Poultry Science*, **54**, 1134–1139.

Debevere, J.M. (1989) The effect of sodium lactate on the shelf life of vacuum-packed coarse liver pate. *Fleischwirtschaft International*, **3**, 68–69.

Delaquis, P.J. & Mazza, G. (1995) Antimicrobial properties of isothiocyanates in food preservation. *Food Technology*, **550**, (11) 73–78.

Delves-Broughton, J. & Gasson, M. J. (1994) Nisin. In *Natural Antimicrobial Systems and Food Preservation* (eds Dillon, V.M. & Board, R.G.), pp. 99–131. Wallingford, Oxon, UK: CAB International.

Demel, R.A., Peelen, T., Siezen, R.J., DeKruijff, B. &

Kuipers, O.P. (1994) Nisin Z, mutant nisin Z and lacticin 481 interactions with anionic lipids correlate with antimicrobial activity: a monolayer study. *European Journal of Biochemistry*, **235**, 267–274.

Denis, F. & Ramet, J.-P. (1989) Antibacterial activity of the lactoperoxidase system on *Listeria monocytogenes* in trypticase soy broth, UHT milk and French soft cheese. *Journal of Food Protection*, **52**, 706–711.

Denyer, S.P. & Hugo, W.B. (eds) (1991) *Mechanisms of Action of Chemical Biocides*. Society for Applied Bacteriology Technical Series No. 27. Oxford: Blackwell Scientific Publications.

Deog-Hwan, O. & Marshall, D.L. (1996) Monolaurin and acetic acid inactivation of *Listeria monocytogenes* attached to stainless steel. *Journal of Food Protection*, **59**, 249–252.

Deuel, H.J., Jr, Alfin-Slater, R., Weil, C.S. & Smyth, H.F., Jr (1954a) Sorbic acid as a fungistatic agent for foods I. Harmlessness of sorbic acid as a dietary component. *Food Research*, **19**, 1–12.

Deuel, H.J., Jr, Calbert, C.E., Anisfeld, L., McKeehan, H. & Blunder, H.D. (1954b) Sorbic acid as a fungistatic agent for foods. II. Metabolism of β-unsaturated fatty acids with emphasis on sorbic acid. *Food Research*, **19**, 13–19.

Dickens, J.A., Lyon, B.G., Whittemore, A.D. & Lyon, C.E. (1994) The effect of an acetic acid dip on carcass appearance, microbiological quality, and cooked breast meat texture and flavor. *Poultry Science*, **73**, 576–581.

Dickens, J.A. & Whittemore, A.D. (1994) The effect of acetic acid and air injection on appearance, moisture, pick-up, microbiological quality, and *Salmonella* incidence on processed poultry. *Poultry Sciences*, **73**, 582–588.

Dickson, J.A. (1992) Acetic acid action on beef tissue surfaces contaminated with *Salmonella typhimurium*. *Journal of Food Science*, **57**, 297–301.

Dillon, R.J. (1994) Antimicrobial agents associated with insects. In *Natural Antimicrobial Systems and Food Preservation* (eds Dillon, V.M. & Board, R.G.), pp. 223–254. Wallingford, Oxon, UK: CAB International.

Dillon, V.M. & Board, R.G. (eds) (1994) *Natural Antimicrobial Systems and Food Preservation*. Wallingford, Oxon, UK: CAB International.

Dillon, V.M. & Cook, P.E. (1994) Biocontrol of undesirable microorganisms in food. In *Natural Antimicrobial Systems and Food Preservation* (eds Dillon V.M. & Board, R.G.), pp. 255–296. Wallingford, Oxon, UK: CAB International.

Doores, S. (1993) Organic acids. In *Antimicrobials in Foods*, 2nd edn (eds Davidson, P.M. & Branen, A.L.), pp. 95–136. New York: Marcel Dekker.

Doyle, M.P. & Marth, E.H. (1975) Thermal inactivation of conidia from *Aspergillus flavus* and *Aspergillus parasiticus*. II. Effects of pH and buffers, glucose, sucrose and sodium chloride. *Journal of Milk and Food Technology*, **38**, 750–758.

Dudman, W.F. (1963) Sorbic hydroxamic acid, an antifungal agent effective over a wide pH range. *Applied Microbiology*, **11**, 262–367.

Dyett, E.J. & Shelley, D. (1966) The effects of sulphite preservative in British fresh sausage. *Journal of Applied Bacteriology*, **29**, 439–446.

Dymicky, M. & Huhtanen, C.N. (1979) Inhibition of *Clostridium botulinum* by *p*-hydroxybenzoic acid *n*-alkyl esters. *Antimicrobial Agents and Chemotherapy*, **15**, 798–801.

Dymicky, M., Bencivengo, M., Buchanen, R.L. & Smith, J.L. (1987) Inhibition of *Clostridium botulinum* 62A by fumarates and maleates and relationship of activity to some physicochemical constants. *Applied and Environmental Microbiology*, **53**, 110–113.

Dziezak, J.D. (1986) Antioxidants—the ultimate answer to oxidation. *Food Technology*, **40** (9), 94–103.

Earnshaw, R.G. & Banks, J.G. (1989) A note on the inhibition of *Listeria monocytogenes* NCTC 11994 in milk by an activated lactoperoxidase system. *Letters in Applied Microbiology*, **8**, 203–205.

Earnshaw, R.G., Banks, J.G., Francotte, C. & Defrise, D. (1990) Inhibition of *Salmonella typhimurium* and *Escherichia coli* in an infant milk formula by an activated lactoperoxidase system. *Journal of Food Protection*, **53**, 170–172.

Eklund, M.W., Pelroy, G.A., Paranjpye, R., Peterson, M.E. & Teeny, F.M. (1982) Inhibition of *Clostridium botulinum* types A and E toxin production by liquid smoke and NaCl in hot-process smoke-flavored fish. *Journal of Food Protection*, **45**, 935–940.

Eklund, T. (1980) Inhibition of growth and uptake processes in bacteria by some chemical food preservatives. *Journal of Applied Bacteriology*, **48**, 423–432.

Eklund, T. (1983) The antimicrobial effect of dissociated and undissociated sorbic acid at different pH levels. *Journal of Applied Bacteriology*, **54**, 383–389.

Eklund, T. (1985) The effect of sorbic acid and esters of *p*-hydroxybenzoic acid on the protonmotive force in *Escherichia coli* membrane vesicles. *Journal of General Microbiology*, **131**, 73–76.

Eklund, T. (1988) Inhibition of microbial growth at different pH levels by benzoic and propionic acids and esters of *p*-hydroxybenzoic acids. *International Journal of Food Microbiology*, **2**, 159–167.

Eklund, T. (1989) Organic acids and esters. In *Mechanisms of Action of Food Preservation Procedures* (ed. Gould, G.W.), pp. 161–200. London: Elsevier Applied Science.

Ekstrand, B. (1994) Lactoperoxidase and lactoferrin. In *Natural Antimicrobial Systems and Food Preservation* (eds Dillon, V.M. & Board, R.G.), pp. 15–63. Wallingford, Oxon, UK: CAB International.

El-Gazzar, F.E., Rusul, G. & Marth, E.H. (1987) Growth

and aflatoxin production of *Aspergillus parasiticus* NRRL 2999 in the presence of lactic acid and at different initial pH values. *Journal of Food Protection*, **50**, 940–944.

El-Gendy, S.M., Nassib, T., Abed-El-Gellel, H. & Nanafy, N-El-Hoda (1980) Survival and growth of *Clostridium* species in the presence of hydrogen peroxide. *Journal of Food Protection*, **43**, 431–432.

El-Kest, S.E. & Marth, E.H. (1988a) Inactivation of *Listeria monocytogenes* by chlorine. *Journal of Food Protection*, **51**, 520–524.

El-Kest, S.E. & Marth, E.H. (1988b) *Listeria monocytogenes* and its inactivation by chlorine: a review. *Lebensmittel Wissenschaft und Technologie*, **21**, 346–351.

El-Kest, S.E. & Marth, E.H. (1988c) Temperature, pH, and strain of pathogen as factors affecting inactivation of *Listeria monocytogenes* by chlorine. *Journal of Food Protection*, **51**, 622–625.

El-Kest, S.E. & Marth, E.H. (1992) Transmission electron microscopy of unfrozen and frozen/thawed cells of *Listeria monocytogenes* treated with lipase and lysozyme. *Journal of Food Protection*, **55**, 687–696.

El-Shenawy, M.A. & Marth, E.H. (1988) Inhibition and inactivation of *Listeria monocytogenes* by sorbic acid. *Journal of Food Protection*, **51**, 842–847.

El-Shenawy, M.A. & Marth, E.H. (1989) Behavior of *Listeria monocytogenes* in the presence of sodium propionate. *International Journal of Food Microbiology*, **8**, 85–94.

El-Shenawy, N.A. & Marth, E.H. (1992) Behavior of *Listeria monocytogenes* in the presence of sodium propionate together with food acids. *Journal of Food Protection*, **55**, 241–245.

Emard, L.O. & Vaughn, R.H. (1952) Selectivity of sorbic acid media for the catalase-negative lactic acid bacteria and clostridia. *Journal of Bacteriology*, **63**, 487–494.

Enfors, S.-O. & Molin, G. (1978) The influence of high concentrations of carbon dioxide on the germination of bacterial spores. *Journal of Applied Bacteriology*, **45**, 279–285.

Erfan, O. (1992) *Method of Preserving Beverages Using Glutathione and Glutamine*. United States Patent US 5 171 597.

Erickson, J.P. & Jenkins, P. (1992) Behavior of psychrotrophic pathogens *Listeria monocytogenes*, *Yersinia enterocolitica* and *Aeromonas hydrophila* in commercially pasteurized eggs held at 2, 6.7 and 12.8°C. *Journal of Food Protection*, **55**, 8–12.

Fang, T.J. & Lo-Wei, Lin (1994) Inactivation of *Listeria monocytogenes* on raw pork treated with modified atmosphere packaging and nisin. *Journal of Food and Drug Analysis*, **2**, 189–200.

Farber, J.M. (1986) Predictive modeling of food deterioration and safety. In *Foodborne Microorganisms and Their Toxins—Developing Methodology* (eds Stern, N.J. & Pierson, M.D.), pp. 57–90. New York: Marcel Dekker.

Field, C.E., Pivarnik, L.P., Barnett, S.M. & Rand, A.G. (1986) Utilization of glucose oxidase for extending the shelf-life of fish. *Journal of Food Science*, **51**, 66–70.

Finne, G. (1982) Modified- and controlled-atmosphere storage of muscle foods. *Food Technology*, **36** (2), 128–133.

Foegeding, P.M. (1983) Bacterial spore resistance to chlorine compounds. *Food Technology*, **37** (11), 100–104, 110.

Foegeding, P.M. (1985) Ozone inactivation of *Bacillus* and *Clostridium* spore populations and the importance of spore coat to resistance. *Food Microbiology*, **2**, 123–134.

Foegeding, P.M. & Busta, F.F. (1983a) Hypochlorite injury of *Clostridium botulinum* spores alters germination responses. *Applied Environmental Microbiology*, **45**, 1360–1368.

Foegeding, P.M. & Busta, F.F. (1983b) Proposed mechanism for sensitization by hypochlorite treatment of *Clostridium botulinum* spores. *Applied Environmental Microbiology*, **45**, 1374–1379.

Foegeding, P.M. & Busta, F.F. (1983c) Effort of carbon dioxide, nitrogen and hydrogen gases on germination of *Clostridium botulinum* spores. *Journal of Food Protection*, **46**, 987–989.

Foegeding, P.M. & Busta, F.F. (1991) Chemical food preservatives. In *Disinfection, Sterilization and Preservation*, 4th edn (ed. Block, S.S.), pp. 802–832. Philadelphia, Pennsylvania: Lea and Febiger.

Franco, D.A., Webb, J. & Taylor, C.E. (1990) Antibiotic and sulfonamide residues in meat: implications for human health. *Journal of Food Protection*, **53**, 178–185.

Frank, H.A. & Willits, C.O. (1961) Prevention of mold and yeast growth in maple syrup by chemical inhibitors. *Food Technology*, **15**, 1–3.

Freese, E. & Levin, B.C. (1978) Action mechanisms of preservatives and antiseptics. *Developments in Industrial Microbiology*, **19**, 207–227.

Freese, E., Sheu, C.W. & Galliers, E. (1973) Function of lipophilic acids as antimicrobial food additives. *Nature London*, **24**, 321–325.

Freybler, L.A., Gray, J.I., Ashghar, A., Booren, A.M., Pearson, A.M. & Buckley, D.J. (1993) Nitrite stabilization of lipids in cured pork. *Meat Science*, **33**, 85–96.

Fukusumi, E. (1972) Preservatives in the future: properties and uses. *Shokuhin Kogyo*, **15**, 40–45.

Fung, D.Y.C., Lin, C.C.S. & Gailani, M.B. (1985) Effect of phenolic antioxidants on microbial growth. *CRC Critical Reviews in Microbiology*, **12**, 153–183.

Gabay, J.E. (1994) Ubiquitous natural antibiotics. *Science*, **264**, 373–374.

Garcia, G.W., Genigeorgis, C. & Lindroth, S. (1987) Risk of growth and toxin production by *Clostridium botulinum* nonproteolytic types B, E, and F in salmon fillets stored under modified atmospheres at low and abused temperatures. *Journal of Food Protection*, **50**, 330–336.

Gardner, W.H. (1972) Acidulants in food processing. In *Handbook of Food Additives*, 2nd edn (ed. Furia, T.E), pp. 225–270. Boca Raton, Florida: CRC Press.

Genigeorgis, C.A. (1985) Microbial and safety implications of the use of modified atmospheres to extend the storage life of fresh meat and fish. *International Journal of Food Microbiology*, **1**, 237–251.

Giese, J. (1994) Antimicrobials: assuring food safety. *Food Technology*, **48** (6), 101–110.

Gill, C.O. & Tan, K.H. (1979) Effect of carbon dioxide on growth of *Pseudomonas fluorescens*. *Applied and Environmental Microbiology*, **38**, 237–240.

Goldberg, H.S. (1964) Non-medical use of antibiotics. *Advances in Applied Microbiology*, **6**, 91–117.

Golden, M.H., Buchanan, R.L. & Whiting, R.C. (1995) Effect of sodium acetate or sodium propionate with EDTA and ascorbic acid on the inactivation of *Listeria monocytogenes*. *Journal of Food Safety*, **15**, 54–65.

Golding, N.S. (1945) The gas requirements of molds. IV. A preliminary interpretation of the growth rates of four common mold cultures on the basis of absorbed gases. *Journal of Dairy Science*, **28**, 737–750.

Gombas, D.E. (1989) Biological competition as a preserving mechanism. *Journal of Food Safety*, **10**, 107–117.

Gooding, C.M. (1945) *Process of Inhibiting Growth of Molds*. US Patent 2 379 294.

Gooding, C.M., Melnick, D., Lawrence, R.L. & Luckmann, E.H. (1955) Sorbic acid as a fungistatic agent for foods. IX. Physicochemical considerations in using sorbic acid to protect foods. *Food Research*, **20**, 639–648.

Goodson, M. & Rowbury, R.J. (1989) Resistance of acid-habituated *Escherichia coli* to organic acids and its medical and applied significance. *Letters in Applied Microbiology*, **8**, 211–214.

Gorman, B.M., Sofos, J.N., Morgan, J.B., Schmidt, G.R. & Smith, G.C. (1995) Evaluation of hand-trimming, various sanitizing agents and hot water spray-washing as decontamination interventions for beef brisket adipose tissue. *Journal of Food Protection*, **58**, 899–907.

Gorman, B.M., Kochevar, S.L., Sofos, J.N., Morgan, J.B., Schmidt, G.R. and Smith, G.C. (1997) Changes on beef adipose tissue following decontamination with chemical solutions or water of 35°C or 74°C. *Journal of Muscle Foods*, **8**, 185–197.

Gould, G.W. (1992) Ecosystem approaches to food preservation. *Journal of Applied Bacteriology*, **73** (Symposium Series No. 21), 58S-68S.

Gould, G.W. (ed.) (1995) *New Methods of Food Preservation*. London: Blackie Academic and Professional.

Gould, G.W. (1996) Industry perspectives on the use of natural antimicrobials and inhibitors for food applications. *Journal of Food Protection*, **59** Suppl. 82–86.

Gourama, H. & Bullerman, L.B. (1988) Effects of potassium sorbate and natamycin on growth and penicillic acid production by *Aspergillus ochraceus*. *Journal of Food Protection*, **51**, 139.

Gray, J.I. & Randall, C.J. (1979) The nitrate/*N*-nitrosamine problem in meats: an update. *Journal of Food Protection*, **42**, 168–179.

Grever, A.B.G. (1974) Minimum nitrite concentrations for inhibition of clostridia in cooked meat products. In *Proceedings of the International Symposium on Nitrite in Meat Products* (eds Krol, B. & Tinbergen, B.J.), pp. 103–109. Wageningen, the Netherlands: Pudoc.

Haas, C.N., Rose, J.B., Gerba, C.P. & Crockett, C.S. (1997) What predictive microbiology can learn from water microbiology. *Food Technology*, **51** (4), 91–94.

Hales, K.C. (1962) Refrigerated transport on shipboard. *Advances in Food Research*, **12**, 147–152.

Hammes, W., Schleifer, K.H. & Kandler, O. (1973) Mode of action of glycine on the biosynthesis of peptidoglycan. *Journal of Bacteriology*, **116**, 1029–1053.

Hammond, S.M. & Carr, J.G. (1876) The antimicrobial activity of SO_2—with particular reference to fermented and non-fermented fruit juices. In *Inhibition and Inactivation of Vegetative Microorganism* (eds Skinner, P.A. & Hugo, W.B.), Society for Applied Bacteriology Symposium Series No. 5, pp. 89–110. London: Academic Press.

Hansen, J.D. & Appleman, M.D. (1955) The effect of sorbic, propionic, and caproic acids on the growth of certain clostridia. *Food Research*, **20**, 92–96.

Hansen, J.N., Banerjee, S. & Buchman, G.W. (1989) Potential of small ribosomally synthesized bacteriocins in design of new food preservatives. *Journal of Food Safety*, **10**, 119–130.

Hardin, M.D., Acuff, G.R., Lucia, L.M., Oman, J.S. & Savell, J.W. (1995) Comparison of methods for decontamination from beef carcasses. *Journal of Food Protection*, **58**, 368–374.

Harmayani, E., Sofos, J.N. & Schmidt, G.R. (1991) Effect of sodium lactate, calcium lactate and sodium alginate on bacterial growth and aminopeptidase activity. *Journal of Food Safety*, **11**, 209–284.

Harmayani, E., Sofos, J.N. & Schmidt, G.R. (1993) Fate of *Listeria monocytogenes* in raw and cooked ground beef with meat processing additives. *International Journal of Food Microbiology*, **18**, 223–232.

Harris, L.J., Daeschel, M.A., Stiles, M.E. & Klaenhammer, T.R. (1989) Antimicrobial activity of lactic acid bacteria against *Listeria monocytogenes*. *Journal of Food Protection*, **52**, 384–387.

Hayatsu, H. & Miura, A. (1970) The mutagenic action of sodium bisulfite. *Biochemical and Biophysical Research Communications*, **39**, 983–988.

Hayatsu, H., Chung, K.G., Kada, T. & Nakajima, T. (1975) Generation of mutagenic compound(s) by a reaction between sorbic acid and nitrite. *Mutation Research*, **30**, 417–419.

Hays, G.L., Burroughs, J.D. & Warner, R.C. (1959) Microbiological aspects of pressure packaged foods. II. The effect of various gases. *Food Technology*, **13**, 567–570.

Herring, H.K. (1973) Effect of nitrite and other factors on the physico-chemical characteristics and nitrosamine formation in bacon. In *Proceedings of the Meat Industry Research Conference*, pp. 47–60. Washington, DC: American Meat Institute.

Hill, C. (1995) Bacteriocins: natural antimicrobials from microorganisms. In *New Methods of Food Preservation* (ed. Gould, G.W.), pp. 22–39. London: Blackie Academic and Professional.

Hintlian, C.B. & Hotchkiss, J.H. (1987) Comparative growth of spoilage and pathogenic organisms on modified atmosphere-packaged cooked beef. *Journal of Food Protection*, **50**, 218–223.

Hobbs, G. (1976) *Clostridium botulinum* and its importance in fishery products. *Advances in Food Research*, **22**, 135–185.

Hoffman, K. (1995) Nitrite in food: consequences for human health. *Fleischeri*, **46** (5), 58, 61–65.

Hollenbeck, C.M. (1979) Liquid smoke flavoring-status of development. *Food Technology*, **33** (5), 88–92.

Holley, R.A. (1981) Prevention of surface mold growth on Italian dry sausage by natamycin and potassium sorbate. *Applied and Environmental Microbiology*, **41**, 422–429.

Hoover, D.G. (1992) Bacteriocins: activities and applications. In *Encyclopedia of Microbiology*, Vol. 1, pp. 181–190. San Diego, California: Academic Press.

Hoover, D.G. & Steenson, L.R. (1993) *Bacteriocins from Lactic Acid Bacteria*. San Diego, California: Academic Press.

Hopkins, E.F. & Loucks, K.W. (1947) The use of diphenyl in the control of stem-end rot and mold in citrus fruits. *Citrus Industry*, **28**, 5–11.

Houtsma, P.C., Heuvelink, A., Dufrenne, J. & Notermans, S. (1994) Effect of sodium lactate on toxin production, spore germination and heat resistance of proteolytic *Clostridium botulinum* strains. *Journal of Food Protection*, **57**, 327–330.

Huffman, D.L. (1974) Effect of gas atmospheres on microbial quality of pork. *Journal of Food Science*, **39**, 723–725.

Hughey, V.L. & Johnson, E.A. (1987) Antimicrobial activity of lysozyme against bacteria involved in food spoilage and food-borne disease. *Applied and Environmental Microbiology*, **53**, 2165–2170.

Hughey, V.L., Wilger, P.A. & Johnson, E.A. (1989) Antibacterial activity of hen egg white lysozyme against *Listeria monocytogenes* Scott A in foods. *Applied and Environmental Microbiology*, **55**, 631–638.

Hugo, W.B. (1967) The mode of action of antibacterial agents. *Journal of Applied Bacteriology*, **30**, 17–50.

Hugo, W.B. (1976a) The inactivation of vegetative bacteria by chemicals. In *Inhibition and Inactivation of Vegetative Bacteria* (eds Skinner, F.A. & Hugo, W.B.), Society for Applied Bacteriology Symposium Series No. 5, pp. 1–11. London: Academic Press.

Hugo, W.B. (1976b) Survival of microbes exposed to chemical stress. In *The Survival of Vegetative Microorganisms* (eds Gray, T.G.R. & Postgate, J.R.), 26th Symposium, Society of General Microbiology, pp. 383–413. Cambridge: Cambridge University Press.

Huhtanen, C.N. (1980) Inhibition of *Clostridium botulinum by* spice extracts and aliphatic alcohols. *Journal of Food Protection*, **43**, 195–196.

Huhtanen, C.N. (1983) Antibotulinal activity of methyl and ethyl fumarates in comminuted nitrate-free bacon. *Journal of Food Science*, **48** (5), 1574–1575.

Huhtanen, C.N., Dymicky, M. & Trenchard, H. (1981) Methyl and ethyl esters of fumaric acids as substitutes for nitrite for inhibiting *Clostridium botulinum* spore outgrowth in bacon. Paper presented at the Annual Meeting of the Institute of Food Technologists, June, Atlanta, Georgia, USA.

Hunter, D.R. & Segel, I.H. (1973) Effect of weak acids on amino acid transport by *Penicillium chrysogenum*: evidence for a proton or charge gradient as the driving force. *Journal of Bacteriology*, **113**, 1184–1192.

Huppert, M. (1957) The antifungal activity of homologous series of parabens. *Antibiotics and Chemotherapy*, **7**, 29–36.

Hurni, H. & Ohder, H. (1973) Reproduction study with formaldehyde and hexamethylenetetramine in beagle dogs. *Food and Cosmetic Toxicology*, **11**, 459–462.

Hurst, A. (1981) Nisin. In *Advances in Applied Microbiology*, Vol. 27 (eds Perlman, D. & Laskin, A.I.), pp. 85–123. New York: Academic Press.

Hurst, A. & Hoover, D.G. (1993) Nisin. In *Antimicrobial in Foods*, 2nd edn (eds Davidson, P.M. & Branen, A.L.), pp. 360–394. New York: Marcel Dekker.

Ingram, M. (1974) The microbiological effects of nitrite. In *Proceedings of the International Symposium on Nitrite in Meat Products* (eds Krol, B. & Tinbergen, B.J.), pp. 63–75. Wageningen, The Netherlands: Pudoc.

Ingram, M. (1976) The microbial role of nitrite in meat products. In *Microbiology in Agriculture, Fisheries, and Food* (eds Skinner, F.A. & Carr, J.G.), pp. 1–18. London: Academic Press.

Ingram, M., Buttiaux, R. & Mossel, D.A.A. (1964)

General microbiological considerations in the choice of antimicrobial food preservatives. In *Microbial Inhibitors in Food* (ed. Molin, N.), pp. 381–392. Stockholm: Almquist and Wiksell.

Insalata, N.F. (1952) CO_2 versus beverage bacteria. *Food Engineering*, **24** (7), 84–85, 190.

IFT (Institute of Food Technologists) (1986) Sulfites as food ingredients. *Food Technology*, **40** (6), 47–52.

IFT (Institute of Food Technologist) (1987) Nitrate, nitrite and nitroso compounds in foods. *Food Technology*, **41** (4), 127–134. 136.

ICMSF (International Commission on Microbiological Specifications for Foods) (1988) *HACCP in Microbiological Safety and Quality*. Oxford, UK: Blackwell Scientific Publications.

ICMSF (International Commission on Microbiological Specifications for Foods) (1996) *Microorganisms in Foods 5: Microbiological Specifications of Food Pathogens*. London: Blackie Academic and Professional.

Ito, K.A. & Bee, G.R. (1980) Microbiological hazards associated with new packaging techniques. *Food Technology*, **34** (10), 78–80.

Ivey, F.J. & Robach, M.C. (1978) Effect of potassium sorbate and sodium nitrite on *Clostridium botulinum* growth and toxin production in canned comminuted pork. *Journal of Food Science*, **43**, 1782–1785.

Ivey, F.J., Shaver, K.J., Christiansen, L.N. & Tompkin, R.B. (1978) Effect of potassium sorbate on toxinogenesis of *Clostridium botulinum* in bacon. *Journal of Food Protection*, **41**, 621–625.

Jacobs, M.B. (1947) *Synthetic Food Adjuncts*. New York: D. Van Nostrand.

Jacobs, M.B. (1958) Vinegar. In *The Chemical Analysis of Foods and Food Products*, 3rd edn, pp. 614–616. Princeton: D. Van Nostrand.

Jarvis, B. & Burke, C.S. (1976) Practical and legislative aspects of the chemical preservatives of food. In *Inhibition and Inactivation of Vegetative Microbes* (eds Skinner, F.A. & Hugo, W.B.), pp. 345–367. London: Academic Press.

Jay, J.M. Antimicrobial properties of diacetyl. *Applied and Environmental Microbiology*, **44**, 525–532.

Jay, J.M. (1982b) Effect of diacetyl on foodborne microorganisms. *Journal of Food Science*, **47**, 1829–1831.

Jay, J.M., Rivers, G.M. & Boisvert, W.E. (1983) Antimicrobial properties of α-dicarbonyl and related compounds. *Journal of Food Protection*, **46**, 325–329.

Jensen, L.B. (1954) *Microbiology of Meats*. Champaign, Illinois: Garrard Press.

Jermini, M.F.G. & Schmidt-Lorenz, W. (1987) Activity of Na-benzoate and ethyl-paraben against osmotolerant yeasts at different water activity values. *Journal of Food Protection*, **50**, 920–927.

Joeng, D.K., Harrison, M.A., Frank, J.F. & Wicker, L. (1992) Trials on the antilisterial effect of glucose oxidase on chicken breast skin and muscle. *Journal of Food Safety*, **13**, 43–49.

Jones, A.H. & Harper, G.S. (1952) A preliminary study of factors affecting the quality of pickles on the Canadian market. *Food Technology*, **5**, 304–308.

Joslyn, M.A. & Braverman, J.B.S. (1954) The chemistry and technology of the pretreatment and preservation of fruit and vegetable products with sulfur dioxide and sulfites. *Advances in Food Research*, **5**, 97–160.

Jung, D.S., Bodyfelt, F.W. & Daeschel, N.A. (1992a) Influence of fat and emulsifiers on the efficacy of nisin in inhibiting *Listeria monocytogenes* in fluid milk. *Journal of Dairy Science*, **75**, 387–393.

Jung, R., Cojocel, C., Muller, W., Bottger, D. & Luecke, E. (1992b) Evaluation of the genotoxic potential of sorbic acid and potassium sorbate. *Food and Chemical Toxicology*, **30**, 1–7.

Junttila, J., Hirn, J., Hill, P. & Nurmi, E. (1989) Effect of different levels of nitrite and nitrate on the survival of *Listeria monocytogenes* during the manufacture of fermented sausage. *Journal of Food Protection*, **52**, 158–161.

Kabara, J. (1981) Food-grade chemicals for use in designing food preservative systems. *Journal of Food Protection*, **44**, 633–647.

Kabara, J.J. (1984) Inhibition of *Staphylococcus aureus* in a model agar–meat system by monolaurin: a research note. *Journal of Food Safety*, **6**, 197–201.

Kabara, J.J. (1993) Medium chain fatty acids and esters. In *Antimicrobials in Food*, 2nd edn (eds Davidson, P.M. & Branen, A.L.), pp. 307–342. New York: Marcel Dekker.

Kada, T. (1974) DNA-damaging products from reaction between sodium nitrite and sorbic acid. *Annual Report of the National Institute of Genetics (Japan)*, **24**, 43–44.

Kantt, C.A. & Torres, J.A. (1993) Growth inhibition by glucose oxidase of selected organisms associated with the microbial spoilage of shrimp (*Pandalus jordani*): *in vitro* model studies. *Journal of Food Protection*, **56**, 147–152.

Karapinar, N. & Gonul, S.A. (1992) Removal of *Yersinia enterocolitica* from fresh parsley by washing with acetic acid or vinegar. *International Journal of Food Microbiology*, **16**, 261–264.

Katz, S.E. & Brady, M.S. (1993) Antibiotic residues and their significance. In *Antimicrobials in Foods*, (eds Davidson, P.M. & Branen, A.L.), pp. 571–596. New York: Marcel Dekker.

Kim, C., Carpenter, C.E., Cornforth, D.P., Mettanant, O. & Mahoney, A.W. (1987) Effect of iron form, temperature, and inoculation with *Clostridium botulinum* spores on residual nitrite in meat and model systems. *Journal of Food Science*, **52**, 1464–1470.

Kim, C.R., Hearnsberger, J.O., Vickery, A.P., White, C.H. & Marshall, D.L. (1995) Extending shelf life of refrigerated catfish fillets using sodium acetate and monopotassium phosphate. *Journal of Food Protection*, **59**, 644–647,

Kimble, C.E. (1977) Chemical food preservatives. In *Disinfection, Sterilization, and Preservation*, 2nd edn (ed. Block, S.S.), pp. 834–858. Philadelphia, Pennsylvania: Lea & Febiger.

King, A.D: & Nagel, C.W. (1967) Growth inhibition of *Pseudomonas* by carbon dioxide. *Journal of Food Science*, **32**, 575–579.

King, A.D. & Nagel, C.W. (1975) Influence of carbon dioxide upon the metabolism of *Pseudomonas aeruginosa*. *Journal of Food Science*, **40**, 362–366.

Kiritaguchi, S., Maraki, M., Mizoguchi, T. & Shida, A. (1973) *Fungicide for Food and Drink*. Japanese Patent 7 303 371.

Klaenhammer, T.R. (1988) Bacteriocins of lactic acid bacteria. *Biochimie*, **70**, 337–349.

Klaenhammer, T.R. (1993) Genetics of bacteriocins produced by lactic acid bacteria. *FEMS Microbiology Reviews*, **12**, 39–86.

Kodicek, E. (1956) The effect of unsaturated fatty acids, of vitamin D and other sterols on Gram-positive bacteria. In *Biochemical Problems Lipids* (eds Popjak, G. & LeBreton, E.), pp. 401–406. London: Butterworths.

Kohler, A.R., Miller, W.H. & Broquist, H.P. (1955) Aureomycin chlortetracycline and the control of poultry spoilage. *Food Technology*, **9**, 151–154.

Kolsarici, N. & Candogan, K. (1995) The effects of potassium sorbate and lactic acid on the shelf-life of vacuum-packed chicken meat. *Poultry Science*, **74**, 1884–1893.

Kono, Y., Shibata, H., Adachi, K. & Tanaka, K. (1994) Lactate-dependent killing of *Escherichia coli* by nitrite plus hydrogen peroxide: a possible role of nitrogen dioxide. *Archives of Biochemistry and Biophysics*, **311** (1), 153–159.

Koser, S.A. & Skinner, W.W. (1922) Viability of the colon-typhoid group in carbonated water and carbonated beverages. *Journal of Bacteriology*, **7**, 111–121.

Kurytowicz, W.A. (ed.) (1976) *Antibiotics: A Critical Review*. Warsaw, Poland: Polish Medical Publishers.

Kuusi, T. & Loytomaki, M. (1972) On the effectiveness of EDTA in prolonging the shelf-life of fresh fish. *Zoological Lebensmittel-Untersuch Forsch.*, **149**, 196–204.

Labots, H. (1977) Effect of nitrite on development of *Staphylococcus aureus* in fermented sausage. In *Proceedings of the Second International Symposium on Nitrite in Meat Products* (eds Tinbergen, B.J. & Krol, B.), pp. 21–27. Wageningen, the Netherlands: Pudoc.

Labuza, T.P., Fru, B. & Taoukis, P.S. (1992) Prediction for shelf-life and safety of minimally processed CAP/MAP chilled foods: a review. *Journal of Food Protection*, **55**, 741–750.

Lattanzio, V., Cardinalli, A. & Palmieri, S. (1994) The role of phenolics in postharvest physiology of fruits and vegetables: browning reactions and fungal diseases. *Italian Journal of Food Science*, **6**, 3–22.

Lechowich, R.V., Brown, W.L., Diebel, R.H. & Somers, I.I. (1978) The role of nitrite in the production of canned cured meat products. *Food Technology*, **32** (5), 45–58.

Lee, J.S., Willett, C.L., Robinson, S.M. & Sinnhuber, R.D. (1967) Comparative effects of chlortetracycline, freezing and radiation on microbial populations of ocean perch. *Applied Microbiology*, **15**, 368–372.

Lehrer, R.I., Ganz, T. & Selsted, M.E. (1991) Defensins: endogenous antibiotic peptides of animal cells. *Cell*, **64**, 229–230.

Leistner, L. (1978) Microbiology of ready to serve foods. *Fleischwirtschaft*, **58**, 2088–2111.

Leistner, L. (1985) Hurdle technology applied to meat products of the shelf stable type and intermediate moisture food types. In *Properties of Water in Foods* (eds Simatos, D. & Multon, J.C.), pp. 309–329. Dordrecht, the Netherlands: Martinus Nijhoff Publishers.

Leistner, L. (1995) Principles and applications of hurdle technology. In *New Methods of Food Preservation* (ed. Gould, G.W.), pp. 1–21. London: Blackie Academic and Professional.

Levin, R.E. (1967) The effectiveness of EDTA as a fish preservative. *Journal of Milk and Food Technology*, **30**, 277–283.

Levinskas, G.J., Ribelin, W.E. & Shaffer, C.B. (1966) Acute and chronic toxicity of pimaricin. *Toxicology of Applied Pharmacology*, **8**, 97–109.

Levy, S.B. (1987) Antibiotic use for growth promotion in animals: ecologic and public health consequences. *Journal of Food Protection*, **50**, 616–620.

Leyer, G.J., Wang, Lih-Ling & Johnson, E.A. (1995) Acid adaptation of *Escherichia coli* 0157:H7 increases survival in acidic foods. *Applied and Environmental Microbiology*, **61**, 3752–3755.

Liewen, M.B. & Marth, E.H. (1985) Growth and inhibition of microorganisms in the presence of sorbic acid: a review. *Journal of Food Protection*, **48**, 364–375.

Lindner, R.L. (1991) *Meat Processing with* Listeria monocytogenes *Reinoculation Control State*. United States Patent US 5 043 174.

Loaharanu, P. (1995) Food irradiation: current status and future prospects. In *New Methods of Food Preservation* (ed. Gould, G.W.), pp. 90–111. London: Blackie Academic and Professional.

Lueck, E. (1976) Sorbic acid as a food preservative. In *International Flavors and Food Additives*, **7** (3), 122–124, 127.

Lueck, E. (1980) *Antimicrobial Food Additives*. Berlin: Springer-Verlag.

Lueck, E. (1992) Food preservatives. *International Food Ingredients*, **3**, 49–56.

Luecke, F.-L. & Earnshaw, R.G. (1991) Starter cultures. In *Food Preservatives*, (eds Russell, N.J. & Gould, G.W.), pp. 215–234. London: Blackie and Son.

Maas, M.R. (1993) Development and use of probability models: the industry perspective. *Journal of Industrial Microbiology*, **12**, 162–167.

Maas, M.R., Glass, K.A. & Doyle, M.P. (1989) Sodium lactate delays toxin production by *Clostridium botulinum* in cook-in-bag turkey products. *Applied and Environmental Microbiology*, **55**, 2226–2229.

Maga, J.A. (1988) *Smoke in Food Processing*. Boca Raton, Florida: CRC Press.

Magee, P.N. & Barnes, J.M. (1967) Carcinogenic nitrosocompounds. *Advances in Cancer Research*, **10**, 163–246.

Makinen, K.K. & Soderling, E. (1981) Effect of xylitol on some food-spoilage microorganisms. *Journal of Food Science*, **46**, 950–951.

Marletta, J. & Stumbo, C.R. (1970) Some effects of ethylene oxide *on Bacillus subtilis*. *Journal of Food Science*, **35**, 627–631.

Marth, E.H. (1966) Antibiotics in foods—naturally occurring, developed and added. *Residue Reviews*, **12**, 65–161.

Marth, E.H., Capp, C.M., Hasenzahl, L., Jackson, H.W. & Hussong, R.V. (1966) Degradation of potassium sorbate by *Penicillium* species. *Journal of Dairy Science*, **49**, 1197–1205.

Matthews, C., Davidson, J., Bauer, E., Morrison, J.L. & Richardson, A.P. (1956) *p* -Hydroxybenzoic acid esters as preservatives. II. Acute and chronic toxicity in dogs, rats, and mice. *Journal of the American Pharmaceutical Association, Scientific Edition*, **45**, 260– 267.

Mayr, G. & Kaemmerer, H. (1959) Fumigation with ethylene oxide. *Food Manufacture*, **34**, 169–170.

Mayr, G.E. & Suhr, H. (1972) Preservation and sterilization of pure and mixed spices. In *Proceedings of the Conference on Spices*, pp. 201–207. London: Tropical Products Institute.

McIver, R., Noren, P. & Tatini, S.R. (1978) Influence of certain food preservatives on growth and production of enterotoxins by *Staphylococcus aureus*. In *Annual Meeting of the American Society of Microbiology*, Abstract No. 187.

McMeekin, T.A., Olley, J.N., Ross, T. & Ratkowsky, D.A. (1993) *Predictive Microbiology, Theory and Application*. Taunton, Somerset, England: Research Studies Press.

McMullen, L.M. & Stiles, M.E. (1996) Potential for use of bacteriocin-producing lactic acid bacteria in the preservation of meats. *Journal of Food Protection*, 1996 (Suppl.), 64–71.

Medina, M., Gaya, P. & Nunez, M. (1989) The lactoperoxidase system in ewe's milk: levels of lactoperoxidase and thiocyanate. *Letters in Applied Microbiology*, **8**, 147–149.

Melnick, D., Luckmann, F.H. & Gooding, C.M. (1954) Sorbic acid as a fungistatic agent for foods. VI. Metabolic degradation of sorbic acid in cheese by molds and the mechanism of mold inhibition. *Food Research*, **19**, 44–58.

Meneely, G.R., Tucker, R.G., Darby, W.J. & Auerbach, S.H. (1953) Chronic sodium chloride toxicity: hypertension, renal and vascular lesions. *Annals of Internal Medicine*, **39**, 991–998.

Meng, J. & Genigeorgis, C.A. (1994) Delaying toxigenesis of *Clostridium botulinum* by sodium lactate in 'sous-vide' products. *Letters in Applied Microbiology*, **19**, 20–23.

Merten, H.L. & Bachman, G.L. (1976) Glutaric acid: a potential food acidulant. *Journal of Food Science*, **41**, 463–464.

Messina, M.C., Ahmad, H.A., Marchello, J.A., Gerba, C.P. & Paquette, M.W. (1988) The effect of liquid smoke on *Listeria monocytogenes*. *Journal of Food Protection*, **51**, 629–631.

Miller, A.J. & Menichillo, D.A. (1991) Blood fraction effects on the antibotulinal efficacy of nitrite in model beef sausages. *Journal of Food Science*, **56**, 1158–1160.

Miller, A.J., Whiting, R.C. & Smith, J.L. (1997) Use of risk assessment to reduce listeriosin incidence. *Food Technology*, **51** (4), 100–103.

Miller, L.G. & Kaspar, C.W. (1994) *Escherichia coli* 0157:H7 and tolerance and survival in apple cider. *Journal of Food Protection*, **57**, 460–464.

Miller, R.K. & Acuff, G.R. (1994) Sodium lactate affects pathogens on cooked beef. *Journal of Food Science*, **59**, 15–19.

Ming, X.T. & Daeschel, M.A. (1993) Nisin resistance of foodborne bacteria and the specific resistance responses of *Listeria monocytogenes* Scott A. *Journal of Food Protection*, **56**, 944–948.

Ming, X.T. & Daeschel, M.A. (1995) Correlation of cellular phospholipid content with nisin resistance of *Listeria monocytogenes* Scott A. *Journal of Food Protection*, **58**, 416–420.

Moir, C.J. & Eyles, M.J. (1992) Inhibition, injury, and inactivation of four psychrotrophic foodborne bacteria by the preservatives methyl *p*-hydroxybenzoate and potassium sorbate. *Journal of Food Protection*, **55**, 360–366.

Montville, T.J. (1989) The evolving impact of biotechnology on food microbiology. *Journal of Food Safety*, **10**, 87–97.

Montville, T.J. & Bruno, M.E.C. (1994) Evidence that dissipation of proton motive force is a common mechanism of action for bacteriocins and other antimicrobial proteins. *International Journal of Food Microbiology*, **24**, 53–74.

Montville, T.J. & Goldstein, P.K. (1989) Sodium bicarbonate inhibition of aflatoxigenesis in corn. *Journal of Food Protection*, **52**, 45–48.

Mortimer, S. & Wallace, C. (1994) *HACCP, A Practical Approach*. London: Chapman & Hall.

Mossel, D.A.A. (1975) *Microbiology of Foods and Dairy Products*. Utrecht: University of Utrecht, Faculty of Veterinary Medicine.

Mossel, D.A.A., Cory, J.E.L., Struijk, C.B. & Baird, R.M. (1995) *Essentials of the Microbiology of Foods*. New York: John Wiley & Sons.

Motlagh, A.M., Johnson, M.C. & Ray, B. (1991) Viability loss of foodborne pathogens by starter culture metabolites. *Journal of Food Protection*, **54**, 873–878.

Mukai, F., Hawryluk, I. & Shapiro, R. (1970) The mutagenic specificity of sodium bisulfite. *Biochemical and Biophysical Research Communications*, **39**, 983–988.

Muriana, P.M. (1996) Bacteriocins for control of *Listeria* spp. in food. *Journal of Food Protection*, 1996 (Suppl.), 54–63.

Nagy, R. (1959) Application of ozone from sterilamp in control of mold, bacteria and odors. In *Ozone Chemistry and Technology* (ed. Leedy, H.A.), Advanced Chemical Series No. 21. Washington, D.C.: American Chemical Society.

Namiki, M. & Kada, T. (1975) Formation of ethylnitrolic acid by the reaction of sorbic acid with sodium nitrite. *Agricultural and Biological Chemistry (Japan)*, **39**, 1335–1336.

Nassar, A., Ismail, M.A. & About-Elala, H.-H (1995). The role of benzoic acid as a fungal decontaminant of beef carcasses. *Fleischnirtschaft*, **75**, 1160–1162.

NACMCF (National Advisory Committee on Microbiology Criteria for Foods) (1992) Hazard analysis and critical control point system. *International Journal of Food Microbiology*, **16**, 1–23.

National Research Council (1981) *The Health Effects of Nitrate, Nitrite and* N-*nitroso Compounds*. Washington, DC: National Academy Press.

National Research Council (1982) *Alternatives to Current Use of Nitrite in Foods*. Washington, DC: National Academy Press.

Natvig, H., Andersen, J. & Rasmussen, E.W. (1971) A contribution of the toxicological evaluation of hexamethylenetetramine. *Food and Cosmetic Toxicology*, **9**, 491–500.

Neal, A.L., Weinstock, J.O. & Lampen, J.O. (1965) Mechanisms of fatty acid toxicity for yeast. *Journal of Bacteriology*, **90**, 126–131.

Nes, I.F. & Eklund, T. (1983) The effect of parabens on DNA, RNA and protein synthesis in *Escherichia coli* and *Bacillus subtilis*. *Journal of Applied Bacteriology*, **54**, 237–242.

Nettles, C.G. & Barefoot, S.F. (1993) Biochemical and genetic characteristics of bacteriocins of food-associated lactic acid bacteria. *Journal of Food Protection*, **56**, 338–356.

Neves, L., Pampulha, M.E. & Loureiro-Dias, M.C. (1994) Resistance of food spoilage yeasts to sorbic acid. *Letters in Applied Microbiology*, **19**, 8–11.

Newberne, P.M. (1979) Nitrite promotes lymphoma incidence in rats. *Science*, **204**, 1079–1081.

Njagi, G.D.E. & Gopalan, H.N.B. (1980) DNA and its precursors might interact with the food preservatives, sodium sulphite and sodium benzoate. *Experientia*, **36**, 413–414.

Notermans, S., Dufrenne, J. & Keybets, M.J.H. (1985) Use of preservatives to delay toxin formation by *Clostridium botulinum* (type B, strain okra) in vacuum-packed, cooked potatoes. *Journal of Food Protection*, **48**, 851–855.

Ogden, S.K., Guerrero, T., Taylor, A.J., Escalona-Buendia, H. & Gallardo, F. (1995) Changes in odour, colour and texture during the storage of acid preserved meat. *Lebensmittlel-Wissenschaft und Technologie*, **28**, 521–527.

Ogilvy, W.S. & Ayres, J.C. (1951) Post-mortem changes in stored meats. II. The effect of atmosphere containing carbon dioxide in prolonging the storage life of cut-up chicken. *Food Technology*, **5**, 97–102.

Ogilvy, W.S. & Ayres, J.C. (1953) Post-mortem changes in stored meats. V. Effects of carbon dioxide on microbial growth on stored frankfurters and characteristics of some microorganisms isolated from them. *Food Research*, **18**, 121–130.

Oka, S. (1964) Mechanism of antimicrobial effect of various food preservatives. In *Microbial Inhibitors in Food* (ed. Molin, N.), pp. 1–15. Stockholm: Almquist and Wiksell.

O'Leary, D.K. & Kralovec, R.D. (1941) Development of *B. mesentericus* in bread and control with calcium acid phosphate and calcium propionate. *Cereal Chemistry*, **18**, 730–741.

Olson, J.C., Jr & Macy, H. (1945) Observations on the use of propionate-treated parchment in inhibiting mold growth on the surface of butter. *Science*, **28**, 701–710.

Ough, C.S. (1993a) Sulfur dioxide and sulfites. In *Antimicrobials in Foods*, 2nd edn (eds Davidson, P.M. & Branen, A.L.), pp. 137–190. New York: Marcel Dekker.

Ough, C.S. (1993b) Dimethyl dicarbonate and diethyl dicarbonate. In *Antimicrobial in Foods*, 2nd edn (eds Davidson, P.M. & Branen, A.L), pp. 343–368. New York: Marcel Dekker.

Owen Fields, F. (1996) Use of bacteriocins in food: regulatory considerations. *Journal of Food Protection*, 1996 (Suppl.), 72–77.

Papageorgiou, D.K. & Marth, E.H. (1989) Behavior of *Listeria monocytogenes* at 4 and 22°C in whey and skim milk containing 6 or 12% sodium chloride. *Journal of Food Protection*, **52**, 625–630.

Pappas, H.J. & Hall, L.A. (1952) Control of thermophilic bacteria. *Food Technology*, **6**, 456–458.

Parekh, K.G. & Solberg, M. (1970) Comparative growth of *Clostridium perfringens* in carbon dioxide and nitrogen atmospheres. *Journal of Food Science*, **35**, 156–159.

Parish, M.E. & Carroll, D.E. (1988) Minimum inhibitory concentration studies of antimicrobic combinations against *Saccharomyces cerevisiae* in a model broth system. *Journal of Food Science*, **53**, 237.

Parke, D.V. & Lewis, D.F.V. (1992) Safety aspects of food preservatives. *Food Additives and Contaminants*, **9**, 561–577.

Parker, M.S. (1969) Some effects of preservatives on the development of bacterial spores. *Journal of Applied Bacteriology*, **32**, 322–328.

Payne, K.D., Rico-Munoz, E. & Davidson, P.M. (1989) The antimicrobial activity of phenolic compounds against *Listeria monocytogenes* and their effectiveness in a model milk system. *Journal of Food Protection*, **52**, 151–153.

Pelroy, G.A., Peterson, M.E., Holland, P.J. & Eklund, M.W. (1994) Inhibition of *Listeria monocytogenes* in cold-process-smoked salmon by sodium lactate. *Journal of Food Protection*, **57**, 108–113.

Phillips, C.R. & Kaye, S. (1949) The sterilizing action of gaseous ethylene oxide. *American Journal of Hygiene*, **50**, 270–279.

Phillips, G.F. & Mundt, J.O. (1950) Sorbic acid as inhibitor of scum yeast in cucumber fermentations. *Food Technology*, **4**, 291–293.

Pierson, M.D. & Corlett, D.A., Jr (1992) *HACCP Principles and Applications*. New York: Van Nostrand Reinhold.

Pierson, M.D., Smoot, L.A. and van Tassel, K.R. (1980) Inhibition of *Salmonella typhimurium* and *Staphylococcus aureus by* butylated hydroxyanisole and the propyl ester of *p*-hydroxybenzoic acid. *Journal of Food Protection*, **43**, 191–194.

Podolak, R.K., Zayas, J.F., Kastner, C.L. & Fung, D.Y.C. (1995) Reduction of *Listeria monocytogenes, Escherichia coli* O157:H7 and *Salmonella typhimurium* during storage on beef sanitized with fumaric, acetic, and lactic acids. *Journal of Food Safety*, **15**, 283–290.

Post, L.S., Lee, D.A., Solberg, M., Furgang, D., Specchio, J. & Graham, C. (1985) Development of botulinal toxin and sensory deterioration during storage of vacuum and modified atmosphere packaged fish fillets. *Journal of Food Science*, **50**, 990–996.

Post, R.C. (1996) Regulatory perspective of the USDA on the use of antimicrobials and inhibitors in foods. *Journal of Food Protection*, 1996 (Suppl.), 78–81.

Prescott, S.C. & Proctor, B.E. (1937) *Food Technology*. New York: McGraw-Hill.

Raccach, M. (1984) The antimicrobial activity of phenolic antioxidants in foods: a review. *Journal of Food Safety*, **6**, 141–170.

Rao, K.V.S.S. & Mathur, B.N. (1996) Thermal death kinetics of *Bacillus stearothermophilus* spores in a nisin supplemented acidified concentrated buffalo milk system. *Milchuissenschaft*, **51**, 186–191.

Ray, B. (1996) *Fundamental Food Microbiology*. Boca Raton, Florida: CRC Press.

Ray, B. & Daeschel, M.A. (1992) *Food Biopreservatives of Microbial Origin*. Boca Raton, Florida: CRC Press.

Ray, B. & Daeschel, M.A. (1994) Bacteriocins of started culture bacteria. In *Natural Antimicrobial Systems and Food Preservation* (eds Dillon, V.M. & Board, R.G.), pp. 133–166. Wallingford, Oxon, UK: CAB International.

Rayman, K., Malik, N. & Hurst, A. (1983) Failure of nisin to inhibit outgrowth of *Clostridium botulinum* in a model cured meat system. *Applied and Environmental Microbiology*, **46**, 1450–1452.

Rayman, M.K., Aris, B. & Hurst, A. (1981) Nisin: a possible alternative or adjunct to nitrite in the preservation of meats. *Applied and Environmental Microbiology*, **41**, 375–380.

Reddish, G.F. (1957) *Antiseptics, Disinfectants, Fungicides, and Chemical and Physical Sterilization*, 2nd edn. Philadelphia, Pennsylvania: Lea & Febiger.

Reed G. (ed.) (1982) *Prescott and Dunn's Industrial Microbiology*, 4th edn. Westport, Connecticut: AVI Publishing.

Reiss, J. (1976) Prevention of the formation of mycotoxins in whole wheat bread by citric acid and lactic acid (mycotoxins in foodstuffs, IX). *Experientia*, **32**, 168–169.

Reiter, B. & Harnulv, G. (1984) Lactoperoxidase antibacterial system: natural occurrence, biological functions and practical applications. *Journal of Food Protection*, **47**, 724–732.

Rekhif, N., Atrih, A. & Lefebvre, G. (1994) Selection and properties of spontaneous mutants of *Listeria monocytogenes* ATCC 15313 resistant to different bacteriocins produced by lactic acid bacteria strains. *Current Microbiology*, **28**, 237–241.

Restaino, L., Lenovich, L.M. & Bills, S. (1982) Effect of acids and sorbate combinations on the growth of four osmophilic yeasts. *Journal of Food Protection*, **45**, 1138–1142.

Rizk, S.S. & Isshak, Y.M. (1974) Thiabendazole as a post harvest disinfectant for citrus fruits. *Agricultural Research Review*, **52**, 39–46.

Robach, M.C. (1978) Effect of potassium sorbate on the growth of *Pseudomonas fluorescens*. *Journal of Food Science*, **43**, 1886–1887.

Robach, M.C. (1979) Influence of potassium sorbate on growth of *Pseudomonas putrefaciens*. *Journal of Food Protection*, **42**, 312–313.

Robach, M.C. & Pierson, M.D. (1978) Influence of *p*-hydroxybenzoic acid esters on the growth and toxin production of *Clostridium botulinum* 10755A. *Journal of Food Science*, **43**, 787–789.

Robach, M.C. & Sofos, J.N. (1982) Use of sorbates in meat products, fresh poultry and poultry products. *Journal of Food Protection*, **44**, 614–622.

Roberts, T. (1989) Human illness costs of foodborne bacteria. *American Journal of Agricultural Economics*, **71**, 468–474.

Roberts, T.A. (1975) The microbial role of nitrite and nitrate. *Journal of Science Food and Agriculture*, **26**, 1755–1760.

Roberts, T.A. (1997) Microbial growth and survival: developments in predictive modeling. *Food Technology*, **51** (4), 88–90.

Roberts, T.A., Gibson, A.M. & Robinson, A. (1981) Prediction of toxin production by *Clostridium botulinum* in pasteurized pork slurry. *Journal of Food Technology*, **16**, 337–355.

Robinson, A., Gibson, A.M. & Roberts, T.A. (1982) Factors controlling the growth of *Clostridium botulinum* types A and B in pasteurized, cured meats. V. Prediction of toxin production: non-linear effects of storage temperature and salt concentration. *Journal of Food Technology*, **17**, 727–744.

Robinson, H.J., Phares, H.F. & Graessle, O.E. (1964) Antimycotic properties of thiabendazole. *Journal of Investigative Dermatology*, **42**, 478–482.

Roland, J.O. & Beuchat, L.R. (1984) Biomass and patulin production by *Byssochlamys nivea* in apple juice as affected by sorbate, benzoate, SO_2 and temperature. *Journal of Food Science*, **49**, 402–406.

Rong-Yu, Z., Huang, Yan-Wen & Beuchat, L.R. (1996) Quality changes during refrigerated storage of packaged shrimp and catfish fillets treated with sodium acetate, sodium lactate or propyl gallate. *Journal of Food Science*, **61**, 241–244.

Rose, A.H. (1993) Sulphur dioxide and other preservatives. *Journal of Wine Research*, **4**, 43–47.

Ross, T. & McMeekin, T.A. (1994) Predictive microbiology. *International Journal of Food Microbiology*, **23**, 241–264.

Roth, N.G. & Halvorson, H.O. (1952) The effect of oxidative rancidity in unsaturated fatty acids on the germination of bacterial spores. *Journal of Bacteriology*, **63**, 429–435.

Rowe, M.T. (1988) Effect of carbon dioxide on growth and extracellular enzyme production by *Pseudomonas fluorescens* B52. *International Journal of Food Microbiology*, **6**, 51–56.

Russell, A.D. (1971) Ethylenediaminetetraacetic acid. In *Inhibition and Destruction of the Microbial Cell* (ed. Hugo, W.B.), pp. 209–224. London, England: Academic Press.

Russell, A.D. (1991) Principles of antimicrobial activity. In *Disinfection, Sterilization and Preservation*, 4th edn (ed. Block, S.S.), pp. 29–58. Philadelphia, Pennsylvania: Lee & Febiger.

Russell, A.D. & Chopra, I. (1996) *Understanding Antibacterial Action and Resistance*, 2nd edn. Chichester: Ellis Horwood.

Russell, A.D. & Fuller, R. (eds) (1979) *Cold-tolerant Microorganisms in Spoilage and the Environment.* Society for Applied Bacteriology Technical Series No. 13. London: Academic Press.

Rusul, G. & Marth, E.H. (1988a) Food additives and plant components control growth and aflatoxin production by toxigenic aspergilli: a review. *Mycopathologia*, **101**, 13–23.

Rusul, G. & Marth, E.H. (1988b) Growth and aflatoxin production by *Aspergillus parasiticus* in a medium at different pH values and with or without pimaricin. *Zoological Lebensmittel Untersuch Forsch.* **1897**, 436–439.

Sahl, H.G., Jack, R.W. & Bierbaum, G. (1995) Biosynthesis and biological activities of antibiotics with unique post-translational modifications. *European Journal of Biochemistry*, **230**, 827–853.

Saitanu, K. & Lund, E. (1975) Inactivation of enterovirus by glutaraldehyde. *Applied Microbiology*, **29**, 571–574.

Sams, W.M., Jr & Carroll, N.V. (1966) Prediction and demonstration of iron chelating ability of sugars. *Nature, London*, **212**, 404–405.

Sauer, F. (1977) Control of yeasts and molds with preservatives. *Food Technology*, **31** (2), 62–67.

Schaftner, D.W. & Labuza, T.P. (1997) Predictive microbiology: where are we and where we are going. *Food Technology*, **51** (4), 95–99.

Schlievert, P.M., Deringer, J.R., Kim, M.H., Projan, S.J. & Novick, R.P. (1992) Effect of glycerol monolaurate on bacterial growth and toxin production. *Antimicrobial Agents and Chemotherapy*, **36**, 626–631.

Schmidt, C.F. (1964) Spores of *Clostridium botulinum*: formation, resistance, germination. In *Botulism, Proceedings of a Symposium* (eds Lewis, K.H. & Cassel, K.), No. 999-FP-1, pp. 69–82. Washington, DC: US Department of Health, Education, and Welfare, Public Health Service.

Schved, F., Pierson, M.D. & Juven, B.J. (1995) Sensitatization of *Escherichia coli* to nisin by maltol and ethyl maltol. *Letters in Applied Microbiology*, **22**, 189–191.

Scott, V.N. & Taylor, S.L. (1981a) Effect of nisin on the outgrowth of *Clostridium botulinum* spores. *Journal of Food Science*, **46**, 117–120, 126.

Scott, V.N. & Taylor, S.L. (1981b) Temperature, pH and spore load effects on the ability of nisin to prevent the outgrowth of *Clostridium botulinum* spores. *Journal of Food Science*, **46**, 121–126.

Sebranek, J.G. & Cassens, R.G. (1973) Nitrosamines: a

review. *Journal of Milk and Food Technology*, **36**, 76–91.

Seiler, D.A.L. (1964) Factors affecting the use of mould inhibitors in bread and cake. In *Microbial Inhibitors in Food* (ed. Molin, N.), pp. 211–220. Stockholm: Almquist and Wiksell.

Seiler, D.A.L. & Russell, N.J. (1991) Ethanol as a food preservative. In *Food Preservatives* (eds Russell, N.J. & Gould, G.W.), pp. 153–171. London, England: Blackie and Son.

Setlow, B. & Setlow, P. (1993) Binding of small, acid-soluble spore proteins to DNA plays a significant role in the resistance of *Bacillus subtilis* spores to hydrogen peroxide. *Applied and Environmental Microbiology*, **59**, 3418–3423.

Shahidi, F. & Pegg, R.B. (1992) Nitrite-free meat curing systems: update and review. *Food Chemistry*, **43**, 185–191.

Shelef, L.A. (1984) Antimicrobial effects of spices. *Journal of Food Safety*, **6**, 29–44.

Shelef, L.A. (1994) Antimicrobial effects of lactates: a review. *Journal of Food Protection*, **57**, 445–450.

Shelef, L.A. & Seiter, J.A. (1993) Indirect antimicrobials. In *Antimicrobials in Foods*, 2nd edn (eds Davidson, P.M. & Branen, A.L.), pp. 539–570. New York: Marcel Dekker.

Shelef, L.A. & Yang, Q. (1991) Growth suppression of *Listeria monocytogenes* by lactate in broth, chicken and beef. *Journal of Food Protection*, **54**, 282–287.

Shibata, T., Tsuji, S., Ito, S.I. *et al.* (1991) Comparison of natamycin and sorbate residue levels and antifungal activities on the surface treatment of Gouda-type cheese. *Journal of Food Hygienic Society Japan*, **32**, 378–401.

Shiralkar, N.D. & Rege, D.V. (1978) Mechanism of action of *p*-hydroxybenzoates. *Indian Food Packer*, **32**, 34–41.

Sholberg, P.L. & Gaunce, A.P. (1995) Fumigation of fruit with acetic acid to prevent postharvest decay. *Hortscience*, **30**, 1271–1275.

Shtenberg, A.J. & Ignat'ev, A.D. (1970) Toxicological evaluation of some combinations of food preservatives. *Food and Cosmetic Toxicology*, **8**, 369–380.

Sieber, R., Buticofer, U. & Bossett, J.O. (1995) Benzoic acid as a natural compound in cultured dairy products and cheese. *International Dairy Journal*, **5**, 227–246.

Silliker, J.H. (1959) The effect of curing salts on bacterial spores. In *Proceeding of the Meat Industry Research Conference*, pp. 51–60. Washington, DC: American Meat Institute.

Silliker, J.H., Greenberg, R.A. & Schack, W.R. (1958) Effect of individual curing ingredients on the shelf stability of canned comminuted meats. *Food Technology*, **12**, 551–554.

Silliker, J.H., Woodruff, R.E., Lugg, J.R., Wolfe, S.K. & Brown, W.D. (1977) Preservation of refrigerated meats with controlled atmospheres: treatment and post-treatment effects of carbon dioxide on pork and beef. *Meat Science*, **1**, 195–204.

Sink, J.D. & Hsu, L.A. (1977) Chemical effects of smoke processing on frankfurter manufacture and storage characteristics. *Journal of Food Science*, **42**, 1489–1491.

Skinner, F.A. & Hugo, W.B. (eds) (1976) *Inhibition and Inactivation* of *Vegetative Microbes*. London, England: Academic Press.

Skirdal, I.M. & Eklund, T. (1993) Microculture model studies on the effect of sorbic acid on *Penicillium chrysogenum, Cladosporium cladosporioides* and *Ulocladium atrum* at different pH levels. *Journal of Applied Bacteriology*, **74** , 191–195.

Skovgaard, N. (1992) Microbiological aspects and technological need: technological needs for nitrates and nitrites. *Food Additives and Contaminants*, **9**, 391–397.

Smith, D.P. & Rollin, N. (1954) Sorbic acid as a fungistatic agent for foods. VII. Effectiveness of sorbic acid in protecting cheese. *Food Research*, **19**, 59–65.

Smith, J.L. & Palumbo, S.A. (1981) Microorganisms as food additives. *Journal of Food Protection*, **44**, 936–955.

Smith, Q.J. & Brown, K.L. (1980) The resistance of dry spores of *Bacillus subtilis* var. *globigii* (NCIB 8058) to solutions of hydrogen peroxide in relation to aseptic packaging. *Journal of Food Technology*, **15**, 169–179.

Smith, W.H. (1963) The use of carbon dioxide in the transport and storage of fruits and vegetables. *Advances in Food Research*, **12**, 96–118.

Smulders, F.J.M., Barendsen, P., van Logtestijn, J.G., Mossel, D.A.A. & van der Marel, G.M. (1986) Review: lactic acid: considerations in favour of its acceptance as a meat decontaminant. *Journal of Food Technology*, **21**, 419–436.

Sofos, J.N. (1981) Nitrite, sorbate and pH interaction in cured meat products. In *Proceedings of the 34th Annual Reciprocal Meat Conference*, pp. 104–120. Chicago, Illinois, USA: National Live Stock and Meat Board.

Sofos, J.N. (1984) Antimicrobial effects of sodium and other ions in foods: a review. *Journal of Food Safety*, **6**, 45–78.

Sofos, J.N. (1985) Improved cooking yields of meat batters formulated with potassium sorbate and reduced levels of NaCl. *Journal of Food Science*, **50**, 1571–1575.

Sofos, J.N. (1986a) Use phosphates in low-sodium meat products. *Food Technology*, **40** (9), 52–69.

Sofos, J.N. (1986b) Antimicrobial activity and functionality of reduced sodium chloride and potassium sorbate in uncured poultry products. *Journal of Food Science*, **51**, 16–19, 23.

Sofos, J.N. (1989a) *Sorbate Food Preservatives*. Boca Raton, Florida: CRC Press.

Sofos, J.N. (1989b) Phosphates in meat products. In *Development in Food Preservation—5* (ed. Thorne, S.), pp. 207–252. Amsterdam: Elsevier Science Publishers.

Sofos, J.N. (1992a) The HACCP system in meat processing and inspection in the United States. *Meat Focus International*, **2**, 217–225.

Sofos, J.N. (1992b) Sorbic acid, mode of action. In *Encyclopedia of Microbiology*, Vol. 4, pp. 43–52. San Diego, California: Academic Press.

Sofos, J.N. (1993) Current microbiological considerations in food preservation. *International Journal of Food Microbiology*, **19**, 87–108.

Sofos, J.N. (1994a) Antimicrobial agents. In *Handbook of Toxicology*, Vol. 1, *Food Additive Technology* (eds Tu, A. & Maga, J.A.), pp. 501–529. New York: Marcel Dekker.

Sofos, J.N. (1994b) Microbial growth and its control in meat, poultry and fish. In *Quality Attributes and Their Measurement in Meat, Poultry and Fish Products* (eds Pearson, A.M. & Dutson, T.R.), pp. 353–403. Glasgow, UK: Chapman and Hall.

Sofos, J.N. & Busta, F.F. (1980) Alternatives to the use of nitrite as an antibotulinal agent. *Food Technology*, **34**, 244–251.

Sofos, J.N. & Busta, F.F. (1981) Antimicrobial activity of serbate. *Journal of Food Protection*, **44**, 614–622.

Sofos, J.N. & Busta, F.F. (1993) Sorbic acid and sorbates. In *Antimicrobials in Foods*, 2nd edn (eds Davidson, P.M. & Branen, A.L.), pp. 49–94. New York: Marcel Dekker.

Sofos, J.N. & Maga, J.A. (1988) Composition and antimicrobial properties of liquid spice smokes. In *The Shelf-life of Foods and Beverages* (ed. Charalambous, G.), pp. 453–472. Amsterdam: Elsevier Science Publishers.

Sofos, J.N. & Raharjo, S. (1994a) Curing agents. In *Handbook of Toxicology*, Vol. 1, *Food Additive Toxicology* (eds Tu, A.T. & Maga, J.A.), pp. 235–267. New York: Marcel Dekker.

Sofos, J.N. & Raharjo, S. (1994b) Salts. In *Handbook of Toxicology*, Vol. 1, *Food Additive Toxicology* (eds Tu, A.T. & Maga, J.A.), pp. 413–430. New York: Marcel Dekker.

Sofos, J.N., Busta, F.F., Bhothipaksa, K. & Allen, C.E (1979a) Sodium nitrite and sorbic acid effects on *Clostridium botulinum* toxin formation in chicken frankfurter-type emulsions. *Journal of Food Science*, **44**, 668–675.

Sofos, J.N., Busta, F.F. & Allen, C.E. (1979b) Sodium nitrite and sorbic acid effects on *Clostridium botulinum* spore germination and total microbial growth in chicken frankfurter emulsions during temperature abuse. *Applied and Environmental Microbiology*, **37**, 1103–1109.

Sofos, J.N., Busta, F.P. & Allen, C.E. (1979c) Botulism control by nitrite and sorbate in cured meats: a review. *Journal Food Protection*, **42**, 739–770.

Sofos, J.N., Busta, F.F. & Allen, C.E. (1979d) *Clostridium botulinum* control by sodium nitrite and sorbic acid in various meat and soy protein formulations. *Journal of Food Science*, **44**, 1662–1667.

Sofos, J.N., Busta, F.F. & Allen, C.E. (1980a) Influence of pH on *Clostridium botulinum* control by sodium nitrite and sorbic acid in chicken emulsions. *Journal of Food Science*, **45**, 7–12.

Sofos, J.N., Busta, F.F., Bhothipaksa, K., Allen, C.E., Robach, M.C. & Paquette, M.W. (1980b) Effects of various concentrations of sodium nitrite and potassium sorbate on *Clostridium botulinum* toxin production in commercially prepared bacon. *Journal of Food Science*, **45**, 1285–1292.

Sofos, J.N., Pierson, M.D., Blocher, J.C. & Busta, F.F. (1986) Mode of action of sorbic acid on bacterial cells and spores. *International Journal of Food Microbiology*, **3**, 1–17.

Sofos, J.N., Maga, J.A. & Boyle, D.L. (1988) Effect of ether extracts from condensed wood smokes on the growth of *Aeromonas hydrophila* and *Staphylococcus aureus*. *Journal of Food Science*, **53**, 1840–1843.

Somers, E.B. & Taylor, S.L. (1987) Antibotulinal effectiveness of nisin in pasteurized process cheese spreads. *Journal of Food Protection*, **50**, 842–848.

Sorrells, K.M., Enigl, D.C. & Hatfield, J.R. (1989) Effect of pH, acidulant, time, and temperature on the growth and survival *of Listeria monocytogenes*. *Journal of Food Protection*, **52**, 571–573.

Spelhaug, S.R. & Harlander, S.K. (1989) Inhibition of foodborne bacterial pathogens by bacteriocins from *Lactococcus lactis* and *Pediococcus pentosaceous*. *Journal of Food Protection*, **52**, 856–862.

Splittstoesser, D.F. & Churney, J.J. (1992) The incidence of sorbic acid-resistant gluconobacters and yeasts on grapes grown in New York state. *American Journal of Ecology and Viticulture*, **43**, 290–293.

Splittstoesser, D.G. & Stoyla, B.O. (1989) Effect of various inhibitors on the growth of lactic acid bacteria in a model grape juice system. *Journal of Food Protection*, **52** (4), 240–243.

Stevens, K.A., Sheldon, B.W., Klapes, N.A. & Klaenhammer, T.R. (1991) Nisin treatment for inactivation of *Salmonella* species and other Gram-negative bacteria. *Applied and Environmental Microbiology*, **57**, 3613–3615.

Stevens, K.A., Sheldon, B.W., Klapes, N.A. & Klaenhammer, T.R. (1992) Effect of treatment conditions on nisin inactivation of Gram-negative bacteria. *Journal of Food Protection*, **55**, 763–766.

Stevenson, K.E. & Shafer, B.D. (1983) Bacterial spore resistance to hydrogen peroxide. *Food Technology*, **37** (11), 111–114.

Stiles, M.E. (1994) Potential for biological control of

agents of foodborne disease. *Food Resources International*, **27**, 245–250.

Sugiyama, H. & Sofos, J.N. (1988) Botulism. In *Developments in Microbiology – 4* (ed. Robinson, R.K.), pp. 77–120. London: Elsevier Applied Science.

Sugiyama, T., Goto, K. & Uenaka, H. (1975) Acute cytogenetic effect of 2-(2-furyl)-3-(5-nitro-2-furyl)-acrylamide (AF-2, a food preservative) on rat bone marrow cells *in vivo*. *Mutation Research*, **31**, 241–246.

Sweet, C.W. (1975) *Additive Composition for Reduced Particle Size Meats in the Curing Thereof*. US Patent No. 3 899 600.

Takayama, S. & Kuwabara, N. (1977) The production of skeletal muscle atrophy and mammary tumors in rats by feeding 2-(2-furyl)-3-(5-nitro-2-furyl) acrylamide. *Toxicology Letters*, **1**, 11–16.

Tanaka, N.E., Traisman, E., Lee, M.H., Cassens, R.C. & Foster, E.M. (1980) Inhibition of botulinum toxin formation in bacon by acid development. *Journal of Food Protection*, **43**, 450–457.

Tanaka, N., Meske, L., Doyle, M.P., Traisman, E., Thayer, D.W. & Johnston, R.W. (1985) Plant trials of bacon made with lactic acid bacteria, sucrose and lowered sodium nitrite. *Journal of Food Protection*, **48**, 679–686.

Tanner, F.W. (1944) *The Microbiology of Foods*, 2nd edn. Champaign, Illinois: Garrard Press.

Tapia-de-Daza, M.S., Aguilar, C.E., Roa, V. & Diaz-de-Tablante, R.V. (1995). Combined stress effects on growth of *Zygosaccharomyces rouxii* from an intermediate moisture papaya product. *Journal of Food Science*, **60**, 356–359.

Tarr, H.L.A. (1941a) The action of nitrites on bacteria. *Journal of Fisheries Research Board, Canada*, **5**, 265–275.

Tarr, H.L.A. (1941b) Bacteriostatic action of nitrites. *Nature, London*, **147**, 417–418.

Tarr, H.L.A. (1942) The action of nitrites on bacteria: further experiments. *Journal of Fisheries Research Board, Canada*, **6**, 74–89.

Tatini, S.R., Lee, R.Y., McCall, W.A. & Hill, W.M. (1976) Growth of *Staphylococcus aureus* and production of enterotoxins in pepperoni. *Journal of Food Science*, **41**, 223–225.

Taylor, S.L., Somers, E.B. & Krueger, L.A. (1985) Antibotulinal effectiveness of nisin-nitrite combinations in culture medium and chicken frankfurter emulsions. *Journal of Food Protection*, **48**, 234–239.

Thakur, B.R., Singh, R.K. & Arya, S.S. (1994) Chemistry of sorbates: a basic perspective. *Food Reviews International*, **10**, 71–91.

Thomas, L.V., Wimpenny, J.W.T. & Davis, J.G. (1993) Effect of three preservatives on the growth of *Bacillus cereus*, Vero cytotoxigenic *Escherichia coli* and *Staphylococcus aureus*, on plates with gradients of pH and sodium chloride concentration. *International Journal of Food Microbiology*, **17**, 289–301.

Tiina, M. & Sandholm, M. (1989) Antibacterial effect of the glucose oxidase–glucose system on food-poisoning organisms. *International Journal of Food Microbiology*, **8**, 165–174.

Todd, E.C.D. (1989) Preliminary estimates of costs of foodborne disease in the United States. *Journal of Food Protection*, **52**, 595–601.

Toledo, R.T., Escher, F.E. & Ayres, J.C. (1973) Sporicidal properties of hydrogen peroxide against food spoilage organisms. *Applied Microbiology*, **26**, 592–597.

Tomasz, A. (1994) Multiple-antibiotic-resistant pathogenic bacteria. *New England Journal of Medicine*, **330**, 1247–1251.

Tomkins, R.G. (1932) The inhibition of the growth of meat-attacking fungi by carbon dioxide. *Journal of the Society of Chemical Industry*, **51**, 261T-264T.

Tompkin, R.B. (1978) The role and mechanism of the inhibition of *C. botulinum* by nitrite – is a replacement available? In *Proceedings of the 31st Annual Reciprocal Meat Conference*, 18–22 June, pp. 135–147. Chicago, Illinois, USA: National Live Stock and Meat Board.

Tompkin, R.B. (1984) Indirect antimicrobial effects in foods: phosphates. *Journal of Food Safety*, **6**, 13–28.

Tompkin, R.B. (1990) The use of HACCP in the production of meat and poultry products. *Journal of Food Protection*, **53**, 795–803.

Tompkin, R.B. (1993) Nitrite. In *Antimicrobials in Foods*, 2nd edn (eds Davidson, P.M. & Branen, A.L.), pp. 191–262. New York: Marcel Dekker.

Tompkin, R.B., Christiansen, L.N., Shaparis, A.B. & Bolin, H. (1974) Effects of potassium sorbate on salmonellae, *Staphylococcus aureus*, *Clostridium perfringens*, and *Clostridium botulinum* in cooked, uncured sausage. *Applied Microbiology*, **28**, 262–264.

Tompkin, R.B., Christiansen, L.N. & Shaparis, A.B. (1980) Antibotulinal efficacy of sulfur dioxide in meat. *Applied and Environmental Microbiology*, **39**, 1096–1099.

Torricelli, A. (1959) Sterilization of empty containers for food industry. In *Ozone Chemistry and Technology* (ed. Leedy, H.A.), Advanced Chemistry Series No. 21. Washington, DC: American Chemical Society.

Tranter, H.S. (1994) Lysozyme, ovotransferrin and avidin. In *Natural Antimicrobial Systems and Food Preservation* (eds Dillon, V.M. & Board, R.G.), pp. 65–97. Wallingford, Oxon, UK: CAB International.

Tricker, A.R. & Kubacki, S.J. (1992) Review of the occurrence and formation of non-volatile *N*-nitroso compounds in foods. *Journal of Food Additives and Contamination*, **9** (1), 39–69.

Troller, J.A. (1965) Catalase inhibition as a possible mechanism of the fungistatic action of sorbic acid. *Canadian Journal of Microbiology*, **11**, 611–617.

Troller, J.A. & Olsen, R.A. (1967) Derivatives of sorbic acid as food preservatives. *Journal of Food Science*, **32**, 228–231.

Tsay, W.I. & Chou, C.C. (1989) Influence of potassium sorbate on the growth of *Yersinia enterocolitica*. *Journal of Food Protection*, **52**, 723–726.

Tsuchido, T., Takano, M. & Shibasaki, I. (1983) Inhibitory effect of sucrose esters of fatty acids on intact and heated bacterial spores. *Journal of Antibacterial and Antifungal Agents*, **11**, 567–573.

Unda, J.R., Molins, R.A. & Walker, H.W. (1991) *Clostridium sporogenes* and *Listeria monocytogenes*: survival and inhibition in microwave-ready beef roasts containing selected antimicrobials. *Journal of Food Science*, **56**, 198–205.

USDA (United States Department of Agriculture) (1979) Acid producing micro-organisms in meat products for nitrite dissipation. *Federal Register*, **44**, 9372–9373.

Vahabzaden, F., Collinge, S.K., Cornforth, D.P., Mahoney, A.W. & Post, F.J. (1983) Evaluation of iron binding compounds as inhibitors of gas and toxin production by *Clostridium botulinum* in ground pork. *Journal of Food Science*, **48**, 1445–1451.

Vandenbergh, P.A. (1993) Lactic acid bacteria, their metabolic products and interference with microbial growth. *FEMS Microbiology Reviews*, **12**, 221–237.

Venugopal, V., Pansare, A.C. & Lewis, N.F. (1984) Inhibitory effect of food preservatives on protease secretion by *Aeromonas hydrophila*. *Journal of Food Science*, **49**, 1078–1081.

Vinter, V. (1970) Germination and outgrowth: effect of inhibitors. *Journal of Applied Bacteriology*, **33**, 50–59.

von Schelhorn, M. (1951) Control of microorganisms causing spoilage in fruit and vegetable products. *Advances in Food Research*, **3**, 429–482.

Wagner, M.K. (1986) Phosphates as antibotulinal agents in cured meats: a review. *Journal of Food Protection*, **49**, 482–487.

Wagner, M.K. & Moberg, L.G. (1989) Present and future use of traditional antimicrobials. *Food Technology*, **43** (1), 143–147, 155.

Walker, H.W. (1977) Spoilage of food by yeasts. *Food Technology*, **31** (2), 57–61, 65.

Walker, J.R.L. (1994) Antimicrobial compounds in food plants. In *Natural Antimicrobial Systems and Food Preservation* (eds Dillon, V.M. & Board, R.G.), pp. 181–204. Wallingford, Oxon, UK: CAB International.

Walker, R. (1985) Sulphiting agents in foods: some risk/benefit considerations. *Food Additives and Contaminants*, **2**, 5–24.

Walters, C.L. (1992) Reactions of nitrate and nitrite in foods with special reference of the determination of *N*-nitroso compounds. *Food Additives and Contaminants*, **9**, 441–447.

Walters, D.M. & Levin, R.E. (1994) Isolation and characteristics of a yeast from preserved fish hydrolysate notably resistant to propionic acid. *Journal of Applied Bacteriology*, **77**, 251–255.

Wang, L.-L. & Johnson, E.A. (1992) Inhibition of *Listeria monocytogenes* by fatty acids and monoglycerides. *Applied and Environmental Microbiology*, **58**, 624–629.

Wang, L.-L., Yang, B.K., Parkin, K.L. & Johnson, E.A. (1993) Inhibition of *Listeria monocytogenes* by monocylglycerols synthesized from coconut oil and milkfat by lipase-catalyzed glycerolysis. *Journal of Agricultural Food Chemistry*, **41**, 1000–1005.

Ward, R.L. & Ashley, C.S. (1980) Comparative study on the mechanisms of rotavirus inactivation by sodium dodecyl sulfate and ethylenediaminetetraacetic acid. *Applied and Environmental Microbiology*, **39**, 1148–1153.

Warth, A.D. (1977) Mechanism of resistance of *Saccharomyces bailii* to benzoic, sorbic and other weak acids used as food preservatives. *Journal of Applied Bacteriology*, **43**, 215–230.

Warth, A.D. (1985) Resistance of yeast species to benzoic and sorbic acids and to sulfur dioxide. *Journal of Food Protection*, **48**, 564–569.

Warth, A.D. (1988) Effect of benzoic acid on growth yield of yeasts differing in their resistance to preservatives. *Applied and Environmental Microbiology*, **54**, 2091–2095.

Warth, A.D. (1989a) Transport of benzoic and propionic acids by *Zygosaccharomyces bailii*. *Journal of General Microbiology*, **133**, 135–138.

Warth, A.D. (1989b) Relationships between the resistance of yeasts to acetic, propionic and benzoic acids to methyl paraben and pH. *International Journal of Food Microbiology*, **8** (4), 343–349.

Warth, A.D. (1989c) Relationships among cell size, membrane permeability and preservative resistance in yeast species. *Applied and Environmental Microbiology*, **55**, 2995–2999.

Warth, A.D. (1991a) Mechanism of action of benzoic acid on *Zygosaccharomyces bailii*: effects on glycolytic metabolite levels, energy production, and intracellular pH. *Applied and Environmental Microbiology*, **57**, 3410–3414.

Warth, A.D. (1991b) Effect of benzoic acid on glycolytic metabolite levels and intracellular pH in *Saccharomyces cerevisiae*. *Applied and Environmental Microbiology*, **57**, 3415–3417.

Wederquist, H.J., Sofos, J.N. & Schmidt, G.R. (1994) *Listeria monocytogenes* inhibition in refrigerated vacuum packaged turkey bologna by chemical additives. *Journal of Food Science*, **59**, 498–500, 516.

Wederquist, H.J., Sofos, J.N. & Schmidt, G.R. (1995) Culture media comparison for the enumeration of *Listeria monocytogenes* in refrigerated vacuum packaged turkey, bologna with chemical additives. *Lebensmittel Wissenschaft und Technologie*, **28**, 455–461.

Welbourn, J. (1994) Developing antimicrobial systems. *Food Technology*, **48** (6), 172.

Wesley, F., Rourke, B. & Darbishire, O. (1965) The formation of persistent toxic chlorohydrins in foodstuffs by fumigation with ethylene oxide and with propylene oxide. *Journal of Food Science*, **30**, 1037–1042.

Whelton, R., Phaff, H.J., Mark, E.M. & Fisher, C.D. (1946) Control of microbiological food spoilage by fumigation with epoxides. *Food Industry*, **18**, 23–25, 174–176, 318–319.

White, R.H., Howard, J.W. & Barnes, C.J. (1971) Determination of polycyclic aromatic hydrocarbons in liquid smoke flavors. *Journal of Agricultural Food Chemistry*, **19**, 143–145.

Whiting, R.C. (1997) Microbial database building: what have we learned? *Food Technology*, **51** (4), 82–86.

Whiting, R.C. & Buchanan, R.L. (1994) Microbial modeling: IFT scientific status summary. *Food Technology*, **48**, 113–119.

Wilkins, K.M. & Board, R.G. (1989) Natural antimicrobial systems. In *Mechanisms of Action of Food Preservation Procedures* (ed. Gould, G.W.), pp. 285–362. London: Elsevier.

Wilkinson, G.S. (1975) Sensitivity to ethylenediaminetetraacetic acid. In *Resistance of* Pseudomonas aeruginosa (ed. Brown, M.R.W.), pp. 145–188. London: J. Wiley & Sons.

Winarno, F.G., Stumbo, C.R. & Hayes, K.M. (1971) Effect of EDTA on the germination and outgrowth from spores of *Clostridium botulinum* 62-A. *Journal of Food Science*, **36**, 781–785.

Wind, C.E. & Restaino, L. (1995) Antimicrobial effectiveness of potassium sorbate and sodium benzoate against *Zygosaccharomyces bailii* in salsa mayonnaise. *Journal of Food Protection*, **58**, 1257–1259.

Winkowski, K., Bruno, M.E.C. & Montville, T.J. (1994) Correlation of bioenergetic parameters with cell death in *Listeria monocytogenes* cells exposed to nisin. *Applied and Environmental Microbiology*, **60**, 4186–4188.

Winkowski, K., Ludescher, R.D. & Montville, T.J. (1996) Physicochemical characterization of the nisin–membrane interaction with liposomes derived from *Listeria monocytogenes*. *Applied and Environmental Microbiology*, **62**, 323–327.

Wong, H.-C. & Chen, Y.-L. (1988) Effects of lactic acid bacteria and organic acids on growth and germination of *Bacillus cereus*. *Applied and Environmental Microbiology*, **54**, 2179–2184.

Woods, L.F.J., Wood, J.M. & Gibbs, P.A. (1981) The involvement of nitric oxide in the inhibition of the phosphoroclastic system of *Clostridium sporogenes* by sodium nitrite. *Journal of General Microbiology*, **125**, 399–406.

Woodzinski, R.S., Labeda, D.P. & Alexander, M. (1978) Effect of low concentrations of bisulfite-sulfite and nitrite on microorganisms. *Applied and Environmental Microbiology*, **35**, 718–723.

Woolford, M.K. (1975) Microbiological screening of food preservatives, cold sterilants, and specific antimicrobial agents as potential silage additives. *Journal of the Science of Food and Agriculture*, **26**, 229–237.

Wuergler, F.E., Schlatter, J. & Maier, P. (1992) The genotoxicity status of sorbic acid, potassium sorbate and sodium sorbate. *Mutation Research*, **283**, 107–111.

Wyss, O. (1948) Microbial inhibition by food preservatives. *Advances in Food Research*, **1**, 373–393.

York, G.K. & Vaughn, R.H. (1954) Use of sorbic acid enrichment media for species of *Clostridium*. *Journal of Bacteriology*, **68**, 739–744.

York, G.K. & Vaughn, R.H. (1955) Resistance of *Clostridium parabotulinum* to sorbic acid. *Food Research*, **20**, 60–65.

Young, J.H. (1989) *Pure Food: Securing the Federal Food and Drugs Act of 1906*. Princeton, New Jersey: Princeton University Press.

Zaika, L.L. (1988) Spices and herbs: their antimicrobial activity and its determination. *Journal of Food Safety*, **9**, 97–118.

Zaika, L.L., Kim, A.H. & Ford, L. (1991) Effect of sodium nitrite on growth of *Shigella flexneri*. *Journal of Food Protection*, **54**, 424–428.

Zhao, T., Doyle, M.P. & Besser, R.E. (1993) Fate of enterohemorrhagic *Escherichia coli* O157:H7 in apple cider with and without preservatives. *Applied and Environmental Microbiology*, **59**, 2526–2530.

CHAPTER 18

Preservation in Specialized Areas

A. PRESERVATION AND DISINFECTION OF PETROLEUM PRODUCTS

1 Microbiology and petroleum

Many of the microbiological problems that arise in the petroleum, engineering and marine industries are a consequence of the microbial spoilage of oil and petroleum products. This may occur during oil extraction and processing, during product distribution and storage, in end-use and in waste discharges.

Very many species of bacteria, yeasts and moulds possess the ability to degrade hydrocarbons and also the additives that are used in petroleum products. Many more microorganisms associate with the primary degraders, utilizing the intermediate degradation products. The microbes colonize a free-water phase, without which significant proliferation is impossible.

This proliferation may be the most significant

factor in system fouling, detrimental chemical and physical changes in product specification, equipment malfunction and accelerated corrosion. The economic consequences are frequently dramatic and expensive and justify detailed appraisals of some of the more important manifestations of microbial growth in petroleum products. Common to many problems is accelerated corrosion; it is frequently the most expensive component of the microbial problem.

2 Microbial corrosion

Microbes may influence corrosion indirectly by destroying corrosion inhibitors. This is an important mechanism during the spoilage of metalworking fluids (MWF) and lubricants. Microorganisms also accelerate normal electrochemical corrosion processes as follows.

1 Most aerobic microorganisms, when they aggregate in slimes or crevices, consume oxygen and create an oxygen-deficient zone around them, which is anodic in relation to relatively oxygen-rich zones, where there are few microbes. Oxygen gradients make electrons flow and anodic corrosion pits develop.

2 Most microbes produce acids that can be directly corrosive. Weak organic acids are usually produced, but a few species (*Thiobacillus* and *Ferrobacillus*) can oxidize sulphides and sulphur to sulphuric acid. *Ferrobacillus* can also oxidize ferrous compounds to ferric compounds. Organic acids corrode aluminium and bronze, this kind of corrosion can occur in aircraft fuel tanks and in lubricating-oil systems. Sulphuric acid will directly attack steel; this corrosion can occur in crude-oil cargo tanks.

3 Many microbes produce hydrogenase enzymes, which remove hydrogen from metal surfaces, thus depolarizing them.

4 Sulphate-reducing bacteria (SRB) produce hydrogen sulphide and ions, such as HS^- and S^{2-}, which are highly aggressive to steel (and copper and its alloys) and characteristic craters form. In carbon-steel corrosion, a skeleton of carbon remains, which is seen as a graphitic (lead-pencil) colour. The bottom of the pit is usually black (ferrous sulphide), although some reoxidation of this may occur at the surface of the metal. At the same time, SRB hydrogenase enzyme, depolarize the steel. The steel progressively becomes more porous and is susceptible to hydrogen ingress. Hydrogen embrittlement is believed to accelerate stress and fatigue corrosion significantly. When ferrous sulphide forms, it is itself cathodic and continues to drive electron flow and anodic pitting, even after the SRB have been killed or have become less active. Corrosion driven by SRB is very pronounced during intermittent aeration, in oxygen gradients or in regular aerobic/anaerobic cycles.

5 Consortia of interdependent microorganisms are involved in SRB corrosion. Many different species may be involved in each consortium, differing not only from system to system but from point to point in the same system. Although many of the organisms (bacteria, yeasts and moulds) can be identified, named and studied individually, those parameters which optimize microbial proliferation and corrosion must relate to a consortium rather than to the individual species. Microenvironments exist and differ millimetre by millimetre in terms of pH, oxygen, electrode potential E_H and chemical composition. They may also change with time, sometimes cyclically. Biofilm is a typical microenvironment for SRB proliferation. The overall microbiological process is usually that oils and occasionally other organic substances first become food for aerobic microorganisms. Partially oxidized compounds are formed and become nutrients for other microorganisms, particularly the SRB. The latter cannot normally feed on hydrocarbons but only on the organic acids, carboxylic acids and alcohols produced by aerobic hydrocarbon degraders. Sulphate-reducing bacteria cannot tolerate molecular or dissolved oxygen but extract and use the oxygen in sulphate to oxidize organic nutrients. They are protected from oxygen by the activity of the aerobic microbes, which locally utilize and deplete the dissolved oxygen; at the same time they change the E_H from 200–300 mV positive to a negative potential; this is another essential parameter for SRB proliferation.

Sulphate in sea water is reduced by SRB to corrosive sulphide; a little of this is assimilated as a nutrient for the reproducing SRB, while the remainder disperses as ions or hydrogen sulphide or reacts with the steel. Many other microorganisms reduce small amounts of sulphate to sulphide but consume most of it as a nutrient. Other

sulphur sources, such as sulphurized oil and sulphonates, occur in crude oil and oil products and can be reduced to yield hydrogen sulphide.
6 With regard to corrosion prevention, the above mechanisms rarely occur in isolation but are in various combinations or in succession. Corrosion rates are dramatically accelerated by microbes in the field but difficult to reproduce in simulators. Any antimicrobial measure developed in the laboratory must be validated in field situations.

3 Product-specific problems

Crude oils and petroleum products have widely different chemical compositions and are transported, stored and used in significantly different physical environments. Nevertheless, their microbial ecology falls into one of the following categories.
1 Water is sparse; the oil or oil product is nutritionally restricted; the oil and water phases are immiscible. This is the situation in distillate fuel. The lack of nutrients in the oil is compensated by short-term contact and frequent turnover of the oil phase and/or supplementary nutrients in the water phase.
2 Water is sparse; the phases are discrete, but agitation tends to disperse water into the oil phase; the oil phase is nutritionally rich. The phases are in long-term contact. This is the situation in lubricating and hydraulic oils. In some hydraulic oils, water is intentionally emulsified into the oil to reduce flammability.
3 Water is abundant; the oil phase is nutritionally rich and emulsified into the water phase. The phases are in long-term contact. This is the situation in MWF.
4 Water is abundant and sometimes nutritionally rich; oil is from spillages and often present as a surface film. Typically, this occurs in bilges, oil tankers carrying water ballast and oily water discharges.

Antimicrobial measures must be appropriate to the category, as defined above, and, if necessary, to the individual product and its specific location. These measures must be cost-effective, safe to implement, environmentally acceptable and in compliance with local, national and international (or European Union (EU)) regulations.

Routine use of antimicrobial chemicals in oily discharges is rare, except to combat corrosion in ships' bilges, and for this application specific anti-SRB activity, for example from Unikorn B (dimetranidazole), may be the only practical option (Hill & Hill, 1993). The first three categories will be addressed in detail in the following sections.

4 Preservation and disinfection of distillate fuels and fuel systems

4.1 The microbial problem

In fuels, the microbial ecology corresponds to the scenario outlined in Section 3(1) above: oil–water mixtures in which water is the minor component (usually *c.* 0.1%), present as a contaminant. The fuel and its additives are the nutrient source and sustain microbes in a lower layer of contaminated water (or water bottom, as it is called) close to the interface. Agitation readily disperses the microbes and their associated polymeric slime into the fuel phase.

In many fuel-contamination problems (Hill, 1978c), the contaminated water bottom is in contact with the oil phase for a relatively short time. As fuel is used or moved on and then replaced, however a fresh nutrient supply is presented to the microorganisms in the residual water bottom on a regular basis. One cannot expect much chemical change to occur in fuel if the contact time with contaminated water is short, and the microbial problem is thus primarily one of fouling and corrosion of tanks and pipes. Microbially produced surfactants may promote water entrainment in the fuel. In stagnant tanks, microbially generated hydrogen sulphide, derived from sulphate in salt-water residues and sulphur-containing fuel components, may be evolved and contribute to corrosion. If there is prolonged contact with the contaminated water, sulphide may become dissolved in the fuel, causing it to become corrosive and/or to fail sulphide-content specifications. Fuel in long-term strategic storage is prone to microbial problems and in such situations, given sufficient time, microbial activity may result in chemical change in the fuel, in addition to problems of fouling and corrosion.

The organisms isolated in fuel water bottoms are predominantly Gram-negative bacteria (particularly *Pseudomonas* spp.), yeasts and moulds. Of the latter, *Hormoconis (Cladosporium) resinae* was once considered the most significant, but the 1990s have seen a considerable increase in the diversity of fungal species spoiling fuels. In modern fuel-spoilage incidents, bacteria producing fouling polymeric slime are often the principal protaganists (Smith, 1988).

Microbial spoilage occurs in marine, automotive and other diesel fuels, in aviation kerosene, paraffin, gas oil, tractor vaporizing oil, heavy fuel oils and heating oils. Heavy residual fuels are prone to microbial contamination, but the consequences are not clear; generally, these are low-quality fuels and microbial fouling will be insignificant compared with other particulate contaminants, although microbially induced corrosion may be a concern. Leaded gasolines were generally not susceptible to microbial spoilage, but the advent of unleaded gasolines has seen an increase in the number of reported gasoline-spoilage incidents. Of concern for the future is the trend towards the use of biodiesels. These are blends of conventional diesel and esters of rape-seed oil, which render the fuel more readily degradable by microbes. This is a distinct advantage in the event of environmental contamination but can present a problem if degradation occurs before or at the point of use. Even small percentages of rape-seed oil esters can significantly increase the susceptibility of fuels to microbial attack (König & Hill, 1996). Common distribution practice, whereby fuel can be comingled, exchanged or blended without full traceability, means that these esters will be found to varying degrees in many storage, distribution and user facilities. Paradoxically, then, it may be that there will be an increased requirement for the use of fuel preservatives, often considered environmentally unfavourable, with the advent of biodiesel.

Early-recognized problems occurred in aircraft-wing tanks containing aviation kerosene. Within the fuel-storage space in the aircraft wings, a water bottom is formed; water, dissolved in fuels, is deposited from solution as the wing tank fuel cools in flight and also condenses from humid air within the cold wing structure. Fuel is turned over on every flight, but the water bottom is drained irregularly. Fouling and spoilage occur, but the principal concern is for pitting corrosion of the internal surface of the lower wing plank, caused by attached proliferating moulds. Obviously, growth cannot occur to any significant extent when the fuel is cold, and microbial growth occurs mostly in warm fuselage tanks and in underutilized aircraft. Luxuriant growth can be anticipated if water bottoms persist in ground-storage installations and was an early feature in warm fuel in supersonic aircraft operations (Hill & Thomas, 1975). Good housekeeping, particularly rigorous water removal, reduced the number of aviation problems and in the 1980s most problems occurred in diesel and gas-oil installations, particularly in ships. Here, there is no 'cold cycle', as there is in aircraft, the water phase is usually salt, not fresh, the turnover is less frequent and 'housekeeping' is generally less satisfactory. In salt caverns used for strategically storing large volumes of fuel, temperatures are more likely to be higher, *c.* 50–55°C. Not surprisingly, the microbial ecology differs from location to location and does not follow that found in aircraft.

4.2 Antimicrobial measures in fuels

4.2.1 General

Undoubtedly, a major factor in the success of antimicrobial measures can be summarized as 'good housekeeping'. The aviation industry has been educated to appreciate the microbial nature of fouling and corrosion, and has significantly improved the design of both ground and aircraft fuel installations to minimize water accumulation. This has been coupled with the introduction of better routines for water draining and fuel testing. However, a recent trend towards the installation of hydrant systems for fuel loading at airports, as opposed to batch delivery by vehicles, has hindered the control of microbial growth in airfield aviation-fuel systems. These systems depend on underground pipelines, which may accumulate contaminated water and release it at a critical stage in the fuel distribution, i.e. just prior to loading onto the aircraft.

The good-housekeeping message has spread rather more slowly to other users of distillate fuels, such as marine engineers and operators of vehicle fleets. Indeed, in ships it is accepted that a water bottom will inevitably be present in fuel-storage tanks, because they are often at the lowest point in the hull, and some vessels have fuel installation systems in which, as the fuel is used, sea water is taken into the tanks to preserve the trim of the vessel.

Where good housekeeping alone fails, antimicrobial chemicals can be used either to preserve fuels or to disinfect fouled fuel systems. Usually, the same active agents are used for both applications but at higher concentrations for disinfection. The requirements for a preservative compared with those for a disinfectant do, however, differ.

4.2.2 Physical methods

Various physical methods can be considered for decontaminating fuels and, where biocide use is not possible for health, environmental or regulatory reasons, they may be the only option. Any process that removes water and/or particulates from fuel is likely to have some beneficial antimicrobial effect. For example, fuel water coalescers will remove microbes from moderately contaminated fuel. However, in the event that fuel is heavily contaminated, there is a risk that the coalescer will become colonized and will then not only cease to function properly but may also actually infect subsequent fuel passing through it. Filtration at 5 μm will remove the majority of microbial aggregates and provide substantial improvement in fuel quality. At < 1 μm, filtration will virtually sterilize fuel. Heat (> 70°C) can also be used to decontaminate fuel and, if combined with vacuum processing, will not only kill microbes but also provide substantial improvement in fuel clarity, probably due to the removal of stable water haze caused by microbial surfactants. Where underutilized vacuum-distillation units are available on refinery sites, these have been successfully used to treat large volumes of fuel economically. Probably the simplest method of removing microbial contaminants is gravitational settlement, the principles of which are governed by Stoke's law. This determines the 'terminal velocity' (V_s) of a falling particle, i.e. the maximum vertical velocity which a particle attains before drag restricts further acceleration.

$$V_s = \frac{pgd^2}{18\mu}$$

in which p = density of particle (g/cm^3), g = acceleration due to gravity (cm/s^2), d = equivalent spherical diameter (cm), μ = viscosity of fluid (g/cm s^{-1}) and V_s = terminal velocity (cm/s).

Note that a non-spherical particle will be subject to greater drag and V_s will be smaller. A 'slip factor' should be applied to very small particles but can be ignored in practice. The density of microbes and microbial debris varies from 0.9 to 1.3 g/cm^3; most wet particles approximate to 1.05 g/cm^3 and 'dry' particles to 1.1 g/cm^3, both considerably greater than the density of normal diesel or kerosene.

To convert this formula to usable figures, for diesel fuel of 4.5cSt viscosity at 25°C, and V_s, expressed as cm/h and particle diameter expressed as μm. For an individual bacterium of 2 μm diameter, a yeast cell or fungal spore of 5 μm diameter and a microbial aggregate of 100 μm diameter (just visible), the values of V_s are 0.18, 1 and 460 cm/h, respectively. Thus, it is obvious from the above that in a quiescent tank not only will microbial aggregates and microbial debris gravitate progressively to the tank bottom but also, as time progresses, any viable microbial units detected in upper fuel will actually be very small units and have reduced fouling significance.

A rule-of-thumb time allowance of one foot tank depth per hour of settlement is often quoted, but this would not suffice for microbial aggregates less than 25 μm in diameter.

Very heavy microbial contamination, accompanied by prolific biosurfactant synthesis, can seriously impede the settlement process. Settlement of small particles can be reversed by fuel movement, such as convection currents. Providing neither of these factors applies, settled particles will accumulate at the fuel/water interface or on the tank bottom, where they can be removed or subjected to supplementary treatment, for example filtration.

The principal drawbacks of physical methods of decontamination are that there is no on-going antimicrobial effect and also that the fuel tank or system is not decontaminated. Physical methods are not readily applied to tank or system decontamination; for example, the use of steam lances rarely provides adequate kill of microbes, due to immense heat losses.

4.2.3 *Antimicrobial chemicals as fuel preservatives*

Typical requirements of a fuel preservative are that the agent should:

- be combustible, leaving no ash or corrosive residues;
- not be surface-active;
- be compatible with the fuel additives and fuel-system components, e.g. sealants;
- not affect the fuel flashpoint;
- not promote oxidation, corrosion or gum formation;
- be safe at in-use concentrations;
- be active against a wide range of microorganisms, particularly Gram-negative bacteria, yeasts and moulds;
- have both fuel and water solubility;
- produce no unacceptable emissions on combustion;
- in the water phase, be neither excessively alkaline or acidic nor corrosive;
- have long-term stability;
- be easily inactivated or safe in the water phase, so as not to present a health hazard (e.g. to personnel operating tank drains) or have an adverse environmental impact;
- be cost-effective when used continuously or semicontinuously.

Rossmore *et al.* (1988) have drawn attention to the various factors that affect the efficacy of biocides for fuel use. The relative solubilities in fuel and water (or partition coefficient) are an important consideration when selecting a fuel preservative. Partition of the preservative into the water phase is essential, so that it may act at the principal site of microbial proliferation. Fuel solubility is desirable for adequate dispersion and to ensure that discrete isolated water pockets are treated. For some preservatives, fuel solubility is imparted by addition of a carrier (e.g. glycol) to the active ingredient. During production and distribution, fuel will contact successive water phases. If the preservative is added early in the distribution chain and has excessive water solubility compared with fuel solubility, it will progressively leach into each contacted water phase and, by the time fuel reaches the end-user, it may no longer be adequately preserved. Fortunately, in storage tanks water volume is usually small compared with fuel volume (typically 1 : 100 or less) and hence, although water-phase concentration will tend to be high, equilibrium concentrations are reached without significant reduction in fuel-phase concentration.

Most biocide-dosing regimes are determined on the basis of total system volume (fuel and water), with little knowledge of the actual volume of water present; consequently, the concentration of preservative accumulating in the water phase can be difficult to predict. For most commercial fuel preservatives, the high degree of water solubility will tend to ensure that water-phase concentration is high and high doses, as calculated per total system volume, are often unnecessary. Even slight overdosing may present a serious health hazard to personnel (e.g. tank-drain operators) exposed to tank water. There may also be a hazard to the environment. Unfortunately, the lack of segregation and traceability of fuels in production and distribution means that a fuel-terminal operator may not always be aware that a fuel has had preservative added. Ideally, preservatives should be easily monitored and easily neutralized in the water phase, when this is drained off to waste. Particular care should be taken where tank water bottoms are passed with site effluent to biotreatment plants, as there is a risk that these may be inactivated, posing further environmental problems. A simple on-site preservative-monitoring device for the water phase is available and can be helpful (Hill & Hill, 1992).

4.2.4 *Antimicrobial chemicals as fuel and fuel-system disinfectants*

Generally, the routine use of chemical antimicrobial agents as fuel preservatives is not widespread and is restricted to situations or facilities which historically have been prone to contamination. More common is the use of antimicrobial chemicals as disinfectants. Often there is a requirement to decontaminate not only the fuel but also all tanks, pipelines and systems with which it has come into contact. Prior desludging or cleaning to remove accumulated biomass and biofilms may be necessary and is a prerequisite to successful decontamination of heavily colonized systems. It is also important to consider that, while biocide treatment will prevent further proliferation of the contaminating microbes, there will be no improvement in the quality of the fuel itself; dead microbes and biomass will still foul the fuel. Hence, where heavy spoilage has occurred, antimicrobial chemicals may need to be used in conjunction with other remedial procedures, such as filtration or settling, to remove biomass. In the worst cases release of dead microbial slimes from tank walls and pipes after biocide treatment can render the fuel unusable.

If the fuel is to be used normally after the use of an antimicrobial chemical as a disinfectant, the criteria in Section 4.2.3 above will apply to the selected agent. Usually, there will be an additional requirement for the agent to be fast-acting; down time of fuel tanks and systems is usually an important cost and operational factor. Fuel and water solubility is again important to maximize dispersion of biocide and treatment of affected areas. Progressive loss of biocide to the water phase is not generally, however, of concern nor is long-term stability. Generally, application of antimicrobial agents as disinfectants is most appropriate at the point of end-use of the fuel, where more control can be exercised over disposal and exposure of personnel and the environment. Disposal of the fuel phase is not a problem; it will be burnt in normal use. Water phases may need special treatment prior to disposal. Where disinfectants are used higher up the fuel distribution chain, environmental and health and safety aspects must be carefully addressed. All parties who may be affected by the presence of the biocide should be notified, although in practice this frequently does not happen. The consequences of this failure of communication are exemplified by an incident on a ship which was subject to a moderate microbial infestation; on refuelling with fuel which, unbeknown to the engineer, contained a biocide, the microbes colonizing the tank walls and pipelines dropped off, fouling the fuel and causing dramatic power loss.

The application of antimicrobial agents that have no fuel solubility can have some limited benefit. In storage-tank water bottoms, microbial proliferation can be prevented by maintenance of a regular dose of a water-soluble preservative. Isolated pockets of water may, however, remain untreated; the efficacy will be best where a permanent large water bottom is maintained, although the deliberate maintenance of a water phase in fuel-storage tanks is contrary to most traditional housekeeping strategies. The principal advantage of the strategy is that the fuel itself is not treated and consequently the inherent risks of biocide treatment are not passed down the fuel-distribution chain.

Water-soluble antimicrobials may also be used to decontaminate fuel systems after they have been drained of fuel and cleaned. However, fuel residues can impair the effectiveness of such treatment. Many water-soluble agents (e.g. sodium hypochlorite) are cheap and easily monitored and, for decontamination of large systems, their use may be the only cost-effective strategy.

4.2.5 Evaluating antimicrobials for fuels

The only current standard method for evaluating the efficacy of antimicrobials in fuels is ASTME 1259-94 (Anon., 1994d). It allows for the impact of fuel/water partitioning and time on the antimicrobial agent, as well as the effect of continual rechallenge. It does not, however, model the effect of biocide loss due to transfer of fuel over successive water phases, an important factor for fuel preservatives, nor does it assess the efficacy of kill within the first few hours of application, often an important factor for fuel and fuel-system disinfectants. Consequently, some modification of the test protocol may be advisable when assessing the suitability of an antimicrobial agent for specific applications.

4.2.6 Use of antimicrobial chemicals in aviation kerosene

Aviation kerosene is traded subject to rigid specification standards; if the specification does not list a biocide, then a biocide addition would render the fuel 'off spec'. This restriction does not apply at the point of use, but antimicrobial agents must be specifically approved by engine builders and users and the high cost of approval has restricted the range of available agents.

Biobor JF (US Borax & Chemical Corp.), a mixture of two organoboron compounds, achieved early market penetration and is still used widely for intermittent treatment, particularly when aircraft are considered to be at risk (such as when grounded for extensive periods) or when contamination is suspected. Biobor JF leaves an ash on combustion and hence, although approved by engine builders, dosing is restricted to 135 parts/10^6 for semicontinuous use or 270 parts/10^6 for occasional shock treatment. Unfortunately, it is not the fastest-acting or most efficacious of antimicrobial agents, but manufacturers of agents that have more potential as fuel biocides have yet to seek the necessary approval, primarily for commercial reasons. A recent development, however, is the granting of engine builders' approval to Kathon FP (Rohm & Haas), a mixture of 5-chloro-2-methyl-4-isothiazolin-3-one and 2-methyl-4-isothiazolin-3-one (see Chapter 2) and rendered fuel-soluble by formulation with propylene glycol. This agent has excellent efficacy and a history of accepted use in many industrial applications and in consumer products, such as cosmetics and toiletries. Water solubility is some 100 times greater than fuel solubility and the implications for health, safety and the environment alluded to above in Section 4.2.3 must be carefully considered.

Ethylene glycol monomethyl ether (EGME), more recently replaced by diethylene glycol monomethyl ether (DEGME), has had considerable success as a dual-purpose aviation-fuel additive, used particularly by military operators. The anti-icing properties of these chemicals are complemented by limited antimicrobial activity, providing an adequate water-phase concentration is maintained. The major deficiencies are that they are only slowly biocidal and hence not suitable as disinfectants, and also that at low concentrations they are readily metabolized by microbes and hence intermittent use may result in promotion rather than prevention of microbial growth. Fortunately, military users normally stipulate that each fuel load should contain DEGME at *c.* 0.15%. However, where the ratio of water to fuel exceeds 1:400, the low water-phase concentration will mean that DEGME is unlikely to be effective.

Alternative strategies for controlling microbial growth in aviation fuel have involved the use of chromates. Traditionally, fuel-tank paints and sealants have contained chromates, which progressively leach into the water phase, where they prevent microbial proliferation. The length of time for which the chromate continues to leach at effective concentrations has not been clearly elucidated. Strontium chromate pellets are sometimes dosed directly into fuel tanks; these can only be active when positioned to be in contact with free water, and this condition is difficult to guarantee. The antimicrobial effectiveness of some formulations has been questionable (Rubridge, 1975).

4.2.7 Use of antimicrobial chemicals in marine fuels and offshore industries

The restrictions for using biocides are, perhaps, less severe in marine and automotive fuels than in aviation fuels, and a variety of biocides have been formulated and tested with varying degrees of success. Those based on isothiazolines (e.g. Kathon FP), oxazolidines (MAR71, Schülke & Mayr), morpholines (Fuelsaver, Angus Chemie) and bromonitropropanediol (Myacide, Boots) are in commercial use. Unlike the aircraft biocides Biobor JF and DEGME, they do not exhibit antifreeze properties and will function at higher ratios of water contamination. Diesel-engine builders are generally prepared to accept their use more readily than aircraft-engine builders.

Many navies operate gas-turbine ships and find it impossible to eliminate water from the fuel-storage tanks. These tanks may be an integral part of the double-bottom structure. Not surprisingly, gas-turbine ships use similar fuel to turbine-engined aircraft. Microbial contamination is often substantial, particularly where the surrounding sea temperature is high. The fuel is pumped up to a service tank and from there fed to the engines and stripped of water by a coalescer unit. Malfunction of this is the usual symptom of microbial contamination. Improved housekeeping is only of limited value; some naval operators with problems have added Biobor to all fuel used, but this expedient is not effective if water content is high. Engine builders may also have reservations on this strategy.

In some turbine ships, and in some offshore-platform fuel-storage facilities, fuel is displaced upwards, as it is used, by sea water. Most attempts at antimicrobial measures under these circumstances have met with only limited success. Measures are usually aimed at adding a biocide to the sea water as it is admitted, but as this water is discharged again on refuelling, often into harbour waters, any biocide must be environmentally acceptable. A temporary solution has been to discharge this biocide-containing sea water into shore tanks for disposal.

In the past decade, there has been a remarkable upsurge in the occurrence of microbial problems in diesel-engined ships. Severe fuel-line and injector fouling has brought ships to a halt throughout the world. Distillate fuels have changed in chemical composition and additive content, and are more supportive of microbial growth.

Ship operators have been reluctant to use fuel preservatives and have favoured a disinfection strategy, activated ideally by a positive fuel microbiological test or a visual assessment, but more commonly by an operational incident. Few biocides have the necessary rapidity of action and spectrum of activity for this application.

4.2.8 Use of antimicrobial agents in fuel for trains and road vehicles

System fouling, filter plugging and serious malfunction of diesel-engine injectors have also been recognized as microbial phenomena in road and rail vehicles. The problems are usually resolved by good housekeeping, and biocides are added only when operational difficulties are experienced. In general, the procedures follow those described for diesel ships. In many cases, the operators have their own storage tanks, and these must be included in decontamination procedures. An increasingly important factor in selecting a suitable agent is the trend towards legislation to reduce environmentally hazardous combustion emissions. Some commercial biocides fell foul of German legislation, which restricts the use of chlorinated additives in automotive fuels. In the USA, comprehensive ecotoxicity data packages have to be presented to obtain approval for additives for automotive fuels.

4.2.9 Heating oils

Although microbial contamination of heating oils is commonplace, associated fouling and corrosion are rarely considered to be of enough significance to warrant antimicrobial measures, other than improved housekeeping. There have, however, been major incidents when heavily fouled heating oil has been distributed to domestic dwellings.

4.3 Monitoring

'Dip-slides' can be used to evaluate contamination in fuel-tank water bottoms, but results are erratic if they are used on the fuel phase. Test kits specifically designed for use with fuels are now available, but these are still not real-time tests (Hill & Hill, 1997). They are, however, useful for determining the requirement for or efficacy of antimicrobial procedures. The issue of what is an acceptable level of contamination is a complex one (Hill & Hill, 1995), and usually in-house standards specific to the use situation or storage conditions need to be set and then used in conjunction with an on-going monitoring programme. The selection of the correct sampling and testing regime is crucial, and the Institute of Petroleum has published guidelines (Anon., 1996). A sample containing water is most easily tested on site; it will give a 'worst-case' estimate of the degree of contamination and so provide early warning of the onset of spoilage. Because the distribution of microbes in fuel is rarely homogenous, a single sample will not provide a representation of the overall degree of contamination in a system. For representative estimates of the extent of contamination in a fuel tank, several samples need to be drawn at different layers; these may be composited for analysis if necessary.

The Biocide Monitor (ECHA Microbiology) is a useful device for assaying biocide concentration in water under biocide-treated fuel.

5 Lubricant and hydraulic oils

5.1 The microbial problem

Here, the problems to be discussed occur in oil–water mixtures in which water is the minor component (usually *c.* 0.1%) and is present as a contaminant. The oil phase is nutritionally rich and capable of sustaining very large populations of microorganisms. The oil may contain up to 20% of additives, some of them incorporating the vital elements nitrogen and phosphorus. More nutrients may be available in the contaminating water, particularly if it has been treated with anticorrosive agents. Although the contamination may initially be restricted to the oil/water interface, contaminated water droplets eventually become dispersed in the oil phase. The problem takes the form of fouling, spoilage and corrosion. Ships' engine crankcase lubricants have been particularly prone to infection (Hill, 1978a,b), as they are inevitably water-contaminated and are maintained at *c.* 38–50°C. Steam-turbine lubricating oils are also prone to water contamination and hence susceptible to infection; microbial problems have also been experienced in a variety of other 'straight' oils, such as cutting, bearing, hydraulic and rust-preventive oils. The phenomenon was rarely apparent before the mid-1970s, probably due to the simpler composition of oils up to that time.

The oil user can experience substantial system fouling, changes in the physical and chemical characteristics of the oil, corrosion and equipment malfunction, sometimes of a catastrophic nature. Additive degradation removes the beneficial properties which they would normally impart; alkalinity (total base number) decreases; microbial surfactants promote stable dispersions of water droplets into the oil. In extreme infections of crankcase oil, bearings may fail and the engine seizes (Hill, 1978a).

Hydraulic oils must be free of particles to function properly and hence are very sensitive to microbial fouling. Oilfields have extensive hydraulic systems, which may be subsea, and positive steps are needed to keep them microbe-free (Hill & Hill, 1996).

5.1.1 Causative microorganisms

'Straight' oils tend to be alkaline, with a reserve of

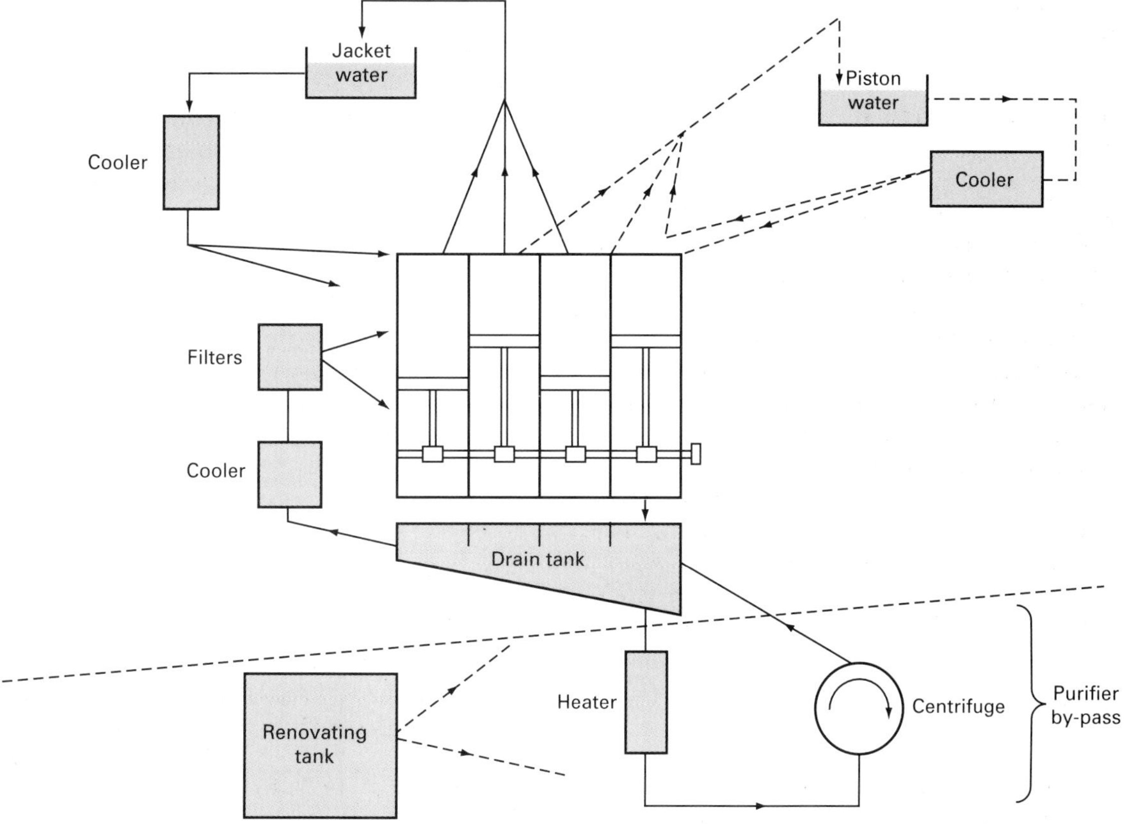

Fig.18.1 Simplified diagram of a marine slow-speed diesel engine. Above broken line: zones of microbial growth. Below broken line: zones of microbial death and/or removal.

alkalinity, and are either maintained at an elevated temperature or become hot during use. These conditions favour the selection of bacteria. Gram-negative bacteria are the predominant spoilage agents in crankcase oils; occasionally thermotolerant moulds, particularly *Aspergillus* spp., cause problems. Yeasts are frequently dominant in hydraulic and bearing oils.

Systems in use are usually well oxygenated. Engine lubricants are agitated; hydraulic oil is less agitated but contains oxygen dissolved under pressure. The microbial population will change when systems cool and become stagnant. Sulphate-reducing bacteria may then flourish.

5.1.2 *Source of microorganisms*

This is often obvious—for example, by filling new oil into dirty systems or passing it through dirty pipes. Frequently, the microbes are already flourishing in the water phase, which leaks into the oil, particularly engine-cooling water and sea water.

5.2 Sampling

Most oil systems run at levels of microbial infection that are negligible or can be tolerated. It is rarely possible to plan logical antimicrobial strategies without taking and testing samples from several parts of a system. This is particularly important when systems incorporate a microbe-limiting device, such as a purifier or a filter. For example, a complete set of samples for the crankcase oil of a large marine diesel engine could be: the bottom of the engine-oil sump; oil before it passes through the heater in the oil purifier and after it exits the purifier centrifuge; the drain from the reserve oil tank; before and after the oil filter for the main engine; engine-jacket cooling water (and the piston-cooling water system, if fitted); and the drain from the tank for renovating the main engine oil by heating and settling, if fitted.

The significance of these locations can be seen by reference to Fig. 18.1. The results must then be interpreted and acted upon if necessary. In Table 18.1, some possible results from tests on oil before and after the purifier are given and interpreted. If the actions listed fail to achieve a satisfactory response, other measures, such as a biocide addition, would have to be considered.

Sampling a hydraulic-oil system is less complex, but at least the system oil and the header-tank

Table 18.1 Tests on oil passing through purifier.

Dip-slide or SMARTGEL Bacteria and/or Yeast							
Before purifier heater (per ml)				After purifier centrifuge (per ml)			
Negative	10^2	10^3	10^4 plus	Negative	10^2	10^3 plus	Action at purifier
√	–	–	–	√	–	–	No action at purifier
–	√	–	–	√	–	–	
–	–	√	–	√	–	–	
–	–	–	√	–	√	–	Confirm heater 75°C plus. Purify continuously
–	√	–	–	–	√	–	Confirm heater 75°C plus. Check turnover is less than 10 h. Check retention time is more than 30 s. The smaller the kill the more urgent and thorough the action taken
–	–	√	–	–	√	–	
–	–	√	–	–	–	√	
–	–	–	√	–	–	√	

Notes. If any moulds are detected after the purifier centrifuge, conduct all of the checks listed for temperature, turnover and retention time. Samples before and after the purifier should be retested 48 h after any adjustments to the purifier. Any detection of viable microorganisms still present after the purifier would prompt a thorough investigation of the system and biocide application if necessary. A thorough investigation would also be indicated if the oil entering the purifier persistently contained large numbers of microorganisms.

drain should be tested and, if possible, the deposit on a filter.

It is obvious that a range of antimicrobial measures could be deployed, both physical and chemical, and expert help might be necessary to devise and implement the most appropriate and safe strategy. In Section 5.3.1, some suggestions are made for complex crankcase-oil problems, many of which can be extrapolated to other oil systems.

5.3 Antimicrobial measures

5.3.1 Crankcase oils

Good housekeeping. Emphasis is placed on water elimination and the correct operation of a purifier, if present. As indicated in Section 5.7, slow-speed diesel-engine crankcase oils are particularly prone to microbial spoilage. Lubricating oils tend to entrain water, and this may only partially be resolved by the normal dewatering procedures of heating and centrifuging. Batch renovation, which involves heating the whole oil charge to *c.* 80°C for 1–2 days, is less common than hitherto but is undoubtedly beneficial for its sterilizing as well as its water-separating function. Considerable data on heating as a key procedure in 'good housekeeping' have been published (Hill & Genner, 1981). High-speed engine lubricants cannot suffer microbial spoilage in use, as the oil temperature achieved effectively pasteurizes the system.

Most large engines have a 'purifier' to remove water; the purifier continuously heats and centrifuges a slipstream of the main lubricant charge. If the heater temperature is kept above 70°C and the flow regulated to achieve a 30 s 'contact' time, the slipstream is continuously decontaminated. Since publication of this knowledge, major crankcase-oil problems rarely occur. However, good housekeeping may lapse when a ship is laid up, and it is advisable to check for microbial contamination before lay-up and before recommissioning. Good housekeeping should extend to the spare oil tank, and condensate water should be regularly drained off.

Preservation. Experience has shown that the use of antimicrobial chemicals as preservatives is of limited success in engine oils. There is often an inherent incompatibility, which restricts active shelf-life, and when the oil is put into use the biocide may be thermally unstable or be washed out of the oil by alternating water ingress and removal. Preservation of hydraulic and bearing oils may be more successful and will be discussed later.

Decontaminating oils in use. Engine-oil contamination is often detected at an early stage by on-board testing, possibly after minor indications of malfunction. Experience has shown that growth of microorganisms in the lubricating oil is at first confined to a water pocket at the bottom of the sump. It can usually be successfully treated by pouring down the sounding pipe of the sump a biocide possessing water and oil solubility. The amount of biocide is estimated from a knowledge of the likely numbers of microorganisms in the pocket and the volume of the pocket.

In some circumstances, particularly where the ship is at sea experiencing some malfunction and microbes have been detected throughout the oil system, it may be considered necessary to treat the whole of the oil charge in use with an oil-soluble biocide.

The biocide used must be selected with great care, as it is imperative that it does not impair the functional properties of the lubricant. In brief, it must not affect the 'wear' properties of the lubricant or its water-shedding capabilities and it must be compatible with lubricant additives. Some procedures for carrying out these tests have been given by Hill (1978b). Any biocide application will result in the release into the oil of dead microbial sludges, which may block filters. Frequent filter changes must be anticipated until these dead sludges are removed. Supplementary purification may be practical to remove the sludges at the purifier centrifuge.

It is sensible at this time to look for and eliminate any obvious sources of microbial contamination and to check on the 'pasteurizing' performance of the purifier. In most cases, it would be unwise to add biocide to a contaminated hydraulic oil until the system can be taken out of use.

Decontaminating systems not in service. At an early stage, it must be decided whether the lubricating-oil charge is to be dumped or retained as still serviceable. This decision may be based on analysis by the oil supplier or a contract laboratory. If it is to be retained, a procedure would be to pump most of the charge up for batch heat sterilization, add oil-soluble biocide to the remainder of the charge and circulate this in the engine for 12–24 h. This would then be dumped and hand-cleaning carried out. The heat-sterilized oil would then be returned to the engine via the purifier, topped up and re-treated with additives if considered necessary. Heat sterilization in a renovating tank must be prolonged and rigorous, as heat losses from the tank walls and bottom reduce the efficacy of this procedure. If the oil has deteriorated substantially, and is considered unserviceable, the whole oil charge can be heavily dosed with an oil-soluble biocide and circulated to sterilize the system before dumping and hand-cleaning. It is greatly preferable to carry out these procedures with hot oil. Depending on the cleanliness achieved, the circulation of a flushing oil may be desirable. In high-risk situations, biocide should be added to the new oil charge, but the protection is likely to be temporary.

In the majority of incidents, microbial proliferation would also take place in the engine-cooling waters (cylinder and piston) and these are a major source of both contaminating water and degradative microbes. These coolants should therefore be discarded when convenient, flushed with aqueous biocide, hand-cleaned and refilled. The cooling waters are invariably treated in use with corrosion-inhibiting chemicals, particularly nitrite–borate formulations or soluble oils, and these support microbial growth.

Biocides cannot be used in coolants in operational use if the coolant is the heat source for the potable-water evaporator.

5.3.2 *Hydraulic-oil systems*

The strategies outlined above may not be appropriate for hydraulic-oil systems. Biocide additions made to systems in use via the header tank will have only a local effect if the system oil does not circulate through the tank. A pump-out and biocide flush may be necessary. In complex systems, microbial growth may be focused at 'slugs' of contaminating water. Even if there is a preservative biocide in the oil, its diffusion across the oil/water interface into the water 'slug' will be very slow under static oil conditions. Nevertheless, a very careful biocide selection procedure, based on laboratory experiments, will indicate the most appropriate chemical preservative agent. Preservation is preferable to decontamination, and Hill & Hill (1996) proposed the following selection criteria for the preservative.

- Soluble in and compatible with the hydraulic oil.
- Soluble in (sea) water.
- Long-term biocide stability in oil and (sea) water.
- Broad antimicrobial activity at slightly alkaline pH.
- Acceptable health and safety/environmental impact.
- Preferably, amenable to on-site monitoring.

Long-term biocide stability was evaluated using the ECHA Biocide Monitor (see Section 6.4). Typical results are given in Tables 18.2 and 18.3. It is of some interest that all of the products listed were sold as oil biocides but only the formulation containing isothiazolin-3-ones (BD) had acceptable long-term activity.

5.3.3 *Other 'straight' mineral oils*

Microbial growth in turbine oils is not uncommon, particularly in electricity-generating units, and the treatment procedures would generally follow those suggested for ships' lubricating oil, always paying due regard to minimum interference with the functional properties of the oil. The water ingress is usually from steam condensate.

Rust-preventive oils pick up contaminated water from residual wash water on the metal components which are to be protected. Strict control of the quality of the wash water is often the best way of preventing local growth and associated corrosion in the preventive oil film. For additional security, an antimicrobial chemical can be added to the rust-preventive oil.

Straight cutting-oil spoilage is initiated by carry-over of infected aqueous MWF from previous machining operations. Periodic bulk heating decontaminates the oil, and the aqueous phase separates and can be drained off.

Stern-shaft lubricants pick up sea water, and the oil is often supplied in a formulation that contains a preservative.

5.4 Biocides for oil

There is a very restricted choice of agents avail-

Table 18.2 Summary of antimicrobial activity changes during storage: residual activity in hydraulic oil %

	Storage time (days)					
Biocide	3	8	17	29	57	86
BP	100	80	60	50	40	40
BCS-8	100	*10*	*16*	21	14	14
		57	36			
PB	100	25	19	19	19	19
BD	*2*	100	*10*	> 89	> 89	*71*
	100		89			84
						86
						> 93
						92
						89
BSL	*2 days*	92	62	> 68	58	55
	100					

BP, formulated mixture of morpholines and dimorpholines; BCS-8, formulation of morpholines and 5-ethyl-l-aza-3,7-dioxabicyclo(3,30) octane; PB, *N*,*N′*-methylene-bis(5-methyloxazolidine); BD, formulation containing isothiazolin-3-ones; BSL, formulation containing thiocyanomethylthiobenzothiazole.

Table 18.3 Summary of antimicrobial activity changes during storage: residual activity in sea water %

	Storage time (days)						
Biocide	1	4	6	13	27	55	83
BP	100	100	100	100	92	73	62
BCS-8	100	100	100	< 84	76	67	59
PB	100	100	100	100	94	94	88
BD	90	100	90	> 100	100	100	95
BSL	100	80	*5*	< 51	32	*56*	10
			100			21	
			6				
			64				

Biocide formulations as for Table 18.2.

able. Compatibility with the oil product is paramount; the cost and time required to determine this are such that there is little incentive to move away from tried and tested products. Those most used have been *NN*-methylene-bis(5-methyl oxazolidine), 4-(2-nitrobutyl)-morpholine, isothiazoline derivatives and formulations and thiocyanomethylthiobenzathiazole.

5.5 Testing

5.5.1 In the laboratory

While the free-water phase can be tested directly with conventional microbiological procedures, including those for SRB, the oil phase must first be converted into an emulsion, by mechanically mixing it with a sterile aqueous solution of a non-toxic, non-ionic emulsifier (Hill, 1975).

5.5.2 On site

Aerobic bacteria, yeasts and moulds in the free water can be assessed with dip-slides. In stagnant systems, a semiquantitative assay for SRB is also essential; three suitable on-site tests for SRB are the Easicult 'S' test (Orion Diagnostica), the Sig Sulphide test (ECHA Microbiology) and the Sani-Check SRB kit (Biosan Laboratories Inc.).

Dip-slides can be used for the oil phase, but they normally grossly underestimate the microbial population, as either the oil fails to remain as a layer on the agar surface or it remains as globules, which do not absorb the aqueous nutrients. The

SMARTGEL technique (Hill & Hill, 1997) yields a quantitative result; a measured oil sample is incorporated directly into a thixotrophic nutritive gel, which is incubated until colonies can be counted.

5.5.3 Interpretation

It is of prime importance that the temperature of incubation is comparable to the temperature of the system. It can then be assumed that any microorganisms detected will be able to flourish at the system temperature. If the system temperature cycles or fluctuates, it is preferable to run replicate tests at a range of temperatures. However, if SRB are present, they are likely to be active in static pockets of water and a single incubation temperature (30–37°C) will be adequate. While numerical values can be attached to warning and action limits for aerobic microorganisms, any detection of SRB is cause for concern.

5.6 Future trends

Without doubt, over the last two decades the incidence of microbial problems in lubricant and hydraulic oils has decreased. In some part, this has been due to better monitoring and early recognition, but a significant factor has been the development of oil products more resistant to microbial spoilage. There is, unfortunately, a backlash to this latter trend, as a vociferous lobby, worried by visible persistent signs of oil spillages, is demanding that oil products should be biodegradable. There is thus a paradox: how can biodegradable oil products retain a resistance to biodeterioration in use? This is as yet unanswered, but one approach is to preserve them with biocides that can be readily neutralized when the product reaches the end of its useful working life. The small size of the market for oil biocides is not conducive to prolonged and expensive research in this area.

6 Preservation and disinfection of metalworking fluids

6.1 The nature of metalworking fluids

Metalworking fluids assist in deforming or cutting metal and function principally as coolants, lubricants and anticorrosion agents. They can be neat oils or water-mix fluids; the latter may be based on emulsified oil or chemical solutions or a combination of both. Water-mix fluids are particularly susceptible to microbial spoilage, neat oils being susceptible only when they become contaminated with water.

6.2 The microbiology of metalworking fluids

Microbial contamination of cutting-oil emulsions has been studied for over 50 years (Lee & Chandler, 1941; Tant & Bennett, 1956) and the economic consequences have been well documented. These oil-in-water (o/w) emulsions are stabilized with a variety of anionic and non-ionic emulsifying agents, and the hydrocarbon content in use varies from *c.* 1 to 15%, depending on the application. They are used to cool and lubricate a wide range of metalworking processes. Other chemicals in the formulation may control viscosity, corrosiveness, extreme pressure lubricity, smell, foaming, colour and microbial infestation. Some formulations, which are coolants rather than lubricants, are inherently oil-free (synthetic fluids) or contain a minor oil content as a microemulsion. Metalworking fluids are sold as concentrates, which are then diluted with water by the user. Many formulations are inherently susceptible to microbial attack; the organisms are free-living in the water phase and metabolize the ingredients in solution, at the oil interface and migrating from the oil phase. Fluid malfunctions are associated with microbial proliferation, particularly emulsion instability and corrosiveness. There may also be unpleasant odours, particularly following plant shut-down (even over a weekend), and there is growing concern about incipient health problems. Opportunistic pathogens can be present and aerosols of endotoxins can be created.

Formulations are normally alkaline (*c.* pH 8–9), and, as they are circulated and hence aerated in use, the initial microbial contamination is normally by aerobic Gram-negative bacteria. However, oxygen deficiencies occur as the flora increases, and it has been found that many of these bacteria are facultative, some by virtue of their ability to reduce nitrite, a cost-effective corrosion inhibitor, but now rarely used in MWF. After some time, tank bottoms may be sufficiently anaerobic to allow SRB to proliferate. An increasing problem is mould growth, particularly in the chemical fluids. Festoons of growth often foul the machine tools and circulatory system. Favourable conditions may be partly due to a fall in pH, due to prior bacterial growth.

Regarding the temperatures likely to be encountered during use, it has been found that the bulk temperature of machine-tool fluids is above ambient, although there are obviously also locally heated areas at the workpiece. Oil emulsions are used in substantial volumes to cool and lubricate rolling-mills; here, the bulk temperature is much higher (*c.* 40–65°C) and a different microbial flora can be expected.

The justification for antimicrobial measures is to minimize fouling, malfunction, smell, short fluid life, corrosion, surface-finish problems and short tool life and also to promote a healthy environment. The latter is encouraged in the UK by publications of the Health and Safety Executive (Anon., 1987, 1991, 1994a,b) and in Germany by the Technische Regelnfür Gefahrstoffe (TRGS) (Anon., 1993b). Antimicrobial chemicals are widely employed, although physical methods are possible.

6.3 Selection of biocides

6.3.1 Preservation of metalworking-fluid concentrates and fluids diluted for use

When preservatives (usually referred to as biocides in the metalworking industry) are being considered to control microbial proliferation, it is necessary to determine their activity towards the initial invading organisms. Preliminary information can be derived from the minimum inhibitory concentrations (MICs) against a range of organisms published in the biocide suppliers' data sheets. It has been found in practice that some of the commonly used biocides, particularly those functioning by virtue of a formaldehyde-release mechanism, have little activity against yeasts and fungi, and these organisms may present a serious secondary-infection hazard after the more vigorously growing bacteria have been suppressed. To guard against this contingency, a mix of biocides may be indicated, but in practice this is rarely carried out.

While it is obvious that effective biocides must exert their activity in the in-use water phase, they are commonly added to the concentrate at manufacture and must disperse in the water phase when this is added by the user. Relative solubility in oil and water is hence an important property of the biocide if the concentrate is an oil phase; the final relative volume of oil to water also influences the all-important equilibrium concentration in the aqueous phase (Carlson & Bennett, 1960). The practice of adding biocide to a concentrate is controversial, as the formulator must assume a dilution ratio over which he/she has no control. Too great a dilution will result in an ineffective aqueous biocide concentration, while too little will be wasteful and in some cases hazardous, if the excessive biocide concentration is irritant to the skin or lungs.

Preserved concentrates are expected to have a long shelf-life and any biocide incorporated must be selected on this basis. Some are unstable and never suitable for preserving concentrates.

As an alternative, biocides can be added to the machine-tool tank or to fluid that has been diluted for addition to the tank. Again, there are critics of this procedure, as target concentrations (often 1000 parts/10^6) are rarely achieved. Volumes of fluid in use are rarely known with certainty. Measuring equipment is sometimes only a bucket and the conduct of the operation is relegated to unskilled staff. A practical compromise is often to rely initially on the activity of the biocide in the concentrate and then to top up by tank-side additions of the same or a complementary biocide.

Fortunately, a strategy has been developed to assay the in-use concentrations of biocide in MWF (Hill *et al.*, 1986) and this will be discussed later.

6.3.2 Cleaning up microbially contaminated systems

The delivery of cutting fluids to the work-face follows two systems. In one, each machine has its individual reservoir and pump; top-up, to replace evaporation, and 'drag-out' (fluid lost by splashing and adherence to the work-piece) can be calculated, and this is carried out for each individual sump. Alternatively, ready-mixed fluid can be drawn from a central mixing tank. In the other system, the fluid is held in a large central reservoir and distributed by a system of pipes to the work-faces of the machines in the shop, being returned by open or closed conduits to the central holding tank.

Biocides have an important valid application as part of the cleansing process, which should be applied to cutting-oil distribution systems between changes of fluid. This procedure is aimed at breaking the sequence of reinfection by carry-over of residual infected fluid to fresh coolant. In this respect, the principles of good manufacturing practice applied to the pharmaceutical and food industries should also be applied here. Methods of doing this are given in detail in the third edition of the Institute of Petroleum's *Code of Practice for Metalworking Fluids* (Anon., 1995). In brief, two basic procedures are used.

1 Discard the original fluid; rinse the reservoirs and distributing systems with water containing cleanser, corrosion inhibitor and biocide, clean manually; circulate aqueous dilute MWF to rinse; recharge with new MWF.

2 Add a high concentration of detergent biocide to the residual fluid; circulate for *c.* 6h: reject this and refill with fresh cutting fluid.

There are obviously many variations to these procedures and the method adopted is very much governed by the time and labour available and the facilities at hand for disposing of the volumes of liquid produced. Descending pipework poses a particular problem and it may be necessary to back up or even reverse the flow, so that pipes can be completely filled with cleansing solution. Floors and stonework around machine tools may become so impregnated with contaminated fluid that they, too, will have to be scrubbed and sterilized.

The cleansing formulation used should ideally posses the following properties: (i) it should be quick-acting; (ii) it should have a broad spectrum of biological activity at the pH and temperature of the fluid; (iii) it should have detergent properties; (iv) it must not be inactivated by slimes or the chemicals in the cutting fluids; (v) it should possess good skin tolerance; (vi) it should not be corrosive; and (vii) it should be disposable.

6.3.3 *Preservation of fluids in use*

Biocides intended for tank-side addition to the dilute MWF fluid, i.e. addition to MWF at the engineering works, will need to have different properties from those added by the fluid manufacturer before delivery to the works. They need not be quick-acting, although they must obviously be capable of coping with continuous recontamination from outside sources, such as carry-over from other microbially contaminated systems, detritus, contaminated rust-preventive and hydraulic oils, contaminated dilution water and airborne contamination. Of prime importance is their compatibility with the formulation components, particularly the oil-emulsifying agents. Incompatibility would soon result in 'cream' formation, i.e. mechanical separation of components by gravity, and ultimately a layer of unemulsified oil would appear on the surface, indicating that the emulsion had 'cracked', i.e. that the emulsion structure had collapsed. For some applications, such as aluminium rolling, the emulsion stability is critically poised and a change to greater emulsion stability is also functionally unacceptable. Hence the biocide should not alter the stability of the emulsion.

The biocide should not inactive the anticorrosive components of the formulation, which it might do by direct inactivation or indirectly by lowering the pH; rust inhibitors work best in alkaline conditions. Other chemical incompatibilities, with dyes, odour masks, extreme-pressure additives and copper passivators, may be experienced. If the user adds a biocide after microbial proliferation has occurred, scums of dead organisms may aggregate at the surface and plug filters. These additions cannot improve a partially spoilt emulsion, but they prevent its further biological deterioration.

6.4 Inactivation and depletion of biocides

Chemical incompatibilities work in both directions, and it is very common to find that the biocide is inactivated by an emulsion constituent. One obvious incompatibility is found between an anionic emulsion and a cationic biocide, and this is the prime reason why quaternary ammonium compounds (QACs, quats) are little used in machine-tool fluids. Many biocides are not persistent and lose their activity progressively in MWF, often within a few days and particularly at above-ambient temperature. This is of particular concern where fluids are mixed in bulk centrally, as any biocide incorporated may be ineffective by the time the fluid has been filled into the machine-tool sumps. Even stable biocides will deplete, as in most cases they are irreversibly bound to those organisms which they have killed.

It cannot be emphasized too strongly that biocide activity can be dramatically decreased by relatively small reductions in concentration, especially if the biocide has a high concentration exponent (Chapter 3).

Many users resort to the process of topping up the biocide concentration, sometimes at hit-or-miss time intervals, sometimes when obvious spoilage is occurring (much too late to be of any value) and sometimes by monitoring the systems. Traditional physicochemical biocide assays have been far too complex for shop-floor use, and it has been more practicable to estimate regularly the bacterial, yeast and fungal populations of the fluids, using 'dip-slides' (Hill, 1975). There is no agreed population level at which addition of further biocide is indicated, but many believe that 10^5 bacteria/ml is a reasonable upper limit. One must accept that modern 'biostable' fluids may continue to function adequately at higher levels of microbial contamination.

Hill (1984) described a new concept for on-site use, the Sig Test. The most useful versions industrially are those which rapidly and semiquantitatively detect nitrite-reducing or sulphide-generating bacteria. Hence, to some extent, the significance of the organisms is emphasized, as well as their numbers. Rapid depletion of nitrite impairs the anticorrosive properties of some grinding fluids. Generation of sulphide, especially the volatile gas hydrogen sulphide, is directly corrosive, as well as being of an offensive odour and a health hazard.

Any method that relies on a microbiological threshold being reached before more biocide is added can be criticized in that this permits some spoilage to occur. An alternative strategy is to repeatedly monitor biocide concentration and to adjust it to an efficacious target concentration. The advantages of this strategy are that biocide concentration is frequently adjusted and spoilage is averted, not 'corrected'. If coupled to microbiological tests, a realistic 'target' biocide concentration can be established and maintained. In large complex systems, we then have some guarantee that a biocide has been dosed at the correct concentration and is adequately dispersed. Experience indicates that different target concentrations may be desirable for the same biocide in different systems.

Simple colorimetric assays for formaldehyde released from donor biocides have been available for some years, but do not seem to be widely used. One problem is that such biocides exert their antimicrobial activity, due both to formaldehyde release and to inherent properties of the parent molecule. The technique is quick and suitable for on-site use, but will require calibrating.

Chemical and physical assays for other biocides usually necessitate initial extraction and/or concentration, followed by assay, using procedures such as high-pressure liquid chromatography (HPLC). The determination may not correlate with known antimicrobial activity, particularly if more than one active agent is present or where biocide activity is potentiated by a formulated component. The techniques are not suitable for on-site use.

There are, of course, a variety of biological techniques for assaying antimicrobial activity, all involving the inhibition of growth of a sensitive microorganism. A simple biological assay was proposed for MWF by Hill *et al.* (1986). The original configuration and sensitivity were modified in an upgraded version in 1996. The assay organism is a *Bacillus* sp. The spores of this organism, plus dried nutrients and a growth-indicating dye, are carried on a pad mounted on a 6 mm×74 mm plastic strip. This is dipped briefly into the fluid to be assayed and incubated overnight at 37°C. The colourless growth indicator turns blue when spore germination and reproduction occur, giving an obvious indication of the presence or absence of an MIC of a chemical inhibitor. The strip can be calibrated against known biocides and biocide mixtures; the MIC so determined is then utilized to assay unknown biocide concentrations in a fluid in use, by testing a range of dilutions. A simple calculation yields the approximate concentration of biocide present.

The device used is referred to as a Biocide Monitor (Echa Microbiology Ltd., Cardiff Workshops, Cardiff). The assay organism is much more sensitive to biocides than are normal spoilage organisms, and hence the MIC determined for the device against a specific biocide is much lower than the target in-use concentration of that biocide. Using this device, it is relatively easy to determine whether target biocide concentrations have been achieved and are being maintained and to adjust concentration if necessary.

Example. An MWF is preserved with biocide *X*; the MIC of the Biocide Monitor for biocide *X* is 100 parts/10^6 and the target concentration is 1000 parts/10^6. A sample is taken and dilutions of 1/5 and 1/10 are tested with the Biocide Monitor. Results are given in Table 18.4. This simple procedure maintains the target concentration and avoids any adverse consequences of biocide overdosing.

Protocols can be developed for checking biocide concentration in MWF concentrates and bulk reservoirs of dilute MWF. The device is also used to monitor residual biocide in effluent discharges. If a rapidly growing thermophilic bacillus is used as the sensitive organism the assay time, at 64°C, can be reduced to 3 h.

6.5 Changes in microflora

There is some evidence that resistant strains of bacteria appear, but in most cases actual biocide assays indicate that the dosage is, in fact, inadequate (Hill *et al.*, 1986). It is, however, common to find, as stated earlier, substantial secondary yeast and fungal contamination occurring even at high pH. This, of course, will necessitate a change in the biocide regime, usually by addition of an antifungal agent tank-side. Some machine shops consider it prudent to alternate biocides routinely.

6.6 The ideal long-term biocide

The desirable properties of a preservative for both the concentrate and diluted emulsion may be summarized as follows.

- Speed of kill sufficient to cope with recontamination.
- Broad spectrum of biological activity at the pH and temperature of the cutting fluids.
- Not inactivated by the cutting-fluid formulation components.
- More soluble in water than oil.
- Good skin and inhalation tolerance.
- No detrimental effect on functional properties of the cutting fluids.
- Safe to handle and easy to monitor.
- Disposable.

6.7 Health hazards from biocides

There is considerable concern about possible health hazards from biocides, and undoubtedly there are occasions when skin irritation has been experienced. The evidence for direct irritancy is not always good, however, and there are often clear indicators that substantial overdosing has often been involved or that the observed effect was due to a complex reaction involving both biocide and fluid. The use of fluids, especially with high-speed tools, may create a fine mist in the atmosphere. This should be borne in mind when contemplating biocide-inhalation toxicity.

The use of MWF (and any biocides subsequently added) is regulated in the UK by the Control of Substances Hazardous to Health Regulations (COSHH) (Anon., 1994c). Any perceived risk from biocides must be balanced against the risk from proliferating opportunistic pathogens, such as *Pseudomonas* and *Legionella* and the risk from inhalation of an endotoxin mist. Nitrosating (nitrite-donating or nitrite-releasing) biocides are not allowed in Germany by the TRGS 611 Regulations (Anon., 1993b), as some MWF contain amines and it is now well known that these can combine slowly with nitrite to form carcinogenic nitrosamines.

Less well known is the fact that formaldehyde

Table 18.4 The Biocide Monitor and its application.

Colour developed		
1/5 Dilution	1/10 Dilution	Action
White	White	None
White	Blue	Add 500 parts/10^6 '*X*'
Blue	Blue	Add 1000 parts/10^6 '*X*'

significantly promotes this reaction. A few biocides are nitrosating agents and also release formaldehyde. A large proportion of biocides used in MWF owe at least part of their activity to the release of formaldehyde. Considerable concern was documented in the USA (Department of Health Education and Welfare (DHEW) National Institute for Occupational Safety and Health (NIOSH) Publication No. 77-126 (Anon., 1976), which has led to restrictions on the use of formaldehyde, particularly in Scandinavian countries, but pressures against formaldehyde vary in different countries at different times.

Health risks from MWF and biocides are high-risk/short-term when handling concentrates and low-risk/long-term for in-use fluids.

6.8 Combination and physical processes

To reduce possible hazards from biocide use or misuse, methods of reducing the concentration required should be mentioned. Increasing biocide activity by heat is one possibility, and rendering microbes more permeable to biocides with sub-lethal doses of ultrasound is another. Both are no more than laboratory curiosities at the moment. When fluids are held in a central tank, a batch pasteurization procedure can be applied to the bulk fluid. In-line pasteurization can also be used (Elsmore & Hill, 1985). Other physical procedures, such as ultrafiltration, show promise as antimicrobial strategies.

The principles of cumulative preservation by introducing a number of 'hurdles' are well known in the food industry and are of relevance to MWF use. 'Hurdles' can be introduced by selecting formulation components that contribute to an antimicrobial environment (Golec *et al.*, 1989; Hill & Hillenbach, 1993).

6.9 Biocides for metalworking fluids

The range of biocides for this purpose is extensive, and a list of compounds that have been or are used is given in Table 18.5. The list is not exhaustive and many active agents are supplied as mixtures. The general properties and chemical structures of some of these agents are considered in Chapter 2 of this volume.

Cresylic acid was an early-used preservative for cutting oils, but its objectionable smell and irritancy and environmental considerations have persuaded most formulators to seek alternatives. Some of these have been phenolic, although there has been a substantial environmental lobby to restrict phenolic discharges in effluent. The formaldehyde releasers (Chapter 2) have been widely used in all areas of preservation, including cutting fluids. The triazines, e.g. hexahydro-1,3,5-triethyl-*s*-triazine, imidazoles and hexamine derivatives are examples. Isothiazolones, oxazolidines and dioxanes are also widely used.

As in all cases when newer compounds are being considered, formulators should ensure that toxicological and environmental hazards are evaluated, as well as in-use efficacy and compatibility with MWF ingredients. Genuinely new antimicrobial agents are in short supply and will remain so because of impending restrictive regulations. An interesting development has been the exploitation of the historic antimicrobial activity of silver. Formulations of silver nitrate and titanium dioxide are available for use in cosmetics but are not yet widely used in MWF. There is sound logic in seeking an enhanced activity and spectrum for preservative systems for MWF by using combinations of two or more biocides chosen from those whose toxicology is well understood.

6.10 Other emulsified fluids

It should be noted that, for some applications, water-in-oil (w/o) emulsions are used, particularly where flame resistance is important, e.g. steel-mill hydraulic fluids. It has been found that incorporation of preservative into the aqueous phase before emulsifying this with the oil is a feasible approach. If a biocide must be added after the emulsion has been made, it must have sufficient oil-solubility to disperse in the continuous oil phase and sufficient water-solubility to pass from there into the entrained water droplets.

6.11 Test methods

Many in-house procedures exist for evaluating biocide efficacy in MWF and two standard methods have been published, ASTM E686-91 and

Table 18.5 Examples of compounds used in the preservation of cutting-oil emulsions.

2-Phenylphenol
p-Chloro-*m*-cresol
2-Bromo-2-nitropropane-1,3-diol
NN-methylene-bis (5-methyl-oxazolidine)
2-*n*-Octyl-4-isothiazolin-3-one
Dichlorophane
6-Acetoxy-2,4-dimethyl-1,3-dioxane
1,3-Di(hydroxymethyl)-5,5-dimethyl-2,4-dioxoimidazole
N,N-methylenebis-5′-(1-hydroxymethyl-2,5,-dioxo-4-imidazolidinyl urea
5-Chloro-2-methyl-4-isothiazolin-3-one mixed with 2-methyl-4-isothiazolin-3-one
cis-1-(3-Chlorallyl-3,5,7-triaza-1-azonia)adamantane chloride
Hexahydro-1,3,5-triethyl-*s*-triazine
1,3-Dichloro-5-dimethyldioxomimidazole
1,2-Benzisothiazolin-3-one
4-(2-Nitrobutyl)-morpholine
Tris(hydroxymethyl)nitromethane
Sodium-2-pyridinethiol-1-oxide
4,4-Dimethyloxazolidine

ASTM D3946-92. Method ASTM E979-91 refers to tests on invert emulsions, such as hydraulic fluids. These methods are often adapted to fit particular fluids and particular situations. The data produced are comparative rather than absolute and field trials usually follow.

The spoilage and performance of MWF is affected by non-microbiological factors, particularly pH, concentration, additive depletion and tramp oil (free surface oil). Efforts have been made to develop monitoring programmes for all parameters, leading to the design of a computer expert system to indicate trends, limits and actions. Modena & Merlino (1989) suggested the principles of such a system based on laboratory testing, as did Moseley and Dobson (1996). An EU-sponsored programme, BRST-CT96-5038, started in 1996 to devise a computer expert system based on on-site monitoring.

6.12 Disposability

With or without preservatives, cutting fluids (whatever the type) have a finite life, determined by solids content, chemical and physical change, performance failure and sometimes merely their acquisition of an objectionable smell. At this point, they must be disposed of in a manner that will satisfy national and local by-laws relating to pollution and waste disposal. This could be by approved dumping or approved effluent discharge, often to the local-authority sewerage. Dilution as a result of mixing with other discharges is often important. Normally, a requirement to separate the emulsion phases by chemical cracking and to remove the oil layer before discharging the aqueous phase would be anticipated. However, local authorities frequently require assurance that, if biocides are present in any product, they are not present in the discharge at a concentration which could inhibit biological sewage-treatment processes. In some cases the 'cracking' process already referred to inactivates the biocide or alters its solubility so that it passes into the oil phase. In other cases, a practical course of action is to dilute the discharge; fortunately, most of the common biocides are biodegradable at appropriate dilution. In practice, the dilemma is considerably eased by anticipating the disposal date and stopping biocide additions during the latter part of the fluid's life. Dutka & Gorrie (1989) have evaluated techniques for monitoring toxic discharges and commented favourably on the Biocide Monitor.

6.13 Future trends and conclusions

There is no doubt that the somewhat cavalier sale and use of biocides in MWF which existed in the 1970s and 1980s have been tempered by increased technical knowledge and a requirement to meet increasing regulation. Yet major incidents of microbial spoilage still occur and sometimes defy efforts to prevent them. New superbiocides are unlikely to arrive. The EU Biocidal Products Directive will eventually be finalized and impose more and costly restrictions on development and supply. Well-tried and established products are already under pressure and some will disappear from the market. At the same time, environmental lobbies press for biodegradable fluids and these will be even harder to protect in use. Effective antimicrobial measures still need to be developed.

The management of MWF systems for maximum functional life will frequently continue to necessitate the use of biocides. Many factors have to be considered for their selection and for designing a treatment regime, and it is only in recent years that the necessary technical knowledge and competence have become available. Environmental and health considerations are rightly playing an increasing role in this field and these and the economic significance of poor system management are highlighted in 26 case histories published by the UK Health and Safety Executive in 1994b.

7 References

Anon. (1976) *Criteria Document: Recommendations for an Occupational Exposure Standard for Formaldehyde*. Publication No. 77-126. US Department of Health Education and Welfare (National Institute for Occupational Safety and Health). Washington: USA.

Anon. (1987) *Nitrosamines in Synthetic Metal Cutting and Grinding Fluids*. EH49. HSE. Sheffield: UK.

Anon. (1991) *Metalworking Fluids: Health Precautions*. EH62. HSE.

Anon. (1993a) *ASTM Standards on Materials and Environmental Microbiology*, 2nd edn. E35-15. Philadelphia: ASTM.

Anon. (1993b) *Technische Regelnfür Gefahrstaffe 611*. Federal Minister for Labour and Social Affairs.

Anon. (1994a) *Health Risks from Metalworking Fluids —Aspects of Good Machine Design*. IND (G) 167L. HSE. Sheffield: UK.

Anon. (1994b) *Management of Metalworking Fluids*, 2nd edn. HSE.

Anon (1994c) *The Control of Substances Hazardous to Health Regulations*. HSE, London: HMSO.

Anon. (1994d) *Standard Test Method for Evaluation of Antimicrobials in Distillate Fuels (Based on Preliminary Screening and Compatibility)*. E 1259-94. Philadelphia: ASTM.

Anon. (1995) *Code of Practice for Metalworking Fluids*, 3rd edn. London: Institute of Petroleum.

Anon. (1996) *Guidelines for the Investigation of the Microbial Content of Fuel Boiling Below 390°C and Associated Water*. London: Institute of Petroleum.

Carlson, V. & Bennett, E.O. (1960) The relationship between the oil–water ratio and the effectiveness of inhibitors in oil-soluble emulsions. *Lubrication Engineering*, **16**, 572–574.

Dutka, B.J. & Gorrie, J.F. (1989) Assessment of toxicant activity in sediments by the Echa Biocide Monitor. *Environmental Pollution*, **57**, 1–7.

Elsmore, R. & Hill, E.C. (1985) The ecology of pasteurised metal-working fluids. *International Biodeterioration*, **22**, 101–109.

Golec, K., Hill, E.C., Kazemi, P. & Sköld, R.O. (1989) Oil/water partition for some hydroxylamines and antimicrobial efficacy in metalworking coolants. *Tribology International*, **22**, 375–382.

Hill, E.C. (1975) Biodeterioration of petroleum products. In *Microbiological Aspects of the Deterioration of Materials* (eds Gilbert, R.J. & Lovelock, D.W.), pp. 127–136. London: Academic Press.

Hill, E.C. (1978a) *Microbial Aspects of Corrosion, Equipment Malfunction and Systems Failure in the Marine Industry*. Technical Research Report TR/069. London: General Council of British Shipping. Reprinted 1983 as TR/104.

Hill, E.C. (1978b) Microbial degradation of marine lubricants—its detection and control. *Transactions, Institute of Marine Engineers*, **90**, 197–216.

Hill, E.C. (1978c) Biodegradation of hydrocarbons in industrial use. In *Developments in Biodegradation of Hydrocarbons*, Vol. 1 (ed. Watkinson, R.J.), pp. 201–225. London: Applied Science Publishers.

Hill, E.C. (1984) Microorganisms—numbers, types, significance, detection. In *Monitoring and Maintenance of Aqueous Metal-Working Fluids* (eds Hill, E.C. & Chater, K.W.A.), pp. 97–112. Chichester: John Wiley & Sons.

Hill, E.C. & Genner, C. (1981) Avoidance of microbial infection and corrosion in slow speed diesel engines by improved design of the crankcase oil system. *Tribology International*, **14**, 67–74.

Hill, E.C. & Hill, G.C. (1992) Microbiological problems in distillate fuels. *Transactions, Institute of Marine Engineers*, **104**, 119–127.

Hill, E.C. & Hill, G.C. (1993) Microbial proliferation in bilges and its relation to pitting corrosion of hull plate of in-shore vessels. *Transactions, Institute of Marine Engineers*, **105**, 175–182.

Hill, E.C. & Hill, G.C. (1996) Prevention of microbiological growth in a sub-sea hydraulic system. In *10th International Colloquium—Tribology* (ed. Bartz, W.J.), pp. 2223–2228. Esslingen: Technische Akademie.

Hill, E.C. & Hillenbach, W. (1993) Dual purpose additives for metalworking fluids. In *Proceedings of the 6th International Congress on Tribology-Eurotrib 93, Budapest*, Vol. 1, pp. 322–326. Budapest: Hungarian Academy of Sciences.

Hill, E.C. & Thomas, A. (1975) Microbiological aspects of supersonic aircraft fuel. In *Proceedings of the 3rd International Biodegradation Symposium* (eds Sharpley, J.M. & Kaplan, A.M.), pp. 157–174. London: Applied Science Publishers.

Hill, E.C., Hill, G.C., Robbins, D.A. & Williams, E. (1986) Sulphide generation in metal-working fluids and its control. In *Additives for Lubricants and Operational Fluids* (ed. Bartz, W.J.), Vol. II, pp. 10.1–10.7 Esslingen: Technische Akademie.

Hill, G.C. & Hill, E.C. (1995) Harmonisation of microbial sampling and testing methods for distillate fuels. In *Proceedings of the 5th International Conference on Stability and Handling of Liquid Fuels*, Rotterdam, the Netherlands, 3–7 October 1994 (ed. Giles, H.N.), Vol. 1, pp. 129–149. Washington, DC: US Department of Energy.

Hill, G.C. & Hill, E.C. (1997) Microbiological quality of fuel—trends, tests and treatments. In *1st International Colloquium on Fuels*, 16–17 January 1997 (ed. Bartz, W.J.), pp. 269–273. Esslingen: Technische Akademie.

König, J.W. & Hill, E.C. (1996) Biodeterioration of green fuels—cause, detection, prevention. Appended to *Papers of the 10th International Biodeterioration and Biodegradation Symposium*, Hamburg, Vol. 133, DECHEMA, 15–18 September 1996.

Lee, M. & Chandler, A.C. (1941) A study of the nature, growth and control of bacteria in cutting compounds. *Journal of Bacteriology*, **41**, 373–386.

Modena, M. & Merlino, G. (1989) Computerized expert system for diagnosis and control of aqueous metalworking fluids. In *Proceedings Update II Aspects of Microbial Control*. London: Institute of Petroleum.

Mosely, L. & Dobson, O. (1996) Knowledge and representation for reasoning: tables, frames and rules in a cutting fluids application. In *Artificial Intelligence for Engineering Design, Analysis and Manufacturing*, pp. 37–45. CUP.

Rossmore, H.W. (1985) Microbial degradation of water based metal-working fluids. In *Comprehensive Biotechnology* (ed. Moo Young, M.), Vol. 14, pp. 249–269. Oxford: Pergamon Press.

Rossmore, H.W. Wireman, J.W., Rossmore, L.A. & Riha, V.F. (1988) Factors to consider in testing biocides for distillate fuels. In *Distillate Fuel: Contamination, Storage and Handling*, ASTM STP 1005 (eds Chesnau, H.L. & Doris, M.M.), pp. 95–104. Philadelphia: American Society for Testing and Materials.

Rubridge, T. (1975) Inadequacy of a strontium chromate formulation for control of fungal growth in a kerosene/water system. *International Biodeterioration Bulletin*, **11**, 133–135.

Smith, R.N. (1988) Bacterial extra-cellular polymers: a major cause of spoilage in middle distillate fuels. *In Biodeterioration 7* (eds Houghton, D.R., Smith, R.N. & Eggins, H.O.W.), pp. 256–262. London: Elsevier Applied Science Publishers.

Tant, C.O. & Bennett, E.O. (1956). The isolation of pathogenic bacteria from used emulsions. *Applied Microbiology*, **4**, 332–338.

B. TEXTILE AND LEATHER PRESERVATION

1 Introduction

Biodeterioration of textile and leather materials refers to a decrease in value of such materials or a reduction in the ability of such products to fulfill the function for which they were intended, due to the biological activities of macro- and/or micro-organisms. It encompasses all biological processes that affect the textile- and leather-processing industries adversely.

Under suitable environmental conditions during textile and leather processing, microbial growth and proliferation may occur on exposed or stored leather or textile substrates, which in turn may result in a variety of spoilage phenomena (e.g. odour production, fibre tendering, strength loss, variegate pigmentation, etc.) and a subsequent devaluation of the substrate. Textile and leather materials may be affected by both aesthetic biodeterioration and chemical assimilatory/dissimilatory biodeterioration. For example, microbes may be found growing on otherwise undamaged textile substrates, utilizing dirt and other extraneous substances, which leads to the development of an unpleasant aesthetic appearance (such as pigment staining) and seriously detracts from its value. Alternatively, the substrate itself may be utilized as a source of nutrient and/or suffer biochemical damage, due to the excretion of waste products.

Reported incidences of biodeterioration in the textile and leather industries are characterized by their sporadic nature. The primary agents of biological attack of such materials are bacteria, fungi and insects. A range of factors are known to affect the incidence and severity of product spoilage (Table 18.6).

A diverse range of chemicals, antimicrobial agents or biocides are applied to textile substrates at different stages of manufacture to prevent microbial degradation and/or insect attack. Biocides may be applied as rot-proofing treatments, to provide temporary protection during processing or as hygienic finishes. Some guidance on the selection of textile preservatives is available. British

Table 18.6 Factors affecting substrate biodeterioration.

Type of substrate
Presence of auxiliaries
Dyeing
pH
Degree of chemical damage
Water activity
Materials in contact
Stage of processing
Length of storage
Light exposure
Mechanical damage
Biodeteriogen distribution
Presence of biocides
Temperature

Standard (BS) 2087 (Anon., 1992a), Parts 1 and 2, deals with methods of treatment and application of a range of textile preservatives, with a guide to the selection of suitable processes and methods of determining the biocide content of treated fabrics. The materials and processes are divided into two classes. Class A processes have been generally accepted and have been in use for some time. Class B processes, although of recognized merit in certain restricted fields, are not yet sufficiently accepted generally to warrant inclusion in class A. The agents are listed in Table 18.7.

There is an increasing focus, as preservative formulations become increasingly complex, to concentrate on performance requirements (Anon., 1991a). Part 3 of BS 2087 is in preparation (to be published in 1997) and will focus on performance requirements for assessing textile preservative treatments.

Table 18.7 Preservatives listed in BS 2087; Part 1: 1992.

Class A
Zinc naphthenate
Copper naphthenate
Cuprammonium hydroxide
Cuprammonium salts
Mineral khaki (insoluble hydrated oxides of iron and chromium)
Pentachlorophenyl laurate
Copper-8-hydroxyquinoline
Dichlorophen
Halogenated diphenylurea derivative
Permethrin
Class B
2-Phenylphenol
2-Thiocyanomethylthiobenzothiazole
Zinc-2-pyridinthiol-*N*-oxide
Dichlorophen mixed ester
Hexahydropyrimidine

Related products/formulations are used in the leather industry; for example, *p*-nitrophenol has been used for military purposes but may in some instances cause discoloration problems. Formaldehyde has been used during the pretanning process, although its use is being reviewed in the light of environmental considerations. Leather may be initially protected from microbial attack by the use of sodium chloride—the 'salting' process. At the tannery, the leather is soaked to remove the salt and additional antimicrobial agents may be applied. Antifungal agents may be applied to the leather in the 'wet blue' state before dyeing. Similarly, additional fungicide may be applied for increased protection during the dyeing process.

The use of selected biocides in the textile and leather industries is currently attracting intense scrutiny because of environmental considerations.

Anthrax, caused by *Bacillus anthracis*, has historically been known as wool-sorters' or Bradford disease. Deaths from anthrax in the nineteenth-century textile industry led to it being listed as a notifiable disease in 1895 (the first occupationally acquired case was recorded in 1847) and to the establishment of the Anthrax Prevention Order (1919). The last confirmed UK textile-related human case occurred in 1991 at a Scottish woollen-mill (Turnbull *et al.*, 1996). The UK Health and Safety Executive issued in 1996 a consultative document entitled *The Proposed Removal of Outdated Textile and Anthrax Prevention Health and Safety Legislation.* The consultative document seeks views on proposals arising from the Health and Safety Commission's Review of Health and Safety Regulation, to repeal or revoke without replacement certain outdated provisions that apply to the textile industry. Countries exporting animal hair are categorized as high-, medium- or low-risk. There are currently two animal-fibre disinfection centres in Europe. In Belgium SA Traitex utilizes a formaldehyde decontamination process, whereas in Germany Frele und Hansetadt operates a vacuum/steam-sterilization system.

2 Recognition of substrate biodeterioration

The importance of and difficulties associated with the recognition of biodeterioration of raw materials and manufactured products have been well documented (Eggins & Oxley, 1980). The following methods have been found most useful in detecting microbial growth on textiles. Similar methods may be applied to leather products. Microbial spoilage may be readily apparent, due to severe pigmentation and fibre tendering. A characteristic fusty odour may be associated with fungal growth and/or bacterial degradation. Detection at this stage normally implies that significant microbial growth has occurred. Sellotape application may, in some instances, be used to recover microbial fragments directly from textile fibres prior to examination. Direct microscopic examination may reveal extensive fibre damage due to bacterial activity or fungal growth on the surface or within the fibre (Greaves & McCarthy, 1991).

Supporting staining methods have been recommended for assisting the detection of microbial activity on substrates. These include: cotton blue–lactophenol; methylene blue G acidified with acetic acid; carbol-fuchsin; safranin; bromthymol blue; and the Pauly stain (McCarty & Greaves, 1988). Similarly, stained areas on wool produced by mildew sometimes fluoresce under ultraviolet (UV) light. However, as various optical brightening auxiliaries also fluoresce, the method is little used. These methods have recently been reviewed in a study relating to archaeological textiles (Peacock, 1996a).

3 Overview of techniques for testing textile materials for resistance to microbial attack

Test methods for assessing the susceptibiliy of textile materials to microbial degradation, or assessing the efficacy of biocides applied to such materials, are generally based on the 'challenge-testing' principle. This involves a method of deliberately infecting the substrate with suitable biodeteriogenic organisms, combined with a method of testing (usually visual assessment or tensile-strength testing) the extent of spoilage. The method selected for testing purposes should reflect the nature of the biocide and its expected in-house performance (McCarthy, 1986).

The major testing procedures may be classified as follows.

3.1 Pure-culture techniques

Samples of material are exposed to attack by a pure culture of a known microorganism under controlled conditions. The processes used for sterilization may modify the substrate (e.g. keratin in wool). The results obtained reflect, of course, growth in a man-made environment.

3.2 Mixed-culture techniques

The advantage of a mixed inoculum is the simultaneous exposure of test samples to a number of organisms, which may possess different susceptibilities to biocides and varied metabolic requirements. However, toxic metabolites may accumulate in the growth medium.

3.3 Perfusion techniques

This method allows the continuous replacement of nutrients and removal of waste metabolic products by perfusion during the incubation period.

3.4 Soil-burial methods

This appears to be the most severe and widely used test method. Test strips are buried in soil in trays or beds under controlled conditions and assessed for loss of strength. Variations in microbial activity will occur with soils from different locations, with time of year, etc.

3.5 Soil-infection method

Test strips are inoculated by partially coating them with a soil suspension thickened with kieselguhr, incubated over water and tested after conditioning. An aqueous suspension of horse dung adjusted to a pH of 5.5 to suppress bacterial growth has also been used. Alternatively, a manure/soil mixture has been used.

4 Laboratory testing techniques for substrate susceptibility and biocide efficacy

Methods selected for testing textile materials for susceptibility to microbial attack or to assess biocide performance will be determined by the nature of the information required (e.g. problem-solving or testing to contract specification). For example, samples of biocide-treated yarn or fabric as received from industrial sources are normally tested 'as received' or after being subjected to various durability procedures. In some instances, conventional chemical assay of the preservative will suffice. In other cases, biological testing may be required.

4.1 Durability testing

The samples may be initially pretreated as follows.
1 Water leaching. Immersed the textile sample in a large beaker or flask of tap water flowing at a rate that will give approximately two to three volume changes per hour. Use an initial liquor ratio of 1:100 (w/w). Continue the process for 24 h. Air-dry the samples at room temperature on a 'washing-line' arrangement, composed of two laboratory clamps and connecting string.
2 Heat ageing. Expose the sample in a dry oven at between 100 and 105°C for 24 h. Ensure that the oven is well ventilated.
3 Light exposure. Expose the samples as specified in method BO2 of BS 1006 (Anon., 1993).
4 Weathering. Expose the samples as specified in method BO4 of BS 1006 (Anon., 1993).

Durability trials are normally required only for very specialized applications (e.g. woollen felt for use in paper-making, military textiles, etc.).

4.2 Application of biocides under laboratory conditions

For laboratory biocide applications, the following standard test cloths may be used.
1 100% worsted flannel (style 526) supplied by Testfabrics Inc., Middlesex, New Jersey, USA.
2 100% wool cloth supplied by the Society of Dyers and Colourists (SDC), Bradford, UK.
3 100% cotton control cloth to confirm inoculum viability, supplied by the British Textile Technology Group, Manchester, UK.

Biocides may normally be applied to the test fabrics in an aqueous solution with a Jeffreys Trial Dyeing rig (or comparable laboratory dyeing equipment). The conditions in the test rig may be adjusted as appropriate to conform to condition in an industrial dyeing winch or scouring set. The system of application will be determined by the nature of the biocide, the particular processing conditions (i.e. duration of process, temperature, etc.), the textile substrate and the degree of protection required. For comparing biocide efficacy, a uniform system (determined by the individual constraints of the industrial problem) is required.

Similarly, biocides may be applied using full-scale processing machinery.

- Application to yarn packages using a Morel conditioning machine.
- Direct application to yarn via a lick roller on conventional spinning machines.
- Incorporation into an oil emulsion applied to loose stock before carding and spinning.
- Direct application via conventional dyeing machines and scouring sets.

4.3 Standard test methods

The most widely used and accepted testing standards employed by government and industry alike in determining antimicrobial effectiveness in textiles are those set forth by the American Association of Textile Chemists and Colorists (AATCC) and by the British Standards Institution (BSI). A wide variety of national and industrial test methods are currently under review by the ISO/TC38 Textiles Committee of the International Organization for Standardization (ISO) and the European Committee for Standardization (CEN) TC 248/SC3/WG5 committee.

The following discussion of the major standard methods aims to provide a practical summary of the techniques involved. For full detailed information, the reader should refer to the standard texts as appropriate. For example, the foreword to BS 6085 (Anon., 1992b) states that the general purpose of these methods is to determine susceptibility of textiles to microorganisms and to evaluate the resistance of treated textiles and textile-containing products to attack by microorganisms. It may be slightly modified to cover leather materials. The standard specifies three areas of testing, whereby specimens of the material under test are subjected to microbial attack by soil burial, by mixed inoculation on an agar plate or in a saturated atmosphere. Biocide efficacy is observed as a significant reduction in strength loss compared with similar material without biocide addition or as prevention of visual surface discoloration.

4.3.1 British Standard 6085: 1992 (Anon., 1992b)

This standard has been revised and now features four test options.

Section 2: soil burial test. This is a very severe test for most textile materials. Fabric or yarn specimens (150 mm × 25 mm or 600 mm, respectively) are buried to a depth of 30–50 mm in John Innes No. 1 potting compost in plastic or metal trays. A loose-fitting lid is required to maintain the moisture content of the soil between 20 and 30%. Glass plates are used to separate neighbouring fabric specimens in the trays. Ten specimens of the material under test are required and five of a cotton control cloth (which should show a strength loss of at least 80% after incubation) for each experiment. The prepared soil trays are placed in an incubator at 28 ± 18°C, with a relative humidity (r.h.) of at least 95%. The cotton control cloths are removed after 7 days' incubation, with particles of soil being removed by gentle agitation and brushing before rinsing with water. The specimens or fragments are then sterilized by soaking in 70% ethanol for 4 h at ambient temperature, allowed to condition (at 20°C and 65% r.h.) and their residual tensile strength (compared with unexposed specimens) determined in accordance with BS 2576 (Anon., 1986) (fabric) or BS 1932: Part 1 (Anon., 1989c). If a strength loss of > 80% has been achieved, incubate the remaining specimens for a full 28 days. Prepare the specimens for testing as above and record as a percentage the observed strength loss between the exposed material and the unexposed controls.

Section 3: agar plate test using fungi. The eight standard test biodeteriogens specified in the standard may be obtained from CAB International, Kew, UK. The cultures may be used only when they are between 14 and 28 days old. However, cultures less than 21 days old may be stored, securely stoppered, in a refrigerator at 6°C for up to 3 months prior to use. Add 15 g agar (Bacto: Difco) per litre of mineral salts solution, and 0.05% (w/v) dioctyl sodium sulphosuccinate to form a mineral salts/wetting-agent solution. Add 30 g/l sucrose to the agar, if necessary, to encourage fungal growth. Gently add 10 ml of mineral salts/wetting agent to each of the eight culture slopes. With a sterile wire look to scrape the surface of the slope to liberate spores without unduly detaching mycelial fragments. Decant the eight suspensions into a 500 ml sterile flask, containing a number of glass beads, and shake vigorously. Filter through a glass filter funnel containing sterile cotton wool to remove large clumps. If a large number of specimens are to be inoculated, pool the suspensions prepared from a number of fungal sets. Centrifuge the mixed spore suspension three times at 3500 *g*, discarding the supernatant and resuspending the spores in sterile mineral-salt solution. Wet out the test specimens (2.5 mm × 2.5 mm for visual assessment, four specimens per sample) and controls by immersing the fabrics in water containing 0.05% dioctyl sodium sulphosuccinate for several minutes. Place each fabric piece on individual mineral-salt agar in Petri dishes and add 0.5 ml of the mixed inoculum to each side of the material. Work in a microbiological safety cabinet when manipulating the cultures. Autoclave and discard unused spore suspensions at the end of the day. Assess the cotton controls after 14 days and the remainng specimens after 28 days. Strength loss may be assessed, as described above. Alternatively, assess specimens visually in accordance with the grading scale listed in the standard.

Section 4: agarplate test using bacteria. This test evaluates the resistance of textiles, particularly woollen articles, to bacterial degradation. The textile provides the sole carbon source and is exposed to pure cultures of bacteria in the presence of a mineral-salt agar. Degradation is assessed by measuring strength loss. The microbes used are *Pseudomonas aeruginosa* (NCIMB 11070) and *Bacillus licheniformis* (NCIMB 10689).

Section 5: saturated atmosphere test. This procedure is intended for textiles that will not come into contact with fungi in the vegetative form but may be contaminated with airborne spores before storage in humid conditions. Inoculate 1 ml of the mixed-spore suspension (prepared as above) on to the cloth or related specimens and controls. Suspend the fabrics above free water (>90% r.h.) in sealed glass Kilner jars. Incubate for 14 days and assess the cotton controls. If the controls are graded 4 or above (against the visual scale), continue the trial and assess the remaining specimens after 28 days.

4.3.2 *AATCC Method 147-1982*

This method—*Detection of Antibacterial Activity of Fabrics: Parallel Streak Method* (Anon., 1993a)—is adaptable for biocide-treated yarns, loose stock and most carpet samples, as well as fabric. The defined objective is the detection of bacteriostatic activity exhibited by textile fabrics. The bacterial species cited in the standard are given below. Similarly, details of maintenance of culture of the test organisms are presented in the standard.

Prepare AATCC bacteriostasis broth as described. Adjust the medium to pH 6.8 with sodium hydroxide. Add 15 g of Bacto (Difco) agar per litre and adjust to pH 7.0–7.2 with sodium hydroxide to prepare AATCC bacteriostasis agar. Prepare the challenge inoculum by transferring 1ml of a 24-h broth culture (37°C) of a test organism to 9 ml sterile distilled-water control. After adequate mixing with a 4 mm inoculating loop, transfer one loopful of diluted inoculum to AATCC agar in a Petri dish; making five approx. 7.5cm-long parallel streaks 1 cm apart without refilling the loop. Locate the textile specimen (normally 1–4 cm diameter) transversely across the inoculum streaks and ensure intimate contact. Small sterile glass weights may be used to prevent the material curling away from the agar. Incubate all samples at 37°C for 24 h.

Results may be evaluated in two ways: (i) Growth-free zone—assess the width (in mm) of the growth-free zone surrounding the test specimens; and (ii) contact inhibition—lift the specimens from the agar surface and, using a low-power binocular microscope, assess the percentage growth-free contact area.

The latter method may be used to provide a rough estimate of biocide efficacy, in that the count of the inoculum will decrease from initial contact on the nutrient agar to the end of the final streak, resulting in increasing degrees of sensitivity. *Staphylococcus aureus* and *Ps. aeruginosa* may be selected as representative test organisms.

4.3.3 *AATCC 30-1993*

This standard—*Antifungal Activity, Assessment on Textile Materials: Mildew and Rot Resistance of Textiles* (Anon., 1993b)—is again arranged as four tests. Test 1 presents a soil-burial method, which may be used as an alternative to BS 6085:1992. The agar-plate—pure culture—sterile-specimen method, which forms the basis of test 2 is for cellulosic materials only and utilizes *Chaetomium globosum* (ATCC 6205). Test 3 is recommended for evaluation of textile specimens where surface-growing organisms are important. The method involves the growth of *Aspergillus niger* (ATCC 6275) on glucose mineral-salt agar. Prepare a spore suspension from 10–14-day-old cultures of the test organism by scraping the fungal mycelia growing on agar slopes into a sterile flask containing 50 ml of sterile water and glass beads. Shake the flask thoroughly to prepare a spore suspension. Prepare the culture medium as described. Autoclave at 121°C for 15 min; wet the specimens (3 cm × 3 cm) in water containing 0.05% (w/v) dioctyl sodium sulphosuccinate (BDH Ltd., Poole, UK); position on the poured medium in a Petri dish and inoculate the surface evenly with 1 ml of the spore suspension, using a sterile dispenser. Incubate the inoculated and control specimens at 28°C for 14 days only. Examine the specimens visually and microscopically for evidence of the growth of *A. niger*.

The initial specimens may be subjected to various pretreatments before testing (e.g. leaching, weathering, exposure to dry heat). Test 1 may be used to demonstrate long-term biocide proofing of material, whereas test 3 may be used to assess biocides applied during processing to provide temporary antifungal protection during manufacture. Test 4 offers a variation on the saturated-atmosphere test (mixed-spore suspension in a humidity jar).

4.3.4 *AATCC 100-1993*

This method—*Assessment of Antibacterial Finishes*

on Fabrics (Anon., 1993c)—presents a qualitative technique for demonstrating bacteriostatic activity. Specimens of treated and control fabrics (3 cm × 3 cm) may be tested qualitatively for antibacterial efficacy, using AATCC 147. For example, streak sufficient agar (AATCC bacteriostasis agar) in Petri dishes with either *Staph. aureus* or *Klebsiella pneumoniae*. Place individual treated or control specimens at right angles to the direction of streak. Examine for clear areas (no growth) either visually or with a low-power microscope.

Those specimens showing activity are then tested quantitatively. Prepare sufficient specimens (4.8 cm diameter) of the test substrate (and controls—made of the same material but untreated) to absorb 1 ml of test inoculum (note the number used). Apply 1 ml of an appropriate dilution of a 24-h culture of the test organism (one of the above), so that recovery at time 0 from the control or the sample is $1–2 \times 10^5$. Dilute, using AATCC broth. Sterilize the samples before the inoculation, using ethylene oxide or intermittent sterilization. Place the discrete sets of specimens in 0.2371 (8 oz) sterile glass jars and apply 1 ml of the inoculum evenly to the specimens, using a sterile dispenser. Include uninoculated but treated controls and seal the containers. For time 0 testing, add 100 ml of AATCC broth (or neutralizer solution, if available) and shake vigorously for 1 min. Make serial dilutions in AATCC broth and plate (in duplicate) on AATCC bacteriostasis agar. Incubate the remaining jars at 378C for 18–24 h and plate out as above. Incubate all plates at 37°C for 24 h. Report bacterial counts as colony-forming units (cfu) of bacteria per fabric sample (i.e. the number in the jar). Calculate percentage reduction of each test organisms for each fabric treatment. Uninoculated samples should be sterile, and increasing numbers of organisms should be observed on the inoculated, untreated control. The method is intended for biocide treatments which may not be detectable by agar-plate techniques (Anon., 1993).

4.3.5 European Committee for Standardization Methods

The CEN/TC248/SC3/WG5 'Determination of resistance of textiles to microbiological attack' committee was established in May 1992. It was given the task of reviewing and assessing established standards and methods. Following round trials and standard drafting, prenormative standards prEN ISO 11721-1 Soil burial test—Part 1 Assessment of rotting retardant finishing and prEN ISO 11721-2 Soil burial test—Part 2 Assessment of rotting retardant finishing (long-term resistance) will be issued during 1998. Further round trials are under way to develop tests to evaluate the action of bacteria and fungi on textiles. A standard 'textiles—evaluation of the action of fungi' is being developed based on prEN ISO 846 1996; 'Plastics—evaluation of the actions of microorganisms'. It will feature mixed and single fungal-culture inoculation, on agar with or without nutrient supplements, and will contain a section using a saturated-atmosphere procedure. Finally, a standard 'Textiles—evaluation of the action of bacteria' is being developed, based on Schweizerische Normen-Vereinigung (SNV) 195 920 1976, *Examination of the Antibacterial Effect of Impregnated Textiles by the Agar Diffusion Test (Using* Staphylococcus aureus *ATCC 6538 and* Escherichia coli *ATCC* 11229) *Contact Inhibition Test* (Anon., 1991b).

The CEN/TC189/WG5 committee has independently produced prENV 12225 'Geotextiles and geotextile-related products—method for determining the microbiological resistance by a soil burial test'.

4.3.6 Bioluminescence techniques applied to biodeterioration

Growth of microorganisms on textile materials may be assessed by the firefly bioluminescent detection and/or assay of adenosine triphosphate (ATP). For a quantitative assessment, prepare a mixed-spore suspension in accordance with BS 6085 (described above). Likewise, prepare all fabric specimens (preweighed and of uniform size) in accordance with Section 3 (agar plate test using fungi) of the standard. The initial stages of the test method were adopted to prepare standard contaminated conditions to encourage fungal growth. Incubate all specimens (three replicates per test material per assay time) at 28°C. At each time interval (normally 3 h intervals throughout the working day), assay the resultant microbial growth (McCarthy, 1989). A Celsis Optocomp luminometer (Celsis plc, Cambridge, UK) and corresponding

Celsis reagents (ATP standards, nucleotide-releasing reagents and luciferin–luciferase mixtures) may be used for ATP assays. Alternatively, samples may be boiled in trichloroacetic acid to extract ATP from the samples (Lundin & Thore, 1975) or immersed in various novel extractants (McCarthy, 1989). Test time zero time samples immediately following addition of the mixed-spore suspension. Inoculate all samples simultaneously and monitor growth of the inoculum at regular intervals over a period of 24–72 h (or longer, if necessary). Express results as an 'activity index', with units of picograms of ATP/0.1 g of test substrate, derived as a mean result from the three replicates. The assay thus provides a rapid non-species-specific test for microbial growth, with significant increases in ATP levels on untreated wool materials. The presence of a biocide applied to fabrics will result in prevention of growth or the rapid killing of the organisms in the inoculum. A positive untreated control (with developing biomass) is required to demonstrate inoculum viability.

4.3.7 *Additional national standards*

The following methods have been proposed for laboratory testing.

- *Performance Requirements for Textile Preservative Treatments Against Microbiological Attack*: UK Ministry of Defence Interim Defence Standard 68–141 (Anon., 1991a).
- Schweizerische Normen-Vereinigung SNV 195 920 1991 *Examination of the Antibacterial Effect of Impregnated Textiles by the Agar Diffusion Test (Using* Staphylococcus aureus *ATCC6538 and* Escherichia coli, *ATCC 11229) Contact Inhibition Test* (Anon., 1991b).
- Schweizerische Normen-Vereinigung SNV 195 921 1976 *Examination of the Antimycotic Effect of Impregnated Textiles by the Agar Diffusion Test (Using* Trichophyton mentagrophytes, *ATCC 9533 and* Candida albicans *ATCC 10259) Contact Inhibition Test* (Anon., 1976).
- Deutsches Institut fur Normung DIN 53 933 1992 Part 1 *Testing of Textiles; Determination of the Resistance of Cellulose Textiles Against Microorganisms (Resistance to Bacteria and Fungi of Soil); Identification of Rotting Retardant Finishing*—relates to soil burial (Anon., 1992c).
- Deutsche Norman DIN 53 931 1992 *Testing of Textiles; Determination of the Resistance of Textiles to Mildew, Growth Test* (Anon., 1992d).

5 Leather

Leather is a product made from skins. It is a proteinaceous, 'readily woven' material, which finds extensive application in footwear, luggage and harness. The treatment to preserve the material and render it pliable and free from the malodour found with raw skins possibly started with simple drying, followed by mechanical manipulation. This was followed by salt treatment, and finally the discovery that leather could be produced by soaking skins in the steep water from certain tree barks, a process called tanning, laid the foundation for the modern process.

Today, leather is produced by soaking skins in an alkaline solution to saponify grease and make dehairing easy. Dehaired hides are tanned, coloured, oiled and finished by a variety of processes.

Leather is at risk of microbial attack during the processing of the skins, when bacteria are the chief source of trouble, and after finishing and making up, when mould growth can be a major hazard. For protection during processing, phenolics, including salicylanilide, 8-hydroxyquinoline and acetic acid have been used. For preservation of the finished product, 4-nitrophenol, 2-naphthol, 2,4-dimethyl-3-chlorophenol, salicylanilide and pentachlorophenol have been recommended.

Under cool conditions, with well-protected skins, sodium chlorite provides good protection of the skin but does not protect the soak liquor. An application rate of 0.1% sodium chlorite solution prevents the build-up of soak-liquor bacteria for at least 24 h but is ineffective at higher temperatures. For prolonged soaking, where high temperatures are involved or where the raw stock is suspect, biocides based on bronopol, methylene bis-thiocyanate or triazine are recommended.

For examples of original publications on this subject see Jordan (1934), Money (1970) and Wessel *et al.* (1964) in the general bibliography.

6 Conclusions

Biocides may be applied to textile and leather substrates to prevent infection (e.g. anthrax), to minimize biodeterioration problems or as hygienic finishes. Commercial formulations of industrial biocides are available to both the textile and the leather industries, with appropriate methods of application and stated compatibility. Such lists will be subject to ever-increasing scrutiny as environmental pressures and resultant legislation evolve. Biocide efficacy may be confirmed by routine chemical assays or by specialized biological testing (primarily challenge testing).

7 References

Anon. (1976) *Examination of the Antimycotic Effect of Impregnated Textiles by the Agar Diffusion Test (Using* Trichophyton mentagrophytes *ATCC 9533 and* Candida albicans *ATCC 10259) Contact Inhibition Test*. Schweizerische Normen-Vereinigung SNV 195 921 1976.

Anon. (1993a) *Activity of Fabrics: Parallel Streak Method*. AATCC Test Method 147-1993. *Detection of Antibacterial* AATCC Technical Manual. Triangle Park, North Carolina: American Association of Textile Chemists and Colorists.

Anon. (1986) *Methods for Determination of Breaking Strength and Elongation (Strip Method) of Woven Fabrics*. British Standard 2576. London: British Standards Institution.

Anon. (1993b) *Antifungal Activity, Assessment on Textile Materials: Mildew and Rot Resistance of Textile Materials*. AATCC Test Method 30-1993. AATCC Technical Manual. Triangle Park, North Carolina: American Association of Textile Chemists and Colorists.

Anon. (1993c) *Assessment of Antibacterial Finishes on Fabrics*. AATCC Test Method 100-1993. AATCC Technical Manual. Triangle Park, North Carolina: American Association of Textile Chemists and Colorists.

Anon. (1989c) *Methods for Determination of Breaking Strength and Breaking Extension*. British Standard 1932, Part 1. London: British Standards Institution.

Anon. (1991a) *Performance Requirements for Textile Preservative Treatments Against Microbiological Attack*. UK Ministry of Defence Interim Defence Standard 68–141.

Anon. (1991b) *Examination of the Antibacterial Effect of Impregnated Textiles by the Agar Diffusion Test (Using* Staphylococcus aureus *ATCC 538 and* Escherichia coli *ATCC 11229) Contact Inhibition Test*. Schweizerische Normen-Vereinigung SNV 195 920 1991.

Anon. (1992a) *Preservative Treatments for Textiles*. British Standard 2087 Parts 1 and 2. London: British Standards Institution.

Anon. (1992b) *Methods of Testing for Determination of the Resistance of Textiles to Microbiological Deterioration*. British Standard 6085. London: British Standards Institution.

Anon. (1992c) *Testing of Textiles; Determination of the Resistance of Cellulose Textiles Against Micro-organisms (Resistance to Bacteria and Fungi of Soil); Identification of Rotting Retardant Finishing*. Deutsches Institut für Normung DIN 53 933 1992 Part 1.

Anon. (1992d) *Testing of Textiles; Determination of the Resistance of Textiles to Mildew, Growth Test*. Deutsche Norm DIN 53 931 1992.

Anon. (1993) *Methods of Testing for Colour Fastness of Textiles and Leather*. BS EN 20105: BO2 (1993) and BO4 (1997) —British Standard 1006. London: British Standards Institution.

Eggins, H.O.W. & Oxley, T.A. (1980) Biodeterioration and biodegradation. *International Biodeterioration Bulletin*, **16**, 53–56.

Greaves, P.H. & McCarthy, B.J. (1991) A microscopical study of severe biodeterioration in a textile floor-covering—a case study. *Journal of the Textile Institute*, **82**, 291–295.

Lundin, A. & Thore, A. (1975) Comparison of methods for extraction of bacterial adenine nucleotides determined by firefly assay. *Applied Microbiology*, **30**, 713–721.

McCarthy, B.J. (1986) Preservatives for use in the wool textile industry. In *Preservatives in the Food, Pharmaceutical and Environmental Industries* (eds Board, R.G., Allwood, M.C. & Banks, J.G.), pp. 75–98. Oxford: Blackwell Scientific Publications.

McCarthy, B.J. (1989) Detection and enumeration of micro-organisms on textiles using ATP luminescence. In *ATP Luminescence: Rapid Methods in Microbiology* (eds Stanley, P.E., McCarthy, B.J. & Smither, R.), pp. 81–86. Oxford: Blackwell Scientific Publications.

McCarthy, B.J.& Greaves, P.H. (1988) Mildew—causes, detection methods and prevention. *Wool Science Review*, **65**, 27–48.

Peacock, E.E. (1996a) Characterization and simulation of water-degraded archaeological textiles: a review. *International Biodeterioration and Biodegradation*, **38**, 35–47.

Peacock, E.E. (1996b) Biodegradation and characterization of water-degraded archaeo logical textiles created for conservation research. *International Biodeterioration and Biodegradation*, **38**, 49–59.

Turnbull, P.C.B., Bowen, J.E., Gillgan, J.S. & Barrett, N.J. (1996) Incidence of anthrax and environmental detection of *Bacillus anthracis* in the UK. *Salisbury Medical Bulletin* (Proceedings of the International Workshop on Anthrax), **87**, 5S–6S.

BIBLIOGRAPHY—GENERAL

Agarwal, P.N. & Nanda, J.N. (1972) Correlation of

tropical room experiments with weathering exposure. In *Biodeterioration of Materials*, Vol. 2 (eds Walters, A.H. & Hueck-van der Plas, E.H.), pp. 179–184. London: Applied Science Publishers.

Anon. (1967) *Resistance to Fungal Attack by* Aspergillus niger *SABS Culture No. 70*. South African Standard Method 472. Pretoria: South African Bureau of Standards.

Anon. (1972a) *Resistance of Textiles to Fungal Growth*. Australian Standard 1157 Part 2. Sydney: Standards Association of Australia.

Anon. (1972b) *Method of Testing for Resistance to Micro-organisms. Surface Growing Fungus Test—Pure Culture*. Canadian Standard CAN 2-4.2-M77. Ottawa: Canadian Government Specification Board.

Anon. (1973) *Resistance of Fungal Attack by Mixed Cultures*. South African Standard Method 484. Pretoria: South African Bureau of Standards.

Armstrong, E.F. (1941) The rot-proofing of sand bags. *Chemistry and Industry*, **60**, 668–674.

Bayley, C.H. & Weatherburn, M.W. (1947a) The effect of weathering on various rot-proofing treatments applied to cotton tentage duck. *Canadian Journal of Research*, **25F**, 92–109.

Bayley, C.H. & Weatherburn, M.W. (1947b) The rotproofing efficacy of metallic naphthenates. *Canadian Journal of Research*, **25F**, 209–220.

Benignus, P.G. (1948) Copper-8-hydroxyquinolinate, industrial preservative. *Industrial and Engineering Chemistry*, **40**, 1426–1429.

Block, S.S. (1953) Humidity requirements for mould growth. *Applied Microbiology*, **1**, 287–293.

Brinj, J.La. & Kauffman, H.R. (1972) Fungal testing of textiles: a summary of co-operative experiments carried out by the working group on textiles of the international biodegradation research group (IBRG). In *Biodeterioration of Materials*, Vol. 2 (eds Walters, A.H. & Hueck-van der Plas, E.H.), pp. 208–217. London: Applied Science Publishers.

Burgess, R. (1924) Bacteriology and mycology of wool. *Journal of the Textile Institute*, **15**, T333–T383.

Burgess, R. (1928) Microbiology of wool. *Journal of the Textile Institute*, **19**, T315–T322.

Burgess, R. (1934) Causes and prevention of mildew on wool. *Journal of the Society of Dyers and Colourists*, **50**, 138–142.

Cavill, G.W.K., Phillips, J.N. & Vincent, J.M. (1949) Relation between fungistatic activity and structure in a series of simple aromatic compounds. *Journal of the Society of Chemical Industry*, **68**, 12–16.

Corry, J.E.L. (1973) The water relations and heat resistance of microorganisms. *Progress in Industrial Microbiology*, **12**, 73–108.

Fargher, R.G., Galloway, L.K.G. & Probert, M.E. (1930) The inhibitory action of certain substances on the growth of mould fungi. *Journal of the Textile Institute*, **21**, T245–T260.

Jordan, I.D. (1934) Troubles in leather manufacture caused by moulds. *Leather Trades Review*, **67**, 197–198.

Kaplan, A.M., Mandels, M. & Greenberger, M. (1972) Mode of action of resins in preventing microbial degradation of cellulosic textiles. In *Biodeterioration of Materials*, Vol. 2 (eds Walters, A.H. & Hueck-van der Plas E.H.), pp. 268–278. London: Applied Science Publishers.

Lloyd, A.O. (1968) The evaluation of rot resistance of cellulosic textiles. *Biodeterioration of Materials* (eds Walters, A.H. & Elphick, J.J.), pp. 170–177. Amsterdam: Elsevier.

Lollar, R.M. (1944) Mould resistant treatment for leather. *Journal of the American Leather Chemists Association*, **39**, 12–24.

Marsh, P.B., Greathouse, G.A., Bollenbacher, K. & Butler M.L. (1944) Copper soaps as rot proofing agents on fabrics. *Industrial and Engineering Chemistry*, **36**, 176–181.

Mills, J., Allsopp, D. & Eggins, H.O.W. (1972) Some new developments in cellulosic material testing perfusion techniques. In *Biodeterioration of Materials*, Vol. 2 (eds Walters, A.H. & Hueck-van der Plas, E.H.), pp. 227–232. London: Applied Science Publishers.

Miller, G. (1972) Tributyltin oxide: some factors influencing its development and application as a preservative. In *Biodeterioration of Materials*, Vol. 2 (eds Walters, A.H. & Hueck-van der Plas, E.H.), pp. 279–285. London: Applied Science Publishers.

Money, C.A. (1970) Short term preservation of hides. *Journal of the American Leather Chemists Association*, **65**, 57–59.

Selby, K. (1968) Mechanism of biodegradation of cellulose. In *Biodeterioration of Materials* (eds Walters, A.H. & Elphick, J.J.), pp. 62–78. London: Elsevier Publishing.

Turner, R.L. (1972) Important factors in the soil burial test applied to rot-proofed textiles. In *Biodeterioration of Materials*, Vol. 2 (eds Walters, H.A. & Hueck-van der Plas, E.H.), pp. 218–226. London: Applied Science Publishers.

Wessel, C.J., Lee, R.W.H. & Janecka, H. (1964) Recent developments in the control of microbial growth on leather and fabrics. *Developments in Industrial Microbiology*, **5** 36–49.

BIBLIOGRAPHY—WOOL

Allsopp, C. & Allsopp, D. (1983) An updated survey of commercial products used to protect materials against biodeterioration. *International Biodeterioration Bulletin*, **19**, 99–146.

Andersen, R.L. (1969) Biological evaluation of carpeting. *Applied Microbiology*, **18**, 180–187.

Anon. (1950) The mildewing of wool: causes and prevention. *Wool Science Review*, **6**, 31–42.

Arnold, L.B. (1984) Antimicrobial activity of carpet. *Carpet and Rug Industry*, **12**, 22–27.

Batson, D.M., Tennisson, D.J. & Porges, N. (1944) Study of a soil burial method for determining rot-resistance of fabrics. *American Dyestuff Reporter*, **33**, 423–454.

Blowers, R. & Wallace, K.R. (1955) The sterilization of blankets with cetyltrimethylamine bromide. *Lancet*, **i**, 1250.

Bobkova, T.S., Zlochevskaya, I.V., Chekunova, L.N., Kirkina, L.I. & Monakhova, R.I. (1975) Use of a rapid method of soil testing for evaluation of the biodeterioration resistance of textile materials. *Vestnik Moskovskoyo Universiteta Biologia, Pochvovedenie*, **30**, 55–59.

Brown, J.C. (1959) The determination of damage to wool fibres. *Journal of the Society of Dyers and Colourists*, **75**, 11–21.

Burgess, R. (1924) Studies on the bacteriology of wool. *Journal of the Textile Institute*, **15**, T575–T583.

Burgess, R. (1934) The use of trypsin for the determination of the resistance of wool fibres to bacterial disintegration. *Journal of Applied Bacteriology*, **17**, 230–245.

Burgess, R. & Galloway, L.D. (1940) *Applied Mycology and Bacteriology*, 2nd edn. London: Leonard Hill.

Burgess, R. & Rimington, C. (1929) A technique for the microscopical examination of wool fibres. *Journal of the Royal Microscopic Society*, **49**, 341–347.

Church, B.D. & Loosli, C.G. (1953) The role of the laundry in the recontamination of washed bedding. *Journal of Infectious Diseases*, **93**, 65–74.

Cody, H.J., Smith, P.F., Blaser, M.J., LaForce, F.M. & Wang, W.L. (1984) Comparison of methods for recovery of *Escherichia coli*, and *Staphylococcus aureus* from seeded laundry fabrics. *Applied and Environmental Microbiology*, **47**, 965–970.

Eggins, H.O.W. (1967) The economics of biodeterioration. *Environmental Engineering*, **29**, 15–16.

Eggins, H.O.W. & Oxley, T.A. (1980) Biodeterioration and biodegradation. *International Biodeterioration Bulletin*, **16**, 53–56.

Eggins, H.O.W., Malik, K.A. & Sharp, R.F. (1968) Some techniques to investigate the colonisation of cellulosic and wood substrates. In *Proceedings of First International Biodeterioration Symposium* (eds Walters, A.H. & Elphick, J.J.), pp. 120–131. London: Elsevier.

English, M.P. (1965) The saprotrophic growth of nonkeratinophilic fungi on keratinized substrata and a comparison with keratinophilic fungi. *Transactions of the British Mycology Society*, **48**, 219–235.

Fraser, R.D.B. & Gillespie, J. (1976) Wool structure and biosynthesis. *Nature*, **261**, 650–654.

Garner, W. (1967) *Textile Laboratory Manual*, 3rd edn, Vol. 6, p. 153. London: Heywood.

Geiger, W.B., Patterson, W.I., Mizell, L.R. & Harris, M. (1941) The nature of the resistance of wool to digestion by enzymes. *Journal of Research of the National Bureau of Standards*, **27**, 459–468.

Georgiewics, G. (1924) *Lehrbuch der Chemisten Technologie der gespinstfasern Deuticke*. Leipzig and Vienna.

Gray, W.D. & Martin, G.W. (1947) Improvements on the soil-burial testing method. *Mycologia*, **39**, 358–369.

Grimm, H. & Kuhne, C. (1969) The standardization of earth rotting tests of the testing of rot-proofing finishes to cellulosic fibres. *Deutscher Textiltechnie*, **19**, 46–49.

Hirst, H.R. (1927) Ultraviolet radiation as an aid to textile analysis. *Journal of the Textile Institute*, **18**, 369–375.

Hughes, W.H. & Davies, R.R. (1970) Bacteria and cadmium-treated fabrics. *British Medical Journal*, **1**, 430.

Ilyichev, V.D. (1979) *Rtitzy-istochnik bioprovrezhdenii*, pp. 47–53. Moscow: Znanie.

Jain, P.C. & Agrawal, S.C. (1980) A note on the keratin decomposing capability of some fungi. *Transactions of the Mycology Society of Japan*, **21**, 513–517.

Kempton, A.G., Maisel, H. & Kaplan, A.M. (1963) Study of the deterioration of fungicide-treated fabrics in soil burial. *Textile Research Journal,* **33** 87–93.

Lashen, E.S. (1971) New method for evaluating antimicrobial activity directly on fabric. *Applied Microbiology*, **21**, 771–773.

Latlief, M.A., Goldsmith, M.T., Friedl, J.L. & Stuart, L.S. (1951) Bacteriostatic, germicidal and sanitising action of quaternary ammonium compounds on textiles. I. Prevention of ammonia formation from urea by *Proteus mirabilis*. *Journal of Paediatrics*, **39**, 730–737.

Lemon, H.M. (1943) A method for collection of bacteria from air and textiles. *Proceedings of the Society of Experimental Biology and Medicine*, **54**, 293–301.

Lewis, J. (1981) Microbial biodeterioration. In *Economic Microbiology*, (ed. Rose, A.H.), pp. 81–130. London: Academic Press.

Lloyd, A.D. (1955) A soil-infection method for the testing of textiles for resistance to microbiological attack. *Journal of the Textile Institute*, **46**, 653–661.

Lloyd, A.D. (1965) An adhesive tape technique for the microscopical examination of surfaces supporting mould growth. *International Biodeterioration Bulletin*, **1**, 10–13.

McCarthy, B.J. (1983a) Biodeterioration in wool textile processing. In *Biodeterioration 5* (eds Oxley, T.A. & Barry, S.), pp. 519–527. London: John Wiley.

McCarthy, B.J. (1983b) Bioluminescent assay of microbial contaminants on textile materials. *International Biodeterioration Bulletin*, **19**, 53–57.

McCarthy, B.J. (1984) Bioluminescent determination of microbial activity on textiles; In *Analytical Applications of Bioluminescence and Chemiluminescence* (eds Kricka, L.J., Stanley, P.E., Thorpe, G.H.G. & Whitehead, T.P.), pp. 46–49. London: Academic Press.

McGee, J.B. & Gettings, R.L. (1985) Method for the evaluation of immobilized antimicrobial agents. In *Book of Papers International Conference of the American Association of Textile Chemists and Colorists*.

McGee, J. & White, W.C. (1984) Evaluations of surface bonded cationic antimicrobials. *Carpet and Rug Industry*, **12**, 24–41.

McQuade, A.B. (1964) Microbiological degradation of wool. *Dermatologia*, **128**, 249–266.

McQuade, A.B. & Sutherland, W.J.A. (1960) An improved device for sampling bacterial populations on blankets. *Journal of Hygiene*, **58**, 157–158.

Mahall, K. (1982) Biodegradation of textile fibres as seen under the microscope—actual case histories. *International Textile Bulletin*, **4**, 280–292.

Majors, P. (1959) Evaluation of the effectiveness of antibacterial finishes for cloth. *American Dyestuff Reporter*, **48**, 91–93.

Mandels, G.R. & Siu, R.G. (1950) Rapid assay for growth: microbial susceptibility and fungistatic activity. *Journal of Bacteriology*, **60**, 249–262.

Mandels, G.R., Stahl, W. & Levinson, H. (1948) Structural changes to wool degraded by ringworm fungus (*Microsporum gypseum*). *Textile Research Journal*, **18**, 224–231.

Mebes, B. (1975) Hygiene finishing in the dyebath. *International Textile Bulletin*, **2**, 122.

Mulcock, A.P. (1965a) *Peyronallaea glomerata*—a fungus growing with the fibres of the unshorn fleece. *Australian Journal of Agricultural Research*, **16**, 691–697.

Mulcock, A.P. (1965b) The fleece as a habitat for microorganisms. *New Zealand Veterinary Journal*, **13**, 87–93.

Nichols, P.S. (1970) Bacteria on laundered fabrics. *American Journal of Public Health*, **60**, 2175–2180.

Nopitsch, M. (1953) Micro-organic attack on textiles and leather. *CIBA Review*, **100**, 3582–3610.

Osborn, J.G.B. (1912) Moulds and mildews: their relation to the damaging of grey cloth and prints. *Journal of the Society of Dyers and Colourists*, **28**, 204–208.

Pauly, H. (1904) Ueber die Konstitution des Histidins (I). *Zeitschrift für Physiologische Chemie*, **42**, 508–518.

Puck, T.T., Robinson, O.H., Wise, H., Loosli, C.G. & Lemon, H.M. (1946) The oil treatment of bedclothes for the control of dust-borne infection. 1. Principles underlying the development and use of a satisfactory oil-in-water emulsion. *American Journal of Hygiene*, **43**, 91–104.

Quinn, H. (1962) A method for the determination of the anti-microbial properties of treated fabrics. *Applied Microbiology*, **10**, 74–78.

Race, E. (1946) Problems in the microbiology of protein fibres. *Journal of the Society of Dyers and Colourists*, **62**, 67–85.

Raschle, P. (1983) Contribution to the examination of the rot resistance of textiles. *International Biodeterioration Bulletin*, **19**, 13–17.

Ruehle, G. & Brewer, C. (1931) *United States Food and Drug Administration Methods of Testing Antiseptics and Disinfectants*. Circular No. 198. Washington: US Department of Agriculture.

Safranek, WW. & Goos, R.D. (1982) Degradation of wool by saprophytic fungi. *Canadian Journal of Microbiology*, **28**, 137–140.

Sankov, E.A., Suchkova, G.C. & Andreeva, K.I. (1972) Investigations of biological wool fibre damage by the dyeing method. *Technical Textiles Industry USSR*, **4**, 152–153.

Seal, K. & Allsopp, D. (1983) Investigative biodeterioration. In *Biodeterioration 5* (eds Oxley, T. & Barry, S.), pp. 528–534. Chichester: John Wiley.

Sherrill, J.C. (1956) The evaluation of bacteriostatic reagents and methods of application to textile fabrics. *Textile Research Journal*, **26**, 342–350.

Thomas, J.C. & Van Den Ende, M. (1941) The reduction of dust-borne bacteria in the air of hospital wards by liquid paraffin treatment of bedclothes. *British Medical Journal*, **1**, 953.

Vigo, T.L. (1978) Antibacterial fibres. In *Modified Cellulosics. Symposium of Cellulose, Paper and Textiles*, pp. 259–284. Division of the American Chemical Society.

Vigo, T.L. & Benjaminson, M.A. (1981) Antibacterial fibre treatments and disinfection. *Textile Research Journal*, **51**, 454.

Von Bergen, W. & Mauersberger, H.R. (1948) *American Wool Handbook*. Textile Book Publishers.

Walton, D.W.H. & Allsopp, D. (1977) A new test cloth for soil burial trials and other studies on cellulose decomposition. *International Biodeterioration Bulletin*, **13**, 112–115.

Wehrner, C. (1902) Stains on textiles caused by *Aspergillus fumigatus*. *Journal of the Society of Dyers and Colourists*, **18**, 112.

Wellman, R.H. & McCallan, S.E.A. (1945) *Office of Strategic Research and Development Report* 5683. Washington: US National Defense Research Communication.

Wiksell, J.C., Pickett, M.A. & Hartmann, P.A. (1973) Survival of microorganisms in laundered polyester cotton sheeting. *Journal of Applied Bacteriology*, **25**, 431–435.

Wilkoff, L.J., Westbrook, L. & Dixon, G.L. (1969) Factors affecting the persistence of *Staphylococcus aureus* on fabrics. *Applied Microbiology*, **17**, 268–274.

C. PAINT AND PAINT FILMS

1 Liquid emulsion paints

Liquid emulsion paints generally contain high proportions of water and inorganic pigments, plus organic constituents, which may include polymer emulsion, emulsion stabilizers, thickeners, surfactants, dispersants, antifoams, coalescing agents, levelling and freeze–thaw stabilizing agents and colour tinters. Without experimentation, it is not possible to predict whether any given material will be inhibitory or stimulatory to microbial growth (Briggs, 1977).

The components of an emulsion paint may be supplied, handled or stored in aqueous dispersion or solution. The factory environment is, of course, not sterile; storage and mixing tanks may be open to the air or, when closed, subject to considerable condensation. It is not uncommon for pipework and equipment to have numerous dead spots, where old or diluted materials may accumulate, washings may be stored or recirculated, and ultimately the paint will most probably be distributed in metal or plastic containers, which may retain a greasy lubricant coating and which will probably undergo temperature cycling during storage. For these reasons, various microbiological problems can occur, leading to deterioration or spoilage of liquid emulsion paint.

Probably the most common form of attack is on the cellulose ether thickening agent of the paint, resulting in a loss of viscosity (and perhaps sedimentation of the solid phase). Alternative mechanisms postulated involve either enzyme-catalysed hydrolysis (Floyd *et al.*, 1966; Winters *et al.*, 1974) or an oxidation process involving bacterial hydrogen peroxide (Winters & Goll, 1976) or redux agents derived from emulsion end-stripping. Other phenomena known to occur include gassing or frothing of paint, malodour and discoloration (perhaps with change in pH, rheological properties or dispersion stability).

There is considerable evidence to link both bacteria and fungi to emulsion paint spoilage (Bravery, 1988; Zyska *et al.*, 1988), and, as already indicated, the source of contamination may be a raw material, a factory process or practice or a storage condition. Problems can best be avoided by a combination of uncontaminated raw materials, resistant formulation, good factory hygiene and effective use of chemical preservation, with particular emphasis being placed on the last in this subchapter.

1.1 Preservation of emulsion paints

Extensive use has been made in the past of organomercurial preservatives, such as phenylmercuric acetate, phenylmercuric dodecyl succinate and others, because these have wide-spectrum antimicrobial activity, are capable of inhibiting a large number of proteins by reaction with protein sulphhydryl groups, especially in enzymes, and can be effective at low concentrations in paint (0.001–0.03% mercury). Such mercurial preservatives tend to be generally toxic, and the coatings industry has been actively phasing out their use.

As alternatives for use in moden compliant paints, a fairly large number of non-mercurial preservatives are available commercially (Smith, 1980; Vore, 1995); however, these have varying chemical, physical and toxicological properties and need to be matched to the formulation in which activity is required. Examples of types include organotins, formaldehyde and formaldehyde-releasing agents, quaternary ammonium compounds (QACs), phenolics, nitrogen and sulphur heterocycles (particular isothiazolinones) and mixtures of various types. Many of these groups are considered in Chapter 2 (also Paulus, 1993). Successful use of non-mercurial preservatives, particularly, requires attention to the points listed below.

1.1.1 *Spectrum of activity*

Aqueous raw materials (e.g. pigment and extender slurries, polymer emulsion, etc.) make-up water and aqueous intermediates present the first possible sources of bacterial, fungal or enzyme contamination. Within the factory, containers of aqueous raw materials, having been opened, may be partially used and then set aside for future use. Thickeners may be dissolved and then stored in solution. Mixing procedures will leave liquid or semisolid accumulations in and on equipment, water and washings will collect and may be recirculated. Frequently condensation will dilute the preservative and possibly wash contamination into the paint. Such circumstances may encourage bacterial or fungal growth (e.g. *Pseudomonas aeruginosa, Pseudomonas putida, Fusarium* spp., *Scopulariopsis* spp.) in or on susceptible materials (Miller, 1973; Keene & Springle, 1976; Briggs, 1978b; Vore, 1995).

An ideal preservative would have antibacterial, antifungal and enzyme-blocking action; however, only heavy-metal compounds appear to be capable of achieving the latter, and then only at impractical levels of addition. The first two requirements are attainable, except that, where the liquid paint is concerned, activity is needed in the aqueous phase (requiring the preservative to be water-soluble), while, in semisolid paint accumulations, water-insolubility may be advantageous to reduce leaching of the preservative by condensation water. Partitioning of preservative between oily and aqueous phases is also an important point to be considered in the preservation of certain pharmaceutical products (Chapter 16).

1.1.2 *Preservative concentration and usage*

Since contamination by microorganisms (and/or their enzymes) can occur at various points before, during and even after paint manufacture, early use of an effective preservative concentration is essential. An initially high preservative concentration added to aqueous raw materials, etc., allows for dilution to a final, economic level in the finished paint. Also, since further dilution will occur in washings and residues, which may be reused, the preservative should either tolerate some dilution or be boosted by further addition.

The 'use concentration' of a preservative is usually estimated by evaluations carried out in paint(s) e.g. in a challenge procedure as described in ASTM: D-2574-86. However, the fully formulated paint is often not a particularly susceptible material (in fact, it is quite possible for an emulsion paint formulation to be toxic or at least inhospitable to bacteria and fungi), suggesting that normal evaluation procedures may not adequately represent the range of in-use situations in which preservative action will be needed (indeed this seems to be the case with ASTM: D-2574-86). Currently the International Biodegradation Research Group (IBRG) is evaluating new methodology.

1.1.3 *Preservative stability*

A preservative being considered for use in a given paint formulation must be stable in the formulation. Despite this, there are occasions when incompatibilities occur. For example, a mercury compound used with sulphide pigment, such as lithopone, may react to produce black mercury sulphide. It is quite common for emulsion paints to be alkaline (pH 8–10), and some preservatives will rapidly hydrolyse under this condition. Again, ammonia may be used to obtain alkalinity, and this may react with certain phenolics or formaldehyde-releasing agents. It is a possibility that redox agent contamination deriving from latex manufacturing, may be a source of preservative degradation (Couquex, 1993). Preservative partition between oil and water phases in the paint can markedly deplete the water phase (Pauli, 1973), although it is not known whether this renders the preservative ineffective. Drastic reduction in active concentration can, however, be caused by, for example, adsorption on to clay extenders or reaction with microbial protein introduced or derived from previous contamination (Smith, 1977; Briggs, 1978a). It seems probable that such deactivation processes, which reduce preservative effectiveness, may well have been mistakenly interpreted as an 'increase in resistance' of microorganisms.

2 Films from emulsion and oil paints

Once applied to a surface, emulsion paints lose water by evaporation and the polymer particles coalesce to form a paint film, which contains pigments plus residues of the various components and additives already mentioned. The presence of these may significantly influence microbial susceptibility of the film, at least while it remains relatively free from organic debris. Oil paints tend to be simpler in formulation, and, although the paint film touch-dries quite quickly by solvent evaporation, it will continue oxidation processes for some considerable time thereafter. The products of oxidation may significantly affect microbial susceptibility of the film (again, while it remains relatively clean).

Given a suitably moist or humid condition, fungal spores present on the surface of a susceptible paint film will germinate to produce mycelial or colonial growth. The organic nutrients required by fungi may come from the paint film or from accumulation of organic debris (e.g. food residues, grease, soil, etc.). It has been reported that distinct colonization sequences tend to occur (Winters *et al.*, 1975), although equally a specific fungus is frequently observed to colonize a particular situation. Fungi commonly isolated include species of the genera *Alternaria, Aspergillus, Aureobasidium, Cladosporium* and *Penicillium*, but this depends on the situation (Skinner, 1972; Hirsch & Sosman, 1976). Where water and light are available (usually soiled exterior surfaces), algal as well as fungal growth may proliferate, and genera such as *Nostoc, Oscillatoria, Pleurococcus, Scytonema, Stichococcus* and *Trentapohlia* have been isolated. Variation in paint-film composition, the nature of the substrate (e.g. wood, plaster, metal, brick, etc.) and the film's environment (e.g. interior, exterior, etc.) will help to determine whether growth occurs and the form it takes.

In the UK, the Clean Air Act has been responsible for revealing many problems of 'dirtiness' as microbial disfigurement. In addition, certain modern building techniques and living habits (e.g. absence of cavity walls; use of poorly insulated precast building slabs; restricted ventilation in kitchens, bathrooms and renovated properties; intermittent cooking and heating systems, particularly those which humidity internal air, etc.) tend to encourage conditions conducive to biological growth (Building Research Establishment, 1981). Thus considerable incentive may exist to try to protect a given surface against fungi or algae, for which application a biocidal paint film may be utilized (probably in conjunction with a disinfectant wash or surface-sterilizing agent). Where an in-service condition causes, or is expected to cause, microbial growth on a coated surface, prevention requires that a number of contributing factors be considered and the most relevant addressed. Broadly, the practical preventative measures are:

- Reduce causal moisture
- Formulate the coating to minimise its susceptibility
- Use chemical biocides which will control or eliminate microbial growth

2.1 Paint-film protection

A paint film applied over a surface may be exploited as a reservoir of biocide (fungicide or algicide), in which a small quantity of active material can be distributed over a wide area. Provided suitable leaching and mobility characteristics are exhibited, continuous protection is possible for a considerable time (although it must be stressed that, as detritus and soiling increase on the paint film, so the biocide's ability to protect will be impaired).

Organomercurial compounds have been used extensively, because of their wide-spectrum activity and relative cheapness; however, such compounds tend to be toxic to higher organisms, are often volatile or water-sensitive and may darken in industrial atmospheres, due to mercury sulphide formation. Alternative fungicides include inorganic and organic compounds of zinc, barium, copper and tin, as well as a number of non-metallic organic materials (Paulus, 1993; Smith & Springle, 1995). Most of the organic biocides are halogen-, nitrogen- and/or sulphur-containing compounds (such as diidomethyl *p*-tolyl sulphone; *N*-(trichloromethyl)-thio-4-cyclohexene-1.2-dicarboximide; 2,4,5,6-tetrachloro-isophthalonitrile; 2-*n*-octyl-4-isothiazolin-3-one; 3-iodo-2-propynyl butylcarbamate) and, especially with newer products, toxicity to mammals and fish tends to be minimized as much as possible, as does persistence in the environment.

Some fungicidal compounds, such as tetramethylthiuram disulphide and tributyltin oxide, also possess algicidal properties and have been used for general protection of exterior paintwork. Other fungicides may well have this ability and, in addition, agricultural herbicides (e.g. triazines, chlorophenyl urea compounds) have found application. In selecting a film biocide, it is advisable to consider the spectrum of action, toxicology and all other technical data available.

An ideal film biocide would have wide-spectrum activity, low mammalian toxicity, resistance to both water leaching and ultraviolet (UV) degradation, compatibility with and stability in different paints and a competitive price. Commercial products have appeared which have suffered from various shortcomings, including retarding oxidative drying of oil paints, such that they remain tacky; colouring white paints, due to degradation intermediates or by reaction with metal ions, such as copper or iron; disturbing the ionic balance of emulsion paints and causing precipitation; and hydrolysing under the alkaline conditions (pH 7.5–9.5) in an emulsion paint and so losing biocidal effectiveness.

Interest in methods of evaluating biocide effectiveness developed along with the appearance of the chemicals themselves, and both natural exposure and laboratory testing have been employed (Springle, 1975; Post *et al.*, 1976; Hoffmann, 1977).

It is usual for film microbicides to require registration and approval in order to be sold commercially. In the United States, EPA legislation controls biocide usage. In Europe, the Biocidal Products Directive (Bell *et al.*, 1998) seems set to be the major influence on the biocides industry in the immediate future. Thus, the selection of an approved biocide for film protection will depend upon a number of factors, including:

- supplier availability
- target organisms
- product performance
- paint compatibility
- incorporation requirements
- toxicology and biodegradability
- cost effectiveness
- technical support.

It has been suggested that only natural exposure can give meaningful assessment. This type of evaluation, however, tends to be expensive, time-consuming, uncontrolled in terms of exposure conditions and often markedly affected by climatic variations. Laboratory exposure conditions (inoculum, temperature, humidity, surface contamination, substrate, film pretreatment, etc.) can be much more closely controlled, and it is possible to simulate an in-use condition of the paint film where this is known.

Laboratory testing can be used to eliminate much time-consuming and expensive natural exposure, although meaningful prediction of performance requires a realistic simulation of in-use conditions. Failure of a paint film to prevent growth under laboratory conditions is a definite indication of its limitation; however, a variety of conditions (involving water leaching, exposure to heat and UV light and contamination of the surface by organic materials) will be needed to represent the range of situations met with in use. Standardization in test methodology is generally considered desirable, and a Paints Working Group operating within the International Biodeterioration Research Group (sponsored by the Organization for Economic Cooperation and Development (OECD), Paris) has evaluated, towards this end, a methodology for testing mould resistance of paint (Barry *et al.*, 1977; Bravery *et al.*, 1978). A standard, BS 3900: Part G6: 1989, has resulted from the collaboration. There is also a US standard ASTM: D-3273-86.

3 Antifouling paint films

Surfaces submerged in the sea tend to accumulate a variety of marine organisms, for example bacteria, fungi, algae, barnacles, hydroids, sea squirts, tube-worms and mussels. When the surface is part of a man-made structure, this 'fouling' can have disastrous results, by causing such problems as increased weight and size, impaired moving parts, blocked or restricted valves, pipework and conduits and increased frictional resistance. This last is of particular importance where ships' hulls are concerned, since the increased drag results in greater fuel consumption to maintain a given service speed, and ultimately means dry-docking the ship for cleaning and repair.

Ships, such as oil-tankers, which operate fairly continuously with few lay-days, have a tendency to foul with algal forms, such as *Enteromorpha* spp. and *Ectocarpus* spp., whereas ships operating in an intermittent manner, with considerable lay-days (e.g. naval ships), tend to foul with animal rather than algal forms. Economic and military implications have stimulated much research into methods of controlling marine fouling. The most practicable and economic method relies on antifouling paint films, from which chemical biocides are released into the water alongside the hull to keep the surface free of fouling for something between 0.5 and 3 years (at present), depending on the paint formulation and exposure conditions involved.

Paints have been developed to work by various mechanisms of biocide release (Furtado & Fletcher, 1987; Mihm & Loeb, 1988). Soluble-matrix paints contain a sea-water-soluble binder component, such as rosin, which dissolves to release the toxicant. Continuous-contact paints contain a greater volume of biocide than the soluble-matrix paints. The binder, such as vinyl or chlorinated rubber, is insoluble and holds the biocide particles closely packed and in continuous contact. Biocide deep within the paint reaches the surface as the biocide above it dissovles in sea water. Diffusion coatings are intended to act as a solid solution of biocide in the binder, which provides a steady supply of biocide at the surface by diffusion through the film. Binders formed as organometallic copolymers are a development in which the organometallic biocide (e.g. an organotin compound) is provided at the surface by slow hydrolysis of the paint film (Atherton, 1978; Mihm & Loeb, 1988). The basic intention of a greater proportion of research into antifouling paints is concerned with the increase of performance life, either by controlling the rate of biocide release from the paint film or by controlling the rate of transport away from the hull (van Londen *et al.*, 1975; Christie, 1978; Lorenz, 1978, Vallee-Rehel, 1998).

Types of biocides that have been used in antifouling paints include copper compounds (mainly cuprous oxide), organotin and organolead compounds, inorganic and organic compounds of mercury, arsenic and zinc, and organic compounds, such as polychlorinated hydrocarbons, phenols, thiadiazoles, nitrothiazoles, dithiocarbamates, chloronaphthoquinones and chlorophenyl urea compounds (de la Court & de Vries, 1973: de la Court, 1977).

The impact of some of these biocides on humans and the environment is a matter of concern and lead to the introduction of restrictions or controls on their usage by certain countries. Studies by various organizations, including the Paint Research Association, have shown that low-toxicity organic antifoulants can be used with some success. The present intention, however, seems to be to accumulate performance data and keep such materials as a reserve armoury of biocides.

4 Acknowledgement

The author wishes to thank the Paint Research Association for permission to publish this chapter.

5 References

Atherton, D. (1978) New development is antifouling, a review of the present state of the art. *American Chemical Society, Division of Organic Coatings and Plastics Chemistry Preprints*, **39**, 380–385.

Barry, S., Bravery, A.F. & Coleman, L.J. (1977) A method for testing the mould resistance of paints. *International Biodeterioration Bulletin*, **13**, 51–57.

Bell, G. & Wilson, G. (1998) *Speciality Chemicals*, **18**, 144–5.

Bravery, A.F. (1988) Biodeterioration of paint—a state-of-the-art comment. In *Biodeterioration 7* (eds Houghton, D.R., Smith, R.N. & Eggins, H.O.W.), pp. 466–485. London: Elsevier Applied Science.

Bravery, A.F., Barry, S. & Coleman, L.J. (1978) Collaborative experiments on testing the mould resistance of paint films. *International Biodeterioration Bulletin*, **14**, 1–10.

Briggs, M.A. (1977) *In-can Preservation: the Cellulase Mechanism of Paint Spoilage*. Paint Research Association Technical Report TR/4/77.

Briggs, M.A. (1978a) *An investigation into the Preservation of a China Clay Slurry*. Paint Research Association Technical Report TR/6/78.

Briggs, M.A. (1978b) *Comparison of Factory Practice and Hygiene with the Available Test Methods of Preservative Efficacy*. Paint Research Association TR/8/78.

Building Research Establishment (1981) *Mould Growth in Buildings*. Proceedings of a joint BRE/Paint RA seminar.

Christie, A.O. (1978) Self-polishing antifouling—a new approach to long term fouling control and hull smoothness. *American Chemical Society, Division of Organic Coatings and Plastics Chemistry Preprints*, **39**, 585–589.

Conquer, L. (1993) Interaction between reagents used in emulsion polymerisation and isothiazolinone biocides. *Polymer, Paint and Colour*, **183**, 421–423.

de la Court, F.H. (1977) Fouling resistant coatings: their functioning and future developments. *Proceeding of 3rd International Conference on Organic Coatings*, pp. 97–137.

de la Court, F.H. & de Vries, H.J. (1973) Advances in fouling prevention. *Progress in Organic Coatings*, **1**, 375–404.

Floyd, J.D., James, W.G. & Wirick, M.G. (1966) Viscosity stability of latex paints containing water-soluble cellulose polymers. *Journal of Paint Technology*, **38**, 398–401.

Furtado, S.E.J. & Fletcher, R.L. (1987) Test procedures for marine antifouling paints. In *Preservatives in the Food, Pharmaceutical and Environmental Industries* (eds Board, R.G., Allwood, M.C. & Banks, J.G.), Society for Applied Bacteriology Technical Series No. 22, pp. 145–163. Oxford: Blackwell Scientific Publications.

Hirsch, S.R. & Sosman, J.A. (1976) A one-year survey of mould growth inside twelve homes. *Annals of Allergy*, **36**, 30–38.

Hoffmann, E. (1977) Techniques for the investigation of the biodeterioration of paints developed at CSIRO, Australia. *Journal of the Oil and Colour Chemists Association*, **60**, 127–136.

Joshi, C.D., Mukunden, U. & Bagool, R.G. (1997) Fungal fouling of architectural paints in India. *Paint India*, **Feb**, 29–34.

Kappock, P. (1997) Conditions that influence the growth of mildew and algae on dry emulsion paint films. *Paint and Coatings Industry*, **July**, 76–78.

Keene, C.R. & Springle, W.R. (1976) *In-can Preservation*. Paint Research Association Technical Report TR/2/76.

Lorenz, J. (1978) Protection against marine growth—the current situation. *Polymers, Paint and Colour Journal*, August, 737–747.

Mihm, J.W. & Loeb, G.I. (1988) The effect of microbial biofilms on organism release by an antifouling paint. In *Biodeterioration 7* (eds Houghton, D.R., Smith, R.N. & Eggins, H.O.W.), pp. 309–314. London: Elsevier Applied Science.

Miller, W.G. (1973) Incidence of microbial contamination of emulsion paint during the manufacturing process. *Journal of the Oil and Colour Chemists Association*, **56**, 307–312.

Pauli, O. (1973) Inter-phase migration of preservatives in latex paints. *Journal of the Oil and Colour Chemists Association*, **56**, 289–291.

Paulus, W. (1993) *Microbiocides for the protection of materials*. London: Chapman and Hall.

Post, M.A., Iverson, W.P. & Campbell, P.G. (1976) Non-mercurial fungicides. *Modern Paint and Coatings*, September, **11**, 31–38.

Skinner, C.E. (1972) Laboratory test methods for biocidal paints. In *Biodeterioration of Materials*, Vol. 2, Part VIII, pp. 346–354. London: Applied Science Publishers.

Smith, A.L. (1980) *Guide to Preservatives for Water-Borne Paints*. Paint Research Association Technical Publication.

Smith, A.L. & Springle, W.R. (1995) *World Guide to Industrial Biocides*. Paint Research Association Technical Publication.

Smith, Q.J. (1977) *In-can Preservation: Bacterial Resistant Strains*. Paint Research Association Technical Report TR/2/77.

Springle, W.R. (1975) Testing biocidal paints. Society for Applied Bacteriology Technical Series 8, Some Methods for Microbiological Assay, pp. 191–201. London: Academic Press.

Vallee-Rehel, K. (1998) A new approach to development and testing of anti-fouling paints. *Journal of Coatings Technology*, **80**, 55–63.

van Londen, A.M., Johnsen, S. & Govers, G.J. (1975) The case of long life antifoulings. *Journal of Paint Technology*, **47**, 62–68.

Vore, R. (1995) Plant hygiene and optimal industrial biocide performance. *Speciality Chemicals*, **15**, 315–321.

Winters, H. & Goll, M. (1976) Non-enzymatic oxidative degradation of hydroxyethyl cellulose thickened latex paints. *Journal of Coating Technology*, **48**, 80–85.

Winters, H., Guidetti, G. & Goll, M. (1974) Growth of a typical paint bacterial isolate in aqueous emulsion paint. *Journal of Paint Technology*, **46**, 69–72.

Winters, H., Isquith, I.R. & Goll, M. (1975) A study of the ecological succession in the biodeterioration of a vinyl acrylic paint film. *Developments in Industrial Microbiology*, **17**, 167–171.

Zyska, J., Cheplik, Z.T., Kwiatkowska, D., Wichary, H.M. & Kozlowska, R. (1988) Fungal colonization of organic coatings in cotton mills. In *Biodeterioration 7* (eds Houghton, D.R., Smith, R.N. & Eggins, H.O.W.), pp. 486–492. London: Elsevier Applied Science.

D. PRESERVATION IN THE CONSTRUCTION INDUSTRY

1 Introduction

A wide variety of materials of organic and inorganic origin is used in the construction industry. Two of the more important, wood, with wood-based products, and paint, are considered individually in separate subchapters of this book (Chapters 18E and 18F, respectively). The present subchapter will therefore be concerned principally with inorganic masonry materials, such as stone, concrete, brick and asbestos cement, with some reference also to preservation requirements for adhesives, sealants and plastics.

2 Masonry materials

Whether stone can be considered the building material first used by early humans in constructing dwellings, enclosures, fortifications and the like is debatable. Certainly, many natural stones are extremely durable and archaeological structures built in natural stone have survived thousands of years. However, natural stones vary widely in their composition and properties (Ashurst & Dimes, 1977). Broadly, igneous rocks, such as granite, are produced from molten magma. They are highly crystalline, silica-rich, dense and of low porosity. Sedimentary rocks are laid down by settlement of eroded particles under water. They include sandstones, consisting mainly of quartz grains bound with iron oxide or calcium carbonate, and limestones, consisting mainly of calcium and magnesium carbonates. They are generally more porous than igneous rocks. Slate and marble building materials are of metamorphic rock, produced by the action of secondary heat and pressure on igneous or sedimentary rocks.

Cementatious materials, such as concrete and mortar, are produced by mixing together, in appropriate proportions, an aggregate of natural sand and gravel with water and cement powder. The latter is a mixture of calcium silicates and aluminates, produced by burning calcium carbonate from chalk or limestone with clay. The chemistry of cement setting is a complex process of recrystallization with water. The porosity and strength of concrete depends upon a number of complex factors, including cement content, the cement : water ratio and the cement : aggregate ratio. The nature of the aggregate, compaction processes and curing time and conditions all play a part. Bricks are produced by baking clays, mostly consisting of aluminium silicates and some calcium silicates. Variation in porosity and hardness results from differing clays, differing compaction and differing firing procedures.

2.1 Durability and biological agencies

The principal degrading agency associated with stone and other masonry materials is the weather. Durability is correlated with the propensity of the stone to absorb and retain water, for the extent of damage depends upon the ability of the stone to resist the solubilizing effects of the water, as well as the stresses, induced by freeze—thaw cycling, and salt recrystallization, induced by the presence of water. Indeed, it is the presence and availability of water which, as with any other ecological niche, is critical in permitting establishment of a population of organisms and, to a degree, in determining the composition of that population (Bravery & Jones, 1977). Studies on the processes of soil formation repeatedly confirm that biological agencies play a significant supporting role to weathering forces in the breakdown of natural stones. Thus a structure built in natural stone or other masonry material presents many of the same ecological 'niches' as occur in the exposed stone of natural cliffs, rock-faces and payements. While the durability and integrity of a stone-built structure depend mainly on the resistance of its stone to weathering forces, there is no doubt that a similar sequence of colonizing organisms can be observed on stone buildings and similar patterns of biologically aided breakdown appear to occur. Furthermore, ecological observations on surfaces of human made, inorganic materials, including concrete, brick and asbestos cement (Lloyd, 1976; Figg *et al.*, 1987), reveal strikingly similar patterns under similar environmental conditions of pH, temperature, illumination, moisture and rates of drying.

Newly exposed surfaces of masonry materials may need preconditioning before any organism can establish itself. Regular wetting is essential, and studies have revealed that it is the duration of the period of wetness that is important rather than the frequency of wetting itself (Bravery & Jones, 1977). The pH, in particular that of new concrete and asbestos cement (which may be as high as 14), will have to be changed to within the pH range 3–9 (Figg *et al.*, 1987).

2.2 Organisms and the nature of the problems

At an early stage of exposure, new surfaces of masonry materials present little nutritional inducement, so that early colonizers must have nutritional independence. Generally, the colonization sequence appears to commence with the establishment of autotrophic bacterial populations. In particular, species of sulphur-oxidizing bacteria, such as *Desulphovibrio desulphuricans*, *Thiobacillus thio-oxidans* and *Thiobacillus thiroparus*, have been isolated (Krumbein & Pochon, 1964; Sadurska & Kawalik, 1966; Pochon & Jaton, 1967; Jaton, 1972, 1973; Paleni & Curri, 1972; Milde *et al.*, 1983; Sand and Bock, 1987). These authors are among the leading authorities who have advanced theories on the sulphur-oxidative mechanism of bacterial action by which sulphuric acid is produced, which in turn has a direct degrading influence on the material. The decay of concrete in sewer pipes by sulphuric acid produced by *Thiobacillus concretivorus* has been cited by Hueck van der Plas (1968), Todd (1974) and Sand & Bock (1987).

Species of the autotrophic oxidizing bacteria *Nitrosomonas* and *Nitrobacter* have also been isolated from decayed stonework (Kauffman, 1952, 1960; Kauffman and Toussaint, 1954; Jaton, 1972, 1973; Eckhardt, 1985), from concrete (Kaltwasser, 1971) and from asbestos cement (Novotny *et al.*, 1973). It has been postulated that ammonia in rainwater and the air, produced by nitrifying bacteria, is oxidized to nitrate, which in turn reacts with calcium carbonate to produce the more soluble calcium nitrate. Subsequent solubilization of the calcium nitrate destroys the integrity of the stone.

Heterotrophic bacteria have been isolated from natural rocks and implicated in degradation by the organic acids they produce (Berthelin, 1983; Krumbein, 1983), solubilizing phosphates, silicates and ions of aluminium, iron and magnesium (Duff *et al.*, 1963; Aristovskaya & Kutuzova, 1968; Sahinkaya & Gurbuzer, 1968; Wood & Macrae, 1972; Dumitru *et al.*, 1976). Heterotrophic bacteria have received comparatively little attention until more recently, but they do appear to have significant decay capability (Eckhardt, 1985; Lewis *et al.*, 1985, 1987, 1988; May & Lewis, 1988).

Though extensively investigated, the role of bacteria in the degradation of stone and masonry remains contentious. However, since these species have been consistently isolated from decayed stonework and they are known to be capable of producing metabolic acids, it seems reasonable to expect them to be of potential significance to the durability of such materials.

2.2.1 *Algae*

Algae, requiring only water and traces of mineral salts, are well able to colonize surfaces of masonry materials when conditions are suitable (Paleni & Curri, 1973; Richardson, 1973). When surfaces become sufficiently wet and remain so for sufficient periods of time, extensive populations of algae are quick to develop. Although the range of species may be large, among those that predominate are the green algae *Stichococcus*, *Pleurococcus*, *Trentepholia* and *Oscillatoria* (Grant, 1982). A number of species of the blue-green algae, the cyanophycetes, are often associated with natural stone and soil. Trotet *et al.* (1973) isolated various cyanophycetes from the surface of a concrete runway and suggested that the algae dissolved calcium carbonate, releasing residual particles of the aggregate to form a slippery mud under wet conditions. As proposed by Bachmann as early as 1915, it seems likely that acidic by-products of algal metabolism induce chemical changes in certain types of masonry materials, although there is in fact little direct evidence. Certainly, the extensive sheets of algal growth that develop under wet conditions will retard subsequent drying of the water responsible for their growth, and this in turn will exacerbate water-induced damage of the underlying masonry. In addition, while the algal growth itself can be unsightly, the appearance is made even worse by the considerable quantities of fine inorganic dust, soot, etc. that become entrapped in the algal mass, particularly in urban environments (Grant, 1982).

2.2.2 *Fungi*

Colonization of external as well as internal surfaces by species of fungi depends upon nutritional preconditioning, in which previously established populations of bacteria and algae may play a major part. Eutrophication also arises from organic debris deposited from wind and rain, and by bird droppings, which may be considerable in certain situations of favoured bird-perching. Fungi have been extensively isolated from wet interior surfaces of plaster- or cement-rendered walls, particularly in relation to food processing, brewing and laundering premises (Flannigan, 1989). Among the commonest are species of *Penicillium*, *Cladosporium*, *Aspergillus* and *Alternaria* (Bravery *et al.*, 1987; Hunter *et al.*, 1988; Grant *et al.*, 1989). In such situations, fungi are more significant as fouling organisms and for potential hazards to human health, rather than for any direct degradation. Their presence is indicative of undesirably high moisture levels, resulting usually from condensation, damp penetration or leakage. Such moisture sources themselves indicate building faults or inadequate ventilation, heating and insulation (Bravery *et al.*, 1987).

Fungi have been studied less extensively in the exterior situation. Ionita (1971, 1974), Krumbein (1972), Paleni & Curri (1972) and Lepidi & Schippa (1973) have isolated a number of fungi from decaying stonework. Lepidi & Schippa (1973) indicated that hyphae were extensively distributed within the decayed stone but penetrated even into that which appeared sound. Production of organic acids by fungi, including oxalic and citric acids, is well known under laboratory conditions (Neculce, 1976) and the ability of such acids to solubilize constituents of stone has also been demonstrated (Henderson & Duff, 1963; Webley *et al.*, 1963; Gaur *et al.*, 1973). Although there is little direct evidence, certain fungi clearly have the potential to contribute to the degradation of masonry materials.

Fungi are also significant in the process of lichenization of algal growths on masonry. Studies on prewashed asbestos-cement panels have revealed lichenization within 12–18 months, even in the urban environment of central London (A.O. Lloyd, personal communication). In the practical context, it is the lichens themselves which are important, rather than the lichen-forming fungi.

2.2.3 *Lichens*

Lichens can apparently develop on almost any surface, with the exception of metallic materials. Their development is well known to be sensitive to local environmental conditions and particularly to atmospheric levels of sulphur dioxide. Indeed, lichens have been used as indicators of air pollution in urban areas. Certainly, the range of species occurring on masonry surfaces is much greater in the cleaner rural environment. The commonest species observed in urban situations are *Lecanora dispersa* and species of *Caloplaca* and of *Candelariella*, including particularly *C. aurella* and *C. vitellina*. Other species common on a variety of masonry materials, especially in rural areas, include *Lecanora conizaeoides*, *Lecanora atra*, *Lecanora muralis*, *Xanthoria parietina* and species of *Physcia*, including *P. caesia*, *P. grisea* and *P. orbicularis*.

While lichen growths are sometimes considered of aesthetic appeal, mellowing the otherwise drab or stark appearance of concrete or stone, they may also have quite serious deleterious effects. In some situations, they are distinctly disfiguring. They are also capable of withstanding prolonged periods of drought, resuming active growth when wet conditions return. Under drought conditions, they desiccate and shrink markedly, inducing shear stresses at the interfere with the masonry. Strong rhizoids, which can penetrate several millimetres even into basaltic granite (Lloyd, 1976), cause shearing and detachment of the outer millimetre or so of material, particularly near the centre of the lichen thallus. Retention of moisture in and on the surface of the structure is potentially degrading, and the thalli, which are difficult to remove completely, can interfere with the bond required in the application of any subsequent recoating, such as masonry paints (Whiteley & Bravery, 1982), renderings or concrete guniting. Extensive lichen growths on asbestos-cement paving cause a slippery walking surface when wet (Barr, 1977), which can be extremely dangerous in gardens or on the maintenance-inspection areas of roofs.

2.2.4 *Mosses, ferns and higher plants*

Mosses, ferns and higher plants may develop wherever there is a potential for root development. Commonest among the mosses are *Tortula muralis*, *Barbula cylindrica*, *Grimmia pulvinata*. *Camptothecium sericeum* and *Rhynchostegiella tenella*. *Asplenium* spp. are common among the ferns, while a wide variety of higher plants occur whose seed dispersal is by wind. Accumulations of fine soils are not an essential prerequisite, as rooting occurs directly into some highly porous stones, such as tufa, or even into an artificial soil, as may be provided by roofing chips.

The action of the earlier colonizers, combined with weathering forces, causes the erosion of small pockets and ledges in stonework, and mixtures of organic and inorganic debris accumulate within them. Spores of mosses and ferns or airborne seeds of higher plants eventually arrive and germinate. Mosses and many ferns do not require extensive rooting support and can become established in profusion with only a very shallow hold on old buildings and structures. Higher plants are more variable and, while grasses and opportunist annuals may abound, even shrubs and trees can be remarkably tenacious. Once again, such vegetation retains large quantities of moisture against the masonry surface. In addition, the stresses caused by powerful penetrating roots can induce physical failure of the materials and even serious instability of the building structure. Pavements, road surfaces and runways may be disrupted, with serious economic and safety consequences.

2.3 Remedial and preventive measures

The presence of organic growths on masonry surfaces is not always regarded as undesirable and damaging, nor is it always necessary or practicable to remove them. The probability of significant biological colonization in relation to the quantities of concrete, brick and natural stone utilized in the 'construction industry', therefore, make pretreatment to preserve them chemically against future biological growths generally impracticable and uneconomic. Preservation of old stonework affected by chemical degradation is a specialized subject, outside the scope of the present book. Incorporation of chemical toxicants into concrete, plaster and mortars has been proposed, but it is not practised on a significant scale.

The potential problems associated with biological growths are being increasingly recognized, and measures to kill and remove contamination of undesirable organisms are being taken as part of normal maintenance procedures (British Standards Institution, 1982). In this sense, then, sterilization of masonry materials is carried out on a growing

Table 18.8 Inorganic chemicals for controlling growths on masonry.

Active chemical	Application rate/ concentration (%)	Product	Application*	Reference
Alkali fluorides			I	Nicot, 1951
Ammonium fluoride			I	Roizin, 1951
Barium metaborate			P	Drisko, 1973
Chromium trioxide			C	Forrester, 1959
Copper (metallic)			C	Forrester, 1959
Copper(II) acetoarsenite (plus many other Cu compounds, including oxychloride)	10		C	Robinson & Austin, 1951
Copper(II) carbonate			C	Gilchrist, 1953
Copper(II) carbonate ammonia in dilute	0.2 5		I	Rechenberg, 1972 Anon., 1992 Genin, 1973
Copper(II) cyanide or arsenate + copper(II) oxide			IE	Norddeutsche Affineric, 1953
Copper(II) naphthenate			E	Stinson, 1956
Copper(II) 8-quinolinolate				Richardson & Ogilvy, 1955
Copper(II) oxide	0.2 (by wt in cement)		EC	Rechenberg, 1972 Lurie & Brookfield, 1948
Copper(II) sulphate	(2 in limewash) 0.1 (by wt in cement)		CE P	Aslam & Singh, 1971 Rechenberg, 1972 Kauffmann, 1960
Disodium octaborate tetrahydrate†	5 4–10	Polybor		Genin, 1973 Anon., 1992 Richardson, 1973
Iron fluoride			I	Roizin, 1951
Mercuric chloride (mercury(II) chloride)			E	Sadurska & Kawalik, 1966
Magnesium fluorosilicate‡	4–10	Lithurin	IE	Genin, 1973 Keen, 1976 Anon., 1992
Potassium permanganate				Rechenberg, 1972
Selenium metal			C	Gilchrist, 1953
Silver nitrate				Sadurska & Kawalik, 1966
Sodium fluoride				Roizin, 1951
Sodium hypochlorite	5	Bleach	CI	Rechenberg, 1972 Keen, 1976 Anon., 1992
Sodium salicylate	2		I	Rechenberg, 1972
Sodium silicofluoride			IC	Roizin, 1951 Gilchrist, 1953
Zinc fluorosilicate‡	4	Lithurin	IE	Genin, 1973 Keen, 1976 Anon., 1992
Zinc naphthenate			E	Stinson & Keyes, 1953
Zinc oxychloride			I	Anon., 1993 Savory, 1980

*C, cement additive; E, toxic wash (exterior use); I, toxic wash (interior use); P, plastics product.

†Borax Consolidated Ltd., Borax House, Carlisle Place, London SW1, UK.

‡Laporte Industries Ltd., General Chemicals Division, Moorfields Road, Widnes WA8 OHE and Chemical Buildings Product Ltd., Cleveland Road, Hemel Hempstead, Herts HP2 7PH, UK.

Masonry biocides are controlled under the Resticides Regulations, 1986. Only approved products can be sold supplied, used, stored or advertised. Publication in this list does not imply approved.

scale, and chemical methods predominate for both interior and exterior situations.

2.3.1 Chemical control

The commonest approach involves chemical solutions as so-called toxic washes (Richardson, 1973; Anon., 1992; Allsopp & Allsopp, 1983). A number of different chemicals have been employed as sterilants and preservatives for masonry, both experimentally and in commercial practice (Tables 18.8 and 18.9). The main types approved for practice (Anon., 1998) (see also Chapter 2) are:
1 sodium hypochlorite (common bleach);
2 sodium pentachlorophenoxide;
3 sodium 2-phenylphenoxide;
4 boric acid;
5 quaternary ammonium compounds (QACs);
6 dodecylamine salicylate and lactate;
7 dichlorophen;
8 tri-*n*-butyl tin oxide;
9 halogenated organic compounds (e.g. sulphamides, thiophthalimides).

The simplest formulations usually contain one of the first seven compounds and are extensively used for initial toxic washing over large surface areas. More complex formulations are available, intended to be more permanent, and they often contain mixtures of one or more of the chemicals, with additives to improve water repellency.

In the main, toxic washes are made up in water on site and applied to flood-affected areas thoroughly, using brushes or spraying and watering equipment. For exterior surfaces, it is desirable wherever possible to apply the toxic wash some 3–14 days before attempting to remove the growths. The washes are more effective when applied to damp surface growths but should not be used immediately after heavy rain or prior to expected rainfall. After prolonged dry periods, growths should be wetted by hosing or spraying with water shortly before applying the toxic wash. Where growths are particularly dense or leathery, penetration and effectiveness of the fluids can be aided if growths are loosened or partially removed by abrading the surface during or immediately prior to treating. Dead and moribund growth is removed using stiff wire brushes, scrapers or powerful water jets. The cleaned surface should be inspected carefully for evidence of residual growths, as certain lichen thalli can be extremely resistant. Residual growth can seriously impair the performance of any subsequent coatings and may also be capable of regeneration. A secondary application of the same, or a more permanent, toxic wash may then be appropriate.

The effective life of exterior toxic washes varies according to the nature of the formulation, the porosity of the surface and the degree of exposure to rain wash. On more porous surfaces somewhat sheltered from the most severe weathering influence, residual control may be obtained for 3 or 4 years. A good-quality, dense concrete surface in exposed conditions may remain protected for only 1 year or less. The application of a colourless water-repellant after the toxic wash has sometimes been advocated. In practice, variable absorptions can lead to a patchy appearance and there can be interference with subsequent applications of coatings. The measure of improved control frequently may not justify the additional costs of the water-repellent and its application. Regular applications of inhibitors may be necessary on prestige buildings or monuments, and care must then be taken to ensure that abrasion of the surfaces does not spoil architectural or artistic detail.

Chemical treatment of interior surfaces may often require special considerations relating to the needs and safety of the occupants of dwellings or the nature of operations in affected areas. Wall coverings and other furnishings may impose limitations, while high condensation in bathrooms and swimming-pools, in addition to surface contamination in kitchens, bakeries, breweries, etc., will make particular demands for permanence and safety of the products and the methods of applying them. Domestic bleach, QACs, dodecylamine salicylate and lactate, as well as dichlorophen, are widely favoured as toxic washes for removing growths on internal surfaces. Growths are washed with a soft brush or absorbent cloth liberally soaked in the sterilant solution, containing also a small quantity of liquid soap to wet the spores. With growths showing prolific sporing, special care is needed to minimize release of spores into the atmosphere, and respiratory protection must be worn. After cleaning, application of a more permanent and penetrating formulation was often advocated, traditionally based on sodium pentachlorophenoxide or sodium 2-phenylphenoxide. There is no published evidence as to whether penetrating formulations or, indeed, the sometimes specified subsequent 'barrier' formulations are necessary. In particularly severe cases of microbial contamination, they may be beneficial. Certainly, penetrating wall sterilants, usually based on sodium pentachlorophenoxide or sodium 2-phenylphenoxide, QACs and zinc oxychloride plaster are used for eliminating the mycelium of the dry-rot fungus *Serpula lacrymans* from within masonry (Anon., 1993; Savory, 1980). In dealing with internal mould contamination, it is desirable to reduce the concentration of spores in the atmosphere. Increasing ventilation reduces both spore concentration and the high humidity which might otherwise facilitate regrowth (Bravery, 1987). Use of disinfectant sprays, even as an adjunct to such measures, is of doubtful value, since potential health risks arise as much from inhalation of the particulate matter in the air (dead or alive) as from any risk of live infections.

Rates of application of chemical solutions, for both interior and exterior use, vary according to the formulations of the different products, and manufacturers' guidance should be followed. Dense growth will require considerably increased amounts of fluid, although with certain materials the dilution may be adjusted. Most commercially available products contain active ingredients at 0.5–5.0% by weight after dilution and are designed for dilution in water at ratios from 1 : 9 to 1 : 20 applied at coverage rates of the order of 1.5–2.5 m^2/l (75–120 sq. ft/gallon). Products are also available in which active chemicals are incorporated into pastes or gels, and these can be useful on vertical surfaces or to provide longer-lasting and deeper-penetrating protection.

Development of improved and safer chemical control agents and requirements for efficacy data for approval purposes have led to a need for standardized, accelerated methods of test. Available techniques have been assessed (Grant & Bravery, 1981a,b) and new methods proposed (Grant & Bravery, 1987).

An alternative chemical approach which has been attempted for certain special applications is that of incorporating toxicants as additives into cementacious materials. Incorporation of pentachlorophenol, copper carbonate, sodium fluorosilicate or even selenium (Gilchrist, 1953) was unsuccessful, despite the compounds being effective in aqueous solution. Keen (1976) has suggested that copper powder (1%), copper sulphate (0.1%) or sodium pentachlorophenate (0.2%) may be effective as additives to concrete, but copper(II) oxide is not only ineffective but may also interfere with normal setting. Robinson & Austin (1951) examined in the laboratory more than 20 compounds of copper, lead and arsenic for their fungicidal effectiveness when incorporated into concrete. They concluded that 10% of copper acetoarsenite was four times as effective as copper oxychloride cement. Although the strength of the concrete was slightly reduced, the process could be economical for special-risk applications, such as flooring in showers, locker-rooms of swimming-pools, kitchens, etc. In similar studies. Bartl & Velecky (1971) found that incorporation of low concentrations of tributyltin acetate into cement and plaster effectively prevented fungal growth. There is no published information on the effectiveness of additives in preventing fouling in practice. Critical factors will be the rates of leaching, the availability of the toxicant to the colonizing organisms and the effects of the toxicants on particular properties of the cement or concrete.

Safety considerations. Biocides used for preservation in the construction industry are pesticides in the context of the definitions given in the Food and Environment Protection Act 1985 (FEPA). The Control of Pesticides Regulations 1986 (CPR), enacted under the powers of FEPA, require that only approved pesticide products shall be sold, supplied, used, stored or advertised. As yet, not all non-agricultural uses of pesticides are subject to equal scrutiny under the provisions of CPR. Masonry biocides certainly are, and the products approved for this use are listed in the Pesticides Safety Directorate/Health and Safety Executive (MAFF/HSE) manual current at any time (currently *Pesticides 1998* (Anon., 1998)).

Applications of preservative products in the construction industry are also subject to control under the Control of Substances Hazardous to Health Regulations 1988. These Regulations lay

Table 18.9 Organic chemicals used to control growths in the construction industry.

Key to coding

A = adhesives
B = bitumen products
C = cement additive
E = toxic wash (exterior use)
F = filters, stoppers, groutings
I = toxic wash (interior use)
J = jointing compounds, scalants, putty
O = wet-state protection concrete additives
P = plastic products
R = rubbers (synthetic and natural)

Active chemical	Application rate/ concentration (%)	Product	Source of supply*	Application	Reference(s)
Aqueous cresol (cresylic acid)		Lysol		I	Rechenberg, 1972 Keen, 1976
Alkoxysilane: 3-(trimethoxysilyl)-propyldimethyl-octadecyl ammonium chloride	0.1	Si-QAC	Dow Corning Corp.	E	Isquith *et al.*, 1972
Benzimidazole derivative + chloracetamide	0.5–2	Mergal 592	Hoechst UK Ltd.	PF	
1,2-Benzisothiazolin-3-one	0.01–0.1	Proxel AB, CRL, HL	ICI Organics	AO	
Benzyl-hemiformals mixture		Preventol D2	Bayer UK	A (liquids)	
Bis(trichloromethyl sulphone)		Chlorosulphone	Tenneco Organics Ltd.	AO	
Chloracetamide + polyglycols + heterocyclic compounds	2–5 0.1–0.3	Mergal K6	Hoechst UK Ltd.	EI A	
Chloracetamine + quaternary ammonium compound + fluorides	0.1–0	Mergal AF	Hoechst UK Ltd.	A	
Cresylic acids	2			R	Pitis, 1972
Copper 8-hydroxyquinolinolate				P	Kaplan *et al.*, 1970
Dichlorophen [2,2′-methylene-bis (4-chlorophenol)]	1 free phenol in isopropanol	Panacide	BDH	EC	Rechenberg, 1972 Keen, 1976
2,3-Dichloro-1,4-naphthoquinone				I	Morgan, 1959
Diisocyanate				I	Sponsel, 1956
Dimethyl benzylammonium chloride		Hyamine 3500	Rohm & Haas (UK) Ltd.	IE	
Dimethyl aminomethyl phenol				R	
3,5-Dimethyltetrahydro-1,3,5-2H-thiadiazine-2-thione			Tenneco Organics Ltd.	AP	
Diquat-1,1-ethylene-2,2-dipyridiylium				ME	Rechenberg, 1972
Dithio-2,2-bisbenzmethylamide	0.2–2	Densil P	ICI Organics	A	
Dithiocarbamates + benzimidazole derivatives	0.05–0.6	Mergal AT30	Hoechst UK Ltd.	AFJ	
Dodecylamine salicylate	2–5	Nuodex 87	Durham Chemicals	EI	
Fluorinated sulphonamide	0.2	Acticide APA	Thor Chemicals Ltd,	F	
Formaldehyde	5 2			IE	Rechenberg, 1972 Keen, 1976

Halogenated acid amide derivatives	0.1–0.3	Parmetol A23	Sterling Industrial	AO	
Halogenated acid amide derivatives + aldehyde + heterocyclic compounds	0.05–0.3	Parmetol K50	Sterling Industrial	O	
Halogenized acid amide derivatives + heterocyclic compounds	1.0–3.0	Parmetol DF12	Sterling Industrial	I	
Hexaminium salt	0.1–0.3	Preventol D1	Bayer UK	A	
2-Hydroxybiphenyl potassium salt	3–20	Acticide 50	Thor Chemicals Ltd.	E	
2-Hydroxydiphenyl sodium salt		Preventol 0N	Bayer UK	A	
5-Hydroxymethoxmethyl-l-aza-3,7-dioxabicyclo (3,3,0) octane + other substituted oxazolidines		Nuosept 95	Durham Chemicals Tenneco Organics Ltd.	AFO	
Lead phenolate and other lead salts of synthetic fatty acids				P	Wexler *et al.*, 1971
3-Methyl-4-chlorophenol		Preventol CMK	Bayer UK	A (powder) F	
Methylene-bisthiocyanate			Tenneco Organics Ltd.	APFO	
2-Mercaptobenzothiazole	0.1–1	Mystox MB	Catomance Ltd.	AO	
2-Mercaptobenzothiazole sodium salt	0.1–0.5	Nuodex 84	Nuodex UK Ltd.; Tenneco Organics Ltd.	A	
N-dimethyl-*N*′-phenyl-(*N*′-fluorodichloromethylthio) sulphamide	1.5–2	Preventol A4	Bayer UK Ltd.	EIJ	
N-(fluordichloromethylthio) phthalimide	1–2	Preventol A3	Bayer UK Ltd.	EIPJ	
N-(trichloromethylthio)phthalimide		Folpet	Murphy Chemical Ltd. (UK)	PEI	Kaplan *et al.*, 1970 Rechenberg, 1972
N-(trichloromethyl)thio-4-cyclohexene-1,2-dicarboximide	0.5–2.5	Captan	Murphy Chemical Ltd. (UK)	P	Kaplan *et al.*, 1970
2,*n*-Octyl-4-isothiazolon-3-one		Kathan 893	Rohm & Haas UK Ltd.	EI	
Organic acid amine	1–5	Nuodex 87	Nuodex Ltd. UK	EI	
Organic-ethoxy compound	0.1–0.5	Acticide BG	Thor Chemicals	AFO	
	0.3–0.8	THP		AO	
Organomercury				I	Nicot, 1951
				R	Zyska *et al.*, 1972
Organotin	0.2–0.5	Acticide FPF	Thor Chemicals	AF	
Orthophenyl phenol				E	
10,10′-Oxybisphenoxarsine				P	Darby & Kaplan, 1968 Cadmus, 1976
Oxyquinoline					Nicot, 1951
Oxyquinoline sulphate					Nicot, 1951

(*Continued p. 592*)

Table 18.9 (*Continued.*)

Active chemical	Application rate/ concentration (%)	Product	Source of supply*	Application	Reference(s)
Paraquat		Gramoxone		E	Powell, 1976
Penthachlorophenol	2	Mystox G	Catomance Ltd.	ECR	Kaplan *et al.*, 1970
	0.1–3			A (starch pastes)	Rechenberg, 1972
					Gilchrist, 1953
					Purkiss, 1972
					Zyska *et al.*, 1972
Pentachlorophenyl laurate	1–3.5	Mystox LPL LSL	Catomance Ltd.	APOR	Zyska *et al.*, 1972
Phenoxy fatty acid polyester	0.4–1.5	Preventol B2	Bayer (UK) Ltd.	JB	
Phenyl mercury acetate			Tenneco Organics Ltd.	A	
Phenyl mercury nonane	0.05–0.3	Aciticide MPM	Thor Chemicals	AO	
Phenyl mercury oleate					Drisko, 1973
Quaternary ammonium compounds	1	Gloquat C	ABM Chemicals; Glover (Chemicals) Ltd.	E I	Keen, 1976 Genin, 1973 Anon., 1992 Richardson, 1973 Nicot, 1951
		Preventol R	Bayer UK Ltd.		
Quaternary ammonium salt: di-isobutyl phenoxyethoxyethyl dimethylbenzyl ammonium chloride monohydrate		Hyamine 10x	Rohm & Haas	IE	Paleni & Curri, 1972
Quaternary ammonium salt: di-isobutyl phenoxyethoxyethyl dimethylbenzyl ammonium chloride monohydrate	0.5	Hyamine 1622	Rohm & Haas	IE	Paleni & Curri, 1972
Quaternary ammonium compound + lauryl pentachlorphenate		Mystox QL	Catomance Ltd.	E	Barr, 1977
Quaternary ammonium salt with tri-*n*-butyl tin oxide		Thaltox Q Stannicide AQ	Wykamol Ltd.; Thomas Swan & Co. Ltd.	E	Genin, 1973 Keen, 1976, Richardson, 1973
Salicylamide	5–8		Bayer UK Ltd.	JP (cable insulation)	Cadmus, 1976
Sodium 2-phenylphenoxide	2	Brunsol conc	Stanhope Chemical Products Ltd	E	Genin, 1973
	2.5				Rechenberg, 1972
					Keen, 1976
	5	Mystox WFA	Catomance Ltd	EI	

Sodium pentachlorophenoxide	2 0.2 on wt of cement	Santobrite	Monsanto Ltd	EI C	Genin, 1973 Rechenberg, 1972 Keen, 1976 Sponsel, 1956
		Preventol PN	Bayer UK Ltd	AFJ	
	2	Brunobrite	Stanhope Chemical Products Ltd	E	Anon., 1992
Sodium salicylanide	1–5 0.5–1.5	Shirlan NA	ICI Ltd	I A	Keen, 1976
2,4,5,6-Tetrachloro-isophthalonitrile	0.5–1.5	Nopeocide N96	Diamond Shamrock UK	APJ	
2,4,5-Tetrachloro-isophthalonitrile (aq.)	0.3–1.8	Nopeocide N54D	Diamond Shamrock AP UK		
3,3,4,4-Tetrachloro-tetrahy drothiophene 1,1-dioxide		Nopeocide 170	Diamond Shamrock UK	EI	
Thiadiazine	0.1–1.0	Thion 66	Thor Chemicals	A	
Thinned tar oil					Rechenberg, 1972 Keen, 1976
Tri-*n*-butyl-tin acetate	0.005–1			C P	Bartl & Velecky, 1971 Cadmus, 1976
Tri-*n*-butyl tin oxide	1	Stannicide M Stannicide A	Thomas Swan & Co. Ltd	IEO	Drisko, 1973 Richardson, 1973 Sadurska & Kawalik, 1966
Tri-*n*-butyltin oxide + non-ionic emulsifier		Stannicide O	Thomas Swan & Co. Ltd.		
Trifluoromethyl-thiophthalimide					Rechenberg, 1972
a,a-Trithiobis (*N*,*N*-dimethylthioformalite)				I	Morgan, 1959
Zinc dithiocarbamate + benzimadazole derivatives	0.5–1.0	Mergal S88	Hoechst UK Ltd.	AFJ	
Zinc-8-hydroxyquinolinolate			Ward Blenkinsop	A	

*ABM Chemicals, Woodley, Stockport, Cheshire, UK.
Bayer (UK) Ltd., Bayer House, Richmond, Surrey TW9 1SJ, UK.
BDH, Poole, Dorset BN12 4NN, UK.
Catomance Ltd., 94 Bridge Road East, Welwyn Garden City A17 1JW, UK.
Diamond Shamrock (UK), 147 Kirkstall Road, Leeds LS3 1JN, UK.
Dow Corning Corporation, Laboratory Division, Stone, Stafford ST15 0BG, UK.
Durham Chemicals, Birtley, Co. Durham DH3 1QX, UK.
Glovers (Chemicals) Ltd., Wortley Low Mills, Whitehall Road, Leeds LS12 4RF, UK.
Hoechst (UK) Ltd., Hoechst House, Salisbury Road, Hounslow TW4 6JH, UK.
ICI Ltd., PO Box 19, Templar House, 81–87 High Holborn, London WCIV 6NP, UK.
ICI Organics, Blackley, Manchester M9 3DA, UK.
Monsanto Ltd., Monsanto House, 10–18 Victoria Street, London SW1H 0NQ, UK.
Murphy Chemicals Ltd., Wheathampstead, St Albans, Herts., UK.
Nuodex (UK) Ltd., Birtley, Co. Durham DH3 1QX, UK.
Rohm & Haas (UK) Ltd., Lennig House, 2 Mason Avenue, Croydon CR9 2NB, UK.
Stanhope Chemical Products, 94 Bridge Road East, Welwyn Garden City A17 1JW, UK.
Sterling Industrial, Chapeltown, Sheffield S30 4YP, UK.
Thomas Swan & Co., Ltd., Consett, Co. Durham DH8 7ND, UK.
Tenneco Organics Ltd, Rockingham Works, Avonmouth, Bristol B11 0YT, UK.
Thor Chemicals Ltd, Ramsgate Road, Margate, Kent, UK.
Ward Blenkinsop, Empire Way, Wembley, London HA9 0LX, UK.
Wykamol Ltd, Tingewick Rd, Buckingham, Bucks, MK18 1AN

Masonry biocides and other specific use of pesticides are controlled under the Control of Pesticides Regulations, 1986. Only approved products can be sold, supplied, used, stored or advertised. Publication in this list does not imply approval.

down essential requirements and a step-by-step approach for the control of hazardous substances and for protecting people exposed to them. The Regulations set out essential measures that employers (and employees) have to take. The basic principles of the COSHH Regulations are:
1 to introduce appropriate measures to control the risk;
2 to ensure that control measures are used;
3 to monitor the exposure of workers and keep their health under surveillance;
4 to inform, instruct and train employees about risks and precautions.

Specific sources of safety guidance are available relating to particular applications but precautions of particular importance are the following.
1 Wear protective gloves, clothes, boots, caps and eye and respiratory protection when mixing and applying toxic products.
2 Do not allow waste fluids, drift, spray or run-off to contact adjacent personnel, vegetation, watercourses or drainage or sewerage-disposal systems or to enter other premises.
3 Dispose of waste containers, washings and contaminated growth safety, as agreed with manufacturers of products and waste-disposal authorities.
4 Never allow untrained personnel to handle toxic products.

Some products may contain chemicals corrosive to flashings, gutters and damp-proof courses, or which may be harmful to certain types of natural stone. Advice and assurances from manufacturers and contractors should be sought at an early stage in specifying work.

Chemical herbicides. Herbicides are sometimes employed for the control of higher plants in certain constructional situations, such as roadways, pavements and the like. It is beyond the scope of the present chapter to consider herbicides in detail. The reader is referred to a short account of higher plants as deteriogens by Allsopp & Drayton (1976), in which three main types of chemical control are recognized:
1 contact herbicides having a corrosive action on plant tissues;
2 systematic herbicides which enter through aerial parts and are translocated within the plant;
3 soil-sterilants which poison the soil and are taken up into the plant through the roots.
Herbicides are available with a range of specificity of target-plant species, and growth-regulating chemicals are also used in plant control. They are all strictly controlled under CPR, and only approved products can be used.

Aquatic control. In special circumstances, control of vegetation may be required under water, e.g. water-drainage and supply structures, retaining walls and weirs. Keen (1976) proposes three approaches, including the use of admixtures and antifouling paints and treatment of the water with algicides. All the systems have serious limitations, because of the high rates of loss by leaching. Toxicity to animal and plant life and effects on potability of water also impose limitations. The use of admixtures is considered earlier in this chapter, and antifouling paints are considered elsewhere in the book. Guidelines are available on the use of herbicides in watercourses and lakes (Anon., 1995).

2.3.2 Non-chemical methods of control

One classic principle of controlling deterioration of materials by organisms is to adjust the environmental conditions to limit growth (Chapter 3). In the context of constructional masonry materials, the source of inoculum is always present, while nutritional requirements and oxygen are likewise rarely limiting. Thus, water-supply becomes the only critical factor capable of providing a potential means of control. Exposure of exterior surfaces to rainfall is largely inevitable, but there is scope for ensuring that water is not concentrated or focused on to particular parts of structures by features of the design and construction, or by inadequate consideration of maintenance needs. Ledges, sills, parapets and similar architectural features can cause localized shedding of water in streaks or sheets, facilitating algal and lichen growth. Poor arrangements for water dispersal from structures or blocked gutters and damaged flashings may permit localized downwash. Regular removal of accumulated dust, silt, leaves and other debris from horizontal surfaces, troughs and gutters can minimize the risk of growth from higher plants.

Interior surfaces are inevitably exposed to the risk of microbial contamination, with water again being the only potential limiting factor. Rising damp, direct water penetration and particularly condensation are the main sources of excessive moisture. Rectification of faults in the waterproofing of the structure is necessary to prevent the first two sources, while elimination of condensation can be much more complex. Requirements will include a combination of improvements in insulation with appropriate installation of vapour barriers, increased ventilation and/or heating. Impermeable wall coverings and non-absorptive paint can often exacerbate the problem of condensation. Restoring absorptive surfaces or the use of anticondensation paints can be beneficial.

Heat sterilization. Heat sterilization has been used in the eradication of the dry-rot fungus *S. lacrymans* from walls. However, the system has fallen from favour, due to the often unacceptably high risk of fire, the high cost and the impracticability of producing sufficiently high temperatures throughout the thickness of the wall. Blowlamp burning can, however, be a convenient method to remove surface growth and colonization if used safely, and paraffin-powered flame guns are commonly used for clearing unwanted higher-plant vegetation from verges, parking spaces, waste ground and the like.

3 Polymeric materials, adhesives and additives

A variety of polymeric materials are used in the construction industry as damp-proofing compounds, sealants, gaskets, adhesives, plastics and wall and floor coverings.

Many of these compounds are manufactured, stored, transported and applied in a 'wet' state as emulsions or suspensions with water, and in this form are highly vulnerable to bacterial, actinomycete or fungal infection. Even in the solid or 'dry' state, many of these materials may be subject to intermittent or permanent dampness, with the attendant risk of colonization by mixed populations of bacteria and mould fungi.

3.1 Water-based mixtures

3.1.1 Problems

Within the scope of this chapter, it is not possible to consider in detail the nature, use and microbial susceptibility of the full range of water-based products used in building and construction. It is possible, however, to simplify matters by considering together the problems of all such materials, because of the similarity in the colonizing microflora and in the basic mechanism of deterioration.

Many cement and concrete additives, adhesives and waterproofing compounds are supplied as mixtures of the active organic chemicals with emulsifiers and surfactants in water, sometimes called 'multiple-phase systems' (Purkiss, 1972). These are vulnerable to forms of microbial fermentation similar to those occurring in emulsion paints, cutting oils and fuel-oil systems. Common among the large numbers of organisms implicated are *Escherichia coli*, *Pseudomonas fluorescens*, *Pseudomonas aeruginosa*, *Micrococcus* spp., *Bacillus subtilis*, *Streptococcus* spp., *Proteus rettgeri*, *Enterobacter* spp. and species of fungi from the genera *Cladosporium*, *Penicillium*, *Paecilomyces* and *Aspergillus*.

Purkiss (1972) has proposed a generalized mechanism of attack of multiple-phase systems in which the microorganisms growing in the water phase oxidize emulsifiers and surfactants, inducing instability of the emulsion. Droplet fusion begins to occur and the organisms may then attack the oil phase itself. Continuing attack leads to continually increasing droplet size, culminating in separation of the system. In addition, generation of gases as by-products of metabolism can cause pressurizing, or even bursting, of containers.

3.1.2 Preservation

The specific chemical constituents, solvents, emulsifiers and surfactants in the various formulations demand particular properties of any preservative agent; thus generalizations are difficult. Biocides need to be compatible with the particular formulation, of low volatility and non-corrosive and to have a broad spectrum of action and suitable chemical stability and water solubility; in particular, the partition coefficients are important. Many emulsions are stabilized at alkaline pH values; thus the biocides must remain stable at pH 8–9. Above all, they must not interfere with the ultimate function of the formulation. The problem of microbial growth in water-based emulsion systems is now widely accepted, and most commercial products contain biocides to prevent in-can spoilage. Some products can confer protection also in the subsequent dry state, although normally the concentration of biocides is increased or an alternative is added which does not lose its activity when the formulation dries or sets. Table 18.9 indicates some of the main chemicals used experimentally and commercially for the different applications.

3.2 Plastics, rubbers, sealants and bitumen

3.2.1 Problems

Natural and synthetic polymers are used as vapour barriers, damp-proof courses, waterproofing products, coatings and sheatings for pipework and cables, rainwater and foul-water pipework, gaskets for pipework and components, as well as jointing and sealing materials between components and cast-concrete sections and for glazing and filling purposes. In almost all of these service situations, the materials are exposed to natural microbial infection from the air, water, sewage, etc., and almost all become wet because of the very nature of their function.

Studies on the fundamental susceptibility to microbial attack of polymer materials and their constituents are numerous (Klausmeier, 1966; Darby & Kaplan, 1968; Dubok *et al.*, 1971; Osmon *et al.*, 1972; Pankhurst *et al.*, 1972; Cadmus, 1976; Zyska, 1981). A recent comprehensive and detailed review has been published by Seal (1988).

Natural and vulcanized rubbers are regarded as generally susceptible to attack by actinomycetes, bacteria and fungi, although they vary in degree (Zobell & Grant, 1942; Zobel & Beckwith, 1944; Rook, 1955; Zyska, 1981; Williams, 1982; Tsuchii *et al.*, 1985). Synthetic rubbers appear to show even more variability in susceptibility to microbes. Polyisoprenes (Tsuchii *et al.*, 1979) and polyisobutadienes (Tsuchii *et al.*, 1978, 1984) show vulnerability to limited degradation by soil bacteria, while most of the available experimental evidence indicates that styrene–butadiene copolymers are resistant (Blake *et al.*, 1955; Dickenson, 1969; Potts, 1978). However, the presence of specific compounding ingredients can decrease the natural resistance of these materials. Acrylonitrile–butadiene rubbers are significantly less susceptible again than styrene–butadienes (Zobell & Beckwith, 1944; Potts *et al.*, 1973). Chloroprene rubbers are considered relatively inert to microbial attack, probably due to the extent of cross-linking and the presence of sulphur (Heap & Morrell, 1968; Dubok *et al.*, 1971; Cundell & Mulcock, 1973). As with other polymer formulations, however, the presence of microbiologically susceptible plasticizers can induce susceptibility (Heap & Morrell, 1968).

Polyurethanes are widely used in construction as adhesives, thin sheet, cable sheathings and, more particularly, rigid and flexible foams. Generally, polyurethanes are susceptible to microbial attack by bacteria and particularly by fungi (Darby & Kaplan, 1970; Kaplan *et al.*, 1970; Wales & Sagar, 1985; Seal & Morton, 1986). Susceptibility is correlated strongly with esterase activity of particular microorganisms (Shuttleworth, 1987) and the nature of the constituent components of the polyurethane (Darby & Kaplan, 1968; Seal & Morton, 1986).

Polysulphide rubbers are used extensively as sealants, mastics and tank linings, and are accepted as being very resistant to microbial attack. Silicone rubbers are extremely inert, although contamination with low-molecular-weight hydrocarbons can permit microbial colonization (Heap & Morrell, 1968). Zobell & Beckwith (1944) observed utilization of silicone rubber by marine microbes, possibly for this reason. Of the two main types of polyesters, aromatic polyesters are regarded as resistant to the growth of microorganisms (Potts, 1978), while aliphatic polyesters have been shown to be biodegradable (Potts *et al.*, 1973; Shuttleworth, 1987). Polyamides are the nylons, which are not used significantly in construction, although in any case they are generally regarded as resistant to microbial attack.

Polyethylenes have been extensively studied and microbial susceptibility shown to be related to molecular weight (Potts *et al.*, 1973). Low-molecular-weight oligomers appear to be utilizable by microbes, but fractions above mol. wt 1000 are non-biodegradable. Direct studies of polyethylenes in soil burial have shown only 1–3% mass loss over periods of 1–8 years (Colin *et al.*, 1981), which was believed to reflect the extent of low-molecular-weight contaminants in the polymer. Hence, it has been concluded that high-molecular-weight polyethylene is resistant to microbial attack (Seal, 1988).

The chemistry of polystyrene provides a highly resistant structure. However, it has been proposed that susceptibility to microorganisms could occur by aromatic-ring degradation mechanisms (Seal, 1988). Certainly, the styrene dimers, trimers and tetramers can be biodegraded (Tshuchii *et al.*, 1997). While mechanisms have been proposed for polystyrene biodeterioration, it is not generally regarded as of major practical significance in construction.

Clearly, microbial resistance of polymers can relate to molecular size, as well as to the amounts and types of primary components, stabilizers, plasticizers, etc. The variation in resistance to attack of some common plasticizers is given in Table 18.10, from data supplied by K.J. Seal (personal communication). Studies with building sealants (Bravery *et al.*, 1977) revealed that in the field a one-part polysulphide sealant was very susceptible to mould, while the two-part polysulphide and acrylic types were less susceptible; a silicone type was almost completely resistant. Three different polyurethane types were resistant, moderately resistant and susceptible, respectively. In laboratory tests, *Epicoccum purpureum* caused significant loss in tensile strength of a polysulphide and a polyurethane sealant prior to weathering, while the other main fungal species isolated from the field tests, *Cladosporium herbarum*, *Mucor racemosus* and *Botrytis cinerea*, only significantly affected the polyurethane. The susceptibility sometimes changed after weathering. Pankhurst *et al.* (1972) concluded that polymers without additives were usually inert, although susceptibility increased with increasing complexity of the material. Polyethylene, polypropylene, epoxy and coal-tar resins were all likely to prove resistant in a soil environment, although bitumen was susceptible. The susceptibility of bitumen for building insulation or coatings of pipes, cables and road surfaces is acknowledged by Pitis & Stanci (1977). Changes caused by microbial attack included asphaltene content, flexibility, surface appearance, resin and oil content.

Table 18.10 Relative resistance of some plasticizers to biodegradation.*

	Plasticizer
Decreasing resistance to biodegradation ↓	Tricresyl phosphate, diiso-octyl phthalate, dinonyl phthalate, didecyl phthalate
	Dioctyl phthalate
	Dibutyl phthalate
	Dinonyl adipate
	Dioctyl adipate
	Dimethyl sebacate
	Diiso-octyl adipate
	Diiso-octyl sebacate
	Butyl stearate
	Dioctyl sebacate
	Dihexyl adipate
	Dibutyl sebacate
	Dicapryl adipate
	Dibenzyl sebacate
	Polypropylene sebacate
	Methyl ricinoleate
	Butyl ricinoleate
	Butoxyethyl stearate
	Zinc ricinoleate

* Based on Petri-dish test using 24 fungi and measuring growth (colony diameters) on agar containing mineral salts and plasticizer (after K.J. Seal, personal communication).

Evidence as to the susceptibility of polymer materials to microbial attack appears sometimes conflicting. For example, Dunkeley (1964) and Dickenson (1969) have contended that natural rubber in pipe rings is resistant to microbial growth, despite the evidence of Heederik (1966) and Hills (1967). Cadmus (1976) states that synthetic polymers are generally very resistant, although susceptibility may increase in certain use situations, such as environments with aggressive microbial populations or in contact with susceptible materials. Klausmeier (1966) offers an explanation for the sometimes conflicting opinions and apparent variations in susceptibility and performance of polymer materials by proposing that certain microorganisms can attack only if additional nutrient is present. This phenomenon is called 'cometabolism', and additional external sources of carbon may be very important. Prediction of likely performance in a given service situation and the potential need for biocidal preservation are complicated by these considerations. The evidence does, however, support the need for specifications to take account of possible biological hazards in service and require assessments to be made of the durability of given materials under conditions representative of those likely to be encountered.

Experience in the methodology needed for such biological testing of polymer materials is already extensive (Walters, 1977).

3.2.2 *Preservation*

Susceptible plastics, rubbers and bitumens can be successfully preserved (Kaplan *et al.*, 1970; Pitis, 1972; Zyska *et al.*, 1972), although biocides and the methods of their application must be carefully selected to be compatible both with the mix during production and with the finished product.

Zyska *et al.* (1972) studied fungicides incorporated into rubber plasticizers and concluded that organomercury compounds were barely effective at 2%, pentachlorophenol was effective at above 2.5% but more than 5% of pentachlorophenol laurate was needed. Cresylic acids at 2% were found effective by Pitis (1972), but efficacy varied according to the type of plasticizer used. Compatibility with the mix and residual effectiveness of the biocide have been referred to by Cadmus (1976), who found poor stability with organotin acetate and salicylate, as well as inactivation by ultraviolet (UV) radiation and hydrolysis. Biocides for polymer materials need some mobility in order to be effective, either by their own vapour pressure or by combination with one of the other constituents, such as the plasticizer (Cadmus, 1976). Captan and folpet, though effective fungicides, tend to be thermally unstable and sometimes do not control surface growths when incorporated into polyvinyl chloride (PVC). Darby & Kaplan (1968) indicate that incorporation of biocides is more difficult in urethanes than in vinyl systems. Both they and Cadmus (1976), however, cite 10,10′-oxybisphenoxarsine as having good compatibility, thermal stability and effectiveness. A number of organometallic, organoarsenical and organosulphur compounds were found useful by Darby & Kaplan (1968). Wexler *et al.* (1971) demonstrated the compatibility and effectiveness of lead phenolate or lead salts of other low-molecular-weight synthetic fatty acids in protecting PVC insulating materials.

A number of chemicals assessed as biocides for the protection of polymer materials are included in Table 18.10, coded to indicate the respective fields of use.

A consequence of continuing extensive studies on the physiological and metabolic mechanisms of microbial attack of polymers is that the improved understanding creates the opportunities for development of microbiologically resistant polymers. This approach, while reducing dependence on toxic preservatives, brings with it the dilemma of disposing of extremely inert polymers.

4 Conclusions

A wide variety of biological problems are encountered in the construction industry capable of inducing significant, even serious, financial loss or wastage. The increasing awareness of the range of problems, organisms and materials involved has generated developments in the chemical industry to produce or adapt biocides for these specific control purposes. In many situations, little is known of the nature of the organisms and their mechanisms of attack, so that chemical control procedures are necessarily pragmatic. Sometimes, although the incidence of microorganisms is recognized, their significance has not been fully investigated.

Many of the materials subject to attack, as well as the biocides themselves, are produced from oil and are energy-intensive to manufacture. Maintenance and repair work occasioned by inadequate performance of materials in service is increasingly expensive, so major cost savings are possible from a better understanding of the significance of biological agencies of deterioration and of strategies for their control. Specifications for building materials and procedures must increasingly take account of potential biodeterioration and demand adequate resistance or protection of materials, as well as requiring designs that minimize the development of conditions conducive to the growth of potentially deteriogenic organisms.

5 References

Allsopp, C. & Allsopp, D. (1983) An updated survey of commercial products used to protect materials against biodeterioration. *International Biodeterioration Bulletin*, **19**, 99–145.

Allsopp, D. & Drayton, I.D.R. (1976) The higher plants as deteriogens. In *Proceedings of the 3rd International Biodeterioration Symposium* (eds Sharpley, J.M. & Kaplan, A.M.), pp. 357–364, London: Applied Science Publishers.

Anon. (1993) *Dry rot: its recognition and control.* Building Research Establishment. Digest No. 299, Walford.

Anon (1995) *Guidelines for the use of herbicides on weeds in or near watercourses and lakes.* Ministry of Agriculture, Fisheries and Food. London: MAFF Publications.

Anon. (1992) *Control of Lichens, Moulds and Similar Growths.* Building Research Establishment. Digest No. 370, London: HMSO.

Anon. (1998) *Pesticides 1991.* MAFF/HSE Reference Book No. 500. London: HMSO.

Aristovskaya, R.V. & Kutuzova, R.S. (1968) Microbial factors in the extraction of silicon from slightly soluble natural compounds. *Soviet Soil Science*, **12**, 1653–1659.

Ashurst, J. & Dimes, F.G. (1977) *Stone in Building: its Use and Potential Today.* London: Architectural Press.

Aslam, M. & Singh, S.M. (1971) Copper sulphate as an algicide in limewash. *Paintindia*, **21**, 21–22.

Bachmann, E. (1915) Kalklösende Algen. *Berichte der Deustchen Botanische Gesellschaft*, **33**, 45–57.

Barr, A.R.M. (1977) *Comparative Studies on the Inhibition of Lichen and Algal Growth on Asbestos Paving Slabs.* International Biodegradation Research Group, Constructional Materials Working Group, April.

Bartl, M. & Velecky, R. (1971) The fungicidal effect of organic tin in cements, limes and plasters. *Cement Technology*, **51**, 54–57.

Berthelin, J. (1983) Microbial weathering processes. In *Microbial Geochemistry* (ed. Krumbein, W.L.), pp. 223–262. Oxford: Blackwell Scientific Publications.

Blake, J.T., Kitchin, D.W. & Pratt, O.S. (1955) Microbiological deterioration of rubber insulation. *Applied Microbiology*, **3**, 35–39.

Bravery, A.F. & Jones, S.C. (1977) Occurrence of biological growths on concrete dams in North Scotland. Unpublished paper. Department of the Environment, Princes Risborough Laboratory. Summary in *Biodeterioration Society Newsletter*, **3**, 1977.

Bravery, A.F., Jones, R.J.R. & Jones, S.C. (1977) Susceptibility to mould growth of some jointing materials. Unpublished report. Building Research Establishment, Princes Risborough Laboratory, Aylesbury, Bucks.

Bravery, A.F., Grant, C. & Sanders, C.H. (1987) Controlling mould growth in housing. In *Proceedings of a Conference on Unhealthy Housing.* University of Warwick, December. Institute of Environmental Health Officers.

British Standards Institution (1982) *Cleaning and Surface Repairs of Buildings Part 1. Natural Stone, Cast Stone and Clay and Calcium Silicate. Brick Masonry.* BS 6270.

Cadmus, E.L. (1976) Biodeterioration in the United States: A review. In *Proceedings of the 3rd International Biodegradation Symposium* (eds Sharpley, J.M. & Kaplan, A.M.), pp. 343–346. London: Applied Science Publishers.

Colin, G., Cooney, J.D., Carlsson, D.J. & Wiles, D.M. (1981) Deterioration of plastic films under soil burial conditions. *Journal of Applied Polymer Science*, **26**, 509–519.

Cundell, A.M. & Mulcock, A.P. (1973) The measurement of the microbiological deterioration of vulcanised rubber. *Material und Organismen*, **8**, 1–15.

Darby, R.T. & Kaplan, A.M. (1968) Fungal susceptibility of polyurethanes. *Applied Microbiology*, **16**, 900–905.

Dickenson, P.B. (1969) Natural rubber and its traditional use in underground pipe sealing rings. *Journal of the Rubber Research Institute of Malaya*, **22**, 165–175.

Drisko, R.W. (1973) *Control of Algal Growths on Paints at Tropical Locations*, US Department of Commerce, National Technical Information Service, Naval Civil Engineering Laboratory, California, December.

Dubok, N.N., Angert, L.G. & Ruban, G.I. (1971) Study of the fungus resistance of rubbers, mix ingredients and vulcanisates. *Soviet Rubber Technology*, 17–20.

Duff, R.B., Webley, D.M. & Scott, R.O. (1963) Solubilisation of minerals and related materials by 2-ketogluconic acid-producing bacteria. *Soil Science*, **95**, 105–114.

Dumitru, L., Popea, F. & Lazar, I. (1976) Investigations concerning the presence and role of bacteria in stone deterioration of some historical monuments from Bucharest, Jassy and Cluj-Napoca. In *Proceedings of the 6th Symposium on Biodeterioration and Climatisation*, p. 67. Bucharest, Rumania: Institul de Cercetari Pentru Industria Electrotechnica.

Dunkeley, W.E. (1964) Die Verwendungsdauer des Kautschuks in Rohren und Leitungen. *Kautschuk—Fontschritt und Entwicklung*, **17**, 98–102.

Eckhardt, F.E.W. (1985) Mechanisms of the microbial degradation of minerals in sandstone monuments, medieval frescos and plaster. In *Proceedings of the 5th International Congress on Deterioration and Conservation of Stone* (ed. Felix, G.), pp. 643–652. Lausanne: Presses Polytechniques Romandes.

Figg, J., Bravery, A.F. & Harrison, W. (1987) *Covenham Reservoir Wave Wall—a Full Scale Experiment on the Weathering of Concrete*, SP-100, pp. 469–492. American Concrete Institute.

Flannigan, B. (1989) Airborne micro-organisms in British houses: factors affecting their numbers and types. In *Airborne Deteriogens and Pathogens* (ed. Flannigan, B.), Biodeterioration Society Occasional Publications No. 6. Kew: CAB International.

Forrester, J.A. (1959) Destruction of concrete caused by sulphur bacteria in a purification plant. *Surveyor*, **118**, 881–884.

Gaur, A.C., Madad, M. & Ostwal, K.P. (1973) Solubilisation of phosphatic compounds by native microflora of rock phosphates. *Indian Journal of Experimental Biology*, **11**, 427–429.

Genin, G. (1973) Control of lichens, fungi and other organisms. *Paint Pigments Vernis*, **49**, 3–6.

Gilchrist, F.M.C. (1953) Microbiological studies of the corrosion of concrete sewers by sulphuric acid-producing bacteria. *South African Industrial Chemist*, **7**, 214–215.

Grant, C. (1982) Fouling of terrestial substrates by algae and implications for control—a review. *International Biodeterioration Bulletin*, **18**, 57–65.

Grant, C. & Bravery, A.F. (1981a) Laboratory evaluation of algicidal biocides for use on constructional materials, 1. An assessment of some current test methods. *International Biodeterioration Bulletin*, **17**, 113–123.

Grant, C. & Bravery, A.F. (1981b) Laboratory evaluation of algicidal biocides for use on constructional materials 2. Use of the vermiculite bed technique to evaluate a quaternary ammonium biocide. *International Biodeterioration Bulletin*, **17**, 125–131.

Grant, C. & Bravery, A.F. (1987) Evaluation of biocides for use on building materials. In *Preservatives in the Food, Pharmaceutical and Environmental Industries* (eds Board, R.G., Allwood, M.C. and Banks, J.G.), pp. 133–144. Oxford: Blackwell Scientific Publications.

Grant, C., Hunter, C.A., Flannigan, B. & Bravery, A.F. (1989) The moisture requirements of moulds isolated from domestic dwellings. *International Biodeterioration*, **25**, 259–284.

Heap, W.M. & Morrell, S.H. (1968) Microbiological deterioration of rubbers and plastics. *Journal of Applied Chemistry*, **18**, 189–193.

Heederik, J.P. (1966) Prüfen von Betonrohren in den Niederlanden. *Beton-Zeitung*, **32**, 635.

Henderson, M.E.K. & Duff, R.B. (1963) The release of metallic and silicate ions from minerals, rocks and soils by fungal activity. *Journal of Soil Science*, **14**, 236–246.

Hills, D.A. (1967) The degradation of natural rubber pipe-joint rings. *Rubber Journal*, **149**, 12–15; 17–77.

Hueck-Van der Plas, E.H. (1968) The microbiological deterioration of porous building materials. *International Biodeterioration Bulletin*, **4**, 11–28.

Hunter, C.A. & Bravery, A.F. (1989) Requirements for growth and control of surface moulds in dwellings. In *Airborne Deteriogens and Pathogens* (ed. Flannigan, B.), pp. 174–182. Biodeterioration Society Occasional Publications No. 6. Kew: CAB International.

Hunter, C.A., Grant, C., Flannigan, B. & Bravery, A.F. (1988) Mould in buildings: the air spora of domestic dwellings. *International Biodeterioration*, **24**, 81–101.

Ionita, I. (1971) Contributions to the study of the biodeterioration of works of art and historic monuments, III. Species of fungi isolated from stone monuments. *Revue Roumaine de Biologie—Serie Botanique*, **16**, 433–436.

Ionita, I. (1974) The involvement of fungi in the stone degradation process of some historical monuments. *Proceedings of the Symposium on Biodeterioration Science (Roumania)*, **4**, 117–122.

Isquith, A.J., Abbot, E.A. & Walters, P.A. (1972) Surface-bonded antimicrobial activity of an organosilicon quaternary ammonium chloride. *Applied Microbiology*, **24**, 859–863.

Jaton, C. (1972) Microbiological changes in the monolithic church of Aubeterre sur Dronne. *Revue d'Ecologie et de Biologie du Sol*, **9**, 471–477.

Jaton, C. (1973) Microbiological aspects of the alteration of stonework of monuments. In *Proceedings of the 1st International Symposium on the Deterioration of Building Stones*, pp. 149–154. La Rochelle: Centre de Recherches et d'Etudes Océanographiques.

Kaltwasser, H. (1971) Destruction of concrete by nitirification. *European Journal of Applied Microbiology and Technology*, **3**, 185–192.

Kaplan, A.M., Greenberger, M. & Wendt, T.M. (1970) Evaluation of biocides for treatment of polyvinyl chloride film. *Polymer Engineering Science*, **10**, 241–246.

Kauffmann, J. (1952) Rôles des bactéries nitrifiantes dans l'altération des pierres calcaires des monuments. *Compterendu*, **234**, 2395–2397.

Kauffman, J. (1960) Corrosion et protection des pierres calcaires des monuments. *Corrosion et Anticorrosion*, **8**, 87–95.

Kauffman, J. & Toussaint, P. (1954) Corrosion des pierres: nouvelles expériences montrant le rôle des bactéries nitrifiantes dans l'altération des pierres calcaires des monuments. *Corrosion et Anticorrosion*, **2**, 240–244.

Keen, R. (1976) *Controlling Algae and Other Growths on Concrete.* Advisory Note 45–020. London: Cement and Concrete Association.

Kerner-Gang, W. (1977) Evaluation techniques for resistance of floor coverings to mildew. In *Biodeterioration Investigation Techniques* (ed. Walters, A.H.), pp. 95–104. London: Applied Science Publishers.

Klausmeier, R.E. (1966) The effects of extraneous nutrients on the biodeterioration of plastics. In *Microbiological Deterioration in the Tropics.* SCI Monograph 23, pp. 232–243. London: Society for Chemical Industry.

Krumbein, W.E. (1972) The role of micro-organisms in the genesis, diagenesis and degradation of rocks. *Revue d'Ecologie et de Biologie du Sol*, **9**, 283–319.

Krumbein, W.E. (1983) *Microbiol Geochemistry.* Oxford: Blackwell Scientific Publications.

Krumbein, W.E. & Pochon, J. (1964) Bacterial ecology of altered stones of monuments. *Annales de l'Institut Pasteur*, **107**, 724–732.

Lepidi, A.A. & Schippa, G. (1973) Some aspects of the growth of chemotrophic and heterotrophic microorganisms on calcareous surfaces. In *Proceedings of the 1st International Symposium on the Biodeterioration of Building Stones*, pp. 143–148. La Rochelle: Centre de Reserches et d'Études Océanographiques.

Lewis, F., May, E. & Bravery, A.F. (1985) Isolation and enumeration of autotrophic and heterotrophic bacteria from decayed stone. In *Proceedings of the 5th International Congress on Deterioration and Conservation of Stone* (ed. Felix, G.), pp. 255–278. Lausanne: Presses Polytechniques Romandes.

Lewis, F., May, E., Daley, B. & Bravery, A.F. (1987) The role of heterotrophic bacteria in the decay of sandstone from ancient monuments. In *Biodeterioration of Constructional Materials* (ed. Morton, L.H.G.), pp. 45–53. Biodeterioration Society Occasional Publication No. 3. Preston: Lancashire Polytechnic.

Lewis, F., May, E. & Greenwood, R. (1988) A laboratory method for assessing the potential of bacteria to cause decay of building stone. In *6th International Congress on Deterioration and Conservation of Stone*, Torun, Poland, pp. 48–58. Vol. 2, *Supplement.* Torun: Nicholas Cupernicus University Press.

Lloyd, A.O. (1976) Progress in studies of deteriogenic lichens. In *Proceedings of the 3rd International Biodegradation Symposium* (eds Sharpley, J.M. & Kaplan, A.M.), pp. 395–402. London: Applied Science Publishers.

Lurie, H.I. & Brookfield, E. (1948) Copper impregnated concrete floors. *South Africa Medical Journal*, **22**, 487–489.

May, E. & Lewis, F. (1988) Strategies and techniques for the study of bacterial populations on decaying stonework. In *6th International Congress on Deterioration and Conservation of Stone*, Torun, Poland, pp. 59–70. Vol. 2, *Supplement.* Torun: Nicholas Cupernicus University Press.

Milde, K., Sand, W., Wolff, W. & Bock, E. (1983) Thiobacilli of the corroded concrete walls of the Hamburg sewer system. *Journal of General Microbiology*, **129**, 1327–1333.

Morgan, O.D. (1959) Chemical control of algae and other nuisance growths on greenhouse benches, pots and potting soil. *Plant Disease Reporter*, **43**, 660–663.

Neculce, J. (1976) Some aspects of fungi in stone biodeterioration. In *Proceedings of the 6th Symposium on Biodeterioration and Climatisation*, pp. 117–123. Bucharest, Rumania: Institul de Cercetari Pentru Industria Electrotechnica.

Nette, I.T., Pomortserva, N.V. & Kozlova, E.I. (1959) Deterioration of rubber by microorganisms. *Microbiologiya*, **28**, 881.

Nicot, J. (1951) Dégradation des murs de plâtre par les moissisures. *Revue Mycologique*, **16**, 168–172.

Norddeutsche Affinerie (1953) Preventing the development of animal and plant life on water-soaked surfaces. German patent 870 340. *Chemical Abstracts*, **52**, (1958), 20775f.

Novotny, J., Wasserbauer, X.Y. & Zadak, Z. (1973) Influence of the biological factors on the destruction of asbestos-cement roofing of stables. In *Symposium on the Deterioration of Building Stones*, pp. 155–156. La Rochelle: Centre de Recherches et d'Études Océanographiques.

Osmon, J.L., Klausmier, R.E. & Jamison, E.I. (1972) Rate limiting factors in biodeterioration of plastics. In *Proceedings of the 2nd International Biodeterioration Symposium*, pp. 66–75. London: Applied Science Publishers.

Paleni, A. & Curri, S. (1972) Biological aggression of works of art in Venice. In *Proceedings of the 2nd International Biodeterioration Symposium*, pp. 392–400. London: Applied Science Publishers.

Paleni, A. & Curri, S. (1973) The attack of algae and lichens on stone and means of their control. In *Proceedings of the 1st International Symposium on the Deterioration of Building Stones*, pp. 157–166. La Rochelle: Centre de Recherches et d'Études Océanographiques.

Pankhurst, E.S., Davies, M.J. & Blake, H.M. (1972) The ability of polymers or materials containing polymers to provide a source of carbon for selected micro-organisms. In *Proceedings of the 2nd International Biodeterioration Symposium*, pp. 76–90. London: Applied Science Publishers.

Pitis, I. (1972) Mycological protection of rubber for industrial products. In *Proceedings of the 2nd International Biodeterioration Symposium*, pp. 294–300. London: Applied Science Publishers.

Pitis, I. & Stanci, A. (1977) Testing of biodeteriorated bitumens. In *Biodeterioration Investigation Techniques*, (ed. Walters, A.H.), pp. 23–40. London: Applied Science Publishers.

Pochon, J. & Jaton, C. (1967) The role of microbiological agencies in the deterioration of stone. *Chemistry and Industry*, 1587–1589.

Potts, J.E. (1978) Biodegradation. In *Aspects of Degradation and Stabilisation of Polymers* (ed. Jellinck, H.H.G.), pp. 617–657. Amsterdam: Elsevier.

Potts, J.E., Glendinning, R.A., Ackart, W.B. & Niegisch, W.D. (1973) The biodegradability of synthetic polymers. In *Polymers and Ecological Problems* (ed. Guillet, J.E.), pp. 61–79. New York: Plenum Press.

Powell, J.M. (1976) Use of gramoxone to control mosses and liverworts in greenhouse pots. *Bi-monthly Research Note*, **31** (5), 35–36. (Department of the Environment of Canada.)

Purkiss, B.E. (1972) Biodeterioration of multiple phase systems. In *Proceedings of the 2nd International Biodeterioration Symposium*, pp. 99–102. London: Applied Science Publishers.

Rechenberg, W. (1972) The avoidance and control of algae and other growths on concrete. *Betontechnische Berichte*, **22**, 249–251.

Richardson, B.A. (1973) Control of biological growths. *Stone Industries*, **8**, 2–6.

Richardson, J.H. & Ogilvy, W.S. (1955) Antimicrobial penetrant sealers. *Applied Microbiology*, **3**, 277–288.

Robinson, R.F. & Austin, C.R. (1951) Effect of copper-bearing concrete on moulds. *Industrial and Engineering Chemistry*, **43**, 2077–2082.

Roizin, M.B. (1951) A whitewash that prevents moulding in storage houses for fruit, vegetables and potatoes. *Doklady Vshesoyuznoy Akademii Nauk imeni V.I. Lenina*, **16**, 39–41. In *Chemical Abstracts*, **46** (1952), 224.

Rook, J.J. (1955) Microbiological deterioration of vulcanised rubber. *Applied Microbiology*, **3**, 302–309.

Sadurska, I. & Kawalik, R. (1966) Experiments on control of sulphur bacteria active in biological corrosion of stone. *Acta Microbiologica Polonica*, **15**, 199–202.

Sahinkaya, H. & Gurbuzer, E. (1968) Study of rock-phosphate dissolving micro-organisms. In *Abstracts Communications: National Conference of General and Applied Microbiology*, Bucharest, p. 98.

Sand, W. & Bock, E. (1987) Simulation of biogenic sulphuric acid corrosion of concrete—importance of hydrogen sulphide, thiosulphate, and methylmercaptane. In *Biodeterioration of Constructional Materials* (ed. Morton, L.H.G.), pp. 29–36. Biodeterioration Society Occasional Publication No. 3. Preston: Lancashire Polytechnic.

Savory, J.G. (1980) Treatment of outbreaks of dry rot *Serpula lacrymans*. *Newsletter, British Wood Preservation Association*, News sheet No. 160, May 1980.

Schwartz, A. (1963) *Microbial Corrosion of Plastics and Their Compounds*. Arbeit Deutscher Akademie der Wissenschatten zu Berlin No. 5.

Seal, K.J. (1988) The biodeterioration and biodegradation of naturally occurring and synthetic plastic polymers. *Biodeterioration Abstracts*, **2**, (4), 295–317.

Seal, K.J. & Morton, L.H.G. (1986) Chemical materials. In *Biotechnology*, Vol. 8: *Microbial Degradation* (ed. Schonborn, W.), pp. 583–606. Weinheim: Verlagsgesellschaft.

Shuttleworth, W.A. (1987) Biodegradation of polycaprolactone polyurethane by *Gliocladium roseum*. PhD thesis, Cranfield Institute of Technology, UK.

Sponsel, K. (1956) Vermeidung von Pilz-und Schimmelbildung in Textilbetrieben. *Zeitschrift für die gesamte Textil-Industrie*, **58**, 596–597.

Stinson, R.F. (1956) Algal growth and the performance of flowering plants in clay pots treated with copper naphthenate. *Proceedings of the American Society of Horticultural Science*, **68**, 564–568.

Stinson, R.F. & Keyes, G.G. (1953) Preliminary report on copper and zinc naphthenate treatments to control algae on clay flower pots. *Proceedings of the American Society of Horticultural Science*, **61**, 569–572.

Todd, J.J. (1974) Blow your problems. *Environment Pollution Management, Classe Chemie, Geologie und Biologie*, **4**, 79–81.

Trotet, G., Dupuy, P. & Grossin, F. (1973) A biological nuisance caused by cyanophycetes. In *Proceedings of the 1st International Symposium on the Deterioration of Building Stones*, pp. 167–170. La Rochelle: Centre de Recherches et D'Études Océanographiques.

Tsuchii, A., Suzuki, T. & Takahara, Y. (1978) Microbial degradation of liquid polybutadiene. *Agricultural and Biological Chemistry*, **43**, 1217–1222.

Tsuchii, A., Suzuki, T. & Takahara, Y. (1979) Microbial degradation of *cis*-1,4-polyisoprene. *Agricultural and Biological Chemistry*, **43**, 2441–2446.

Tsuchii, A., Suzuki, T. & Fukuoka, S. (1984) Bacterial degradation of 1,4-type polybutadiene. *Agricultural and Biological Chemistry*, **48**, 621–625.

Tsuchii, A., Suzuki, T. & Takeda, K. (1985) Microbial degradation of natural rubber vulcanizates. *Applied and Environmental Microbiology*, **50**, 965–970.

Wales, D.S. & Sagar, B.F. (1985) The mechanism of polyurethane biodeterioration. In *Biodeterioration and Biodegradation of Plastics and Polymers*, Proceedings of the Annual Meeting of the Biodeterioration Society (ed. Seal, K.J.), pp. 56–59. Kew: CMI.

Walters, A.H. (1977) *Biodeterioration Investigation Techniques*. London: Applied Science Publishers.

Webley, D.M., Henderson, M.E.K. & Taylor, I.F. (1963) The microbiology of rocks and weathered stones. *Journal of Soil Science*, **14**, 102–112.

Wexler, T., Ortenberg, E. & Pitis, I. (1971) New fungistatic agents and their behaviour in PVC mixtures. *Chimica Industriale, Chimica Generale*, **104**, 201–206.

Whiteley, P. & Bravery, A.F. (1982) Masonry paints and cleaning methods for walls affected by organic growths. *Journal of the Oil and Colour Chemists Association*, **65**, 25–27.

Williams, G.R. (1982) The breakdown of rubber polymers by micro-organisms. *International Biodeterioration*, **18**, 31–36.

Wood, P.A. & Macrae, I.C. (1972) Microbial activity in sandstone deterioration. *International Biodeterioration Bulletin*, **8**, 25–27.

Zobell, C.E. & Beckwith, J.D. (1944) The deterioration of rubber products by micro-organisms. *Journal of the American Water Works Association*, **36**, 439–453.

Zobell, C.E. & Grant, C.W. (1942) The bacterial oxidation of rubber. *Science*, **96**, 379–380.

Zyska, H. (1981) Rubber. In *Microbial Biodeteriorations: Economic Microbiology*, Vol. 6 (ed. Rose, A.H.), pp. 323–385. London: Academic Press.

Zyska, B.J., Rytych, B.J., Zankowicz, L.P. & Fudalej, D.S. (1972) Microbiological deterioration of rubber cables in deep mines and the evaluation of some fungicides in rubber. In *Proceedings of the 2nd International Biodeterioration Symposium*, pp. 256–267. London: Applied Science Publishers.

Chapter 18

E. WOOD PRESERVATION

1 Introduction

Wood is destroyed, or deteriorates, by action of fungi, bacteria, insects and chemical and physical agents, including weather, fire and mechanical wear. Economically, decay by fungi or insects is most serious and wood preservation is primarily aimed at its prevention.

Some fungi feed on wood substances (cellulose, hemicellulose and lignin), thereby causing massive decay (wet rot or dry rot). Other fungi and some bacteria have a more limited ability to attack wood, and cause deterioration but not massive decay (sap-stain fungi discolour and reduce impact resistance, bacteria increase permeability). Yet other fungi (moulds) feed on material within the cells without affecting the main structure.

Insects simply eat the wood; attack in temperate climates is mainly by the larvae of Coleoptera (beetles) but in the tropics and subtropics Isoptera (termites) are major destroyers of wood.

Wood preservation is the protection of wood from decay by treatment with chemicals. Both the preservative used and the process used to apply it are important in determining the degree of protection. The choice and use of wood preservatives are now widely affected by health, safety and environmental considerations. In most countries, they are subject to regulation.

2 Deterioration

2.1 Fungi

Fungi require food, warmth and water to grow. Wood is food and warmth is almost any ambient temperature, so that the liability of wood to fungal decay parallels its liability to get wet. Buried in, or in contact with, the ground, wood will certainly get wet, infection is immediate and continuous and decay is certain. It is most rapid in the wet, warm tropics. Outdoors, exposed to the weather, wood will get wet intermittently; drying out is very varied, so that, while wood in this situation is always at risk, occurrence is variable, especially when partly protected by design, or when a surface finish restricts drying more than wetting. Inside a building, wood should remain dry unless there is faulty design or construction, or failure in the integrity of the outer skin, damp-proofing, plumbing and the like, coupled with lack of maintenance. Experience shows that decay due to one or more of these causes is sufficiently frequent, or of such consequence with some components, to justify preservation. Accordingly, the need to protect wood inside a building is based on experience.

2.1.1 *Fungal decay*

The fungi causing massive wood decay are Basidiomycetes. Decay may be wet rot or dry rot. Wet rot is by far the most common form of decay, both inside buildings and outside; commonly attacked wood is soft, wet and pulpy. Many species cause wet rot; some are brown rots and some white rots (Table 18.11). Optimum wood-moisture content for different species of wet-rot fungi range from 30–40% (*Coniophora puteana*) to 50–70% (*Paxillus panuoides*) (Bech-Andersen, 1985). The moisture content was based on the dry weight of wood. Growth is substantially confined to the wet part of any piece of wood.

Dry rot in the UK is caused by a single, somewhat unique species, *Serpula lacrymans*, with an optimum moisture content for growth of 20–30% and not growing above 55% (Bech-Andersen, 1985). It produces sufficient water to sustain further growth, is able to transport water and nutrients over some distance and so is able to spread into drier wood and over non-nutrient bases such as masonry to infect timber distant from the first outbreak (Coggins, 1976; Jennings, 1981; Bravery & Grant, 1985). In damp walls, these strands can survive for a long time, possibly as long as 9 years.

Table 18.11 Wood-decay fungi.

Latin name	Common name	Woods attacked	Occurrence
Wet rots			
Brown rots			
Coniophora puteana	Cellar fungus	Softwoods and hardwoods	Widely, especially in wood soaked by water leakage
Amyloporia xantha	–	Softwoods	Common, especially in warmer parts of buildings (*Amyloporia xantha*, *Poria placena*, *Fibroporia vaillantii*)
Poria placena	–	Softwoods	
Fibroporia vaillantii	White pore or mine fungus	Softwoods	
Paxillus panuoides			
White rots			
Phellinus contiguus	–	Softwoods and hardwoods	External joinery
Donkioporia expansa	–	Hardwoods, especially oak	Near leaks or in beam-ends, with death-watch beetle
Pleurotus osteatus	Oyster fungus	Hardwoods	
Asterostroma spp.	–	Softwoods	Chipboard, etc. e.g. skirting boards, generally limited spread, exceptionally very wide
Dry rot			
Brown rot			
Serpula lacrymans	Dry-rot fungus	Any	In buildings only

The need to kill them, so that they do not regrow to start a new outbreak, adds considerably to the difficulties and cost of eradicating dry rot.

Serpula is important in the UK; it has some importance in parts of continental Europe, locally in parts of North America and in Honshu province in Japan (Doi, 1983) and in parts of southern Australia (Thornton, 1989). It has a low upper temperature threshold for growth and is consequently unknown in the tropics and places with summer temperatures above about 27°C (Hegarty, *et al.*, 1986). Growth ceases at this temperature, and death occurs if subjected to temperatures above 35°C (Miric & Willitner, 1984), even for only a few hours.

Infected, decayed wood generally looks dry—hence the name. Appearance alone is not, however, an indication of dry rot; any decayed timber that becomes dry cracks and looks dry. In countries outside Britain, other fungi may be referred to as dry rot if the decayed timber has this appearance.

Dry rot occurs only in buildings and, while less common than wet rot, individual outbreaks are usually more extensive and more expensive to eradicate.

Some fungi destroy cellulose preferentially, leaving the lignin largely intact. Decayed wood is brown and these fungi are called brown rots. White rots also attack the lignin, leaving the wood white or light-coloured (Table 18.11).

The micromorphology of the two types of fungi is different. In both, the hyphae penetrate into the lumen and lie on the inner cell wall. With white rot, lysis occurs along the line of contact, while, with brown rot, erosion of the cell wall is more general (Levy, 1987). This is due to the extent to which the enzymes diffuse away from the hyphae (Green, 1980).

With timber buried in the soil, or in very wet conditions, decay is commonly by microfungi (Ascomycetes, Fungi Imperfecti). While these destroy wood substance, attack is confined to a zone near the wood surface and only develops deeper as the outer layers are destroyed. Such decay is referred to as soft rot (Savory, 1955). Because of the severity of the conditions, decay is none the less rapid.

Soft-rot hyphae penetrate into the cell wall and form cavities in the centre of the cell wall. Some soft-rot fungi can, at high temperatures (35–40°C), grow at moisture contents down to 15% (Morton & Eggins, 1976).

Under abnormal conditions, such as are found in the ground below the water-table, destruction may be due to bacteria and anaerobic fungi (Boutelje & Goransson, 1971).

Decay, in some situations, is the result of a complex process of a succession of organisms, involving many species of fungi and other micro-organisms, with competition between different species and with stimulation or inhibition of one by another.

Typically, new timber is initially invaded by a random range of bacterial and fungal spores. Early bacterial development causes little damage but opens up the way to fungal invasion. The first fungi to develop are the microfungi—soft rot, moulds and sap stainers. Commonly, these are then overtaken by the Basidiomycetes. Many accounts give overall details or examine specific aspects (Findlay & Savory, 1954; Savory, 1954; Levy, 1965, 1987; Butcher, 1971; Dickinson & Levy, 1979; Levy & Dickinson, 1980; Smith, 1980; Carey, 1981, 1982).

2.1.2 Non-decaying fungi

Some fungi grow on wood without causing any great decay. These are moulds and blue stain.

Moulds such as *Penicillium* spp., *Aspergillus* spp. and *Cladosporium* spp. feed on free sugars or surface dirt of damp wood; they are unsightly but cause no real damage. Moulds occur both indoors and outdoors. Outdoor timber may also support slime moulds, known collectively as Myxomycetes.

Blue stain or sap stain is the name given to fungi which grow in sapwood, causing discoloration. Hyphae permeate throughout the sapwood, penetrating cell walls through very fine boreholes, but they do little harm other than to discolour the wood. The impact strength may be reduced but the timber is suitable for all but the most demanding uses (Cartright & Findlay, 1958). The discoloration reduces the value of new timber and mars the appearance of transparent finishes. For sap-staining fungi to grow, moisture content must be above fibre saturation but below complete saturation, i.e. with both air and water in the lumen. Over 260 species have been reported as causing sap stain; some continue growth below freezing (Land *et al.*, 1985). Some sap-stained woods were sought after to form decorative inlay for cabinet-making. Sap stain commonly develops in freshly felled timber while it is drying out, but, if timber in service reaches similar moisture contents, it may also be attacked. Common species in the two situations are different. Those most common in service are *Aureobasidium pullulans, Schlerophoma pithyophila, Diplodia* spp. and *Cladosporium* spp. Most commonly, these grow under paints and other surface finishes, and the most noticeable effect is on the finish.

2.2 Insects

Throughout the world, seasoned wood in use is liable to be attacked by insects. Only a few species attack wood; in all parts of the world, the larvae of some beetles (Coleoptera) live in and feed on wood. Adults emerge from wood solely to mate and lay eggs, often flying away to spread infestation (Hickin, 1963).

In the UK and much of the temperate region, the most important species are the common furniture beetle or woodworm, *Anobium punctatum* (De Geer); the death-watch beetle, *Xestobium rufovillosum* (De Geer); lyctus or powder-post beetles, *Lyctus linearis* (Goeze), *Lyctus brunneus* (Stephens) and other *Lyctus* spp.; and the house longhorn beetle, *Hylotrupes bajulus* (Linneaus). All these occur in northern Europe, America, South Africa, Australia, New Zealand and elsewhere, but their relative importance varies.

In the UK, the woodworm is by far the most common, most older houses being infested to some extent. Incidence in houses built after 1960 appears to be as low as 1%, possibly due to changes in design, construction or heating practice or better maintenance (Bravery *et al.*, 1995). Death-watch is the most notorious; it favours old, damp hardwoods, such as are most common in churches and other historic buildings. It knocks its head on the wood to attract a mate, and this sound has given rise to morbid superstitions of an approaching death. House longhorn has a very limited distribution in the UK, being common only around Camberley. It is more widespread in continental Europe and also occurs in South Africa.

Different woods differ in their susceptibility to insect attack, but use and location are less significant than with fungi. Structural timber, furniture, tool handles or anything made of wood may become infested, and, while very dry wood is less likely to be attacked than damp, moisture content is not critical, most economic damage being to wood that is 'ordinarily' dry.

Weevils may attack timber when it is wet and slightly decayed, and perhaps sometimes when it is not. Generally these are regarded as minor pests, but in parts of the UK they are becoming more common (Hum *et al.*, 1980).

Many more beetles and some other insects, including wasps, attack fallen wood in the forest; occasionally, these insects may attack timber in use. Pinhole borers attack newly felled wood, but attack dies out as soon as the wood is seasoned. Boreholes, usually surrounded by a dark stain, caused by symbiotic fungi, may be seen in such woods.

In the tropics, by far the most damaging timber pests are termites. There are about 1500 species of termite, several hundred of which attack wood (Harris, 1971; Hickin, 1971). Termites are social insects, building nests with thousands, or even millions, of individuals. The main groups are: (i) subterranean termites, building nests in the ground and foraging for wood; (ii) dry-wood termites, building nests in wood; and (iii) damp-wood termites, inhabiting old stumps and damp wood. Termites occur in southern Europe, with isolated pockets in some more northern towns (e.g. Paris, Hamburg); only a single established infestation (*Reticulitermes lucifugis*) has been found in the UK, and this recently (Bravery *et al.*, 1995).

Ants (*Camponotus* spp.) damage sound wood in nest-building in some countries, e.g. Sweden (Butovitsch, 1976), Canada and the USA (Hickin, 1985).

2.3 Marine

Timber in the sea is subject to fungal attack by marine species and is also subject to damage by marine borers, such as *Teredo* spp. (shipworm) and *Limnoria* (gribble) (Ray, 1959; Jones & Eltringham, 1968).

2.4 Weather

On exposure to the weather, wood is subject to a variable cocktail of physical, chemical and biological agents (Hilditch & Woodbridge, 1985; Hilditch, 1987). These cause deterioration at the surface and may pave the way for deeper decay.

Principal agents are radiation from the sun, wetting by rain or dew, changes in atmospheric humidity, changing temperature, wind and wind-borne particles, atmospheric chemicals and fungal, algal and bacterial infection.

Wood exposed to the weather constantly goes through wetting and drying cycles, these changes causing repeated shrinking and swelling. Changes are greater near the surface than at depth, thereby setting up strains that lead to physical separation of fibres. There may also be direct degradation of the wood substance by water. Light, both ultraviolet and visible, causes breakdown of both cellulose and lignin. Protection against the weather is by use of paints, wood stains and similar finishes (Hilditch & Crookes, 1981).

3 Preservation

The main sectors of timber preservation are as follows.

1 Preventive (pre)treatment, being the treatment of timber before it is installed to prevent decay or insect attack.

2 Remedial or curative treatment, being the treatment of timber in place, in buildings or elsewhere, to cure decay or insect attack and to prevent recurrence.

Industrial pretreatment and remedial treatment by specialists are major, worldwide industries. There is also substantial treatment of timber, for either purpose, by private individuals ('do-it-yourself' (DIY)), craftsmen or tradesmen and on estates and farms.

3.1 Prevention

In principle, there are two approaches to preserving wood: to impregnate the whole of the wood with a preservative or to impregnate the outer zone of each piece so as to create a toxic barrier, or 'cordon sanitaire', around the rest of the wood. In practice, because of the resistance of wood to liquid penetration, it is seldom, if ever, possible to treat the whole of the wood, and a compromise has to be accepted with maximum achievable penetration giving a thick toxic barrier. The effectiveness of such a treatment depends on its resistance to fungal penetration and on its life and integrity. For many situations, more limited penetration provides adequate protection, allowing use of less preservative and more convenient or economical treatment methods.

Wood has two parts, heartwood and sapwood. Heartwood is the inner part of the tree trunk and, in some but not all species, contains resins and extractives, which give it a high natural durability. In most species, heartwood is difficult to impregnate. Sapwood, which is the outer part of the trunk in which sap moves in the living tree, is of low natural durability. Treatability of sapwood is species-specific, some readily accepting treatment and others not. For specific uses, both treatability and natural durability must be considered. Essentially, if the sapwood is permeable and the heartwood durable, the timber can be treated for use in a high-hazard situation, but, if the sapwood is impermeable and the heartwood perishable, then the timber cannot be treated for any but low-hazard situations.

Theoretically, any preservative can be applied by almost any method. However, when the intrinsic properties of the preservative, the achievement of the different methods of application and economics are all taken to account the market splits along technical lines (Table 18.12).

3.1.1 Industrial

Current practice for preventive pretreatment in industry falls into several groups (Anon., 1986c).

1 The application of creosote under pressure. This is the main treatment for railway sleepers and transmission poles; it is also used for some farm and estate timbers.

2 Application of water-borne salts under pressure. This process competes with creosote in the treatment of poles and posts but is also used to treat building timbers. It is little used on dimensioned timbers, such as window-frames and other joinery, because of the risk of distortion.

Table 18.12 Fields of use.

Application	Preservative		
	Creosote	Water-borne	Organic solvent
Pressure	Sleepers, posts and poles	Posts and poles	Not used in UK, poles in USA
Double-vacuum/ double-vacuum + pressure	Not used	Limited use	Building timbers, especially external joinery
Immersion	Fence panels	Not used	Building components, garden timbers
Spray	Amateur	Not used	Remedial, amateur
Brush	Amateur	Not used	Amateur

3 Double-vacuum or double-vacuum pressure treatment with organic solvent preservatives is mainly used for window-frames and other dimensioned components, including prefabricated roof trusses, where the absence of any dimensional effect is the main consideration.
4 Some industrial pretreatment is by simple immersion of timber in an organic solvent preservative.

3.1.2 Trade and amateur

Do-it-yourself, trade maintenance or craft construction uses organic solvent preservatives or, for fences and similar uses, creosote. Application is mostly by brush and sometimes by spray or immersion. These are the least effective of the methods of treatment, but, using organic solvent preservatives which have superior penetrating powers, adequate protection for all but the most demanding situations can be obtained. Much domestic fencing is treated with low-price aqueous, pigmented, stains; these offer little or no protection again decay.

Whenever timber is worked, treatment cannot be effectively carried out until after working is complete; methods of treatment , other than brush, dip or spray, are often not practicable.

3.2 Eradication

Most dwellings and many other buildings world wide are part wood and at some time in their life will suffer insect attack or decay. Commonly, this is of limited extent, and repair, depending on the type and extent of deterioration, is a combination or replacement and curative treatment.

The basic principles of eradicating insect attack and decay are quite different.

3.2.1 Insects

For the eradication of insects, the dominant use in the last 60 years has been of organic solvent preservatives, containing an insecticide with contact and stomach action. These are applied to the surface of the infected timber, into which they penetrate typically 4–10 mm. In badly infested wood much deeper penetration will occur through the galleries bored by the insect larvae.

Any larvae within the zone of penetration are killed immediately, both solvent and insecticide having effect. Some kill below this zone may result from fumigant action, but insects deep inside the wood are not killed at the time of application. Kill will follow when, as is necessary to complete their life cycle, the larvae tunnel towards the surface.

The technique is effective for eradication of insects in 'ordinary'-size timbers, but can be less than fully effective with large timbers.

Several other methods may be used selectively, including drilling and injection of fluid and the use of pastes. There is substantial use of emulsions for woodworm eradication.

Remedial treatments are carried out by many specialist firms, by the building trade and by private individuals (DIY). Professional application is mostly by spray, but DIY usage is more often by brush. Often, insect attack is, in the initial stages, very localized. Local treatment by the householder is fully adequate and considerably cheaper.

3.2.2 *Fungi*

To speak of eradicating fungal attack from timber is somewhat misleading. Preservatives of the sort used for preventive treatment will kill any fungus when they contact it. However, to achieve sufficient penetration to kill all the fungal mass pervading infected wood is not practical, except (and then not always reliably) where decay and infection are only shallow or by using special techniques, only suitable for museums.

Eradication of fungal decay from a building is a combination of measures: (i) to cut out decayed and infected timber and remove or eradicate any other source of infection; (ii) to eliminate the dampness, without which decay would not have occurred; (iii) to apply preservative to remaining sound timbers as an additional safeguard against recurrence; and (iv) to replace, with pretreated timber, timbers that have been cut out.

In taking these measures, there is a major difference between wet rot and dry rot. With wet rot, infection spreads little, if at all, beyond the visible decay. With dry rot, there may be some infection of the wood beyond the obvious, and there is commonly massive growth over and into walls, often for some metres from the wood. Treatment of dry rot must therefore include sterilization of the wall. This is done by irrigating the infected parts with fungicide, mostly in aqueous solution.

4 Wood preservatives

Wood preservatives are liquids with fungicidal and/or insecticidal components which will remain active over many years, so as to give long-term protection. The common types are categorized (Anon., 1975) as tar oil (creosote), water-borne and organic solvent. For the last two, the liquid in which the preservative components are dissolved is water or an organic solvent, respectively. Emulsions, mainly oil-in-water, are increasingly used.

4.1 Creosote

Creosote is obtained by distillation of coal tar, which in turn is obtained by the destructive distillation of coal. Creosote is the fraction collected between about 200°C and 400°C.

Originally, the prime processing of coal was to produce coal gas for lighting and heating. Creosote was one of several by-products. Currently, processing is mainly to produce smokeless fuels or blast-furnace coke.

The exact composition of creosote varies with the coal from which it is obtained and the process used for its manufacture. Essentially, it is a mixture of tar acids, tar bases and neutral materials. Tar acids are mixed phenol, cresol, xylenols and higher homologues (Chapter 2). Tar bases include pyridine, quinoline, acridine, etc. Neutral compounds are mainly hydrocarbons, such as naphthalene, anthracene, fluorene (diphenylene methane) and phenanthracene (van Groenou *et al.*, 1951; McNeil, 1952).

Commercially, creosote is available in heavy grades, which must be applied hot, and in low-viscosity grades, which can be applied cold by brush or dip (Anon., 1973a). The difference between the two is mainly in the proportion boiling above 355°C. In the UK and elsewhere, there is now a limit on the content of water-soluble phenols and benz pyrenes, for some market sectors, on health grounds.

Despite having been in use since at least 1838 (Bethell, 1838), creosote is still one of the most effective preservatives known. It is also one of the cheapest, but is a dark variable brown, is oily and has a strong odour. These make it unacceptable for building and many other uses. Its main uses are for the pressure treatment of wooden railway sleepers and telegraph and fence posts (Anon., 1973b) and for dip treatment of fence panels and DIY retreatment of them, with some use on farm and estate timbers.

4.2 Water-borne

Many water-soluble inorganic salts are effective fungicides. Used as timber preservatives, they are liable to be leached out if the timber is put into a wet location. Water-borne preservatives in use today follow developments from the 1930s, based on the use of mixtures of salts, which, after impregnation into the wood, undergo a change so that the residual preservative is insoluble and therefore leach-resistant. Most fall into one of two groups. Foremost are those using dichromate, which causes a reaction with the wood, and those based on ammonia, evaporation of which leaves a residue insoluble in water.

Water attaches to the wood cellulose by hydrogen bonding; these bondings cause the cell wall to expand, and the whole wood to swell as it gets wet and shrink as it dries. Treatment with water-borne preservatives may therefore cause distortion.

Water-borne preservatives do not naturally penetrate readily into seasoned timber and are therefore applied only by pressure processes. Because of the amount of water absorbed (150–300 l/m^3), timber needs redrying for some uses. The cost and/or time of drying can be a restriction on its use.

4.2.1 *Copper chrome arsenate*

The most widely used water-borne preservative is copper chrome arsenate (CCA), known in America as chromated copper arsenate. It consists of a mixture of copper, arsenic and dichromate salts, for example:

Copper sulphate ($CuSO_4{\cdot}5H_2O$)	32–35%
Sodium dichromate ($Na_2Cr_2O_7{\cdot}2H_2O$)	41–45%
Arsenic pentoxide ($As_2O_5{\cdot}2H_2O$)	26–20%
	(Anon., 1987a)

or

Chromium trioxide (CrO_3)	65.5%
Cupric oxide (CuO)	18.1%
Arsenic pentoxide (As_2O_5)	16.4%
	(Anon., 1981)

Argument has gone on for years over the relative merits of the two types and on the effect of changes in the ratio of components. There does not seem to be any good evidence of significant differences between products of the first (salt) type and those of the second (oxide) type in their effectiveness in preserving wood. The electrical conductivity of wood treated with salt-type formulations is much higher and the rate of corrosion of metals (under conditions where both types cause corrosion) is also higher with the salt type (Cross *et al.*, 1989). Variation in ratios, especially of copper : dichromate, have a modifying effect on fixation (Wallace, 1964). Currently, most commercial products are of the oxide type. At ambient temperature, fixation takes, typically, 3 weeks. During this period, there is a pollution risk from washing off and a hazard to the worker, if used prematurely. Accelerated fixation processes have been developed, and are now used to reduce this time to a few hours (Anon., 1991e; Coggins, 1991; Connell *et al.*, 1995).

Some countries place restrictions on the use of arsenic-containing preservatives in buildings and some other places. Many alternatives have been proposed; several are used in various parts of the world, but few, if any, fully match in performance (Tillott & Coggins, 1981).

Preservatives that fix by dichromate reaction, but that do not contain arsenic, include CCB (Wolman, 1958), based on copper, dichromate and boric acid, typically 34% $CuSO_4{\cdot}5H_2O$, 38% $K_2Cr_2O_7$, 26% H_3BO_3 (Wolman, 1975). Chromium is now also regarded as hazardous; materials free from both arsenic and chromium are being introduced (Cornfield *et al.*, 1993).

4.2.2 *Ammoniacal preservatives*

Preservatives fixing by evaporation of ammonia are less used, although there is renewed interest, since they offer a route to fixed preservatives not containing either arsenic or chromium, both of which are viewed as a health hazard. Preservatives in use include ammoniacal copper arsenate (ACA), made by dissolving cuprous oxide and arsenic pentoxide in approximately equal amounts (calculated as Cu_2O and As_2O_5) in ammonia solution in the presence of air (Anon., 1974a). Other compositions have used, in addition to copper and ammonia, pentachlorophenol (Hagar, 1954), caprylic acid (Hagar, 1972) or various branched-chain carboxylic acids (Hilditch, 1977a). Ammonia, at high concentrations, presents a hazard to health and is very corrosive to plant. Alternatives, but with a similar rationale, include copper alkanolamines, usually with other ingredients, for example quaternary ammonium compounds (McCarthy, 1978).

4.3 Organic solvent preservatives

Organic solvent preservatives are solutions of an active ingredient in an organic liquid, currently almost always petroleum-derived. There are two types. One type uses a light volatile paraffinic solvent, with boiling range typically 140–270°C, which, after application, dries leaving a clean, paintable surface (Anon., 1979a). The other type is based on a non-volatile solvent, similar to gas oil or diesel oil, boiling range 180–370°C (Anon., 1979b).

Organic solvents penetrate more readily than any other type, enabling use of less onerous methods of application. They do not form any bond to wood, so that treatment does not cause any dimensional change. Thus they are used for the treatment of wood that has already been shaped (Hilditch, 1964). Organic solvent products also have the advantage of being clean and quick-drying, but they are the most expensive of the preservatives. Use is therefore mainly where these features are of most benefit.

In addition to the main solvent, auxiliary solvents are needed, with some active ingredients to give stable solutions. Aromatic solvents, some esters and alcohols have been used. Crystalline active ingredients also require an antibloom agent to stop formation of crystals on the surface during drying; non-volatile esters, oils and resins are used.

Depending on the specific intended use of the preservative, the active ingredient is a fungicide or an insecticide, or both. Fungicides in use in the past 25 years are: pentachlorophenol 5%, tributyltin oxide 1%, a combination of the two (1.75% and 0.44%, respectively) and copper naphthenate, 2% or 2.75% Cu (Anon., 1979a). Pentachlorophenol and tributyltin oxide are now widely restricted on health or environmental grounds. They are being replaced by newer materials, which include zinc carboxylates (Anon., 1979a), trihexyleneglycol biborate, triazoles and other organic compounds. Lindane has been the main insecticide, but is now being partly superseded by synthetic pyrethroids, such as permethrin and cypermethrin.

Environmental objectives to reduce the discharge of organic solvents to the atmosphere generally, but especially in the workplace and in occupied buildings, are leading to recovery and recycling systems in industrial use and to replacement by emulsion formulations for remedial application.

4.3.1 Copper and zinc carboxylates

The copper and zinc salts of naphthenic acid were first used as wood preservatives in Denmark in 1911 under the trade name Cuprinol. Naphthenic acid is a mixture of saturated cyclic carboxylic acids, occurring naturally in crude petroleum.

In the UK, both naphthenates were long used in DIY and industrial preservatives (Bulman, 1955; Hilditch, 1964, 1977b). In the USA, copper naphthenate in heavy oil is used for pressure preservation of heavy structural timbers (Barnes & Hein, 1988); it gives good service, especially in soil. For this and similar uses, it is increasingly replacing pentachlorophenol, because of environmental considerations.

Metal salts of synthetic organic acids, especially those produced by the 'oxo' and 'Koch' processes, have come into wide use (Sparks, 1978; Hilditch *et al.*, 1983). These are cleaner and more consistent than the naphthenates, but otherwise have broadly similar properties. Acypetacs–zinc is a combination of the zinc salts of C_8–C_{10} oxo and Koch acids (Hilditch *et al.*, 1978). Zinc versatate is a combination of zinc with a Koch acid only. These materials are widely used for joinery treatment and in retail products.

4.3.2 Pentachlorophenol

Pentachlorophenol (PCP) was developed from 1930 (Carswell & Nason, 1938) and has become more used than any other active ingredient for organic solvent preservatives. Application is by any of the main processes—double-vacuum, immersion, brush or spray for pretreatment of building components and for remedial treatment of wet or dry rot. In the USA, it is also used for pressure treatment of heavy constructional timbers. It gives excellent results, even in the ground (Cockroft, 1974).

The sodium salt of PCP in water is used to treat green timber to prevent sap staining between felling and seasoning, and for wall sterilization in dry-rot control. Pentachlorophenol and its salts have many other uses and, as a combined result, has become widely distributed in the environment (Rango Rao, 1977; Anon., 1987b). Restrictions on its use are widespread, and use in the UK is now minimal (Anon., 1991a).

4.3.3 *Tributyltin oxide*

Tributyltin oxide (TBTO) came into use as a wood preservative in the 1960s (Richardson, 1988) and from 1968 became the most widely used preservative for the treatment of window joinery in the UK. The main advantage of TBTO for this purpose is ready acceptance, without any adverse effect of paint. It does not perform well in soil contact and its adequacy in other situations, including joinery, has been questioned. Established instances of failure in service are, however, few.

Tributyltin oxide was also extensively used in marine antifouling paints. Pollution of waters and its effects on fish resulted in its prohibition for this use, and restrictions of its use as a wood preservative have been introduced in the UK (following some restriction elsewhere). Some industrial use, by, for example, double vacuum, remains but is diminishing.

4.3.4 *Triazoles*

These fungicides have been used as wood preservatives for 10–15 years. Azaconazole came first, but has been largely superseded by propiconazole (Goodwine, 1990) or tebuconazole (Bayer). Typically both are used at 1.75–0.9%. Synergism has been claimed for a 1:1 mixture. Tebuconazole is also used, with copper and boron, in water-based preservatives (Williams & Ryan, 1996).

4.3.5 *Other fungicides*

Dichlorfluanid is mainly used in wood stains and the like for protection against blue stain. 3-Iodo-2-propynylbutylcarbamate (IPBC) has been used for over 10 years, mainly in the USA, with little use in Europe or the UK.

4.3.6 *Lindane*

Lindane is the pure γ-isomer of hexachlorocyclohexane (HCH) (Biegel, 1988). It is a powerful insecticide with good persistence, and is extensively used in wood preservatives, at 0.5% for prevention or 1% for eradication.

Lindane is called γ-benzene hexachloride (BHC) in the USA and elsewhere. This has given rise to confusion with benzene, to which it is unrelated. Confusion also exists between the pure lindane and crude mixed isomers.

Lindane has become widely distributed in the environment, as a result of agricultural use, and there is concern about its effects on marine life and on human health. There is controversy around its use as a wood preservative, in particular because of its fatal effect on bats, which often roost in places that are treated to eradicate woodworm.

Other chlorinated hydrocarbon insecticides, such as dieldrin, aldrin and chlordane, have been used in wood preservatives, but their use is now minimal, because of concern about their health and environmental effects.

4.3.7 *Synthetic pyrethroids*

Permethrin, cypermethrin and deltamethrin belong to a group of synthetic chemicals related to the naturally occurring pyrethrum. They have become widely used in place of lindane in wood preservatives (Carter, 1984) and are generally regarded as environmentally acceptable. New insecticides include flufenoxuron, a benzoyl urea compound, acting as a growth regulator on insects (Wegen *et al.*, 1996).

4.4 Emulsions

Historically, emulsions were only used for short-term protection, such as the prevention of pinhole borers in the forest or of lyctus in timber yards and sawmills. Following concern for potential health effects of solvent use in dwellings and factories and the need to reduce solvent discharge to atmosphere, there has been much development and re-evaluation of emulsion systems. They have less odour and present less fire hazard.

Most are conventional oil-in-water emulsions,

containing 10–20% solvent. Some are microemulsions, in which the oil droplet size is below 0.1 μm. Some advantages are claimed for microemulsions—better penetration and prevention of emergence. Both fall short of solvent products, but are generally of adequate performance for insect eradication, so that, when health and environmental considerations are taken into account, they are now widely preferred for *in situ* insect treatment (Dawson & Czipri, 1991; Czipri *et al.*, 1993; Dawson, 1993). There is some *in situ* use as fungicidal treatments, but this is less well substantiated. There is also some use for pretreatment by the double-vacuum process.

Pastes (see Section 5.5) based on organic solvent preservatives are oil-in-water emulsions, with up to 80% disperse phase. The active ingredients are the same as those used in solvent preservers.

5 Preservation processes

Several methods are used to apply preservatives, ranging from a prolonged treatment under pressure, to force deep penetration, to a simple, short dip or brush treatment, resulting in relatively shallow penetration (Hunt & Garratt, 1953; Nichols, 1973; Wilkinson, 1979; Anon., 1986c).

5.1 Pressure processes

Timber is placed in a closed vessel, the vessel is flooded with preservative, a pressure of around 14 bar is applied to the liquid and held typically for 4 h, to force preservative into the wood.

There are two basic types of process—full-cell and empty-cell. In the full-cell process, the pressure is released, preservative pumped out of the treatment vessel and the timber taken out. In the empty-cell process, a vacuum is applied to draw out some of the preservative. The two processes achieve similar penetration but the empty-cell process uses less preservative and leaves a cleaner surface. There are several varieties of both processes, some using an initial vacuum to increase preservative uptake.

As with all processes, the achievement is different with different timbers. With a readily treatable timber, such as European redwood or Scots pine (*Pinus sylvestris*), all sapwood will be fully penetrated and there will be some penetration into the heartwood. Preservative usage is high, typically 300 l/m^3 for full-cell treatment and 150 l/m^3 for empty-cell. Because of this high usage, with potentially high cost, only water-borne preservatives and creosote are applied by these processes. With impermeable woods, such as spruce (*Picea abies*), penetration may be only a few millimetres.

With either creosote or CCA, both processes are very effective, giving service lives in the 50–100-year range.

5.2 Double-vacuum/double-vacuum pressure processes

Timber is placed in a closed vessel and a vacuum drawn to pull air out of the wood. The vessel is filled with preservative and the vacuum released. Preservative is drawn into the timber. After a short period for completion of absorption, a second vacuum is applied to draw some preservative out. The amount used is reduced, giving a cleaner, quicker-drying treatment. The process is used for light or medium treatment of permeable softwoods, such as European redwood, for example, in window-frames.

For treatment of less permeable woods or for higher levels of treatment in permeable ones, further absorption is forced by applying a positive pressure of between 1 and 2 bar, held for 15–60 min (double-vacuum pressure process).

Only organic solvent-type preservatives are widely applied by this process; fluid usage is typically 25–50 l/m^3.

5.3 Immersion treatment

Timber is simply immersed totally in the preservative fluid. Organic-solvent preservatives and creosote are applied this way.

The efficiency of the process is totally dependent on the immersion time. As generally practised, this is 3–10 min; at this level, the process is somewhat less effective than double-vacuum, but is still adequate for many purposes. Extended to several hours, as used on some estates and by amateurs, and provided the right products are used, the process gives long-term protection, even to timbers in ground contact.

5.4 Brush and spray

Topical application with a brush or spray uses less preservative and achieves less penetration than other methods. It is thus the least effective. Spraying is extensively used for professional, remedial treatment of timbers *in situ*. Brushing and, to a lesser extent, spraying are used for both preventive and remedial treatment by amateurs. Using organic solvent preservatives or low-viscosity creosote, and providing care is taken to ensure application to all surfaces of the wood, adequate protection is obtained for most purposes, where there is no ground contact. Where there is exposure to the weather, exposed surfaces should be periodically re-treated.

Brushing is also used to treat cut ends and other worked surfaces on timber treated by other processes prior to working.

5.5 Miscellaneous methods

Several other methods are used to apply wood preservatives in specific situations. These include the following procedures.

In hot and cold soak, whereby timber is heated in a bath of preservative and, while still in the bath, allowed to cool, the contraction of air in the wood sucks in preservative. This method was much used for butt treatment of fence posts.

Injection of preservative directly into the timber is used for remedial treatment of large timbers in insect eradication, e.g. death-watch or termites, of early decay in window-frames, for ground-line treatment of transmission and other poles. Several techniques are used.

Pastes, either of water-diffusible salts or of organic solvent preservatives are applied thickly to the surface of the wood. They provide a reservoir of preservative that will continue to penetrate into the timber for several days or more. Both pastes and injection techniques aim at getting deep penetration into timbers in existing structures and are used against both insects and decay.

Some timber is treated while green (unseasoned), by diffusion or sap-displacement methods. The two commonest are boron diffusion, whereby wood is dipped in a bath of hot, concentrated solution of borax and boric acid, lifted out and stacked under cover, to prevent drying until the borax has diffused throughout the timber. This is one of the few techniques that achieves full penetration, even into heartwood, but, because the borax remains water-soluble, it cannot be used in wet situations or be exposed to the weather. The second of the common methods is the Boucherie process. This is used in France and some other countries to treat green poles for use as transmission posts. One end of the pole is capped, and preservative (copper sulphate solution) is fed into the cap from a tank at the top of a tower. Over a few days, the solution will diffuse down the length of the pole.

6 Testing

Testing a wood preservative involves demonstrating the chemical's ability to kill or inhibit wood-destroying organisms and to demonstrate that this activity will be retained by the treated wood in service over many years. Further testing must determine the effect, if any, that treatment will have on all the properties of wood and any working or further processing, finishing, etc. to which the treated wood may be subjected. Extensive testing to evaluate health and environmental risks, in using the preservative or treated wood, is now essential.

Present practices in fungal testing have been reviewed (Hilditch & Mendes, 1987). The commonest laboratory test is to treat small blocks of wood with serial concentrations of preservative and then expose them to assault by single species of wood-destroying fungi. Separate tests with different species must be done to give a useful picture. Standard methods (Anon., 1982, 1985a) must be used when testing is for official approval, although many variations in block size and culture conditions are used for other purposes.

Similar principles are followed in testing for effectiveness against insects (Anon., 1989a,b,c,d).

To get an indication of permanence, either fungal or insect tests may be preceded by submitting the wood blocks to artificial leaching (Anon., 1989f) or evaporation (Anon., 1989e).

Such tests examine the resistance of wood preservatives to specific, single assault. They in no way mimic the multiple assault or complex succession of organisms that are encountered in real situations (Hilditch & Mendes, 1987; Levy, 1987). No accelerated laboratory test yet devised does this in full. Some approach is made in tests similar to those already described, but these incubate the treated wood in natural, not sterile, soil. These tests have much value but have the major disadvantage of poor reproducibility.

Laboratory tests as currently used examine the effectiveness of chemicals, not of the total treatment. To evaluate properly the practical performance of a treatment—depending, as it does, partly on the chemicals employed and partly on the method of application used—field tests in which treated timber is exposed to natural conditions are essential. There are two disadvantages: firstly, the time, 15–25 or more years, and, secondly, the fact that any one test relates only to the specific conditions under which it is carried out.

The commonest of the field tests is the burial of stakes (Anon., 1974b), while a variety of tests have been used for natural evaluation under out-of-ground situations (Hilditch & Mendes, 1987).

Tests are based on practical principles, as much as on scientific rules. They seek to reflect performance under specific real conditions, for which the basic scientific details have yet to be fully elucidated. Long-term evaluation, under practical conditions, and the accumulation of service data are essential for the newer materials now in use.

7 Health, safety and the environment

Wood preservatives are designed to kill or prevent the development of wood-destroying fungi or insects. They can, in varying degrees, present a hazard to humans and/or have detrimental effects on the environment. Most countries now control use under a range of legislation (Anon., 1985b, 1986b).

Long experience shows harmful effects to occur only when there is gross disregard for even simple precautions, such as should be taken in using any chemical. There are now detailed recommendations for use and the training of users (Anon., 1989g, 1991b,c,d, 1990a,b). Nonetheless, as an understanding of the more subtle relations between human health and the environment evolves, there is a need to introduce new materials with less effect on non-target organisms and to determine and reduce risks associated with any stage of the manufacture and application of wood preservatives and the long-term use of treated timber. Much current development has this as a cornerstone.

Considerations include both the chemicals used and the design of plant and methods for their application.

8 Conclusion

For the construction of dwellings and many other structures there is no sensible alternative to wood. Wood decay is natural and unavoidable. The practice and science of wood preservation are well established. Yet many current materials and practices are facing challenge, resulting from the general concern about the indiscriminate use of chemicals, especially as pesticides. To take the science and practice of wood preservation forward, a higher level of research into all aspects of use and towards and development of new materials is essential. The basis for this input exists.

9 References

Anon. (1973a) *Specification for Coal Tar Creosote for the Preservation of Timber*. British Standard 144:1973. London: British Standards Institution.

Anon. (1973b) *Specification for Wood Preservation by Means of Pressure Creosoting*. British Standard 913: 1973. London: British Standards Institution.

Anon. (1974a) *Wood Preservation. P5–72. Standards for Water-borne Preservatives*. Standard 080. Rexdale, Ontario: Canadian Standards Association.

Anon. (1974b) *Standard Method of Evaluating Wood Preservatives by Field Test with Stakes*. Standard D–1758–74. Philadelphia, Pennsylvania: American Society for Testing and Materials.

Anon. (1975) *Guide to the Choice, Use and Application of Wood Preservatives*. British Standard BS 1282: 1975. London: British Standards Institution.

Anon. (1979a) *Solutions of Wood Preservatives in Organic Solvent*. (Part 1. *Specification for Solutions for General Purpose Applications, Including Timber that is to be Painted*. British Standard BS 5707: 1979, Part 1. London: British Standards Institution.

Anon. (1979b) *Solutions of Wood Preservatives in Organic Solvent. Specification for Pentachlorophenol Wood Preservative for Use on Timber that is not Required to be Painted*. British Standard BS 5707: 1979, Part 2. London: British Standards Institution.

Anon. (1981) *Standards for Waterborne Preservatives*. Standard P5-81. Washington, DC: American Wood-Preserver's Association.

Anon (1982) *Wood Preservatives. Determination of Toxic Values Against Wood Destroying Basidiomycetes Cultured on an Agar Medium.* British Standard BS 6009: 1982. London: British Standards Institution.

Anon. (1985a) *General Introductory Document on European (or CEN) Methods of Test for Wood Preservatives.* British Standard BS 6559: 1985. London: British Standards Institution.

Anon. (1985b) *Food and Environmental Protection Act 1985*, Chapter 48. London: HMSO.

Anon. (1986a) *Specification for Biocides.* Standard 2.0. London: British Wood Preserving Association.

Anon. (1986b) *Pesticides. The Control of Pescticides Regulations 1986.* Statutory Instrument 1986, No. 1510. London: HMSO.

Anon. (1986c) *Timber Preservation.* London: Timber Research and Development Association and British Wood Preserving Association.

Anon. (1987a) *Wood Preservation by Means of Copper/Chrome/Arsenic Compositions.* Part 1. *Specification for Preservatives.* British Standard 4072: 1987: Part 1. London: British Standards Institution.

Anon. (1987b) *Environmental Health Criteria. 71: Pentachlorophenol.* Geneva: World Health Organization.

Anon. (1989a) *Wood Preservatives: Determination of the Toxic Values Against* Anobium punctatum *(De Geer) by Larval Transfer (Laboratory Method).* British Standard BS 5218: 1989. London: British Standards Institution.

Anon. (1989b) *Wood Preservatives: Determination of Preventative Action Against Recently Hatched Larvae of* Hylotrupes bajulus (Linnaeus) (Laboratory Method). British Standard BS 5434: 1989. London: British Standards Institution.

Anon. (1989c) *Wood Preservatives: Determination of Toxic Values Against Larvae of* Hylotrupes bajulus *(Linnaeus) (Laboratory Method).* British Standard BS 5435: 1989. London: British Standards Institution.

Anon. (1989d) *Wood Preservatives: Determination of eradicant action against larvae of* Anobium punctatum *(De Geer) (Laboratory Method).* British Standard BS 5436: 1989. London: British Standards Institution.

Anon. (1989e) *Wood Preservatives: Accelerated Aging of Treated Wood Prior to Biological Testing.* Part 1: *Evaporative Aging Procedure.* British Standard BS 5761: 1989, Part 1. London: British Standards Institution.

Anon. (1989f) *Wood Preservatives: Accelerated Aging of Treated Wood Prior to Biological Testing.* Part 2: *Leaching Procedure.* British Standard BS 5761: 1989, Part 2. London: British Standards Institution.

Anon. (1989g) In-situ *Timber Treatment Using Timber Preservatives.* Guidance Note GS 46. Health and Safety Executive.

Anon. (1990a) *Recommendations for Training Users of Non-Agricultural Pesticides.* Health and Safety Commission.

Anon. (1990b) *Environmental Protection Act 1990.* London: HMSO.

Anon. (1991a) Restrictions on the marketing and use of certain dangerous substances and preparations. Council Directive 91/173/EEC 21 March 1991 amending for the ninth time Directive 76/769/EEC. *Official Journal of the European Communities*, L85. S April 1991, pp. 34–36. Luxemburg: Office for Official Publications.

Anon. (1991b) *The Safe Use of Pesticides for Non-agricultural Purposes.* Health and Safety Commission, HMSO.

Anon. (1991c) *Remedial Treatment of Timber in Buildings.* Health and Safety Executive, HMSO.

Anon. (1991d) *Secretary of State's Guidance—Chemical Treatment of Timber and Wood Based Products.* PG6/3 (91). Department of the Environment.

Anon. (1991e) *Publications CFT 100*, Castleford: Hicksons Timber Products.

Barnes, H.M. & Hein, R.W. (1988) Treatment of steam-conditioned pine poles with copper naphthenate in hydrocarbon solvent. In *Record of the 1988 Annual Convention of the British Wood Preserving Association*, pp. 3–24. London: British Wood Preserving Association.

Bayer (n.d.) *Information on Wood Protection, Preventol A8.*

Bech-Andersen, J. (1985) Basische Baustoffe und begrenzte Feuchtigkeit-Verhaltnisse Antworten auf die Frage, wasum der echte Nausschwamm nur in Hausern vorkommt. *Material und Organismen*, **20**, 301–309.

Bethell, J. (1938) *Rendering Wood, Cork and Other Articles More Durable, etc.* British Patent 7731/1838. London: Her Majesty's Patent Office.

Biegel, W. (ed.) (1988) *Lindane: Answers to Important Questions.* Brussels: Centre International d'Etudes du Lindane.

Boutelje, J.B. & Goransson, B. (1971) Decay in wood construction below the ground water table. In *Biodeterioration of Materials* (eds Walters, A.H. & Hueck-van der Plas, E.H.), Vol. 2, pp. 311–318. London: Applied Science Publishers.

Bravery, A.F. & Grant, C. (1985) Studies on the growth of *Serpula lacrymans* (Schumacher ex Fr.) Gray. *Material und Organismen*, **20**, 171–191.

Bravery, A.F., Berry, R.W., Carey, J.K., Miller, E.R. & Orsler, R.J. (1995) Progress in wood protection at the BRE. In *Record of the 1995 Convention of the British Wood Preserving and Damp-proofing Association.* London: British Wood Preserving and Damp Proofing Association.

Bulman, R.A. (1955) The development and use of naphthenates for timber preservation. In *Record of the 1955 Annual Convention of the British Wood Preserving Association*, pp. 36–46. London: British Wood Preserving Association.

Butcher, J.A. (1971) Analysis of the fungal population in wood. In *Biodeterioration of Materials* (eds Walters, A.H. & Hueck-van der Plas, E.H.), Vol. 2, pp. 319–325. London: Applied Science Publishers.

Butovitsch, V.V. (1976) Uber Vorkommen und Schadwirkung der rossameisen *Camponotus herculeanus und C. ligniperda* in Gebauden in Schweden. *Material und Organismen*, **11**, 160–170.

Carey, J.K. (1981) Colonisation of wooden joinery. In *Biodeterioration* (eds Oxley, T.A. & Barry, S.), Vol. 5, pp. 13–25. Chichester: John Wiley & Sons (this paper was presented in 1981, but published in 1983).

Carey, J.K. (1982) Assessing the performance of preservative treatments for window joinery. *Holz als Rohund Werkstoff*, **40**, 269–274.

Carswell, T.S. & Nason, H.K. (1938) Properties and uses of pentachlorophenol. *Industrial and Engineering Chemistry*, **30**, 622–626.

Carter, S.W. (1984) The use of synthetic pyrethroids as wood preservatives. In *Record of the 1984 Annual Convention of the British Wood Preserving Association*, pp. 32–41. London: British Wood Preserving Association.

Cartright, K.St.G. & Findlay, P.F.K. (1958) *Decay of Timber and its Prevention*. London: HMSO.

Cockroft, R. (1974) *The Performance of Pentachlorophenol in a Stake Test in the United Kingdom*. Watford: Building Research Establishment, Department of the Environment.

Coggins, C.R. (1976) Growth patterns of *Serpulia lacrimans*, the dry rot fungus. In *Record of the 1976 Annual Convention of the British Wood Preserving Association*, pp. 73–83. London: British Wood Preserving Association.

Coggins, C.R. (1991) Improvements in safety and environmental protection at timber treatment plants, accelerated fixation and other new systems. In *Record of the 1991 Convention of the British Wood Preserving and Damp-proofing Association*. London: British Wood Preserving and Damp Proofing Association.

Connell, M., Baldwin, W.J. & Smith, T. (1995) Controlled fixation technology. In *3rd International Wood Preservation Symposium 1995*. Stockholm: International Research Group on Wood Preservation.

Cornfield, J.A., Connell, M. & Williams, G.R. (1993) A new timber preservative. In *Record of the 1993 Convention of the British Wood Preserving and Damp-proofing Association*. London: British Wood Preserving and Damp-proofing Association.

Cross, J.N., Bailey, G. & Schofield, M.J. (1989) Performance of metal fastenings in CCA treated timber. In *Record of the 1989 Annual Convention of the British Wood Preserving Association*, pp. 3–6. London: British Wood Preserving Association.

Czipri, J.J., Dawson, H.B., Lankford, W.T., Fitzsimons P.J. & Woodhouse, L.B. 1992 Nanosol and microemulsions: emulsions—unique high performance, water-based, wood preservatives. In *Record of the 1992 Convention of the British Wood Preserving and Damp-proofing Association*. London: British Wood Preserving and Damp Proofing Association.

Dawson, H.B. (1993) Microemulsions for timber treatment. In *Record of the 1993 Convention of the British Wood Preserving and Damp-proofing Association*.

Dawson, H.B. & Czipri, J.J. (1991) Microemulsions—a new development for the wood treatment industry. *Wood Protection*, **1**, 55–60.

Dickinson, D.J. & Levy, J.F. (1979) Mechanisms of decay and its prevention. In *Record of the 1979 Annual Convention of the British Wood Preserving Association*, pp. 33–37. London: British Wood Preserving Association.

Doi, S. (1983) *The Evaluation of Survey of Dry Rot Damage in Japan*. Document IRG/WP/1179. Stockholm: International Research Group on Wood Preservation.

Findlay, W.P.K. & Savory, J.G. (1954) Decomposition of wood by lower fungi. *Holz als Roh-und Werkstoff*, **12**, 293–296.

Goodwine, W.R. (1990) Suitability of Propiconazole as a new generation wood preserving fungicide. *Proceedings, American Wood Preservers Association*. Washington. D.C.

Green, N.B. (1980) The biochemical basis of wood decay micro-morphology. *Journal of the Institute of Wood Science*, **8**, 221–228.

Hagar, B.O. (1954) *Improvements in or Relating to Preserving Agents for Timber or Other Organic Material*. British patent 808277. London: Her Majesty's Patent Office.

Hagar, B.O. (1972) *Improvements Relating to Materials and Processes Applicable to Treatment of Wood and Similar Materials*. British Patent 1379095. London: Her Majesty's Patent Office.

Harris, W.V. (1971) *Termites, Their Recognition and Control*, 2nd edn. London: Longman.

Hegarty, B., Buckwald, G., Cymorek, S. & Willeitner, H. (1986) Der Echte Hausschwamm—immer noch ein Problem? *Material und Organismen*, **21**, 87–99.

Hickin, N.E. (1963) *The Insect Factor in Wood Decay*. London: Hutchinson.

Hickin, N.E. (1971) *Termites: A World Problem*. London: Hutchinson.

Hickin, N.E. (1985) *Pest Animals in Buildings*. London: George Godwin.

Hilditch, E.A. (1964) Modern developments in organic solvent wood preservers. In *Record of the 1964 Annual Convention of the British Wood Preserving Association*, pp. 41–53. London: British Wood Preserving Association.

Hilditch, E.A. (1977a) *Compositions Containing Preservative Metals and their Use for Preservation of Wood and Like Materials and as a Fungicide*. British Patent 1,574,939. London: Her Majesty's Patent Office.

Hilditch, E.A. (1977b) Wood preservative naphthenates. *Timber Trades Journal*, 22 October.

Hilditch, E.A. (1987) Protecting wood against the weather. In *Wood and Cellulosics* (eds Kennedy, J.F., Phillips, G.O. & Williams, P.A.), pp. 545–552. Chichester: Ellis Horwood.

Hilditch, E.A. & Crookes, J.V. (1981) Exterior wood stains, varieties performance and appearance. In *Record of the 1981 Annual Convention of the British Wood Preserving Association*, pp. 59–67. London: British Wood Preserving Association.

Hilditch, E.A. & Mendes, F. (1987) Wood preservation —fungal testing. In *Preservatives in the Food, Pharmaceutical and Environmental Industries* (eds Board, R.G., Allwood, M.C. & Banks, J.G.), Society for Applied Bacteriology Technical Series No. 22, pp. 115–131. Oxford: Blackwell Scientific Publications.

Hilditch, E.A. & Woodbridge, R.J. (1985) Progress in timber finishing in Great Britain. *Journal of the Oil and Colour Chemists Association*, **68**, 217–228.

Hilditch, E.A., Hambling, R.E., Sparks, C.R. & Walker, DA. (1978) *Anti-fungal Compositions and Methods of Preserving Materials Therewith*. European Patent 5361. London: European Patent Office.

Hilditch, E.A., Sparks, C.R. & Worringham, J.H.M. (1983) Further developments in metal soap-based preservatives. In *Record of the 1983 Annual Convention of the British Wood Preserving Association*, pp. 61–72. London: British Wood Preserving Association.

Hum, M., Glasser, A.E. & Edwards, R. (1980) Wood-boring weevils of economic importance in Britain. *Journal of the Institute of Wood Science*, **8**, 201–207.

Hunt, G.M. & Garratt, G.A. (1953) *Wood Preservation*. New York: McGraw-Hill.

Jennings, D.H. (1981) Recent studies on translocation in the dry rot fungus *Serpula lacrimans*. In *Record of the 1981 Annual Convention of the British Wood Preserving Association*, pp. 19–25. London: British Wood Preserving Association.

Jones, E.B.G. & Eltringham, S.K. (1968) *Marine Borers and Fouling Organisms of Wood*. Paris: Organization for Economic Cooperation and Development.

Land, C.J., Banhidi, Z.G. & Albertsson, A-C. (1985) Surface discoloring and blue staining filamentous fungi on outdoor softwood in Sweden. *Material und Organismen*, **20**, 133–156.

Levy, J.F. (1965) The soft rot fungi, their mode of action and significance in the degradation of wood. In *Advances in Botanical Research* (ed. Preston, R.D.), pp. 323–357. London: Academic Press.

Levy, J.F. (1987) The natural history of the degradation of wood. *Philosophical Transactions of the Royal Society, London*, **A321**, 423–433.

Levy, J.F. & Dickinson, D.J. (1980) Wood protection research at Imperial College. In *Record of the 1980 Annual Convention of the British Wood Preserving Association*, pp. 67–73. London: British Wood Preserving Association.

McCarthy, D.F. (1978) Australian Patent application 35221/78.

McNeil, D. (1952) Some notes on the chemical composition of coal tar creosote. In *Record of the 1952 Annual Convention of the British Wood Preserving Association*, pp. 147–161. London: British Wood Preserving Association.

Mirie, M. & Willitner, H. (1984) *Lethal Temperatures for Some Wood Destroying Fungi with Respect to Heat*. Document IRG/WP/1229. Stockholm: International Research Group on Wood Preservation.

Morton, L.H.G. & Eggins, H.O.W. (1976) The effect of moisture content in wood on the surface growth and penetration of fungi. *Material und Organismen*, **11**, 279–294.

Nichols, D.D. (1973) *Wood Preservation and its Prevention by Preservative Treatment*, 2 vols. Syracuse, New York: Syracuse University Press.

Rango Rao, K. (ed.) (1977) *Pentachlorophenol: Chemistry, Pharmacology and Environmental Toxicology*. New York: Plenum Press.

Ray, D.L. (ed.) (1959) *Marine Boring and Fouling Organisms*. Seattle, Washington: University of Washington Press.

Richardson, B.A. (1988) Organotin wood preservatives: activity and safety in relation to structure. In *Proceedings, American Wood-Preserver's Association 1988*, pp. 56–69. Stephensville, Maryland: American Wood-Preserver's Association.

Savory, J.G. (1954) Breakdown of timber by Ascomycetes and Fungi Imperfecti. *Annals of Applied Biology*, **41**, 336–347.

Savory, J.G. (1955) The role of microfungi in the decomposition of wood. In *Record of the 1955 Annual Convention of the British Preserving Association*, pp. 3–20. London: British Wood Preserving Association.

Smith, D.N.R. (1980) Study of decay of preservative-treated wood in soil. *Journal of the Institute of Wood Science*, **8**, 194–200.

Sparks, C.R. (1978) A new brand of metallic chemical for use in wood preservation. In *Record of the 1978 Annual Convention of the British Wood Preserving Association*, pp. 48–51. London: British Wood Preserving Association.

Thornton, J.D. (1989) *The Restricted Distribution of* Serpula lacrymans *in Australian Buildings*. Document IRG/WP/1382. Stockholm: International Research Group on Wood Preservation.

Tillott, R.J. & Coggins, C.R. (1981) Non-arsenical

water-borne preservatives—a review of performance and properties. In *Record of the 1981 Annual Convention of the British Wood Preserving Association*, pp. 32–48. London: British Wood Preserving Association.

van Groenou, H.B., Rischen, H.W.L. & van den Berge, J. (1951) *Wood Preservation During the Last 50 Years*. Leiden: A.W. Sijthoff Uitgeversmaatschappij N.V.

Wallace, E.M. (1964) Factors affecting the permanence of wood preservatives and some of the problems arising therefrom. In *Record of the 1964 Annual Convention of the British Wood Preserving Association*, pp. 131–150. London: British Wood Preserving Association.

Wegen, H.W., Platen, A. & Hollbacher, G., (1996) Suitability of benzoyl urea compounds as insecticides in a new generation of wood preservatives. In *Record of the 1996 Convention of the British Wood Preserving and Damp-proofing Association*. London: British Wood Preserving and Damp Proofing Association.

Wilkinson, J.G. (1979) *Industrial Timber Preservation*. London: Associated Business Press.

Williams, G.R. & Ryan, N.P. (1996) The protection of wood with copper azole preservative. In *Record of the 1996 Convention of the British Wood Preserving and Damp-proofing Association*. London: British Wood Preserving and Damp Proofing Association.

Wolman (1958) Allgemeine Holzimpragnierung Dr Wolman GmbH. *Wood Preserving Agents*. British Patent 911519. London: Her Majesty's Patent Office.

Wolman (1975) Dr Wolman Gmbh. *Wood Preservative Solution Containing a Dye*. British Patent 1,531,868. London: Her Majesty's Patent Office.

F. PRESERVATION OF MUSEUM SPECIMENS

1 Introduction

Conservation, the science of preserving artefacts in a museum, can be defined as 'the means by which the true nature of an object is preserved'. The true nature of an object includes evidence of its origins, its original construction, the materials of which it is composed and information as to the technology used in its manufacture (UKIC, 1984). Conservation is, however, frequently confused with restoration, which is not directly concerned with preservation but with improvements to the appearance of a deteriorated object.

Museums, libraries and historic houses can contain a wide range of historic and aesthetic objects collected from activities in the sciences and arts, and this diversity is reflected in the many branches of conservation. Practitioners are often generalists, treating and preserving collections of natural history, archaeology, social history, fine and decorative art and even buildings. Conservation practice draws on the knowledge and experience of many disciplines, adapting them and using them to their best effect. As a preservation science in its own right, it has only developed in any substance since the 1950s and come of age in the last few years.

The aim of conservation, which is to preserve objects for perpetuity, is patently unachievable. The size and variety of collections often only allow a broad preservation policy to slow down deterioration, and only in significant cases—such as the Lindow Bog Man, preserved in a peat bog since its ritual burial there in the first century, or the *Mary Rose*, the flagship of Henry VIII excavated and lifted from Portsmouth Harbour in 1982—can detailed and specific remedial action be taken.

2 Degradation of historic and artistic material

It is known that materials deteriorate through a number of complex mechanisms. In the case of aesthetically appreciated objects, that deterioration may not be degradation but a surface despoiling, such as mould growth or soiling. However, the major factors causing deterioration are a combination of chemical, physical and biological agents, which although their actions are interlinked, can be considered separately (Thomson, 1986).

2.1 Environmental destructive factors

2.1.1 Temperature

Most artefacts are, by their very nature, relatively stable at normal ambient temperatures. However, temperature changes can affect some objects through a number of mechanisms, such as phase change, expansion/contraction cycles, etc. Wax-faced dolls and entomological specimens embedded in wax have been damaged irreparably by the radiant heat of spotlights, while poorly glazed pottery can develop 'crazing' caused by the incompatible expansion coefficients. Temperature also affects the rate of reactions, according to the Arrhenius equation:

$$k = A \exp(-E/RT)$$

where k is the rate constant, R the gas constant, T the temperature, A the frequency factor and E the activation energy.

As a general rule of thumb, a 10°C rise in temperature is considered to double the rate of chemical reaction (see also Chapter 3). As a consequence, vulnerable material is stored at low temperature, with costume and other textiles often stored at around 15°C, while colour photographs are recommend to be stored at 2°C. Low-temperature storage inhibits the growth of biological systems and thus is effective in controlling insect pests, fungal growth and small pest mammals, such as mice. Chemical activity, such as metal corrosion and light-catalysed oxidation of organic polymers (paints, varnishes, plastics, rubbers, wood-based materials, etc.), is slowed down. As an economic preservative tool, it has much to recommend it for long-term care; however, its effective use is often counteracted by the higher temperatures demanded by visitors and researchers.

2.1.2 *Humidity*

Relative humidity (r.h.) is defined as:

$$\frac{\text{The amount of water in a given quantity of air}}{\text{The maximum amount of water which that air can hold at that temperature}} \times 100\%$$

and this is thus expressed as a percentage. It represents the degree of saturation of the air at a particular temperature. All organic materials, under normal circumstances, contain loosely bound water in their structures, which is in dynamic equilibrium with the r.h. of the surrounding air. To a lesser degree, most porous inorganic materials, such as pottery, stone and some metals, are in the same equilibrium.

A rise or fall in the r.h. of the microclimate surrounding an object induces it to gain or lose moisture to restore the equilibrium. In most organic materials, the absorption of atmospheric moisture is within the fibrous structure of the cells. For instance, in wood (Fig. 18.2), the cellular fibre-saturation point is reached at approximately a 25% equilibrium moisture content, which corresponds to an r.h. of around 100%. Below the fibre-saturation point, the effect of fluctuating moisture

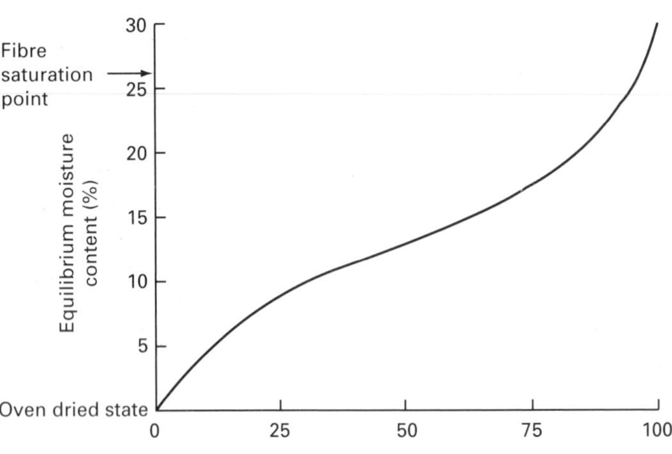

Fig. 18.2 The relationship between relative humidity and moisture content of wood.

content tends to cause dimensional changes in organic materials (Hoadley, 1978).

Where movement is restricted, by the anisotropy of the material and/or by the method of construction, the cellular structure becomes permanently damaged and cracks, splits, shakes, warps, etc. can develop, through plastic deformation (Buck, 1972). Low humidities (40% r.h.) are especially damaging, as the loss of moisture causes embrittlement of the structure. High humidities (65–70% r.h.) are associated with enhanced biological action through bacterial, fungal and insect attack, and chemical deterioration is also increased.

Porous inorganic materials, such as some stonework and pottery, can be damagingly affected by fluctuating humidities. Absorbed hygroscopic salts can concentrate on or near the surface, causing disfiguring salt growths or spalling (splintering and cracking) of the surface layers (Torraca, 1988).

Current conservation practice in assessing suitable storage environments considers a number of factors both scientific and pragmatic. A knowledge of the environmental history of the object is important, as it may have achieved a long-term stability by acquiring an equilibrium with seemingly non-ideal conditions. The long-term preservation of fine furniture in damp castles, for instance, would be jeopardized by resiting that furniture into stores at lower humidities to inhibit the possibilities of biological growth.

Very low humidities are recognized as slowing down many chemical and biological deteriogens, and thus might be considered advantageous. However, other factors, such as the concomitant increase in fragility through embrittlement at low humidities, thus increasing the danger of mechanical damage, may legislate against its use.

A common, economically acceptable, compromise solution for determining storage conditions is to use environmentally buffered stores and displays, which avoid large fluctuations in conditions and maintain an r.h. of the annual mean inside level. In the UK and other temperate climates this is usually 50–60% r.h., in tropical climates 60–70% r.h. and in cooler, northern countries, such as Canada, 40–50% r.h. Where special conditions are required, air-conditioning or mechanical humidification/dehumidification systems can be used for large areas, while small, well-sealed showcases and storage containers can be well controlled using hygroscopic materials, such as silica gel. The silica gel is preconditioned to provide a moisture reservoir which will effectively maintain the container in which it is put at a specified humidity.

2.1.3 Light

Visible light and the associated infrared and ultraviolet (UV) radiations are major deteriogens of museum objects, although their actions vary. Infrared radiation (radiant heat) causes damage through its heating effect, leading to temperature damage. The shorter wavelengths of visible light and UV radiation cause chemical damage, notably oxidative reactions and breakdown of polymeric materials, through a number of complex pathways, believed to be based on peroxide and free-radical formation (Brill, 1980). Thus, where R is an organic molecule excited by light energy, h is Planck's constant and hv the energy of a photon of light of frequency v,

$$R + hv \rightarrow R^*$$

Free radical formation ensues:

$$R^* \rightarrow R^0$$

Reaction with oxygen follows to form the highly reactive, strongly oxidizing peroxy radical:

$$R^0 + O_2 \rightarrow RO_2^0$$

The observed deterioration from light attack is familiar as fading of dyestuffs and pigments, embrittlement and breaking of textile threads and yellowing of newspapers.

Light-induced damage is limited by dark storage and low-level-lighting illuminance of displays. Commonly used limits are: (i) a maximum of 50 lux illuminance for sensitive material, such as textiles and watercolours; and (ii) a maximum of 200 lux illuminance for less sensitive material, such as polychromed wood and oil paintings. Normally, all UV radiation is eliminated by careful choice of illuminants and by UV screening.

2.1.4 Pollution

Museums and their contents are at a heightened

risk from pollution damage, because of the extreme length of exposure. Chronic deterioration may become apparent only after considerable periods of time have elapsed, even with low pollution levels (Baer & Banks, 1985).

Particulate pollution from combustion products, such as smoke and soot, is normally acidic and hygroscopic, and can be oily and sticky. It causes deterioration through soiling and chemical attack, particularly on carbonate rocks (limestone, marble), where the damage is evident as surface blackening and increased erosion. Drying plaster and cement can produce aerosols of alkaline particles, which are known to attack oil-painting varnishes.

Gaseous pollution is divided between that generated externally, such as the oxides of sulphur and nitrogen, and that generated locally within the museum. The protective envelope of containers, showcases and buildings limits the effect of external pollutants but can contain and intensify the damaging effect of indoor sources. Sulphur dioxide from space heating can tarnish metals, damage paints, pigments and dyes and weaken organic materials, such as paper, leather and textiles. Hydrogen sulphide from rubber, from some plastic and dyes and from wool can tarnish metals and photographic emulsions. Ozone from electrical discharges in machinery (e.g. some photocopiers) can cause colour changes in pigments, degrade cellulose, etc.

Damage from pollution is limited by excluding external sources by having well-sealed buildings, filtered air-handling systems and protected storage and display conditions; by minimizing pollution sources by removing non-vented heating systems, sealing surfaces with non-emitting coatings and testing all storage and display materials for their stability; and by the rational use of absorbers, corrosion inhibitors, etc., such as charcoal-weave cloth as a local absorbent of pollutant gases.

2.1.5 Biological agents

As with any object with a natural organic content, museum artefacts are at risk from attack by fungi, insect pests and other biological agents. In the expected climatic conditions that exist within museum and art galleries only insect pests are normally a hazard. Wood and wood-based material, such as paper and board, can be attacked by the larvae of wood-boring beetles, especially the Anobiidae, which include the most commonly damaging species—*Anobium punctatum* (common furniture beetle) and *Xestobium rufovillosum* (death-watch beetle)—but also the Lyctidae, Bostrychidae, Cerambycidae and Curculionidae. Keratinous-based materials, such as wood, fur, feathers, horn, hide, etc., are commonly attacked by a number of insect species, especially the Dermestidae (carpet beetles, etc.), Tineidae (clothes moth) and Oecophoridae (house moths). A number of other species can attack museum material and all organic-based material is at risk.

Elimination of insect pests was traditionally done as a reactive measure on sighting damage or insects, and regular routine use of insecticides was often carried out on buildings and contents alike. Current practice is now based on preventive measures and insect monitoring, rather than reactive treatments. The introduction of pests into the museum is minimized by having well-sealed buildings that are well maintained, to remove for instance bird's nests, accumulated rubbish, etc. Preventive measures to minimize the risk of any infestation developing is based on the good housekeeping measures of effective cleaning and inspection. Monitoring for the presence of insects is usually through careful inspection, assisted by sticky 'blunder-type' traps, sometimes augmented with pheromone attractants.

Where infestations have become established and a treatment to kill the pests is necessary, traditional toxic insecticides are now rarely used. Museums have developed effective non-toxic measures, including temperature modification (deep-freezing and high-temperature treatments), and anoxic-gas fumigation (using nitrogen and carbon dioxide). Where residual insecticidal activity is required, desiccant dusts have been successfully used, and residual liquid-based treatments based on the synthetic pyrethroids (Pinniger, 1994).

3 Preservation of organic archaeological material

Historical material from buried environments presents particular conservation problems on its excavation, owing to the rapid change in ambient conditions. Objects are frequently mechanically damaged before burial, and invariably some aerobic decomposition has taken place through insect or microbial attack.

Insects cause mechanical damage to organic materials, especially wood tissues. The principal insect classes responsible for damage in seasoned wood are the Anobiidae, Cerambycidae, Lyctidae and Curculionidae. The larval stage of the insects attacks the wood by extensive boring into the interior sapwood or heartwood, reducing it to a fine powder.

Microorganisms, including the Basidiomycotina, Ascomycotina, Deutoromycotina and bacteria, can colonize and decompose wood, primarily if conditions of temperature, moisture content and pH are suitable. Mould fungi of the Ascomycotina type are not responsible for biodeterioration, being essentially surface colonies. However, soft-rot fungi and brown-rot fungi can break down cellulose and brown-rot fungi can also break down lignin, eventually causing the total decomposition of the wood. Other organic materials are similarly degraded (Young, 1988).

On burial in an anaerobic environment, insect attack ceases and fungal attack is strongly inhibited. It is thought that some bacterial action can continue, but at a very low level. Objects maintain their dimensional stability through bulking, i.e. filling, by water. On excavation, objects are normally in a highly fragile state and in danger of collapsing on desiccation. The abnormal shrinkage noted in drying out biodegraded waterlogged objects is due to cell collapse when the bulking water is removed (Kaarik, 1974).

Immediate conservation treatment for excavated waterlogged material is water immersion or spraying in holding-tanks. Further biodegradation can be retarded by the use of biocides, but, where this may hinder future analysis (for ^{14}C dating), chilled water is preferred. Treatments for preservation involve dehydrating the wood without cell collapse to consolidate the object sufficiently for handling. Early treatments involved dehydration with acetone followed by impregnation with resin—an expensive, dangerous and often unsuccessful technique. Present methods concentrate on freeze-drying, followed by consolidation with polyethylene glycol (PEG), a water-soluble synthetic wax of various molecular weights. Timbers from the *Mary Rose* were treated by initial washing, followed by pretreatment with disodium edetate to remove iron salts precipitated within the wood. The wood is then immersed in baths of PEG 3400 (PEG of average molecular weight 3400) of increasing concentrations over a period of months until a 50% solution is reached. Excess water is sublimated out of the wood by freeze-drying at –20°C, when the wood is removed and stored at a relative humidity of 50–60%.

Other organic materials are treated similarly. Lindow Man, a first century human body excavated from a waterlogged peat bog in 1984, was initially placed in cold storage to minimize biodeterioration. After cleaning and microbiological monitoring to determine the presence of pathogens or deteriogens, the body was consolidated in a 15% aqueous solution of PEG 400 and then freeze-dried (Omar *et al.*, 1989).

4 Preservation of natural-history collections

Museums have a long tradition of collecting natural history material, and tried-and-tested methods of preservation have grown up, based on desiccation or on fluid immersion. Stricter legislation on the use of biocides and a greater awareness of the degradation effects of some preservatives on objects have led to a re-evaluation of methods (Stansfield, 1984)

4.1 Preservation through desiccation

Drying of organisms may be sufficient to ensure their long-term preservation, by lowering the moisture content below that necessary to support fungal and bacterial deteriogens. The drying mechanisms follow a number of courses.

4.1.1 Taxidermy

Birds and animals have traditionally been preserved by the taxidermist's art in removing the skin (and other structural and relevant material, such as bones, skull and claws) of an animal. The skin is defleshed and all fat removed, and then is preserved either by desiccation (through natural drying or with desiccants) or, in the case of larger mammals, by pickling or tanning. The treated skin is then mounted over a framework in a lifelike pose. Further attack by biodeteriogens is prevented by fungicides and insecticides.

4.1.2 *Freeze-drying*

Owing to the expense and time required for the specialist art of taxidermy, small birds and mammals are increasingly preserved by freeze-drying. Advantages are the preservation of internal organs and the dry preservation of specimens previously only preservable by total fluid immersion.

4.1.3 *Desiccation*

Entomological collections and other suitable natural-history material, such as eggshells, molluse shells and herbariums, are regularly preserved by drying out under normal ambient r.h. Occasionally, biocides are used to prevent any further biodegradation.

4.1.4 *Total immersion*

The need to preserve delicate natural history material which would ordinarily be destroyed by air-drying is often fulfilled by immersion in a preserving fluid. Traditionally, soft-bodied mammals, invertebrates and some botanical material have been 'fixed' in formaldehyde solution and then transferred to ethanol solution (70–80%) for preservation by the replacement of internal water with the alcohol solution. Recently, 'safer' solvents, such as isopropanol and propylene phenoxetol have been used, but with less success in the long term.

4.2 Ultradeep-freezing

In some specialist institutions, where collecting of natural-history material is done specifically for research or where traditional methods of preservation are inappropriate, deep-freezing at –40°C and lower of tissue samples, etc. is currently used.

5 Conclusions

The traditional methods of museum preservation tended to concentrate on the use of adhesives, consolidants and protective surface coatings and the ubiquitous use of biocides. The inevitable deterioration was masked by heavy restoration methods, disguising or replacing damaged areas. Modern conservation techniques stress the importance of static conditions, with the objects in equilibrium with their environment. Intrusive preservation methods are evaluated for their effect on the object, as well as their toxicity or hazardous nature, and the treatments are designed to be, as far as possible, invisible and reversible. Old damage and deterioration are accepted as part of the history of the object, and conservation is concerned with the long-term preservation of objects for future generations.

6 References

Baer, N.S. & Banks, P.N. (1985) Indoor air pollution: effects on cultural and historic materials. *International Journal of Museum Management and Curatorship*, **4**, 9–20.

Brill, T.B. (1980) *Light: its Interaction with Art and Antiquities*, London: Plenum Press.

Buck, R.R. (1972) Some applications of rheology to the treatment of panel paintings. *Studies in Conservation*, **17**, 1–11.

Hoadley, R.B. (1978) The dimensional response of wood to variation in relative humidity. In *Conservation of Wood in Painting and the Decorative Arts*, IIC (Oxford Congress), pp. 1–6.

Kaarik, A.A. (1974) Decomposition of wood. In *Biology of Plant Litter Decomposition* (eds Dickinson, C.H. & Pugh, G.F.), pp. 129–174. London: Academic Press.

Omar, S., McCord, M. & Daniels, V. (1989) The conservation of bog bodies by freeze-drying. *Studies in Conservation*, **34**, 101–109.

Pinniger, D. (1994) *Insect Pests in Museums*. London: Archetype Publications.

Stansfield, G. (1984) Conservation and storage: biological collections. *Manual of Curatorship*, pp. 289–295. London: Butterworths/Museum Association.

Thomson, G. (1986) *The Museum Environment*. London: Butterworths.

Torraca, G. (1988) *Porous Buildings Materials*. Rome: ICCROM.

UKIC (United Kingdom Institute for Conservation) (1984) *Guidance for Conservation Practice*. London: UKIC.

Young, A.M. (1988) An assessment of the fungal populations within the timbers of the Tredunnock boat. BSc archaeological conservation thesis, University of Wales.

PART III

Sterilization and Pasteurization

Parts I and II considered the inactivation of microorganisms by chemical agents, although heat as a disinfecting agent was perforce referred to where relevant, e.g. in Chapters 7 and 10G. In Part III, the principles of pasteurization by heat and of sterilization, involving the inactivation of microorganisms by thermal methods, radiation and gaseous procedures and their removal by filtration, are discussed in Chapters 19–22, together with the applications in medical and food areas. New and emerging technologies are described in Chapter 23, a contentious issue (the reuse of disposables) in Chapter 24 and finally sterility assurance in Chapter 25.

CHAPTER 19

Heat Sterilization

A. STERILIZATION AND DISINFECTION BY HEAT METHODS

1 Introduction

Traditionally, heat in one form or another has been employed as a major sterilization procedure (Hugo, 1991, 1995; Olson, 1997). It still occupies a key role, and heat, in particular as a process employing steam, is the sterilization method of choice wherever possible. Furthermore, high temperatures have been used in conjunction with other antimicrobial agencies, such as chemicals and ionizing radiation, for the purposes of synergistic sterilization (Olson, 1997; Russell *et al.*, 1997; Russell, 1998). Low-temperature steam (LTS) with formaldehyde (LTSF) comes into this latter category (Alder & Simpson, 1992). Kowalski (1993) has produced an interesting paper on the selection of a sterilization method.

Disinfection or decontamination may be achieved by hot water at temperatures below 100°C.

Here, the principles of these processes will be considered. Subsequent parts of this chapter will examine the response of bacterial spores to moist and dry heat (Chapter 19B), the medical applications of thermal processes (Chapter 19C) and the applications of thermal processing in the food industry (Chapter 19D). Although a certain amount of overlapping is inevitable, this should enhance, rather than detract from, the overall concept of heat as an important sterilization and disinfection procedure, with wide application. Useful reviews that provide additional invaluable information are those by Russell (1982, 1991a, 1993, 1998), Gould (1989), Dewhurst & Hoxey (1990), Haberer & Wallhaeusser (1990), Soper & Davies (1990), Gardner & Peel (1991a,b), Wood (1991, 1993), Medical Devices Directorate (1993), Owens (1993), Young (1993), Brown (1994) and Denyer & Hodges (1998).

2 Sterilization and disinfection by moist heat

Heating in the presence of moisture has for many years been used as a method of sterilization or, where relevant, disinfection. Temperatures below, at or above 100°C have been employed for various purposes.

2.1 Terminology

Several terms are widely used to measure the sensitivity of microorganisms to thermal processes.

1 The D-value (decimal reduction time (DRT)), which is defined as the time in minutes at a particular temperature to reduce the viable population by 1 log cycle, i.e. to 10% or by 90%. The D-value is independent of inoculum size and decreases at higher temperatures.
2 Inactivation factor (IF), which is the degree of reduction in the viable population and which is calculated from the initial viable count (N_0)/final viable count (N_t) at t min.
3 The z-value, which is defined as the temperature (°C) to bring about a 10-fold reduction in D-value; it is obtained from the slope of the curve in which the D-value on a logarithmic scale is plotted against temperature (arithmetic scale; see Chapter 19D, Fig. 19.7).
4 F-value, which expresses heat treatment at any temperature as equal to that effect produced by a certain number of minutes at 121°C; F_0 is the F-value when z is 10°C. The *British Pharmacopoeia* (1998) generally requires a minimum F_0 value of 8 from a steam-sterilization process. As pointed out by Denyer & Hodges (1998), the temperature–time combination in the *British Pharmacopoeia* (1998) of 121°C for 15min equates to an F_0-value of 15, but this relates to the sterilization of material that may contain large numbers of thermophilic bacterial spores. They add that an F_0 of 8 is appropriate when the bioburden is low, mesophilic spores are likely to be present and the process has been validated microbiologically.

The F_0-values can be calculated graphically by the 'area under the curve' method, as depicted in Fig. 19.10 in Chapter 19D. Alternatively, F_0 can be calculated from the equation

$$F_0 = A_t \Sigma\ 10^{(T-121)/z}$$

in which A_t is the time interval between temperature measurements, T is the product temperature at time t and z is assumed to be 10°C.

2.2 Microbial susceptibility to moist heat

Microorganisms show wide variation in their response to moist heat. Non-sporulating bacteria are usually destroyed at temperatures of 50–60°C, although enterococci are more resistant (Gardner & Peel, 1991a; Bradley & Fraise, 1996). The vegetative forms of yeasts and moulds show a similar response to most vegetative bacteria (Soper & Davies, 1990). Many viruses are sensitive to moist heat at 55–60°C (Russell & Hugo, 1987; Alder & Simpson, 1992), but Gardner & Peel (1991a) point out that boiling or autoclaving is recommended for the inactivation of viruses in association with blood and tissues, e.g. human immunodeficiency virus (HIV) and hepatitis B virus (HBV), although HIV in small amounts of blood will still be inactivated at recommended temperatures, e.g. 70°C for 3 min. Although the vegetative cells (trophozoites) of amoeba, such as *Acanthamoeba polyphaga*, are sensitive to temperatures of 55–60°C, the cyst forms survive for long periods and higher temperatures are needed to inactivate them (Kilvington, 1989). Low-temperature steam (dry, saturated steam) at 73°C for not less than 10 min is a disinfection process that inactivates vegetative microorganisms and heat-sensitive viruses (Medical Devices Directorate, 1993). Boiling water inactivates non-sporulating microbes, fungi, viruses and some mesophilic spores (Medical Devices Directorate, 1993).

Prions are highly resistant to moist heat (Taylor, 1987; Chapter 7). Of the 'typical' microorganisms, thermophilic bacterial spores, e.g. *Bacillus stearothermophilus*, are the most resistant (Russell, 1982). Although spores are considered in detail later (Chapter 19B), their possible responses to moist heat are presented in Fig. 19.1, curves A–D.

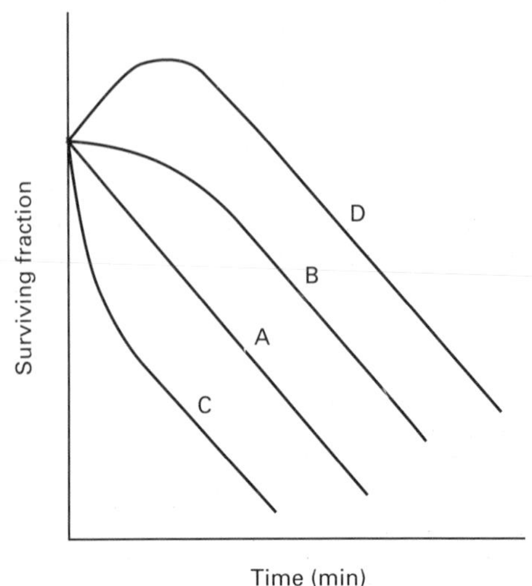

Fig. 19.1 Inactivation of microorganisms by moist heat.

The usual responses are depicted in curves B and D; in the former, an initial shoulder precedes exponential inactivation, whereas in the latter the initial apparent increase in viable numbers occurs as a consequence of heat activation (Gould, 1989).

2.3 Sterilization by moist heat

2.3.1 Quality of steam

Sterilization in an autoclave by moist heat depends upon four properties of dry, saturated steam, namely high temperature, wealth of latent heat, ability to form water of condensation and instantaneous contraction in volume, which occurs during condensation (Bowie, 1955; Young, 1993). These properties are present at optimal level in steam on the phase boundary between itself and the condensate at the same temperature (Fig. 19.2, Table 19.1). Steam at any point on the phase boundary has the same temperature as the boiling water from which it was produced but holds an extra load of latent heat, which, without drop in temperature, is available for transfer when it condenses on to a cooler surface. Superheated steam is hotter than dry saturated steam at the same pressure and is less efficient, becoming equivalent to dry heat (Section 3). Superheated steam behaves as a gas and only slowly yields its heat to cooler objects. A small degree of superheating (maximum 5°C), is permitted i.e. the steam temperature must not be greater than 5°C higher than the phase-boundary temperature at that particular pressure (Fig. 19.2).

When air is present in a space with steam, the air will carry part of the load, so that the pressure of the steam is reduced. In the context of Dalton's law of partial pressures (using P to denote pressure), $P_{total} = P_{steam} + P_{air}$. The temperature achieved in the

Table 19.1 Temperature and pressure relationships in steam sterilization.

	Steam pressure	
Temperature (°C)	kPa	psi
121	103	15
126	138	20
134	207	30

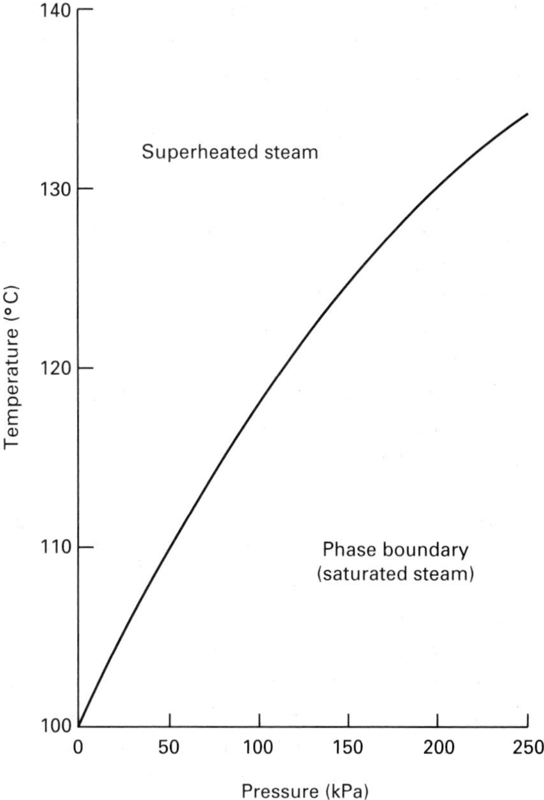

Fig. 19.2 Temperature–pressure relationship for steam.

pressence of air will thus reflect the contribution made by the steam and may be less than that associated with the total pressure recorded, although large volumes of air trapped in an autoclave load are not necessarily associated with reduced temperatures. However, the heating-up period will be prolonged. Such times are considerably reduced when an efficient air-displacement system is used (Scruton, 1989). The removal of air is thus important in ensuring efficient autoclaving; the presence of air in packages of porous materials, such as surgical dressings, hinders the penetration of steam, thereby preventing sterilization from being achieved (Alder & Gillespie, 1957). This aspect will be considered again below (Section 2.3.3).

2.3.2 Time–temperature relationships

A series of time–temperature relationships is authorized by the *British Pharmacopoeia* (1998).

These holding periods (Fig. 19.3) are presented in Table 19.2. The lethality of the process includes not only the holding period (BC in Fig. 19.3), but also the heating-up and cooling-down periods (respectively, AB and CD in Fig. 19.3). The F_0-value (see Section 2.1) is used to express the lethality of the whole process as an equivalent holding period at 121°C. At the higher temperatures presented in Table 19.2, the lethal effect is considerably greater, calculated F_0 values at 121°C (15 min), 126°C (10 min) and 134°C (3 min) being 15, 31 and 59, respectively (Dewhurst & Hoxey, 1990). At 115°C for 30 min, the calculated F_0 value is 8.1 (Dewhurst & Hoxey, 1990).

2.3.3 *Design of sterilizers*

Since various types of objects are sterilized by means of autoclaving, it is not surprising that different sterilizers have been designed. Steam sterilization is employed as a terminal process for bottled fluids, previously cleaned items, unwrapped instruments and utensils, wrapped goods and porous loads, and a British Standard (BS 3970, Parts 1–4, 1990 and 1991) is available that describes appropriate types of equipment (Part 5 of BS 3970 providing a specification for low-temperature steam disinfectors). Additionally, BS 2646 (1988) provides a specification for the design and construction of laboratory autoclaves, and BS EN 554 (EN 554) (1994) describes the validation and control of heat sterilization.

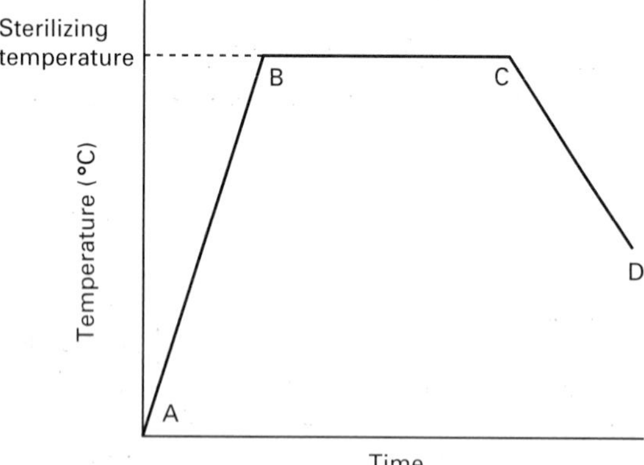

Fig. 19.3 Stages in moist-heat sterilization process. AB, heating up; BC, holding; CD, cooling.

Table 19.2 Time–temperature relationships in thermal sterilization process. (*British Pharmacopoeia* (1998) recommendations; see also *United States Pharmacopoeia* (1995) and *European Pharmacopoeia* (1997).)

Process	Temperature (°C)	Holding period (min)
Moist heat (autoclaving)	121 126 134	15 10 3
Dry heat	Minimum of 160 170 180	Not less than 120 60 30

Porous-load (high, prevacuum) sterilizers are used for sterilizing wrapped goods and porous materials. Air removal is vital and this is achieved by evacuation and steam injection; a vacuum of 4–6 kPa absolute is followed by a series of steam injections and evacuations. The procedure is monitored routinely with the Bowie–Dick test (Bowie *et al.* (1963), the basis of which is a uniform colour change of a temperature-sensitive indicator. An air detector ensures the absence of air in the sterilizer.

Downward-displacement (instrument and utensil) sterilizers rely upon displacement of air by steam admitted from a separate steam source or generated within the sterilizing chamber. Despite the terminology, steam generated within the chamber may, in fact, ensure upward displacement of air (Dewhurst & Hoxey, 1990).

Both of the sterilizers described above rely on direct contact between steam and the product being sterilized. In contrast, bottled-fluids sterilizers act in a different manner; here, steam condenses on the surface of the containers, followed by heat transfer across the container walls, so that the contents are raised to the sterilizing temperature. The pressure within the sealed container will rise; this may be counteracted by the strength of the container and the pressure of steam within the chamber. The chamber pressure may be increased by the addition of sterile air (air ballasting) to prevent breakage of glass containers or deformation of polymeric ones. After the holding period has been completed, the cooling period can be accelerated by spray-cooling with water (sterile, to prevent the possibility of contamination).

Further information about the uses of these

types of sterilizers is provided in Table 19.3, and Fig. 19.4 illustrates a large-scale steam sterilizer, operating on dry saturated steam from a separate boiler, for routine hospital or industrial use.

2.3.4 *Validation and monitoring*

Validation of steam sterilizers is achieved by determining the inactivation of heat-resistant spores, e.g. *B. stearothermophilus* (D_{121} 1.5 min, z 10°C). In contrast, biological indicators have no role in monitoring steam sterilization. Functional performance tests involve physical (thermometric) measurement of the conditions (Dewhurst & Hoxey, 1990; Graham, 1991; Bruch, 1993; Graham & Boris, 1993; Medical Devices Directorate, 1993; Hodges, 1995). Chemical indicators provide a visual assessment that a process has been

Table 19.3 Types of steam sterilizers (based on Dewhurst & Hoxey, 1990, and Medical Devices Directorate, 1993).

Type of steam sterilizer	Sterilization conditions	Use
Porous load	134–138°C, 3 min	Unwrapped instruments, dressings and utensils
Fluid cycle	121°C, 15 min	Fluids in sealed containers, e.g. injections in ampoules
Unwrapped instruments	134–138°C, 3 min	Unwrapped instruments and utensils
LTSF*	73°C, 3 h	Heat-sensitive equipment

* Doubts have been expressed about the efficiency of low-temperature steam with formaldehyde (LTSF) as a sterilization process; see Section 2.4.

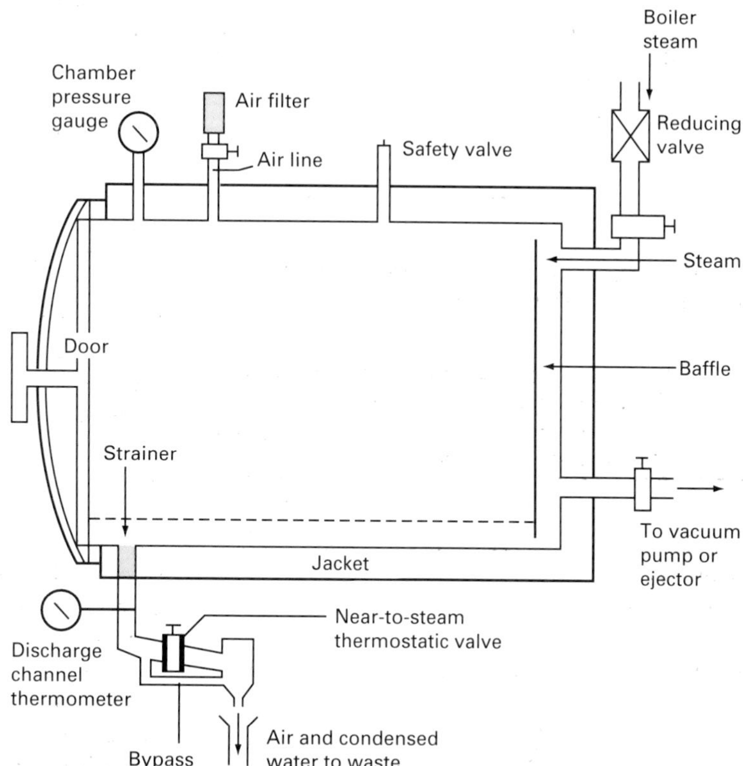

Fig. 19.4 A large-scale steam sterilizer (autoclave) for routine hospital or industrial use, operating on dry saturated steam from a separate boiler (reproduced by courtesy of Albert Browne Ltd., Leicester, UK).

undertaken, but provide no guarantee as to sterility. The specific use of the Bowie–Dick test was referred to in Section 2.3.3.

A comprehensive discussion is provided in Chapter 25.

2.4 Sterilization by low-temperature steam and formaldehyde

Low-temperature steam at subatmospheric pressure was developed originally for disinfecting heat-sensitive materials. At 80°C, LTS was found to be much more effective than water at the same temperature and the addition of formaldehyde to LTS to produce LTSF achieved a sporicidal effect (Alder & Gillespie, 1961; Alder *et al.* 1966, 1971a,b; Line & Pickerill, 1973; Gibson, 1977, 1980; Alder, 1987). As a sterilization procedure, LTSF has been reviewed by Dewhurst & Hoxey (1990), Soper & Davies (1990), Hoxey (1991), Alder & Simpson (1992) and Denyer & Hodges (1998).

Generally, LTSF operates in a temperature range of 70–80°C, with a formaldehyde concentration per sterilization chamber volume of approx. 14 mg/l. The design of an LTSF sterilizer is similar to that of a porous-load steam sterilizer (see Section 2.3), the main differences being its operation at subatmospheric pressure and the injection of formaldehyde gas. Further detailed information will be found in Chapter 21.

Recent papers have been published on the activity of LTSF against the spores of the thermophile, *B. stearothermophilus* (Wright *et al.*, 1995, 1996, 1997), the most interesting aspect of which was the finding that treated spores could be revived by an appropriate postexposure heat shock (Wright *et al.*, 1997). This implies that spores may not, after all, be inactivated by LTSF and some doubt has thus been cast on the efficacy of this combined treatment. It is to be hoped that this matter can be resolved, since, in principle, LTSF is potentially a useful process.

2.5 Sterilization by heating with a bactericide

The activity of a chemical agent is normally increased when the temperature at which it acts is raised. At ambient temperatures, the chlorinated phenol, chlorocresol, and the organomercurials, phenylmercuric nitrate (PMN) and phenylmercuric acetate (PMA), are sporistatic rather than sporicidal (Russell, 1991a,b, 1997). At elevated temperatures, however, they are sporicidal, a property that suggested to Berry *et al.* (1938) that these agents might find usage as sterilization procedures. They accordingly proposed a new method of 'heating with a bactericide' (chlorocresol or PMN) for the sterilization of some types of parenteral products, which was incorporated into the fourth addendum to the 1932 *British Pharmacopoeia*. The underlying procedure was also invoked as one that was allowed officially in the UK for the sterilization of eye-drops, the bactericides being PMN, PMA, chlorhexidine diacetate and benzalkonium chloride. It is interesting to note that relatively low numbers of *Bacillus subtilis* spores were found to survive heating with chlorocresol (Davies & Davison, 1947) or PMN (Davison, 1951). It must, however, be pointed out that the containers used in these experiments consisted of screw-capped bottles with rubber liners; both chlorocresol and, to a greater extent, PMN are absorbed into rubber, thereby reducing their concentration and efficacy (Sykes, 1958).

Heating with a microbicidal agent is no longer permitted as an official method of sterilization of injectables or eye-drops in the UK, having been deleted from the 1988 British Pharmacopoeia and finding no place in the current edition (*British Pharmacopoeia*, 1998).

2.6 Disinfection by moist heat

Inactivation of microorganisms by moist heat has been practised for many years. For example, the pasteurization of milk is based upon Louis Pasteur's observations that spoilage of wines could be prevented by heating at temperatures of 50–60°C. Likewise, the inactivation of bacteria in killed bacterial vaccines may be achieved by similar temperatures, although generally an agent such as phenol is nowadays employed (Sheffield, 1998).

Disinfection with LTS is achieved by using an automatically controlled disinfector under conditions that ensure the removal of air and subsequent exposure to subatmospheric, dry, saturated steam at 73°C for not less than 10 min. Details of the equipment, monitoring procedure, uses and monitoring are provided by BS 3970 (1990, Parts 1 and 5), Babb (1993), Medical Devices Directorate (1993) and Health Technical Memorandum No. 2010 (1994). The process kills most vegetative microorganisms and viruses.

Disinfection may also be achieved by means of soft-water boiling at normal atmospheric pressure at 100°C for 5 min or more. Articles to be disinfected in this manner must be precleaned. Details of the equipment required and its operation and maintenance, together with the disadvantages of the process, are described by the Medical Devices Directorate (1993).

Washer disinfectors (BS 2745, 1993; Health Technical Memorandum No. 2030, 1995) achieve disinfection by a combination of physical cleaning and thermal effects. A temperature of about 80°C is employed and the process inactivates all microorganisms except bacterial spores. The Medical Devices Directorate (1993) provides additional information. Babb (1993) considers the process options, using moist-heat temperatures of 65–100°C for various implants. *Enterococcus faecalis* may be employed as a biological indicator of thermal disinfection.

2.7 Mechanisms of microbial inactivation

In general, moist heat sterilization and disinfection processes act by heat-catalysed hydrolytic changes. There are several targets in vegetative microorganisms and in bacterial spores that are susceptible to a high level of damage when exposed to moist heat (Gould, 1989). Such targets include the cytoplasmic membrane, enzymes, deoxyribonucleic acid (DNA), ribonucleic acid (RNA) and protein. The possible sites and types of damage are considered more fully in Chapters 19B and 19D.

3 Sterilization by dry heat

Sterilization by dry heat is a physical process, carried out in the absence of moisture. It is a less efficient process than moist heat.

3.1 Terminology

Definitions of *D*-value, *z*-value and were given for moist heat in Section 2.1 and apply equally here. The *F*-value concept utilized in steam-sterilization processes has an equivalent in dry-heat sterilization, although, as pointed out by Denyer & Hodges (1998), its application has been limited. This equivalent, F_H, describes the lethality in terms of the equivalent number of minutes at 170°C. Russell (1982, 1998) has demonstrated that higher *D*-values and *z*-values are found with dry heat than with moist heat and in dry-heat calculations a *z*-value of 20°C is considered to be suitable.

3.2 Microbial susceptibility to dry heat

Dry heat will inactivate all microorganisms, although bacterial spores are the most resistant (Russell, 1982). Resistance depends on the degree of dryness of the cells (Ababouch *et al.*, 1995). Prions are not inactivated by microwave irradiation and are only inactivated by radiant heat at very high temperatures (Chapter 7).

3.3 Sterilization by dry heat

3.3.1 *Principles*

A variety of methods can be used to achieve dry-heat sterilization. They include the most widely employed procedure (hot air) and sterilizing tunnels, which utilize infrared irradiation to achieve heat transfer. The underlying principle of dry heat sterilization is to raise the temperature of the object to be sterilized to the sterilization temperature and to maintain it at that level for the desired period of time.

3.3.2 *Design of sterilizers*

As pointed out above (Section 3.3.1), a hot-air oven is usually employed to effect dry heat sterilization. The sterilizer consists of an insulated, polished, stainless-steel chamber, which contains perforated shelving to permit circulation of hot air. Sterilization depends upon heat transfer from a gas (hot air) to cooler objects and it is essential that even temperature distribution throughout the sterilization chamber is achieved. In practice, this is done by the inclusion of a fan unit at the rear of the oven, which ensures forced air circulation. The items that are to be sterilized must be cleaned and dried before commencement of the process. Further information is to be found in BS 3970 (1990), Medical Devices Directorate (1993) and Health Technical Memorandum No. 2010 (1994), as well as useful discourses on dry-heat sterilization by Gardner & Peel (1991b) and Wood (1991, 1993).

Infrared heaters have also been used to achieve dry heat sterilization. Infrared rays are characterized by long wavelengths and very low levels of radiant energy. They depend upon the fact that the radiant energy is converted to heat when it is absorbed by solids or liquids. Infrared rays have the ability to raise rapidly the surface temperature of objects that they strike, with the interior temperature raised by conduction.

Microwave radiations are also characterized by long wavelengths and very low levels of radiant energy. Although microwave radiation has been considered for sterilization purposes (Rohrer & Bulard, 1985; Lohmann & Manique, 1986; Jeng *et al.*, 1987), the major problem with its use has been the uneven heating achieved. It has also been applied to the inactivation of microorganisms in suspension (Latimer & Matsen, 1977; Fujikawa *et al.*, 1992; Fujikawa & Ohta, 1994) and in infant formula preparations (Kindle *et al.*, 1996), although the microwaves are not operating here, of course, as a source of dry heat. *Mycobacterium bovis* dried on to scalpel blades was destroyed after 4 min of microwave exposure (Rosaspina *et al.*, 1994). Microwaves have been used for the disinfection of contact lenses and urinary catheters (Douglas *et al.*, 1990).

The problems associated with the use of infrared

Table 19.4 Principles of sterilization by moist heat.

Parameter	Explanation
Properties of steam	Wealth of latent heat given up when steam condenses on cooler object until temperature equilibrium attained
Quality of steam	Dry saturated steam on phase boundary (Fig. 19.2); superheated and supersaturated steam to be avoided
Air removal from load	Air removal is essential, otherwise steam is unable to act properly as sterilizing agent
Microbial inactivation	Several target sites: at high steam temperatures, degradation of DNA and RNA, inactivation of enzymes, membrane damage, protein coagulation, damage to spore germination system

Table 19.5 Principles of sterilization by dry heat.

Parameter	Explanation
Properties of dry heat	Heat transfer to cooler objects (a) Hot-air oven:* transfer from gas (b) Infrared radiation: surface increase in temperature, interior temperature raised by conduction
Effectiveness of process	Hot-air oven: forced circulation of hot air essential, correct packaging. Infrared radiation: suitable for small packages
Microbial inactivation	Probably oxidative processes; efficacy depends upon water content of microorganisms

*See BS 3421 (1961).

and microwave radiations are well discussed by Gardner & Peel (1991b).

3.3.3 Validation and monitoring

Validation can be achieved by determining the inactivation of a suitable dry-heat-resistant organism, such as spores of a non-toxigenic *Clostridium tetani* strain. As with steam sterilization, routine monitoring is undertaken by thermometric measurement. Chemical indicators provide a visual check that a process has taken place, but give no guarantee of sterility (see also Chapter 25).

3.4 Mechanisms of microbial inactivation

Dry heat probably inactivates bacterial spores and vegetative microorganisms by an oxidative process (Russell, 1982). The water content of the cells themselves plays an important role in this inactivation, as discussed more fully in Chapter 19B, Section 5.1.

4 Conclusions

Both moist heat and dry heat (summarized in Tables 19.4 and 19.5, respectively), particularly the former, have an important role to play in the field of sterilization. The principles underlying their efficacy are, however, different (see Chapter 19B). Applications of thermal methods of sterilization remain widespread (see Chapter 19C,D).

5 References

Ababouch, L.H., Grimit, L., Eddafry, R. & Busta, F.F. (1995) Thermal inactivation kinetics of *Bacillus subtilis* spores suspended in buffer and in oils. *Journal of Applied Bacteriology*, **78**, 669–676.

Alder, V.G. (1987) The formaldehyde/low temperature steam sterilizing procedure. *Journal of Hospital Infection*, **9**, 194–200.

Alder, V.G. & Gillespie, W.A. (1957) The sterilization of dressings. *Journal of Clinical Pathology*, **10**, 299–306.

Alder, V.G. & Gillespie, W.A. (1961) Disinfection of woollen blankets in steam at subatmospheric pressure. *Journal of Clinical Pathology*, **14**, 515–518.

Alder, V.G. & Simpson, R.A. (1992) Heat sterilization. A. Sterilization and disinfection by heat methods. In *Principles and Practice of Disinfection, Preservation and Sterilization*, 2nd edn (eds Russell, A.D., Hugo, W.B. & Ayliffe, G.A.J.), pp. 483–498. Oxford: Blackwell Scientific Publications.

Alder, V.G., Brown, A.M. & Gillespie, W.A. (1966) Disinfection of heat-sensitive material by low-temperature steam and formaldehyde. *Journal of Clinical Pathology*, **19**, 83–89.

Alder, V.G., Boss, E., Gillespie, W.A. & Swann, A.J. (1971a) Residual disinfection of wool blankets treated with formaldehyde. *Journal of Applied Bacteriology*, **34**, 757–763.

Alder, V.G., Gingell, J.C. & Mitchell, J.P. (1971b) Disinfection of cystoscopes by subatmospheric steam and formaldehyde at 80°C. *British Medical Journal*, **iii**, 677–680.

Babb, J.R. (1993) Methods of cleaning and disinfection. *Zentralblatt Sterilization*, **1**, 227–237.

Berry, H., Jensen, E. & Silliker, F.K. (1938) The sterilization of thermolabile substances in the presence of bactericides. *Quarterly Journal of Pharmacy and Pharmacology*, **11**, 729–735.

Bowie, J.H. (1955) Modern apparatus for sterilization. *Pharmaceutical Journal.*, **174**, 473–477.

Bowie, J.H., Kelsey, J.C. & Thompson, R. (1963) The Bowie and Dick autoclave tape test. *Lancet*, **i**, 586–587.

Bradley, C.R. & Fraise, A.P. (1996) Heat and chemical resistance of enterococci. *Journal of Hospital Infection*, **34**, 191–196.

British Pharmacopoeia (1998) London: The Stationery Office.

Brown, K.L. (1994) Spore resistance and ultra heat treatment processes. *Journal of Applied Bacteriology Symposium Supplement*, **76**, 67S–80S.

Bruch, C.W. (1993) The philosophy of sterilization validation. In *Sterilization Technology* (eds Morrissey, R.F. & Phillips, G.B.), pp. 17–35. New York: Van Nostrand Reinhold.

BS 3421 (1961) *Specification for Performance of Electrically Heated Sterilizing Ovens*. London: British Standards Institute.

BS 2646 (1988) *Autoclaves for Sterilization in Laboratories*. Part 1: *Specification for Design and Construction*. London: British Standards Institute.

BS 3970 (1990) *Sterilizing and Disinfecting Equipment for Medical Products*. Part 1: *Specification for General Requirements*; Part 3: *Specification for Steam Sterilizers for Wrapped Goods and Porous Loads*; Part 4: *Specification for Transportable Steam Sterilizers for Unwrapped Instruments and Utensils*; Part 5: *Specification for Low-temperature Steam Disinfectors*. London: British Standards Institute.

BS 3970 (1991) *Sterilizing and Disinfecting Equipment for Medical Products*. Part 2: *Specification for Steam Sterilizers for Aqueous Fluids in Rigid Sealed Containers*. London: British Standards Institute.

BS 2745 (1993) *Washer Disinfectors*. Parts 1–3. London: British Standards Institute.

BS EN 554 (EN 554) (1994) *Validation and Control of Moist Heat Sterilization*. London: British Standards Institute.

Davies, G.E. & Davison, J.E. (1947) The use of antiseptics in the sterilization of solutions for injection. Part I. The efficiency of chlorocresol. *Quarterly Journal of Pharmacy and Pharmacology*, **20**, 212– 218.

Davison, J.E. (1951) The use of antiseptics in the sterilization of solutions for injection. Part II. The efficiency of phenylmercuric nitrate. *Journal of Pharmacy and Pharmacology*, **3**, 734–738.

Denyer, S.P. & Hodges, N.A. (1998) Principles and practice of sterilization. In *Pharmaceutical Microbiology*, 6th edn (eds Hugo, W.B. & Russell, A.D.), pp. 385–409. Oxford: Blackwell Scientific Publications.

Dewhurst, E. & Hoxey, E.V. (1990) Sterilization methods. In *Guide to Microbiological Control in Pharmaceuticals* (eds Denyer, S.P. & Baird, R.M.), pp. 182–218. Chichester: Ellis Horwood.

Douglas, C., Burke, B., Kessler, D.L. & Bracken, R.B. (1990) Microwave: practical cost-effective method for sterilizing urinary catheters in the home. *Urology*, **35**, 219–222.

Fujikawa, H. & Ohta, K. (1994) Patterns of bacterial destruction in solutions by microwave irradiation. *Journal of Applied Bacteriology*, **76**, 389–394.

Fujikawa, H., Ushioda, H. & Kudo, Y. (1992) Kinetics of *Escherichia coli* destruction by microwave irradiation. *Applied and Environmental Microbiology*, **58**, 920–924.

Gardner, J.F. & Peel, M.M. (1991a) Principles of heat sterilization. In *Introduction to Sterilization, Disinfection and Infection Control*, pp. 47–59. Edinburgh: Churchill Livingstone.

Gardner, J.F. & Peel, M.M. (1991b) Sterilization by dry heat. In *Introduction to Sterilization, Disinfection and Infection Control*, pp. 60–69. Edinburgh: Churchill Livingstone.

Gibson, G.L. (1977) Processing urinary endoscopes in a low-temperature steam and formaldehyde autoclave. *Journal of Clinical Pathology*, **30**, 269–274.

Gibson, G.L. (1980) Processing heat-sensitive instruments and materials by low-temperature steam and formaldehyde. *Journal of Hospital Infection*, **1**, 95–101.

Gould, G.W. (1989) Heat-induced injury and inactivation. In *Mechanisms of Action of Food Preservation Procedures* (ed. Gould, G.W.), pp. 11–42. London: Elsevier Applied Science.

Graham, G.S. (1991) Biological indicators for hospital and industrial sterilization. In *Sterilization of Medical Products* (eds Morrissey, R.F. & Prokopenks, Y.I.), Vol. V, pp. 54–71. Morin Heights: Polyscience Publications.

Graham, G.S. & Boris, C.A. (1993) Chemical and biological indicators. In *Sterilization Technology* (eds Morrissey, R.F. & Phillips, G.B.), pp. 36–69. New York: Van Nostrand Reinhold.

Haberer, K. & Wallhaeusser, K.-H. (1990) Assurance of sterility by validation of the sterilization process. In *Guide of Microbiological Control in Pharmaceuticals* (eds Denyer, S.P. & Baird, R.M.), pp. 219–240. Chichester: Ellis Horwood.

Health Technical Memorandum No. 2010 (1994) *Sterilizers*. London: Department of Health.

Health Technical Memorandum No. 2030 (1995) *NHS Estates*. Part 1. London: HMSO.

Hodges, N. (1995) Reproducibility and performance of endospores as biological indicators. In *Microbiological Quality Assurance: A Guide towards Relevance and Reproducibility of Inocula* (eds Brown, M.R.W. & Gillespie, P.), pp. 221–233. Boca Raton: CRC Press.

Hoxey, E.V. (1991) Low temperature steam formaldehyde. In *Sterilization of Medical Products* (eds Morrissey, R.F. & Prokopenko, Y.I.), Vol. V, pp. 359–364. Morin Heights: Polyscience Publications.

Hugo, W.B. (1991) A brief history of heat and chemical preservation and disinfection. *Journal of Applied Bacteriology*, **71**, 9–18.

Hugo, W.B. (1995) A brief history of heat, chemical and radiation preservation and disinfection. *International Biodeterioration Biodegradation*, **36**, 197–218.

Jeng, D.K.H., Kaczmarek, K.A., Wodworth, A.G. & Balasky, G. (1987) Mechanism of microwave sterilization in the dry state. *Applied and Environmental Microbiology*, **53**, 2133–2137.

Kilvington, S. (1989) Moist heat disinfection of pathogenic *Acanthamoeba* cysts. *Letters in Applied Microbiology*, **9**, 187–189.

Kindle, G., Busse, A., Kampa, D., Meyer-König, U. & Daschner, F.D. (1996) Killing activity of microwaves in milk. *Journal of Hospital Infection*, **33**, 273–278.

Kowalski, J.B. (1993) Selecting a sterilization method. In *Sterilization Technology* (eds Morrissey, R.F. & Phillips, G.B.), pp. 70–78. New York: Van Nostrand Reinhold.

Latimer, J.M. & Masten, J.M. (1977) Microwave oven irradiation as a method for bacterial decontamination in a clinical microbiology laboratory. *Journal of Clinical Microbiology*, **6**, 340–342.

Line, S.J. & Pickerill, J.K. (1973) Testing a steam formaldehyde sterilizer for gas penetration efficiency. *Journal of Clinical Pathology*, **26**, 716–720.

Lohmann, S. & Manique, F. (1986) Microwave sterilization of vials. *Journal of Parenteral Science and Technology*, **40**, 25–30.

Medical Devices Directorate (1993) *Sterilization, Disinfection and Cleaning of Medical Equipment*. London: HMSO.

Olson, W.P. (1977) Synergistic sterilization: a brief history. *PDA Journal of Pharmaceutical Science and Technology*, **51**, 116–118.

Owens, J.E. (1993) Sterilization of LVPs and SVPs. In *Sterilization Technology* (eds Morrissey, R.F. & Phillips, G.B.), pp. 254–285. New York: Van Nostrand Reinhold.

Rohrer, M.D. & Bulard, R.A. (1985) Microwave sterilization. *Journal of the American Dental Association*, **110**, 194–198.

Rosaspina, S., Salvatorelli, G. & Anzanel, D. (1994) The bactericidal effect of microwaves on *Mycobacterium bovis* dried on scalpel blades. *Journal of Hospital Infection*, **26**, 45–50.

Russell, A.D. (1982) *The Destruction of Bacterial Spores*. London: Academic Press.

Russell, A.D. (1991a) Fundamental aspects of microbial resistance to chemical and physical agents. In *Sterilization of Medical Products* (eds Morrissey, R.F. & Prokopenko, Y.I.), Vol. V, pp. 22–42. Morin Heights: Polyscience Publications.

Russell, A.D. (1991b) Bacterial spores and chemical sporicidal agents. *Clinical Microbiology Reviews*, **3**, 99–119.

Russell A.D. (1993) Theoretical mechanisms of microbial inactivation. In *Industrial Sterilization Technology* (eds Morrissey, R.F. & Phillips, G.B.), pp. 3–16. New York: Van Nostrand Reinhold.

Russell, A.D. (1997) Microbial susceptibility and resistance to chemical and physical agents. In *Topley & Wilson's Microbiology and Microbial Infections*, 9th edn, Vol. 2 (eds Balows, A. & Duerden, B.I.), pp. 149–184. London: Arnold.

Russell, A.D. & Hugo, W.B. (1987) Chemical disinfectants. In *Disinfection in Veterinary and Farm Animal Practice* (eds Linton, A.H., Hugo, W.B. & Russell, A.D.), pp. 12–42. Oxford: Blackwell Scientific Publications.

Russell, A.D., Furr, J.R. & Maillard, J.-Y. (1997) Synergistic sterilization. *PDA Journal of Pharmaceutical Science and Technology*, **51**, 174–175.

Scruton, M.W. (1989) The effect of air with steam on the temperature of autoclave contents. *Journal of Hospital Infection*, **14**, 249–262.

Sheffield, F.W. (1998) The manufacture and quality control of immunological products. In *Pharmaceutical Microbiology*, 6th edn (eds Hugo, W.B. & Russell, A.D.), pp. 304–320. Oxford: Blackwell Scientific Publications.

Soper, C.J. & Davies, D.J.G. (1990) Principles of sterilization. In *Guide to Microbiological Control in Pharmaceuticals* (eds Denyer, S.P. & Baird, R.M.), pp. 156–181. Chichester: Ellis Horwood.

Sykes, G. (1958) The basis for 'sufficient of a suitable bacteriostat' in injections. *Journal of Pharmacy and Pharmacology*, **10**, 40T–45T.

Taylor, D.M. (1987) Autoclaving standards for Creutzfeldt–Jakob disease agent. *Annals of Neurology*, **22**, 557–558.

Wood, R.T. (1991) Dry heat sterilization. In *Sterilization of Medical Products* (eds Morrissey, R.F. & Prokopenko, Y.I.), Vol. V, pp. 365–375. Morin Heights: Polyscience Publications.

Wood, R.T. (1993) Sterilization by dry heat. In *Sterilization Technology* (eds Morrissey, R.F. & Phillips, G.B.) pp. 81–119. New York: Van Nostrand Reinhold.

Wright, A.M., Hoxey, E.V., Soper, C.J. & Davies, D.J.G. (1995) Biological indicators for low temperature steam and formaldehyde sterilization: the effect of defined media on sporulation, growth index and formaldehyde resistance of spores of *Bacillus stearothermophilus* strains. *Journal of Applied Bacteriology*, **79**, 432–438.

Wright, A.M., Hoxey, E.V., Soper, C.J. & Davies, D.J.G. (1996) Biological indicators for low temperature steam and formaldehyde sterilization: investigation of the effect of change in temperature and formaldehyde concentration on spores of *Bacillus stearothermophilus* NCIMB 8224. *Journal of Applied Bacteriology*, **80**, 259–265.

Wright, A.M., Hoxey, E.V., Soper, C.J. & Davies, D.J.G. (1997) Biological indicators for low temperature steam formaldehyde and sterilization: effect of variations in recovery conditions on the response of spores of *Bacillus stearothermophilus* NCIMB 8224 to low temperature steam and formaldehyde. *Journal of Applied Microbiology*, **82**, 552–556.

Young, J.H. (1993) Sterilization with steam under pressure. In *Sterilization Technology* (eds Morrissey, R.F. & Phillips, G.B.), pp. 120–151. New York: Van Nostrand Reinhold.

Chapter 19

B. DESTRUCTION OF BACTERIAL SPORES BY THERMAL METHODS

1 Introduction

Several thermal methods are employed in large-scale sterilization processes. These procedures include autoclaving using saturated steam or high-pressure water (Ernst, 1968; Brennan *et al.*, 1969), high-temperature–short-time sterilization, using steam injection or heat-exchanging systems (Ashton, 1977), and continuous sterilization, with either superheated steam (metal cans: Denny & Matthys, 1975; Quast *et al.*, 1977) or short-wave infrared radiation (glass vessels: Molin, 1976). The various heating methods have many technical differences, but as far as bacterial spores are concerned they are relatively similar. However, apart from the time/temperature cycle, there is one major difference, namely whether the method is based on moist (wet) heat or on dry heat. Moist heat is by definition a condition where the water activity (A_w) is 1.0 and dry heat thus represents all conditions where the A_w is less than 1.0 (Pflug & Schmidt, 1968). Thermal processing is widely employed in the pharmaceutical and food industries (Gould, 1995; Brown, 1994; Russell, 1998).

The heat-inactivation kinetics of bacterial spores is strongly dependent on whether the spores are exposed to moist or dry heat.

Whatever heat-sterilization method is used, the most important consideration when evaluating the effectiveness of a specific heating cycle is the A_w value. The inactivation rate of spores exposed to heat in a certain sterilization process can thus be calculated on the basis of heat-resistance data achieved from inactivation studies at a defined A_w. The heat resistance of the spores is not, however, solely influenced by the A_w, but also by a number of other parameters. These parameters, on the other hand, are not necessarily directly linked to a specific sterilization method, but rather to the nature of the substrate or material with which the spore is associated.

In the present review, an account of the various parameters which influence the heat resistance of bacterial spores is given and discussed in the light of current ideas concerning the heat-inactivation mechanisms of spores.

2 Kinetics

Microorganisms are generally considered to be heat-inactivated in geometric regression, where in each equal successive time interval the same fraction of remaining viable cells is destroyed. This process can be described as in equation (19.1):

$$\log N_T = -\frac{T}{D} + \log N_0 \qquad (19.1)$$

where N_0 is the initial viable cell number, D is the microbial inactivation rate (the time needed to reduce the population by 90% at a certain temperature) and N_T is the viable cell number after T minutes of heating. If the logarithmic number of surviving cells is plotted versus time, the resulting curve ('survivor curve' or 'inactivation curve') is a straight line. This equation can also be presented as

$$\log N_0 - \log N_T = \frac{T}{D}$$

or

$$\log \frac{N_0}{N_T} = \frac{T}{D} \qquad (19.2)$$

Equation (19.2) gives a measure of the inactivation factor.

Furthermore, the relationship between the inactivation rate and the temperature can be represented by a straight line (thermal-resistance curve). This empirically found phenomenon was first observed by Bigelow (1921). The temperature coefficient, D_r, of Bigelow is described in equation (19.3):

$$\log D_r = \frac{1}{z}(T_0 - T) + \log D_{r_0} \qquad (19.3)$$

where T_0 is the initial temperature, D_{r_0} is specified and T is the new temperature corresponding to D_r. As seen from equation (19.3), the z value is a measure of the slope of the straight line and the number of degrees (°C) of temperature change necessary to change to D-value by a factor of 10.

The logarithmic order of inactivation and the temperature-coefficient model of Bigelow are in general considered to be valid for both moist- and dry-heat inactivation of bacterial spores.

Deviations from the logarithmic order of inactivation are frequently reported in the literature. The course of the non-linear inactivation curves has been explained by experimental artefacts (Stumbo, 1965), the multiple critical sites theory (Rahn, 1943; Moats, 1971) and heterogeneity of spore heat resistance (Han, 1975; Han *et al.*, 1976; Cerf, 1977; Sharpe & Bektash, 1977). Nevertheless, it should be borne in mind, when inactivation data are evaluated, that the logarithmic inactivation model imposes a number of restrictions on an experimental programme. According to Pflug (1973), these are:

1 the spores of the sample being evaluated must be genetically, chemically and physically uniform;

2 the conditions of the heat-inactivation tests must be constant on a test-to-test basis;

3 the overall handling procedures, media, incubation temperature and recovery method must be constant.

Common types of deviations from linearity are a shoulder or a sudden drop at the beginning of the inactivation curve and a 'tailing' of the later portion of the curve. All types have been reported in both moist and dry heat inactivation studies, e.g. in moist heat by Russell (1971, 1982) and in dry heat by Fox & Pflug (1968), Alderton & Snell (1969) and Staat & Beakley (1969). Tailing has been extensively discussed by Cerf (1977).

Several workers have pointed out that the linear relationship obtained between the inactivation rate and temperature is an approximation only valid in narrow temperature ranges (Rahn, 1945; Amaha, 1953; Levine, 1956) and the Arrhenius analysis is sometimes proposed as an alternative to the temperature-coefficient model of Bigelow. Deviations from the model of Bigelow have been reported to occur in moist heat by, for example, Wang *et al.* (1964) and Edwards *et al.* (1965a) at temperatures >120°C, and in dry heat at temperatures >160°C by Oag (1940). However, in dry heat at low A_w, Molin (1977c) showed that the thermal-resistance curve of *Bacillus subtilis* spores was straight (constant z-value) in the temperature interval of 37–190°C. This supports the accuracy of the Bigelow model at conditions of low A_w values. With moist heat, on the other hand, neither the Bigelow model nor the Arrhenius model seems to fit when applied over a wide temperature range (Davies *et al.*, 1977; Jonsson *et al.*, 1977).

Table 19.6 Some *D*- and *z*-values for spores heated in phosphate buffer (pH 7) or in water (see also Russell, 1982).

Bacillus/Clostridium species	Strain	Investigated temperature range (°C)	*D*-value (min)	*z*-value (°C)	Reference
B. cereus 1	–	104–121	$D_{121} = 0.03$	9.9	Bradshaw *et al.*, 1975
B. cereus 2	–	116–129	$D_{121} = 2.4$	7.9	
B. coagulans	604	115–125	$D_{120} = 2.3$	7.2	Daudin & Cerf, 1977
B. globisporus	ATCC 23301	85–90	$D_{90} = 11$	7.8	Michels & Visser, 1976
B. megaterium	ATCC 19213	85–100	$D_{92} = 1$	6.3	
B. psychrosaccharolyticus	ATCC 23296	81–90	$D_{90} = 4.5$	8.5	Bender & Marquis, 1985
B. stearothermophilus	NCIB 8923	115–130	$D_{120} = 5.8$	13	Scholefield & Abdelgadir, 1974
B. stearothermophilus	NCIB 8919	115–130	$D_{120} = 5.3$	11	
B. stearothermophilus	NCIB 8924	115–130	$D_{120} = 1.0$	8.9	
B. stearothermophilus	ATCC 7953	111–125	$D_{121} = 2.1$	8.5	Jonsson *et al.*, 1977
B. stearothermophilus	–	110–121	$D_{121} = 3.4$	7.6	Pflug & Smith, 1977
B. stearothermophilus	ATCC 7953	110–120	$D_{118} = 10$	5.7	Bender & Marquis, 1985
B. subtilis	5230	77–121	$D_{121} = 0.5$	14	Fox & Eder, 1969
B. subtilis	NCIB 8054	85–95	$D_{90} = 4.8$	9.3	Härnulv & Snygg, 1972
B. subtilis var. *niger*	–	90–100	$D_{94} = 10$	6.6	Bender & Marquis, 1985
Cl. aerofoetidium	NCTC 505	80–95	$D_{90} = 139$	6.8	Roberts *et al.*, 1966a
Cl. botulinum	–	104–127	$D_{101} = 5.5$	8.5	Stumbo *et al.*, 1950
Cl. botulinum	62A	104–113	$D_{113} = 1.7$	11	Alderton *et al.*, 1976
Cl. botulinum	–	110–115	$D_{110} = 1.2$	10	Odlaug *et al.*, 1978
Cl. histolyticum	NCIB 503	70–90	$D_{90} = 12$	10	Roberts *et al.*, 1966b
Cl. perfringens	NCTC 8238	80–100	$D_{90} = 120$	9	Roberts, 1968
Cl. perfringens	NCTC 8797	80–100	$D_{90} = 15$	12–24	
Cl. perfringens	NCTC 8798	80–100	$D_{90} = 36$	16	
Cl. perfringens	NCTC 3181	80–100	$D_{90} = 5.0$	6	
Cl. perfringens	NCTC 8084	80–100	$D_{90} = 4.5$	7	
Cl. perfringens	NCTC 8798	99–116	$D_{101} = 2.3–3.3$	10–12	Bradshaw
Cl. perfringens	NCTC 10240	99–116	$D_{101} = 1.4–5.2$	9.5–12	*et al.*,1977
Cl. sporogenes	PA 3679	104–132	$D_{101} = 37$	9.8	Stumbo *et al.*, 1950
Cl. sporogenes	NCTC 532	70–90	$D_{90} = 34$	13	Roberts *et al.*, 1966b
Cl. sporogenes	NCTC 532	105–115	$D_{103} = 43$	9.0	Pflug & Smith, 1977

3 Inherent heat resistance

3.1 Moist heat

The heat resistance varies between spores of different species and strains. The magnitude of this genetically determined variation is often difficult to estimate, due to the influence of a wide spectrum of other parameters critical to the apparent heat resistance (see below). However, the order of magnitude of the moist heat resistance for a range of organisms is indicated in Table 19.6.

It has been shown by Warth (1978) that the heat resistance of the spores of different *Bacillus* spp. increased with an increasing optimum growth temperature for the vegetative cells of the organism. Thus, the spores of organisms with a high optimum temperature (55–67°C), e.g. *B. coagulans*, *B. stearothermophilus* and *B. caldolyticus*, had the highest moist heat resistance. *Bacillus stearothermophilus* is also a commonly used indicator organism for the biological controlling of moist heat-sterilization processes (Kereluk & Gammon, 1973; Heintz *et al.*, 1976). However, the calculated *z*-values (Table 19.6) indicate that *Clostridium* spp. are often the most heat-resistant spores at higher inactivation temperatures (> 140°C). The D_{100} values among different species were found to span 600-fold or 3000-fold by Beaman *et al.* (1982) and Beaman & Gerhardt (1986), respectively. In both cases, *B. stearothermophilus* was the most resistant species, while *Bacillus cereus* spores were among the most heat-sensitive ones.

It should be noted that the genetic variation in moist heat resistance among different strains of the same species may be of a considerable magnitude. For example, Roberts (1968) found that the D_{90} value for seven strains of *Clostridium perfringens* had a maximum variation of 48 times (*z*-value 4 times) and Bradshaw *et al.* (1975) reported the D_{121} value of two strains of *B. cereus* to vary by a factor of 78 (*z* value 1.2).

Spores of proteolytic, Group I, strains of *Clostridium botulinum* are heat-resistant and these strains produce toxins of type A, B or F. Group 2 strains of *C. botulinum* are non-proteolytic and form toxins of type B, E or F. Spores of these strains are less heat-resistant but are able to survive some heat treatment between 65 and 95°C (Lund & Peck, 1994). It has been pointed out (Lund & Peck, 1994) that, in most studies with non-proteolytic strains of *Cl. botulinum*, no attention has been paid to the incorporation of lysozyme into the recovery medium. This aspect will be considered later (Section 6.3).

3.2 Dry heat

Some data taken from the literature concerning the dry heat resistance of spores of different organisms are shown in Table 19.7.

As can be seen, the variations in data for the same species, in some cases even within the same investigation, are so large that it is almost impossible to draw any conclusions about the significance of the differences in heat resistance between the different species and strains. For example, the *z* values reported for *B. subtilis* var. *niger* spores vary from 13°C to 139°C. This can be compared to the variation in *z* value of 6.8°C to 24°C in moist heat, including all organisms listed in Table 19.6. The main reason for the large discrepancy in the dry heat-resistance data may be that the different studies have been performed at different A_w values. The A_w is fixed for all inactivation studies in moist heat, but can have an infinite number of values between 0.0 and 1.0 in dry heat. However, in a standardized test system, Molin (1977a) attempted to evaluate the magnitude of the inherent genetic differences in dry heat resistance between nine different *Bacillus* strains (including seven different species). The highest *D* values were recorded for *B. subtilis* var. *niger* spores and the lowest for *B. cereus* spores. The difference was about 10-fold in the whole temperature range investigated. The highest *z*-value (31°C) was obtained for *B. coagulans* and the lowest (19°C) for a strain of *B. stearothermophilus*. It should be pointed out that the difference in dry-heat resistance between the different *Bacillus* spores tested in this investigation was relatively small, compared with the variations reported in the literature, especially with respect to the *z*-value.

Generally, *B. subtilis* var. *niger* is considered to be a suitable indicator organism for the biological control of dry heat sterilization processes (Bruch *et al.*, 1963; Craven *et al.*, 1968; Costin & Grigo, 1974).

Table 19.7 Some *D*- and *z*-values for spores inactivated by dry heat (see also Russell, 1982).

Bacillus/Clostridium species	Strain	Investigated temperature range (°C)	*D*-value (min)	*z*-value (°C)	Reference
B. cereus	NCIB 9373	140–160	D_{160} = 0.03	22	Molin, 1977a
B. coagulans	NCIB 9365	140–170	D_{160} = 0.18	31	
B. megaterium	NCIB 9376	150–170	D_{160} = 0.06	21	
B. polymyxa		145–182	D_{177} = 0.1	28	Collier & Townsend, 1956
B. polymyxa	NCIB 8158	150–170	D_{160} = 0.27	22	Molin, 1977a
B. pumilus	NCTC 10337	150–180	D_{160} = 0.23	25	
B. strearothermophilus	1518	160–180	D_{177} = 0.1	26	Collier & Townsend, 1956
B. stearothermophilus	1518	121–160	D_{160} = 0.35	24	Bruch *et al.*, 1963
B. strearothermophilus	NCA 1518	100–160	D_{160} = 3.2–27	14–22	Alderton & Snell, 1969
B. stearothermophilus		100–160	D_{160} = 5	40	Niepokojczycka & Zakrzewski, 1972
B. stearothermophilus	ATCC 7953	150–170	D_{160} = 0.08	19	Molin, 1977a
B. stearothermophilus	NCTC 10339	150–180	D_{160} = 0.16	26–29	
B. subtilis	5230	121–160	D_{160} = 1.4–1.7	18	Pheil *et al.*, 1967
B. subtilis	5230	124–140	D_{110} = 47–95	17–55	Fox & Pflug, 1968
B. subtilis	5230	95–152	D_{112} = 10	17	Fox & Eder, 1969
B. subtilis	NCIB 8054	105–145	D_{112} = 12–150	13–19	Härnulv & Snygg, 1972
B. subtilis	NCIB 8054	150–170	D_{160} = 0.25	23	Molin, 1977a
B. subtilis	ATCC 6633	120–180	D_{160} = 0.43	23	Molin & Östlund, 1975
B. subtilis	1–12	95–110	D_{110} = 2–100	10–70	Kooiman & Jacobs, 1977
B. subtilis var. *niger*		121–160	D_{160} = 1.8	27	Bruch *et al.*, 1963
B. subtilis var. *niger*		105–160	D_{125} = 78–3200	13–32	Angelotti *et al.*, 1968
B. subtitlis var. *niger*		200–300	D_{210} = 0.02–0.03	29, 139	Bruch & Smith, 1968
B. subtilis var. *niger*		115–135	D_{125} = 2–220	13–22	Wang, 1968
B. subtilis var. *niger*		120–150	D_{150} = 0.23–0.35	18–23	Filho, 1975
B. subtilis var. *niger*	ATCC 9372	120–190	D_{160} = 0.3–0.8	22	Molin & Östlund, 1976
B. xerothermodurans	ATCC 27380	125–150	D_{150} = 150	15	Bond & Favero, 1975
Cl. sporogenes	PA 3679	148–177	D_{177} = 0.1	60	Collier & Townsend, 1956
Cl. sporogenes	PA 3679	124–160	D_{160} = 1.0–3.9	18–21	Augustin & Pflug, 1967
Cl. sporogenes	PA 3679	121–160	D_{160} = 1.9–2.4	22	Pheil *et al.*, 1967

4 Preheating history

4.1 Sporulation medium

Components of the sporulation medium which affect spore formation include carbohydrates, amino acids, fatty acids, cations and phosphates. The effects of these are reflected in the number of spores produced and also in the properties of the spores, for example, their heat resistance. The influence of these and other nutrients on moist heat resistance has been thoroughly reviewed by Roberts & Hitchins) 1969) and Russell (1971, 1982).

An attempt to estimate the importance of medium composition on the dry heat resistance of *B. subtilis* spores was made by Molin & Svensson (1976). *Bacillus subtilis* spores were investigated on 20 different media. The yield varied by a factor of 10^6 and the variation of the D_{160} value was about 10-fold. However, the main part of the tested media gave spores with a D_{160} value in the range of 40–150 s, i.e. that heat resistance changed by a factor of about 4.

A factor that is usually not considered is the source of the water used in the preparation of culture media. Knott *et al.* (1997) have shown that the source of water can influence greatly the germination and outgrowth of spores, as well as procedures adopted for the production of spores themselves.

4.2 Sporulation temperature

The moist heat resistant of *Bacillus* spores, as seen from the *D*-value, has in some investigations been found to increase when the spores were produced at higher temperatures (El-Bisi & Ordal, 1956; Lechowitch & Ordal, 1960; Cook & Gilbert, 1968b). El-Bisi & Ordal (1956) showed that, although the *D*-value increased at increasing growth temperatures, the *z*-value decreased.

Yokoya & York (1965) and Rey *et al.* (1975) tested the influence of incubation temperature on *B. coagulans* and *Cl. perfringens*, respectively, but noted no effect on the heat resistance. Sugiyama (1951) studied *Cl. botulinum* spores and reported that the highest resistance was obtained at a sporulation temperature of 37°C. On the other hand, Beaman & Gerhardt (1986) demonstrated that an increasing sporulation temperature causes reductions in protoplast water content between limits of *c.* 57% and 28% (wet-weight basis), thereby increasing sporal heat resistance. Furthermore, a heat shock of dormant spores does not necessarily break the dormancy in all exposed spores (so-called heat activation). Some spores may become only partly activated, which can actually increase their resistance by a factor of 2.6 (Beaman *et al.*, 1988).

It should be noted that the reports mentioned deal with the influence of incubation temperature on the moist heat resistance of spores. There is a lack of data concerning the relations between sporulation temperature and dry heat resistance of spores.

4.3 Chemical state

The 'chemical state' of bacterial spores can be manipulated by *in vitro* chemical pretreatments between a heat-sensitive and a heat-resistant state (Alderton & Snell, 1963; Alderton *et al.*, 1964; Ando & Tsuzuki, 1983; Bender & Marquis, 1985). The change in resistance, under certain circumstances, may also occur during the course of heat treatment.

The bacterial spore has a reversible cation exchange system, which, when loaded with Ca^{2+} ions, gives a spore of high resistance (resistant state) and, when loaded with hydronium ions, gives a spore of low resistance (sensitive state). The change in moist heat resistance (*D*-value) between spores of the two states can be more than 10-fold (Alderton *et al.*, 1976). The phenomenon has also been shown to exist in dry heat (Alderton & Snell, 1969, 1970).

It should be stressed that, even if the *D*-values at lower temperatures are decreasing by mineralization with hydronium ions, the *z*-value of H-spores is higher (Bender & Marquis, 1985). Thus, the difference in heat resistance between spores of the two chemical states decreases with increasing inactivation temperature.

5 Heating conditions

5.1 Water activity

The heat resistance of bacterial spores is generally considerably higher in dry heat ($A_w < 1.0$) than in moist heat ($A_w = 1.0$). It was shown by Murrell & Scott (1966) that the heat resistance (*D*-value) of *Bacillus megaterium* spores heated at constant A_w varied by a factor greater than 1000 in the A_w range of 0.0–1.0. The highest *D*-value was reported at A_w values of 0.2–0.4. These findings have since been confirmed by Angelotti *et al.* (1968), Alderton & Snell (1970) and Härnulv &

Snygg (1972) in studies on spores of *B. subtilis* var. *niger*, *B. stearothermophilus* and *B. subtilis* (NCIB 8054), respectively. It was further shown by Brannen & Garst (1972) that, even in very dry systems ($A_w < 0.013$), changes in the A_w influenced the heat resistance of *B. subtilis* spores. Brannen & Garst (1972) found that in the A_w range of 6×10^{-5} to 1×10^{-2} the highest *D*-value was obtained at 1×10^{-2} and the lowest at 7×10^{-4}.

The investigations mentioned above have been carried out at constant A_w values. Such constant conditions in A_w can hardly be achieved in dry heat sterilization under actual working conditions where the A_w is changing with temperature and treatment time during the course of the heat exposure. Thus, in a system with no control of A_w, the available amount of water present in the spores during heating is dependent on the initial water content of the spores, the water level of the heating environment and the desiccation (or sorption) rate of the spores during the heat treatment. The desiccation rate, which has been shown to be critical for heat resistance (Angelotti, 1968), is strongly dependent on whether the heating system is open or closed, i.e. if the spores are enclosed within a limited space or if they are surrounded by an 'infinite' space. The influence of the water content of spores heated in open systems has been studied by Fox & Pflug (1968), Hoffman *et al.* (1968) and Drummond & Pflug (1970), among others.

Hoffman *et al.* (1968) showed that the D_{160} value was changed about three times, depending on whether the spores before heating were equilibrated to the relative humidity (r.h.) of 11% or 85%. The difference in *D*-value increased with decreasing temperature. It has also been shown that spores equilibrated to a high moisture content generally have a higher dry-heat resistance in open systems, as seen from the *D*-value, than spores equilibrated to a low initial water content (Hoffman *et al.*, 1968; Drummon & Pflug, 1970).

It has been proposed by Alderton & Snell (1970) that anomalous discrepancies in *z*-values obtained in some dry heat inactivation studies, e.g. Angelotti *et al.* (1968) and Bruch & Smith (1968), are due to changes in A_w of the spores during heating. Thus, the obtained *D*-values in such a system are dependent not only on the temperature but also on the A_w, which is changing with the temperature and either diminishing or reinforcing the temperature effect on the inactivation rate: see Pfeifer & Kessler (1994).

5.2 pH and ionic environment

It is well documented that factors such as pH, buffer components, sodium chloride (NaCl) and cations in the suspending menstruum can influence the heat resistance of bacterial spores (Roberts & Hitchins, 1969; Russell, 1971, 1982). For example, the resistance of *B. stearothermophilus* spores heated in acetate buffer was successively increased from a pH value of 3.0 ($D_{100} = 23$ min) to one of 6.0 ($D_{100} = 14$ h). At a pH value of over 8.0, the resistance started to decrease again (Anderson & Friesen, 1974). According to Löwik & Anema (1972), the *z*-value is independent of pH.

Phosphates generally seem to decrease the moist-heat resistance of spores (Cook & Gilbert, 1968b, Adams, 1973; Steinbuch, 1977), the magnitude of influence depending on the spore strain. Adams (1973) found that the heat resistance (D_{100}) of three different *Clostridium* spp. was, respectively, 1.4, 2.0 and 41 times higher in water than in 60 mmol/l sodium phosphate buffer (pH 7). López *et al.* (1996) found that the *D*-values of strains of *B. stearothermophilus* increased as phosphate concentrations in heating solutions increased.

Sodium chloride in smaller concentrations is reported to have a weak sensitizing effect (Anderson *et al.*, 1949) or no effect at all (Roberts *et al.*, 1966b). In contrast, Härnulv & Snygg (1972) demonstrated that the D_{95} value of *B. subtilis* spores decreased by a factor of about 6 when heated in 26% NaCl ($A_w = 0.78$), compared with water vapour at the same A_w. More recently, it has been found that even low concentrations (0.06% w/v) of NaCl in the heating menstruum reduced the heat resistance of *B. stearothermophilus* strains (López *et al.*, 1996).

Calcium ions have been reported to protect spores from moist heat (Steinbuch, 1977), which contradicts earlier findings by Sugiyama (1951). However, in the light of newer findings on the importance of the chemical state of spores, it is obvious that Ca^{2+} ions can improve the heat resistance of insufficiently Ca-loaded spores. Bender &

Marquis (1985) showed that the heat resistance of remineralized H-spores increased in the order K < Mg < Mn < Ca. Remineralization with Na^+ ions yielded spores with an even lower heat resistance than the H-spores.

5.3 Organic substances

Proteins (e.g. serum albumin) and carbohydrates (e.g. sucrose) are known to increase the heat resistance of bacterial spores (Amaha & Sakaguchi, 1954; Roberts & Hitchins, 1969; Russell, 1971; Smelt *et al.*, 1977). However, under certain conditions, some sugars seem to have the ability to decrease the heat resistance. The D_{160} value of *B. subtilis* spores in dry heat was decreased by a factor of 3 when heated in the presence of glucose or fructose. On the other hand, the D_{160} value of the same spores was increased to the same degree in sucrose (Molin, 1977b).

Furthermore, the concentration of viable spores at the start of heat exposure may affect the measured *D*-value. This has been shown in both moist heat (Casolari, 1974) and in dry heat (Molin & Östlund, 1976).

Spores heated in the presence of lipids have a higher heat resistance than spores heated in pure phosphate buffer (Molin & Snygg, 1967; Senhaji & Loncin, 1977). It has been argued that this effect is due solely to a reduction in A_w by the added lipid (Russell, 1971). This assumption was also supported by a numerical simulation of results obtained from spores heated in soya-bean oil (Senhaji, 1977). However, when the effect of different lipids on the spore resistance was measured in dry heat, i.e. all spores were heated at the same low A_w, regardless of their being enclosed in lipid or not, it was shown that different lipids increased the heat resistance in the order: olive oil < triolein < soya-bean oil < tricaprin < trilaurin (Molin, 1977b). Spores heated in the presence of tricaprin or trilaurin had a significantly higher heat resistance than the controls (clean spores), while spores heated in soya-bean oil had about the same resistance as the controls. It may be pointed out that in the above study only the *D*-values were influenced by the lipids. The *z*-value was not affected.

5.4 Chemical inhibitors

The inclusion of chemical inhibitors in the medium in which spores are heated has been studied over many years. The reduction in heat resistance of bacterial spores was utilized as a means of sterilizing some types of pharmaceutical products (Russell, 1982), but this process has been discontinued (Russell, 1998) and is no longer an official method for the sterilization of parenteral or ophthalmic solutions (*British Pharmacopoeia*, 1998, 1993; Russell *et al.*, 1997).

The presence of sodium benzoate (0.1% w/v), potassium sorbate (0.1% w/v) or sodium nitrite (125 parts/10^6, 0.0125% w/v) in the heating menstruum did not reduce the heat resistance of spores of several strains of *B. stearothermophilus* (López *et al.*, 1996).

5.5 Gas atmosphere

The effect of various gas atmospheres on the dry-heat resistance of spores has been studied by Pheil *et al.* (1967) and Filho (1975), among others. These studies show only a minor influence of the gas atmosphere (CO_2, O_2 or N_2) on heat resistance. Thus, it seems that no significant advantages, with respect to the inactivation rate, are to be gained by exchanging the air with, for instance, O_2 or CO_2 in dry heat sterilization processes.

5.6 Supporting material

Spores exposed to dry heat on carriers of different materials can show differences in heat resistance (Bruch *et al.*, 1963; Angelotti *et al.*, 1968; Bruch & Smith, 1968). Bruch *et al.* (1963), for example, found that the *D*-value of spores heated on three different carriers decreased in the order: sand >glass >paper. Angelotti *et al.* (1968) and Alderton & Snell (1970) suggested that drastic differences in heat resistance between spores applied on (or in) different materials are due to differences in the A_w of the microenvironment of spores during heating, and not to any unknown characteristic of the material.

Sugimoto *et al.* (1996) have described the recovery of bacterial spores dried on aluminium strips.

6 Recovery and revival

6.1 Medium

Heat-damaged spores are sometimes more exacting in their growth requirements than are unheated spores. The composition of the recovery medium may thus affect the apparent resistance of heat-treated spores. The influence of the recovery medium on the moist-heat resistance of bacterial spores is complex, but has been relatively well studied (reviewed by Roberts & Hitchins, 1969; Roberts, 1970; Russell, 1971, 1982). Campbell *et al.* (1965) proposed that the requirements for heat-damaged spores were for germination and not outgrowth. Edwards *et al.* (1965a,b) found that a known germination stimulant, calcium dipicolinate, stimulated the numbers of heat-stressed *B. subtilis* spores that were able to form colonies.

Heat-injured spores are also highly sensitive to the presence of inhibitors in recovery agar (Russell, 1982; Williams & Russell, 1992).

Little information is available concerning the effect of the composition of the recovery medium on the dry-heat resistance of spores. Augustin & Pflug (1967) reported that the apparent dry-heat resistance of *Clostridium* spores varied on different recovery media. The D_{149} value varied by a factor of about two among seven different media tested. The z-value varied in the range of 18.3–21.7°C. The corresponding values in moist heat were a factor of three (D_{121} value) and 9.6–11°C (z value). Other useful information can be obtained by consulting Gurney & Quesnel (1980) and Russell (1982).

6.2 Temperature

Data on the influence of incubation temperature on the recovery of heat-damaged spores are scanty. There are indications that the recovery of moist heat-treated spores is more effective at temperatures somewhat below the optimum growth temperature of the organism (Williams & Reed, 1942; Edwards *et al.*, 1965b; Cook & Gilbert, 1968a; Futter & Richardson, 1970; Gonzalez *et al.*, 1995).

The temperature interval giving maximum recovery seems to be narrower for heated than for unheated spores. There are also indications that it is not the germination that is critical for recovery but the outgrowth (Prentice & Clegg, 1974), although this would appear to go against the currently accepted view (see Section 7) that the germination system may be a key element in spore inactivation.

6.3 Specific role of lysozyme

Incorporation of lysozyme or of an extracellular protein, termed initiation protein (IP) and produced by vegetative cells of *Cl. perfringens*, into recovery media increases the counts of heat-treated *Cl. perfringens* type A (Cassier & Sebald, 1969) and types B, C and D (Labbe & Chang, 1995) spores. Lysozyme also aids the recovery of heated *Cl. botulinum* spores, types B, G and F (Sebald & Ionescu, 1972; Peck *et al.*, 1992a,b, 1993, 1995; Stringer *et al.*, 1997).

D-values of *Cl. perfringens* types B, C and D are greater when lysozyme is included in the recovery medium (Table 19.8; Labbe & Chang, 1995). A diphasic response has been observed with *Cl. botulinum* (Fig. 19.5), with about 1–2% of heat-treated spores responding to lysozyme, thus indicating the presence of lysozyme-permeable and lysozyme-impermeable spores in the population (Lund & Peck, 1994). Treatment of heated spores with sodium thioglycollate prior to plating increases the number of colonies on agar containing lysozyme (Lund & Peck, 1994), the spores becoming more permeable to the enzyme as a consequence of the breakage of disulphide bonds in the coats (Fig. 19.6).

Table 19.8 Effect of lysozyme (1 µg/ml) on $D_{90°C}$ of spores of *Clostridium perfringens* types B,C and D.

Type	Strain	$D_{90°C}$ ratio*†
B	PS49	2.6
C	5388	2.5
	PS51	2.0
D	738	2.8
	748	2.3
	PS52	2.3

*Ratio of *D*-value in presence of lysozyme : *D*-value in absence of lysozyme.
†Calculated from the data of Labbe & Chang (1995).

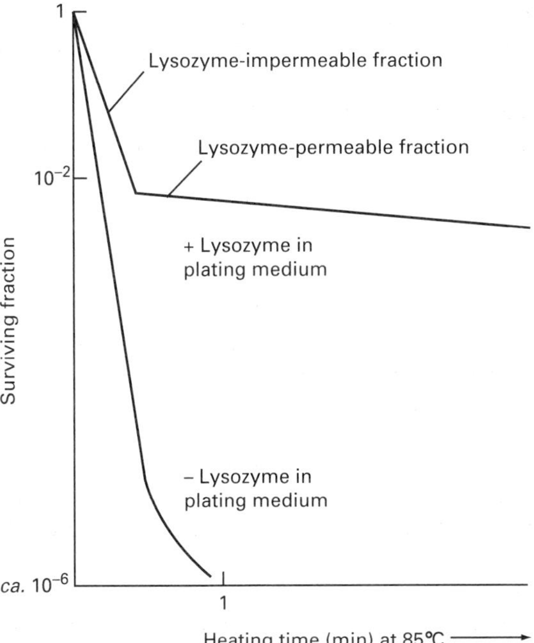

Fig. 19.5 Effect of lysozyme (10 μg/ml) in the recovery plating medium on the estimated heat resistance of *Cl. botulinum* 17B at 85°C (based on Peck *et al.*, 1992a; Lund & Peck, 1994).

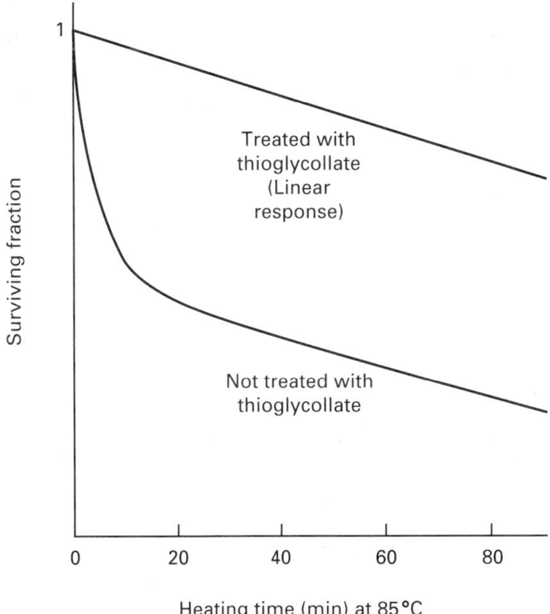

Fig. 19.6 Pretreatment of heated spores of *Cl. botulinum* with alkaline thioglycollate prior to plating on recovery medium containing lysozyme (10 μg/ml.) (based on Peck *et al.*, 1992b; Lund & Peck, 1994).

7 Mechanisms of spore inactivation by heat

It is highly unlikely that thermal inactivation results from a single event in a vegetative cell or a spore. There are several potential target sites in non-sporulating bacteria, ranging from the outer membrane of Gram-negative bacteria to the cytoplasmic membrane, ribonucleic acid (RNA) breakdown and protein coagulation (Allwood & Russell, 1970; Russell, 1984; 1998; Gould, 1989). Pellon & Sinskey (1984) pointed out that virtually all structures and functions can be damaged by heat but that repair to non-deoxyribonucleic acid (DNA) structures can occur only if DNA remains functional, thereby providing the necessary genetic information. A considerable body of evidence implicates the involvement of DNA in heat damage, probably as a result of enzymatic action after thermal injury (Pellon & Sinskey, 1984; Gould, 1989).

Brannen (1970) presented experimental evidence in favour of the assumption that the principal mechanism for moist heat inactivation of spores is DNA denaturation. This, however, somewhat contradicts the findings of Flowers & Adams (1976), who suggest that the site of injury is the spore structure destined to become the cell membrane or cell wall. In bacterial spores, thermal injury has, in fact, been attributed also to denaturation of vital spore enzymes, impairment of germination and outgrowth, membrane damage (leading to leakage of calcium dipicolinate), increased sensitivity to inhibitory agents, structural damage (as demonstrated by electron microscopy) and damage to the spore chromosome (shown by mutations or DNA strand breaks) (Russell, 1998). Effects on DNA are much more pronounced during dry heating, which generates a high level of mutants in spore populations (Gould, 1989).

Deficiencies in DNA repair mechanisms render spores more heat-sensitive (Hanlin *et al.*, 1985). Thus, the ability to repair DNA after heating must be an important aspect of heat tolerance. Likewise, *B. subtilis* spores pretreated with ethidium bromide are rendered heat-sensitive, the reason being an inability of the cells to repair heat-damaged DNA during outgrowth (Hanlin & Slepecky, 1985).

The germination system itself may, however, be a key element of heat inactivation (Gould, 1989). Heated spores may be unable to initiate germination; with heated clostridia, the presence of lysozyme in the recovery media aids revival, as pointed out in Section 6.3. Lysozyme induces germination by hydrolysing cortex peptidoglycan. Other workers (reviewed by Russell, 1982) have demonstrated that artificial germinants, such as calcium dipicolinate, have a similar effect on heated spores.

For earlier information on the thermal death of bacteria and spores, the interested reader is referred to the publications by Rahn (1945), Charm (1958), Pflug & Schmidt (1968) and Corry (1973).

Dry heat inactivation has generally been considered to be primarily an oxidation process (Rahn, 1945; Sykes, 1965; Ernst, 1968; Wang, 1968). However, this contradicts the findings of Pheil *et al.* (1967), which showed the dry heat resistance of spores to be somewhat higher in oxygen than in air. Similar results have been reported by Rowe & Koesterer (1965) and Fox & Pflug (1968), who compared the resistance in air with that in nitrogen, finding that the resistance in air was higher than that in nitrogen.

Considering the strong influence of A_w on the dry heat resistance of spores, a possible explanation of dry heat inactivation could be the removal of bound water, critical for maintaining the helical structure of proteins. This belief is stressed in investigations that show that a certain level of water is necessary for the maintenance of heat stability in spores. If the spores were strongly desiccated by high-vacuum drying, they would be sensitized to heat (Soper & Davies, 1971, 1973). Furthermore, it has been shown that *B. subtilis* spores heated at lower A_w are inactivated in accordance with a constant *z*-value (23°C) over the temperature interval of 37–190°C (Molin, 1977c). Thus, in a dry environment the spores were inactivated at growth temperature ($D_{37} = 44\,d$) and this inactivation followed the same inactivation model as the one valid at high temperatures (140–190°C).

8 Mechanisms of spore resistance to heat

Earlier theories about the possible mechanisms of spore resistance to thermal processes were discussed by Roberts & Hitchins (1969), Russell (1971, 1982), Gould (1977) and Gerhardt & Murrell (1978). The resistance of spores to dry heat differs considerably from the resistance to moist heat, concerning both inactivation rate (*D*-value) and temperature coefficient (*z*-value).

Several factors contribute to the resistance of spores to moist heat (Hodges, 1995). The resistance of spores to moist heat can be manipulated over several orders of magnitude by exposure to extreme pH values or cationic-exchange treatment (respectively, the H- or Ca-form: Alderton & Snell, 1963; Alderton *et al.*, 1980). The content and location of water in the spore core have an important role to play, but spore coats do not contribute to thermal resistance. Spores have a low internal water content and Gould and his colleagues (Gould & Dring, 1975; Gould, 1989) found that resuspension of newly germinated spores in high concentrations of non-permeating solutes (sucrose or NaCl, but not glycerol) restored resistance to heat (or to ionizing radiation). In this osmoregulatory mechanism, the cortex would maintain a uniform pressure upon, and thereby control, the water content of the spore core. Heat resistance undoubtedly arises from dehydration of the core (Beaman *et al.*, 1984; Koshikawa *et al.*, 1984; Nakashio & Gerhadt, 1985). An alternative theory to account for this was the 'anisotrophic swollen cortex by enzymatic cleavage' put forward by Warth (1977, 1978).

Warth (1985) proposed three types of mechanisms which would contribute to protein stability in spores, namely: they could be intrinsically stable; substances might be present which could help in stabilizing them; and the removal of water could alter their stability. The role of calcium dipicolinate in heat resistance has yet to be fully determined (Gould, 1989).

Several spore properties, however, are now well known to be important for the heat resistance of spores. These are protein thermotolerance, dehydration, mineralization, thermal adaptation and cortex function (Murrell, 1981; Beaman & Gerhardt, 1986; Beaman *et al.*, 1988, 1989; Gerhardt & Marquis, 1989; Marquis *et al.*, 1994). Calcium dipicolinate may be involved in the establishment and maintenance of dormancy (Mallidis & Scholefield, 1987). In addition, small acid-soluble spore proteins (SASPs), found in the spore core (Setlow, 1994), may have a role to play. SASPs are of two types:

1 α/β-type associated with spore DNA;

2 γ-type, not associated with any spore macromolecule.

Spores lacking α/β-type SASPs are more thermosensitive than wild-type spores, implicating DNA damage in spore inactivation (Setlow, 1994; see also Section 7). However, heat resistance during sporulation is attained well after their synthesis, and SASPs are thus not a major determinant of spore resistance to moist heat (Setlow, 1994).

Heat resistance during sporulation is an intermediate event and occurs after the development of resistance to some chemicals but before the onset of resistance to lysozyme or glutaraldehyde (Power *et al.*, 1988; Shaker *et al.*, 1988; Knott *et al.*, 1996).

The water content of spores is an important factor in their response to dry heat. It has been postulated (Rowe & Silverman, 1970) that only a relatively small amount of water is needed to protect the heat-sensitive site in spores and that resistance to dry heat depends mainly on the location, rather than on the amount, of water in the spore and on its association with other molecules.

Spores are also more resistant to heat when suspended in oils than in buffer (Ababouch *et al.*, 1995).

9 Conclusions

Bacterial spores are considerably more resistant to both moist- and dry heat than are non-sporulating bacteria. Although the exact mechanisms for this high resistance have yet to be elucidated, the content and location of water in the core are important and controlled by the cortex, with several contributory factors.

Spore inactivation by moist heat probably involves damage to a key element of the germination system. Studies on the specific role of lysozyme in the revival of heat-treated clostridial spores have played an important part in this context, as well as providing valuable information in food microbiology.

10 Acknowledgement

The author acknowledges Dr G. Molin for his contribution in writing the original version of this chapter.

11 References

Ababouch, L.H., Grimit, L., Eddafry, R. & Busta, F.F. (1995) Thermal inactivation kinetics of *Bacillus subtilis* spores suspended in buffer and in oils. *Journal of Applied Bacteriology*, **78**, 669–676.

Adams, D.M. (1973) Inactivation of *Clostridium perfringens* type A spores at ultra high temperatures. *Applied Microbiology*, **26**, 282–287.

Alderton, G. & Snell, N. (1963) Base exchange and heat resistance in bacterial spores. *Biochemical and Biophysical Research Communications*, **10**, 139–143.

Alderton, G. & Snell, N. (1969) Chemical states of bacterial spores: dry heat resistance. *Applied Microbiology*, **17**, 745–749.

Alderton, G. & Snell, N. (1970) Chemical states of bacterial spores: heat resistance and its kinetics at intermediate water activity. *Applied Microbiology*, **19**, 565–572.

Alderton, G., Thompson, P.A. & Snell, N. (1964) Heat adaptation and ion exchange in *B. megaterium* spores. *Science*, **143**, 141–143.

Alderton, G., Ito, K.A. & Chen, J.K. (1976) Chemical manipulation of the heat resistance of *Clostridium botulinum* spores. *Applied and Environmental Microbiology*, **31**, 492–498.

Alderton, G., Chen, J.K. & Ito, K.A. (1980) Heat resistance of the chemical resistance forms of *Clostridium botulinum* 62A spores over the water activity range 0 to 0.9. *Applied and Environmental Microbiology*, **40**, 511–515.

Allwood, M.C. & Russell, A.D. (1970) Mechanisms of thermal injury in non-sporulating bacteria. *Advances in Applied Microbiology*, **12**, 89–119.

Amaha, M. (1953) Heat resistance of Cameron's putrefactive anaerobe 3679 in phosphate buffer (*Clostridium sporagenes*). *Food Research*, **18**, 411–420.

Amaha, M. & Sakaguchi, K.-I. (1954) Effects of carbohydrates, proteins, and bacterial cells in the heating media on the heat resistance of *Clostridium sporogenes*. *Journal of Bacteriology*, **68**, 338–345.

Anderson, E.E., Esselen, W.B. & Fellers, C.R. (1949) Effect of acids, salt, sugar, and other food ingredients on thermal resistance of *Bacillus thermoacidurans*. *Food Research*, **14**, 499–510.

Anderson, R.A. & Friesen, W.T. (1974) The thermal resistance of *Bacillus stearothermophilus* spores: the effects of temperature and pH of the heating medium. *Pharmaceutica Acta Helvetiae*, **49**, 295–298.

Ando, Y. & Tsuzuki, T. (1983) Mechanism of chemical manipulation of the heat resistance of *Clostridium perfringens* spores. *Journal of Applied Bacteriology*, **54**, 197–202.

Angelotti, R. (1968) Protective mechanisms affecting dry heat sterilization. In *Sterilization Techniques for Instruments and Materials as Applied to Space Research* (ed. Sneath, P.H.A.), COSPAR Technique Manual Series. No. 4, pp. 59–74. Paris: COSPAR Secretariat.

Angelotti, R., Maryanski, J.H., Butler, T.F., Peeler, J.T. & Campbell, J.E. (1968) Influence of spore moisture content on the dry heat resistance of *Bacillus subtilis* var. *niger*. *Applied Microbiology*, **16**, 735–745.

Ashton, T.R. (1977) Ultra-high-temperature treatment of milk and milk products. *World Animal Review*, **23**, 37–42.

Augustin, J.A.L. & Pflug, I.J. (1967) Recovery patterns of spores of putrefactive anaerobe 3679 in various subculture media after heat treatment. *Applied Microbiology*, **15**, 266–276.

Beaman, T.C. & Gerhardt, P. (1986) Heat resistance of bacterial spores correlated with protoplast dehydration, mineralization, and thermal adaptation. *Applied and Environmental Microbiology*, **52**, 1242–1246.

Beaman, T.C., Greenamyre, J.T., Corner, T.R., Pankratz, H.S. & Gerhardt, P. (1982) Bacterial spore heat resistance correlated with water content, wet density, and protoplast/sporoplast volume ratio. *Journal of Bacteriology*, **150**, 870–877.

Beaman, T.C., Koshiikawa, T., Pankratz, H.S. & Gerhardt, P. (1984) Dehydration partioned within core protoplast accounts for heat resistance of bacterial spores. *FEMS Microbiology Letters*, **24**, 47–51.

Beaman, T.C., Pankratz, H.S. & Gerhardt, P. (1988) Heat shock affects permeability and resistance of *Bacillus stearothermophilus* spores. *Applied and Environmental Microbiology*, **54**, 2515–2520.

Beaman, T.C., Pankratz, H.S. & Gerhardt, P. (1989) Low heat resistance of *Bacillus sphaericus* spores correlated with high protoplast water content. *FEMS Microbiology Letters*, **58**, 1–4.

Bender, G.R. & Marquis, R. (1985) Spore heat resistance and specific mineralization. *Applied and Environmental Microbiology*, **50**, 1414–1421.

Bigelow, W.D. (1921) The logarithmic nature of thermal death time curves. *Journal of Infectious Diseases*, **29**, 528–536.

Bond, W.W. & Favero, M.S. (1975) Thermal profile of a *Bacillus* species (ATCC 27380) extremely resistant to dry heat. *Applied Microbiology*, **29**, 859–860.

Bradshaw, J.G., Peeler, J.T. & Twedt, R.M. (1975) Heat resistance of ileal loop-reactive *Bacillus cereus* strains isolated from commercially canned food. *Applied Microbiology*, **30**, 943–945.

Bradshaw, J.G., Peeler, J.T. & Twedt, R.M. (1977) Thermal inactivation of ileal loop-reactive *Clostridium perfringens* type A strains in phosphate buffer and beef gravy. *Applied and Environmental Microbiology*, **34**, 280–284.

Brannen, J.P. (1970) On the role of DNA in wet heat sterilisation of micro-organisms. *Journal of Theoretical Biology*, **27**, 425–432.

Brannen, J.P. (Garst, D.M. (1972) Dry heat inactivation of *Bacillus subtilis* var. *niger* spores as a function of relative humidity. *Applied Microbiology*, **23**, 1125–1130.

Brennan, J.G., Butters, J.R., Cowell, N.D. & Lilly, A.E.V. (1969) *Food Engineering Operations*. Amsterdam: Elsevier.

British Pharmacopoeia (1988) London: HMSO.

British Pharmacopoeia (1998) London: HMSO.

Brown, K.L. (1994) Spore resistance and ultra heat treatment processes. *Journal of Applied Bacteriology Symposium Supplement*, **76**, 67S–80S.

Bruch, C.W., Koesterer, M.G. & Bruch, M.R. (1963) Dry-heat sterilization: its development and application to components of exobiological space probes. *Developments in Industrial Microbiology*, **4**, 334–342.

Bruch, M.K. & Smith, F.W. (1968) Dry heat resistance of spores of *Bacillus subtilis* var. *niger* on kapton and teflon film at high temperatures. *Applied Microbiology*, **16**, 1841–1846.

Campbell, L.L., Richards, C.M. & Sniff, E.E. (1965) Isolation of strains of *Bacillus stearothermophilus* with altered requirements for spore germination. In *Spores III* (eds Campbell, L.L. & Halvorson, H.O.), pp. 55–63. Ann Arbor: American Society for Microbiology.

Casolari, A. (1974) Non-logarithmic behaviour of heat-inactivation curves of P.A. 3679 spores. In *Proceedings, IV International Congress of Food Science and Technology*, Vol. 3, pp. 86–92.

Cassier, M. & Sebald, M. (1969) Germination lysozyme-dependante des spores de *Clostridium perfringens* ATCC 3624 apres traitment thermique. *Annales de l'Institut Pasteur, Paris*, **117**, 312–314.

Cerf, O. (1977) A review: tailing of survival curves of bacterial spores. *Journal of Applied Bacteriology*, **42**, 1–19.

Charm, S.E. (1958) The kinetics of bacterial inactivation by heat. *Food Technology*, **12**, 4–8.

Collier, C.P. & Townsend, C.T. (1956) The resistance of bacterial spores to superheated steam. *Food Technology*, **10**, 477–481.

Cook, A.M. & Gilbert, R.J. (1968a) Factors affecting the heat resistance of *Bacillus stearothermophilus* spores. I. The effect of recovery conditions on colony count of unheated and heated spores. *Journal of Food Technology*, **3**, 285–293.

Cook, A.M. & Gilbert, R.J. (1968b) Factors affecting the heat resistance of *Bacillus stearothermophilus* spores. II. The affect of sporulating conditions and nature of the heating medium. *Journal of Food Technology*, **3**, 295–302.

Corry, J.E.L. (1973) The water relations and heat resistance of microorganisms. *Progress in Industrial Microbiology*, **12**, 75–108.

Costin, I.D. & Grigo, J. (1974) Bioindikatoren zur autoklavierungskontrolle einige theoretische aspekte und praktische erfahrungen bei der entwicklung und anwendung. *Zentralblatt für Bakteriologie, Parasitenkunde, Infektionskrankheiten und Hygiene. Abtellung I. Originale*, **A227**, 483–521.

Craven, C.W., Stern, J.A. & Erwin, G.F. (1968) Planetary quarantine and space vehicle sterilization. *Astronautics and Aeronautics*, **6**, 18–48.

Daudin, J.D. & Cerf, O. (1977) Influence des echoes thermiques sur la destruction des spores bacteriénnes par la chaleur. *Lebensmittel-Wissenschaft und Technologie*, **10**, 203–207.

Davies, F.L., Underwood, H.M., Perkin, A.G. & Burton, H. (1977) Thermal death kinetics of *Bacillus stearothermophilus* spores at ultra high temperatures. I. Laboratory determination of temperature coefficients. *Journal of Food Technology*, **12**, 115–129.

Denny, C.B. & Matthys, A.W. (1975) *NCA Tests on Dry Heat as a Means of Sterilization of Containers, Lids, and a Closing Unit for Aseptic Canning*. Final report No. RF 4614. Washington DC: National Canners Association.

Drummond, D.W. & Pflug, I.J. (1970) Dry heat destruction of *Bacillus subtilis* spores on surfaces: effect of humidity in an open system. *Applied Microbiology*, **20**, 805–809.

Edwards, J.L., Jr, Busta, F.F. & Speck, M.L. (1965a) Thermal inactivation characteristics of *Bacillus subtilis* spores at ultrahigh temperatures. *Applied Microbiology*, **13**, 851–857.

Edwards, J.L., Jr, Busta, F.F. & Speck, M.L. (1965b) Heat injury of *Bacillus subtilis* spores of ultrahigh temperatures. *Applied Microbiology*, **13**, 858–864.

El-Bisi, H.M. & Ordal, Z.J. (1956) The effect of sporulation temperature on the thermal resistance of *Bacillus coagulans* var. *thermoacidurans*. *Journal of Bacteriology*, **71**, 10–16.

Ernst, R.R. (1968) Sterilization by heat. In *Disinfection, Sterilization and Preservation* (eds Lawrence, C.A. & Block, S.S.), pp. 703–740. Philadelphia: Lea & Febiger.

Filho, L.P.G. (1975) Die Thermische Abtötung von Sporen von *Bacillus subtilis* var. *niger* ATCC 9372 in Gasphasen mit einer Wasseraktivität < 1.0. *Lebensmitel-Wissenschaft und Technologie*, **8**, 29–33.

Flowers, R.S. & Adams, D.M. (1976) Spore membrane(s) as the site of damage within heated *Clostridium perfringens* spores. *Journal of Bacteriology*, **125**, 429–434.

Fox, K. & Eder, B.D. (1969) Comparison of survivor curves of *Bacillus subtilis* spores subjected to wet and dry heat. *Journal of Food Science*, **34**, 518–521.

Fox, K. & Pflug, I.J. (1968) Effect of temperature and gas velocity on the dry-heat destruction rate of bacterial spores. *Applied Microbiology*, **16**, 343–348.

Futter, B.V. & Richardson, G. (1970) Viability of clostridial spores and the requirements of damaged organisms: I. Method of colony count, period and temperature of incubation, and pH value of the medium. *Journal of Applied Bacteriology*, **33**, 321–330.

Gerhardt, P. & Marquis, R.E. (1989) Spore thermoresistance mechanisms. In *Regulation of Procaryotic Development* (eds Smith, I., Slepecky, R. & Setlow, P.), pp. 17–63. Washington, DC: American Society for Microbiology.

Gerhardt, P. & Murrell, W.G. (1978) Basis and mechanism of bacterial spore resistance. *Spore Newsletter*, **6** (March), 1–21.

Gonzalez, I., Lopez, M., Mazas, M., Gonzalez, J. & Bernardo, A. (1995) The effect of recovery conditions on the apparent heat resistance of *Bacillus cereus* spores. *Journal of Applied Bacteriology*, **78**, 548–554.

Gould, G.W. (1977) Recent advances in the understanding of resistance and dormancy in bacterial spores. *Journal of Applied Bacteriology*, **42**, 297–309.

Gould, G.W. (1989) Heat-induced injury and inactivation. In *Mechanisms of Action of Food Preservation Procedures* (ed. Gould, G.W.), pp. 11–42. London: Elsevier Applied Science.

Gould, G.W. (1995) *New Methods of Food Preservation*. London: Blackie Academic & Professional.

Gould, G.W. & Dring, G.J. (1975) Role of expanded cortex in resistance of bacterial endospores. In *Spores VI* (eds Gerhardt, P., Costilow, R.N. & Sadoff, H.L.), pp. 541–546. Washington, DC: American Society for Microbiology.

Gurney, T.R. & Quesnel, L.B. (1980) Thermal activation and dry heat inactivation of spores of *Bacillus subtilis* MD2 and *Bacillus subtilis* var. *niger*. *Journal of Applied Bacteriology*, **48**, 231–247.

Han, Y.W. (1975) Death rates of bacterial spores: non-linear survivor curves. *Canadian Journal of Microbiology*, **21**, 1464–1467.

Han, Y.W., Zhang, H.I. & Krochta, J.M. (1976) Death rates of bacterial spores: mathematical models. *Canadian Journal of Microbiology*, **22**, 295–300.

Hanlin, J.H. & Slepecky, R.A. (1985) Mechanism of heat sensitization of *Bacillus subtilis* spores by ethidium bromide. *Applied and Environmental Microbiology*, **49**, 1396–1400.

Hanlin, J.H., Lombardi, S.J. & Slepecky, R.A. (1985) Heat and UV light resistance of vegetative cells and spores of *Bacillus subtilis* Rec$^-$ mutants. *Journal of Bacteriology*, **163**, 774–774.

Härnulv, B.G. & Snygg, B.G. (1972) Heat resistance of *Bacillus subtilis* spores at various water activities. *Journal of Applied Bacteriology*, **35**, 615–624.

Heintz, M.-T., Urban, S., Schiller, I., Gay, M. & Bühlman, X. (1976) The production of spores of

Bacillus stearothermophilus with constant resistance to heat and their use as biological indicators during the development of aqueous solutions for injection. *Pharmaceutica Acta Helvetiae*, **51**, 137–143.

Hodges, N.A. (1995) Reproducibility and performance of endospores as biological indicators. In *Microbiological Quality Assurance: A Guide Towards Relevance and Reproducibility of Inocula* (eds Brown, M.R.W. & Gilbert, P.), pp. 221–233. Boca Raton: CRC Press.

Hoffman, R.K., Gambill, V.M. & Buchanan, LM. (1968) Effect of cell moisture on the thermal inactivation rate of bacterial spores. *Applied Microbiology*, **16**, 1240–1244.

Jonsson, U., Snygg, B.G., Härnulv, B.G. & Zachrisson, T. (1977) Testing two models for the temperature dependence of the heat inactivation rate of *Bacillus stearothermophilus* spores. *Journal of Food Science*, **42**, 1251–1252, 1263.

Kereluk, K. & Gammon, R. (1973) A comparative study of biological indicators for steam sterilization. *Developments in Industrial Microbiology*, **15**, 411– 419.

Knott, A.G., Dancer, B.N., Hann, A.C. & Russell, A.D. (1997) Non-variable sources of pure water and the germination and outgrowth of *Bacillus subtilis* spores. *Journal of Applied Microbiology*, **82**, 267–272.

Kooiman, W.J. & Jacobs, R.P.W.M. (1977) The heat resistance of *Bacillus subtilis* 1–12 in relation to the water activity during pre-equilibration and during exposure to heat. In *Spore Research 1976* (eds Barker, A.N., Wolf, J., Ellar, D.J., Dring, G.J. & Gould, G.W.), pp. 477–485. London: Academic Press.

Koshikawa, T., Beaman, T.C., Pankratz, H.S., Nakashio, S., Corner, T.R. & Gerhardt, P. (1984) Resistance, germination, and permeability correlates of *Bacillus megaterium* spores successively divested of integument layers. *Journal of Bacteriology*, **159**, 624–632.

Labbe, R.G. & Chang, C.-A. (1995) Recovery of heat-injured spores of *Clostridium perfringens* types B,C and D by lysozyme and an initiation protein. *Letters in Applied Microbiology*, **21**, 302–306.

Lechowitch, R.V. & Ordal, Z.J. (1960) The influence of sporulation temperature on the thermal resistance and chemical composition of endospores. *Bacteriological Proceedings*, pp. 44–45.

Levine, S. (1956) Determination of the thermal death rate of bacteria. *Food Research*, **21**, 295–301.

López, M., Mazas, M., González, I., González, J. & Bernardo, A. (1996) Thermal resistance of *Bacillus stearothermophilus* spores in different heating systems containing some approved food additives. *Journal of Applied Bacteriology*, **23**, 187–191.

Löwick, J.A.M. & Anema, P.J. (1972) Effect of pH on the heat resistance of *Clostridium sporogenes* spores in minced meat. *Journal of Applied Bacteriology*, **35**, 119–121.

Lund, B.M. & Peck, M.W. (1994) Heat resistance and recovery of spores of non-proteolytic *Clostridium botulinum* in relation to refrigerated, processed foods with an extended shelf-life. *Journal of Applied Bacteriology Symposium Supplement*, **76**, 115S–118S.

Mallidis, C.G. & Scholefield, J. (1987) Relation of the heat resistance of bacterial spores to chemical composition and structure I. Relation to core components. *Journal of Applied Bacteriology*, **62**, 65–69.

Marquis, R.E., Sim, J. & Shin, S.Y. (1994) Molecular mechanisms of resistance to heat and oxidative damage. *Journal of Applied Bacteriology Symposium Supplement*, **76**, 40S–48S.

Michels, M.J.M. & Visser, F.M.W. (1976) Occurrence and thermoresistance of spores of pyschrophilic and psychrotrophic aerobic sporeformers in soils and food. *Journal of Applied Bacteriology*, **41**, 1–11.

Moats, W.A. (1971) Kinetics of thermal death of bacteria. *Journal of Bacteriology*, **105**, 165–171.

Molin, G. (1976) Infra-red sterilization of glass packaging for aseptic processing. In *22nd European Meeting of Meat Research Workers*, Congress Documentation, Vol. II, J8: pp. 3–7.

Molin, G. (1977a) Inherent genetic differences in dry heat resistance of some *Bacillus* spores. In *Spore Research 1976* (eds Barker, A.N., Wolf, J., Ellar, D.J., Dring, G.J. & Gould, G.W.), pp. 487–500. London: Academic Press.

Molin, G. (1977b) Dry heat resistance of *Bacillus subtilis* spores in contact with serum albumin, carbohydrates or lipids. *Journal of Applied Bacteriology*, **42**, 111–116.

Molin, G. (1977c) Inactivation of *Bacillus* spores in dry systems at low and high temperatures. *Journal of General Microbiology*, **101**, 227–231.

Molin, G. & Östlund, K. (1975) Dry heat inactivation of *Bacillus subtilis* spores by means of infra-red heating. *Antonie van Leeuwenhoek Journal of Microbiology and Serology*, **41**, 329–335.

Molin, G. & Östlund, K. (1976) Dry heat inactivation of *Bacillus subtilis* var. *niger* spores with special reference to spore density. *Canadian Journal of Microbiology*, **22**, 359–363.

Molin, G. & Svensson, M. (1976) Formation of dry heat resistant *Bacillus subtilis* var. *niger* spores as influenced by the composition of the sporulation medium. *Antonie van Leeuwenhoek Journal of Microbiology and Serology*, **42**, 387–395.

Molin, N. & Snygg, B.G. (1967) Effect of lipid materials on heat resistance of bacterial spores. *Applied Microbiology*, **15**, 142–146.

Murrell, W.B. (1981) Biophysical studies on the molecular mechanisms of spore heat resistance and dormancy. In *Sporulation and Germination* (eds Levinson, H.S., Sonenshein, A.L. & Tipper, D.J.), pp. 64–77. Washington, DC: American Society for Microbiology.

Murrell, W.B. & Scott, W.J. (1966) The heat resistance

of bacterial spores at various water activities. *Journal of General Microbiology*, **43**, 411–425.

Nakashio, S. & Gerhardt, P. (1985) Protoplast dehydration correlated with heat resistance of bacterial spores. *Jounal of Bacteriology*, **162**, 571–578.

Niepokojezycka, E. & Zakrzewski, K. (1972) Alumina-attached spores of *Bacillus stearothermophilus* for the control of sterilization process. *Acta Microbiologica Polonica* (Ser. B), **4**, 141–153.

Oag, R.K. (1940) The resistance of bacterial spores to dry heat. *Journal of Pathology and Bacteriology*, **51**, 137–141.

Odlaug, T.E., Pflug, I.J. & Kautter, D.A. (1978) Heat resistance of *Clostridium botulinum* type B spores grown from isolates from commercially canned mushrooms. *Journal of Food Protection*, **41**, 351–353.

Peck, M.W., Fairbain, D.A. & Lund, B.M. (1992a) The effect of recovery medium on the germinated heat-inactivation of spores of non-proteolytic *Clostridium botulinum. Letters in Applied Microbiology*, **15**, 146–151.

Peck, M.W., Fairbain, D.A. & Lund, B.M. (1992b) Factors affecting growth from heat-treated spores of non-proteolytic *Clostridium botulinum. Letters in Applied Microbiology*, **15**, 152–155.

Peck, M.W., Fairbain, D.A. & Lund, B.M. (1993) Heat resistance of spores of non-proteolytic *Clostridium botulinum* estimated on a medium containing lysozyme. *Letters in Applied Microbiology*, **16**, 126–131.

Peck, M.W., Lund, B.M., Fairbain, D.A., Kaspersson, A.S. & Underland, P.C. (1995) Effect of heat treatment on survival of, and growth from, spores of non-proteolytic *Clostridium botulinum* at refrigeration temperatures. *Applied and Environmental Microbiology*, **61**, 1780–1785.

Pellon, J.R. & Sinskey, A.J. (1984) Heat-induced damage to the bacterial chromosome and its repair. In *The Revival of Injured Microbes* (eds Andrew, M.H.E. & Russell, A.D.), Society for Applied Bacteriology Symposium Series No. 12, pp. 105–125. London: Academic Press.

Pfeifer, J. & Kessler, H.G. (1994) Effect of relative humidity of hot air on the heat resistance of *Bacillus cereus* spores. *Journal of Applied Bacteriology*, 77, 121–128.

Pflug, I.J. (1973) Heat sterilization. In *Industrial Sterilization* (eds Phillips, G.B. & Miller, W.S.), pp. 239–282. Durham, North Carolina: Duke University Press.

Pflug, I.J. & Schmidt, C.F. (1968) Thermal destruction of microorganisms. In *Disinfection, Sterilization and Preservation* (eds Lawrence, C.A. & Block, S.S.), pp. 63–105. Philadelphia: Lea & Febiger.

Pflug, I.J. & Smith, G.M. (1977) Survivor curves of bacterial spores heated in parenteral solutions. In *Spore Research 1976* (eds Barker, A.N., Wolf, J., Ellar, D.J., Dring, G.J. & Gould, G.W.), pp. 501–525. London: Academic Press.

Pheil, C.G., Pflug, I.J., Nicholas, R.C. & Augustin, J.A.L. (1967) Effect of various gas atmospheres on destruction of microorganisms in dry heat. *Applied Microbiology*, **15**, 120–124.

Power, E.G.M., Dancer, B.N. & Russell, A.D. (1988) Emergence of resistance to glutaraldehyde in spores of *Bacillus subtilis* 168. *FEMS Microbiology Letters*, **50**, 223–226.

Prentice, G.A. & Clegg, L.F.L. (1974) The effect of incubation temperature on the recovery of spores of *Bacillus subtilis* 8057. *Journal of Applied Bacteriology*, **37**, 501–513.

Quast, D.G., Leitao, M.F.F. & Kato, K. (1977) Death of *Bacillus stearothermophilus* 1518 spores on can covers exposed to superheated steam in a Dole aseptic canning system. *Lebensmittel-Wissenschaft und Technologie*, **10**, 198–202.

Rahn, O. (1943) The problem of the logarithmic order of death in bacteria. *Biodynamica*, **4**, 81–130.

Rahn, O. (1945) Physical methods of sterilization of microorganisms. *Bacteriological Reviews*, **9**, 1-47.

Rey, C.R., Walker, H.W. & Rohrbaugh, P.L. (1975) The influence of temperature on growth, sporulation and heat resistance of spores of six strains of *Clostridium perfringens. Journal of Milk and Food Technology*, **38**, 461–465.

Roberts, T.A. (1968) Heat and radiation resistance and activation of spores of *Clostridium welchii. Journal of Applied Bacteriology*, **31**, 133–144.

Roberts, T.A. (1970) Recovering spores damaged by heat ionizing radiations or ethylene oxide. *Journal of Applied Bacteriology*, **33**, 74–94.

Roberts, T.A. & Hitchins, A.D. (1969) Resistance of spores. In *The Bacterial Spore* (eds Gould, G.W. & Hurst, A.), pp. 611–670. London, New York: Academic Press.

Roberts, T.A., Gilbert, R.J. & Ingram, M. (1966a) The heat resistance of anaerobic spores on aqueous suspension. *Journal of Food Technology*, **1**, 227–235.

Roberts, T.A., Gilbert, R.J. & Ingram, M. (1966b) The effect of sodium chloride on heat resistance and recovery of heated spores of *Clostridium sporogenes* (PA $3679/S_2$). *Journal of Applied Bacteriology*, **29**, 549–555.

Rowe, A.J. & Silverman, G.J. (1970) The absorption–desorption of water by bacterial spores and its relation to dry heat resistance. *Developments in Industrial Microbiology*, **11**, 311–326.

Rowe, J.A. & Koesterer, M.G. (1965) Dry heat resistance of *Bacillus subtilis* under several heated gaseous environments. In *Bacteriological Proceedings*, p. 8.

Russell, A.D. (1971) The destruction of bacterial spores. In *Inhibition and Destruction of the Microbial Cell* (ed. Hugo, W.B.), pp. 451–612. London: Academic Press.

Russell, A.D. (1982) *The Destruction of Bacterial Spores*. London: Academic Press.

Russell, A.D. (1984) Potential sites of damage in microorganisms exposed to chemical or physical agents. In *The Revival of Injured Microbes* (eds Andrew, M.H.E. & Russell, A.D.), Society for Applied Bacteriology Symposium Series No. 23, pp. 1–18. London: Academic Press.

Russell, A.D. (1998) Microbial sensitivity and resistance to chemical and physical agents. In *Topley & Wilson's Microbiology and Microbial Infections*. Vol. 2: *Systematic Bacteriology* (eds A. Balows & B.I. Duerden) 9th edn, pp. 149–184. London: Arnold.

Russell, A.D., Furr, J.R. & Maillard, J.-Y. (1997) Synergistic sterilization. *PDA Journal of Pharmaceutical Science and Technology*, **51**, 174–175.

Scholefield, J. & Abdelgadir, A.M. (1974) Heart resistance characteristics of spore of rough and smooth variants of *B. stearothermophilus*. In *Proceedings of the IV International Congress of Food Science and Technology*, Vol. 3, pp. 71–78.

Sebald, M. & Ionescu, H. (1972) Germination 1zP-dépendante des spores de *Clostridium botulinum* type E. *Comptes Rendues Académie de Science Paris (Serie D)*, **275**, 2175–2177.

Senhaji, A.F. (1977) The protective effect of fat on the heat resistance of bacteria (II). *Journal of Food Technology*, **12**, 217–230.

Senhaji, A.F. & Lonein, M. (1977) The protective effect of fat on the heat resistance of bacteria (I). *Journal of Food Technology*, **12**, 203–216.

Setlow, P. (1994) Mechanisms which contribute to the long-term survival of spores of *Bacillus* species. *Journal of Applied Bacteriology Symposium Supplement*, **76**, 49S–60S.

Shaker, L.A., Dancer, B.N., Russell, A.D. & Furr, J.R. (1988) Emergence and development of chlorhexidine resistance during sporulation of *Bacillus subtilis* 168. *FEMS Microbiology Letters*, **51**, 73–76.

Sharpe, K. & Bektash, R.M. (1977) Heterogeneity and the modelling of bacterial spore death: the case of continuously decreasing death rate. *Canadian Journal of Microbiology*, **23**, 1501–1507.

Smelt, J.P.P.M., Santos Da Silva, M.J. & Haas, H. (1977) The combined influence of pH and water activity on the heat resistance of *Clostridium botulinum* types A and B. In *Spore Research 1976* (eds Barker, A.N., Wolf, J., Ellar, D.J., Dring, G.J. & Gould, G.W.), pp. 469–476. London: Academic Press.

Soper, C.J. & Davies, D.J.G. (1971) The effect of high vacuum drying on the heat response of *Bacillus megaterium* spores. In *Spore Research 1971* (eds Barker, A.N., Gould, G.W. & Wolf, J.), pp. 275–288. London: Academic Press.

Soper, C.J. & Davies, D.J.G. (1973) The effects of rehydration and oxygen on the heat resistance of high vacuum treated spores. *Journal of Applied Bacteriology*, **36**, 119–130.

Staat, R.H. & Beakley, J.W. (1969) Dry heat inactivation characteristics of *Bacillus subtilis* var. *niger* spores. *Bacteriological Proceedings* Vol. 17, p. 17.

Steinbuch, E. (1977) The acid sensitization of heat resistant bacterial spores. In *Spore Research 1976* (eds Barker, A.N., Wolf, J., Ellar, D.J., Dring, G.J. & Gould, G.W.), pp. 451–468. London: Academic Press.

Stringer, S.C., Fairbairn, D.A. & Peck, M.W. (1997) Combining heat treatment and subsequent incubation temperature to prevent growth from spores of non-proteolytic *Clostridium botulinum*. *Journal of Applied Microbiology*, **82**, 128–136.

Stumbo, C.R. (1965) *Thermobacteriology in Food Processing*. New York: Academic Press.

Stumbo, C.R., Murphy, J.R. & Cochran, J. (1950) Nature of thermal death time curves for P.A. 3679 and *Clostridium botulinum*. *Food Technology*, **4**, 321–326.

Sugimoto, E.E., Raasch, A.J. & Ehioba, R.M. (1996) Recovery of bacterial spores dried on aluminum strips. *Journal of Applied Bacteriology*, **80**, 147–152.

Sugiyama, H. (1951) Studies on factors affecting the heat resistance of spores of *Clostridium botulinum*. *Journal of Bacteriology*, **62**, 81–96.

Sykes, G. (1965) *Disinfection and Sterilization*, 2nd edn. London: Chapman & Hall.

Wang, D.I.C., Scharer, J. & Humprey, A.E. (1964) Kinetics of death of bacterial spores at elevated temperatures. *Applied Microbiology*, **12**, 451–454.

Wang, J.-S. (1968) Alternation of dry heat resistivity of *Bacillus subtilis* var. *niger* by intracellular and extracellular water. Thesis, Massachusetts Institute of Technology, Boston.

Warth, A.D. (1977) Molecular structure of the bacterial spore. *Advances in Microbial Physiology*, **17**, 1–45.

Warth, A.D. (1978) Relationship between the heat resistance of spores and the optimum and maximum growth temperatures of *Bacillus* species. *Journal of Bacteriology*, **124**, 699–705.

Warth, A.D. (1985) Mechanisms of heat resistance. In *Fundamental and Applied Aspects of Bacterial Spores* (eds Dring, G.J., Ellar, D.J. & Gould, G.W.), pp. 209–225. London: Academic Press.

Williams, N.D. & Russell, A.D. (1992) Increased susceptibility of injured spores of *Bacillus subtilis* to cationic and other stressing agents. *Letters in Applied Microbiology*, **15**, 253–255.

Williams, O.B. & Reed, J.M. (1942) The significance of the incubation temperature of recovery cultures in determining spore resistance to heat. *Journal of Infectious Diseases*, **71**, 225–227.

Yokoya, F. & York, G.K. (1965) Effect of several environmental conditions on the 'thermal death rate' of endospores of aerobic, thermophilic bacteria. *Applied Microbiology*, **13**, 993–999.

C. MEDICAL APPLICATIONS OF THERMAL PROCESSES

1 Parenteral products

All parenteral products must be sterile when administered. Whenever possible, aqueous injections are terminally sterilized by autoclaving, the exception being products containing heat-labile drugs. Pharmacopoeial methods in Europe recommend moist-heat sterilization at a minimum temperature of 121°C maintained throughout the load during a holding period of 15min. Other combinations of time and temperature can be used, but the crucial requirement is that the cycle delivers an adequate level of 'lethality' to the product. In practice, many manufacturers apply the F_0 principle (see Chapter 18D) to autoclave processing, an F_0 of 8 being the usual minimum lethality acceptable. However, in some instances of poor heat tolerance of a product, an F_0 value as low as 4 can be employed. It is essential in all cases to ensure a low presterilization bioburden and the absence of heat-resistant spores, especially when the F_0 approach is employed. In addition to the requirement for sterility, all parenteral products must be free from excessive numbers of particles and be non-pyrogenic (see Groves, 1973, and the *Pharmaceutical Codex*, 1993, for a detailed discussion of these issues).

The current approach to parenterals is to consider not only the injection (formulation, sterility, etc.) but also the safest means of delivery to the patient. Consequently, there have been significant developments in the packaging of parenterals to improve this safe delivery. Because this has led to the wide use of plastic materials to fabricate such delivery systems, the applicability of thermal processing has been compromised in many instances. It is important to ensure that the introduction of less heat-stable packaging does not substantially reduce the sterility assurance of the final product.

1.1 Small-volume injections

Parenteral preparations of potent heat-stable drugs are distributed into, and sterilized in, glass or plastic ampoules. Glass ampoules are made by extrusion of tubular borosilicate glass. They may be made under clean-room conditions and supplied sealed ready for filling, resealing and sterilization. The most critical operation during the preparation of glass ampoules is the ampoule-sealing process (Brizell & Shatwell, 1973). To detect leakage, the most convenient method is to immerse ampoules in a heat-stable dye solution during autoclaving. Any seal failure will lead to loss of air from the ampoule during heating up and consequent ingress of dye during cooling, which is easily seen on inspection. For a detailed analysis of leak testing, see Anon. (1986). Injections can also be manufactured in polyethylene or polypropylene ampoules, using blow–fill–seal technology, for example the Rommelag process, in which the ampoule is formed, filled, sealed and heat-sterilized in one continuous process (Sharpe, 1988).

1.2 Multidose injections

A small number of injections are still required in multidose containers, comprising glass vials with an aluminium ring holding the rubber closure tightly on the bottle neck. Multidose injections must include a preservative unless the drug is intrinsically antimicrobial (Allwood, 1978). However, none of the multidose injections that remain acceptable to Licensing Authorities, such as insulin, some vaccines and heparins, are heat-sterilized.

1.3 Fat emulsions

It is possible to prepare a stable fat emulsion for parenteral administration, which is sterilized by autoclaving. Such emulsions consist of 10–20% oil in water, stabilized by lecithin. The droplet size is in the range 0.2–0.4 μm diameter. These emulsions are used as an energy source in parenteral nutrition (fat contains more than twice the calorie content of carbohydrates, compared on a weight basis, and yet does not increase the tonicity of the injection). Emulsions can also be used as a vehicle for poorly water-soluble drugs, such as fat-soluble vitamins and the intravenous anaesthetic propofol. It is also possible to use fat emulsions to target drugs to particular organs, such as the liver.

1.4 Oily injections

Thermostable drugs prepared in anhydrous vehicles intended for parenteral administration are sterilized by dry heat, using a cycle of 180°C for 30 min, or its equivalent time/temperature combination (*British Pharmacopoeia*, 1998). As with aqueous injections, the F_0 approach is now commonly applied to the sterilization of anhydrous products. These oily injections are normally packed in single-dose ampoules.

1.5 Large-volume parenterals

Large-volume aqueous injections (> 100 ml) have a variety of clinical uses (Allwood, 1998). These include restoration of electrolyte balance (for example, saline or glucose infusion), fluid replacement, large-volume infusions containing a therapeutic agent (for example, chlormethiazole) and concentrated solutions of amino acids used in parenteral nutrition. Such preparations are prepared in glass or plastic containers. The manufacturing process for large-volume parenterals (LVPs) is designed to ensure that a particle- and pyrogen-free solution with low microbial content is filled into clean containers. Controls designed to achieve this end, however, may be nullified by poor container design or manufacture. Therefore, the choice, quality and method of manufacture of the packaging are critical to the quality of the finished product.

1.5.1 Rigid containers

Rigid containers manufactured from borosilicate glass were widely used for large-volume sterile fluids in the past, but have now been largely superseded by plastic containers. However, glass bottles are still used for some products, such as amino acid infusions, some blood substitutes and agents such as the hypnotic, chlormethiazole. Such products are sterilized by autoclaving. Borosilicate glass is more resistant to thermal and chemical shock.

Bottles are closed using a rubber (elastomer) plug secured by an aluminium ring, which holds the rubber plug tightly on to the bottle rim. The major microbial risk to a product autoclaved in a glass bottle sealed with a rubber plug results from seal failure under the physical stress exerted on the closure during the autoclaving cycle. For a typical glass infusion container, the combined effect of steam under pressure and air at 121°C, together with the compression of the head-space due to water expansion, creates a pressure in the bottle of approximately 2.9 bar (56 p.s.i.) greater than the chamber pressure. This internal pressure exerts considerable stress on the rubber closure, already softened by the high temperature. Seal failure can occur because of poor manufacturing tolerances of the bottle neck or rim, inadequate torque applied to the rubber plug by the aluminium cap, incorrect hardness of rubber or poor closure design. The consequence of seal failure is air loss from the bottle during the heating-up stage of autoclaving (Allwood *et al.*, 1975) and subsequent ingress of water during spray-cooling (Beverley *et al.*, 1974). The entry of spray-cooling water poses the greatest risk, since it may contain viable microorganisms (Coles & Tredree, 1972). Even if the spray-cooling water is sterile, it remains contaminated with particulate matter, trace metals and pyrogens. The incidence of closure failure may be reduced by improved closure design (Hambleton & Allwood, 1976a). There is little evidence to suggest that an insert-type closure offers greater seal effectiveness than flat liners of the correct thickness and rubber hardness. The bottle-neck quality and variations in neck dimensions are especially important factors. The degree of torque applied to the rubber closure via the aluminium crimp-on cap is also significant. Glass containers are no longer considered the most suitable container for parenterals, especially as plastic containers provide a product more cheaply with less risk of contamination and lower particulate levels.

1.5.2 Flexible containers

The choice of a suitable plastic to package LVPs is largely governed by the thermal stability of the material (Wickner, 1973). However, a number of factors must be considered. These include the ease of production of a suitable design which is particle- and pyrogen-free, is easily filled under clean-room conditions and does not impart significant quantities of extractables, leached from the material of the container itself to the contents. For example, it is well recognized that plasticizers in polyvinyl chloride (PVC), such as phthalate salts, can leach from poor-quality film into aqueous solutions (Hambleton & Allwood, 1976b). Plastic containers can be formed into a completely sealed pouch or bottle before autoclaving. Therefore, there is no danger of spray-cooling water or air entering the contents during autoclaving, provided there is no seam failure or pinholing (these faults are normally detected by leakage of the contents). Since plastic films become more flexible on heating, the pressure increase in the container during autoclaving is far less than in a rigid container. However, in order to prevent flexible plastic containers from bursting, it is essential that autoclaving be conducted in an air–steam mixture to counterbalance pressure differences (Schuck, 1974). Plastic LVP containers are discussed by Petrick *et al.*, (1977), Turco & King (1987) and Allwood (1990). The most commonly used plastics for sterile products are PVC, polyethylene, polypropylene and non-PVC containing laminates. The relative merits of each are discussed by Hambleton & Allwood (1976b) and Turco & King (1987). One significant point of relevance to sterilization is that PVC-fabricated packs can be placed in an outer wrap before autoclaving. Also, PVC is able to withstand higher temperatures (up to 115–117°C) than polyethylene (112–114°C).

2 Non-parenteral sterile fluids

Sterile fluids suitable for clinical use (Table 19.9) are required in increasing quantity. These include non-injectable water, for use in theatres and wards when sterile fluids are required to wash open wounds or for peritoneal dialysis, for fluids for antiseptic solutions in ready-to-use dilution in critical-risk areas and for diluents for drugs used in nebulizers. All of these applications required the sterile fluid to be packaged in such a way that it can be used without becoming contaminated. For example, non-injectable water is required in a rigid bottle that allows pouring of a sterile liquid; antiseptic solutions should be transferable to a sterile container at the bedside without contamination. Peritoneal fluids must be packaged in order to allow convenient delivery into the peritoneum via suitable administration sets. This requires a flexible-walled container that collapses on emptying.

Most producers manufacture non-injectable water in rigid polypropylene bottles. The bottle may be sealed using a screw cap, with tear-off hermetic overseal, or a snap-break closure of a fully moulded container. Peritoneal dialysis fluids are packaged in flexible PVC pouches or rigid polypropylene bottles. Smaller-volume antiseptic solutions and nebulizer solutions may be packaged in plastic ampoules, PVC or laminate sachets. All these preparations should be autoclavable (Table 19.9).

Table 19.9 Uses of moist heat as a sterilization process.

Product or equipment	Comment
Metal instruments (including scalpels)	Dry heat preferred method; cutting edges to be protected from mechanical damage
Rubber gloves	γ-Radiation preferred method; if autoclave used, care with drying at end of process (little oxidative damage when high-vacuum autoclave used)
Respirator parts	Recommended method. If disinfection required, low-temperature steam or hot water at 80°C to be used
Surgical dressings	Choice of sterilization method depends upon stability of dressings material to stress applied and nature of dressings components
Parenteral products	Autoclaving is the approved method for sterilization of thermostable products
Non-parenteral sterile fluids	Sterile fluids suitable for clinical use; autoclaving process wherever possible
Ophthalmic solutions (eye-drops)	Autoclaving is the approved method for sterilization of thermostable products

3 Ophthalmic preparations

All ophthalmic preparations must be sterile to avoid the introduction of infecting microorganisms on to the surface of the eye. Under certain circumstances, such as postoperatively or after trauma, the cornea and conjunctiva are very susceptible to infection. Eye-drops are available in single and multidose presentations. The former method of packaging is clearly preferable, since the risks inherent in repeated-use preparations are removed. Traditionally, eye-drops have been prepared in glass containers (see below), although it is now far more common to use plastic. Single-dose packs are available in which the solutions can be sterilized by autoclaving in air-ballasted autoclaves. These solutions can therefore be formulated without a preservative. One example is the Minim (Smith & Nephew Ltd.), in which the package is made from polypropylene film with a removable cap for ease of use. This is placed in an outer wrap prior to autoclaving. Each Minim contains 0.5 ml.

Eye-drops are sterilized by autoclaving, whenever the stability of the therapeutic agent permits. Multidose preparations must contain an antimicrobial preservative to prevent proliferation of contaminants during use and support the maintenance of sterility. Examples of preservatives are phenylmercuric nitrate or acetate (0.002% w/v) chlorhexidine acetate (0.01% w/v) or benzalkonium chloride (0.01% w/v). Choice is to some extent dependent upon the active ingredient and the formulation. Preservatives can, however, migrate into both plastic and rubber components of the packaging (Allwood, 1990). Most types of rubber absorb preservatives (Allwood, 1978). It is therefore necessary to compensate for this loss by pre-equilibrating rubber closures with the particular preservative in the formulation. Benzalkonium chloride may be incompatible with natural rubber (Anon., 1966) and therefore synthetic rubber teats should be substituted, silicone rubber being recommended. However, moisture loss through silicone rubber occurs rapidly during storage, thus limiting the shelf-life of such a package (Shaw *et al.*, 1972). This is sometimes overcome by supplying the dropper separately from the bottle, the dropper being applied to the bottle immediately before use. Eye-drops are also commonly prepared in plastic dropper bottles, using filter-sterilized solutions and aseptic processing into presterilized containers.

The sealing of eye-dropper bottles during autoclaving can be improved by substituting metal for bakelite caps (Richards *et al.*, 1963). Other suggestions have been made for improving this type of packaging (Norton, 1962). Similar problems relate to containers for eye lotions, except that the closure does not incorporate a rubber teat. Eye lotions are normally treated as single-dose items and a preservative is not included. In contrast, contact-lens solutions, as well as being prepared as sterile preparations, preferably terminally sterilized by autoclaving, contain antimicrobial combinations to act as preservatives, since they are multidose preparations (Davies, 1978).

4 Dressings

4.1 Dressing sterilizers

Traditionally, gravity (downward-displacement autoclaves) has been used to sterilize dressings (Anon, 1959; Fallon & Pyne, 1963; Knox & Pickerill, 1964); however, this technology is now considered obsolete and high-vacuum porous-load steam sterilizers are the method of choice (Anon., 1993). In both cases, the essential requirements are for total removal of air from the load and the prevention of excessive condensation within the dressing packs during the cycle. If air is not removed, sterilizing conditions throughout the load will not be attained. If excessive condensation occurs, the dressing will become unusable. Condensation may also interfere with heat penetration. Porous-load autoclaves for dressing sterilization are described in British Standard BS 3970.

The essential difference between the traditional downward-displacement systems and high-vacuum air removal is the use of a far greater vacuum applied in the chamber to remove almost all of the air in the air space and trapped within the dressing packs. It is essential that air leaks into the chamber are prevented (Fallon, 1961). This vacuum must be below 20 mmHg absolute, which will remove more than 95% of the air in the chamber and load almost instantaneously. As the initial pressure is very low, steam is less likely to condense on the load material during the initial heating-up phase. This also depends on packing, and will vary in mixed loads; in fact, to ensure complete air removal from the load, it is usual to employ a rapid-pulsing evacuation procedure before the final heating-up stage, taking 6–8 min in all. The minimum holding time of 3 min at 134–138°C, a saturated-steam pressure equivalent to 2.2 bar or 32 p.s.i., is followed by steam removal, by condenser or vacuum, and drying, which can be shortened to 3–4 min for most loads packaged in paper or linen. Therefore, the total cycle time is about 28–35 min.

It is essential to ensure that the steam is dry and saturated, containing $\ngtr 5\%$ by weight of water as condensed droplets. If the steam is too wet, it will soak dressings, causing them to trap air. The other danger to be avoided is superheating. This can be caused by the lagging of reducing valves, by exothermic reactions related to greases in valves etc., by too high a jacket temperature or by retention of air in the load. Superheating can also occur within the load from the heat of hydration of very dry (< 1% moisture content) cotton fabrics (Bowie, 1961; Sykes, 1965). This can be avoided by allowing fabrics to equilibrate with normal levels of humidity (> 50% relative humidity (r.h.)) before sterilization.

4.2 Surgical dressings

It is essential that surgical dressings are sterile. Most dressings are sterilized by moist heat (Table 19.9). Correct packaging of each item is vital to allow sterilization and avoid contamination during application. The nature of the packaging must allow complete steam penetration into the dressing, as well as post-sterilization drying, and must be designed to allow the item to be removed aseptically. In general, all dressings are double-wrapped so that items can be taken through a contamination barrier into a clean area, during which the dressing and its immediate packaging remain sterile. Also, items are usually packed individually or in dressing kits (all the required items for one procedure are packed into one outer wrapping (Hopkins, 1961)). Fortunately, packaging developments have proceeded apace with improvements in autoclave technology. Improvements in the design of the autoclave cycle have allowed the use of improved packaging materials and methods of packaging. Thus introduction of the high-prevacuum autoclave cycle has not only provided a much shorter cycle period and improved sterilization performance, but also provided greater flexibility in the use of packaging techniques.

Any packaging material must allow steam and air to penetrate but still maintain its resistance to heat and breakage, especially when wet (Hunter *et al.*, 1961). It should be an adequate barrier to prevent entry of dust or microorganisms during storage. There is a considerable choice of material available, including metal, calico (muslin), cardboard, paper and plastic films. Traditionally, stainless-steel dressing drums have been used for the routine packing of dressings. However, these have now been superseded, especially with the use of high-prevacuum autoclaves, although metal boxes are being reintroduced. It is now usual practice to pack each item in paper, and then overwrap it in paper or fabric; alternatively, they may be placed in cardboard boxes (Hopkins, 1961), although other packaging materials are also available. In general, steam- and air-permeable paper packs are relatively easily sterilized, either by gravity or high-prevacuum steam control. In addition, the material is cheap and readily disposed of, and each pack is sealed with self-adhesive autoclave tape. Cardboard cartons can serve as outer rigid containers and are reusable. It is, however, important to maintain the steam in a dry state during autoclaving or the cardboard will disintegrate. Fabrics, such as calico, are suitable for gravity-steam penetration and the material often proves to be a reasonably effective air filter. However, fabrics are less resistant to bacterial penetration than paper (Standard *et al.*, 1973). They are reusable but require laundering. Some plastic-film materials can be employed, provided the material is steam-penetrable. Cellophane is often suitable for small items but tends to become brittle during autoclaving and therefore cannot be used in high-temperature autoclaves. The method of packing is often critical, especially in gravity-displacement autoclaves. Packs must be arranged so that the critical steam flow is not impeded between dressings. The use of high-prevacuum cycles largely overcomes the problem of steam penetration, provided the packing is sufficiently loose to allow good air and steam circulation inside and between packs and packaging material.

5 Uses of dry heat sterilization

Dry heat as a means of sterilization is reserved for those products and materials that contain little or no water and cannot be saturated with steam during the heating cycle (Table 19.10). It is used for dry powdered drugs, heat-resistant containers (but not rubber items), certain terminally sterilized preparations, some types of surgical dressings and

Table 19.10 Uses of dry heat as a sterilization process.

Product or equipment*	Comment
Syringes (glass)†	Dry heat is preferred method using assembled syringes
Needles (all metal)	Preferred method
Metal instruments (including scalpels)	Preferred to moist heat
Glassware	Recommended method
Oils and oily injections	Autoclaving clearly unsuitable
Powders	One of four methods (others are ethylene oxide, γ-radiation, filtration) recommended by *British Pharmacopoeia* (1993)

*Dry heat may also be used at high temperatures (220°C) for the depyrogenation of glassware.

†Now mainly replaced by disposable syringes, sterilized by γ-radiation (see Chapter 20A).

surgical instruments. The instruments include metal scalpels, other steel instruments and glass syringes (although most syringes now consist of plastic and are disposable). The advantage offered by dry heat sterilization of syringes is that they can be sterilized fully assembled in the final container (Anon., 1962). The difficulties associated with autoclaving syringes include lack of steam penetration, enhanced by the protective effect of lubricant, and the need to assemble them after sterilization. Examples of pharmaceutical products subjected to dry heat sterilization include implants (Cox & Spanjers, 1970), eye-ointment bases, oily injections (usually sterilized in ampoules) and other oily products (silicone used for catheter lubrication, liquid paraffin, glycerine). Dressings sterilized by dry heat include paraffin gauze and other oily-impregnated dressings.

The recommended treatment is maintenance of the item at 160°C for 2 h. This may be limited by the heat stability of the particular item and therefore some dispensation is accepted, e.g. human fibrin foam is sterilized at 130°C for 3 h. Sutures may be sterilized at 150°C for 1 h in a non-aqueous solvent. However, after this treatment, the suture material must be transferred to aqueous tubing fluid to render the material flexible and restore its tensile strength. Ionizing radiation is now the preferred method of sterilization of sutures, as it minimizes the loss of tensile strength.

6 References

Allwood, M.C. (1978) Antimicrobial agents in single- and multi-dose injections. *Journal of Applied Bacteriology*, **44**, Svii–Sxiii.

Allwood, M.C. (1998) Sterile pharmaceutical products. In *Pharmaceutical Microbiology*, 6th edn (eds Hugo, W.B. & Russell, A.D.), pp. 410–425. Oxford: Blackwell Scientific Publications.

Allwood, M.C. (1990) Package design and product integrity. In *Guide to Microbiological Control in Pharmaceutical*, (eds Denyer, S. & Baird, R.) pp. 341–355. Chichester: Ellis Horwood.

Allwood, M.C., Hambleton, R. & Beverley, S. (1975) Pressure changes in bottles during sterilization by autoclaving. *Journal of Pharmaceutical Sciences*, **64**, 333–334.

Anon. (1959) *Medical Research Council, Report by Working Party on Pressure-Steam Sterilization*. London: HMSO.

Anon. (1962) *The Sterilization, Use and Care of Syringes*. MRC Memorandum No. 14. London: HMSO.

Anon. (1966) *Pharmaceutical Society Laboratory Report*, P/66/7.

Anon. (1986) *The Prevention and Detection of Leaks in Glass Ampoules*. Technical Monograph No. 1. Swindon: Parenteral Society Publications.

Anon. (1993) *Sterilisation, Disinfection and Cleaning of Medical Equipment: Guidance on Decontamination*. Microbial Advisory Committee to Department of Health Medical Devices Directorate. London: HMSO.

Beverley, S., Hambleton, R. & Allwood, M.C. (1974) Leakage of spray cooling water into topical water bottle. *Pharmaceutical Journal*, **213**, 306–308.

Bowie, J.H. (1961) The control of heat sterilisers. In *Sterilization of Surgical Materials*, pp. 109–142. London: Pharmaceutical Press.

British Pharmacopoeia (1998) London: HMSO.

Brizell, I.G. & Shatwell, J. (1973) Methods of detecting leaks in glass ampoules. *Pharmaceutical Journal*, **211**, 73–74.

Coles, J. & Tredree, R.L. (1972) Contamination of autoclaved fluids with cooling water. *Pharmaceutical Journal*, **209**, 193–195.

Cox, P.H. & Spanjers, F. (1970) The preparation of sterile implants by compression. *Overdurk Mit Pharmaceutisch Weekblad*, **105**, 681–684.

Davies, D.J.G. (1978) Agents as preservatives in eye drops and contact lens solutions. *Journal of Applied Bacteriology*, **44**, Sxix–Sxxxiv.

Fallon, R.J. (1961) Monitoring of sterilization of dressing in high vacuum pressure-steam sterilizers. *Journal of Clinical Pathology*, **14**, 666–669.

Fallon, R.J. & Pyne, J.R. (1963) The sterilization of surgeons' gloves. *Lancet*, **i**, 1200–1202.

Groves, M.J. (1973) *Parenteral Products*. London: Heinemann.

Hambleton, R. & Allwood, M.C. (1976a) Evaluation of a new design of bottle closure for non-injectable water. *Journal of Applied Bacteriology*, **14**, 109–118.

Hambleton, R. & Allwood, M.C. (1976b) Containers and closures. In *Microbiological Hazards of Infusion Therapy* (eds Phillips, I., Meers, P.D. & D'Arcy, P.F.), pp. 3–12. Lancaster: MTP Press.

Hopkins, S.J. (1961) Central sterile supply in Cambridge hospitals. In *Sterilization of Surgical Materials*, pp. 153–166. London: Pharmaceutical Press.

Hunter, C.L.F., Harbord, P.E. & Riddett, D.J. (1961) Packaging papers as bacterial barriers. In *Sterilization of Surgical Materials*, pp. 166–172. London: Pharmaceutical Press.

Knox, R. & Pickerill, J.K. (1964) Efficient air removal from steam sterilized dressing without the use of high vacuum. *Lancet*, **i**, 1318–1321.

Norton, D.A. (1962). The properties of eye-drop bottles. *Pharmaceutical Journal*, **189**, 86–87.

Petrick, R.J., Loucas, S.P., Cohl, J.K. & Mehl, B. (1977) Review of current knowledge of plastic intravenous fluid containers. *American Journal of Hospital Pharmacy*, **34**, 357–362.

Pharmaceutical Codex (1993) London: Pharmaceutical Press.

Richards, R.M.E., Fletcher, G. & Norton, D.A. (1963) Closures for eye drop bottles. *Pharmaceutical Journal*, **191**, 655–660.

Schuck, L.J. (1974) Steam sterilization of solutions in plastic bottles. *Developments in Biological Standards*, **23**, 1–5.

Sharpe, J.R. (1988) Validation of a new form–fill–seal installation. *Manufacturing Chemist and Aerosol News*, **59**, 22, 23, 27, 55.

Shaw, S., Hayward, J. & Edlongton, M. (1972) Eye drop bottles. *Journal of Hospital Pharmacy*, April, 108.

Standard, P.G., Mallison, G.F. & Mackel, D.C. (1973) Microbial penetration through three types of double wrappers for sterile packs. *Applied Microbiology*, **26**, 59–62.

Sykes, G. (1965) *Disinfection and Sterilization*, 2nd edn. London: E. & F.N. Spon.

Turco, S. & King, R.E. (1987) *Sterile Dosage Forms*, 3rd edn. Philadelphia: Lea & Febiger.

Wickner, H. (1973) Hospital pharmacy manufacturing of sterile fluids in plastic containers. *Svensk Farmaceutisk Tidskrift*, **77**, 773–777.

D. APPLICATION OF THERMAL PROCESSING IN THE FOOD INDUSTRY

1 Introduction

1.1 Aims of thermal processing of foods

Thermal processing for the sterilization of high-pH (low-acid), high-water-activity (A_w) foods for ambient stability aims to inactivate the spore forms of all those bacteria that could otherwise grow in those products. Pasteurization processes aim to inactivate mainly vegetative spoilage or pathogenic microorganisms, with subsequently limited product shelf-life, or with longer shelf-life if the growth of any surviving microorganisms is inhibited, e.g. by low-temperature storage, by the addition of preservatives or due to the intrinsic properties of a particular food.

If an otherwise unpreserved food is to be stable during indefinite storage at ambient temperatures, all microorganisms capable of growth in that food must be eradicated and reinfection from extraneous sources prevented. If the ambient temperatures expected during the life of the food include those typical of tropical conditions, the thermal process must be sufficient to inactivate spores of those organisms able to grow at high temperatures (thermophiles), such as *Bacillus stearothermophilus* and *Clostridium thermosaccharolyticum*. Such thermophilic bacteria produce the most resistant types of spores, so the required processes are severe. On the other hand, if the food is destined for temperate regions, complete eradication of thermophiles is not necessary, since they cannot grow at the lower temperatures, and milder thermal processes are adequate. Such foods therefore need not be sterile. However, they must be heated sufficiently to be free from the spores of spoilage and toxinogenic microorganisms that are capable of growth under the temperate ambient conditions. This is sometimes referred to as 'commercial sterility'. Special attention is given to the eradication of any spores of proteolytic strains of *Clostridium botulinum* that may be present, because these are the most heat-resistant of the toxinogenic spores and their survival and growth can result in particularly severe food poisoning.

If foods are formulated in such a way that spoilage and toxinogenic spore-formers are inhibited from growing, for instance by reduction in pH value or A_w or by the addition of preservatives, then it may be unnecessary to inactivate the spores. Milder, pasteurization, processes may then be adequate to ensure stability and safety. Finally, for some foods that are unpreserved and yet stored for limited periods of time or at well-controlled low temperatures, pasteurization may likewise be sufficient. Requirements for sterilization are therefore clearly defined (see below), whereas requirements for pasteurization vary according to product characteristics and intended storage life.

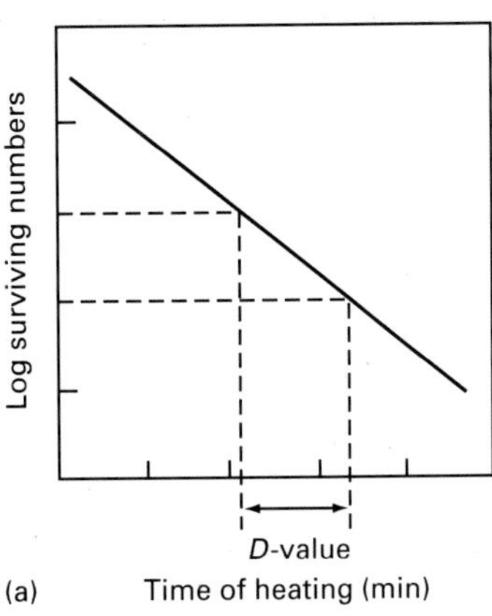

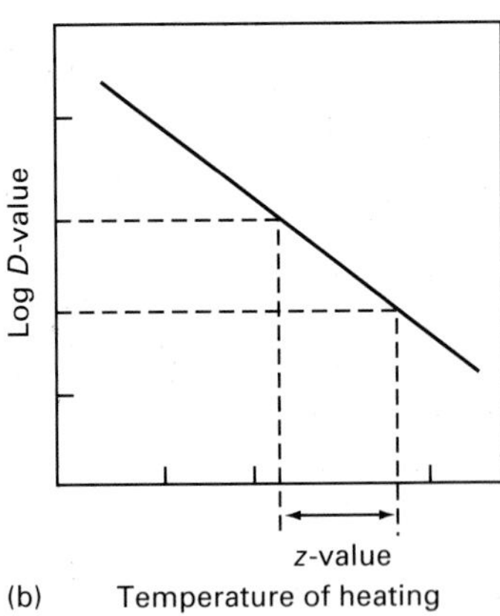

Fig. 19.7 Idealized heat-inactivation curves of bacterial spores showing: (a) exponential decline in numbers of survivors during heating at constant temperature and the derivation of the *D*-value; (b) exponential decline in *D*-value with rise in temperature and the derivation of the *z*-value.

1.2 Kinetics of heat inactivation of microorganisms

The numbers of viable cells in a population of spores of a single strain of a microorganism heated at constant temperature are generally regarded to decrease exponentially with time (Fig. 19.7a). This is often assumed to result from 'single-hit' kinetics, with each individual spore having the same intrinsic heat resistance and having the same chance of inactivation per unit time. The slope of the inactivation curve is designated *D* in minutes (the time taken for one decimal reduction). The rate of inactivation increases with temperature such that *D* decreases exponentially with rise in temperature, and the slope of this curve is designated *z* in degrees (Fig. 19.7b; see also Chapter 19B).

These relationships form the basis for the thermal processing of foods, despite the fact that many experimental observations have cast doubt on the universal validity of the simplicity of these relationships. Various explanations for deviations from linearity have been proposed (Roberts & Hitchins, 1969; Pflug & Holcomb, 1977; Russell, 1982; Gould, 1989). For example, it has been suggested that survivor curves with shapes like 'b' in Fig. 19.8 result from multihit processes (Moats *et al.*, 1971). Alternatively, the presence of large numbers of clumps of cells in a suspension may result in a delay before the numbers of colony-forming units (cfu) begin to fall. An initial rise in count (curve 'c') or a shoulder may result from a requirement of the spores to be heat-activated before they are able to germinate. Tailing (curve 'd')

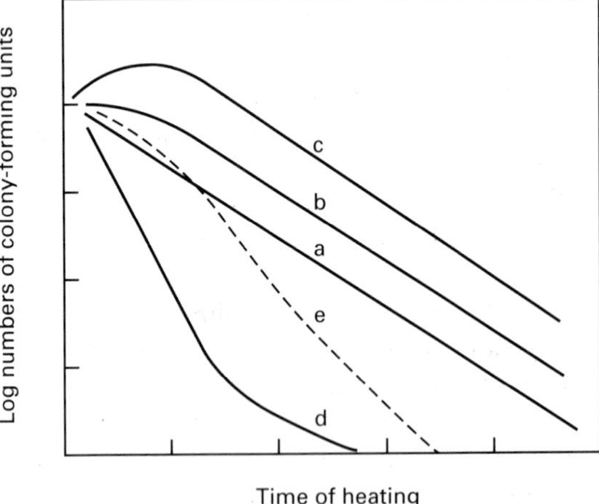

Fig. 19.8 Varieties of experimentally derived heat-inactivation curves (b–e) that differ from the idealized kinetics (a) summarized in Fig. 19.7. For proposed explanations, see text. (From Gould, 1989.)

is often seen and may result from the presence of small numbers of large clumps in the suspension, from a variation in the heat resistances of individual spores within the population (Cerf, 1977; Sharpe & Bektash, 1977) or from an increase in spore heat resistance occurring during the heating process itself (heat adaptation; Han *et al.*, 1976). A mixture of these effects will be expected to lead to the commonly observed sigmoidal type of curve ('e').

At the very high temperatures of ultraheat treatment (UHT) processing, when inactivation rates are very high, accurate data are difficult to obtain. Consequently, extrapolations have been made to small values of *D*, assuming constant *z* over the whole temperature range (Fig. 19.7b). Experiments using spores of *Cl. botulinum* at temperatures in excess of 140°C have indicated that inactivation kinetics are close to those that would be expected by extrapolation from lower temperatures (Brown & Gaze, 1988). The most confidently acquired data therefore suggest that there has not been an underestimate of required heat processes, and theoretical considerations indicate that any deviations within the practicably useful range of temperatures should be small (McKee & Gould, 1988).

If the vegetative forms of bacteria are heated at sublethal temperatures, then their resistance to subsequent heating at a higher temperatures may increase, due to the phenomenon of heat adaptation, or the heat-shock response. This is part of a complex series of stress responses that many types of microorganism, plant and animal cells undergo (Schlessinger *et al.*, 1982). The extent to which the synthesis of heat-shock proteins that occurs within the stressed cells and the consequent thermal adaptation are important in food preservation is arguable, because most practical uses of heat, in sterilization and pasteurization procedures, involve relatively rapid heating rates, so that the opportunity for adaptation does not arise. However, some slow cooking procedures are used, e.g. for large-bulk products, and cooking in the home may sometimes involve long, slow heating, so that it has been suggested that heat adaptation may be significant in a limited number of cases, e.g. with respect to the survival of organisms such as *Salmonella*, which contaminate many foods of animal origin and in which the effect can be quite large (Fig. 19.9).

However, in spite of the many reported deviations from exponential kinetics for the inactivation of vegetative and spore forms of bacteria, the simple relationships shown in Fig. 19.7 still form the basis for the calculation of thermal processes in the food industry, and with an excellent track record of efficacy and safety.

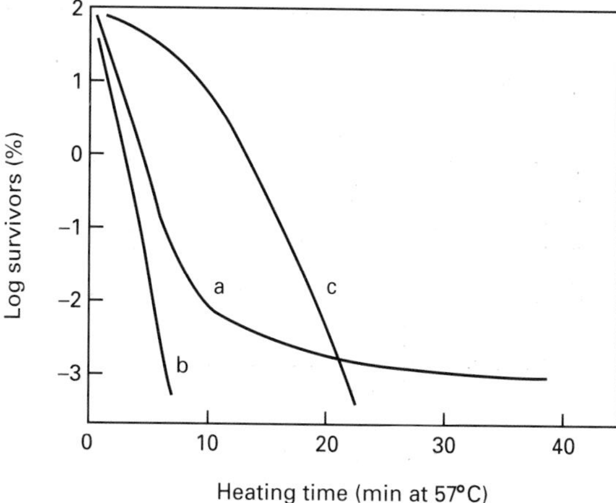

Fig. 19.9 Non-exponential inactivation kinetics and heat adaptation of vegetative cells. Survivor curves of *Salmonella typhimurium* heated at 57°C: heated in ground beef (a); heated in broth medium without a prior heat shock (curve b) or following a heat shock (curve c) at 48°C for 30 min. (From Mackey & Derrick, 1986, and Thompson *et al.*, 1979.)

2 Thermal processing

2.1 Basic requirements

The basic requirement for food-sterilization processes remains the reduction of the chance of survival of spores of mesophilic strains of *Cl. botulinum* by a sufficiently large factor. The accepted magnitude of the 'sufficiently large factor' derives from studies undertaken over 70 years ago by Esty & Meyer (1922), who proposed standards for food sterilization equivalent to a reduction of spore numbers by a factor of about 10^{12}-fold, and by Hicks (1961), who argued that destruction of spores of *Cl. botulinum* by this extent (the '12*D* concept') was necessary to ensure an acceptable degree of safety for low-acid, thermally processed foods.

Since the *z*-value (Fig. 19.7b) allows comparison of the lethal effects of heating at different temperatures, it is useful for practical purposes to choose a reference temperature to which the effects of other temperatures can be related. This is done with the *F*-value, which expresses a heat treatment in terms of the equivalent effect of a stated number of minutes at some standard temperature, assuming a particular *z*-value. A reference temperature of 121.1°C (250°F) and a *z*-value of 10°C (18°F) for spores of mesophilic *Cl. botulinum* are adopted by the food industries and, under these conditions, *F* is designated F_0. Based on the heat-inactivation kinetics of *Cl. botulinum* spores in phosphate buffer, an F_0-value of 2.45 min is accepted as the heat treatment necessary to achieve a 10^{12}-fold reduction in numbers. In some foods, *D*-values slightly higher than those in buffers have been found (Murrell & Scott, 1966; Verrips & Kwast, 1977; Alderton *et al.*, 1980), so the required F_0 is commonly taken as 3.0 min in order to ensure the expected lethality.

In pasteurization processes, *P*-values, analogous to *F*-values but with reference temperatures more relevant to the lower heat processes (e.g. 60°C or 71°C; Shapton *et al.*, 1971; Wojchiechowski, 1981), are sometimes used. There have been arguments in favour of abandoning this parameter in favour of using *D*- and *F*-values instead (Corry, 1974; Verrips & Kwast, 1977; Smelt & Mossel, 1982). However, for non-sterilizing thermal processes, where the *D*-and *z*-values of a particular target microorganism are confidently known, it is widely agreed to be appropriate to retain the use of *P*-values.

2.2 Process calculation

In order to determine the correct conditions for foods thermally processed in sealed containers, temperatures are usually measured using thermocouples during heating and cooling at the slowest heating point within containers the retort. The *F*-value delivered is calculated from the lowest integrated time–temperature curve registered, and the required minimal treatment is based on this. A consequence of using the minimum-heat point is that most of the food in a batch is usually substantially overprocessed. Biological indicators (e.g. spores of *B. stearothermophilus*; Pflug *et al.*, 1980) have sometimes been used to check the validity of processes.

Guidelines for setting processes are covered in several standard texts (see Stumbo, 1973; Hersom & Hulland, 1980; Pflug, 1982a,b). All rely on integration to determine the total *F*-value of the process, having chosen the values of *D* and *z*, and there are a variety of ways of doing this. In the

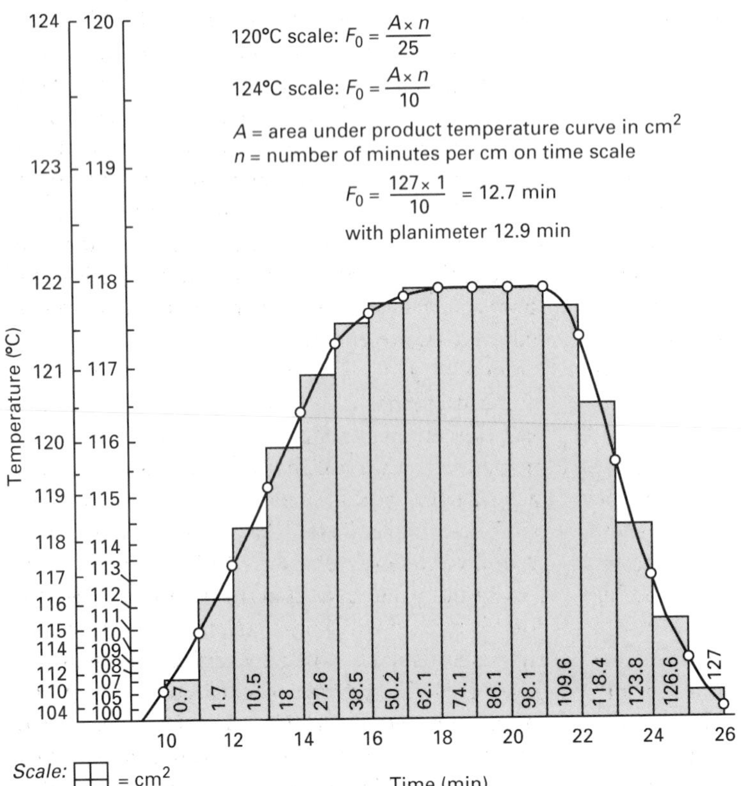

Fig. 19.10 Graphical determination of F_0 values from measured temperatures (°C) during a thermal process. The numbers within the rectangles represent their cumulative areas and therefore the cumulative lethality of the process, when adjusted by the appropriate scale factor (see inset). (From Smelt & Mossel, 1982.)

graphical method, the lethal rate per minute, at a particular temperature, is represented by length on the vertical axis of '*F*-reference paper' (Fig. 19.10). Time is plotted linearly on the horizontal axis. The area beneath the curve is then a measure of the *F*-value, and can be calculated by multiplication by the appropriate scale factor (see inset to Fig. 19.10). In the addition method, the lethal rate per minute at each specific temperature is read from a table (Table 19.11), and the F_0-value calculated from the sum of the lethal effects (rates) multiplied by the appropriate time factor in minutes.

The precision of the two basic methods is similar and has been further improved by the availability of user-friendly software, allowing quicker and more confident computer-aided integration of lethality (Tucker & Clark, 1989; Tucker, 1990). Changing the *z*-values and reference temperatures allows the programmes to be used for pasteurization processes and also allows determination and control of 'cook values' (see Section 2.5). Process control has likewise become increasingly precise with the use of modern temperature recorder-controllers, which have been developed to the point where they are complete process controllers themselves (Hamilton, 1990).

2.3 Combination treatments

The combination of other factors with thermal processes can allow a reduction in the degree of heating necessary to achieve product stability. The most widely employed is the combination with acidification, such that foods with pH values below 4.5 do not require a full 'botulinum cook'. This is because any spores of *Cl. botulinum* that may be present and survive in such 'acid-canned' foods cannot grow at such a low pH.

Combinations with reduced A_w, with or without pH reduction, were first shown by Braithwaite & Perigo (1971) to lead to a variety of options for combinations of pH, A_w and F_0 that ensure stability. Some of these options are now widely used for the preservation of ambient or long-chill-stored products. Particularly successful examples include the shelf-stable products (SSPs)—meat-based and other products promoted by the 'hurdle technology' concept of Leistner and his colleagues Leistner *et al.*, 1981; Leistner, 1995a). These pH- and A_w-adjusted products, some with additional preservation due to the presence of nitrite or other adjuncts, receive mild heat treatments in sealed packs. They contain surviving spores. These slowly germinate during storage, but they are unable to grow and therefore die, steadily reducing in numbers as time passes (autosterilization; Leistner, 1995b).

Combinations of heating with chill storage are widely employed to extend the shelf-life of mildly heated, and therefore high quality, food products. Much attention has been given to determining the level of heating necessary to control pathogens in such foods. There is now general agreement that the safety of mildly heated products that are intended to have a short shelf-life, and that are otherwise unpreserved, can be assured by a minimum heat treatment and a tight restriction of shelf-life (Anon., 1989). Such products are therefore given heat treatments sufficient to inactivate vegetative pathogens, e.g. in excess of a 10^6-fold reduction in numbers of *Listeria monocytogenes*, which can be achieved by 70°C for 2 min or a heat process of equivalent lethality assuming a *z*-value between 6 and 7.4°C (Gaze *et al.*, 1989), or in excess of 10^8-fold, achieved by a 72°C, 2-min process (Mossel & Struijk, 1991). However, these processes are insufficient to inactivate spores of psychrotrophic strains of *Cl. botulinum*, some of which are able to grow slowly at temperatures as low as 3.3°C. The processes are therefore acceptable only if the temperatures of storage are sufficiently low and the storage times sufficiently short to prevent growth from any of these spores that may be present (Anon., 1989).

There is general agreement that, for products intended to have a long shelf-life, and which are otherwise unpreserved, heat processing must be more severe. It must be sufficient to achieve a large, i.e. 10^6-fold reduction of spores of psychrotrophic *Cl. botulinum* if storage below 3.3°C cannot confidently be assured (ACMSF, 1992). It is generally agreed that a temperature–time combination of 90°C for 10 min or a process of equivalent lethality will achieve this, although it is recognized that additional data are still required (Notermans *et al.*, 1990; Lund & Peck, 1994; Gould, 1996). These chilled food products, which have been mildly heated in hermetically sealed

Table 19.11 Lethal rates for the thermal processing of foods (from Smalt & Mossel, 1982, and National Food Processors Association, n.d.).

T	LR	T	LR	T	LR	T	LR
88.0	0.001	109.4	0.068	115.4	0.269	120.0	0.774
92.0	0.001	109.7	0.073	115.5	0.275	120.1	0.791
93.0	0.002	110.0	0.077	115.6	0.281	120.2	0.809
95.0	0.002	110.2	0.080	115.7	0.287	120.3	0.828
95.2	0.003	110.4	0.084	115.8	0.294	120.4	0.848
96.5	0.003	110.6	0.088	115.9	0.301	120.5	0.868
96.7	0.004	110.8	0.093	116.0	0.308	120.6	0.888
97.5	0.004	111.0	0.097	116.1	0.315	120.7	0.909
97.8	0.005	111.2	0.102	116.2	0.322	120.8	0.930
98.3	0.005	111.4	0.107	116.3	0.330	120.9	0.951
98.5	0.006	111.6	0.112	116.4	0.338	121.0	0.974
99.0	0.006	111.8	0.117	116.5	0.346	121.1	0.998
99.4	0.007	112.0	0.122	116.6	0.354	121.2	1.022
99.7	0.007	112.1	0.124	116.7	0.362	121.3	1.046
100.0	0.008	112.2	0.128	116.8	0.370	121.4	1.070
100.6	0.009	112.3	0.131	116.9	0.379	121.5	1.094
101.1	0.010	112.4	0.134	117.0	0.388	121.6	1.118
101.4	0.011	112.5	0.137	117.1	0.397	121.7	1.144
101.7	0.011	112.6	0.141	117.2	0.406	121.8	1.172
102.0	0.012	112.7	0.144	117.3	0.416	121.9	1.199
102.2	0.013	112.8	0.148	117.4	0.426	122.0	1.227
102.5	0.014	112.9	0.151	117.5	0.436	122.1	1.256
102.8	0.015	113.0	0.154	117.6	0.446	122.2	1.286
103.0	0.016	113.1	0.158	117.7	0.456	122.3	1.317
103.3	0.017	113.2	0.162	117.8	0.466	122.4	1.347
103.6	0.018	113.3	0.166	117.9	0.477	122.5	1.377
103.9	0.019	113.4	0.170	118.0	0.488	122.6	1.408
104.2	0.020	113.5	0.174	118.1	0.499	122.7	1.441
104.4	0.022	113.6	0.178	118.2	0.511	122.8	1.475
104.7	0.023	113.7	0.182	118.3	0.523	122.9	1.510
105.0	0.024	113.8	0.186	118.4	0.536	123.0	1.546
105.3	0.026	113.9	0.190	118.5	0.549	123.1	1.582
105.6	0.028	114.0	0.194	118.6	0.562	123.2	1.619
105.9	0.030	114.1	0.198	118.7	0.574	123.3	1.657
106.1	0.032	114.2	0.203	118.8	0.587	123.4	1.695
106.4	0.034	114.3	0.208	118.9	0.601	123.5	1.732
106.7	0.036	114.4	0.213	119.0	0.615	123.6	1.770
107.0	0.038	114.5	0.218	119.1	0.630	123.7	1.809
107.2	0.041	114.6	0.223	119.2	0.645	123.8	1.858
107.5	0.043	114.7	0.228	119.3	0.660	123.9	1.900
107.8	0.046	114.8	0.234	119.4	0.675		
108.0	0.049	114.9	0.239	119.5	0.691		
108.3	0.053	115.0	0.245	119.6	0.707		
108.6	0.056	115.1	0.251	119.7	0.723		
108.9	0.060	115.2	0.257	119.8	0.740		
109.2	0.064	115.3	0.263	119.9	0.757		

The lethal rates (LR) are shown for temperatures (T) from 88.0 to 123.9°C, assuming a z-value of 10°C.

packages, or heated and packaged without recontamination, include refrigerated processed foods of extended durability ('REPFEDs'): Mossel *et al.*, 1987; Notermans *et al.*, 1990), 'sous vide' products (Livingston, 1985) and other products with pasteurization and preservation combinations that deliver extended shelf-lives under chill storage (Brown & Gould, 1992). 'Sous vide' refers to a process in which foods are vacuum-packed prior to cooking for long periods of time at relatively low pasteurization temperatures, so as to deliver high quality with respect to texture and retention of flavour.

Combination of mild heat processing with high hydrostatic pressure is being suggested as a further means of reducing heat damage to foods. While this combination works well, it is still not sufficiently effective to match the safety requirements of traditional thermal processing for long-ambient-stable foods (see Chapter 23). Likewise, combinations of heat with ultrasonication and slight overpressure ('manothermosonication') are in the early stages of development, but may eventually offer practical methods for pasteurizing or sterilizing liquid products using thermal treatments less than those currently required (see Chapter 23).

2.4 Product quality

The temperature coefficients of the chemical and physical reactions that cause quality loss of foods, leading to changes in taste, texture, appearance and nutritional value, are such that it is usually advantageous to process foods at as high a temperature, and consequently for as short a time, as possible. This has led to the consideration of 'cook values' (*c*-values), analogous to *z*-values but for quality parameters rather than for microbial ones. For example, Ohlsson (1980a) found values as high as 33°C for the deterioration of various parameters of product quality, and used the data he derived to define optimum processes for quality retention in foods thermally processed in flat containers (Ohlsson, 1980b) and in cylindrical cans (Ohlsson, 1980c). High-temperature–short-time processing is, of course, less easy to achieve in container-packaged than in free-flowing foods, so that liquid products, such as milk, custards, sauces, soups and drinks, have benefited most from HTST pasteurization processing or UHT sterilization processing.

2.5 Process hygiene

Postprocess contamination of thermally treated foods may occur through defective packaging, defects in sealing or aseptic filling operations or through damage to otherwise intact packs. Since the consequent leaker spoilage results from the ingress of microorganisms from the external environment, the types involved may be diverse. Spoilage resulting from leakage through seams is most important (Segner, 1979), and avoidance demands a high degree of postprocess hygiene. In particular, the major contributor to leaker spoilage is unhygienic handling of processed packs while they are still wet. Clean handling is especially critical during cooling, when pressure changes encourage leaks. Dependable, non-destructive, in-line, leak-detection methods are available for some types of packages, and a variety of biotest methods (challenging packs with high concentrations of microorganisms externally; Michels & Schram, 1979) allow statistical estimates of the incidence of potential leakers to be made.

3 Alternative means for heat delivery and control

Recent developments in the thermal processing of foods have targeted improvements in product quality through: (i) reducing heat-induced damage by aiming for HTST processing, particularly through aseptic processing; (ii) using new forms of packaging that allow more rapid and more uniform heat transfer into and out of packed foods during processing; (iii) delivering heat in new ways (e.g. ohmic, microwave; see below); and (iv) controlling processes more tightly so as to achieve minimal processing and so avoid the extreme overprocessing that often occurs within batches of conventionally thermally processed foods.

Progress with aseptic processing has been substantial. The high-temperature treatments are normally delivered to foods in plate or tubular heat exchangers if the products are liquid or viscous, or in scraped-surface heat exchangers if the products tend to congeal on the exchanger surfaces or contain particulates, which can be up to about 1.5cm in diameter. Typically, temperatures are in the range 135–145°C and holding times are less than 5s. It is not possible to measure continuously the temperature within a food particle as it moves through a heat exchanger, so the F_0 delivered must be estimated from the thermal properties of the food materials and the kinetics, residence times, etc. within the system. The process can then usefully be verified using biological methods (Dignan *et al.*, 1989). Such methods have involved the use of 'biological thermocouples', consisting of spores sealed into small glass bulbs (Hersom & Shore, 1981) or entrained within gel particles, such as beads of calcium alginate (Dallyn *et al.*, 1977).

Most of the filling systems in aseptic processes make use of hot hydrogen peroxide to sterilize packs or webs of packaging material prior to dosing the sterilized (or pasteurized) product. These procedures can regularly achieve inactivation of spores on packaging by factors in excess of 10^8-fold. However, rigorous control of the whole system is essential. This is illustrated by the statistics quoted by Warwick (1990), who found, in a survey of 120 users of aseptic systems in Europe, that nearly 50% of installations experienced more than one non-sterile pack per 10 000, and that these resulted from contamination, not from failure of the thermal process *per se*.

The major changes in packaging that allow improved, more uniform, heat penetration into products have involved the development of new flexible pouches and polypropylene rigid containers. Cartons and thermoformed containers are the most-used forms of packaging for aseptically processed foods, but any kind of pack that can be hermetically sealed can be used. Materials now include tin-free steel, aluminium, aluminium foil and a wide variety of foil–plastic combinations in addition to glass and tin plate (Bean, 1983). Packs that do not have the strength of conventional cans or jars require special handling techniques to avoid damage and are often retailed in overwraps or carton outers to protect them and avoid recontamination during distribution (Turtle & Alderson, 1971; Aggett, 1990).

New heat-delivery systems include a number of alternatives to steam heating, including direct application of flame to containers, heating by passing alternating electric currents through products (ohmic heating) prior to aseptically packaging them, and heating using microwave energy. In particular, much development work has been undertaken on electrical-resistance heating procedures and commercial developments have been tested and applied in some countries (Goddard, 1990).

Electrical-resistance heating allows liquids and contained particulates to heat at the same rate and very rapidly, giving the potential for minimal thermal damage and high product quality. The physical basis of the process, but well understood so that results are closely predictable from first principles (Fryer, 1995). Microwave processing also has the advantage over conventional thermal processing that heat can be delivered very rapidly, and to solid food products, and volumetrically, so that heat transfer within the food can be much faster than processes that rely on conduction (Mullin, 1995). The slow take-up of microwaves for commercial food sterilization reflects technical barriers to confident large-scale control of heat distribution, as well as marketing constraints.

4 Conclusions and future developments

The various developments which aim to raise the quality of food products by minimizing heat damage to their components, while at the same time ensuring that the correct F_0 is delivered, will probably remain the most important targets in the near future. These will include the further exploitation of the newer heat-delivery and packaging systems, but also improved, tighter, control of conventional processes. Combination treatments, in which the thermal process is reduced and yet compensated for by other 'hurdles' are already used and probably set to find wider use, as confidence in the procedures grows. Finally, radically new approaches, such as some of those summarized in Chapter 23, will probably continue to be more widely exploited in growing niche markets.

5 References

Aggett, P. (1990) New niche for processables. *Food Manufacture*, **65**(6), 43–46.

Alderton, G., Chen, J.K. & Ito, K.A. (1980) Heat resistance of the chemical resistance forms of *Clostridium botulinum* 62A over the water activity range 0 to 0.9. *Applied and Environmental Microbiology*, **40**, 511–515.

ACMSF (1992) *Report on Vacuum Packaging and Associated Processes*. London: HMSO.

Anon (1989) *Chill and Frozen: Guidelines on Cook–Chill and Cook–Freeze Catering Systems*. London: HMSO.

Bean, P.G. (1983) Developments in heat treatment processes for shelf-stable products. In *Food Microbiology: Advances and Prospects* (eds Roberts, T.A. & Skinner, F.A.), pp. 97–112. London: Academic Press.

Braithwaite, P.J. & Perigo, J.A. (1971) The influence of pH, water activity and recovery temperature on the heat resistance and outgrowth of *Bacillus* spores. In *Spore Research 1971* (eds Barker, A.N., Gould, G.W. & Wolf, J.), pp. 189–302. London: Academic Press.

Brown, K.L. & Graze, J.E. (1988) High temperature resistance of bacterial spores. *Dairy Industries International*, **53**(10), 37–39.

Brown, M.H. & Gould, G.W. (1992) Processing. In *Chilled Foods: a Comprehensive Guide* (eds Dennis, C. & Stringer, M.F.), pp. 111–146. London: Ellis Horwood.

Cerf, O. (1977) Trailing of survival of bacterial spores. *Journal of Applied Bacteriology*, **42**, 1–19.

Corry, J.E.L. (1974) The effect of sugars and polyols on the heat resistance of salmonellae. *Journal of Applied Bacteriology*, **37**, 31–43.

Dallyn, H., Falloon, W.C. & Bean, P.G. (1977) Method for the immobilization of bacterial spores in alginate gel. *Laboratory Practice*, **26**, 773–775.

Dignan, D.M., Berry, M.R., Pflug, I.J. & Gardine, T.D. (1989) Safety considerations in establishing aseptic processes for low-acid foods containing particulates. *Food Technology*, **43**(3), 112–118, 131.

Esty, J.R. & Meyer, K.F. (1922) The heat resistance of the spores of *B. botulinus* and allied anaerobes. XI. *Journal of Infectious Diseases*, **31**, 650–663.

Fryer, P. (1995) Electrical resistance heating of foods. In *New Methods of Food Preservation* (ed. Gould, G.W.), pp. 205–235. Glasgow: Blackie Academic and Professional.

Gaze, J.E., Brown, G.D., Gaskell, D.E. & Banks, J.G. (1989) Heat resistance of *Listeria monocytogenes* in homogenates of chicken, beef steak and carrot. *Food Microbiology*, **6**, 251–259.

Goddard, R. (1990) Developments in aseptic packaging. *Food Manufacture*, **65**(10), 63–66.

Gould, G.W. (1989) Heat-induced injury and inactivation. In *Mechanisms of Action of Food Preservation Procedures* (ed. Gould, G.W.), pp. 11–42. London: Elsevier.

Gould, G.W. (1996) Conclusions of ECFF botulinum working party. In *Proceedings of the 2nd European Symposium on Sous Vide*, pp. 173–180. Leuven: Katholieke Universiteit.

Hamilton, R. (1990) Heat control in food processing. *Food Manufacture*, **65**(6), 33–36.

Han, Y.W., Zhang, H.I. & Krochta, J.M. (1976) Death rates of bacterial spores: mathematial models. *Canadian Journal of Microbiology*, **22**, 295–300.

Hersom, A.C. & Hulland, E.D. (1980) *Canned Foods: Thermal Processing and Microbiology*, 7th edn. London: Churchill Livingstone.

Hersom, A.C. & Shore, D.T. (1981) Aseptic processing of foods comprising sauce and solids. *Food Technology*, **35**(5), 53–62.

Hicks, E.W. (1961) Uncertainties in canning process calculations. *Journal of Food Science*, **26**, 218–226.

Leistner, L. (1995a) Use of hurdle technology in food: recent advances. In *Food Preservation by Moisture Control: Fundamentals and Applications* (eds Barbosa-Canovas, G.V. & Welti-Chanes, G.), pp. 377–396. Lancaster, Pennsylvania: Technomic Publishing.

Leistner, L. (1995b) Principles and applications of hurdle technology. In *New Methods of Food Preservation* (ed. Gould, G.W.) pp. 2–21. Glasgow: Blackie Academic and Professional.

Leistner, L., Rodel, W. & Krispien, K. (1981) Microbiology of meat and meat products in high and intermediate-moisture ranges. In *Water Activity: Influences on Food Quality* (eds Rockland, L.B. & Stewart, G.F.), pp. 855–916. New York: Academic Press.

Livingston, G.E. (1985) Extended shelf life chilled prepared foods. *Journal of Food Service Systems*, **3**, 221–230.

Lund, B.M. & Peck, M.W. (1994) Heat resistance and recovery of spores of non-proteolytic *Clostridium botulinum* in relation to refrigerated, processed foods with an extended shelf life. *Journal of Applied Bacteriology, Symposium Supplement*, **76**, 115S–128S.

McKee, S. & Gould, G.W. (1988) A simple mathemetical model of the thermal death of microorganisms. *Bulletin of Mathematical Biology*, **50**, 493–501.

Mackey, B.M. & Derrick, C.M. (1986) Elevation of the heat resistance of *Salmonella typhimurium* by sublethal heat shock. *Journal of Applied Bacteriology*, **61**, 389–393.

Michels, M.J.M. & Schram, B.L. (1979) Effect of handling procedures on the post-process contamination of retort pouches. *Journal of Applied Bacteriology*, **47**, 105–111.

Moats, W.A., Dabbah, R. & Edwards, V.M. (1971) Interpretation of non-logarithmic survivor curves of heated bacteria. *Journal of Food Science*, **36**, 523–526.

Mossel, D.A.A. & Struijk, C.A. (1991) Public health implications of refrigerated pasteurized ('sous-vide') foods. *International Journal of Food Microbiology*, **13**, 187–206.

Mossel, D.A.A., van Netten, P. & Perales, I. (1987) Human listeriosis transmitted by food in a general medical-microbiological perspective. *Journal of Food Protection*, **50**, 894–895.

Mullin, J. (1995) Microware processing. In *New Methods of Food Preservation* (ed. Gould, G.W.), pp. 112–134. Glasgow: Blackie Academic and Professional.

Murrell, W.G. & Scott, W.J. (1966) The heat resistance of bacterial spores at various water activities. *Journal of General Microbiology*, **43**, 411–425.

National Food Processors Association (n.d.) *Laboratory Manual for Food Canners and Processors*. Westport, Connecticut: AVI Publishing.

Notermans, S., Dufrenne, J. & Lund, B.M. (1990) Botulism risk of refrigerated processed foods of extended durability. *Journal of Food Protection*, **53**, 1020–1024.

Ohlsson, T (1980a) Temperature dependence of sensory quality changes during thermal processing. *Journal of Food Science*, **45**, 836–839, 847.

Ohlsson, T. (1980b) Optimal sterilization temperature for flat containers. *Journal of Food Science*, **45**, 848–852, 859.

Ohlsson, T. (1980c) Optimal sterilization temperatures for sensory quality in cylindrical containers. *Journal of Food Science*, **45**, 1517–1522.

Pflug, I.J. (1982a) *Textbook for an Introductory Course in the Microbiology and Engineering of Sterilization Processes*. Minneapolis: Environmental Sterilization Laboratory.

Pflug, I.J. (1982b) *Selected Papers on the Microbiology and Engineering of Sterilization*, 4th edn. Minneapolis: Environmental Sterilization Laboratory.

Pflug, I.J. & Holcomb, R.G. (1977) Principles of thermal destruction of microorganisms. In *Disinfection, Sterilization and Preservation* (ed. Block, S.S.), pp. 933–994. Philadelphia: Lea and Febiger.

Pflug, I.J., Smith, G., Holcomb, R. & Blanchet, R. (1980) Measuring sterilization values in containers. *Journal of Food Protection*, **43**, 119–123.

Roberts, T.A. & Hitchins, A.D. (1969) Resistance of spores. In *The Bacterial Spore* (eds Gould, G.W. & Hurst, A.), pp. 611–670. London: Academic Press.

Russell, A.D. (1982) *The Destruction of Bacterial Spores*. London: Academic Press.

Schlessinger, M.J., Ashburner, M. & Tissieres, A. (eds) (1982) *Heat Shock: from Bacteria to Man*. New York: Cold Spring Harbour.

Segner, W.P. (1979) Mesophilic aerobic spore forming bacteria in the spoilage of low acid canned foods. *Food Technology*, **33**(1), 55–59, 80.

Shapton, D.A., Lovelock, D.W. & Laurito-Longo, R. (1971) The evaluation of sterilization and pasteurization processes from measurements in degrees Celsius (°C). *Journal of Applied Bacteriology*, **34**, 491–500.

Sharpe, K. & Bektash, R.M. (1977) Heterogeneity and the modelling of bacterial spore death: the cause of continuously decreasing death rate. *Canadian Journal of Microbiology*, **23**, 1501–1507.

Smelt, J.P.P.M. & Mossel, D.A.A. (1982) Applications of thermal processing in the food industry. In *Principles and Practice of Disinfection, Preservation and Sterilization* (eds Russell, A.D., Hugo, W.B. & Ayliffe, G.A.J.), pp. 478–512. London: Blackwell Scientific Publications.

Stumbo, C.R. (1973) *Thermobacteriology and Food Processing*, 2nd edn. New York: Academic Press.

Thompson, W.S., Busta, F.F., Thompson, D.R. & Allen, C.E. (1979) Inactivation of salmonellae in autoclaved ground beef exposed to constantly rising temperatures. *Journal of Food Protection*, **42**, 410–415.

Tucker, G.S. (1990) Evaluating thermal processes. *Food Manufacture*, **65**(6), 39–40.

Tucker, G.S. & Clark, P. (1989) *Computer Modelling for the Control of Sterilization Processes*. Technical Memorandum No. 529. Campden Food and Drink Research Association.

Turtle, B.I. & Alderson, M.G. (1971) Sterilizable flexible packaging. *Food Manufacture*, **45**, 23, 48.

Verrips, C.T. & Kwast, R.H. (1977) Heat resistance of *Citrobacter freundii* in media with various water activities. *European Journal of Applied Microbiology*, **4**, 225–231.

Warwick, D. (1990) Aseptics: the problems revealed. *Food Manufacture*, **65**(6), 49–50.

Wojchiechowski, J. (1981) Charakteristik und Bewertung der Technologischen Verwendbarkeit thermobakteriologischer Pasteurisierungstests von Fleischkonserven 2. Mitteilung: Charakteristik der hitzewider Standigkeit der Aerobier, Pasteurisierungswert und kritische Punkte von Halbkonserven. *Fleischwirtschaft*, **61**, 437–442.

CHAPTER 20

Radiation Sterilization

A. IONIZING RADIATION

1 Introduction

Studies during the past three decades or so have revealed that ionizing radiation is a powerful process for inactivating various types of microorganisms. As such, it can be used for the sterilization of those pharmaceutical or medical products that are too thermolabile to withstand conventional heat-sterilization procedures, provided that these products suffer no harmful effects when exposed to high doses of radiation.

Numerous studies have also been undertaken that provide considerable information about those factors that influence microbial sensitivity to radiation, together with valuable data about the mechanisms involved in the inactivation of microorganisms, the reasons for the above-average resistance of certain types of bacteria and the way in which microbial enzyme-repair systems operate.

During the 1960s and 1970s, rapid growth in the usage of ionizing radiation as a sterilization procedure took place in Europe, the USA and Australia, such that it is nowadays a widely used process, often as an alternative to gaseous sterilization methods (Chapter 21).

In this chapter, the effects of radiation on microorganisms will be discussed, its actual and potential uses considered and control of the process described. Ionizing radiation is listed in the *British Pharmacopoeia* (BP, 1998), *United States Pharmacopoeia* (USP, 1995) and *European Pharmacopoeia* (EP, 1997) as one of the major methods for producing terminally sterilized products. Russell (1991) has described the fundamental aspects of microbial response to chemical and physical agents, including radiation, and Rakitskya *et al.* (1991) the theoretical and practical aspects of the radioresistance of microorganisms.

2 Radiation energy

Radiation is generally classified into two groups, namely electromagnetic and particulate (Table 20.1). Electromagnetic radiation is exemplified by γ-rays, X-rays, ultraviolet (UV) and visible light, infrared rays and microwave energy, is non-particulate and travels at the speed of light. Particulate radiation is exemplified by α-rays, β-rays, neutrons and protons; however, such particulate radiations have less penetrative power than

Table 20.1 Electromagnetic and particulate radiation.

Type of radiation	Example	Properties
Electromagnetic	γ-Rays	Low-wavelength ionizing radiation, high energy and penetrating power
	X-Rays	Low-wavelength ionizing radiation, high energy and penetrating power
	Ultraviolet light	Excitation of atoms; non-ionizing radiation
	Infrared*	Long wavelength, very low levels of radiant energy
	Microwaves*	Long wavelength, very low levels of radiant energy
Particulate	α-Rays	Helium nuclei, charged and heavy, little penetrating power
	β-Rays	Electrons: when accelerated to very high speeds, gain energy and penetrating power

*See Chapter 19A.

the electromagnetic γ-rays or X-rays. In practice, only γ-rays and high-speed electrons (β-rays) have found usage as sterilization methods (see Section 3); α-rays are charged and heavy and have little penetrative power.

Ionizing radiation strips off electrons from the atoms of the material through which it passes. Essentially all the chemical effects that occur are produced by these electrons. Ultraviolet light causes excitation of atoms, i.e. an alteration of electrons within their orbits, but does not possess enough energy to eject an electron to produce an ion, and is thus not an ionizing radiation. Ultraviolet radiation is considered further later (Chapter 20B). Infrared radiations have the ability to raise rapidly the temperature of objects which they strike and may thus be employed for their heating effects (see Chapter 19A). Microwaves also generate heat, but a major problem to date is the uneven heating effect (Chapter 19A).

X-rays and γ-rays consist of very short wavelengths; X-rays are produced from machines, and γ-rays from radioactive sources, such as cobalt-60 (^{60}Co) and caesium-137 (^{137}Cs). High-speed electrons were originally produced from radioactive isotopes but had little penetrative power; subsequently, various machines were developed which accelerated atomic particles, thereby giving them the energies for penetrating deeply (Stewart & Hawcroft, 1977; Phillips, 1987; Gardner & Peel, 1991; Silverman, 1991).

The energy of all these ionizing radiations is expressed as electron volts (eV). This is defined as the energy gained by an electron moving through a potential difference of 1 volt.

The energy absorbed, i.e. the absorbed dose, is measured by the unit gray (Gy), which is defined as 1 joule (J) of energy absorbed per kilogram of material irradiated. The original unit was the rad; this is still sometimes used and will certainly be found in older books and papers. The rad was defined as 100 erg of energy absorbed per gram of material irradiated, i.e. 10^{-2} J/kg. Thus, 1 Gy = 100 rad, or 25 kGy = 2.5 Mrad, the usual sterilizing dose (see Section 6).

3 Radiation sources

Radiation sterilization has been used commercially for more than 40 years (Artandi & Van Winkle, 1959). The basic physical and chemical processes by which ionizing radiation interacts with matter are complex and have been reviewed by Wilski (1987, 1990). The earliest industrial-scale radiation sterilizers in the USA used electron accelerators to sterilize sutures, whereas in the UK, Australia and France processing with radioisotopes commenced in the early 1960s (Herring &

Saylor, 1993). The source of γ-rays in these countries was ^{60}Co (Beers, 1990).

Only ^{137}Cs and ^{60}Co have met the criteria laid down by Herring & Saylor (1993) and been found to be suitable for sterilization by γ-rays. These criteria are: (i) availability of γ-emitting isotopes in large quantity; (ii) provision of γ-ray emission with sufficient energy to penetrate deeply; and (iii) possessing the property to have a half-life ($t_{1/2}$) sufficiently long to maintain a reasonably steady processing rate. All γ-irradiators have a radiation shield, a radioisotope source, a shield for the source and a product-conveying system, whereby products to be sterilized are exposed to the source.

High-energy electrons, like γ-rays and X-rays, have energies above 10^6MeV and can penetrate sufficiently into products for sterilization to be produced. Accelerators can provide intense electron beams, which are used for sterilization purposes as well as having other industrial uses (Cleland *et al.*, 1993). High-intensity electron beams provide short exposure times, with minimal degradation of product materials, but the dose distribution is less uniform than with γ-rays (Cleland *et al.*, 1993).

4 Radiation sensitivity and resistance of microorganisms

4.1 General aspects

Bacterial spores are generally the most resistant bacterial types to radiation, although *Deinococcus radiodurans* is the most resistant organism known (Moseley, 1989), other than prions (see Chapter 7). Among the clostridial spores, *Clostridium botulinum* types A and B are the most resistant, with type E being highly sensitive. Among *Bacillus* spp., *B. pumilus* E601 is probably the most resistant (Table 20.2; Russell, 1998).

In general, multicellular organisms are more sensitive to radiation than are unicellular organisms. Gram-negative bacteria are more sensitive than Gram-positive ones. The most radiation-resistant fungi are about as resistant as those bacterial spores having moderate radiation resistance, and the viruses in general are more resistant than bacteria. Some viruses are among the living systems with the highest radiation resistance known (for detailed information for special purposes, see the International Atomic Energy Agency's (IAEA's) *Manual on Radiation Sterilization*, 1973, see also Table 20.2).

Microorganisms with a low resistance will not survive an exposure to a dose of radiation efficient enough to have a measurable influence on a very resistant microorganism, even when the number of sensitive cells is high. It must, however, be noted that enzymes, pyrogens, toxins and antigens of microbial origin are in general very radiation-resistant, compared with living cells. Therefore, the number of microorganisms present prior to a radiation sterilization is of importance when dealing with medical products, regardless of the radiation resistance of the contaminating population (Christensen *et al.*, 1992).

4.2 Dose–response aspects

Various types of dose–response curves are obtained when microorganisms are exposed to ionizing

Table 20.2 Relative sensitivities of microorganisms to ionizing radiation (based on Thornley, 1963; Russell, 1982; Phillips, 1987; Gardner & Peel, 1991; Farkas, 1994).

Radiation response	Examples
Sensitive	Non-sporulating bacteria, especially *Pseudomonas aeruginosa*, *Salmonella* spp.; *Sarcina lutea* and *Streptococcus pygenes* rather more resistant
Moderately resistant	Moulds and yeasts
Resistant	Bacterial spores *Deinobacter* spp. Most viruses *Enterococcus faecium* (dried from serum broth)
Highly resistant	*Deinococcus radiodurans* Foot-and-mouth disease virus

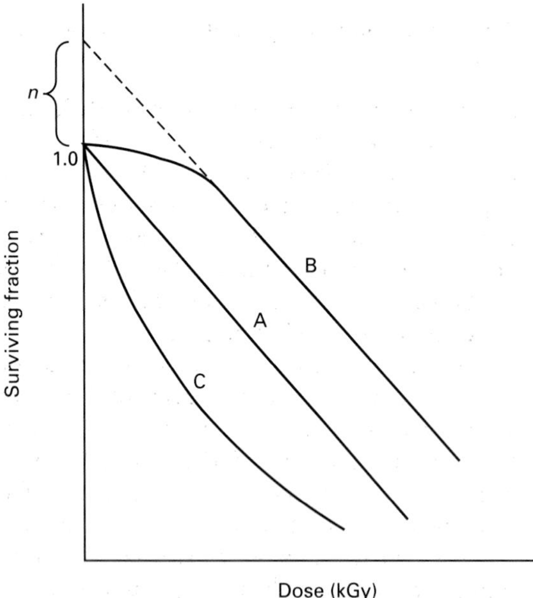

Fig. 20.1 Types (A,B,C) of inactivation curves. n, Extrapolation number.

radiations (Fig. 20.1A–C). In Fig. 20.1, curve A represents a straight-line or exponential rate of inactivation, which has been found with certain types of spores and with several types of non-sporulating bacteria (Thornley, 1963; Goldblith, 1971; Russell, 1982; Silverman, 1991; Christensen *et al.*, 1992).

Mathematically, this type A curve can be represented by the equation

$$N_t/N_0 = e^{-kD} \tag{20.1}$$

in which N_0 and N_t are the numbers of viable cells at time zero and t, respectively, i.e. the surviving fraction after an absorbed dose of radiation D, and k is the inactivation rate constant.

A more usual type of response is depicted in Fig. 20.1B, in which an initial shoulder on the curve is followed by an exponential death rate. This pattern is found with various types of spores and with *D. radiodurans* and, under certain conditions, with *Enterococcus faecium* (Christensen & Kjems, 1965; Bridges, 1976; Moseley & Williams, 1977; Russell, 1982; Moseley, 1984; Gardner & Peel, 1991; Silverman, 1991; Christensen *et al.*, 1992).

Mathematically, the type B can be represented by the following equation (20.2), which is derived on the basis that a single hit is necessary on more than one target to achieve cell inactivation (see also Section 5.2)

$$N_t/N_0 = 1-(1-e^{kD})^n \tag{20.2}$$

where n is the number of targets. Below a surviving fraction of 0.1, this equation approximates closely to

$$N_t/N_0 = ne^{-kD} \tag{20.3}$$

or

$$\log (N_t/N_0) = \log n - kD/2.303 \tag{20.4}$$

in which n represents the intercept with the log N_t/N_0 axis of the extrapolated linear portion of the survivor curve (Soper & Davies, 1990; Fig. 20.1). Equations have also been derived on the basis that more than one hit, i.e. multihits, on a single susceptible target is necessary to achieve cell inactivation (Grecz, 1965; Soper & Davies, 1990).

The response depicted in Fig. 20.1C, in which an exponential rate of kill is followed by a decreasing rate of spore inactivation, is encountered less frequently, although such 'tailing-off' phenomena have been observed for sporing and non-sporulating bacteria (Russell, 1982). The reasons for such an effect are unknown, but it may result from the production of radiation-resistant mutants or from non-homogeneous resistance in the microbial population. For practical sterilization purposes, the type C response is considered to be atypical.

4.3 Terminology

The D-value, usually expressed in kGy, is the dose necessary to reduce the initial microbial population by 90%, i.e. to 10%. The D-value can be read directly from the dose–survival curve, but where an initial shoulder occurs (Fig. 20.1, curve B) the D-value is calculated from the exponential part of the graph, together with the extrapolation number (n-value).

The D-value can also be obtained from the following equation:

$$D\text{-value} = \text{radiation dose}/\log N_0 - \log N \tag{20.5}$$

where N_0 and N represent a 1–log difference in viable numbers.

D-values differ greatly among different types of microorganisms (Russell, 1982), with occasionally considerable variation among different strains of the same organism. Radiation response also depends upon external conditions (see Section 4.4).

The D_{37}–value is the dose of radiation which reduces the microbial population to 37% of its original value; 0.5 is the logarithm (base 10) corresponding to 37% of survival. The term is thus based on the halfway point (0.5) of the $\log_{10}$ scale.

The inactivation factor (IF) is defined as the initial number of viable cells divided by the final number. It can also be calculated from the following equation:

$$\text{IF} = \text{radiation dose}/D\text{-value} \quad (20.6)$$

Finally, the degree of sterility can be calculated from

$$\text{IF/average number of organisms per article sterilized} \quad (20.7)$$

4.4 Factors influencing sensitivity of irradiated spores

Several factors, summarized in Table 20.3, affect the sensitivity of bacterial spores, and of other organisms, to ionizing radiation. One of the most important factors is the inoculum size, since the choice of sterilizing dose (see Section 6) is based upon a knowledge of the numbers of organisms (bioburden) present on items before they are subjected to the sterilization process.

The preirradiation treatment is also important, and organisms (especially *E. faecium*) dried from serum broth are much more resistant to radiation (Christensen & Kjems, 1965), a factor of some importance in Scandinavian countries when choosing a suitable sterilization dose (Section 6).

Spores under anoxic conditions are more resistant to radiation than are spores irradiated in the presence of oxygen or air (Tables 20.3 and 20.4). Since irradiation is carried out under the latter conditions, then this problem is negated. The

Table 20.3 Factors affecting the sensitivity of irradiated bacterial spores (based on Russell, 1982, 1998, and Farkas, 1994).

Parameter	Effect
Inoculum size	The higher the initial population, the greater is the radiation dose needed to inactivate
Type and strain of organism	Differences within *Bacillus* spp. (*B. pumilus* E601 is most resistant) and *Clostridium* spp. (*Cl. botulinum* types A and B are most resistant)
Preirradiation treatment	
Freeze-drying from sugars	Radioprotective effect may occur due to presence of a 'glass'
Drying in various media	Greatest resistance after suspension and drying in serum broth
Oxygen effect	Effects on spores of gaseous environment during and after radiation are complex (see text and Table 20.4)
Environment	
Suspending medium	Generally, spores more sensitive when irradiated in phosphate buffer than in various foodstuffs
pH of suspending medium	Possibly, little effect (except below 5.0)
Additives	Radiation sensitivity may be increased or decreased (see Tables 20.4 and 20.8)
Temperature	Effects are complex and occasionally paradoxical (see Table 20.8)

Table 20.4 Effects of 'additives' on the efficacy of ionizing radiation.

Presence of	Response to radiation
Antimicrobial agents	
Nisin or tylosin	Increased sensitivity
Sodium chloride, sodium nitrate, sodium nitrite, EDTA	Increased sensitivity
Sensitizers and protectors	
Oxygen during or after radiation	Increased sensitivity
Ketonic agents of differing electron affinities*	Increased sensitivity
Ketonic agent plus •OH scavenger (tertiary butanol)*	Maximum amount of sensitization almost eliminated
Hydrogen peroxide	Increased sensitivity
Nitrous oxide	Radiosensitization
Nitrous oxide plus tertiary butanol	Complete reversal of radiosensitization

*See Tallentire & Jacobs (1972).
EDTA, ethylenediamine tetraacetic acid.

'oxygen effect' is itself complex and three categories of mechanisms (reviewed by Russell, 1982) leading to lethal damage in the standard air-dried spore have been summarized as: (i) oxygen-independent, temperature-independent, occurring during irradiation in nitrogen; (ii) oxygen-dependent, temperature-dependent, involving very short-lived chemical species; and (iii) oxygen-dependent, involving long-lived free radicals.

Temperature can affect radiation (see Section 8), as can the presence of additives in the form of antimicrobial agents (Table 20.4; Section 8) and other chemicals, where radiosensitization may occur (Table 20.4). Ketonic agents (acetone, acetophenone and *p*-nitroacetophenone (PNAP)) sensitize spores in anoxic buffer suspension to subsequent radiation (reviewed by Russell, 1982). Hydroxyl radical (•OH) scavengers, such as tertiary butanol, greatly reduce this sensitization.

5 Mechanisms of lethal action

5.1 Microbial target site

The major target site in microorganisms that is susceptible to ionizing radiation is deoxyribonucleic acid (DNA). Evidence for this has come from two sources: first, substitution of thymine by 5-bromouracil sensitizes bacteria to radiation in proportion to the extent of substitution (Opara-Kubinska *et al.*, 1961); second, the isolation of mutants of wild-type bacteria that are more sensitive to radiation because they lack the ability to repair damage to DNA (Moseley & Williams, 1977; Moseley, 1984, 1989).

5.2 Target theory

With an exponential rate of microbial inactivation (Fig. 20.1, curve A), it is presumed that a single 'hit' on the sensitive target site, DNA, is responsible for cell death, whereas with survival curves of type B in Fig. 20.1, multihits on DNA are deemed to be necessary to inactivate DNA. However, this target theory does not take into account the fact that several bacteria possess the ability to repair damage to DNA (see Section 5.4) at lower doses of radiation (Moseley, 1984, 1989) and such repair may, in fact, account for the initial shoulder seen in type B dose–survivor curves.

5.3 Deoxyribonucleic acid damage

Ionizing radiations induce structural damage in microbial DNA, which, unless repaired, will inhibit DNA synthesis or cause some error in protein synthesis, leading to cell death (Hutchinson, 1985).

The primary event in ionizing radiation is the

ejection of an electron (leading to the production of a positively charged ion), with further chemical reactions taking place within cells, leading ultimately to their destruction. In the bacterial cell, ionizations occur principally in water, with the production of highly reactive, short-lived hydroxyl radicals (HO•). These cause breakage of phosphodiester bonds in DNA and hence single-strand breaks (SSB) or double-strand breaks (DSB). Damage to DNA sugar or to DNA bases may also occur, e.g. the production of 5,6-dihydroxythymine. These events are depicted in Figs 20.2 and 20.3, respectively; see also Table 20.5.

The state of DNA in microbial cells has an influence on sensitivity to radiation. As pointed out earlier, spores are generally more resistant to ionizing radiation than are non-sporulating bacteria. There are several possible reasons for this.

1 Bacterial spores contain a radioprotective substance, although there is no evidence to support this contention.

2 Spore coats confer protection to core DNA; however, coatless spores are no less resistant to radiation than 'normal' spores (Russell, 1998).

3 DNA exists in a different state in spores. In spores, DNA is in the A-form, associated with a low water activity (A_w) value, and it is true that DNA in the intact spore is more resistant to SSB or DSB than is DNA in the intact cell. However, DNA extracted from spores shows the same response *in vitro* to ionizing radiation as DNA extracted from non-sporulating bacteria. Additionally, newly germinated spores exposed to ionizing radiation in a high-osmotic-pressure environment (high sucrose but not high glycerol concentrations) again become heat- and radiation-resistant (Gould, 1984, 1989).

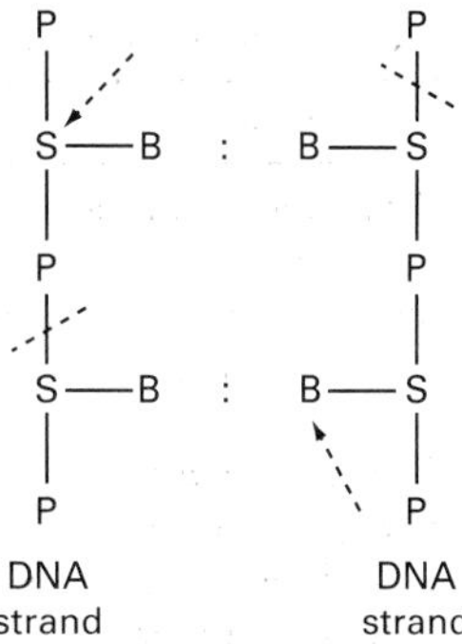

Fig. 20.2 Effects of ionizing radiation on microbial DNA. Dotted arrows or lines signify DNA strand breakage (single-strand breaks, SSB; double-strand breaks, DSB) or base damage. S, sugar; B, base; P, phosphate.

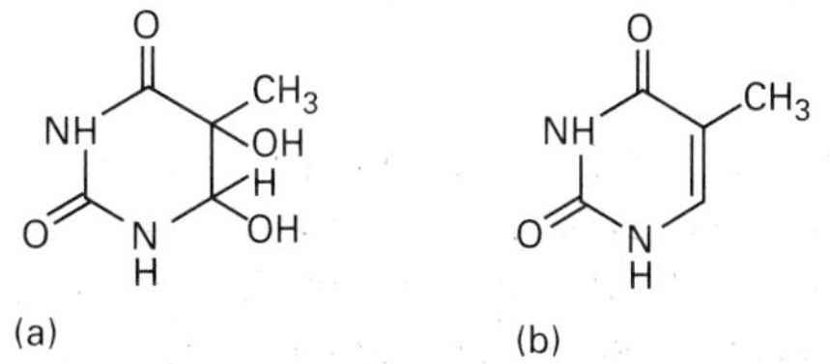

Fig. 20.3 Formation of (a) 5,6-dihydroxy-5,6-dihydrothymine from (b) thymine.

About 20% of the protein in the dormant spore is in the form of a group of small acid-soluble proteins (SASPs; Setlow, 1994). These exist as two types, namely α, β-types, associated with spore DNA, and γ-type, not associated with any macromolecule. During germination, these proteins are rapidly degraded. The α/β-types have some role to play in conferring heat resistance and appear to be

Table 20.5 Mechanisms of damage induced by ionizing radiation in microorganisms.

Type of organism	Damage
Non-sporulating bacteria	DNA: SSB, DSB, base or sugar damage (see Figs 20.2 and 20.3)
Bacterial spores	Loss of dipicolinic acid (DPA), but only after significant lethal effect Loss of optical density DNA: SSB and DSB occur, but DNA more resistant than DNA in non-sporulating bacteria

essential for spore UV resistance, but neither α/β nor γ-type SASPs are involved in γ-radiation resistance (Setlow, 1994).

Double-strand breaks are more lethal than SSB and are more difficult for a cell to repair. Although several radiolysis products of pyrimidines have been detected, the major one was described above (Fig. 20.3) and was first detected in radiation-exposed *D. radiodurans* (Hariharan & Cerutti, 1972).

5.4 Deoxyribonucleic acid repair

Deoxyribonucleic acid repair will be considered first in non-sporulating bacteria and then in bacterial spores (Table 20.6).

5.4.1 *Non-sporulating bacteria*

Several *Escherichia coli* mutants, with increased sensitivity to ionizing radiation, have been useful in studies of repair of SSB in DNA (Lindahl, 1982; Moseley, 1984, 1989; Sancar & Sancar, 1988; Nickoloff & Hoekstra, 1997). Two major pathways for enzymic repair are known. The first, a fast, growth-medium-independent pathway, requires DNA polymerase I, the product of the *polA* gene, since *polA* mutants are more radiation-sensitive than wild-type *E. coli*. In the second pathway, a slow, growth-medium-dependent repair, involving recombination, occurs only under conditions permitting bacterial growth; *recA*, *recB* and *recC* gene products are all required.

Double-stranded breaks are, of course, more difficult to repair. Very few DSB are tolerated in organisms such as *E. coli*, but they are much more likely to occur in radiation-resistant bacteria, such as *D. radiodurans* (Table 20.6), with recombination being involved in the repair of a multiplicity of DSB.

5.4.2 *Bacterial spores*

Farkas (1994) has pointed out that repair enzymes may be present in an inactive state in dormant spores, being activated during germination. Furthermore, Durban *et al.* (1974) observed that rejoining of SSB in DNA occurred under anaerobic conditions during or immediately after irradiation in radiation-resistant but not radiation-sensitive spores of *Cl. botulinum*.

Such repair mechanisms could have a major bearing on spore sensitivity, as exemplified by the dose–survivor responses depicted in Fig. 20.1.

Table 20.6 Repair of DNA damage in irradiated cells (based on Russell, 1982, and Moseley, 1984, 1989).

Organism(s)	Examples of repair mechanisms†
Non-sporulating bacteria	
Escherichia coli	SSB repaired in radiation-resistant B/r strain but not in radiation-sensitive B_{s-1} strain (mutation in *lexA* gene responsible for inability to repair)
	polA mutants: more sensitive than wild-type strain, DNA polymerase I involved in repair of SSB
	recA, *recB* and *recC* mutants: corresponding gene products all required in repair of SSB
Deinococcus radiodurans	Recombination may lead to repair of DSB
	Removal of damaged bases by exonuclease activity of DNA polymerase I
Bacterial spores	Repair of SSB during postirradiation germination
	In radiation-resistant (but not radiation-sensitive) *Cl. botulinum*, rejoining of DNA SSB under anaerobic conditions during or immediately after irradiation

6 Choice of radiation dose

The Medical Devices Directorate (1993) states that the delivery of a radiation dose in excess of 25 kGy (2.5 Mrad) is accepted as providing adequate assurance of sterility. The dose of 25 kGy is based upon a consideration of the radiation resistance of microorganisms. Soper & Davies (1990), for example, calculate that a dose of 18 kGy is necessary to achieve an IF of 10^6 against *B. pumilus* NCIB 8982 (ATCC 14884), the reference strain, so that 25 kGy would be a safe, effective dose in practice.

One of the factors influencing radiation efficacy is inoculum size (see Table 20.3), i.e. the number of organisms, or bioburden, present on a product before irradiation. Clearly, the lower the bioburden, the more effective the process. Gardner & Peel (1991) point out that a dose of 25 kGy would be sufficient provided that the bioburden does not exceed 100 microorganisms per item and that the organisms are not more resistant than *B. pumilus* (*D*-value here and in the example above 3 kGy under anoxic conditions, so that approximately an $8 \times D$ reduction would be obtained.)

Some Scandinavian countries recommend a dose of up to 45 kGy (4.5 Mrad), which is much higher than the dose of 25 kGy used in the UK, the USA and many other countries. One of the reasons for the choice of this higher sterilization dose has been the isolation in those countries of organisms with above-average resistance, including *E. faecium*, although this is resistant only under specialized conditions, i.e. when dried from serum broth (Christensen & Kjems, 1965), as well as organisms isolated from dust samples (Christensen, 1977).

In practice, a dose of 25 kGy has been found to be perfectly acceptable, although Hansen (1993) has noted that there are products that require a dose in excess of 25 kGy to achieve a sterility assurance level (SAL) of 10^{-6}. She adds that the use of 25 kGy as an overkill dose is no longer acceptable without validation to prove the achievement of the desired SAL. Hanson (1993) drew attention to the dose-setting methods proposed by the Association for the Advancement of Medical Instrumentation (AAMI) in the USA, which are also considered by Bruch (1993).

Whitby (1979, 1991) comments that the AAMI methods were developed to provide a means to extrapolate from the behaviour of a microbial population that yields a 10^{-2} SAL to a 10^{-6} SAL. These were based, at least in part, on the studies of Tallentire and his colleagues (Tallentire *et al.*, 1971; Tallentire, 1973; Khan *et al.*, 1977), who employed sterility tests to devices subjected to incremental doses of radiation. Whitby (1991) observed that a flexible radiation-dosing system could be adopted to produce reasonable assurance that desired standards were met. Under some conditions, sterilization doses below 25 kGy are feasible, based upon low presterilization microbial contamination. Such dose-setting methods have not been universally accepted (Dewhurst & Hoxey, 1990).

It is imperative that the radiation dose chosen has no harmful effect on the product (USP, 1995). Ishigaki *et al.* (1991) have discussed the effects of radiation on polymeric materials.

7 Control procedures

Biological indicators (BIs; bioindicators) are preparations of microorganisms selected for their above-average resistance to a particular process and thus employed to validate that process (Haberer & Wallhaeusser, 1990). Suitable BIs are available for validating steam sterilizers, dry-heat sterilization and gaseous sterilization. For ionizing radiation, *B. pumilus* has been recommended as the reference organism, although certain other microorganisms are known to be more resistant (Section 4). The choice of *B. pumilus* for validating ionizing radiation sterilization has been discussed by Graham (1991) and Graham & Boris (1993), and the choice of a suitable sterilization dose was considered in Section 6. Validation based upon the dose-setting methods recommended by the AAMI involve an evaluation of the resistance of naturally occurring microorganisms on the product when exposed to a series of subprocess doses of radiation (Bruch, 1993).

Biological indicators are not used for routine monitoring of ionizing radiation. The control of the irradiation plant must ensure that the recommended dose is delivered to all points within the product being sterilized (Medical Devices Directorate, 1993). The UK Panel on Gamma and Electron Irradiation (1989) provides full details of dose-monitoring systems. Radiation is accurately monitored by exposure of dosimeters within the load (Dewhurst & Hoxey, 1990; Haberer & Wallhaeusser, 1990).

8 Uses of ionizing radiation

The major uses of ionizing radiation are for the sterilization of thermolabile medical items, as demonstrated in Table 20.7. Radiation sterilization has thus proved to be an invaluable industrial procedure. However, it must be pointed out that deleterious changes may occur in irradiated products, especially preparations in aqueous solutions. Here, radiolysis of water contributes to the damage. Glass or plastic, such as polypropylene, can also be damaged. For these reasons, radiation sterilization is usually reserved for articles in the dried state.

The use of radiations for sterilizing foodstuffs remains a contentious issue. In the early 1980s, the World Health Organization (WHO) and the Food and Agriculture Organization (FAO) approved the use of radiation for treatment of food with doses lower than an average 10 kGy (WHO, 1981; FAO and WHO, 1984). This official international recognition caused renewed interest in the method (IAEA, 1989). Decontamination of most food products for human consumption by means of radiation must obviously be combined with efficient precautions against recontamination and against growth of surviving organisms, if the method is to find general application (Christensen *et al.*, 1992). Of other procedures of practical value, decontami-

Table 20.7 Actual and potential uses of radiation-sterilization procedures.

Type of product	Comment
Medical and pharmaceutical	Ionizing radiation suitable for Disposable syringes Sutures Some types of powders Adhesive and other dressings Intravenous infusion sets
Foodstuffs	Ionizing radiation currently forbidden, but regulations may be relaxed at some point in future

Table 20.8 Synergistic sterilization methods involving ionizing radiation.

Process*	Result
Aseptic process plus low-dose γ-irradiation (TPN solutions irradiated at different doses)	As low a dose as 1.5 kGy improved SALs from 10^{-3} to $<10^{-9}$
Radiation plus salts	Radiation dose required to inactivate *Cl. botulinum* reduced
Preheating plus irradiation	Little effect on radiation response
Preirradiation plus heating	Possible effect: sensitization to heat
Thermoradiation (simultaneous heat and irradiation)	Radiation sensitivity† of *Cl. botulinum* type A increases with rise in temperature in range −50°C to +30°C; between 30 and 80°C, increase in radioresistance (thermorestoration) Synergy noted with ionizing radiation plus dry heat

*Based in part on Olson (1997) and Russell *et al.* (1997).
†Not all authors agree with these findings and thermorestoration is not always found: see Russell (1982).
TPN, total parenteral nutrition.

nation of spices by radiation, as a substitute for decontamination by toxic gases, and the sterilization or decontamination of food for laboratory animals can be mentioned. Summaries on radiation microbiology relative to food irradiation have been published by Josephson & Peterson (1982, 1983).

Finally, the possibility of using ionizing radiation in combination with other procedures must be mentioned. Examples are provided in Table 20.8, from which it can be seen that radiation doses may be decreased in certain circumstances.

9 Conclusions

Ionizing radiation has been shown, over several decades, to be a safe and effective process for sterilizing various types of medical and pharmaceutical devices. Although some organisms, e.g. *D. radiodurans* (by virtue of an efficient repair mechanism), are more resistant than others, this has not been found to be a problem in practice.

The sterilization procedure and sterilizing dose can be monitored accurately by appropriate physical methods. Microbial inactivation is brought about by SSB and, especially, DSB in DNA, although DNA base and sugar damage contributes to the lethal effects.

Irradiation of foodstuffs has met with much public resistance but may be accepted in due course.

10 References

Artandi, C. & Van Winkle, W. (1959) Electron-beam sterilization of surgical sutures. *Nucleonics*, **17**, 86–90.

Beers, E. (1990) Innovations in irradiator design. *Radiation Physics and Chemistry*, **35**, 539–546.

Bridges, B.A. (1976) Survival of bacteria following exposure to ultraviolet and ionising radiation. In *The Survival of Vegetative Microbes* (eds Gray, T.R.G. & Postgate, J.R.), pp. 183–208. Cambridge: Cambridge University Press.

British Pharmacopoeia (BP) (1993) Methods of sterilisation. Vol. II, A264–A253. London: HMSO.

Bruch, C.W. (1993) The philosophy of sterilization validation. In *Sterilization Technology* (eds Morrissey, R.F. & Phillips, G.B.), pp. 17–35. New York: Van Nostrand Reinhold.

Christensen, E.A. (1977) The role of microbiology in commissioning a new facility and in routine control. In *Sterilization by Ionizing Radiation* (eds Gaughran, E.R.L. & Goudie, A.J.), Vol. II, pp. 50–64. Montreal, Quebec, Canada: Multiscience Publishers.

Christensen, E.A. & Kjems, E. (1965) The radiation resistance of substrains from *Streptococcus faecium* selected after irradiation of two different strains. *Acta Pathologica et Microbiologica Scandinavica B*, **63**, 281–290.

Christensen, E.A., Kristensen, H. & Miller, A. (1992) Radiation sterilization. A. Ionizing radiation. In *Principles and Practice of Disinfection, Preservation and Sterilization* (eds Russell, A.D., Hugo, W.B. & Ayliffe, G.A.J.), 2nd edn, pp. 528–543. Oxford: Blackwell Scientific Publications.

Cleland, M.R., O'Neill, M.T. & Thompson, C.C. (1993) Sterilization with accelerated electrons. In *Sterilization Technology* (eds Morrissey, R..F. & Phillips, G.B.) pp. 218–253. New York: Van Nostrand Reinhold.

Dewhurst, E. & Hoxey, E.V. (1990) Sterilization methods. In *Guide to Microbiological Control in Pharmaceuticals* (eds Denyer, S.P. & Baird, R.M.), pp. 182–218. Chichester: Ellis Horwood.

Durban, E., Grecz, N. & Farkas, J. (1974) Direct enzymatic repair of DNA single strand breaks in dormant spores. *Journal of Bacteriology*, **118**, 129–138.

European Pharmacopoeia (EP) (1997) Sterilization procedures. 3rd edn, pp. 283–288. Strasburg: Council of Europe.

FAO and WHO (1984) Codex general standard for irradiated foods and recommended international code of practice for the operation of radiation facilities used for the treatment of goods. *Codex Alimentarius Commission*, Vol. XV, 1st ed. Rome: FAO, WHO.

Farkas, J. (1994) Tolerance of spores to ionizing radiation: mechanisms of inactivation, injury and repair. *Journal of Applied Bacteriology, Symposium Supplement*, **76**, 81S–90S.

Gardner, J.F. & Peel, M.M. (1991) *Introduction to Sterilization, Disinfection and Infection Control*, 2nd edn. Edinburgh: Churchill Livingstone.

Goldblith, S.A. (1971) The inhibition and destruction of the microbial cell by radiations. In *Inhibition and Destruction of the Microbial Cell* (ed. Hugo, W.B.), pp. 285–305. London: Academic Press.

Gould, G.W. (1984) Injury and repair mechanisms in bacterial spores. In *The Revival of Injured Microbes* (eds Andrew, M.H.E. & Russell, A.D.), Society for Applied Bacteriology Symposium Series No. 12, pp. 199–220. London: Academic Press.

Gould, G.W. (1989) Heat-induced injury and inactivation. In *Mechanisms of Action of Food Preservation Procedures* (ed. Gould, G.W.), pp. 11–42. London: Elsevier Applied Science.

Graham, G.S. (1991) Biological indicators for hospital and industrial sterilization. In *Sterilization of Medical*

Products (eds Morrissey, R.F. & Prokopenko, Y.I.), Vol. V, pp. 54–71. Morin Heights: Polyscience Publications.

Graham, G.S. & Boris, C.A. (1993) Chemical and biological indicators. In *Sterilization Technology* (eds Morrissey, R.F. & Phillips, G.B.), pp. 36–69. New York: Van Nostrand Reinhold.

Grecz, N. (1965) Biophysical aspects of clostridia. *Journal of Applied Bacteriology*, **28**, 17–35.

Haberer, K. & Wallhaeusser, K.-H. (1990) Assurance of sterility by validation of the sterilization process. In *Guide to Microbiological Control in Pharmaceutical* (eds Denyer, S.P. & Baird, R.M.), pp. 219–240. Chichester: Ellis Horwood.

Hansen, J.M. (1993) AAMI dose setting: ten years experience. In *Sterilization of Medical Products* (ed. Morrissey, R.F.), Vol. VI, pp. 273–281. Morin Heights: Polyscience Publications.

Hariharan, P.V. & Cerutti, P.A. (1972) Formation and repair of γ-ray-induced thymine damage in *Micrococcus radiodurans*. *Journal of Molecular Biology*, **66**, 65–81.

Herring, C.M. & Saylor, M.C. (1993) Sterilization with radioisotopes. In *Sterilization Technology* (eds Morrissey, R.F. & Phillips, G.B.), pp. 196–217. New York: Van Nostrand Reinhold.

Hutchinson, F. (1985) Chemical changes induced in DNA by ionizing radiation. *Progress in Nucleic Acid Research and Molecular Biology*, **32**, 115–154.

IAEA (1973) *Manual on Radiation Sterilization of Medical and Biological Materials*. Technical Report Series No. 159. Vienna: IAEA.

IAEA (1989) *Acceptance, Control of and Trade in Irradiated Foods*. Conference Proceedings, Geneva, 1988. STI/PUB/788. Vienna: IAEA.

Ishigaki, I., Yoshii, F., Makuuchi, K. & Tamura, N. (1991) Radiation effects on polymeric materials. In *Sterilization of Medical Products* (eds Morrissey, R.F. & Prokopenko, Y.I.), Vol. V, pp. 308–321. Morin Heights: Polyscience Publications.

Josephson, E.S. & Peterson, M.S. (1983) *Preservation of Food by Ionizing Radiation*, Vols I, II & III. Florida: CRC press.

Khan, A.A., Tallentire, A. & Dwyer, J. (1977) Quality assurance of sterilized products: verification of a model relating frequency of contaminated items and increased radiation dose. *Journal of Applied Bacteriology*, **43**, 205–213.

Lindahl, T. (1982) DNA repair enzymes. *Ann. Rev. Biochem.*, **51**, 61–87.

Medical Devices Directorate (1993) *Sterilization, Disinfection and Cleaning of Medical Equipment*. London: HMSO.

Moseley, B.E.B. (1984) Radiation damage and its repair in non-sporulating bacteria. In *The Revival of Injured Microbes* (eds Andrew, M.H.E. & Russell, A.D.), Society for Applied Bacteriology Symposium Series No. 12, pp. 147–174. London: Academic Press.

Moseley, B.E.B. (1989) Ionizing radiation: action and repair. In *Mechanisms of Action of Food Preservation Procedures* (ed. Gould, G.W.), pp. 43–70. London: Elsevier Applied Science.

Moseley, B.E.B. & Williams, E. (1977) Repair of damaged DNA in bacteria. *Advances in Microbial Physiology*, **14**, 99–156.

Nickoloff, J.A. & Hoekstra, M.F. (1997) *DNA Damage and Repair*. Vol. I: *DNA Repair in Prokaryotes and Lower Eukaryotes*. Totowa, New Jersey: Humana Press.

Olson, W.P. (1997) Synergistic sterilization: a brief history. *PDA Journal of Pharmaceutical Science and Technology*, **51**, 116–118.

Opara-Kubinska, Z., Lorkiewicz, Z. & Szybalski, W. (1961) Genetic transformation studies. II. Radiation sensitivity of halogen-labelled DNA. *Biochemical and Biophysical Research Communications*, **4**, 288–292.

Phillips, J.E. (1987) Physical methods of veterinary disinfection and sterilization. In *Disinfection in Veterinary and Farm Animal Practice* (eds Linton, A.H., Hugo, W.B. & Russell, A.D.), pp. 117–143. Oxford: Blackwell Scientific Publications.

Rakitskaya, G.A., Samoilenko, I.I., Pavlov, Ye.P., Ramkova, N.V., Zykova, S.V. & Saribekian, V.V. (1991) Radioresistance of microorganisms: theoretical and practical aspects. In *Sterilization of Medical Products* (eds Morrissey, R.F. & Prokopenko, Y.I.), Vol. V, pp. 296–307. Morin Heights: Polyscience Publications.

Russell, A.D. (1982) *The Destruction of Bacterial Spores*. London: Academic Press.

Russell, A.D. (1991) Fundamental aspects of microbial resistance to chemical and physical agents. In *Sterilization of Medical Products* (eds Morrissey, R.F. & Prokopenko, Y.I.), Vol. V, pp. 22–42. Morin Heights: Polyscience Publications.

Russell, A.D. (1998) Microbial susceptibility and resistance to chemical and physical agents. In *Topley & Wilson's Microbiology and Microbial Infections*, 9th edn, Vol. 2 (eds Balows, A. & Duerden, B.I.), pp. 149–184. London: Arnold.

Russell, A.D., Furr, J.R. & Maillard, J.-Y. (1997) Synergistic sterilization. *PDA Journal of Pharmaceutical Science and Technology*, **51**, 174–175.

Sancar, A. & Sancar, G.B. (1988) DNA repair enzymes. *Annual Review of Biochemistry*, **57**, 29–67.

Setlow, P. (1994) Mechanisms which contribute to the long-term survival of spores of *Bacillus* species. *Journal of Applied Bacteriology, Symposium Supplement*, **76**, 49S–60S.

Silverman, G.J. (1991) Sterilization and preservation by ionizing radiation. In *Disinfection, Sterilization and*

Preservation (ed. Block, S.S.), 4th edn, pp. 566–579. Philadelphia: Lea & Febiger.

Soper, C.J. & Davies, D.J.G. (1990) Principles of sterilization. In *Guide to Microbiological Control in Pharmaceuticals* (eds Denyer, S.P. & Baird, R.M.), pp. 156–181. Chichester: Ellis Horwood.

Stewart, J.C. & Hawcroft, D.M. (1977) *A Manual of Radiobiology*. London: Sedgwick and Jackson.

Tallentire, A. (1973) Aspects of microbiological control of radiation sterilization. *International Journal of Radiation Sterilization*, **1**, 85–103.

Tallentire, A. & Jacobs, G.P. (1972) Radiosensitization of bacterial spores by ketonic agents of different electron affinities. *International Journal of Radiation Biology*, **21**, 205–213.

Tallentire, A., Dwyer, J. & Ley, F.J. (1971) Microbiological quality control of sterilized products: evaluation of a model relating the frequency of contaminated items with increasing radiation treatment. *Journal of Applied Bacteriology*, **34**, 521–534.

Thornley, M.J. (1963) Radiation resistance among bacteria. *Journal of Applied Bacteriology*, **26**, 334–345.

UK Panel on Gamma and Electron Irradiation (1989) Code of Practice for the validation and routine monitoring of sterilization by ionizing radiation. *Radiation Physics and Chemistry*, **33**, 245–249.

United States Pharmacopoeia (USP) (1995) Sterilization and sterility assurance of compendium articles. Vol. 23, pp. 1976–1981. Rockville, Maryland: USP Convention.

Whitby, J.L. (1979) Radiation resistance of microorganisms comprising the bioburden of operating room packs. *Radiation Physics and Chemistry*, **14**, 285–288.

Whitby, J.L. (1991) Resistance of microorganisms to radiation and experiences with dose setting. In *Sterilization of Medical Products* (eds Morrissey, R.F. & Prokopenko, Y.I.), Vol. V, pp. 344–352. Morin Heights: Polyscience Publications.

WHO (1981) *Wholesomeness of Irradiated Food*. Report of a joint FAO/IAEA/WHO Expert Committee, World Health Organization, Technical Report Series 659. WHO: Geneva.

Wilski, H. (1987) The radiation-induced degradation of polymers. *Radiation Physics and Chemistry*, **29**, 1–14.

Wilski, H. (1990) Radiation stability of polymers. *Radiation Physics and Chemistry*, **35**, 186–189.

B. ULTRAVIOLET RADIATION

1 Introduction

Ultraviolet (UV) radiation has a wavelength range between about 328 and 210 nm (3280 and 2100 Å). Its maximum bactericidal effect is listed as 240–280 nm (Sykes, 1965), 265 nm (Thimann, 1963; Morris, 1972; Schechmeister, 1983) and 254–280 nm (McCulloch, 1945). Modern mercury-vapour lamps emit more than 90% of their radiation at 253.7 nm (Morris, 1972), which is at, or near to, the maximum for microbicidal activity. The quantum of energy liberated is low, so that UV radiation has less penetrating ability and is less effective as a microbicidal agent than other radiations (Gardner & Peel, 1991; Russell, 1998).

There are several reviews dealing with the action and uses of UV radiation, notably those of Hollaender (1955), Roberts & Hitchins (1969), Smith & Hanawalt (1969), Witkin (1969, 1976), Russell (1971, 1982, 1990a,b, 1993), Morris (1972), Howard-Flanders (1973), Bridges (1976), Moseley & Williams (1977), Alper (1979), Gould (1983, 1984, 1985), Hanawalt *et al.* (1979), Harm (1980), Haseltine (1983), Schechmeister (1983); Moseley (1984), Phillips (1987), Thurman & Gerba (1988), Gardner & Peel (1991) and Setlow (1994). This chapter will compare the susceptibility of different types of microorganisms to UV radiation, examine the factors influencing these responses, discuss the theoretical aspects of inactivation and repair and finally consider the practical uses of UV light as a sterilizing or disinfecting agent. Additional information will be found in chapters dealing with viruses (Chapter 6), unconventional agents (Chapter 7) and protozoa (Chapter 8).

2 Survival curves

Survival curves of bacteria or bacterial spores exposed to UV light are generally of two types.

1 A straight-line response (Fig. 20.4A), as noted with *Salmonella typhimurium* (Moseley & Laser, 1965), *Escherichia coli* B_{S-1} (Haynes, 1966) and the *E. coli* K12 strain AB2480 *uvr*$^-$ *rec*$^-$ (Tyrell *et al.*, 1972).

2 An initial shoulder, followed by exponential death (Fig. 20.4B), as found with vegetative cells (a very slight shoulder) and dormant spores (much

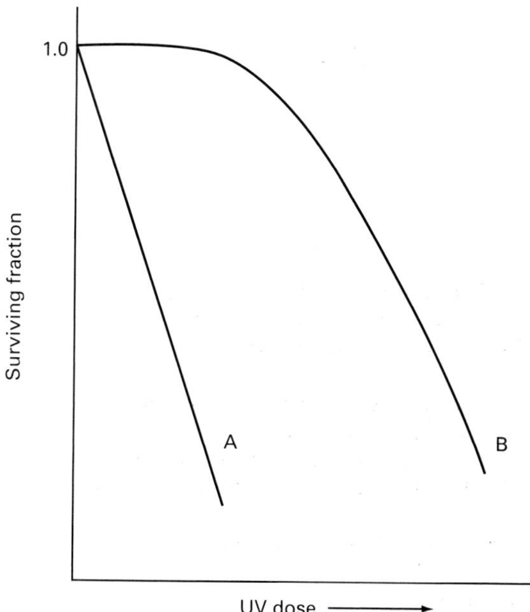

Fig. 20.4 Survival curves for UV-exposed bacteria. A: some non-sporulating bacteria (not *D. radiodurans*); B: bacterial spores and *D. radiodurans*.

greater initial shoulder) of *Bacillus megaterium* (Donnellan & Stafford, 1968). A large initial shoulder has also been noted for UV-irradiated *E. coli* B/r (Haynes, 1964, 1966), *E. coli* K12 strain, AB1157 *uvr*$^+$ *rec*$^+$ (Tyrrell *et al.*, 1972), *Staphylococcus aureus* and *Micrococcus lysodeikticus* (Haynes, 1964). The classic example, however, is undoubtedly *Deinococcus radiodurans*, which is highly resistant to both UV and ionizing radiations; survival curves for this organism against both types of radiation have large initial shoulders, wtih high extrapolation numbers (Moseley & Laser, 1965; Moseley, 1967). Organisms that are resistant to UV radiation may possess efficient repair processes and thus can survive quite high doses; see Section 3.8. Ability to repair UV-induced damage to deoxyribonucleic acid (DNA) is probably the single most important factor in determining microbial response to UV light.

3 Factors influencing activity of ultraviolet radiation

Ultraviolet radiation has several uses, but unfortunately is also subject to several limitations. It is important, therefore, to consider the various factors that affect its activity.

3.1 Type of organism

According to McCulloch (1945), Gram-negative rods are the most easily killed by UV light, followed (in this order) by staphylococci, streptococci and bacterial spores, with mould spores being the most resistant. This early classification is inevitably somewhat out of date, because it takes no account of viruses, protozoa and prions or of non-sporulating bacteria that possess the ability to repair UV-induced injury. *Legionella pneumophila* and other species of legionellae are very sensitive to low doses of UV light (Table 20.9).

Bacterial spores are generally more resistant to UV radiation than are vegetative cells (Sykes, 1965; Ashwood-Smith & Bridges, 1967; Russell,

Table 20.9 Relative resistances of microorganisms to ultraviolet radiation (based on Morris, 1972; Johansen & Myhrstad, 1978; Latarjet, 1979; Rice & Hoff, 1981; Gilpin, 1984; Chang *et al.*, 1985; Knudsen, 1985; Muraca *et al.*, 1985; Rodgers *et al.*, 1985; Committee, 1986; Farr *et al.*, 1988; Department of Health, 1989; Report, 1990).

Resistance level	Examples of microorganisms
High	Prions
	Deinococcus radiodurans
	Bacillus subtilis/*Bacillus globigii* spores*
	Sarcina lutea†
Intermediate	*M. sphaeroides*
	Salmonella typhimurium
	Saccharomyces spp.
	Streptococcus lactis
	Protozoa
Low	Legionellae
	HIV?
	Vaccinia virus
	Escherichia coli
	Staphylococcus aureus
	Proteus vulgaris
	Brewer's yeast
	T3 coliphage

**Bacillus pumilus* E601 (ATCC 27142) spores are considered to be highly UV-resistant and to be suitable organisms for monitoring the effectiveness of UV radiation (Abshire *et al.*, 1980).

†High resistance is possibly the result of a screening effect produced by cell aggregates.

1982, 1998), although the degree of sporulation can influence the sensitivity (Section 5).

Viruses are also inactivated by UV light (Morris & Darlow, 1971); they are less resistant than bacterial spores but are often more resistant than non-sporulating bacteria (Morris, 1972). Ultraviolet radiation at doses below 5×10^3 J/m^2 may not eliminate all infectious human immunodeficiency virus (HIV; Report, 1990). Unenveloped animal viruses are more resistant to UV light than enveloped ones (Watanabe *et al.*, 1989), but conventional virus types are considerably more susceptible than the unconventional or so-called slow viruses, the prions. Creutzfeldt–Jakob disease (CJD) agent is highly resistant to UV radiation (Committee, 1986; Rappaport, 1987); the agents of kuru and scrapie are likewise insusceptible (Latarjet, 1979). Morphological changes induced in human rotaviruses have been described (Rodgers *et al.*, 1985).

Protozoa such as *Giardia lamblia* cysts are more UV-resistant than non-sporulating bacteria (Rice & Hoff, 1981).

Examples of relative susceptibilities to UV radiation are provided in Table 20.9.

3.2 Inoculum size

As would be expected, the greater the inoculum size, the greater is the UV dose necessary to effect an equivalent lethality (Morris, 1972).

3.3 Stage of growth or germination

Tyrrell *et al.* (1972) investigated the variation in UV sensitivity of four K12 strains (AB2480 *uvr*$^-$ *rec*$^-$, AB1886 *uvr*$^-$ *rec*$^-$, AB2463 *uvr*$^+$ *rec*$^-$ and AB1157 *uvr*$^+$ *rec*$^+$) of *E. coli* as a function of their growth phase. The smallest changes in sensitivity were found in the double mutant, the excision-deficient and recombination-deficient AB2480 *uvr*$^-$ *rec*$^-$, and in the excision-deficient mutant AB1886 *uvr*$^-$ *rec*$^+$. With the recombination-deficient mutant, AB2463 *uvr*$^+$ *rec*$^-$, UV sensitivity increased during the early exponential growth phase, and decreased after 5 h. With the mutant (AB115 *uvr*$^+$ *rec*$^+$) possessing the full complement of repair genes, a sharp decrease in UV sensitivity was observed in the early exponential phase, followed by a large increase and later a decrease.

At certain times in their germination, spores of *Bacillus cereus* (Stuy, 1956), *Bacillus subtilis* (Irie *et al.*, 1965; Donnellan & Stafford, 1968; Stafford & Donnellan, 1968) and *B. megaterium* (Donnellan & Stafford, 1968; Stafford & Donnellan, 1968) become much more resistant to UV radiation. This phase is followed by one in which the sensitivity to UV light of the germinating spores increases, and eventually these forms become more sensitive than the dormant spores. The possible reasons for this phenomenon are discussed later (Section 5).

3.4 Type of suspension

Bacillus subtilis spores are more resistant to UV radiation when tested in the form of a 'dust suspension' than when they are exposed as an aerosol (Sykes, 1965). Likewise, a small but significant increase in UV irradiation is required for a 90% or 98% disinfection level of dried droplets, as opposed to wet droplets, of *Bacillus globigii* spores and of non-sporulating organisms (Morris, 1972).

3.5 Effect of organic matter

Morris (1972) has shown that the presence of peptone, egg, milk and especially blood and serum means that the UV dose required for 90% inactivation of *Serratia marcescens* increased markedly when compared with buffer suspensions of this organism. Thus, surfaces infected with these fluids would need greater UV irradiation to ensure disinfection.

3.6 Effect of temperature

Most organisms (a notable exception is *D. radiodurans*) appear to be supersensitive to UV radiation at low temperatures (Ashwood-Smith & Bridges, 1967; Bridges *et al.*, 1967), although this increase in sensitivity occurs only when the bacteria are frozen; under such conditions the number of thymine dimers (Fig. 20.5) is reduced considerably. Another thymine-containing photoproduct accumulates, which appears to be less susceptible to repair by the bacterial cell (see Sections 3.8, 4.1, 4.2 and 4.3).

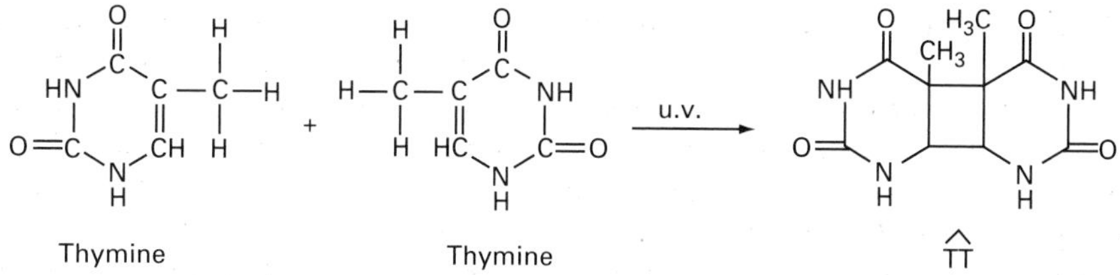

Fig. 20.5 Formation of thymine dimer (TT) in UV-irradiated DNA.

3.7 Wavelength of ultraviolet radiation

Ultraviolet lamps are normally employed at 253.7 nm. There is, however, a peak of activity at 250–280 nm, with negligible activity above a wavelength of 300 nm (Setlow & Boling, 1965).

3.8 Repair processes

Many bacterial species can, under appropriate conditions, repair the damage induced by UV radiation. The repair processes involve light repair (photoreactivation) and dark repair (excision and recombination), and organisms capable of repairing damage are obviously likely to be more resistant to UV radiation than those that lack these repair systems. The isolation of mutants that are defective in one or more of these systems has been responsible for a much better understanding of the nature of UV-induced damage at the molecular level and of the ways in which organisms achieve repair. These aspects are considered in more detail later (Sections 4.2 and 4.3).

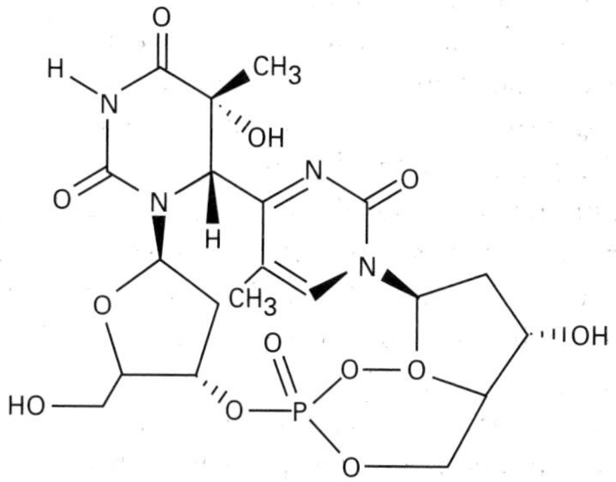

Fig. 20.6 Pyrimidine-(6-4)-pyrimidone photoproduct.

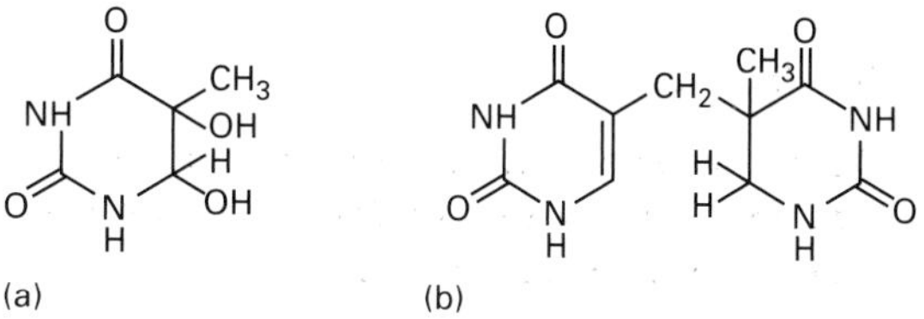

Fig. 20.7 (a) 5,6-Dihydroxydihydrothymine; (b) 5-thyminyl-5,6-dihydrothymine (TDHT).

4 Effect of ultraviolet radiation on non-sporulating bacteria

4.1 Target site and inactivation

The major target site for UV radiation is undoubtedly DNA. Several types of damage have been found to occur in UV-treated bacteria; low numbers of phosphodiester strand breaks and DNA intrastrand cross-links occur at high UV doses. Nucleic acid–protein cross-links are also induced, but their significance in microbial inactivation is uncertain. The most important event is the accumulation of photoproducts (Bridges, 1976; Moseley, 1984; Figs 20.5–20.7).

In vegetative bacteria and yeasts, purine and pyrimidine dimers are formed between adjacent molecules in the same strand of DNA. This is exemplified in Fig. 20.5 by the formation of thymine dimers (TT), the most widely studied phenomenon, in UV-irradiated DNA. Ultraviolet radiation is absorbed most strongly by nucleic acids, especially the wavelength (253.7 nm) which forms the output of most lamps (Bridges, 1976).

Another type of photoproduct (5,6-dihydroxydihydrothymine; Fig. 20.7a) is found in *D. radiodurans*. In bacterial spores, yet another photoproduct (5-thyminyl-5,6-dihydrothymine

(TDHT); Fig. 20.7b) is induced. This is considered in more detail later (Section 5).

Unless removed, these photoproducts form non-coding lesions in DNA and cell death occurs. In the frozen state, UV-treated non-sporulating bacteria accumulate a photoproduct (presumably TDHT; see Fig. 20.7b) which appears to be identical to that found in the DNA of UV-exposed bacterial spores. The photoproduct TDHT is not repairable in non-sporing organisms and, under such conditions, the cells are supersensitive to UV radiation. The yield of cyclobutane-type dimers is greatly reduced and photoreactivation (PR; see Section 4.3) is ineffective.

A less well-known and less frequent type of photoproduct is pyrimidine-(6–4)-pyrimidone ((6–4)PP; Fig. 20.6). This is the relevant lesion involved in the toxic and mutagenic effects of UV (Mitchell & Nairn, 1989; Koehler *et al.*, 1996).

4.2 Repair mechanisms

In *E. coli*, most of the inducible genes that code for DNA repair proteins belong to one of two major regulatory networks that are induced as a consequence of DNA injury. These are: (i) the SOS network, controlled by the RecA and LexA proteins; and (ii) the adaptive-response network, controlled by the Ada protein (Walker, 1985).

The SOS network controls the expression of genes whose products play roles in, for example, excision repair, daughter-strand gap repair and double-strand break repair. When *E. coli* is exposed to agents (UV and other) that damage DNA or interfere with DNA replication, a diverse set of physiological responses, the SOS responses, is induced. These include an increased capacity to reactivate UV-irradiated phage, the induction of mutations, filamentous growth and the increased capacity to repair double-strand breaks. The SOS responses pertinent to the repair of UV-induced injury are considered in Section 4.3.

The adaptive response network differs from the SOS. *Escherichia coli* cells exposed to low concentrations of methylating mutagens become resistant to the mutagenic and lethal effects of higher concentrations. This induced resistance results from the formation of a set of induced repair processes independent of the SOS network and controlled by production of the *ada* gene. Ultraviolet light and most of the other agents that induce an SOS response do not induce the adaptive response. For detailed information on revival and repair, see Andrew & Russell (1984).

Repair mechanisms in non-sporulating bacteria exposed to UV radiation are of three major types. These are: (i) light repair (PR), in which a photoreactivating enzyme (photolyase; Sancar & Sancar, 1988) becomes activated when UV-treated cells are exposed to light of a higher wavelength; (ii) dark repair (excision), in which the non-coding lesion is excised and replaced; and (iii) dark repair (postreplication recombination), which involves recombination between two sister DNA strands.

During the first 30 min following a moderate UV dose, (6–4)PP are removed at a higher rate than pyrimidine dimers by repair-proficient *E. coli* cells, but less rapidly than by cultured mammalian cells (Koehler *et al.*, 1996).

4.3 Radiation mutants of *Escherichia coli*

Several radiation-sensitive and resistant mutants of *E. coli* have been described over the years. The sensitive mutants have a block in one or more of the pathways involved in DNA repair. Some of the best-known types of these mutants are described briefly below.

1 The *phr* gene: *phr*$^-$ mutants lack the ability to photoreactivate, because the PR enzyme is absent. Kelner (1949a,b) found that the exposure of UV-irradiated *Streptomyces griseus* or *E. coli* to suitable visible light, below 510 nm, resulted in the recovery of a large portion of the cells from what would otherwise have been death. This phenomenon, PR, has since been defined (Jagger, 1958) as the reversal with near-UV or visible light of UV-radiation damage to a biological system, or as the restoration of UV-radiation lesions in a biological system with light of wavelength longer than that of the damaging radiation. The process of photoreactivation is depicted in Fig. 20.8, from which it can be seen (Fig. 20.8a) that the PR enzyme brings about a monomerization *in situ* of the thymine dimers, resulting in repair of the damage to DNA (Fig. 20.8b).

In *E. coli*, the DNA photolyase binds equally well to UV-irradiated supercoiled and relaxed,

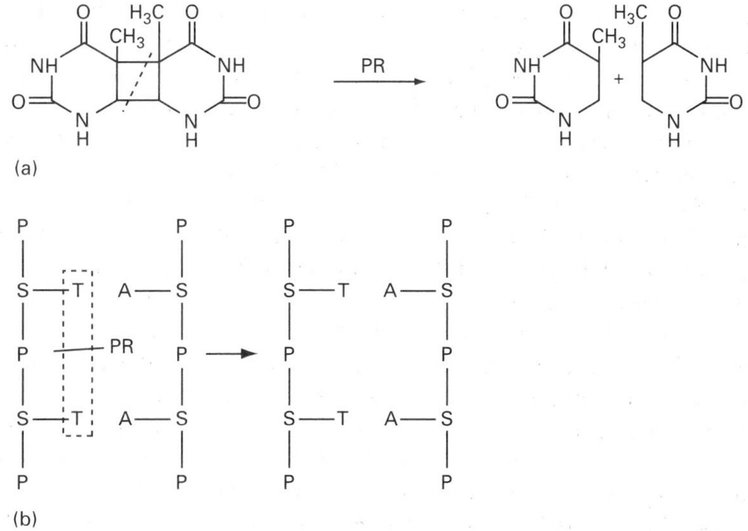

Fig. 20.8 Photoreactivation (PR) by photoreactivating enzyme: (a) monomerization of thymine dimer; (b) formation of TT in DNA and photoreversal. P, phosphate; S, sugar; T, thymine; A, adenine.

double-stranded DNA; the enzyme does not unwind the helix to a significant degree upon binding (Sancar & Sancar, 1988).

It must be added that there is a wide divergence among bacteria in their PR capability. Bacterial spores cannot be photoreactivated, whereas vegetative cells of bacilli can (Stuy, 1955). Sporulating cultures of *B. cereus* completely lose their PR ability at the same time as UV resistance increases (Romig & Wyss, 1957).

As pointed out in Section 4.1, bacteria in the frozen state are usually more sensitive to UV radiation, because of a reduction in the yield of cyclobutane-type pyrimidine dimers and the formation of TDHT, a photoproduct insusceptible to the action of DNA photolyase.

2 The *uvr* gene: mutants *uvrA*$^-$ and *uvrB*$^-$ lack the UV-specific endonuclease involved in dark repair and are unable to excise pyrimidine dimers from their DNA or from irradiated phage. They are thus unable to carry out host-cell reactivation of UV-irradiated phage and, in addition to being *uvr*$^-$ mutants, they are thus also termed *Hcr*$^-$. These mutants do not, however, show an increased sensitivity to ionizing radiation. Mutations in *uvrA*, *uvrB* or *uvrC* genes render cells extremely sensitive not only to UV radiation but also to mitomycin C, nitrous acid and other genotoxic agents (Sancar & Rupp, 1983; Sancar & Sancar, 1988). *uvrD* also interferes with the excision repair of pyrimidine dimers, but differs from the other three *uvr* mutations in that a mutation at the *uvrD* locus can also cause a considerable increase in spontaneous mutation rate (Walker, 1985).

3 The *polA* gene: polymerase-deficient mutants lack the activity of DNA polymerase I and show a 10-fold increase in sensitivity to UV radiation and a threefold increase in sensitivity to ionizing radiation (Bridges, 1976). These mutants are also *Hcr*$^-$.

The excision mechanism (dark repair) for the removal of UV-induced thymine dimers is a multienzyme process, which involves (Fig. 20.9) a single-strand incision by a UV-specific endonuclease in the region of TT, an excision of the dimer and adjacent bases (by means of the exonucleolytic activity of DNA polymerase I or a UV-specific exonuclease), a repolymerization with DNA polymerase I of the single-strand gap, using the complementary strand as a template, and finally a joining of the single-strand break by means of a polynucleotide ligase. Thus, mutants, such as *uvr*$^-$ and *pol*$^-$, which lack some part of the dark-repair (excision) mechanism show an increased sensitivity to UV light.

4 The *rec* gene: this gene is lacking in recombination-deficient mutants. The *recA* mutants show no genetic recombination, whereas mutants lacking *recB* or *recC* genes have a lowered genetic recombination. For a general review of recombination, see Cox & Lehman (1987).

In postreplication recombination repair (Fig.

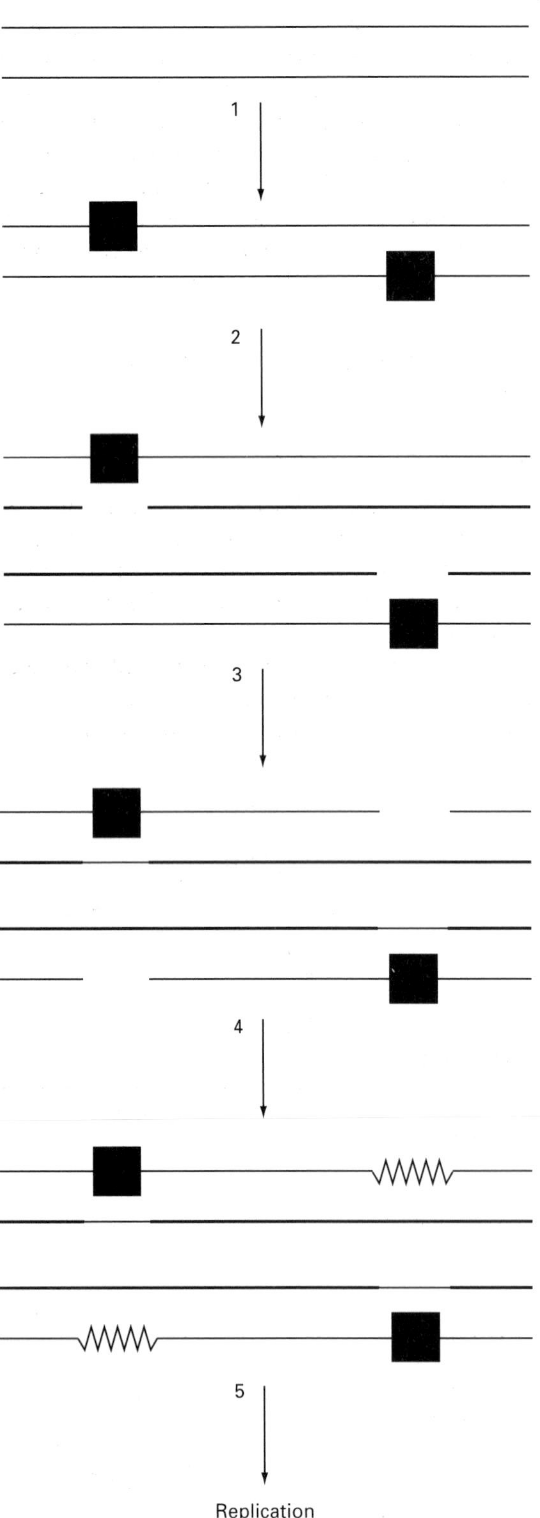

20.9), DNA replication continues normally until it reaches an unexcised dimer which is a non-coding lesion, and so a gap is left opposite. Replication then recommences at a new initiation site some distance from the dimer. Since cyclobutane-type dimers are likely to occur in both parental strands, the gaps left opposite them will also be present in both daughter strands, and so full coding potential is lacking in all four DNA strands. Thus, soon after synthesis, the new DNA strands occur in relatively short pieces, whereas after further incubation the pieces become longer, until they eventually attain the normal length. This disappearance of the gaps is attributed to crossovers (Witkin, 1976). Postreplication repair is eliminated by *recA* mutations which abolish this crossing over.

The most sensitive of all mutants to UV radiation are the *uvr*$^-$ *recA*$^-$ double mutants, which lack both of the dark-repair (excision and recombination) mechanisms.

5 The *exr* (*lex*) gene: an important *recA*$^+$-dependent pathway is known as error-prone repair. A characteristic effect of UV radiation is the induction of mutants among the survivors, these mutants arising as errors during posttreatment repair of DNA damage. Bacteria lacking the *exr* gene show no radiation mutagenesis, since the *exr* mutant blocks this error-prone pathway active in postreplication repair (Setlow & Carrier, 1972). There is increased DNA degradation in these strains, which show an increased sensitivity to UV radiation (15-fold) and to ionizing radiation (threefold); see Bridges (1976).

6 The *lon* (*fil*) gene: some strains of *E. coli*, e.g. strain B, show a loss in viability when exposed to UV radiation, even though growth and nucleic acid synthesis are normal. The cells form long, non-septate filaments, which eventually lyse. Radiation-sensitive mutants, designated *lon*$^-$, produce filaments and are about 10 times as sensitive

Fig. 20.9 Post-replication recombination repair (after Witkin, 1976). Stage 1, induction of thymine dimers (■) in u.v.-irradiated DNA; Stage 2, replication; Stage 3, recombinational exchange; Stage 4, repair replication and ligase sealing; Stage 5, replication (thymine dimers, ■, still present). —— parent DNA; —— daughter DNA; VVVV DNA polymerised as a result of repair replication.

to UV light and three times as sensitive to ionizing radiation (Bridges, 1976). The first radiation-resistant mutant (B/r) of *E. coli* B possesses a suppressor (designated *sul*) for *lon*.

For further information on the various repair processes, the interested reader should consult Fig. 20.10 and the following references: Stuy (1955, 1956a,b) Boyce & Howard-Flanders (1964), Howard-Flanders & Boyce (1966), Howard-Flanders (1973), Hanawalt & Setlow (1975), Bridges (1976), Witkin (1976), Haseltine (1983), Moseley (1984), Walker (1985), Cox & Lehman (1987) and Sancar & Sancar (1988).

4.4 *Deinococcus radiodurans*

Deinococcus radiodurans is the organism most resistant to ionizing and UV radiations. It appears to possess a remarkable ability to repair damage inflicted on its DNA by both types of radiation (Bridges, 1976), especially by excision repair, although why this is more efficient than with other organisms is currently unknown.

It is of interest to note that, whereas most bacteria in the frozen state become more sensitive to UV radiation (Section 3.6), *D. radiodurans* shows no difference in sensitivity at temperatures down to –60°C and actually becomes more resistant between –60°C and –196°C, presumably because it can repair damage resulting from the formation of another thymine photoproduct (Ashwood-Smith & Bridges, 1967).

5 Effect of ultraviolet radiation on bacterial spores

5.1 Inactivation and repair

It was pointed out above (Sections 3.1 and 3.3) that bacterial spores are more resistant than vegetative bacteria to UV radiation, and that at certain times during germination spores become much more resistant.

When bacterial spores are irradiated, thymine-containing photoproducts (TDHT; Varghese, 1970; see Fig. 20.7b and postulated formation in

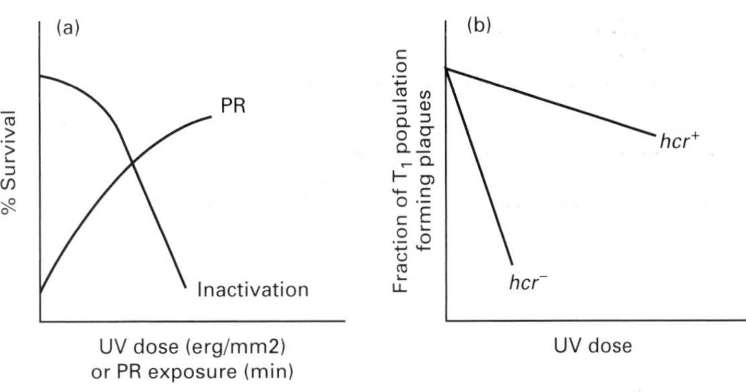

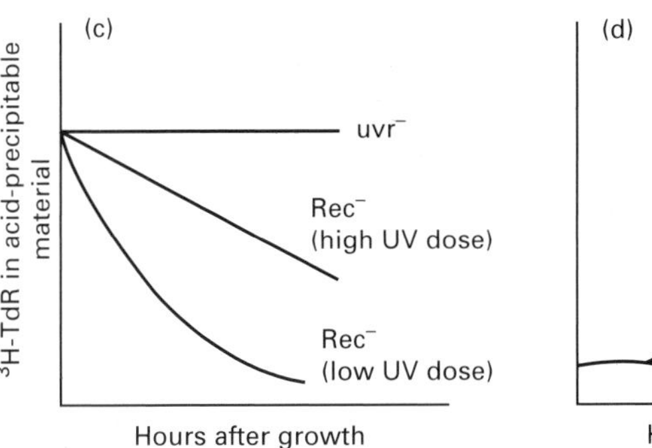

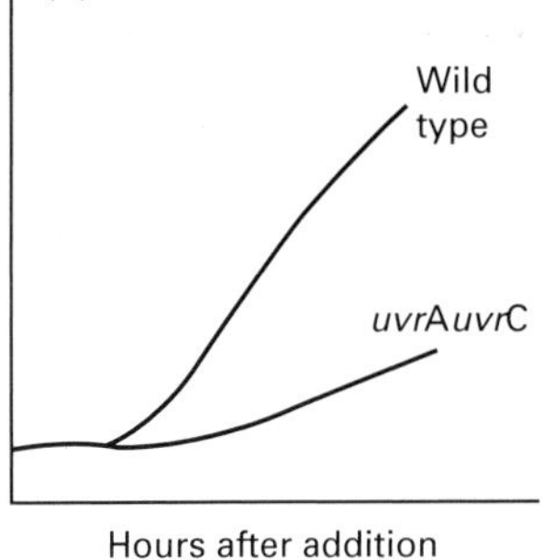

Fig. 20.10 Summary of responses to UV radiation. (a) Photoreactivation (PR); (b) host-cell reactivation (*hcr*); (c) postirradiation DNA degradation; (d) postirradiation DNA synthesis. *rec*⁻, recombination-deficient strains; *uvr*⁻, mutant lacking UV-specific endonuclease. In (c), the organisms are grown in media containing ^{3}H-thymidine (^{3}H-TdR), then irradiated and subsequently suspended in unlabelled medium containing thymine, to minimize reincorporation of any ^{3}H-TdR released. In (d), the irradiated cells are transferred to a suitable medium containing ^{3}H-TdR; the ordinate scale (*y*-axis) is as depicted for (c).

Fig. 20.11) accumulate which are different from the thymine-containing cyclobutane dimers (Fig. 20.5) produced in vegetative cells (Donnellan & Setlow, 1965). In spores, these non-cyclobutane photoproducts do not disappear after a photoreactivation process, but are eliminated from DNA by a dark-repair mechanism which is different from that found for thymine dimers in non-sporulating bacteria (Donnellan & Stafford, 1968).

During germination of *B. megaterium* spores (Stafford & Donnellan, 1968), the peak resistance to UV light occurs at 3 min, and at this point the amount of thymine-containing photoproducts is only a fraction of that found in vegetative cells or dormant spores. During germination, the amount of spore photoproduct falls rapidly but for the 3-min period there is little or no vegetative cell photoproduct (thymine dimer) formation. After this 3-min period, spore photoproduct falls slightly, but $\widehat{UT}$ and $\widehat{TT}$ dimers rapidly begin to appear, coinciding with an increase in UV sensitivity. The changes in sensitivity during germination have been explained (Stafford & Donnellan, 1968) in terms of:

1 changes in spore-type and cyclobutane-type photoproducts;

2 absence of both types at 3min being responsible for the extreme resistance of spores at that point.

The transition in UV resistance from dormant spores to vegetative cell over an extended time scale was reinvestigated by Nokes & Powers (1977), who found that the major peak of UV resistance occurred after about 60 min incubation at 25°C, with a secondary peak of resistance at *c.* 20 min. It was suggested that the reason for this latter phenomenon was linked to DNA conformation, since the DNA in spores, in germinating spores and in vegetative cells may exist in different environments —at one extreme the 'dry' DNA of spores and at the other the 'wet' DNA of vegetative cells.

The spore photoproduct (TDHT; Figs 20.7b and 20.11) is, in fact, identical to a photoproduct that accumulates in hydrolysates of DNA exposed dry or as a frozen solution to UV radiation (Rahn & Hosszu, 1968; Varghese, 1970). The sensitivity of spore-core DNA to UV light varies with the water content of the core (Germaine *et al.*, 1973).

It was stated earlier (Sections 3.6 and 4.4) that vegetative cells (except *D. radiodurans*) in the frozen state were supersensitive to UV light, and (Section 3.6) that another photoproduct, presumably TDHT, accumulated which was less susceptible to repair. The logical question is, therefore, why spores in which TDHT is induced by UV radiation should be so much more resistant to UV than non-sporing organisms. Clues are provided from the studies of Munakata & Rupert (1972, 1974), who showed that UV-sensitive mutants of UV-resistant *B. subtilis* spores formed the same thymine-containing photoproduct (TDHT) and to the same extent for a given UV dose as the resistant spores; thus the ability to remove TDHT must be linked to resistance. Two genetically controlled mechanisms were described for this removal: the first involved the early elimination of TDHT during germination, although vegetative growth was not required; the second, demonstrated in a mutant lacking the first mechanism, required

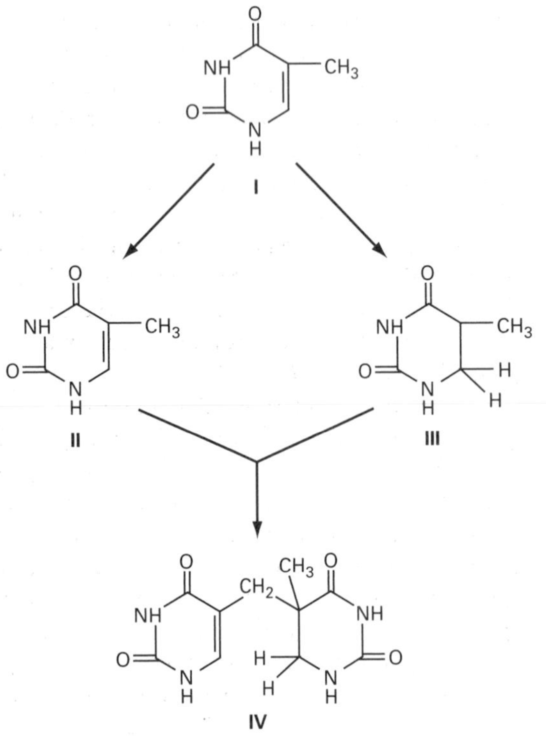

Fig. 20.11 Postulated formation of spore photoproduct (5-thyminyl-5,6-dihydrothymine (TDHT) (after Varghese, 1970). I, thymine; II, thyminyl radical; III, thymyl radical; IV, TDHT.

further development towards the vegetative cell for operation, and was an excision–resynthesis mechanism. In spores of high UV sensitivity, in which both mechanisms were blocked, TDHT was not removed (Munakata & Rupert, 1972). During germination, spores possessing the 'spore repair' process can change the TDHT into a harmless product. This appears to be a direct, enzymatic, dark repair, where by TDHT is converted to thymine, with the result that the DNA backbone is left intact (Van Wang & Rupert, 1977).

5.2 Role of small, acid-soluble spore proteins

Some 10–20% of the protein in the core of the dormant spore occurs in the form of a group of small, acid-soluble spore proteins (SASPs; Setlow, 1988, 1994). These SASPs comprise:

1 α, β types, which are associated with DNA. They are the products of a multigenic family and are synthesized around the third hour (t_3) of sporulation;

2 γ types, which are not associated with any macromolecule. They are the products of a single gene and are also synthesized at around t_3 of sporulation.

During germination, SASPs are rapidly degraded and are thus not found in vegetative cells of spore-forming species. They are important because of their relationship to spore resistance to UV radiation (Setlow; 1988, 1992, 1994; Fairhead & Setlow, 1992; Setlow *et al.*, 1992; Fairhead *et al.*, 1993; Fajardo-Cavazos *et al.*, 1993; Sanchez-Salas & Setlow, 1993; Setlow & Setlow, 1993a) and to hydrogen peroxide (Setlow & Setlow, 1993b) and sodium hypochlorite (Sabli *et al.*, 1996), but not to ionizing radiation (Setlow, 1988, 1994).

The α, β-type SASPs appear to coat the DNA in wild-type spores of *B. subtilis*. Spores ($\alpha^-\beta^-$) lacking such SASPs are significantly more sensitive to UV light (Mason & Setlow, 1986), even more so than vegetative cells (Setlow, 1992). The reason for the increased sensitivity of α^-, β^- spores is the reduced generation of spore photoproduct but the production of significant levels of thymine dimers.

During sporulation, UV resistance is acquired in parallel with α, β-type SASPs. The forespores are, in fact, more UV-resistant than the dormant spores. A possible reason for this is because dipicolinic acid (DPA), which sensitizes spore DNA to UV, is synthesized later in sporulation.

During spore germination, DPA is lost well before SASP degradation occurs. Thus, during the first few minutes of germination, UV resistance increases above the level found in dormant spores. Subsequently, as α, β-type SASPs are degraded, UV sensitivity ensues. During germination, SASP degradation is initiated by a germination endoprotease (GPR), which cleaves SASP. If a mutation occurs in GPR, α, β-type SASP degradation is slowed, so that the hyper-resistance to UV radiation persists for a longer period during germination (Sanchez-Salas & Setlow, 1993).

This fascinating insight into the role of SASPs in protecting DNA does much to explain the earlier phenomena, reported in Section 5.1, of the phase responses of spores and germinating cells to UV radiation.

5.3 Ultraviolet radiation and hydrogen peroxide

Although bacterial spores are more resistant to UV light and to hydrogen peroxide than non-sporulating bacteria, simultaneous treatment of spores with far-UV radiation and peroxide produces a greatly enhanced rate of kill (Bayliss & Waites, 1979a,b; Waites & Bayliss, 1984; Waites *et al.*, 1988). The most effective wavelength is around 270 nm, and it has been postulated that the action of the UV radiation in the combination is not directly on spore DNA but rather on the production of free hydroxyl radicals from hydrogen peroxide (Waites *et al.*, 1988).

One mechanism of sporicidal action of hydrogen peroxide is the generation of hydroxyl radicals, which cleave the DNA backbone (Imlay & Linn, 1988). The α, β-type SASPs saturate the spore chromosome and protect the DNA backbone against hydroxyl-radical cleavage. The α^-, β^- spores are much more sensitive than wild-type spores to peroxide (Setlow, 1994). It would be interesting to compare the sensitivities of wild-type and mutant spores to a UV–peroxide combination.

6 Practical uses of ultraviolet radiation

Ionizing radiations, such as X-rays, γ-rays and high-speed electrons (β-rays), strip off electrons from the atoms of the material through which the radiations pass and essentially all the chemical effects are produced by these stripped-off electrons. In contrast, UV light causes excitation of atoms, i.e. there is an alteration of electrons within their orbits, but insufficient energy is possessed for electron ejection to produce an ion; UV radiation is not therefore, an ionizing radiation. Ultraviolet radiation has little penetrative power through solids and is extensively absorbed by glass and plastics. Sterilization is achieved only by irradiation levels beyond the limits of practicability (Morris, 1972; Gardner & Peel, 1991).

It would nevertheless be incorrect to state that UV radiation serves no useful purpose as a disinfection procedure. It has been employed in the disinfection of drinking-water (Sykes, 1965; Angehrn, 1984), as a possible means of obtaining pyrogen-free water (Cook & Saunders, 1962) and especially in air disinfection, notably in hospitals (wards and operating theatres; Lidwell, 1994), in aseptic laboratories and in ventilated safety cabinets in which dangerous microorganisms are being handled (Morris, 1972).

In air disinfection of rooms, UV irradiation is directed towards the upper portion of the rooms to protect any personnel working in these areas. In contrast to this indirect irradiation, continuous irradiation from wall- or ceiling-fixed UV lamps can be employed, but any personnel present must wear protective clothing and adequate eye shields. One of the best methods of achieving air sterilization is to use a combination of air filtration and UV radiation.

The value of UV irradiation of operating theatres has been shown to be rather uncertain, the overall infection rate being unaffected, although some reduction in the sepsis of clean wounds has been noted (National Research Council, 1964). A possible reduction in the cross-infection of chickenpox has been claimed with the use of UV barriers over doors (McMath & Hussain, 1960).

An important offshoot of molecular biological aspects of excision–repair mechanisms in bacteria has been a better understanding of a disease (xeroderma pigmentosum) in humans, characterized by an abnormal sensitivity of the skin to sunlight and the likely development of malignant tumours. In a most interesting review of the repair processes for photochemical damage in mammalian cells, Cleaver (1974) has likened such people to *uvr*$^-$ and *Hcr*$^-$ bacterial mutants. The repair of DNA in mammalian cells has also been dealt with comprehensively by Hanawalt *et al.* (1979).

7 Conclusions

This brief chapter has dealt with the factors influencing the activity of UV radiation and its actions, uses and limitations. There is no doubt that UV light is much less useful as a sterilizing/disinfecting agent than ionizing radiation, but it is nevertheless of some value in air disinfection. Molecular biology studies, especially on repair processes, have yielded exciting new information, with at least one important application to human welfare (Nickoloff & Hoekstra, 1997a,b).

The role of SASPs in spore resistance to UV radiation is now well documented and researched and helps explain the long-known phenomenon of changes in UV sensitivity during sporulation and germination.

8 References

Abshire, R.L., Bain, B. & Williams, T. (1980) Resistance and recovery studies on ultraviolet-irradiated spores of *Bacillus pumilus. Applied and Environmental Microbiology*, **39**, 695–701.

Alper, T. (1979) *Cellular Radiobiology*. Cambridge: Cambridge University Press.

Andrew, M.H.E. & Russell, A.D. (eds) (1984) *The Revival of Injured Microbes*. Society for Applied Bacteriology Symposium Series No. 12. London: Academic Press.

Angehrn, M. (1984) Ultraviolet disinfection of water. *Aqua*, **2**, 109–115.

Ashwood-Smith, M.J. & Bridges, B.A. (1967) On the sensitivity of frozen micro-organisms to ultraviolet radiation. *Proceedings of the Royal Society of London, Series B*, **168**, 194–202.

Bayliss, C.E. & Waites, W.M. (1979a) The synergistic killing of spores of *Bacillus subtilis* by hydrogen peroxide and ultraviolet light irradiation. *FEMS Microbiology Letters*, **5**, 331–333.

Bayliss, C.E. & Waites, W.M. (1979b) The combined effects of hydrogen peroxide and ultraviolet light irradiation on bacterial spores. *Journal of Applied Bacteriology*, **47**, 263–269.

Boyce, R.P. & Howard-Flanders, P. (1964) Release of ultraviolet light-induced thymine dimers from DNA in

E. coli K12. *Proceedings of the National Academy of Sciences, USA*, **51**, 293–300.

Bridges, B.A. (1976) Survival of bacteria following exposure to ultraviolet and ionizing radiations. In *The Survival of Vegetative Microbes* (eds Gray, T.G.R. & Postgate, J.R.), 26th Symposium of Society for General Microbiology, pp. 183–208. Cambridge: Cambridge University Press.

Bridges, B.A., Ashwood-Smith, M.J. & Munson, R.J. (1967) On the nature of the lethal and mutagenic action of ultraviolet light on frozen bacteria. *Proceedings of the Royal Society of London, Series B*, **168**, 203–215.

Chang, J., Ossoff, S., Lobe, D. *et al.* (1985) UV inactivation of pathogenic and indicator organisms. *Applied and Environmental Microbiology*, **49**, 1361–1365.

Cleaver, J.E. (1974) Repair processes for photochemical damage in mammalian cells. *Advances in Radiation Biology*, **4**, 1–75.

Committee (1986) Committee on Health Care Issues, American Neurological Association. Precautions in handling tissues, fluids and other contaminated materials from patients with documented or suspected Creutzfeldt–Jakob disease. *Annals of Neurology*, **19**, 75–77.

Cook, A.M. & Saunders, L. (1962) Water for injection by ion-exchange. *Journal of Pharmacy and Pharmacology*, **14**, 83T–86T.

Cox, M.M. & Lehman, I.R. (1987) Enzymes of general recombination. *Annual Review of Biochemistry*, **56**, 229–262.

Department of Health (1989) *Report of the Expert Advisory Committee on Biocides*. London: HMSO.

Donnellan, J.E. & Setlow, R.B. (1965) Thymine photoproducts but not thymine dimers found in ultraviolet-irradiated bacterial spores. *Sciences, New York*, **149**, 308–310.

Donnellan, J.E. & Stafford, R.S. (1968) The ultraviolet photochemistry and photobiology of vegetative cells and spores of *Bacillus megeterium*. *Biophysical Journal*, **8**, 17–28.

Fairhead, H. & Setlow, P. (1992) Binding of DNA to α/β-type small, acid-soluble proteins from spores of *Bacillus* or *Clostridium* species prevents formation of cytosine dimers, cytosine-thymine dimers and bipyrimidine photoadducts upon ultraviolet irradiation. *Journal of Bacteriology*, **174**, 2874–2880.

Fairhead, H., Setlow, B. & Setlow, P. (1993) Prevention of DNA damage in spores and *in vitro* by small, acid-soluble proteins from *Bacillus* species. *Journal of Bacteriology*, **175**, 1367–1374.

Fajardo-Cavazos, P., Salazar, C. & Nicholson, W.L. (1993) Molecular cloning and characterization of the *Bacillus subtilis* spore photoproduct lyase (*spl*) gene, which is involved in repair of ultraviolet radiation-induced DNA damage during spore germination. *Journal of Bacteriology*, **175**, 1735–1744.

Farr, B.M., Gratz, J.C., Tartaglino, J.C., Getchell-White, S.I. & Groschel, D.H.M. (1988) Evaluation of ultraviolet light for disinfection of hospital water contaminated with legionella. *Lancet*, **ii**, 669–672.

Gardner, J.F. & Peel, M.M. (1991) *Introduction to Sterilization and Disinfection*. Edinburgh: Churchill Livingstone.

Germaine, G.R., Goggiola, E. & Murrell, W.G. (1973) Development of ultraviolet resistance in sporulating *Bacillus cereus* T. *Journal of Bacteriology*, **116**, 823–831.

Gilpin, R.W. (1984) Laboratory and field applications of UV light disinfection on six species of *Legionella* and other bacteria in water. In *Legionella: Proceedings of the Second International Symposium* (eds Thornsberry, C., Balows, A., Feeley, J.C. & Jakubowski, W.), pp. 337–339. Washington, DC: American Society for Microbiology.

Gould, G.W. (1983) Mechanisms of resistance and dormancy. In *The Bacterial Spore* (eds Hurst, A. & Gould, G.W.), Vol. 2, pp. 173–209. London: Academic Press.

Gould, G.W. (1984) Injury and repair mechanisms in bacterial spores. In *The Revival of Injured Microbes* (eds Andrew, M.H.E. & Russell, A.D.), Society for Applied Bacteriology Symposium Series No. 12, pp. 199–220. London: Academic Press.

Gould, G.W. (1985) Modification of resistance and dormancy. In *Fundamental and Applied Aspects of Bacterial Spores* (eds Dring, D.J., Ellar, D.J. & Gould, G.W.), pp. 371–382. London: Academic Press.

Hanawalt, P.C. & Setlow, R.B. (1975) *Molecular Mechanisms for the Repair of DNA*. New York: Plenum Press.

Hanawalt, P.C., Cooper, P.K., Ganesan, A.K. & Smith, C.A. (1979) DNA repair in bacteria and mammalian cells. *Annual Review of Biochemistry*, **48**, 783–836.

Harm, W. (1980) *Biological Effects of Ultraviolet Radiation*. IUPAB Biophysics Series I. Cambridge: Cambridge University Press.

Haseltine, W.A. (1983) Ultraviolet light repair and mutagenesis revisited. *Cell*, **33**, 13–17.

Haynes, R.H. (1964) Role of DNA repair mechanisms in microbial inactivation and recovery phenomena. *Photochemistry and Photobiology*, **3**, 429–450.

Haynes, R.H. (1966) The interpretation of microbial inactivation and recovery phenomena. *Radiation Research Supplement*, **6**, 1–29.

Hollaender, A. (1955) *Radiation Biology*, Vol. 2. New York: McGraw-Hill.

Howard-Flanders, P. (1973) DNA repair and recombination. *British Medical Bulletin*, **29**, 226–235.

Howard-Flanders, P. & Boyce, R.P. (1966) DNA repair and genetic recombination studies of mutants of

Escherichia coli deficient in these processes. *Radiation Research. Supplement*, **6**, 156–184.

Imlay, J.A. & Linn, S. (1988) DNA damage and oxygen radical toxicity. *Science*, **240**, 1302–1309.

Irie, R., Yano, N., Morichi, T. & Kembo, H. (1965) Temporary increase in UV resistance in the course of spore germination of *Bacillus subtilis*. *Biochemical and Biophysical Research Communications*, **20**, 389–392.

Jagger, J. (1958) Photoreactivation. *Bacteriological Reviews*, **22**, 99–142.

Johansen, E.S. & Myhrstad, J.A. (1978) Factors influencing the use of UV irradiation as a water disinfectant. *NIPH Annual*, **1**, 3–10. (National Institute of Public Health, Oslo, Norway.)

Kelner, A. (1949a) Effect of visible light on the recovery of *Streptomyces griseus* conidia from ultraviolet irradiation injury. *Proceedings of the National Academy of Sciences, USA*, **35**, 73–79.

Kelner, A. (1949b) Photoreactivation of ultraviolet-irradiated *Escherichia coli* with special reference to the dose-reduction principle and to ultraviolet-induced mutation. *Journal of Bacteriology*, **58**, 511–532.

Knudsen, G.B. (1985) Photoreactivation of UV-irradiated *Legionella pneumophila* and other *Legionella* species. *Applied and Environmental Microbiology*, **49**, 975–980.

Koehler, D.R., Courcelle, J. & Hanawalt, P.C. (1996) Kinetics of pyrimidine (6–4) pyrimidone photoproduct repair in *Escherichia coli*. *Journal of Bacteriology*, **178**, 1347–1350.

Latarjet, R. (1979) Inactivation of the agents of scrapie, Creutzfeldt–Jakob disease and kuru by radiations. In *Slow Transmissible Diseases of the Nervous System* (eds Prusiner, S.B. & Hadlow, W.J.), Vol. 2, pp. 387–407. London: Academic Press.

Lidwell, O.M. (1994) Ultraviolet radiation and the control of airborne contamination in the operating room. *Journal of Hospital Infection*, **28**, 245–248.

McCulloch, E. (1945) *Disinfection and Sterilization*. London: Kimpton.

McMath, W.E.T. & Hussain, K.K. (1960) Investigation of ultraviolet radiation in the control of chicken pox cross-infection. *British Journal of Clinical Practice*, **14**, 19–21.

Mason, J.M. & Setlow, P. (1986) Evidence for an essential role for small, acid-soluble, spore proteins in the resistance of *Bacillus subtilis* spores to ultraviolet light. *Journal of Bacteriology*, **167**, 174–178.

Mitchell, D.L. & Nairn, R.S. (1989) The biology of the (6–4) photoproduct. *Photochemistry and Photobiology*, **49**, 805–819.

Morris, E.J. (1972) The practical use of ultraviolet radiation for disinfection purposes. *Medical Laboratory Technology*, **29**, 41–47.

Morris, E.J. & Darlow, H.M. (1971) Inactivation of viruses. In *Inhibition and Destruction of the Microbial Cell* (ed. Hugo, W.B.), pp. 637–702. London: Academic Press.

Moseley, B.E.B. (1967) Repair of ultraviolet radiation damage in sensitive mutants of *Micrococcus radiodurans*. *Journal of Bacteriology*, **97**, 647–652.

Moseley, B.E.B. (1984) Radiation damage and its repair in non-sporulating bacteria. In *The Revival of Injured Microbes* (eds Andrew, M.H.E. & Russell, A.D.), Society for Applied Bacteriology Symposium Series No. 12, pp. 147–174. London: Academic Press.

Moseley, B.E.B. & Laser, H. (1965) Similarity of repair of ionizing and ultraviolet radiation damage in *Micrococcus radiodurans*. *Journal of Bacteriology*, **97**, 647–652.

Moseley, B.E.B. & Williams, E. (1977) Repair of damaged DNA in bacteria. *Advances in Microbial Physiology*, **16**, 99–156.

Munakata, N. & Rupert, C.S. (1972) Genetically controlled removal of 'spore photoproduct' from deoxyribonucleic acid of ultraviolet-irradiated *Bacillus subtilis* spores. *Journal of Bacteriology*, **111**, 192–198.

Munakata, N. & Rupert, C.S. (1974) Dark repair of DNA containing 'spore photoproduct' in *Bacillus subtilis*. *Molecular and General Genetics*, **130**, 239–250.

Muraca, P., Stout, J.E. & Yu, V.L. (1985) Comparative assessment of chlorine, heat, ozone and light for killing *Legionella pneumophila*, within a modern plumbing system. *Applied and Environmental Microbiology*, **53**, 447–453.

National Research Council (1964) Post-operative wound infection. *Annals of Surgery*, Supplement No. 2.

Nickoloff, J.A. & Hoekstra, M.F. (1997a) *DNA Damage and Repair*. Vol. I: *DNA Repair in Prokaryotes and Lower Eukaryotes*. Totowa, New Jersey: Humana Press.

Nickoloff, J.A. & Hoekstra, M.F. (1997b) *DNA Damage and Repair*. Vol. II: *DNA Repair in Higher Eukaryotes*. Totwa, New Jersey: Humana Press.

Nokes, M.A. & Powers, E.L. (1977) Sensitivity of bacterial spores to UV during germination and outgrowth. *Photochemistry and Photobiology*, **25**, 307– 309.

Phillips, J.E. (1987) Physical methods of veterinary disinfection and sterilisation. In *Disinfection in Veterinary and Farm Animal Practice* (eds Linton, A.H., Hugo, W.B. & Russell, A.D.), pp. 117–143. Oxford: Blackwell Scientific Publications.

Rahn, R.O. & Hosszu, J.L. (1968) Photoproduct formation in DNA at low temperatures. *Photochemistry and Photobiology*, **8**, 53–63.

Rappaport, E.B. (1987) Iatrogenic Creutzfeldt–Jakob disease *Neurology*, **37**, 1520–1522.

Report (1990) *HIV–The Causative Agent of AIDS and Related Conditions*. Second Revision of Guidelines. Advisory Committee on Dangerous Pathogens.

Rice, E. & Hoff, J. (1981) Inactivation of *Giardia lamblia* cysts by ultraviolet irradiation. *Applied and Environmental Microbiology*, **42**, 546–547.

Roberts, T.A. & Hitchins, A.D. (1969) Resistance of spores. In *The Bacterial Spore* (eds Gould, G.W. & Hurst, A.), pp. 611–670. London: Academic Press.

Rodgers, F.G., Hufton, P., Kurzawska, E., Molloy, C. & Morgan, S. (1985) Morphological response of human rotavirus to ultraviolet radiation, heat and disinfectants. *Journal of Medical Microbiology*, **20**, 123–130.

Romig, W.R. & Wyss, O. (1957) Some effects of ultraviolet radiation on sporulating cultures of *Bacillus cereus*. *Journal of Bacteriology*, **74**, 386–391.

Russell, A.D. (1971) The destruction of bacterial spores. In *Inhibition and Destruction of the Microbial Cell* (ed. Hugo, W.B.), pp. 451–612. London: Academic Press.

Russell, A.D. (1982) *The Destruction of Bacterial Spores*. London: Academic Press.

Russell, A.D. (1990a) Bacterial spores and chemical sporicidal agents. *Clinical Microbiology Reviews*, **3**, 99–119.

Russell, A.D. (1990b) The effects of chemical and physical agents on microbes: disinfection and sterilization. In *Topley & Wilson's Principles of Bacteriology, Virology and Immunity*, 8th edn, Vol. 1 (eds Linton, A.H. & Dick, H.M.), pp. 71–103. London: Edward Arnold.

Russell, A.D. (1993) Theoretical aspects of microbial inactivation. In *Sterilization Technology* (eds Morrissey, R.F. & Phillips, G.B.), pp. 3–16. New York: Van Nostrand Rheinhold.

Russell, A.D. (1998) Microbial susceptibility and resistance to chemical and physical agents. In *Topley & Wilson's Microbiology and Microbial Infections*, 9th edn, Vol. 2 (eds Balows, A. & Duerden, B.I.), pp. 149–184. London: Edward Arnold.

Sabli, M.Z.H., Setlow, P. & Waites, M.W. (1996) The effect of hypochlorite on spores of *Bacillus subtilis* lacking small acid-soluble proteins. *Letters in Applied Microbiology*, **22**, 405–407.

Sancar, A. & Rupp, W.D. (1983) A novel repair enzyme: uvrABC excision nuclease of *Escherichia coli* cuts a DNA strand on both sides of the damaged region. *Cell*, **33**, 249–260.

Sancar, A. & Sancar, G.B. (1988) DNA repair enzymes. *Annual Review of Biochemistry*, **57**, 29–67.

Sanchez-Salas, J.-L. & Setlow, P. (1993) Proteolytic processing of the protease which initiates degradation of small, acid-soluble, proteins during germination of *Bacillus subtilis* spores. *Journal of Bacteriology*, **175**, 2568–2577.

Schechmeister, I.L. (1983) Sterilization by ultraviolet irradiation. In *Disinfection, Sterilization and Preservation*, 3rd edn (ed. Block, S.S.), pp. 106–124. Philadelphia: Lea & Febiger.

Setlow, B. & Setlow, P. (1993a) Dipicolinic acid greatly enhances the production of spore photoproduct in bacterial spores upon ultraviolet irradiation. *Applied and Environmental Microbiology*, **59**, 640–643.

Setlow, B. & Setlow, P. (1993b) Binding of small, acid-soluble spore proteins to DNA plays a significant role in the resistance of *Bacillus subtilis* spores to hydrogen peroxide. *Applied and Environmental Microbiology*, **59**, 3418–3423.

Setlow, B., Sun, D. & Setlow, P. (1992) Studies of the interaction between DNA and α/β-type small, acid-soluble spore proteins: a new class of DNA binding protein. *Journal of Bacteriology*, **174**, 2312–2322.

Setlow, J.K. & Boling, M.E. (1965) The resistance of *Micrococcus radiodurans* to ultraviolet radiation. II Action spectra for killing, delay in DNA synthesis and thymine dimerization. *Biochimica et Biophysica Acta*, **108**, 259–265.

Setlow, P. (1988) Small acid-soluble, spore proteins of *Bacillus* species: structure, synthesis, genetics, function and degradation. *Annual Reviews of Microbiology*, **42**, 319–338.

Setlow, P. (1992) I will survive: protecting and repairing spore DNA. *Journal of Bacteriology*, **174**, 2737–2741.

Setlow, P. (1994) Mechanisms which contribute to the long-term survival of spores of *Bacillus* species. *Journal of Applied Bacteriology, Symposium Supplement*, **76**, 495–605.

Setlow, R.B. & Carrier, J.K. (1972) The disappearance of thymine dimers from DNA: an error-correcting mechanism. *Proceedings of the National Academy of Sciences, USA*, **51**, 226–231.

Smith, K.C. & Hanawalt, P.C. (1969) *Molecular Photobiology, Inactivation and Recovery*. London: Academic Press.

Stafford, R.S. & Donnellan, J.E. (1968) Photochemical evidence for conformation changes in DNA during germination of bacterial spores. *Proceedings of the National Academy of Science, USA*, **59**, 822–828.

Stuy, J.H. (1955) Photoreactivation of ultraviolet-inactivated bacilli. *Biochemica et Biophysica Acta*, **17**, 206–211.

Stuy, J.H. (1956a) Studies on the mechanism of radiation inactivation of micro-organisms. II. Photoreactivation of some bacilli and of the spores of two *Bacillus cereus* strains. *Biochimica et Biophysica Acta*, **22**, 238–240.

Stuy, J.H. (1956b) Studies on the mechanism of radiation inactivation of micro-organisms. III. Inactivation of germinating spores of *Bacillus cereus*. *Biochimica et Biophysica Acta*, **22**, 241–246.

Sykes, G. (1965) *Disinfection and Sterilization*, 2nd edn. London: E. & F.N. Spon.

Thumann, K. (1963) *The Life of Bacteria*, 2nd edn. New York: Macmillan.

Thuman, R.B. & Gerba, C.P. (1988) Molecular mechanisms of viral inactivation by water disinfectants. *Advances in Applied Microbiology*, **33**, 75–105.

Tyrrell, R.M., Moss S.H. & Davies, D.J.G. (1972) The variation in UV sensitivity of four K12 strains of *Escherichia coli* as a function of their stage of growth. *Mutation Research*, **16**, 1–12.

Van Wang, T.-C. & Rupert, C.S. (1977) Evidence for the monomerization of spore photoproduct to two thymines by the light-independent 'spore repair' process in *Bacillus subtilis. Photochemistry and Photobiology*, **25**, 123–127.

Varghese, A.J. (1970) 5-Thyminyl-5,6-dihydrothymine from DNA irradiated with ultraviolet light. *Biochemical and Biophysical Research Communications*, **38**, 484–490.

Waites, W.M. & Bayliss, C.E. (1984) Damage to bacterial spores by combined treatments and possible revival and repair processes. In *The Revival of Injured Microbes* (eds Andrew, M.H.E. & Russell, A.D.), Society for Applied Bacteriology Symposium Series No. 12, pp. 221–240. London: Academic Press.

Waites, W.M., Harding, S.E., Fowler, D.R., Jones, S.H., Shaw, D. & Martin, M. (1988) The destruction of spores of *Bacillus subtilis* by the combined effects of hydrogen peroxide and ultraviolet light. *Letters in Applied Microbiology*, **7**, 139–140.

Walker, G.C. (1985) Inducible DNA repair systems. *Annual Review of Biochemistry*, **54**, 425–457.

Watanabe, Y., Miyata, H. & Sato, H. (1989) Inactivation of laboratory animal RNA-viruses by physicochemical treatment. *Experimental Animals*, **38**, 305–311.

Witkin, E.M. (1969) Ultraviolet-induced mutation and DNA repair. *Annual Review of Genetics*, **3**, 525–552.

Witkin, E. (1976) Ultraviolet mutagenesis and inducible DNA repair in *Escherichia coli. Bacteriological Reviews*, **40**, 869–907.

CHAPTER 21

Gaseous Sterilization*

1 Introduction

Chemical agents in gaseous form have been used for fumigation for over 100 years. Early applications were for disinfection (Aronson, 1897) and disinfestation (Cotton & Roark, 1928), or to lower microbial populations in spices and gums (Griffith & Hall, 1940). Early reports of the use of gaseous chemicals for sterilization relate to the use of ethylene oxide in the 1930s (Gross & Dixon, 1937).

*The opinions expressed in this chapter are those of the authors and should not be presumed to represent the policies of the Medical Devices Agency.

Despite this long experience with gaseous sterilants, the methods of choice for sterilization in medical applications are the use of elevated temperatures, as either moist or dry heat, or the use of ionizing radiation (Dewhurst & Hoxey, 1990). Sterilization processes employing physical agents are preferred because of their relative simplicity; the conditions required to achieve sterility can be closely defined and directly measured. As a result, procedures are relatively straightforward, both for demonstrating that a defined process is capable of sterilizing a specified product (validation) and for control and monitoring to show that the validated process has been routinely reproduced (see Chapter 25).

For gaseous sterilization processes, however, not only do physical conditions, such as temperature and pressure, need to be controlled and monitored, but also a variety of chemical variables must be taken into account. Means must be available to deliver the gaseous sterilant, in the appropriate chemical form, to all parts of a sterilization load. Attention must be paid to achieving both the required concentration of sterilant and the distribution of the sterilant throughout the sterilizer chamber and load. The sterilant must also penetrate into the product item itself. Generally, achievement of these chemical conditions cannot be demonstrated by direct measurements. The validation of gaseous sterilization processes invariably includes studies in which reference microorganisms deposited on to carriers (biological indicators (BIs)) are exposed to fractions of the defined sterilization process. Additionally, routine control often requires the use of further BIs, together with continuous monitoring of the physical-process variables.

By their nature, gaseous sterilants can be toxic. Some gaseous sterilants are inflammable and/or explosive and have the potential to cause environmental damage. Furthermore, residues of sterilant may remain within products after sterilization. As a result, the use of gaseous sterilants may require particular safety precautions, controls of the emission of sterilant after processing and special provision to remove residues from product items.

However, physical sterilization methods, using elevated temperatures or ionizing radiation, are not universally applicable. Not all products needing to be sterilized can tolerate exposure to temperatures in excess of 100°C, and ionizing radiation can produce undesirable chemical changes in some materials. There is thus a continuing need for methods of sterilization that are suitable for heat sensitive items and that do not influence the properties of sterilized items adversely.

Traditionally, gaseous sterilants have been employed to sterilize products which are not compatible with moist heat, dry heat or ionizing radiation. Ethylene oxide and formaldehyde are the most commonly used gaseous sterilants, but these agents have recognized limitations and problems associated with their use. Hence, alternative gaseous sterilants have been developed to a stage at which they are being applied in either industrial facilities or health-care establishments.

2 General principles

2.1 Features of an ideal gaseous sterilant

There are a number of features that are ideal for a gaseous sterilization process. These include:

1 high microbicidal activity against bacteria, including bacterial spores, fungi and viruses;
2 extrapolation of microbial inactivation kinetics to predict the level of sterility assurance attained by a defined process;
3 capability to control and monitor all variables within the sterilization process;
4 capability to penetrate inside packages;
5 compatibility with a wide range of products and materials;
6 absence of residues in sterilized products;
7 operation below 65°C;
8 absence of hazards to operators of the sterilization process;
9 short processing time;
10 defined regulatory requirements;
11 low cost.

None of the available gaseous sterilization processes exhibits all these features. Selecting an appropriate gaseous sterilization process thus requires balancing the advantages and disadvantages of the available options. In this chapter, we shall consider the extent to which the available gaseous sterilants possess these desirable features.

2.2 Types of gaseous sterilant

Gaseous sterilizing agents can be categorized into

alkylating agents and oxidizing agents, based on their mechanism of microbicidal action.

Alkylating agents include the two most widely used gaseous sterilants, ethylene oxide and formaldehyde. Other alkylating agents are propylene oxide (Bruch & Koesterer, 1961), β-propiolactone (Hoffman & Warshowsky, 1958) and methyl bromide (Kolb & Schneitner, 1950). These agents are not commonly used for the sterilization of medical products and will not be considered further.

Oxidizing agents include gas plasmas, hydrogen peroxide, peracetic acid, ozone and chlorine dioxide. Reports of the microbicidal properties of these chemicals have been available for some time, but application as sterilants is relatively recent.

The properties of a number of gaseous sterilants are summarized in Table 21.1. Table 21.2 gives some basic information about their safe use.

2.3 Mechanisms of action

2.3.1 *Alkylating agents*

Alkylating agents are highly reactive chemicals, which will interact with a number of cellular constituents. Phillips (1949) reported that the microbicidal activity of a group of gaseous alkylating agents was related directly to the alkylating activity of each chemical. Possible reaction sites include amino, sulphydryl and hydroxyl groups of proteins and purine nucleosides of nucleic acids (Phillips, 1952; Hoffman, 1971; Adams *et al.*, 1981).

Formaldehyde reacts irreversibly with nucleic acids and this causes inhibition of germination (Trujillo & David, 1972). Formaldehyde reacts with nucleotides, ribonucleic acid (RNA) and denatured deoxyribonecleic acid (DNA) to give monomethylol derivatives and with proteins and nucleic acids to give methylene cross-links, forming nucleic acid–protein cross-links (Wilkins & MacCloud 1976; Bedford & Fox 1981; Benyajati *et al.*, 1983). Formaldehyde will not react with natural DNA unless the interstrand hydrogen bonds are broken first (Chattoraj, 1970; Kozlov & Debabov, 1972). Spicher & Peters (1976, 1981) and Wright *et al.* (1997) have reported revival of spores treated with aqueous formaldehyde and low-temperature steam with formaldehyde (LTSF) by postprocessing heat treatment. This suggests that the mechanism of action of formaldehyde is complex. Interestingly, sodium hydroxide can also cause the revival of glutaraldehyde-treated spores (Dancer *et al.*, 1989), suggesting that the precise mechanism of action of alkylating agents remains unexplained.

2.3.2 *Oxidizing agents*

Oxidizing agents used as gaseous sterilants are also highly reactive and may interact with a number of cellular constituents. Once again, the precise mechanism of action has not been identified.

Hydrogen peroxide is probably the oxidizing agent that has been studied in greatest detail. Turner (1983) suggested that its action is due to the production of the hydroxyl radical, which reacts

Table 21.1 Summary of properties of gaseous sterilants.

Sterilant	Chemical formula	Alternative names	Molecular weight	Boiling point (°C)
Ethylene oxide	C_2H_4O	Dimethylene oxide, oxirane	44.05	10.8
Formaldehyde	CH_2O	Methanal	30.03	–19.1
Hydrogen peroxide	H_2O_2	–	34.02	150.2
Peracetic acid	CH_3COOOH	Peroxyacetic acid Ethaneperoxoic acid	76.05	110
Ozone	O_3	–	48	–111.35
Chlorine dioxide	ClO_2	–	67.45	11

Table 21.2 Summary of health and safety information on gaseous sterilants.

Sterilant	Review of toxicity	Type of exposure limit	Long-term exposure limit* (parts/10^6)	Short-term exposure limit† (parts/10^6)
Ethylene oxide	International Agency for Research on Cancer (1994)	MEL‡	5	15§
Formaldehyde	International Programme on Chemical Safety (1991a)	MEL‡	2	2
Hydrogen peroxide	International Agency for Research on Cancer (1985)	OES‖	1	2
Peracetic acid		Not set	–	–
Ozone	International Programme on Chemical Safety (1990)	OES‖	0.1	0.3
Chlorine dioxide	International Programme on Chemical Safety (1991b)	OES‖	0.1	0.3

* The long-term exposure limit is specified as an 8 h time-weighted average (Health and Safety Executive, 1996).
† The short-term exposure limit is specified over a 15 min reference period (Health and Safety Executive, 1996).
‡ A maximum exposure limit (MEL) is established taking socioeconomic factors into account and a residual risk to health may remain (Health and Safety Executive, 1996).
§ No short-term exposure limit is cited, therefore this limit is taken as three times the long-term exposure limit (Health and Safety Executive, 1996).
‖ An occupational exposure standard (OES) is a level at which there is no indication of a risk to health (Health and Safety Executive, 1996).

with membrane lipids, nucleic acids and other cellular components. Jacobs (1989) and Mecke (1992) reported the interaction of free radicals produced within a plasma with essential cellular components, such as enzymes, nucleic acids and the cell membrane.

Bacterial destruction by ozone may occur as a result of action at the cell surface, leading to disintegration of the bacterial cell wall (National Research Council, 1980). Ozone attacks glycoprotein, glycolipid and certain amino acids within the bacterial membrane. Ozone also disrupts cellular enzymatic activity by reacting with sulfhydryl groups. It also acts on nucleic acids within the cell by modifying the purine and pyrimidine bases (Greene *et al.*, 1993).

The primary target for the inactivation of poliovirus by chlorine dioxide is the viral genome (Alvarez & O'Brien, 1982), although subsequent studies with f2 bacteriophage (Hauchman *et al.*, 1986), ϕ174 bacteriophage and poliovirus 1 (Hauchman, 1983) indicate that the nucleic acid remains infectious after treatment with chlorine dioxide. Noss *et al.* (1986) report that the protein component of f2 virus appears to be the site of the lethal lesion produced by chlorine dioxide.

2.4 Principal features of sterilizing equipment

Although detailed equipment specifications depend upon the sterilant employed, all sterilizing equipment must be designed to contain toxic and potentially environmentally hazardous sterilants and to avoid the risk of fires or explosions. An international standard specifying safety requirements for sterilizers using toxic gases is in preparation (International Electrotechnical Commission, 1996). In addition, a specific standard for a sterilizer employing LTSF is available (British Standards Institution, 1990) and a standard for an ethylene oxide sterilizer is nearing publication (Comité Européen de Normalisation, 1994a).

The essential features of a sterilizer for a gaseous sterilization process are: sterilizer chamber; automatic controller; recorder for process variables, i.e. temperature, time, sterilant concentration, humidity; vacuum system; and means of generating gaseous sterilant and, if necessary, humidity.

2.4.1 *Sterilizer chamber*

Items are exposed to a gaseous sterilant in a sealed chamber. The chamber is generally heated to obtain a controlled and uniform temperature during exposure. The most common method of heating is by surrounding the chamber with a jacket through which heated water or heated air is circulated. Smaller chambers may be heated electrically, provided that this does not lead to an explosion hazard.

Sterilizer chambers are usually considered as pressure vessels, because most sterilization cycles include stages operating either above or below atmospheric pressure. They must be designed and manufactured to comply with pressure-vessel regulations (International Electrotechnical Commission, 1996).

Sterilizer chambers may vary in size from 150 l to 30 m^3 or larger. The size of the chamber is influenced by the nature of the sterilant gas and by the volume of goods to be sterilized. Larger chambers may require a recirculation system to achieve and maintain a uniform distribution of sterilant gas throughout the chamber and load.

2.4.2 *Controller and recorder*

Sterilizers using sterilant gases are fitted with automatic controllers to reproduce the sterilization cycle consistently and to operate safely. The automatic controller takes the sterilizer through the sequence of operating stages which comprise the sterilization cycle. The critical cycle variables are recorded continuously throughout the sterilization cycle. This recording function should be independent of the automatic controller. It should not just log the functioning of the controller; it should provide an independent check on the critical parameters, such that a single fault, for example in a sensor, cannot result in an unsatisfactory cycle being accepted as satisfactory.

2.4.3 *Vacuum system*

Sterilizers using gaseous sterilants are fitted with evacuation systems to remove air from the chamber and load at the beginning of the sterilization cycle. This assists penetration of the sterilant throughout the load and prevents the occurrence of potentially inflammable or explosive air/sterilant mixtures within the chamber.

At the end of the sterilization cycle, sterilant gas is removed from the chamber and load, so that the load can be removed safely. This is generally achieved by evacuating the chamber. In some circumstances, alternate pulses, consisting of evacuation followed by air or inert-gas admission, are employed to improve the removal of sterilant from the load. Sterilant gas removed from the chamber at the end of the sterilization cycle has to be disposed of safely, and regulations may restrict the release of sterilant gases into the environment (Brandys, 1993).

2.4.4 *Vaporization and humidification*

The gaseous sterilant may be generated *in situ* or may be supplied: (i) as a solid; (ii) as a liquid or solution; or (iii) as a liquefied gas in pressurized cylinders. In the last three cases, it is usual to pass the sterilant through a heated vaporizer. The effective operation of the vaporizer is monitored for each sterilization cycle, as the admission of unvaporized sterilant can lead to an ineffective sterilization cycle and present a safety hazard.

Humidity control within the chamber is needed for some gaseous sterilants whose effectiveness is humidity-dependent. The preferred method of raising the humidity is to admit steam into the chamber. The alternative method of admitting nebulized water presents a risk of microbiological contamination of the load (Comité Européen de Normalisation, 1994b). When steam is generated from an external source, the source of the steam has to be controlled to ensure that the steam is neither too wet nor too dry to be effective in humidifying the load. Furthermore, any additives in the water-supply from which the steam is raised have to be controlled to ensure that they do not carry over in the steam and contaminate the load. Chapter 19A, dealing with sterilization by moist heat, provides more information.

2.5 Biological indicators

Biological indicators are used to assess the effectiveness of a gaseous sterilant in inactivation of microorganisms during process development, as part of validation and for routine monitoring of the sterilization process. They are positioned throughout the load, including locations which are judged the most difficult for the gaseous sterilant to reach. A process-challenge device may be used. This is constructed to represent the worst-case product for the sterilization process. For routine monitoring, BIs are often placed in positions from which they can be readily retrieved.

A BI consists of a known number of specific reference microorganisms, usually resistant spores, deposited on to a carrier material. The most commonly used carrier is paper, although other materials, such as metal, silk threads and glass tubes, have been employed.

For process development or validation, indicator organisms may be deposited directly on to a product. One advantage of direct inoculation is that it permits access to locations in the product into which a BI will not fit. However, the inoculation of product can be difficult to control; uneven disposition of the inoculum, for example as clumps, alters the apparent resistance of the microorganisms on the inoculated product.

Requirements for BIs for the testing of sterilization processes, such as ethylene oxide and LTSF, are specified in European standards (Comité Européen de Normalisation, 1995a,b,c,d). Some key features of a BI are incorporated into these standards, including: a pure strain of a specific microorganism; a known population of this defined microorganism; known resistance to the defined sterilization process, expressed as the decimal reduction time (*D*-value); a suitable carrier that can withstand transportation and handling and the sterilization process for which it is intended, can be readily located within a load and does not retain any substance (such as sterilant residues) that inhibits the growth of surviving organisms; a primary pack to prevent contamination and damage and for ease of handling; and a means of recovering any surviving microorganisms, including defined culture conditions (medium and incubation temperature). Table 21.3 illustrates the test organisms commonly used in BIs for gaseous sterilization processes.

2.6 Validation

A sterilization process must be validated before it is put into routine use (Commission of the European Communities, 1993). Validation is the demonstration that a specified process, operated within defined tolerances, will consistently pro-

Table 21.3 Examples of biological indicators for gaseous sterilization processes.

Sterilization process	Test organism
Ethylene oxide	*Bacillus subtilis*
Low-temperature steam and formaldehyde (LTSF)	*Bacillus stearothermophilus*
Hydrogen peroxide gas plasma	*B. subtilis*
Peracetic acid	*B. subtilis* or *B. stearothermophilus*
Chlorine dioxide	*B. subtilis*
Ozone	*B. subtilis*

duce product complying with a predetermined specification. The key factors that need to be demonstrated in validation of a sterilization process are that the products are indeed sterile and that they perform as intended without presenting a hazard to the patient or the user. An international standard specifying general requirements for characterizing a sterilizing agent and for the validation and routine control of a sterilization process is in preparation (International Standards Organization, 1997). This standard will apply to any sterilization process for which a specific standard has not been prepared; currently, the only specific standards that have been published for a gaseous sterilization process relate to the use of ethylene oxide (Comité Européen de Normalisation, 1994b; International Standards Organization, 1994).

Process development is undertaken prior to validation, in order to define the process variables and the acceptable tolerances. Validation of sterilization processes has two distinct stages: installation qualification (or commissioning) and performance qualification (Comité Européen de Normalisation, 1994b; International Standards Organization, 1994).

Installation qualification is the demonstration that the sterilizing equipment meets its specification and performs as intended when installed and operated at its point of use. It is undertaken either with the sterilizing equipment empty or using homogeneous reference material. It demonstrates the correct functioning of the equipment and the ability to deliver the specified physical conditions. An element of installation qualification for a gaseous sterilization process is the determination of the temperature distribution across the empty sterilizer chamber.

Next comes performance qualification, which uses the installed equipment to demonstrate that the specified process is capable of producing sterile items that are safe and perform as intended. This can be further subdivided into two elements: physical-performance qualification and microbiological-performance qualification.

Physical-performance qualification is the demonstration of the consistent attainment of the specified conditions throughout the loaded sterilizer chamber. Sensors, for example, for temperature and humidity, must be placed at selected locations within products. Data generated during installation qualification are used in selecting the locations to be monitored in physical-performance qualification.

Microbiological-performance qualification uses BIs to demonstrate that the sterilization process can inactivate a defined challenge of reference microorganisms. It is undertaken by distributing BIs throughout the sterilization load and then exposing the load to a process that is a fraction of that to be used routinely. At the end of the fractional exposure, the BIs are removed from the load and cultured for survivors. From the data obtained, a prediction can be made as to the probability of a reference microorganism surviving a complete sterilization process. Broadly, there are two approaches to making this prediction:

1 estimating the number of microroganisms surviving the fractional exposure and extrapolating, based on the initial number of microorganisms and the number of survivors;

2 employing a fractional exposure after which no BIs show growth and then adding a safety factor, usually doubling the exposure time from which no survivors were obtained (Comité Européen de Normalisation, 1994b; International Standards Organization, 1994).

Product evaluation is undertaken in parallel with validation studies to show that the products continue to comply with their specification after processing and that any residues of the sterilant remaining within products are below predetermined limits.

The outcome of validation is a process specification that can be used for the routine control and monitoring of the sterilization process.

2.7 Routine control and monitoring

Routine control and monitoring demonstrate that the validated sterilization process has been delivered within defined tolerances. This demonstration provides the evidence that product items processed in a particular sterilization process are sterile and, in this regard, fit for their intended use.

Routine control comprises the activities which ensure that the specified process is delivered and the monitoring provides the documentary evidence that this has occurred. The elements of routine control include: provision of documented procedures for the handling of product items before and after sterilization; calibration of instrumentation used to control and monitor the sterilization process; planned, preventive maintenance for the sterilizing equipment and any associated plant; and specification of the sterilization process, including the tolerances around the process variables.

Routine monitoring involves the measurement and recording of the process variables, including temperature, pressure, humidity and admission of gaseous sterilant. If all the variables of the sterilization process can be directly monitored and recorded, the resulting records provide sufficient evidence that the validated sterilization cycle has been reproduced. In this situation, product items can be released following sterilization on the basis of these records (Hoxey, 1989). This is termed parametric release. Requirements for parametric release of products following ethylene oxide sterilization have been included in standards for validation and routine control of ethylene oxide sterilization (Comité Européen de Normalisation, 1994b; International Standards Organization, 1994).

For gaseous sterilization processes, direct monitoring of sterilant concentration and the distribution and penetration of the sterilant throughout the load is not always practical. Parametric release, therefore, is not often used at present (see also Chapter 25). More commonly, monitoring of the physical-cycle variables is supplemented by placing BIs in the sterilization load. At the end of the sterilization cycle, the BIs are removed and cultured. Products can be released following sterilization, if the records show that the cycle has been delivered within the defined limits and no survivors are recovered from the BIs.

2.8 Residues of gaseous sterilants

Traces of sterilant remaining in products after sterilization are called residues and may subsequently desorb slowly from the product, posing a risk to the patient. Residues from gaseous sterilization processes are of particular concern because of the toxicity of many gaseous sterilants. The International Standards Organization is preparing a general standard for the determination of allowable limits for process residues, using health-based assessment (International Standards Organization, 1995).

The level of residues in a particular product will depend upon the materials from which the product is constructed and the sterilant used and will be influenced by the sterilization cycle employed. To accelerate the desorption of residues, a sterilization process may include an aeration phase, in which the product is exposed to increased temperature, increased air flow or a combination of these two. The conditions specified for aeration should be shown to achieve a predetermined residue level and should be monitored as part of the sterilization process (Comité Européen de Normalisation, 1994b; International Standards Organization, 1994).

If a gaseous sterilant breaks down readily and the breakdown products do not present a risk, residues do not present a problem. Examples are: (i) plasmas, which re-form as the source gas; (ii) hydrogen peroxide, which breaks down to oxygen and water; (iii) peracetic acid, which breaks down to acetic acid and water; and (iv) ozone, which breaks down to oxygen. However, the kinetics of the breakdown of the sterilant will be product-dependent and require individual consideration; for example, Ikarashi *et al.* (1995) report residues of hydrogen peroxide in a variety of materials at levels capable of inducing a cytotoxic effect.

The gaseous sterilant for which the issue of residues has been considered in greatest detail is ethylene oxide (Page, 1993). The residues concerned are ethylene oxide itself and the principal transformation products formed by reactions during the sterilization process; ethylene chlorohydrin, formed by reactions with inorganic chlorine; and ethylene glycol, formed by reactions with water. An international standard has been published (International Standards Organization, 1996) which provides a means of determining the allowable limits for ethylene oxide residues, based upon the likely extent of exposure of an individual to those residues over the individual's lifetime, balancing the risk of the exposure to the residues against the benefits of the medical intervention. A revision of this standard is currently under way.

Formaldehyde residues can occur as paraformaldehyde on the surface and/or as absorbed formaldehyde in the material (Handlos, 1977). The levels of residues in various materials following exposure to gaseous formaldehyde have been investigated (Handlos, 1977, 1979, 1984; Profumo & Pesavento, 1986; Vink, 1986). Handlos (1984) concluded that the amounts of formaldehyde dissolved within plastics materials will be small compared with ethylene oxide, if the sterilization process is designed to remove paraformaldehyde from the surface of product items by steam pulsation. Vink (1986), however, reported that some formaldehyde-sterilized materials appeared to be toxic in a screening test for acute toxicity.

Little has been published on residues of chlorine dioxide following sterilization. Jeng & Woodworth (1990a) reported on the feasibility of chlorine dioxide as a sterilant for oxygenators; oxygenators present particular problems for residues because all the patient's blood is circulated through the product. From a limited study, they concluded that chlorine dioxide did not pose problems of acute toxicity, hypersensitivity or mutagenicity.

3 Alkylating agents

3.1 Ethylene oxide

3.1.1 Historical perspective

Cotton & Roark (1928) reported that concentrations of 3.2–32 mg/l ethylene oxide killed a variety of insect pests. The bactericidal activity of ethylene oxide was reported in a patent application by Schrader & Bossert (1936), but they did not provide supporting data for this activity. A subsequent patent application by Gross & Dixon (1937) included reports of tests using 48 different microorganisms in moist cotton, sugar cystals and moist-cut tobacco. Griffith & Hall (1940) were also granted a patent on the use of ethylene oxide as a sterilant for foodstuffs. The basic evaluation of the microbicidal effectiveness of ethylene oxide was performed by Phillips & Kaye (Kaye, 1949; Kaye & Phillips, 1949; Phillips, 1949; Phillips & Kaye, 1949).

Further work was undertaken to increase the understanding of the microbicidal action of ethylene oxide and to develop an accepted sterilization process using automated sterilizers, for application both in industry and in health-care facilities (Ernest & Shull, 1962a,b; Ernst & Doyle, 1968). In addition to studies on the inactivation of bacteria and bacterial spores (Bruch, 1961; Kereluk *et al.*, 1970), the inactivation of fungi by ethylene oxide (Liu *et al.*, 1968; Blake & Stumbo, 1970; Dadd & Daley, 1980) and its viricidal effectiveness (Klarenbeek & Van Tongeren, 1954) have been investigated.

More recently, standards for ethylene oxide sterilizers and for the validation and routine control of ethylene oxide sterilization have been prepared (Comité Européen de Normalisation, 1994a,b; International Standards Organization, 1994). However, no standard set of conditions for sterilization by ethylene oxide has been adopted and each individual sterilization process is developed and its performance qualified microbiologically for the product to be sterilized (Hoxey, 1989).

3.1.2 Applications

Ethylene oxide is used extensively to sterilize products that are sensitive to heat, moisture or radiation. Although it has been applied for sterilization of a wide range of products (Bruch, 1961), the major application today is for the sterilization of single-use medical devices made of plastics. It is also used for the sterilization of some empty plastic containers for subsequent aseptic filling with pharmaceutical products. Ethylene oxide also has applications in health-care establishments for the sterilization of reusable medical devices, for example certain flexible endoscopes, which will not withstand exposure to moist heat.

Increased awareness of the need to prevent exposure to ethylene oxide, together with the phasing out of ethylene oxide–chlorofluorocarbon-12 (CFC-12) mixtures (see Section 3.1.3) and the stringent safety requirements for the operation of sterilizers using pure ethylene oxide, has led many users to reappraise their use of ethylene oxide. There has been an increasing use of specialist sterilization subcontractors, the redesign of products to be compatible with other methods of sterilization and interest in other forms of gaseous sterilization, leading to the closure of many in-house sterilization facilities. Despite these trends, ethylene oxide remains the most common method of gaseous sterilization and will probably continue to be so for the foreseeable future.

3.1.3 *Physical and chemical properties*

At room temperature and pressure, ethylene oxide is a colourless gas and has been reported as having a sweet, ether-like odour at concentrations above approximately 430 parts/10^6 (Amoore & Hauttala, 1983).

Ethylene oxide is both inflammable and explosive, with an inflammable concentration range in air of 3–100% v/v. It is supplied as a pressurized gas in cylinders for use as a pure gas, with specific safety precautions for the installation, or mixed with an inert diluent, such as carbon dioxide or hydrochlorofluorocarbon (HCFC) to provide a non-flammable and nonexplosive blend. Historically, the most common diluent gas was CFC-12, but this has been phased out, because of the environmental impact from its ozone-depleting properties (United Nations Environment Programme, 1987; Jorkasky, 1993). Ethylene oxide–HCFC mixtures have been introduced as an interim replacement for ethylene oxide–CFC-12. While HCFCs have significantly less ozone-depleting potential than CFCs, they still have an environmental impact. Ethylene oxide–HCFC mixtures are subject to specific regulation in Europe (Commission of the European Communities, 1994) and are scheduled to be phased out worldwide by 2030 (United Nations Environment Programme, 1987). Replacements with zero ozone depleting potential are under development.

The properties of, and some health and safety information related to, ethylene oxide are summarized in Tables 21.1 and 21.2.

3.1.4 *Factors affecting microbicidal activity*

Temperature. Temperature has the most pronounced influence on the effectiveness of ethylene oxide as a sterilant. Increasing temperature increases the rate of inactivation of microorganisms; a number of investigators have reported that a temperature increase of 10°C approximately doubles the rate of inactivation, with the exact value of the increase influenced by the ethylene oxide concentration (Phillips, 1949; Ernst & Shull, 1962a; Kereluk *et al.*, 1970). Clearly, the inverse also applies and a decrease in temperature of 10°C will approximately halve the rate of inactivation. It can be seen, therefore, that a spread of temperature of 10°C across a sterilization load will lead to a 100% difference in the rate of inactivation between the hottest and coldest locations.

Sterilant concentration. Increasing the concentration of ethylene oxide increases the rate of microbial inactivation, up to a plateau concentration above which further concentration increases do not lead to increased effectiveness (Ernst & Shull, 1962a; Kereluk *et al.*, 1970). Ernst & Shull (1962a) reported that the plateau concentration depends upon the temperature employed; at 30–50% relative humidity, plateau concentrations have been reported as 800 mg/l at 30°C and 500 mg/l at 54°C.

Humidity. Kaye & Phillips (1949) reported the critical influence of humidity on the effectiveness of ethylene oxide. Winano & Stumbo (1971) suggested that the presence of water was critical for the alkylation reaction to proceed. The moisture content of a microorganism is related directly to the humidity of its surrounding environment and the microenvironment adjacent to the microorganism is critical in determining its resistance to ethylene oxide (Kereluk *et al.*, 1970). Once microorganisms become dehydrated, their resistance to ethylene oxide increases and it can take a significant period of equilibration with high humidity to reverse this effect (Gilbert *et al.*, 1964). Dadd *et al.* (1985) noted that the application of a high vacuum in an ethylene oxide sterilization cycle would cause dehydration of microorganisms and hence increased resistance; the need for a stage in the sterilization cycle to rehydrate the microorganisms was stressed.

The optimal humidity for microbicidal effectiveness has been reported as 35% (Ernst & Shull, 1962b; Gilbert *et al.*, 1964), but in practice most ethylene oxide sterilization processes operate between 40 and 80% relative humidity, because of the significant amount of moisture-absorbing material, such as packaging materials, included in a sterilization load. Care must be taken, however, to avoid the presence of excess free water, as this can lead to the formation of inactive ethylene glycol or ethylene oxide dissolving in the free water, reducing the ethylene oxide concentration (Dadd *et al.*, 1985).

3.1.5 *Sterilization process*

The process used for ethylene oxide sterilization generally consists of three distinct phases: (i) preconditioning; (ii) the sterilization cycle; and (iii) aeration. Modern installations operate on a 'cell' system, with separate chambers for the three phases. Product is transferred automatically from one cell to the next, reducing the potential for operator exposure to ethylene oxide.

A wide variety of conditions have been employed for ethylene oxide sterilization (Table 21.4). The recent trend has been to decrease the concentration of ethylene oxide in order to reduce the levels of residues in product items at the end of the sterilization cycle, thereby reducing the time required for aeration.

Preconditioning. Preconditioning takes place at atmospheric pressure prior to the product being transferred into the sterilizer chamber, in order to raise the temperature and humidity of the load to the levels required for sterilization. The duration of the sterilization cycle is reduced and the throughput of the sterilization process increased if this is done before the product is put into the sterilizer chamber.

Raising the temperature of a large, dense load can take a significant time, particularly for processes operating at 50–55°C. Preconditioning may take 12–18 h.

Table 21.4 Summary of the range of conditions used for ethylene oxide sterilization.

Process variable	Range encountered
Exposure time	1–24 h
Ethylene oxide concentration	250–1200 mg/l
Temperature	25–65°C
Humidity	30–85%

Sterilization cycle. The sterilization cycle itself takes place in a sealed chamber and consists of a series of stages under the control of an automatic controller. The stages are: (i) air removal; (ii) leak test; (iii) conditioning; (iv) sterilant admission; (v) exposure; (vi) sterilant removal; (vii) flushing; and (viii) air break (Comité Européen de Normalisation, 1994a). These stages are illustrated in Fig. 21.1.

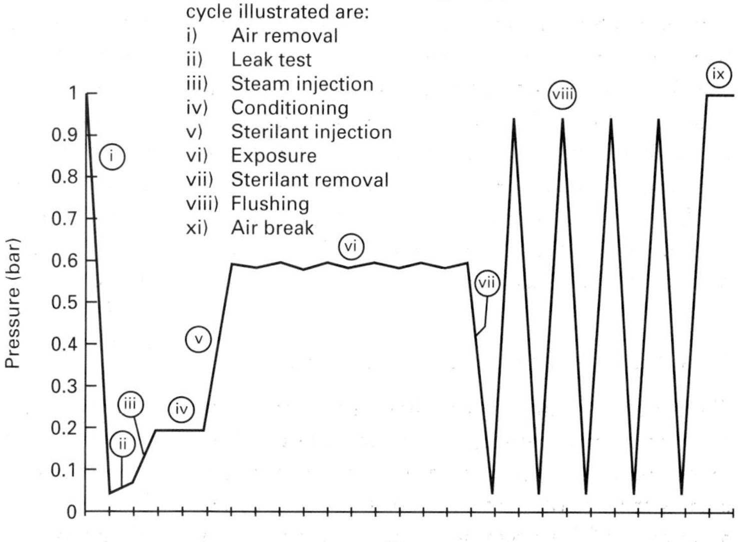

Fig. 21.1 Illustration of an ethylene oxide sterilization cycle operating below atmosphere pressure.

During the air-removal stage, a vacuum is drawn to a preset level to remove air from the chamber and load. The vacuum system is then turned off and the pressure in the chamber monitored for a preset period; if the pressure rises by more than a defined amount, it indicates that there is a leak into the chamber and the cycle is terminated.

Steam is then admitted to the chamber to a preset pressure, selected to achieve the required humidity during conditioning. The conditioning stage serves to replace the moisture in the chamber and load that was removed during air removal. Penetration of moisture into the load is assisted by the reduced pressure.

Following conditioning, sterilant is admitted to the chamber, via a vaporizer, until the preset pressure required to achieve the specified concentration of ethylene oxide is reached. This pressure will also depend upon the sterilant mixture used; pure ethylene oxide cycles, together with cycles using ethylene oxide mixed with nitrogen or HCFC, operate at subatmospheric pressure, whereas ethylene oxide–carbon dioxide mixtures operate at 2–6 bar above atmospheric pressure. The correct functioning of the vaporizer is monitored, usually by measuring the temperature of the sterilant gas as it enters the chamber, to ensure that only gaseous ethylene oxide is admitted. The concentration is checked independently by one of the following: (i) the reduction in weight of the sterilant cylinders; (ii) a measure of the volume of liquid ethylene oxide flowing to the vaporizer; or (iii) analysis of the concentration of ethylene oxide in the chamber (Comité Européen de Normalisation, 1994a,b; International Standards Organization, 1994).

The product items are exposed to ethylene oxide for a defined time. During exposure, the pressure in the chamber is monitored. As ethylene oxide is adsorbed by the load, the pressure in the chamber falls. Further ethylene oxide may be admitted during the exposure period to maintain the specified pressure; these admissions are called 'make-ups'.

The sterilant-removal and flushing stages remove ethylene oxide from the chamber and load, allowing the chamber to be unloaded safely. Sterilant is first removed by evacuation and the subsequent flushing stage consists of pulses comprising admission of air or an inert gas, followed by evacuation. This is repeated a defined number of times. Following the flushing stage, air is admitted to return the chamber to atmospheric pressure. It is important that products are then removed and not left in a sealed chamber because ethylene oxide will slowly desorb from the load and accumulate within the chamber. This can produce a safety hazard (International Electrotechnical Commission, 1996).

Aeration. The purpose of aeration is to desorb ethylene oxide and any reaction products from the product items in order to attain predetermined levels of residues. This is generally achieved by holding the load at elevated temperature for a defined time, with an increased flow of air to improve desorption. Matthews *et al.* (1989) reported that the application of microwaves increased desorption of ethylene oxide residues.

3.1.6 *Validation and routine control*

Requirements for the validation and routine control of sterilization by ethylene oxide have been published in an international standard (International Standards Organization, 1994) and a European standard (Comité Européen de Normalisation, 1994b). This standard describes the approaches for physical and microbiological qualification and provides guidance on practical details, including: numbers of sensors or BIs to be used; their placement during qualification studies; and acceptance criteria.

The validation of ethylene oxide sterilization includes all of the elements described in the general section of this chapter: installation qualification, physical-performance qualification and microbiological-performance qualification.

If parametric release is to be used routinely, microbiological-performance qualification is required to generate a knowledge of the inactivation of BIs by the specified process. This may be achieved in one of two ways: either by the construction of a survival curve for reference microorganisms on BIs, or by the estimation of the *D*-value of the reference microorganism. A method for determining the *D*-value by the most probable number (MPN) technique is specified, as described by Pflug & Holcomb (1983).

For routine control with parametric release, all the process variables must be monitored directly: time, temperature (including the temperature within the load), pressure, humidity and sterilant concentration. Product may be released if all the process variables are within specified limits (Sordellini, 1997). Alternatively, if BIs are to be used as an element of routine monitoring, microbiological-performance qualification may use a 'half-cycle' approach. In this approach, no survivors are obtained from a cycle in which the exposure time has been reduced to half that to be used routinely.

For routine control with BIs, time, chamber temperature and pressure still have to be monitored and recorded, but humidity may be interpreted from the records of temperature and pressure and sterilant concentration inferred from the pressure rise on sterilant admission, together with either the weight loss from the sterilant cylinders or the volume of ethylene oxide vaporized.

3.2 Formaldehyde

3.2.1 Historical perspective

Early investigations into the bactericidal properties of formaldehyde were reported by Loew (1886), and its use as a vapour-phase decontaminant for rooms dates from the 1890s (Aronson, 1897). A system for disinfection in a heated vacuum chamber at 80–90°C with an exposure time of 30 min, using formaldehyde generated by heating formaldehyde solution, was documented by Sprague (1899). The method was reported as inactivating spores of *Bacillus anthracis*, but no precise quantification was carried out. Nordgren (1939) extensively reviewed the history of formaldehyde as a disinfecting agent and investigated its bactericidal effectiveness. He concluded that formaldehyde had a strong bactericidal action but had only a limited capacity to sterilize without elevated temperatures and reduced pressure to aid penetration through narrow orifices.

The activity of formaldehyde against a wide range of microorganisms, including vegetative bacteria, fungi and viruses, has been demonstrated (Spicher & Peters, 1976; Ide, 1979).

Alder & Gillespie (1961) investigated the use of steam at subatmospheric pressure for the disinfection of woollen blankets and subsequently demonstrated that the addition of formaldehyde with the steam produced a sporicidal combination (Alder *et al.*, 1966). They concluded that the LTSF combination, operating at 80°C, was cheap, efficient and easy to control. Subsequent work (Pickerill, 1975; Hurrell *et al.*, 1983; Robertshaw, 1983) further refined the process, and automated sterilizers were developed, which have been widely used in health-care facilities, particularly in Scandanavia, Germany and the UK.

3.2.2 Applications

Low-temperature steam with formaldehyde has been widely used in health-care facilities, particularly in northern Europe, for the sterilization of reusable medical devices which will not withstand moist-heat sterilization. It has been used for endoscopic equipment, such as laparoscopes, telescopes and fibre-optic leads (Hoxey, 1991). However, LTSF has not been in common use for industrial applications or in health-care facilities in North America.

3.2.3 Physical and chemical properties

Pure, dry formaldehyde is a colourless gas with a characteristic, pungent odour; it polymerizes at room temperature to produce a white film of polyoxymethylene glycols. Formaldehyde gas is irritating to the eyes, nose and throat at levels as low as 0.05–0.5 parts/10^6 (Sintim-Damoa, 1993). Formaldehyde gas is inflammable and forms an explosive mixture with air at compositions of 7–72% v/v; however, the concentration of formaldehyde used in gaseous sterilization processes is well below the explosive range and is nonflammable.

Formaldehyde is supplied as a solution (formalin) or as a polymeric hydrate (paraformaldehyde).

In solution, formaldehyde is present as the monohydrate, methylene glycol ($CH_2(OH)_2$) and a series of low molecular weight polyoxymethylene. increases with increasing formaldehyde concentration. Formalin contains 37–40% w/v formaldehyde and 10–15% w/v methanol to inhibit polymerization.

Paraformaldehyde is a mixture of polyoxymethylene glycols, containing 90–99% formaldehyde with a balance of free and combined water. Paraformaldehyde gradually vaporizes, generating monomeric formaldehyde gas; this depolymerization is accelerated by increasing temperature.

Gaseous formaldehyde for use as a sterilant can be produced by heating either formalin or paraformaldehyde. Alternatively, for fumigation of rooms, gaseous formaldehyde can be generated by initiating an exothermic reaction with the addition of a strong oxidizing agent, such as potassium permanganate, to formalin (Walker, 1964).

The properties of, and some health and safety information related to, formaldehyde are summarized in Tables 21.1 and 21.2.

3.2.4 *Factors affecting microbicidal activity*

Temperature. Nordgren (1939) evaluated the effect of temperature over the range 10–70°C on the inactivation rate of microorganisms and observed an increasing inactivation rate with increasing temperature. The Public Health Laboratory Service (1958), however, reported little difference in inactivation rate with increasing temperature between 0 and 30°C.

Preliminary investigations into the effect of temperature on LTSF sterilization at a concentration of 14 mg/l indicated that a reduction in temperature from 80 to 70°C produced only a slight decrease in the rate of inactivation, but that a further decrease to 65°C produced a significant reduction in the rate of inactivation (Hoxey, 1984). Wright *et al.* (1996), however, later reported that, at a concentration of 12 mg/l, increasing temperature from 63 to 83°C did not produce an increased rate of inactivation.

Humidity. The effect of humidity on microbial inactivation by formaldehyde has been investigated by a number of workers. Nordgren (1939) showed increased microbicidal effect with increasing humidity up to 50% relative humidity, but little further increase up to 95%. This has generally been confirmed (Cross & Lach, 1990), although the Public Health Laboratory Service (1958) identified an optimum relative humidity of 80–90% and Spiner and Hoffman (1971) reported that a relative humidity in excess of 50% was essential.

Concentration. As would be expected, the activity of formaldehyde has been reported as increasing with concentration. Nordgren (1939) showed a significant increase in activity with increasing concentration from 0.1 to 1.3 mg/l. The Public Health Laboratory Service (1958) reported a linear relationship between concentration and rate of inactivation between 0.04 and 0.31 mg/l, and Spiner & Hoffman (1971) came to a similar conclusion for the concentration range 1.1–10.6 mg/l.

Investigations into the effect of formaldehyde concentration on LTSF sterilization at 80°C suggested that increasing concentration over the range 6–20 mg/l has only a small effect on the rate of inactivation; a further increase in concentration to 27 mg/l had a marked effect (Hoxey, 1984). Later work by Wright *et al.* (1996), however, reported that, at 73°C, an increasing rate of inactivation was observed with increasing concentration from 3 to 12 mg/l, but that there was no further increase in rate of inactivation from 12 to 18 mg/l.

3.2.5 *Sterilization process*

Low-temperature steam with formaldehyde sterilization cycles have been investigated at temperatures between 60 and 80°C, but the most common operating temperature is 73 ± 2°C, selected to balance material compatibility with ease of temperature control (Pickerill, 1975; Alder, 1987). Formaldehyde concentrations of 8–16 mg/l formaldehyde are generated by vaporizing 0.5–1 ml formalin/30 l chamber volume (Hurrell *et al.*, 1983), although the use of higher concentrations has been reported (Pickerill, 1975; Alder, 1987).

The sterilization cycle consists of a series of stages: (i) initial vacuum; (ii) steam flush; (iii) formaldehyde–steam pulsing; (iv) hold period; (v) sterilant removal; and (vi) air break. This is illustrated in Fig. 21. 2.

The initial vacuum is pulled to remove air from the chamber and load. This is followed by steam admission to the chamber with the vacuum pump still running, to purge the chamber of air and to heat the load.

The next stage of the cycle is a series of pulses.

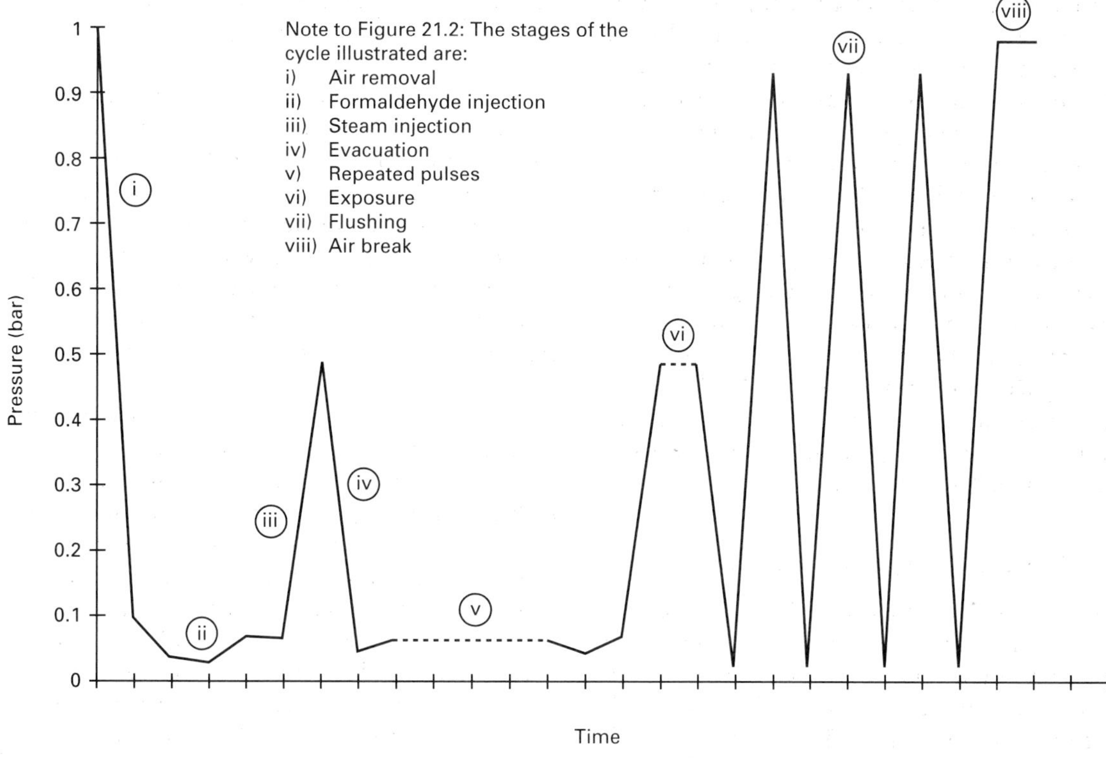

Fig. 21.2 Illustration of an LTSF sterilization cycle.

A set volume of formalin is admitted into the vaporizer and the resultant formaldehyde gas admitted to the chamber. After a 2-min hold period to allow the formaldehyde to penetrate the load, steam is admitted to the chamber to the pressure required to obtain the operating temperature. A vacuum is then pulled again and formaldehyde admission repeated. The number of repetitions of this stage may vary up to a total of 20 pulses.

The pulsing stage may be followed by a hold period, in which formaldehyde, followed by steam, is admitted to the required pressure and these conditions are maintained for a set period. This stage is not always included, as it has been shown that the formaldehyde concentration declines rapidly during this holding period (Handlos, 1979; Marcos & Wiseman, 1979; Hurrell *et al.*, 1983).

Formaldehyde is removed from the sterilizer and load by repeated alternate evacuation and flushing with steam or air. Handlos (1979) showed a reduced level of residues when steam pulsing was used in this phase, but such pulsing requires the subsequent inclusion of an extended drying stage under vacuum to dry the load. The cycle concludes by the admission of air to atmospheric pressure.

3.2.6 Validation and routine control

Procedures for the validation and routine control of LTSF have been published (Department of Health, 1994).

For validation, the procedures initially parallel the requirements for qualifying a steam sterilizer or a low-temperature steam disinfector (see Chapters 19A and 25). These physical measurements demonstrate the acceptable performance of the sterilizer in assuring steam penetration and achieving the required temperatures throughout the load. These studies are then followed by microbiological-performance qualification of the LTSF cycle. This consists of replicate cycles to demonstrate distribution and penetration. To show distribution, BIs containing 10^6 spores of *Bacillus stearothermophilus* of defined resistance (Comité Européen de Normalisation, 1995c) are removed from their individual packages and suspended on threads from a frame within the chamber. In addition, two process-challenge devices are used to demonstrate penetration. The process-challenge device used is stainless-steel tubing coiled into a helix, with a small chamber at one end into which a BI can be placed (Line & Pickerill, 1973). These challenge devices are exposed to the operating cycle and no growth must be observed on incubation of the BIs.

For routine control, the records are examined to check that the physical-cycle variables have been reproduced within the defined tolerances. In addition, each cycle contains a Line–Pickerill helix incorporating a BI. At the end of the cycle, the BI is transferred to growth media and incubated; the absence of growth on incubation confirms that the cycle was satisfactory.

4 Oxidizing agents

4.1 Gas plasma

4.1.1 Historical perspective

A gas-plasma sterilization process was patented in 1968 (Menashi, 1968). The patent reports a method for the sterilization of parenteral vials by production of a high-voltage frequency discharge from a wire introduced into the vial. The process was able to inactivate 10^6 spores in vials in less than 1 s. A subsequent patent (Ashman & Menashi, 1972) was granted for the sterilization of container surfaces using low-temperature halogen plasmas under low pressures. A flow-through plasma sterilization system for medical devices was developed by the Boeing Company in 1974 (Fraser *et al.*, 1974, 1976).

Sterilization of vials using a plasma induced by a laser was first reported by Tensmeyer (1976). In 1981, a system was developed in which the life of the plasma was sustained by a microwave field, without the introduction of any object into the vial (Tensmeyer *et al.*, 1981). This was further developed by Peeples & Anderson (1985a,b) to establish a system to simplify the initiation and prolong the life of the plasma. The sterilization of empty 10 ml vials was reported, together with some bacterial endotoxin destruction.

Further patents were issued on 'seeded plasma', a combination of plasma and aldehydes (Gut Boucher, 1980), and sterilization through sealed porous packaging with pressure pulsing of plasma to enhance sporicidal activity in apertures and narrow lumens (Bithell, 1982a,b).

The use of hydrogen peroxide gas to seed a plasma in a chamber was reported as a sterilization process by Addy (1991). This was the basis for a gas plasma system for the sterilization of instruments within the health-care setting, which became commercially available in the early 1990s. More recently, a sterilizer utilizing a secondary plasma has also been made available. The plasma species, created by electromagnetic radiation in the plasma-generating chamber, flows downstream into the sterilization chamber (Caputo *et al.*, 1993). The precursor for this system is peracetic acid.

4.1.2 Applications

Gas-plasma sterilization systems are intended primarily for the reprocessing of medical devices used in the health-care environment. They have been in use in the USA and parts of Europe, particularly Germany, since the early 1990s, although still in their infancy.

Gas plasma is suitable for reprocessing instruments and devices that cannot withstand elevated temperatures (greater than 60°C) and is seen as an alternative to ethylene oxide and liquid chemical disinfectants, particularly for flexible endoscopes, although gas plasma is unable to penetrate long narrow lumens, such as those within an endoscope. A special adaptor containing the precursor has to be inserted into any lumened device so that the plasma is generated *in situ*.

Items for reprocessing must be thoroughly dry, as moisture interferes with the ability to obtain the required vacuum. Certain materials, such as cellulose packaging material, absorb hydrogen peroxide and cannot be processed, due to the subsequent changes in pressure this causes.

Gas plasma is being considered for the sterilization of certain medical devices, because it is perceived as having advantages with respect to material compatibility, compared with existing sterilization processes.

4.1.3 *Physical and chemical properties*

Gas plasmas are considered to be a fourth state of matter, distinct from solids, gases and liquids. Plasmas occur naturally, as in the northern lights, or can be generated at a low temperature, as in fluorescent lighting. Plasmas consists of ions, electrons and neutral species (Bell, 1974; Addy, 1991).

Commercially, plasma is created in a sealed chamber under vacuum, using radiofrequency or microwave energy to generate the strong electric or magnetic fields required to excite the gas. The gas is ionized by the electric field, and the electrically charged particles produced (ions and electrons) are subsequently accelerated by the electric field and collide to produce further ionization and molecular dissociation. This produces free radicals, electrons, ions and excited radicals, which give the plasma its reactivity. These gas plasmas are classified as low-temperature plasmas and are also known as non-equilibrium or glow-discharge gas plasmas.

4.1.4 *Factors affecting microbicidal activity*

Plasma source. Addy (1991) reported that hydrogen-peroxide-seeded plasma had greater sporicidal activity than plasma produced from the precursors water vapour, hydrogen, oxygen or nitrous oxide. This is thought to be due to the lower energy required to create hydroxyl radicals than for most other precursors and the fact that the reactive species generated from hydrogen peroxide are among the most reactive.

Sporicidal activity was found to decrease as the distance from the generation source increased for the precursor gases oxygen, hydrogen, nitrous oxide and nitrogen dioxide (Addy, 1991). Sporicidal activity increases with radiofrequency power, as does the temperature (Addy, 1991).

Concentration. Increasing the concentration of hydrogen peroxide precursor was found to increase sporicidal activity (Addy, 1991).

4.1.5 *Sterilization process*

A typical sterilization cycle for the hydrogen peroxide gas-plasma system comprises: (i) air removal; (ii) hydrogen peroxide injection; (iii) diffusion; (iv) gas plasma; and (v) aeration. This is illustrated in Fig. 21.3.

The sterilization chamber is evacuated to around 0.3 mbar. The time taken for the required vacuum conditions may be up to about 20 min but will depend on the moisture content of the load, and for this reason items should be placed into the chamber dry. Excess moisture will prevent the required conditions from being attained and the cycle will abort.

Once the required vacuum is attained, a small volume of the precursor, hydrogen peroxide solution (58% w/v), is dispensed from a cassette, vaporized and injected into the sterilization chamber. The hydrogen peroxide vapour diffuses throughout the chamber and the load. Radiofrequency energy is applied to the vapour-phase hydrogen peroxide within the chamber to generate a gas plasma.

After the required plasma stage, the chamber is flushed with air and the chamber restored to atmospheric pressure by the introduction of filtered air.

4.1.6 *Validation and routine control*

There are no specific standards for the validation and routine control of sterilization using gas-plasma systems. For a particular application, validation and routine control protocols have to be prepared, based on the standard giving general requirements for the validation and routine control of sterilization processes, which is under development (International Standards Organization, 1997).

The cycle is subject to automatic control and monitoring. Factors to be monitored include pressure, temperature, plasma initiation, admission of the specified quantity of seed gas and duration of each stage of the cycle. A record of the parameters for the cycle is generated and compared with the cycle specification.

A BI and a chemical indicator are available for use with the hydrogen-peroxide-plasma system. The BI consists of spores of *Bacillus subtilis*,

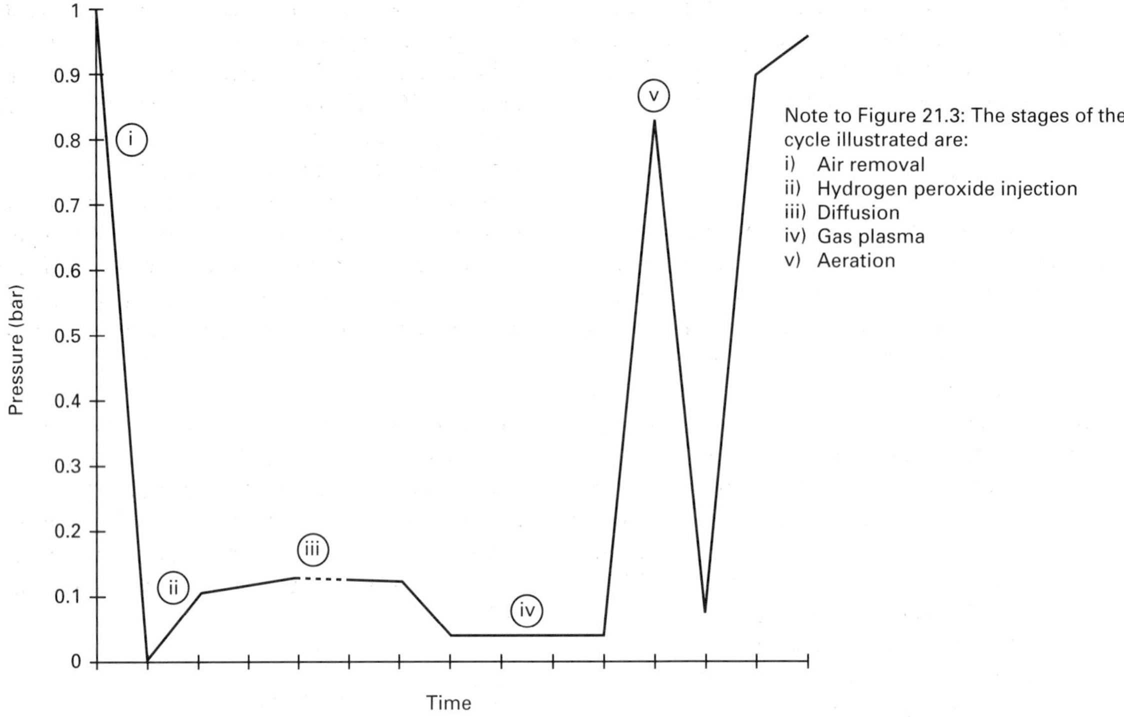

Fig. 21.3 Illustration of a hydrogen peroxide gas-plasma sterilization cycle.

located at the blind end of a lumened device, to be positioned at the point within the chamber posing the greatest challenge to the process. The chemical indicator is placed within the chamber to indicate the presence of hydrogen peroxide.

4.2 Hydrogen peroxide

4.2.1 Historical perspective

The microbicidal activity of hydrogen peroxide has been recognized for over 100 years. The early applications were reviewed by Curran *et al.* (1940), and it has been used in the food industry for the sterilization of filters and piping since 1916 (Schumb *et al.*, 1955).

Investigations into the microbicidal effectiveness of hydrogen peroxide have been undertaken in both liquid and vapour phases. It has been demonstrated as being sporicidal by a number of authors (Swartling & Lindgren, 1968; Toledo *et al.*, 1973; Stevenson & Shafer, 1983: see also Chapter 10C).

Two more recent applications of hydrogen peroxide have been as a 'seed gas' for a gas-plasma sterilization system (see Section 4.1) and as a vapour-phase hydrogen peroxide process (VPHP) (Rickloff & Graham, 1989; Klapes & Vesley, 1990; Johnson *et al.*, 1992; Chapter 10C). The VPHP has been developed with three modes: (i) a deep-vacuum system, operating with admission of vaporized hydrogen peroxide into an evacuated chamber; (ii) a 'flow-through' mode, using a mixture of vaporized hydrogen peroxide and filtered air as a carrier gas; and (iii) a combined 'deep-vacuum, flow-through' system for items of equipment that can act as their own chambers, such as freeze-driers or isolators (Klapes & Vesley, 1990; Johnson *et al.*, 1992). Klapes & Vesley (1990) reported the inactivation of 10^6 *B. subtilis* spores at some but not all locations in a centrifuge after exposure for 32 min, using a combined 'deep-vacuum, flow-through' process at 4°C. Johnson *et al.* (1992) investigated the decontamination of freeze-driers with VPHP. They noted no appreciable difference in lethality when comparing a 'deep-vacuum' process with the combined 'deep-vacuum, flow-through' mode and reported on the problems of penetration of vapour into dead-legs in the system.

4.2.2 *Applications*

The use of hydrogen peroxide has increased with the growing application of aseptic packaging operations in the food, pharmaceutical and medical devices industries. Hydrogen peroxide may be applied as a liquid, or as a vapour or aerosol.

A system of fogging with an aerosol of hydrogen peroxide, followed by hot-air drying, for applications in the aseptic packaging of foods has been described (Posey *et al.*, 1988; Posey & Swank, 1989). The applicability of hydrogen peroxide for the decontamination of spacecraft components has also been reported (Wardle & Renninger, 1975).

The VPHP process in various modes has been proposed as suitable for sterilizing medical products, such as endoscopes, and for decontaminating equipment for aseptic processes, such as isolators, pipework or freeze-driers, and contaminated equipment, such as centrifuges, incubators, safety cabinets or glove boxes (Rickloff & Graham, 1989; Klapes & Vesley, 1990; Johnson *et al.*, 1992). However, the VPHP system cannot be used with cellulosic materials, including paper-based packaging materials, and some material damage has been reported with nylon, some anodized aluminium surfaces and some epoxides (Rutala & Weber, 1996).

4.2.3 *Physical and chemical properties*

In a pure form, hydrogen peroxide is a colourless liquid, but it is generally encountered as a solution in concentrations up to 50% w/v. It breaks down readily to water and oxygen. The properties of, and some health and safety information related to, hydrogen peroxide are summarized in Tables 21.1 and 21.2.

4.2.4 *Factors affecting microbicidal activity*

Temperature. Temperature exerts a marked effect on the activity of hydrogen peroxide in solution, a 10°C temperature increase approximately doubling the rate of inactivation (Curran *et al.*, 1940; Swartling & Lindgren, 1968; Toledo *et al.*, 1973). Johnson *et al.* (1992) concluded that a temperature between 10 and 50°C was required for feasible sterilizing conditions, reporting little difference in inactivation over this temperature range, but a reduced inactivation at 60°C. They concluded that this reduced inactivation was due to the higher temperatures promoting decomposition of the hydrogen peroxide. Klapes & Vesley (1990), however, reported acceptable sporicidal activity at 4°C.

Concentration. Increasing concentration in hydrogen peroxide solution leads to increasing rates of inactivation (Swartling & Lindgren, 1968). The concentration that can be achieved reliably in the vapour phase, however, is limited, and typical vapour concentrations used for sterilization are 1–5 mg/l.

4.2.5 *Sterilization process*

The VPHP process in deep-vacuum mode uses the vacuum to pull a 30% solution of hydrogen peroxide through a heated vaporizer into the sterilizer chamber, where it diffuses throughout the chamber and the load. The process operates at 55–60°C and has a cycle time of approximately 90 min.

In the 'flow-through' mode, the VPHP process uses a portable vapour generator to vaporize a 30% hydrogen peroxide solution. The solution is metered into a vaporization chamber through spray nozzles. The vaporization chamber is heated to 105°C to provide rapid vaporization without fractioning the hydrogen peroxide solution and leaving the peroxide behind (Johnson *et al.*, 1992). The vapour is then mixed with a carrier gas, such as filtered air, and admitted into the enclosed space to be decontaminated.

The combined 'deep-vacuum, flow-through' mode, as its name implies, uses a combination of these two approaches. The equipment to be sterilized, such as a centrifuge rotor or freeze-drier, is evacuated and the portable vapour generator is used to inject hydrogen peroxide vapour, followed by the controlled admission of a small volume of air. After a defined time interval, there are a series of further admissions of hydrogen peroxide vapour and air, while a vacuum is pulled to draw the vapour through the equipment. This is followed by a series of subatmospheric pulses of alternate evacuation and admission of filtered air (Johnson *et al.*, 1992).

4.2.6 *Validation and routine control*

There are no specific standards for the validation and routine control of sterilization using vaporized hydrogen peroxide. The standard for general requirements (see Section 2.6) should be used as the basis for specific protocols for validation and routine control (International Standards Organization, 1997).

A process-development exercise should be undertaken to define an appropriate process for a defined product or range of products. The validation of the process should then include installation qualification to demonstrate that the equipment has been installed and is capable of delivering the defined process reproducibly, followed by performance qualification.

Physical-performance qualification should demonstrate the delivery of the defined process by measuring the physical factor such as: (i) level of vacuum and the rate at which it is attained; (ii) pressure rise(s) on admission(s) of sterilant; (iii) operating temperature of vaporizer; (iv) temperature distribution; (v) weight of liquid hydrogen peroxide used; (vi) pressure changes during degassing phase.

Microbiological-performance qualification should be BIs of *B. stearothermophilus*. Routine monitoring of the process should include measurements to demonstrate compliance with the physical-process specification used in performance qualification, supplemented with the use of BIs of *B. stearothermophilus*.

4.3 Peracetic acid

4.3.1 *Historical perspective*

The microbicidal activity of aqueous solutions of peracetic acid was reported in the 1950s. A broad spectrum of action against bacteria (Gershenfeld & Davis, 1952; Baldry, 1983), bacterial spores (Jones *et al.*, 1967), fungi (Lowings, 1956) and viruses (Briefman-Kline & Null, 1960) was demonstrated. The initial evaluation of vapour-phase peracetic acid was attributed to Greenspan and colleagues in 1951 by Portner & Hoffman (1968), who themselves evaluated the sporicidal effect of the vapour.

Evaluation of the properties of peracetic acid has continued primarily in aqueous solution for waste-water treatment (Sanchez-Ruiz *et al.*, 1995) and for health-care applications (Malchesky, 1993).

4.3.2 *Applications*

The practical application of peracetic acid has been limited by its corrosive nature (Portner & Hoffman, 1968; Malchesky, 1993). A buffered solution of peracetic acid has been developed for the sterilization of endoscopes (Malchesky, 1993). In the vapour phase, peracetic acid has been used: (i) as a seed gas for a gas plasma (see Section 4.1); and (ii) to sterilize isolators and other enclosed spaces, using a spray of dilute solution (Davenport, 1989).

4.3.3 *Physical and chemical properties*

Peracetic acid is formed by reaction between hydrogen peroxide and acetic acid and exists in solution as an equilibrium mixture of peracetic acid, acetic acid, hydrogen peroxide and water. Peracetic acid is commercially available as a 35% w/v solution. Vapour-phase peracetic acid is generated by heating a solution of 2–5% peracetic acid stabilized with 10–20% hydrogen peroxide; hence systems using peracetic acid inevitably also have hydrogen peroxide present as well. Peracetic acid has a pungent odour and is irritating to the mucous membranes.

The properties of peracetic acid are summarized in Table 21.1.

4.3.4 *Factors affecting microbicidal activity*

Portner & Hoffman (1968) investigated the sporicidal effect of vapour-phase peracetic acid. Using a concentration of 1 mg/l and a temperature of 25°C, they reported the inactivation of up to 8×10^5 spores of *B. subtilis* in 10 min at relative humidities between 40 and 80%. The optimum humidity was 80% and inactivation was reduced significantly at 20% relative humidity.

4.3.5 Sterilization process

Technologies for using vapour-phase peracetic acid have been developed for specific applications. For example, Davenport (1989) devised a spray system to deliver a controlled atomized spray of peracetic acid.

4.3.6 Validation and routine control

There is no standard describing the procedures for the validation and routine control of vapour-phase peracetic acid. For each individual application, separate protocols for validation and routine control and monitoring have to be established, based on the standard giving general requirements (International Standards Organization, 1997) (see Section 2.6).

4.4 Ozone

4.4.1 Historical perspective

Calmette (1899) reported the destruction of bacteria when the water supply of Lille, France, was treated with ozone and, since the early 1900s, ozone has been used to treat domestic drinking-water supplies (Symons, 1980).

The microbicidal effectiveness of gaseous ozone was demonstrated by Elford & van den Ende (1942). Leiguarda *et al.* (1949) reported the destruction of spores of *Clostridium perfringens* and *B. anthracis* by exposure to ozone, and Kietzmann (1957) described the effectiveness of low concentrations of ozone against airborne bacteria, but not against surface contaminants or in the presence of organic matter. Ozone has been found to be effective against Gram-negative and Gram-positive bacteria, including spore-formers and amoebae (Symons, 1980).

Ingram & Barnes (1959) reported that fungi were as at least as resistant to ozone as bacteria, while Sulzer *et al.* (1959) indicated that yeasts were less resistant. Studies have also shown ozone to be effective against a number of different virus types (Kessel, 1943; Majumdar, 1973; Snyder & Chang, 1974; Burleson *et al.*, 1975; Sproul & Majumdar, 1975; Farooq & Akhlaque, 1983; Vaughn *et al.*, 1987).

4.4.2 Applications

Ozone is primarily used for the treatment of water, in particular, water for domestic use, and for the disinfection of sewage effluent. It is not widely used in the health-care environment, but two sterilizers have been reported (Karlson, 1989; Stoddart, 1989) and it is used in the pharmaceutical industry to treat deionized water systems. It was first used in 1987 in the preparation of dialysing solution (Bommer & Ritz, 1987) and has been proposed for the disinfection of regenerated capillary dialysers (Gal *et al.*, 1992). In combination with ultraviolet (UV) radiation, ozone has also been used to produce a pharmacopoeial standard for purified water (Lee *et al.*, 1990). Other uses of ozone include the decontamination of contact lenses (Kamiki & Kikkawa, 1976).

The effects of short-term (24 h and long-term (100 h exposure of medical and optical devices, electronics, plastics and metal instruments to 8% ozone were studied by Karlson (1989). Most items were not affected, but copper and iron were oxidized and plastic gloves, polyurethane and polystyrene were affected after prolonged exposure, due to the destruction by ozone of such weakly bonded natural rubber and plastics.

4.4.3 Physical and chemical properties

In a pure form, ozone is a blue gas. It is relatively stable in dry air but decomposes rapidly at high humidities. It is produced by passing dry air or oxygen between high-voltage electrodes, which produce a corona discharge, or by UV irradiation of air or oxygen. It has to be produced at the point of use because of its instability. Ozone is produced from the disassociation of oxygen molecules, which collide with other oxygen molecules to create triatomic oxygen, with one loosely bonded O atom; this readily attaches to other molecules and makes ozone a powerful oxidizing agent.

The properties of, and some health and safety information related to, ozone are summarized in Table 21.1 and 21.2.

4.4.4 *Factors affecting microbicidal activity*

The destruction of bacteria and viruses within the range pH 5.6–9.8 has been reported. (Masschelein, 1982; Singer, 1990). In combination with UV radiation, the activity of ozone increases, due to the formation of reactive hydroxyl radicals (Lee *et al.*, 1990).

While the rate of microbial inactivation by ozone remains under debate, its action has been shown to be time-dependent, and its effectiveness decreases over time (Dahi, 1976). An increase in relative humidity from 45% to 60 or 80% increases the biocidal effect of ozone (Busta & Foegeding, 1983). German *et al.* (1966) reported that desiccated spores and bacteria wee highly resistant to ozone, while gauges contaminated with *Staphylococcus aureus* and *Escherichia coli* were sterilized in a moist environment.

Ozone has a limited ability for penetration.

4.4.5 *Sterilization process*

An ozone sterilizer has been described with a cycle of three stages (Karlson, 1989). Oxygen is delivered to the ozone generator during the first stage, where it is converted into ozone of a high concentration. The gaseous ozone displaces the air in the sterilizer chamber. During the second stage, the ozone is continuously passed through the chamber for a defined period of time. A cooling system maintains the ozone generator at a defined temperature, which contributes to the control of the ozone concentration. The ozone level within the chamber is continuously monitored. At the end of the second stage, the generation of ozone is switched off, but the oxygen flow continues in order to flush out the ozone. When the level of ozone approaches zero, the cycle is considered complete.

An alternative system (Stoddart, 1989) delivers ozone at a concentration of 10–12%. The sterilization cycle is performed under vacuum and takes between 30 and 60 min, including aeration. Following exposure, the ozone is purged, filtered and converted back into oxygen. The sterilizer is monitored by an automated control system.

4.4.6 *Validation and routine control*

There is no standard describing the specific procedures for the validation and routine control of ozone. For each individual application, separate protocols for validation and routine control and monitoring have to be established, based on the standard giving general requirements (International Standards Organization, 1997) (see Section 2.6).

4.5 Chlorine dioxide

4.5.1 *Historical perspective*

Chlorine dioxide has been used for the treatment of water-supplies in Europe since the 1850s and as a bleaching agent in the paper and textile industries since the 1920s (Benarde *et al.*, 1965; Jeng & Woodworth, 1990b).

McCarthy (1944) reported chlorine dioxide to be an effective germicide in water with a low organic content. In the same year, the use of chlorine dioxide as a disinfectant in drinking-water treatment was reported from the Niagara Falls Water Treatment Plant (Syvan *et al.*, 1944). Subsequent studies indicated that chlorine dioxide was as at least as effective as chlorine (Trakhtman, 1946; Ridenour & Ingols, 1947), although the data are considered to be of questionable value (Benarde *et al.*, 1965). Liquid chlorine dioxide has been reported as an effective bactericide (Ridenour & Ingols, 1947; Ridenour & Armbruster, 1949; Benarde *et al.*, 1965), a viricide (Cronier, 1977) and a sporicide at a concentration of approximately 0.2 mg/l (Masschelein, 1979; Ridenour *et al.*, 1949).

The sporicidal activity of chlorine dioxide in its gaseous form was not demonstrated until relatively recently (Orcutt *et al.*, 1981). This has been further supported in the literature and patents (US Patent 4 504 442, March 1985; Knapp *et al.*, 1986; Rosenblatt *et al.*, 1987; Kowalski *et al.*, 1988; Jeng & Woodworth, 1990a,b). Chlorine dioxide gas was estimated to be 1075 times more potent than ethylene oxide as a sterilant at temperature of 30°C and similar relative humidity (Jeng & Woodworth, 1990b).

4.5.2 *Applications*

Chlorine dioxide is used for the control of taste and odours in water-supplies (Walker *et al.*, 1986; White, 1986), due to its property as a powerful oxidizing agent. Chlorine dioxide has also been investigated for the control of legionellae in a hospital water system (Walker *et al.*, 1995). It has been used as a surface sanitizer in the food industry and in the health-care environment as a gaseous or liquid chemical sterilant. In gaseous form, it has been used for the sterilization of oxygenators on an industrial scale (Jeng & Woodworth, 1990b). Jeng & Woodworth (1990b) indicated that chlorine dioxide gas could penetrate packaging materials using: (i) sealed polyvinyl chloride tubes; and (ii) rigid polyvinyl chloride medical-device containers (approximately 0.03 mm thickness) with spun-bonded polyolefin covers.

4.5.3 *Physical and chemical properties*

Chlorine dioxide is an orange-green gas with a pungent odour similar to that of chlorine. The odour threshold is around 0.1 parts/10^6. It is highly soluble in water and, in an aqueous medium, it forms a non-ionizing stable radical (Wagner, 1962).

Chlorine dioxide is explosive at concentrations above 10% v/v in air (Haller & Northgraves, 1955) but is non-explosive and non-flammable at the concentrations used for sterilization. Chlorine dioxide is relatively unstable and, as a result, and also because of its explosivity at high concentration, it has to be generated *in situ* (Aieta & Berg, 1986). Chlorine dioxide is produced from chlorine or the action of acid on sodium chlorite.

4.5.4 *Factors affecting microbicidal activity*

Concentration. The sporicidal activity of chlorine dioxide gas was found to be concentration-dependent (Jeng & Woodworth, 1990b). Activity against spores of *B. subtilis* var. *niger* at ambient relative humidity (20–40%) and at room temperature (23°C) was greater at a higher gas concentration.

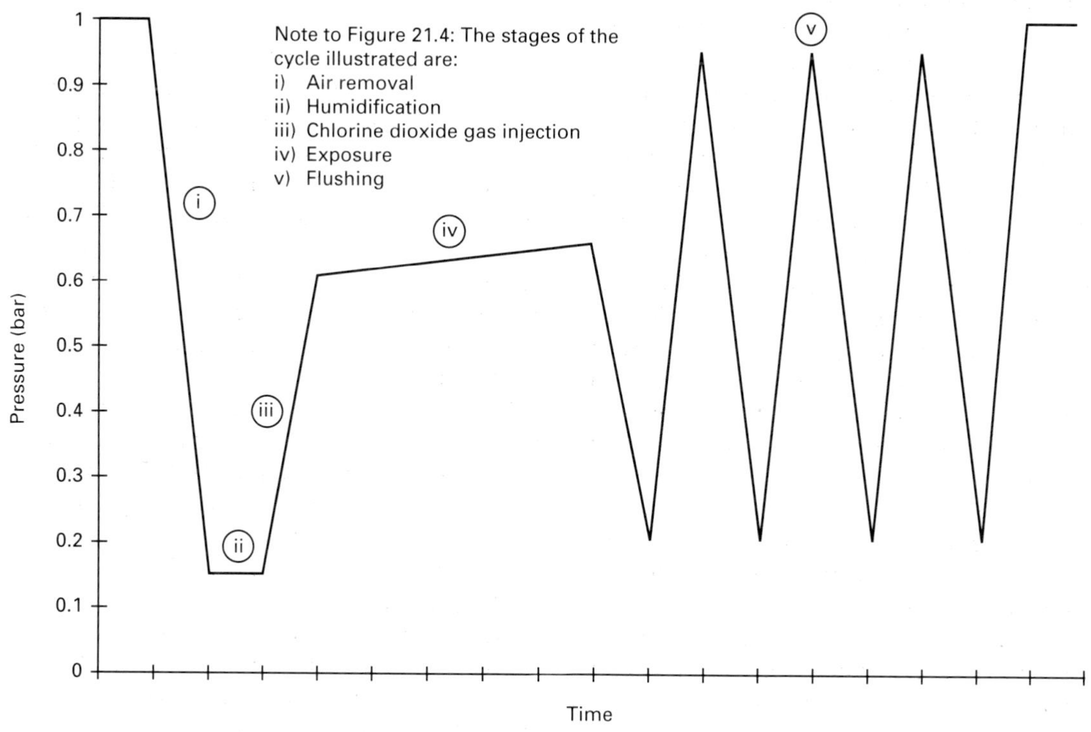

Fig. 21.4 Illustration of a chlorine dioxide sterilization cycle.

Humidity. Jeng & Woodworth (1990b) reported that prehumidification to 70–75% relative humidity greatly enhanced the effectiveness of chlorine dioxide and confirmed previous reports on the importance of prehumidification to the sporicidal activity of chlorine dioxide (Rosenblatt *et al.*, 1985, 1987; Knapp *et al.*, 1986).

4.5.5 *Sterilization process*

A system for sterilizing health-care devices using gaseous chlorine dioxide was developed in the 1980s. Figure 21.4 shows a typical gaseous chlorine dioxide sterilization cycle. A typical cycle operates at ambient temperature (between 25 and 30°C), at a relative humidity of 70–90%. Chlorine dioxide is generated *in situ*, from dry sodium chlorite and chorine gas in a nitrogen carrier. The chlorine dioxide gas is then drawn into the evacuated chamber and the pressure rises to just below atmospheric pressure, to achieve the required sterilant concentration. The conditions are maintained for the required exposure time. Further chlorine dioxide is admitted to the chamber during the exposure stage to maintain the required concentration. At the end of the cycle, the chamber is evacuated and the exhaust gas is passed through a chemical column to absorb the chlorine dioxide. The cycle time ranges from 3 min to 2 h using between 10 and 50 mg/l chlorine dioxide (Janssen & Schneider, 1993; Sintim-Damoa, 1993).

4.5.6 *Validation and routine control*

There is no specific standard for the validation and routine control of sterilization by gaseous chlorine dioxide. For each individual application, separate protocols for validation and routine control and monitoring have to be established, based on the standard giving general requirements (International Standards Organization, 1997; see Section 2.6).

The physical-process variables that require routine control and monitoring include the gas concentration (this may be measured spectrophotometrically from an in-line system, which draws continuous samples of gas); relative humidity; pressure, temperature and exposure time.

The BI *B. subtilis* var. *niger* spores are used for the microbiological-performance qualification of the process.

5 References

Adams, R.L.P. Burdon, R.H., Campbell, A.M., Leader, D.P. & Smellie, R.M.S. (1981) *The Biochemistry of Nucleic Acids*, 9th edn. London: Chapman and Hall.

Addy, T.O. (1991) Low temperature plasma: a new sterilization technology for hospital applications. In *Sterilization of Medical Products*, Vol. V (eds Morrissey, R.F. & Prokopenko, Y.I.), pp. 89–95. Morin Heights, Canada: Polyscience Publications.

Aieta, E.M. & Berg, J.D. (1986) A review of chlorine dioxide in drinking water treatment. *Journal of the American Water Works Association*, **78**, 62–72.

Alder, V.G. (1987) The formaldehyde/low temperature steam sterilizing procedure. *Journal of Hospital Infection*, **9** 194–200.

Alder, V.G. & Gillespie, W.A. (1961) Disinfection of woollen blankets in steam at sub-atmospheric pressure. *Journal of Clinical Pathology*, **14**, 515–518.

Alder, V.G., Brown, A.M. & Gillespie, W.A. (1966) Disinfection of heat sensitive material by low temperature steam and formaldehyde. *Journal of Clinical Pathology*, **19**, 83–89.

Alvarez, M.E. & O'Brien, R.T. (1982) Mechanisms of inactivation of poliovirus by chlorine dioxide and iodine. *Applied and Environmental Microbiology*, **44**, 1064–1071.

Amoore, J.E. & Hautala, E. (1983) Odor as an aid to chemical safety: odor thresholds compared with threshold limit values and volatilities for 214 industrial chemicals in air and water dilution. *Journal of Applied Toxicology*, **3**, 272–290.

Aronson, H. (1897) Über eine neue Methode zur Desinfection von grosseren Raumen mittels Formalin. *Zeitschrift für Hygiene*, **25**, 168–178.

Ashman, L.E. & Menashi, W.P. (1972) *Treatment of Surface with Low-pressure Plasmas*. US Patent 3 701 628.

Baldry, M.G.C. (1983) The bactericidal, fungicidal and sporicidal properties of hydrogen peroxide and peracetic acid. *Journal of Applied Bacteriology*, **54**, 417–423.

Bedford, P. & Fox, B.W. (1981) The role of formaldehyde in methylene dimethanesulphonate-induced DNA cross-links and its relevance to cytotoxicity. *Chemical–Biological Interactions*, **38**, 119–126.

Bell, A.T. (1974) Fundamentals of plasma chemistry. In *Techniques and Applications of Plasma Chemistry*. New York: Wiley-Interscience.

Benarde, M.A., Israel, B.M., Olivieri, V.P. & Granstrom, M.L. (1965) Efficiency of chlorine dioxide as a bactericide. *Applied Microbiology*, **13**, 776–780.

Benyajati, C., Place, A.R. & Sofer, W. (1983) Formaldehyde mutagenesis in *Drosophila*: molecular analysis of ADH-negative mutants. *Mutation Research*, **111**, 1–7.

Bithell, R.M. (1982a) *Package and Sterilizing Process for Same*. US Patent 4 321 232.

Bithell, R.M. (1982b) *Plasma Pressure Pulse Sterilization*. US Patent 4 348 357.

Blake, D.F. & Stumbo, C.R. (1970) Ethylene oxide resistance of micro-organisms important in spoilage of acid and high-acid foods. *Journal of Food Science*, **35**, 26–29.

Bommer, J. & Ritz, E. (1987) Water quality—a neglected problem in hemodialysis. *Nephron*, **46**, 1–6.

Brandys, R.C. (1993) Regulations on worker safety and the environment. In *Sterilization Technology* (eds Morrissey, R.F. & Phillips, G.B. (pp. 491–509. New York: Van Nostrand Reinhold.

Briefman-Kline, L. & Null, R.N. (1960) The viricidal properties of peracetic acid. *American Journal of Clinical Pathology*, **33**, 30–33.

British Standards Institution (1990) *BS 3970 Specifications for Sterilizers and Disinfectors for Medical Purposes*. Part 6. *Specification for Low Temperature Steam with Formaldehyde Sterilizers*. London: British Standards Institution.

Bruch, C.W. (1961) Gaseous sterilization. *Annual Review of Microbiology*, **15**, 245–262.

Bruch, C.W. & Koesterer, M.G. (1961) The microbicidal activity of gaseous propylene oxide and its application to powdered or flaked foods. *Journal of Food Science*, **26**, 428–435.

Burleson, G.R., Murray, T.M. & Pollard, M. (1975) Inactivation of viruses and bacteria by ozone, with and without sonication. *Applied Microbiology*, **29**, 340–344.

Busta, F.F. & Foegeding, P.M. (1983) Chemical food preservatives. In *Disinfection, Sterilization and Preservation*, 3rd edn (ed. Block, S.S.), pp. 657–694. Philadelphia: Lea and Febiger.

Calmette, A. (1899) Rapport sur la sterilisation industrielle des eaux potables. *Annales de l'Institut Pasteur*, **13**, 344–357.

Caputo, R.A., Fisher, J., Jarzynski, V. & Martens, P.A. (1993) Validation testing of a gas plasma sterilization system. *Medical Device and Diagnostic Industry*, January, 132–138.

Chattoraj, D.K. (1970) Formaldehyde induced changes of heat denatured DNA. *Zeitschrift für Naturforschung*, **256**, 1316–1319.

Comité Européen de Normalisation (CEN) (1994a) *pr EN 1422 Sterilizers for Medical Purposes—Ethylene Oxide Sterilizers—Requirements*. Brussels: CEN.

Comité Européen de Normalisation (CEN) (1994b) *EN 550 Sterilization of Medical Devices—Validation and Routine Control of Sterilization by Ethylene Oxide*. Brussels: CEN.

Comité Européen de Normalisation (CEN) (1995a) *pr EN 866-1 Biological Systems for Testing Sterilizers and Sterilization Processes—Part 1: General Requirements*. Brussels: CEN.

Comité Européen de Normalisation (CEN) (1995b) *pr EN 866-2 Biological Systems for Testing Sterilizers and Sterilization Processes—Part 2: Particular Systems for Use in Ethylene Oxide Sterilizers*. Brussels: CEN.

Comité Européen de Normalisation (CEN) (1995c) *per EN 866-5 Biological Systems for Testing Sterilizers—Part 5: Particular Systems for Use in Low Temperature Steam and Formaldehyde Sterilizers*. Brussels: CEN.

Comité Européen de Normalisation (CEN) (1995d) *pr EN 866-8 Biological Systems for Testing Sterilizers and Sterilization Processes—Part 8: Particular Requirements for Self-contained Biological Indicator Systems for Use in Ethylene Oxide Sterilizers*. Brussels: CEN.

Commission of the European Communities (1993) Directive concerning medical devices 93/42/EEC. *Official Journal of the European Communities*, **L169**, 1–43.

Commission of the European Communities (1994) Council Regulation (EC) No. 3093/94 of 15 December 1994 on substances that deplete the ozone layer. *Official Journal of the European Communities*, **L333**, 1–19.

Cotton, R.T. & Roark, R.C. (1928) Ethylene oxide as a fumigant. *Industrial and Engineering Chemistry*, **20**, 805.

Cronier, S.D. (1977) Destruction by chlorine dioxide of viruses and bacteria in water. MS thesis, University of Cincinnati, Ohio.

Cross, G.L.C. & Lach, V.H. (1990) The effects of controlled exposure to formaldehyde vapour on spores of *Bacillus globigii* NCTC 10073. *Journal of Applied Bacteriology*, **68**, 461–469.

Curran, H.R., Evans, F.R. & Leviton, A. (1940) The sporicidal action of hydrogen peroxide and the use of crystalline catalase to dissipate residual peroxide. *Journal of Bacteriology*, **40**, 423–434.

Dadd, A.H. & Daley, G.M. (1980) Resistance of micro-organisms to inactivation by gaseous ethylene oxide. *Journal of Applied Bacteriology*, **49**, 89–101.

Dadd, A.H., Town, M.M. & McCormick, K.E. (1985) The influence of water on the resistance of spores to inactivation by gaseous ethylene oxide. *Journal of Applied Bacteriology*, **58**, 613–621.

Dahi, E. (1976) Physicochemical aspects of disinfection of water by means of ultrasound and ozone. *Water Research*, **10**, 677–684.

Dancer, B.N., Power, E.G. & Russell, A.D. (1989) Alkali-induced revival of *Bacillus* spores after inactivation by glutaraldehyde. *FEMS Microbiology Letters*, **48**, 345–348.

Davenport, S.M. (1989) Design and use of a novel peracetic acid sterilizer for absolute barrier sterility testing chambers. *Journal of Parenteral Science and Technology*, **43**, 158–166.

Department of Health (1994) *Health Technical Memorandum 2010 Part 3: Validation and Verification—Sterilization*. London: Her Majesty's Stationery Office.

Dewhurst, E. & Hoxey, E.V. (1990) Sterilization methods. In *Guide to Microbiological Control in Pharmaceuticals* (eds Denyer, S. & Baird, R.), pp. 182–218. London: Ellis Horwood.

Elford, W.J. & van den Ende, J. (1942) An investigation of the merits of ozone as an aerial disinfectant. *Journal of Hygiene*, **42**, 240–265.

Ernst, E.R. & Doyle, J.E. (1968) Sterilization with gaseous ethylene oxide: a review of chemical and physical factors. *Biotechnology and Bioengineering*, **10**, 1–31.

Ernst, E.R. & Shull, J.J. (1962a) Ethylene oxide gaseous sterilization. I. Concentration and temperature effects. *Applied Microbiology*, **10**, 337–341.

Ernst, E.R. & Shull, J.J. (1962b) Ethylene oxide gaseous sterilization. II. Influence of method of humidification. *Applied Microbiology*, **10**, 342–344.

Farooq, S. & Akhlaque, S. (1983) Comparative response of mixed cultures of bacteria and viruses to ozonation. *Water Research* **17**, 809–812.

Fraser, S.J., Gillette, R.B. & Olson, R.L. (1974) *Sterilizing and Packaging Process Utilizing Gas Plasma*. US Patent 3 851 436.

Fraser, S.J., Gillette, R.B. & Olson, R.L. (1976) *Sterilizing Process and Apparatus Utilizing Gas Plasma*. US Patent 3 948 601.

Gal, G., Kiss, E., Foldes, J. & Dombi, A. (1992) Disinfection of regenerated dialyzers with ozone. *International Journal of Artificial Organs*, **15**, 461–464.

German, A., Panouse-Perin, J. & Gurin, B. (1966) Sterilization with ozone. *Annales Pharmaceutiques Françaises*, **24**, 693–701.

Gershenfeld, L. & Davis, D.E. (1952) The effect of peracetic acid on some thermoaciduric bacteria. *American Journal of Pharmacy*, **124**, 337–342.

Gilbert, G.L., Gambill, V.M., Spiner, D.R., Hoffman, R.K. & Phillips, C.R. (1964) Effect of moisture on ethylene oxide sterilization. *Applied Microbiology*, **12**, 496–503.

Greene, A.K., Few, B.K. & Serafini, J.C. (1993) A comparison of ozonation and chlorination for the disinfection of stainless steel surfaces. *Journal of Dairy Science*, **76**, 3612–3620.

Griffith, C.L. & Hall, L.A. (1940) *Sterilizing Colloid Materials*. US Patent 2 189 949.

Gross, P.M. & Dixon, L.F. (1937) *Method of Sterilizing*. US Patent 2 075 845.

Gut Boucher, R.M. (1980) *Seeded Gas Plasma Sterilization Method*. US Patent 4,207,286.

Haller, J.F. & Northgraves, W.W. (1955) Chlorine dioxide and safety. *TAPP*, **38**, 199–202.

Handlos, V. (1977) Formaldehyde sterilization I. Determination of formaldehyde residuals in autoclave-sterilized materials. *Archives of Pharmaceutical Chemistry and Scientific Education*, **5**, 163–169.

Handlos, V. (1979) Formaldehyde sterilization II. Formaldehyde-steam sterilization; the process and its influence on the formaldehyde residuals. *Archives of Pharmaceutical Chemistry and Scientific Education*, **7**, 1–11.

Handlos, V. (1984) Technical aspects of gaseous formaldehyde as a sterilant. *Biomaterials*, **5**, 81–85.

Hauchman, F.S. (1983) Inactivation of viruses with chlorine dioxide. PhD thesis, Johns Hopkins University, Baltimore, Maryland.

Hauchman, F.S.I., Noss, C.I. & Olivieri, V.P. (1986) Chlorine dioxide reactivity with nucleic acids. *Water Research*, **20**, 357–361.

Health and Safety Executive (1996) *EH 40/96 Occupational Exposure Limits 1996*. Sheffield: Health and Safety Executive.

Hoffman, R.K. (1971) Toxic gases. In *Inhibition and Destruction of the Microbial Cell* (ed. Hugo, W.B.), pp. 225–258. London and New York: Academic Press.

Hoffman, R.K. & Warshowsky, B. (1958) Beta-propiolactone vapor as a disinfectant. *Applied Microbiology*, **6**, 358–362.

Hoxey, E.V. (1984) Bacterial spores as biological indicators for sterilization by low temperature steam and formaldehyde. PhD thesis, University of Bath.

Hoxey, E.V. (1989) The case for parametric release. In *Proceedings of the Eucomed Conference on Ethylene Oxide Sterilization* (21–22 April 1989, Paris), pp. 45–47. Brussels: Eucomed.

Hoxey, E.V. (1991) Low temperature steam formaldehyde. In *Sterilization of Medical Products* (eds Morrissey, R.F. & Prokopenko, Y.I.), pp. 359–364. Morin Heights, Canada: Polyscience Publications.

Hurrell, D.J., Line S.J. & Cutts, D.W. (1983) Isolating samples in the chamber of a steam–formaldehyde sterilizer. *Journal of Applied Bacteriology*, **55**, 135–142.

Ide, P.R. (1979) The sensitivity of some avian viruses to formaldehyde fumigation. *Canadian Journal of Comparative Medicine*, **43**, 211–216.

Ikarashi, Y., Tsuchiya, T. & Nakamura, A. (1995) Cytotoxicity of medical materials sterilized with vapour-phase hydrogen peroxide. *Biomaterials*, **16**, 177–183.

Ingram, M. & Barnes, E.M. (1959) Sterilization by means of ozone. *Journal of Applied Bacteriology*, **17**, 246–271.

International Agency for Research on Cancer (IARC) (1985) *Hydrogen Peroxide*. IARC Monograph. Geneva: World Health Organization.

International Agency for Research on Cancer (IARC) (1994) *Ethylene Oxide*. IARC Monograph. Geneva: World Health Organization.

International Electrotechnical Commision (IEC) (1996) *IEC FDIS 1010-2-042 Safety Requirements for Electrical Equipment for Measurement, Control and Laboratory Use. Particular Requirements for Autoclaves Using Toxic Gas for the Treatment of Medical Materials, and for Laboratory Processes*. Geneva: IEC.

International Programme on Chemical Safety (IPCS) (1990) *Ozone*. IPCS Chemical Safety Card, Vol. 68. Geneva: World Health Organization.

International Programme on Chemical Safety (IPCS) (1991a) *Formaldehyde*. IPCS Health and Safety Guide, Vol. 57. Geneva: World Health Organization.

International Programme on Chemical Safety (IPCS) (1991b) *Chlorine Dioxide*. IPCS Safety Card, Vol. 127. Geneva: World Health Organization.

International Standards Organization (ISO) (1994) *ISO 11135 Sterilization of Medical Devices—Validation and Routine Control of Industrial Ethylene Oxide Sterilization*. Geneva: ISO.

International Standards Organization (ISO) (1995) *ISO CD 14538 Method for the Establishment of Allowable Limits for Residues in Medical Devices Using Health-based Risk Assessment*. Geneva: ISO.

International Standards Organization (ISO) (1996) *ISO 10993-7 Biological Evaluation of Medical Devices—Part 7: Ethylene Oxide Sterilization Residuals*. Geneva: ISO.

International Standards Organization (ISO) (1997) *ISO CD 14937 Sterilization of Healthcare Products—General Requirements for Characterization of a Sterilizing Agent, and the Development, Validation and Routine Control of a Sterilization Process*. Geneva: ISO.

Jacobs, P.T. (1989) Plasma sterilization. *Journal of Healthcare Material Management*, 7, 49.

Janssen, D.W. & Schneider, P.M. (1993) Overview of ethylene oxide alternative sterilization technologies. *Zentral Sterilisation*, **1**, 16–32.

Jeng, D.K. & Woodworth, A.G. (1990a) Chlorine dioxide gas sterilization of oxygenators in an industrial scale sterilizer: a successful model. *Artificial Organs*, **14**, 361–368.

Jeng, D.K. & Woodworth, A.G. (1990b) Chlorine dioxide gas sterilization under square wave conditions. *Applied and Environmental Microbiology*, **56**, 514–519.

Johnson, J.W., Arnold, J.F., Nail, S.L. & Renzi, E. (1992) Vaporized hydrogen peroxide sterilization of freeze dryers. *Journal of Parenteral Science and Technology*, **46**, 215–225.

Jones, L.A. Jr, Hoffman, R.K. & Philips, C.R. (1967) Sporicidal activity of peracetic acid and β-propiolactone at subzero temperatures. *Applied Microbiology*, **15**, 357–362.

Jorkasky, J.F. (1993) Special considerations for ethylene oxide: chlorofluorocarbons. In *Sterilization Technology* (eds Morrissey, R.F. & Phillips, G. B.), pp. 391–401. New York: Van Nostrand Reinhold.

Kamiki, T. & Kikkawa, Y. (1976) Ozone sterilization technique of hydrophillic contact lenses. *A 20th Congress Paper. Contact*, **20**, 16–18.

Karlson, E.K. (1989) Ozone sterilization. *Journal of Healthcare Material Management*, 7, 43–45.

Kaye, S. (1949) The sterilizing action of gaseous ethylene oxide. III. The effect of ethylene oxide and related compounds upon bacterial aerosols. *American Journal of Hygiene*, **50**, 289–295.

Kaye, S. & Phillips, C.R. (1949) The sterilizing action of gaseous ethylene oxide. IV. The effect of moisture. *American Journal of Hygiene*, **50**, 296–306.

Kietzmann, U. (1957) Über die Wirkung von Ozon gegen Bakterien in der Lebensmittel und Fischindustrie. *Archiv für Lebensmittelhygiene*, **8**, 35–37.

Kereluk, K., Gammon R.A. & Lloyd R.S. (1970) Microbiological aspects of ethylene oxide sterilization. II Microbial resistance to ethylene oxide. *Applied Microbiology*, **19**, 152–156.

Kessel, J.F., Allison, D.K., Moore, F.J. & Kaime, M. (1943) Comparison of chlorine and ozone as virucidal agents of poliomyelitis virus. *Proceedings of the Society for Experimental Biology and Medicine*, **53**, 71–73.

Klarenbeek, A. & Van Tongeren, H.A.E. (1954) Viricidal action of ethylene oxide gas. *American Journal of Hygiene*, **52**, 525–528.

Klapes, N.A. & Vesley, D. (1990) Vapour-phase hydrogen peroxide as a surface decontaminant and sterilant. *Applied and Environmental Microbiology*, **56**, 503–506.

Knapp, J.E., Rosenblatt, D.H. & Rosenblatt, A.A. (1986) Chlorine dioxide as a gaseous sterilant. *Medical Device and Diagnostic Industry*, 8, 48–51.

Kolb, R.W. & Schneitner, R. (1950) The germicidal and sporicidal efficacy of methyl bromide for *Bacillus anthracis*. *Journal of Bacteriology*, **59**, 401–412.

Kowalski, J.B., Hollis, R.A. & Roman, C.A. (1988) Sterilization of over wrapped foil suture packages with gaseous chlorine dioxide. In *Developments in Industrial Microbiology*, Vol. 29 (ed. Pierce, G.), pp. 239–245. Amsterdam: Elsevier Science Publishers.

Kozlov, Y.I. & Debabov, V.G. (1972) Change in matrix properties of native DNA treated with formaldehyde. *Biochemistry USSR*, **37**, 304–311.

Lee, M.G., Ireland, D.S., Hunt, P., Vallor, J., Francis, P. & Gothard, A. (1990) Water purification using ozone and UV radiation in combination. *Pharmaceutical Journal*, **245**, 674–675.

Leiguarda, R.H., Peso, D.A. & de Palazzolo, A. (1949) Accion bactercida del ozono. *Annales de la Asociacion Quimica Argentina*, **37**, 165.

Line, S.J. & Pickerill, J.K. (1973) Testing a steam–formaldehyde sterilizer for gas penetration efficiency. *Journal of Clinical Pathology*, **26**, 716–719.

Liu, T.S., Howard, G.L. & Stumbo, C.R. (1968) Dichlorodifluoromethane–ethylene oxide mixture as a sterilant at elevated temperatures. *Food Technology*, **22**, 86–89.

Loew, O. (1886) Über Formaldehyd und dessen Condensation. *Journal für Praktische Chemie Chemiker Zeitung*, **33**, 321–351.

Lowings, P.H. (1956) The fungal contamination of kentish strawberry fruits in 1955. *Applied Microbiology*, **4**, 84–88.

McCarthy, J.A. (1944) Bromine and chlorine dioxide as water disinfectants. *Journal of the New England Water Works Association*, **58**, 55–68.

Majumdar, S.B., Ceckler, W.H. & Sproul, O.J. (1973) Inactivation of poliovirus in water by ozonation. *Journal WPCF*, **45**, 2433–2443.

Malchesky, P.S. (1993) Peracetic acid and its application to medical instrument sterilization. *Artificial Organs*, **17**, 147–152.

Marcos, D. & Wiseman, D. (1979) Measurements of formaldehyde concentrations in a sub-atmospheric steam–formaldehyde autoclave. *Journal of Clinical Pathology*, **32**, 567–575.

Masschelein, W.J. (1979) Industrial applications of chlorine dioxide and sodium chlorite. In *Chemistry and Environmental Impact of Oxychlorine Compounds* (ed. Rice, R.G.), pp. 147–183. Ann Arbor, Michigan: Ann Arbor Science Publishers.

Masschelein, W.J. (1982) *Ozonization Manual for Water and Wastewater Treatment*. New York: John Wiley & Sons.

Matthews, I.P., Gibson, C. & Samuel, A.H. (1989) Enhancement of the kinetics of the aeration of ethylene oxide sterilized polymers using microwave radiation. *Journal of Biomedical Material Research*, **23**, 143–156.

Mecke, P. (1992) Hydrogen peroxide plasma—an interesting microbiocidal concept. *Hygiene und Medizin*, **17**, 537–543.

Menashi, W.P. (1968) *Treatment of Surfaces*. US Patent 3 383 163.

National Research Council (1980) *Drinking Water and Health*, Vol. 2. Washington, DC: National Research Council.

Nordgren, G. (1939) Investigations on the sterilization efficacy of gaseous formaldehyde. *Acta Pathologica et Microbiologica Scandinavica*, Supplement XL, 1–165.

Noss, C.I., Hauchman, F.S. & Olivieri, V.P. (1986) Chlorine dioxide reactivity with proteins. *Water Research*, **20**, 351–356.

Orcutt, R.P., Otis, A.P. & Alliger, H. (1981) Alcide TM: an alternative sterilant to peracetic acid. In *Recent Advances in Germfree Research. Proceedings of the VIIth International Symposium on Gnotobiology* (eds Sasaki, S., Ozawa, A. & Hashioto, K.), pp. 79–81. Tokyo: Japan: Tokai University Press.

Page B.F.J. (1993) Special considerations for ethylene oxide: product residues. In *Sterilization Technology* (eds Morrissey, R.F. & Phillips, G.B.), pp. 402–420. New York: Van Nostrand Reinhold.

Peeples, R.E. & Anderson, N.R. (1985a) Microwave coupled plasma sterilization and depyrogenation I. System characteristics. *Journal of Parenteral Science and Technology*, **39**, 2–8.

Peeples, R.E. & Anderson, N.R. (1985b) Microwave coupled plasma sterilization and depyrogenation II. Mechanisms of action. *Journal of Parenteral Science and Technology*, **39**, 9–15.

Pflug, I.J. & Holcomb, R. (1983) Principles of thermal destruction of microorganisms. In *Disinfection, Sterilization and Preservation*, 3rd edn (ed. Block, S.S.), pp. 51–810. Philadelphia: Lea and Febiger.

Phillips, C.R. (1949) The sterilizing action of gaseous ethylene oxide. II Sterilization of contaminated objects with ethylene oxide and related compounds: time, concentration and temperature relationships. *American Journal of Hygiene*, **50**, 280–288.

Phillips, C.R. (1952) Part IX. Relative resistance of bacterial spores and vegetative bacteria to disinfectants. *Bacteriological Reviews*, **16**, 135–138.

Phillips, C.R. & Kaye, S. (1949) The sterilizing action of gaseous ethylene oxide. I. Review. *American Journal of Hygiene*, **50**, 270–279.

Pickerill, J.K. (1975) Practical system for steam–formaldehyde sterilizing. *Laboratory Practice*, **24**, 401–404.

Portner, D.M. & Hoffman, R.K. (1968) Sporicidal effect of peracetic acid vapour. *Applied Microbiology*, **16**, 1782–1785.

Posey, J.L. & Swank, R.W. (1989) *Apparatus for Sterilizing Film and Like Packaging Material*. US Patent 4 888 155.

Posey, J.L., Swank, R.W., Sliva, M.E. & Picken, J.E. (1988) *Apparatus for Removing Liquid and Residue from a Web of Film*. US Patent 4 783 947.

Profumo, A. & Pesavento, M. (1986) Extraction and gas chromatographic determination of residual formaldehyde in micro-surgical materials. *Analyst*, **111**, 241–242.

Public Health Laboratory Service (1958) Disinfection of fabrics with gaseous formaldehyde by the committee on formaldehyde disinfection. *Journal of Hygiene, Cambridge*, **56**, 488–515.

Rickloff, J.R. & Graham, G.S. (1989) Vapour phase hydrogen peroxide sterilization. *Journal of Healthcare Material Management*, **7**, 45–49.

Ridenour, G.M. & Armbruster, E.H. (1949) Bactericidal effect of chlorine dioxide. *Journal of the American Water Works Association*, **41**, 537–550.

Ridenour, G.M. & Ingols, R.S. (1947) Bactericidal properties of chlorine dioxide. *Journal of the American Water Works Association*, **39**, 561–567.

Ridenour, G.M., Ingols, R.S. & Armbruster, E.H. (1949) Sporicidal properties of chlorine dioxide. *Water and Sewage Works*, **96**, 279–283.

Robertshaw, R.G. (1983) Low temperature steam and formaldehyde sterilization. *Journal of Hospital Infection*, **4**, 305–314.

Rosenblatt, D.H., Rosenblatt, A.A. & Knapp, J.E. (1985) *Use of Chlorine Dioxide Gas as a Chemosterilizing Agent*. US Patent 4 504 442.

Rosenblatt, D.H., Rosenblatt, A.A. & Knapp, J.E. (1987) *Use of Chlorine Dioxide Gas as a Chemosterilizing Agent*. US Patent 4 681 739.

Rutala, W.A. & Weber, D.J. (1996) Low temperature sterilization technologies: do we need to redefine 'sterilization'? *Infection Control and Hospital Epidemiology*, **17**, 87–91.

Sanchez-Ruiz, C., Martinez-Royano, S. & Tejero-Monzon, I. (1995) An evaluation of the efficiency and impact of raw wastewater disinfection with peracetic acid prior to ocean discharge. *Water Science and Technology*, **32**, 159–166.

Schrader, H. & Bossert, E. (1936) *Fumigant Composition*. US Patent 2,037,439.

Schumb, W.C., Satterfield, C.N. & Wentworth, R.L. (1955) *Hydrogen Peroxide*. New York: Reinhold.

Singer, P.C. (1990) Assessing ozonation research needs in water treatment. *Journal of the American Water Works Association*, **84**, 78–88.

Sintim-Damoa, K. (1993) Other gaseous methods. In *Sterilization Technology* (eds Morrissey, R.F. & Phillips, G.B.), pp. 335–347. New York: Van Nostrand Reinhold.

Snyder, J.E. & Chang, P.W. (1974) Relative resistance of eight human enteric viruses to ozonation in Saugatucket River water. In *Proceedings of the International Ozone Institute Workshop on Aquatic Applications of Ozone*, pp. 82–99. Boston: International Ozone Institute.

Sordellini, P.J. (1997) Speeding ethylene oxide-sterilized products to market with parametric release. *Medical Device and Diagnostic Industry*, **19**, 67–80.

Spicher, G. & Peters, J. (1976) Microbial resistance to formaldehyde I. Comparative quantitative studies in some selected species of vegetative bacteria, bacterial spores, fungi, bacteriophages and viruses. *Zentralblatt für Bakteriologie, Parasitenkunde, Infektions-Krankheiten und Hygiene, I. Abteilung Originale, Reihe B*, **173**, 188–196.

Spicher, G. & Peters, J. (1981) Heat activation of bacterial spores after inactivation by formaldehyde: dependence of heat activation on temperature and duration of action. *Zbl. Bakt. Hyg. I Abt. Orig. B* **173**, 188–196.

Spiner, D.R. & Hoffman, R.K. (1971) Effect of relative humidity on formaldehyde decontamination. *Applied Microbiology*, **22**, 1138–1140.

Sprague, E.K. (1899) Formaldehyde disinfection in a vacuum chamber. *Public Health Reports*, **14**, 1549–1559.

Sproul, O.J. & Majumdar, S.B. (1975) Poliovirus inactivation with ozone in water. In *Proceedings of the 1st International Symposium on Ozone Water Wastewater Treatment 1973* (eds Rice, R.G. & Browning, M.E.), pp. 288–295. Waterbury, Connecticut: International Ozone Institute.

Stevenson, K.E. & Shafer, B.D. (1983) Bacterial spore resistance to hydrogen peroxide. *Food Technology*, **37**, 111–114.

Stoddart, G.M. (1989) Ozone as a sterilizing agent. *Journal of Healthcare Material Management*, **7**, 42–43.

Sulzer, F., Ramadan, F. & Wuhrmann, K. (1959) Studies on the germicidal action of ozone. *Schweiz. Z. Hydrol.* **21**, 112–122.

Swartling, P.& Lindgren, B. (1968) The sterilizing effect against *Bacillus subtilis* spores of hydrogen peroxide at different temperatures and concentrations. *Journal of Dairy Research*, **35**, 423–428.

Symons, J.M. (1980) Ozone, chlorine dioxide and chloramines as alternatives to chlorine for disinfection of drinking water: generation and usage of alternate disinfectants. In *Ozone and Chlorine Dioxide Technology for Disinfection of Drinking water*. (ed. Katz, J.), pp. 4–12. Park Ridge, New Jersey: Noyes Data Corporation.

Syvan, J.F., MacMahon, J.D. & Vincent, G.P. (1944) Chlorine dioxide—a development in the treatment of potable water. *Water Works and Sewerage*, **91**, 423–426.

Tensmeyer, L.G. (1976) *Method of Killing Microorganisms in the Inside of a Container Utilizing a Laser Beam Induced Plasma*. US Patent 3,955,921.

Tensmeyer, L.G., Wright, P.E., Fegenbush, D.O. & Snapp, S.W. (1981) Sterilization of glass containers by laser initiated plasmas. *Journal of Parenteral Science and Technology*, **35**, 93–96.

Toledo,R.T., Escher, F.E. & Ayres, J.C. (1973) Sporicidal properties of hydrogen peroxide against food spoilage organisms. *Applied Microbiology*, **26**, 592–597.

Trakhtman, N.N. (1946) Chlorine dioxide in water disinfection. *Giegiena i Sanit*, **11**, 10–13.

Trujillo, R. & David, T.J. (1972) Sporostatic and sporicidal properties of aqueous formaldehyde. *Applied Microbiology*, **23**, 618–622.

Turner, F.J. (1983) Hydrogen peroxide and other oxidant disinfectants. In *Disinfection, Sterilization and Preservation*, 3rd edn (ed. Block, S.S.), pp. 240–250. Philadelphia: Lea and Febiger.

United Nations Environment Programme (UNEP)

(1987) *Montreal Protocol on Substances that Deplete the Ozone Layer.* Final act, Nairobi. New York: UNEP.

Vaughn, J.M., Chen, Y.S., Lindburg, K. & Morales, D. (1987) Inactivation of human and simian rotaviruses by ozone. *Applied and Environmental Microbiology*, **53**, 218–2221.

Vink, P. (1986) Residual formaldehyde in steam–formaldehyde sterilized materials. *Biomaterials*, **7**, 221–224.

Wagner, E.L. (1962) Bond character in XYm-type molecules: chlorine–oxygen compounds. *Journal of Chemistry and Physics*, **37**, 751–759.

Walker, G.S., Lee, F.P. & Aieta, E.M. (1986) Chlorine dioxide for taste and odour control. *Journal of the American Water Works Association*, **78**, 84–93.

Walker, J.F. (1964) *Formaldehyde.* ACS Monograph No. 159. New York: Reinhold.

Walker, J.T., Mackerness, C.W., Malloin, D., Makin, T., Williets, T. & Keevil, C.W. (1995) Control of *Legionella pneumophila* in a hospital water system by chlorine dioxide. *Journal of Industrial Microbiology*, **15**, 384–390.

Wardle, M.D. & Renninger, G.M. (1975) Bactericidal effect of hydrogen peroxide on spacecraft isolates. *Applied Microbiology*, **30**, 710–711.

White, G.C. (1986) *Handbook of Chlorination*, 2nd edn. New York: Van Nostrand Reinhold.

Wilkins, R.J. & MacLeod, H.D. (1976) Formaldehyde induced DNA–protein crosslinks in *Escherichia coli. Mutation Research*, **36**, 11–16.

Winarno, F.G. & Stumbo, C.R. (1971) Mode of action of ethylene oxide on spores of *Clostridium botulinum* 62A. *Journal of Food Science*, **36**, 892–895.

Wright, A.M., Hoxey, E.V., Soper, C.J. & Davies, D.J.G. (1996) Biological indicators for low temperature steam formaldehyde sterilization: investigation of the effect of change in temperature and formaldehyde concentration on spores of *Bacillus stearothermophilus* NCIMB 8224. *Journal of Applied Bacteriology*, **80**, 259–265.

Wright, A.M., Hoxey, E.V., Soper, C.J. & Davies, D.J.G (1997) Biological indicators for low temperature steam formaldehyde sterilization: effect of variations in recovery conditions on the response of spores of *Bacillus stearothermophilus* NCIMB 8224 to low temperature steam formaldehyde. *Journal of Applied Bacteriology*, **82**, 552–556.

CHAPTER 22

Filtration Sterilization

1 Historical introduction

It was stated in Chapter 1 that ancient historical writers recognized the clear and drinkable quality of water trickling through a river or lake bank, although the source was foul-tasting and clouded. Certain ancient purveyors of wine, Rhodian for example, were renowned for producing a crystal-clear product, although, like other wise technologists, they did not make their secret available to others, but it was believed that a filtration process was involved.

Early attempts to purify water were made by allowing it to percolate through beds of sand, gravel or cinders and a complex ecosystem developed on these filters. An increasing knowledge of bacteriology and an awareness of the involvement of water-borne bacteria (*Vibrio cholerae*, enterobacteria and pathogenic protozoa and worms, in disease and epidemics, eventually led to a more thorough study of filtration devices.

Chamberland, a colleague of Louis Pasteur, invented a thimble-like vessel, made by sintering a moulded kaolin and sand mix. These so-called Chamberland candles were the first fabricated filters and represent another example of the inventive output from the Pasteur school (Chamberland, 1884). Later to be made by the English firm of Doulton and other ceramic manufacturers, they were essentially of unglazed porcelain. These filters enjoyed a great vogue in the pharmaceutical industry until the advent of membrane filters (Section 2.4) rendered them practically obsolete in this area.

2 Filtration media

The ideal filter medium to remove microorganisms from solutions destined for parenteral administration should offer the following characteristics:
- efficient removal of particles above a stated size;
- acceptably high flow rate;
- resistance to clogging;
- steam-sterilizable;
- flexibility and mechanical strength;
- low potential to release fibres or chemicals into the filtrate;

- low potential to sorb materials from liquids being sterilized;
- non-pyrogenic and biologically inert.

Additionally, when such a medium is mounted in a holder or support, it must be amenable to *in situ* sterilization and integrity testing. The medium most frequently employed, and which most nearly approaches the ideal, is the polymeric membrane, usually in the format of a flat disc or a pleated cartridge (Section 2.4). As a consequence this medium is by far the most important in current use, but several other filter media have been used in the past, which are deficient in one or more of the above and yet retain limited and specialized applications (Sections 2.2 and 2.3).

2.1 Filters of diatomaceous earth

Diatomaceous earth, added to liquid products to form a suspended slurry, has been widely used as a filter aid in the pharmaceutical industry. The slurry is deposited on porous supports and the liquid then passes through, leaving coarse particulate matter entrained within the retained filter cake. Such an approach is employed in rotary-drum vaccum filters (Dahlstrom & Silverblatt, 1986), as used in antibiotic manufacture for instance, where the drum rotates within the slurry, pulling filtered liquid through the retained cake under vacuum and leaving the cell debris behind.

2.2 Fibrous-pad filters

Originally constructed of asbestos fibres, until the toxicity of asbestos was recognized, microfibres of borosilicate glass are now employed to create these filters. They have found widespread application in filter presses and as prefilters for clarification of pharmaceutical solutions. It is usual to employ such filters with a membrane filter (Section 2.4) downstream to collect any shed fibres.

Other materials used in the construction of this type of filter include paper, nylon, polyester, cellulose-acetate fibres and woven-wool fibres.

2.3 Sintered or fritted ware

This type of filter was made by taking particles of glass or metal (stainless steel or silver), assembling them in suitable holders and subjecting them to a heat process, so that the particles melted or softened on their surfaces and, on cooling, fused together. It is clear that a complete melting would defeat the object of the technology and this partial melting, followed by surface fusion, was called sintering or frittering. Such a process will give rise to a porous sheet of material, which can then act as a filter (Smith, 1944). This process differs from the sintering process used in the manufacture of unglazed porcelain, in that the latter contains several components and the process is accompanied by chemical changes in the constituents.

2.3.1 Sintered glass filters

Their invention is attributed to the German glass manufacturers Scholt u Gen. of Jena (Prausnitz, 1924).

Their application to bacteriology was described by Morton & Czarnatzky (1937), where a disc of porosity 3 surmounted by one of porosity 5, suitably retained in a funnel, was used to sterilize culture media. It was also shown that broth cultures of several microbial species, including *Serratia marcescens*, were sterilized by passing through this system. The pore size of the filters is controlled by the general particle size of the glass powder used to fabricate them.

Sintered-glass filters are easily cleaned, using back-washing or oxidizing chemicals, such as hypochlorite or nitric/sulphuric acid; they have low sorption properties and do not shed particles into the solution they are filtering. On the other hand, their size is constrained by their nature and they are fragile and relatively expensive.

2.3.2 Sintered metal filters

Metal particles can be fabricated into porous sheets by the same process as for glass. Bronze, cupronickel, stainless steel and silver have been used. Sintered silver is a potential sterilizing filter, combining, as it does, its filtering facility with its potential oligodynamic action.

2.4 Membrane filters

Membrane filter technology has had over 80 years

in which to develop, since the first description, by Zsigmondy & Bachmann in 1918, of a method suitable for producing cellulose membrane filters on a commercial scale. The full potential of membrane filters was not recognized until their successful application in the detection of contaminated water-supplies in Germany during the Second World War (Gelman, 1965). Following their commercial exploitation in the 1950s and 1960s, a number of large international companies evolved which now offer the potential user an ever-increasing but bewildering array of filters and associated equipment from which to choose. Undoubtedly, the role played by membrane filters continues to expand, both in the laboratory and in industry, and they are now routinely used in water analysis and purification, sterility testing and sterilization. Their future is assured, at least in the pharmaceutical industry, unless other, as yet undiscovered, techniques emerge, since they represent the most suitable filtration medium currently available for the preparation of sterile, filtered parenteral products to a standard accepted by all the various regulatory authorities.

2.4.1 Methods of manufacture

There are four major methods of membrane-filter manufacture currently employed on an industrial scale. These involve either a gelling and casting process, an irradiation-etch process, an expansion process or a procedure involving the anodic oxidation of aluminium. Each method produces membranes with their own particular characteristics.

Gelling and casting process. This is perhaps the most widely used process, and all the major filter manufacturers offer filters prepared by this method. Cast polymeric membranes, as they are known, are principally derived from pure cellulose nitrate, mixed esters of acetate and nitrate or other materials offering greater chemical resistance, e.g. nylon 66 (Kesting *et al.*, 1983), polyvinylidine fluoride (PVDF) or polytetrafluoroethylene (PTFE) (Gelman, 1965).

In essence, the process still utilizes the principles outlined by Zsigmondy & Bachmann in 1918, where the polymer is mixed with a suitable organic solvent or combination of solvents and allowed to gel (Ehrlich, 1960). In the modern process, a minute quantity of hydrophilic polymer may be present as

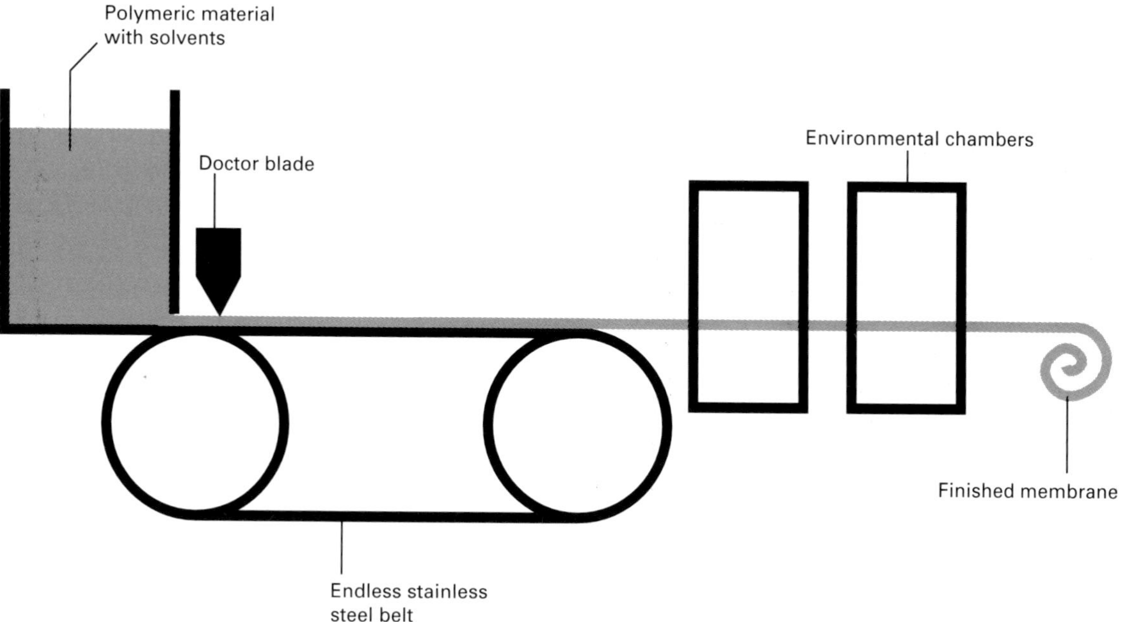

Fig. 22.1 Membrane manufacture—the casting process.

a wetting agent, ethylene glycol may be added as a 'pore-former' and glycerol is often included to afford flexibility to the finished membrane. The mixture is then cast on to a moving, perfectly smooth, stainless-steel belt, to give a film 90–170 μm thick (Fig. 22.1). By carefully controlling the temperature and relative humidity, the solvents are slowly evaporated off, leaving a wet gel of highly porous, three-dimensional structure, which dries to give a membrane of considerable mechanical strength (Fig. 22.2). Pore size and other membrane characteristics are determined by the initial concentration of the polymer, the mixing process, including the solvents added, and the environmental drying conditions.

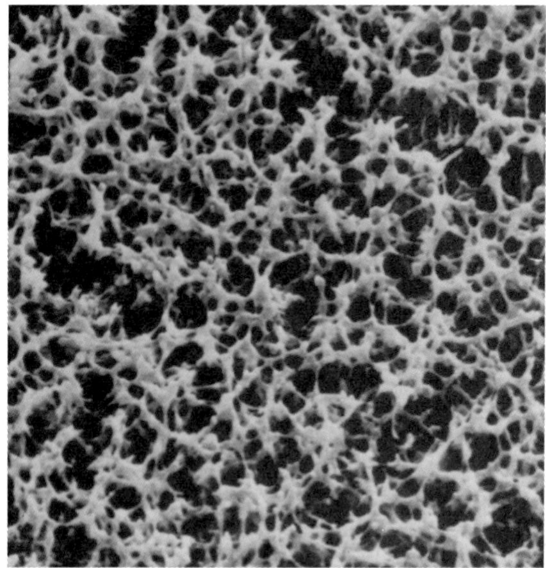

Fig. 22.2 Scanning electron micrograph (4000×) of the surface of a 0.22 μm pore-size cast cellulose membrane filter.

Track-etch (irradiation-etch) process. Developed from the method of Fleischer *et al.* (1964) and originally patented with the Nuclepore Corporation, this process is operated in two stages. First, a thin film (5–10 μm thick) of polycarbonate or polyester material is exposed to a stream of charged particles in a nuclear reactor; this is followed by a second stage, where the fission tracks made through the film are etched out into round, randomly dispersed cylindrical pores (Fig. 22.3). Pore density and pore size are controlled by the duration of exposure of the film within the reactor and

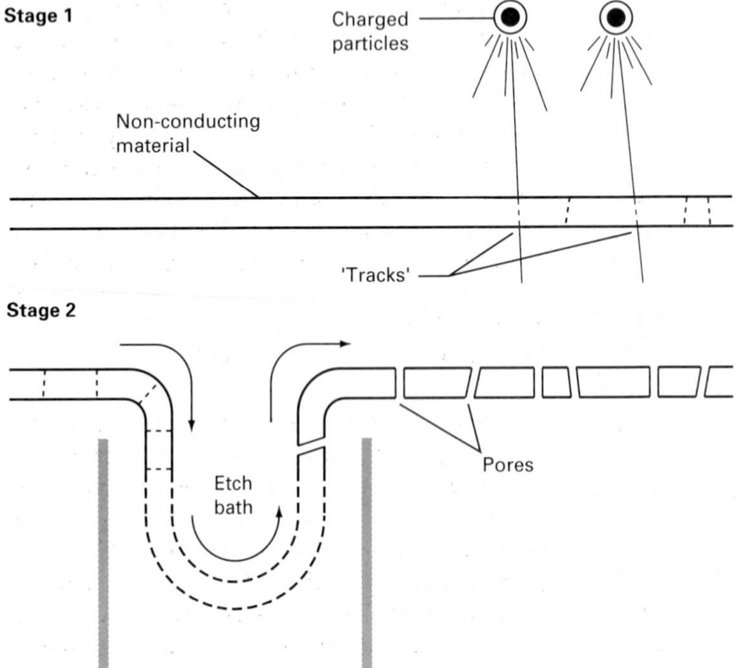

Fig. 22.3 Membrane manufacture—the irradiation-etch process (see text for details of stages 1 and 2).

by the etching process, respectively. The finished track-etched membranes are thin, transparent, strong and flexible (Fig. 22.4).

Expansion process. Stretching and expanding of fluorocarbon sheets, e.g. PTFE, along both axes is sometimes undertaken to provide porous, chemically inert membranes. A support of polyethylene or polypropylene is usually bonded to one side of the membrane to improve handling characteristics. Their hydrophobic nature ensures that these filters are widely employed in the filtration of air and non-aqueous liquids.

An alternative method of production for PTFE filters is by a process that forms a continuous mat of microfibres, fused together at each intersection to prevent shedding into the filtrate. These filters usually have no supporting layer to reduce their chemical resistance.

Anodic oxidation of aluminium. This procedure is employed to produce ultrathin membranes, with a honeycomb-pore structure, in which the pores have a narrow size distribution (Jones, 1990). These membranes are hydrophilic and offer several advantages over polymeric membranes, including very high temperature stability (up to 400°C) and minimal levels of extractable materials, because monomers, plasticizers and surfactants are not used in the production process.

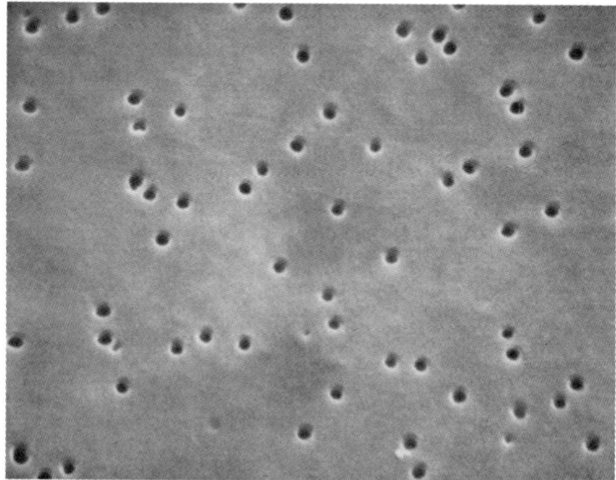

Fig. 22.4 Scanning electron micrograph (10000×) of the surface of a 0.2-μm pore-size polycarbonate track-etch membrane filter.

Other methods of filter construction. Other methods of manufacture include solvent leaching of one material from a cast mixture, leaving pores and the production of bundles of hollow fibres.

2.4.2 The mechanisms of membrane filtration

Membrane filters are often described as 'screen' filters and are thereby contrasted directly with filter media that are believed to retain particles and organisms by a 'depth' filtration process. By this simple definition, filters made from sintered glass, compressed fibre or ceramic materials are classified as depth filters, while membranes derived from cast materials, stretched polymers and irradiated plastics are classified as screen filters. In essence, during depth filtration, particles are trapped or adsorbed within the interstices of the filter matrix, while screen filtration involves the exclusion (sieving out) of all particles larger than the rated pore size (Fig. 22.5).

Unfortunately, classification of membrane filters is not nearly as simple as this scheme might suggest. It is now recognized that the filtration characteristics of many membrane filters cannot be accounted for in terms of the sieve-retention theory alone. In 1963, Megaw & Wiffen pointed out that, although membrane filters would be expected to act primarily by sieve retention, they did possess the property of retaining particles that were much smaller than the membrane pore size, larger particles being trapped by impaction in the filter pores. (This aspect is discussed in more detail below). A more precise classification might be expected to take into consideration the considerable variation in membrane filter structure (see Section 2.4.1) and the subsequent influence that this may have on the mechanism of filtration.

The influence of membrane-filter structure on the filtration process. Several studies have reported a marked difference between the pore structure of the upper and lower surfaces of cellulose membrane filters. Of particular note are the works of Preusser (1967), Denee & Stein (1971) and Marshall & Meltzer (1976). These workers have all shown one surface to have a greater porosity than the other. This phenomenon can be used to advantage in filtrations, since it confers a depth-like filtration

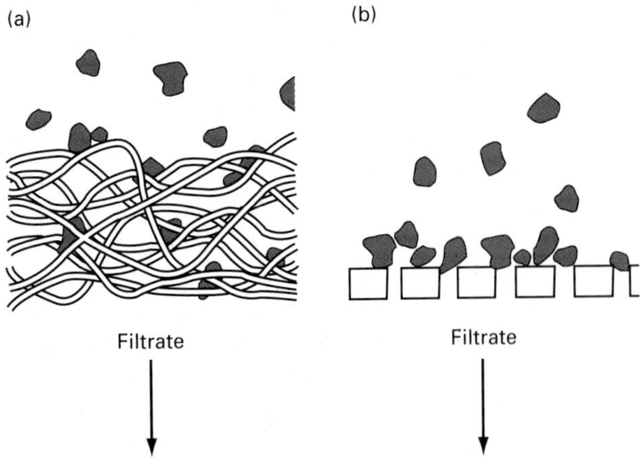

Fig. 22.5 Comparison between (a) depth, and (b) screen filtration.

characteristic on the cellulose membranes when used with the more open side upstream. Particles can now enter the interstices of the filter, increasing the time to clogging. The variation in flow rate and total throughput resulting from the different directions of flow can exceed 50%. Most filter manufacturers recognize the asymmetry of their membranes; indeed, several emphasize it in their technical literature and ensure that all filters are packed in the preferred flow direction (top to bottom). Highly anisotropic membranes, with superior filtration characteristics to those of conventional mixed-ester membranes, have been described (Kesting *et al.*, 1981; Wrasidlo & Mysels, 1984).

A membrane filter can be further characterized by its pore-size distribution and pore numbers. Manufacturers give their membranes either a 'nominal' or 'absolute' pore-size rating, usually qualified by certain tolerance limits. 'Nominal' pore size implies that a certain percentage of contamination above that size is retained, e.g. if the initial inoculum is 10^6 bacteria, a 99.999% retention efficiency for an organism above the pore size means that 10 bacteria pass into the filtrate Wallhausser, 1976). Graphs depicting pore-size distribution have been offered by several filter manufacturers (Fig. 22.6). It must be remembered that the techniques used to establish pore size vary from manufacturer to manufacturer, and the values obtained are not necessarily comparable (Brock, 1983).

Jacobs (1972) described the distribution of pore diameters in graded ultrafilter membranes and dis-

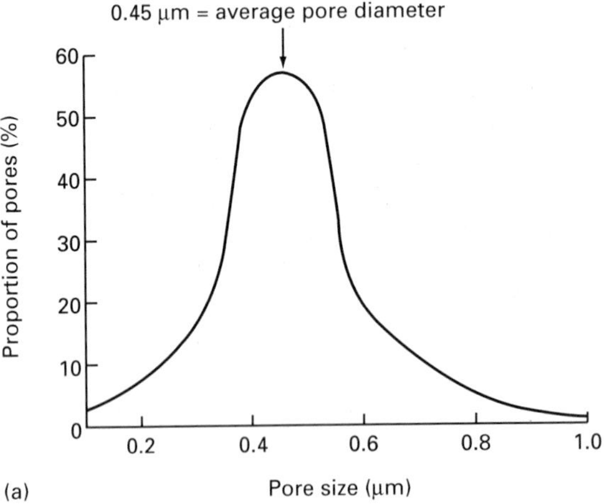

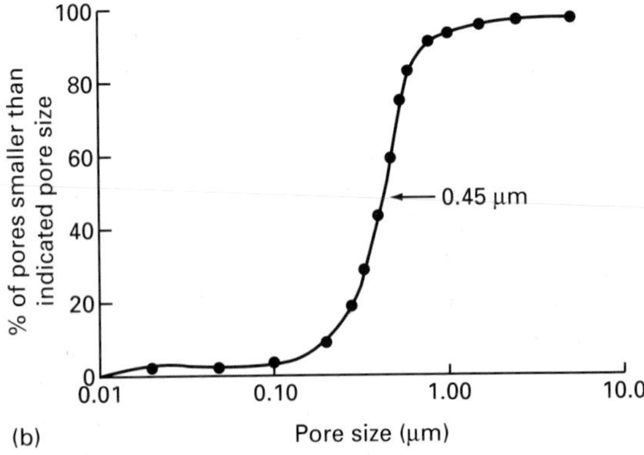

Fig. 22.6 Typical pore-size distribution curves for some commercially available 0.45 μm rated cellulose membrane filters. (a) Schleicher & Schüll type BA85; (b) Oxoid Nuflow. These data were obtained from mercury intrusion tests. (Reproduced by courtesy of the companies concerned.)

cussed the maximum pore diameters and average pore diameters of various commercially available membranes. Subsequently, other workers were unable to confirm a pore size distribution of ±0.03 μm about a mean value, as is claimed for certain 0.45 μm filters (Pall, 1975; Marshall & Meltzer, 1976). While it has long been established that track-etched filters normally possess a greater uniformity than cast polymeric membranes, it is, nevertheless, clear that track-etched filters may not be entirely free from irregularities in pore size and shape (Pall, 1975; Alkan & Groves, 1978). A broader pore-size distribution within a membrane filter is not necessarily considered a failing, since it offers resistance to early clogging occasioned by too close a match between the dominant pore size and the prevailing particle size.

Cellulosic filters (available in a range of pore sizes from around 12 μm down to 0.025 μm) possess between 10^7 and 10^{11} pores/cm^2, the number increasing as the pore size decreases. This contrasts with the 10^5 to 6×10^8 pores/cm^2 offered by a similar size range of track-etched filters. The number of pores and their size distribution will contribute to the overall porosity (void volume) of the filter system, which is considered to be approximately 65–85% for cellulose filters (decreasing with decreasing pore size) and only 5–10% for the track-etched product. Overall fluid-flow characteristics are similar for both types of filter (Ballew *et al.*, 1978), however, since the greater thickness of cellulose filters (≃150 μm) and their tortuous pore system afford approximately 15 times more resistance to flow than the 10-μm-thick track-etched filter.

There appears little justification for assuming a uniform pore structure, at least within the cast polymeric membranes, and the simple capillary pore model (Fig. 22.5) does not describe correctly the typical membrane filter. Duberstein (1979) states that the bacterial-removal efficiency of membrane filters depends on the membrane pore size distribution and on the thickness of the membrane; the latter is in disagreement with the sieve theory (see below), which relies solely on retention associated with the pore size of the surface pores. Furthermore, these two factors are not the only ones that have a bearing on the bacterial-removal efficacy; both the tortuosity of the pores through the membrane and its chemical composition (and hence its surface charge) will influence the extent of removal.

For the thin track-etched membrane, the contribution made by the thickness of the filter towards the retention process may be considered small, especially in the light of their relatively uncomplicated pore structure, and the term 'screen' filter may adequately described this type of membrane (Heidam, 1981). The thicker cast polymeric membranes, as exemplified by the cellulose filters, however, offer characteristics between those of a true depth filter and those of a true screen filter and may best be described as membrane 'depth' filters. With these filters, very small particles will be retained by adsorption, but a point must be reached beyond which the smallest particle confronting any filter is larger than that filter's largest pore, in which case the sieve mechanism can adequately describe the filtration phenomenon.

By accepting this distinction within the group of membrane filters, it is possible to understand why the useful lifetime of track-etched filters can sometimes be extended by 'back-flushing'. During any filtration process, as particles are removed from suspension and deposited on the filter, a gradual increase in pressure is required to maintain the same filtration rate. At a certain point, this pressure becomes unacceptably high and the membrane can then be said to be effectively plugged. The reversal of fluid flow easily dislodges particles from the membrane surface, satisfactorily unplugging screen filters, but it cannot remove those particles trapped within the interstices of the membrane 'depth' filter, which generally remains blocked.

The removal of microorganisms from liquids by filtration. It would be logical to assume that the pore size of sterilizing membrane filters is a major factor in determining whether bacteria are retained by the filter or can pass through into the filtrate. Such a premise is based on the sieve-retention theory of filtration, with a direct relationship between the largest pore in the filter and the smallest particle present (Brooks, 1979). The bubble-point method commonly used as an indication of pore size (Section 4; see also Rogers & Rossmore, 1970; Lukaszewiez *et al.*, 1978) is considered to be a useful guide to the ability of a filter element to remove bacteria, although it is deficient in some respects (Pall, 1975). Lukaszewicz & Meltzer (1979a) and Trasen (1979) likewise opine that this method serves as an index of retentivity.

Sterile filtration—the absolute removal of bacteria, yeasts and moulds—should by definition be able to deliver a sterile effluent independently of the challenge conditions, even when these are severe (Reti, 1977). In practice, this can be achieved by means of a 0.22 (or 0.2)-μm filter, although various authors have, in fact, shown that this filter is not absolute. Bowman *et al.* (1967) described the isolation of an obligate aerobe (cell diameter < 0.33 μm), then termed a *Pseudomonas* sp. ATCC 19146 (later called *Ps. diminuta*, now *Brevundimonas diminuta*), which could pass through a 0.45-μm membrane filter (see below); this poses a severe challenge to sterilization by filtration. The idea that sterile filtration is independent of the challenge condition is untenable. One of the prerequisites for successful filtration is an initial low number of organisms; as the number of *Br. diminuta* in the test challenge increases, the probability of bacteria in the filtrate increases (Wallhausser, 1976). An early report (Elford, 1933) had likewise shown that a filter's ability to retain organisms decreased as the number of test organisms (in this case, *Serr. marcescens*) increased and as the filter's pore-size rating increased. Approximately 0–20 *Pseudomonas* organisms/l can pass through even so-called absolute filters (Wallhausser, 1979); the extent of the passage of *Br. diminuta* through membrane filters is encouraged by increasing pressures (Reti & Leahy, 1979).

Leptospira species, together with other waterborne bacteria, have also been reported in the filtrate of well water that had passed through a 0.2-μm-rated membrane (Howard & Duberstein, 1980), and even the larger cells of *Serr. marcescens* can also pass through a 0.2-μm filter, although to a much smaller extent than *Br. diminuta* (Wallhauser, 1979). Mycoplasmas, which lack rigid cell walls and consequently have a more plastic structure than bacteria, can pass through 0.22-μm filters (Lukaszewicz & Meltzer, 1979b), and such an organism, *Acholeplasma laidlawii*, has been used to validate 0.1-μm-rated sterilizing filters (Bower & Fox, 1985).

Wallhausser (1979) emphasizes the pore-size distribution of filter materials, which may be heterogeneous in form and composition, and the fact that pore size itself cannot be taken as an absolute yardstick for sterile filtration. It is to be expected, therefore, that two filters with the same nominal pore size can have markedly different filtration efficiencies, not only because the number, tortuosity and sorption characteristics of the channels within them may vary, but also because they have been characterized using different methods. The Food and Drugs Administration (FDA, 1987) has defined a sterilizing filter as one which, when challenged with *Br. diminuta* at a minimum concentration of 10^7 organisms cm^2 of filter surface area, will produce a sterile filtrate. Different manufacturers, however, may adopt alternative, and possibly markedly less severe, criteria; Osumi *et al.*, (1991) identified four manufacturers among whom the range of maximum bacterial challenges used to demonstrate a sterile filtrate was from $10^9/cm^2$ down to $10^4/cm^2$. Clearly therefore, care must be exercised in selecting a filter, particularly in an industrial setting, when there are several alternatives of the same nominal grade to choose from. There are dangers in attempting to select on the basis of price alone.

The reduction in bacterial concentration used as a parameter of filter efficiency is normally termed the titre reduction value (Tr). Because it is the ratio of the number of organisms challenging the filter to the number of organisms that pass through, the production of a sterile filtrate will, axiomatically, give a Tr of infinity. Under these circumstances, convention places '>' in front of the challenge number, so that a sterile filtrate resulting from a challenge of 10^7 is represented as a Tr of $> 10^7$. The Tr may also be represented as its logarithmic value, i.e. 7, when it is called a log removal factor.

The foregoing thus suggests that sieve retention is only one mechanism responsible for sterile filtration. Other contributing factors include van der Waals forces and electrostatic interactions (Lukaszewicz & Meltzer, 1979b). Tanny *et al.* (1979) showed that many *Br. diminuta* cells could be removed from suspension by adsorptive sequestration, using a 0.45-μm membrane filter, and postulated that an organism could actually enter the pore but be retained there by this mechanism.

The retention mechanisms operating during

membrane filtration are elegantly illustrated in the scanning electron micrographs of Todd & Kerr (1972), where the screen-filter action of a track-etched filter is clearly contrasted with the depth-filter characteristics of a cellulose membrane filter. Similarly, Osumi *et al.* (1991) published scanning electron micrographs clearly showing that many of the pores in a 0.2-μm-rated membrane were much larger than the *Br. diminuta* cells that were entrapped within them, and that the bacteria were usually retained by the membrane within the first 30 μm of the filter depth. The dominance of adsorptive effects during the filtration of plasma proteins and influenza vaccine through 0.22-μm and 0.45-μm membrane filters, respectively, has been recognized (Hawker & Hawker, 1975; Tanny & Meltzer, 1978). Track-etched filters show few adsorptive properties and this can be attributed to their thinness, lack of tortuous channels and hence purely sieve-like properties. Adsorptive sequestration is not an inherent quality of a filter, but rather describes the ability of that filter to capture organisms of a given size (Lukaszewicz *et al.*, 1978; Lukaszewicz & Meltzer, 1979a). Depth-type filters, with a broad distribution of pore sizes, are believed to retain organisms largely by adsorption (Lukaszewicz & Meltzer, 1979a). Bobbit and Betts (1992) compared bacterial retention at a range of pore sizes on both screen-type polycarbonate membranes and cellulose-ester membranes. They observed that the former exhibited a much more distinct size threshold at which no further cells would pass through the membrane, and so had greater potential for the selective removal of bacteria from suspension according to size.

Specific developments in membrane filter materials have led to the creation of positively charged filters (Hou & Zaniewski, 1980), with the capacity to remove viral, pyrogen (Baumgartner *et al.*, 1986; Hou *et al.*, 1990; Van-Doorne, 1993) and bacteriophage contaminants from liquids. These contaminants are retained by electrostatic attraction within the matrix of the filter; their dimensions would not allow removal by sieving. The efficiency of charged filters can be influenced by operational conditions (Carazzone *et al.*, 1985). Aranah-Creado *et al.* (1996) have demonstrated that hydrophilic PVDF membrane filters in the form of discs or cartridges are capable of producing a Tr of at least 10^6 for viruses larger than 50 nm, irrespective of the carrier fluid, and even Tr values of 10^4 or more for very small viruses, e.g. poliovirus (28–30 nm) when suspended in water. Greater Tr values, of the order of 4×10^9, have been reported by Parks *et al.* (1996) for MS-2 coliphage during the operating of air filters, but the phage were generated as aerosols, with droplet sizes which were much greater than the dimensions of the individual phage particles (23 nm).

Thus, sieve retention may yet be the most important mechanism whereby sterile filtration is achieved, but it is unlikely to be the sole contributory factor. Although many membrane filters can no longer be considered to act simply as sieves, their thinness and greater uniformity of pore size give them several advantages over conventional depth filters (Section 2.4.4), a fact that is widely exploited in filtration technology.

Perhaps the most widely accepted description of a membrane filter would be that it has a thin, continuous and homogeneous polymeric structure, from which no parts can be shed. As such, it would comply with the definition laid down by the FDA in the USA for a non-fibre-releasing filter which 'after any appropriate pre-treatment such as washing or flushing, will not continue to release fibres into the drug product or component which is being filtered' (Elias, 1975). In addition, it would meet the requirements for a sterilizing filter as laid down by the *United States Pharmacopoeia* (1995) and the *European Pharmacopoeia* (1997).

2.4.3 Membrane filters used for sterilization

A typical size distribution of particles within a fluid is illustrated in Fig. 22.7, where, despite the broad range of sizes, the highest concentration of particles exists in the submicrometre range. Superimposed upon the graph are curves comparing the reduced particulate burden of the filtrate following passage through a 1.0-μm nominal-depth filter and a 1.0-μm absolute membrane filter.

The most suitable pore size for a sterilizing-grade filter is chosen, in part, by considering the minimum dimension (frequently less than 1 μm) of the microorganism to be retained (Fig. 22.7). The efficient removal of all bacteria from contaminated solutions may sometimes require a 0.1-μm-rated

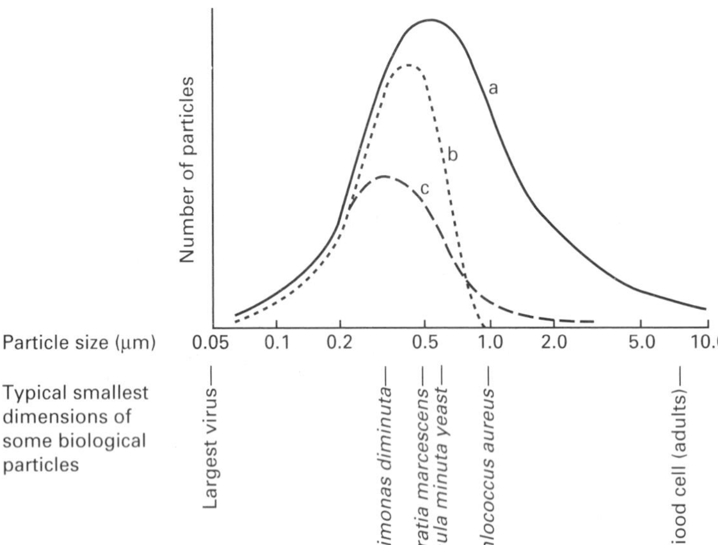

Fig. 22.7 A typical distribution of particle sizes within a fluid. (a) Unfiltered particle size distribution; (b) distribution after passage through a 1-μm absolute membrane filter; (c) distribution after passage through a 1-μm nominal-depth filter.

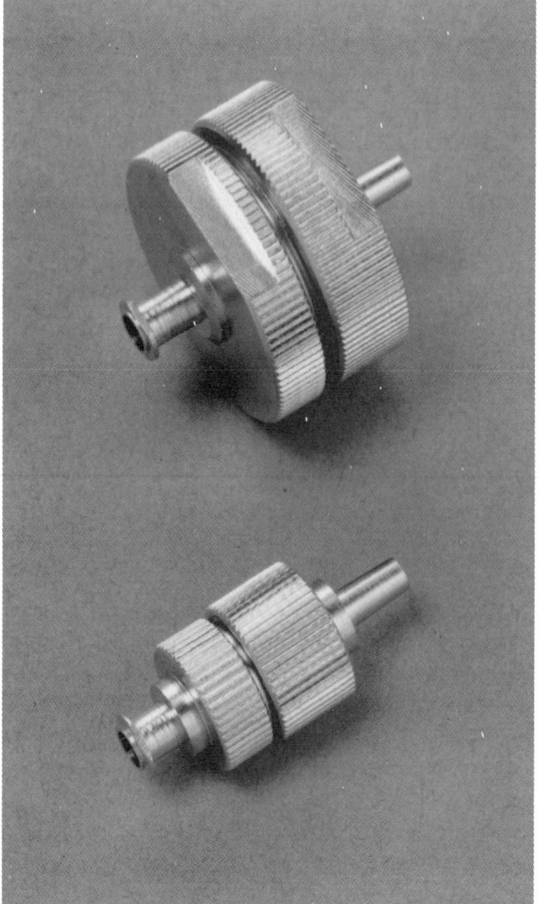

(a)

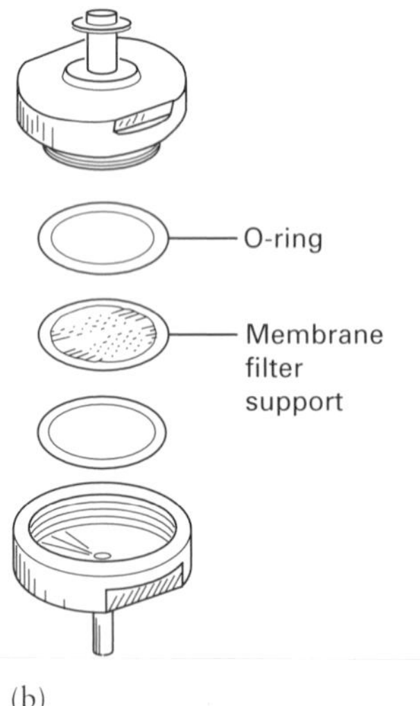

(b)

Fig. 22.8 13-mm and 25-mm stainless-steel filter holders designed for filtering small volumes of fluid from a syringe.

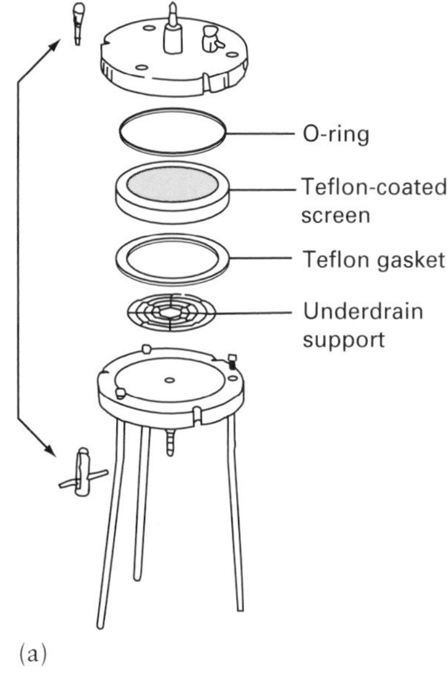

(a)

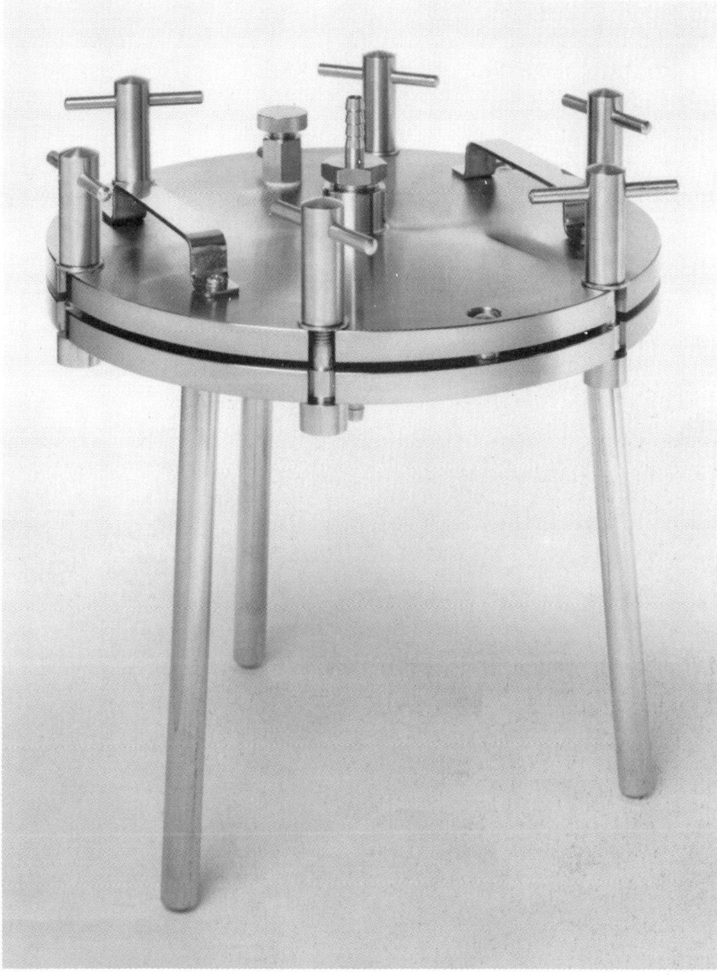

(b)

Fig. 22.9 293-mm stainless-steel filter holder.

membrane filter (Howard & Duberstein, 1980). Certainly, the exclusion of mycoplasmas from certain tissue-culture preparations is achieved by the use of such a filter (Lukaszewicz & Meltzer, 1979b). Experience has shown, however, that, under normal pharmaceutical good manufacturing practice (GMP) conditions (Anon., 1989; Rules, 1997), the sterilization of pharmaceutical and blood products can be assured by their passage through a 0.2–0.22-μm membrane filter, but part of the process validation must include regular sterility tests.

In other areas, where the likely contaminants are known or additional filtrative mechanisms are at play, a membrane filter of larger pore size may be considered sufficient to ensure sterility. For

Table 22.1 Effect of filter diameter on filtration volumes.

Filter diameter (mm)	Effective filtration area* (cm^2)	Typical batch volume† (l)
13	0.8	0.01
25	3.9	0.05–0.1
47	11.3	0.1–0.3
90	45	0.3–5
142	97	5–20
293	530	20

* Taken from one manufacturer's data and to some extent dependent on the type of filter holder used. Values may well vary from manufacturer to manufacturer.

† For a low-viscosity liquid.

instance, the sterilization of air and gases during venting or pressurizing procedures can often be assured by passage through filters of 0.45–0.8-μm-rated pore size. The removal of yeast during the stabilization of beers and wines can be effected by a 0.6-μm membrane filter. In general, however, such filters are only employed in systems where a reduction in bacterial numbers and not complete sterilization is demanded. An ideal example of this is the routine filtration through a 0.45-μm-rated filter of parenteral solutions that are later to be terminally sterilized. This reduces the likelihood of bacterial growth and pyrogen production prior to autoclaving.

An absolute filter cannot distinguish between particle types and, as a consequence, filtration sterilization will ensure the removal of all particles (in addition to microorganisms) with dimensions in excess of the rated pore size. This is of obvious benefit in the pharmaceutical production of sterile parenteral fluids, in which the presence of particulate matter can have serious consequences (Turco & Davis, 1973a).

Sterilizing membrane filters are available in discs

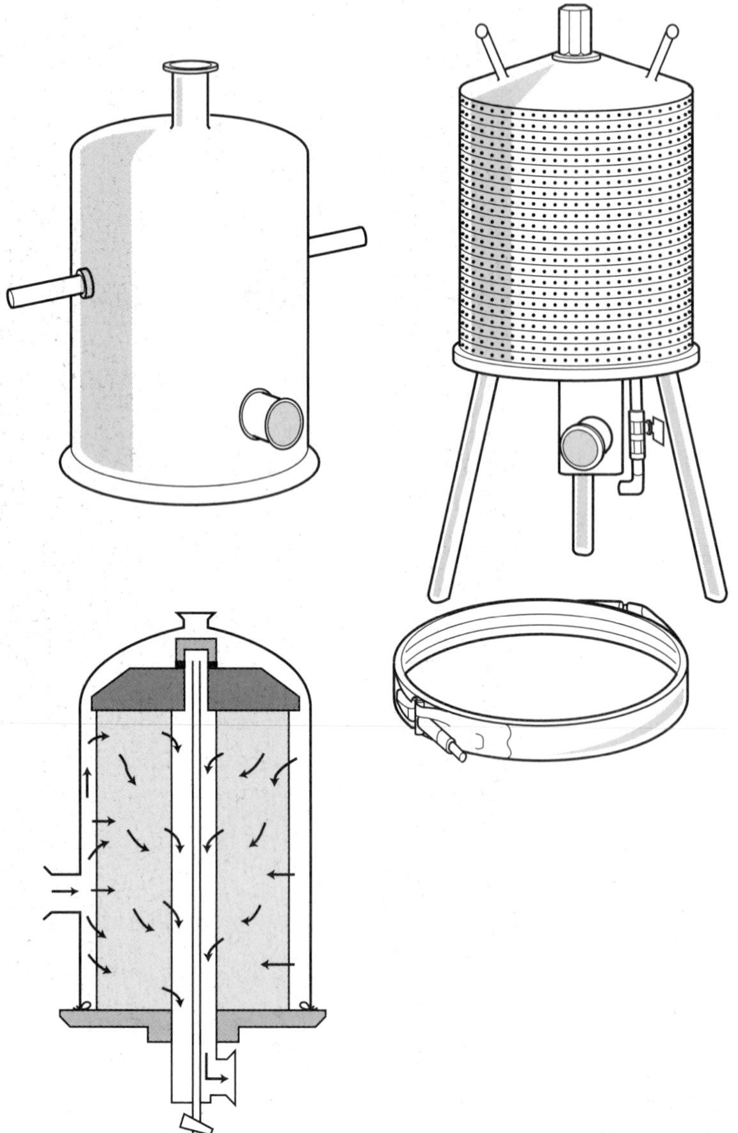

Fig. 22.10 A typical multiple-plate filtration system, with inset showing the fluid-flow path during filtration.

ranging from 13 to 293 mm in diameter and are designed for assembly into filter holders of the types illustrated in Figs 22.8 and 22.9. Their filtrative capacities make them the ideal choice for the small- and medium-scale processes normally encountered in the laboratory or hospital pharmacy (Table 22.1).

The flow rate of a clean liquid through a membrane filter (volume passed per unit time) is a function of that liquid's viscosity, the pressure differential across the filter and the filtration area and is given by:

$$Q = C\frac{AP}{V} \quad (21.1)$$

where Q = volumetric flow rate, A = filtration area, V = viscosity of the liquid, P = pressure differential across the membrane and C = resistance to fluid flow offered by the filter medium, governed in part by the size, tortuosity and number of pores.

The industrial manufacturer of sterile fluids needs to filter very large volumes and, as a consequence, demands a flow rate far beyond the capabilities of the largest available membrane disc. To provide the filtration area needed, multiple-plate filtration systems have been employed, where up to 60 flat filter discs of 293 mm diameter, separated by screens and acting in parallel, can be used to provide a total surface area of $3.0\,m^2$. A typical multiple-plate filtration system is illustrated in Fig. 22.10.

A second approach can be to use cartridge filters (Cole *et al.*, 1979). These are essentially hollow cylinders formed from a rigid perforated plastic core, around which the membrane filter, supported by a suitable mesh and sometimes protected by a prefilter, is wound. An outer perforated plastic sleeve provides protection against back-pressure and is held in place by bonded end-caps. The cartridge filter combines the advantages of increased filtration area with ease of handling. Since the filter is no longer in the form of a fragile disc, it can be easily installed in special holders. Multiple cartridge units are available, which may contain, for example, up to 20 79-cm filter tubes (of 5.7 cm diameter), giving a maximum filtration area of approximately $2.4\,m^2$.

The most common filter format for use in large-scale filtration systems is the pleated-membrane cartridge. Early devices were manufactured from a flexible acrylic polyvinylchloride copolymer membrane, incorporating a nylon web support (Conacher, 1976); other membranes have now evolved, which can also be pleated without damage (Meltzer & Lukaszewicz, 1979), and the range of materials includes cellulose esters, PVDF PTFE, nylon, acrylic and polysulphone. The pleated configuration of the membrane ensures a far greater surface

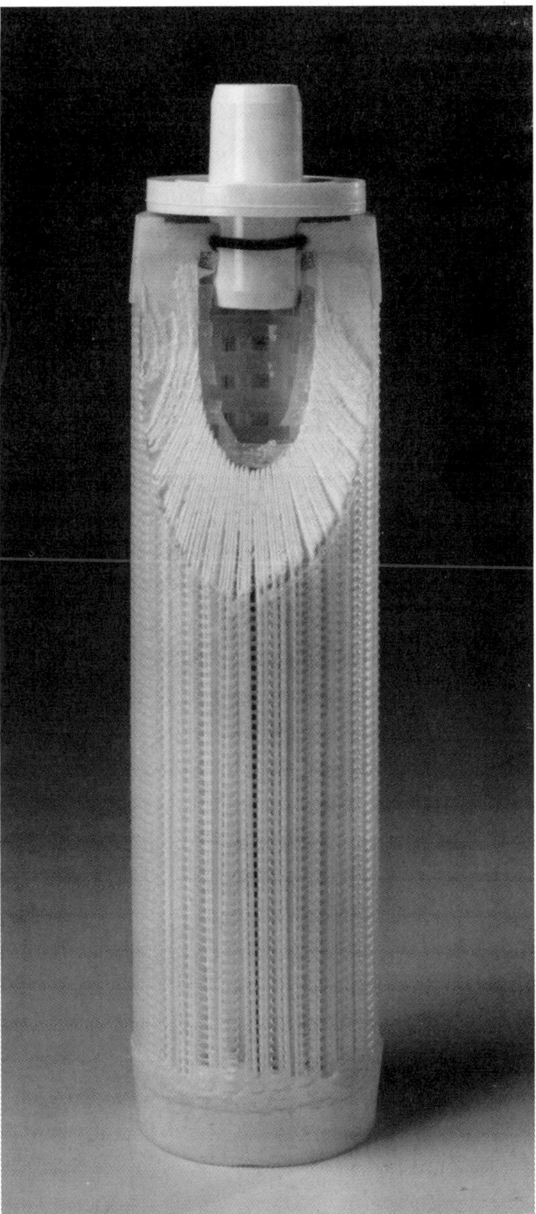

Fig. 22.11 Cutaway showing the construction of a pleated polycarbonate membrane cartridge filter.

area for filtration than a normal cartridge filter of similar dimensions. For comparison, a single standard pleated-polycarbonate membrane cartridge of 24.8 cm length and 6.4 cm diameter, such as that illustrated in Fig. 22.11, can offer a filtration area approaching 1.7m^2, approximately 30 times that afforded by a typical 293-mm membrane disc; the effective area can be increased even further by connecting these cartridges in series. Pleated cartridges are also manufactured as units in sealed plastic capsules, which are disposable and convenient to use, but relatively expensive. Figure 22.12 shows the diverse range of cartridges and capsules currently available.

To ensure the widest application for their filters, manufacturers offer their membranes in a wide variety of constituent materials and formats (Fig. 22.12). This permits the selection of a suitable filter type for use with most of the commonly encountered solvent systems (Gelman, 1965; Brock, 1983). Extensive chemical-compatibility lists are included in the catalogues of most manufacturers

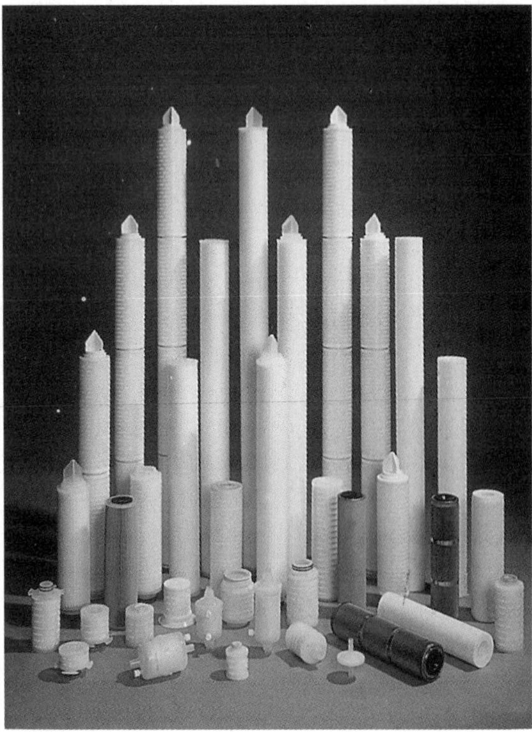

Fig. 22.12 A selection of cartridge and capsule filters, which illustrate the variety available from a major manufacturer.

and further guidance can often be obtained through their technical-support services. Subtle changes in filter structure do occur, however, when processing mixtures of liquids, the complex fluid presenting entirely different solvent properties to the membrane from what could be predicted from compatibility studies involving the individual liquid components. In a number of instances, these changes have resulted in filter failure, and compatibility tests should always be undertaken when mixed-solvent systems are to be processed (Lukaszewicz & Meltzer, 1980). It is as well to remember, also, that any system is only as compatible as its least resistant component, and attention must be paid to the construction materials of the filter holder, seals, tubing and valves.

Hydrophobic filters (e.g. PTFE) are available for the sterile aeration of holding tanks and fermentation vessels in the beverage and biotechnology industries, for the supply of fermentation tanks with sterilized gas, for the filtration of steam and for the removal of water droplets from an oily product. They can be used to filter aqueous solutions by first wetting the membrane with a low-molecular-weight alcohol, such as ethanol. Hydrophobic-edged filters, derived from cellulose nitrate or acetate, whose rims have been impregnated to a width of 3–6 mm with a hydrophobic agent can also be obtained. These find wide application in filtrations requiring that no residual solution remains trapped under the sealing ring of the filter holder, e.g. during the sterility testing of antibiotics. They also have the advantage that air or gas trapped behind a filter can escape through the rim and thus prevent airlocks or dripping during a filtration process.

To ensure the production of a sterile filtrate, the final filter and its holder, together with any downstream distribution equipment, must be sterilized. To minimize aseptic manipulations, it is customary to sterilize the membrane filter after mounting it in the filter holder. The sterilization method is usually selected from among the following: autoclaving, in-line steaming, dry heat, ethylene oxide and γ-irradiation. The choice depends largely upon the heat resistance of the filter and its ancillary equipment, and, before embarking upon any sterilizing procedure, it is first necessary to confirm their thermal stability. In extreme cases, chemical sterilization—for example, by immersion in a 2–3% formaldehyde solution for 24 h—may be the only satisfactory method.

Most filter types will withstand autoclaving conditions of 121°C for 20–30 min and, as a result, the routine autoclaving of assembled small-scale filtration equipment is common practice. Similarly, in-line steaming is a widely used process, in which moist steam is forced through the assembled filter unit (and often the entire filtration system) under conditions sufficient to ensure an adequate period of exposure at 121°C or other appropriate temperature (Kovary *et al.*, 1983; Chrai, 1989). This method is of particular value in large systems employing cartridge filters. It has the added advantage that the complete system can be sterilized, thereby lowering the bacterial contamination upstream from the final bacteria-proof filter. Voorspoels *et al.* (1996) undertook temperature mapping and process-lethality determinations at different locations within assembled cartridge filters, and their findings are particular pertinent to the design of *in situ* sterilization-validation protocols. If the sterilization temperature or time exceeds the limits which are imposed by the manufacturer, 'pore collapse' may occur, with a subsequent reduction in membrane porosity. Frequently, cartridge filters are validated for a fixed number of resterilizations, e.g. four exposures, each of 15 min at 121°C. For this reason, dry heat sterilization is rarely used, since the conditions employed are often too severe. For convenience, certain membrane filters may be obtained in a presterilized form, either individually packed or ready-assembled into filter holders, as single-use devices. Sterility is, in this case, usually achieved by ethylene oxide treatment or γ-irradiation.

2.4.4 Advantages and disadvantages of membrane filters

Membrane filters have several advantages over conventional depth-filtration systems, a conclusion emphasized by the technical literature supplied by the major membrane-filter companies. Table 22.2 summarizes the more important characteristics of membrane filters and compares them with conventional depth filters. Several features require further discussion, since they have considerable bearing on the quality of the final filtered product.

Table 22.2 Characteristics of membrane and depth filters.

Characteristic	Membrane	Depth
1 Filtration (retention efficiency for particles > rated pore size (see Fig. 22.7)	100%	< 100%
2 Speed of filtration	Fast	Slow
3 Dirt-handling capacity	Low	High
4 Duration of service (time to clogging)	Short	Long
5 Shedding of filter components (media migration)	No	Yes
6 Grow-through of microorganisms	Rare (see text)	Yes
7 Fluid retention	Low	High
8 Solute adsorption	Low	High
9 Chemical stability	Variable (depends on membrane)	Good
10 Mechanical strength	Considerable (if supported)	Good
11 Sterilization characteristics	Good	Good
12 Ease of handling	Generally poor	Good
13 Disposability	Yes	Not all types
14 Leaching of extractables	Variable (depends on membrane)	Unlikely

A problem usually associated only with conventional depth filters is that of 'organism grow-through'. If a bacterial filter is used over an extended period of time, bacteria lodged within the matrix can reproduce and successive generations will penetrate further into the filter, eventually emerging to contaminate the filtrate. The extent of this phenomenon will be a function of, at least in part, the nutritional status of the medium being filtered and the nutritional requirements of the contaminant. This problem is no longer considered to be exclusive to conventional depth filters and has been recognized to occur with some 0.45-μm membrane 'depth' filters (Section 2.4.2) (Rusmin *et al.*, 1975). For this reason, it is recommended that the duration of filtration be as short as possible (Lukaszewicz & Meltzer, 1979a; *United States Pharmacopoeia*, 1995).

Solute adsorption by filter is rarely a major problem in large-scale industrial processes, but it can be of greater consequence in the filtration of small volumes containing medicaments at high dilution. Conventional depth-filtration media have been implicated in the adsorption of antibiotics from solution (Wagman *et al.*, 1975), while the thinner membrane filters appear to suffer less from this disadvantage (Rusmin & DeLuca, 1976). Nevertheless, Naido *et al.* (1972) have reported the retention of appreciable quantities (11–17%) of benzalkonium chloride on a 0.45-μm cellulose membrane filter after passing 30 ml of an ophthalmic solution containing 0.02% w/v of the preservative through that filter. S.P. Denyer (unpublished results) has observed a similar loss (38%) of tetradecyltrimethylammonium bromide after filtration of 10 ml of a 0.001% w/v solution through a 0.22-μm cellulose membrane filter. Drug sorption has been reported by De Muynck *et al.* (1988), and a method for its control suggested by Kanke *et al.* (1983). Presumably, adsorption sites are rapidly saturated in these thin membranes, and the passage of additional solution would probably occur without further loss. Nevertheless, it emphasizes the need to select the most compatible filter material and to discard, if at all possible, the first few millilitres of solution run through any filtration system. Flushing through to remove downstream particles is often an integral part of the filtration process anyway.

Care should be taken in the choice of filter in special operations, particularly where the loss of high-value material could be of significant economic importance. For instance, proteins (in particular those of high molecular weight) are readily removed from solution on passage through cellulose-nitrate and mixed-ester filters, and nylon (Hawker & Hawker, 1975; Olson *et al.*, 1977; Akers *et al.*, 1993). This is not so evident for fluorocarbon and cellulose-acetate filters, which would therefore be more suitable for filtration of pharmaceutical protein preparations (Pitt, 1987). The conformational changes elicited in proteins by filtration through filter media have been highlighted by Truskey *et al.* (1987).

A further problem associated with some membrane filters is the leaching of extractives, some of which may be potentially toxic (Brock, 1983; Kristensen *et al.*, 1985). Surfactants, glycerol and other extractable materials added during the manufacturing process may leach from these filters during use, and limited flushing beforehand has been recommended (Olson *et al.*, 1980). As an alternative to flushing, a leaching process has been suggested, which requires boiling the new filter for 5–10 min in two changes of apyrogenic water. The level of extractable material ranges from 0% to 15% of the filter weight and varies according to filter type and filter manufacturer. Special low-water-extractability filters, e.g. those constructed of anodized aluminium (Jones, 1990), are available for use in highly critical applications involving sensitive biological systems, e.g. tissue-culture work, or very small volumes of filtrate. Track-etched membranes yield no leachable material and need not be treated before use.

One problem associated with membrane filters of all types, and of considerable economic importance, is the rapidity with which they clog when a large volume of solution or highly contaminated fluid is processed. To overcome this, it is possible to introduce a depth filter, as a prefilter, into the system, the high 'dirt'-handling capacity of which will remove much of the initial solids and complement the filtering efficiency of the final (sterilizing) membrane filter (Lukaszewicz *et al.*, 1981a). Such a prefilter is generally constructed of bonded borosilicate glass fibre and is available from most manufacturers in sizes and grades compatible with their membrane filters. For use on a large scale, prefilters are often supplied as cartridges. In the critical area of parenteral-product filtration, cellulose-webbing prefilters that do not shed particles are available. By selecting the correct grade of prefilter, the throughput characteristics for any membrane-filtration assembly can be improved significantly (Fig. 22.13).

The correct matching or prefilter grade with membrane pore-size rating does not, on its own, provide the most economical and efficient system. Consideration must also be given to the prefilter membrane surface-area ratio, since too small a prefilter area will result in premature plugging with usable life still remaining in the membrane. Conversely, if the area of the prefilter is too large, it will be left only partly used when the membrane becomes blocked. The ideal ratio will make for the most economic filtration and must be determined for each new system.

3 Applications and limitations of filtration

3.1 Filtration sterilization

Sterilization by filtration is widely used industrially and in hospitals. In brief, it may be employed for the sterilization of thermolabile solutions and soluble solids, as well as in the sterilization of air and other gases. Air sterilization is of particular importance in areas involving the aseptic production of many pharmaceutical products (Fare, 1987; Stockdale, 1987; Anon., 1989; Hargreaves, 1990; *Rules*, 1997; Denyer, 1998), in surgical theatres and in hospital wards specially designed for patients with a low resistance to infection. It would, however, be erroneous to imply that filtration sterilization has no disadvantages or limitations, and these will also be considered where appropriate.

3.1.1 *Sterilization of liquids*

Wherever possible, solutions should be sterilized by heating in an autoclave, because this eliminates the contamination risks associated with the transfer of filtered liquid to sterilized containers. Some solutions are unstable when heated and consequently an alternative sterilizing procedure has to be sought. Ionizing radiation has been studied extensively, but, unfortunately, many substances that can be sterilized by this process in the solid state are unstable when irradiated in solution. Filtration is an obvious choice, although it must be added that another alternative for substances thermostable in the solid form but unstable in solution (even at ambient temperatures) is to sterilize the solid by dry heat and prepare the solution aseptically immediately before use.

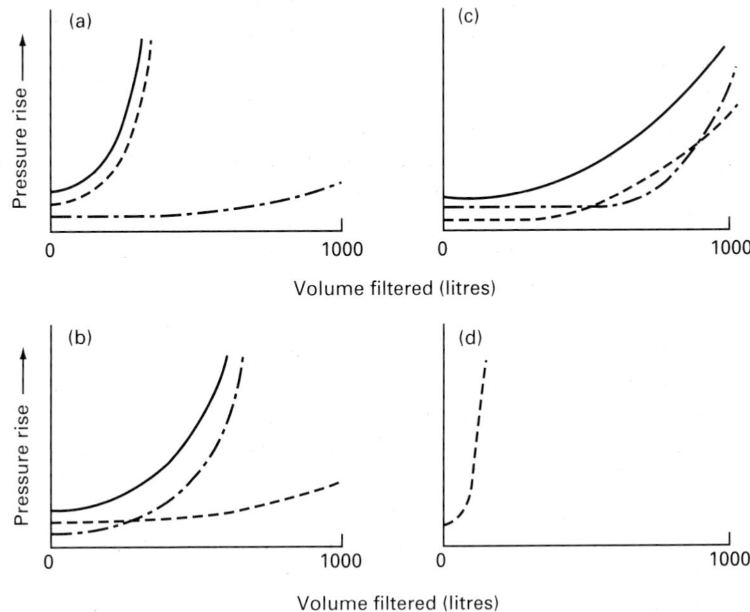

Fig. 22.13 Effect of prefilter characteristics on the volume filtered and filtration pressure. ——, Combination of membrane filter + prefilter; ·—·—·, prefilter alone; - - - - -, membrane filter alone. (a) Prefilter too coarse; insufficient preseparation, membrane filter clogs rapidly, pressure rises rapidly. (b) Prefilter too fine: prefilter clogs faster than membrane filter, poor effective filter life. (c) Correct prefilter: prefilter and membrane filter exhaust themselves approx. simultaneously, optimum effective filter life. (d) Membrane filter without prefilter: rapid rise in pressure, short effective filter life.

Wallhausser (1979) has, however, queried whether filtration can, in fact, be regarded as being a true sterilization process. Admittedly, it will remove microorganisms (see Section 2.4.2 for a discussion of the possible mechanisms of filtration), but the filtration process must then be followed by an aseptic transference of the sterilized solution to the final containers, which are then sealed, and recontamination at this stage remains a possibility.

Sterility assurance levels for products that have been filter-sterilized and aseptically filled are typically of the order of 10^{-3} (Gilbert & Allison, 1996), and it is for this reason that such products are much more heavily reliant on tests for sterility than heat-processed ones, which have sterility assurance levels of, at least, 10^{-6} and usually much better than this. Persuasive arguments, based on a statistical appraisal of the information conventional sterility tests can supply, have been put forward for their abandonment as a means of monitoring thermal-sterilization processes, the tendency now being to validate these processes by biological indicators (see Chapter 25; Brown & Gilbert, 1977). Nevertheless, although there might be much scientific merit in their abandonment, they do form an additional defence in the case of litigation following trauma from a suspected contaminated product, and sterility testing should always be carried out on samples of any batch prepared by an aseptic method. This would mean, in essence, that a solution which can be sterilized rapidly by filtration should ideally not be used until the test sample has passed the sterility test, which may take several days. In an emergency, however, it may well be that clinical judgment has to come down in favour of a hospital-prepared product which has not yet passed a test for sterility, if failure to use it poses a greater risk to the patient.

Despite these criticisms, filtration sterilization is performed on a wide range of liquid preparations (McKinnon & Avis, 1993; Avis, 1997) and routinely on liquid parenteral products (including sera) and on ophthalmic solutions. It is often the only method available to manufacturers of products that cannot be sterilized by thermal processes. Information as to the actual procedures may be found in the *United States Pharmacopoeia* (1995), *British Pharmacopoeia* (1998) and other national and international pharmacopoeias. It must be emphasized that membrane filters are almost exclusively used in this context and that filtration with a filter of 0.22 (or 0.2)-μm pore size, rather than one of 0.45μm, is recommended for this purpose.

Membrane filters find an equally important application in the small-scale intermittent preparation of sterile radiopharmaceuticals and intravenous additives. As a result of the special circumstances surrounding the preparation and use of such products, disposable, sterile filters attached to a syringe are generally used. Preparation of these products is best performed under laminar air flow (LAF) conditions (Section 3.1.3).

The use of sterilizing-grade filters in parenteral therapy is not confined to the production stage alone. In-line terminal membrane filtration has been widely advocated as a final safeguard against the hazards associated with the accidental administration of infusion fluids contaminated with either particles or bacteria (Maki, 1976; Lowe, 1981; McKinnon & Avis, 1993; Voorspoels *et al.*, 1996). These filtration units, generally of 0.22 μm rating, may comprise an integral part of the administration set or form a separate device for introduction proximal to the cannula. In addition to affording some protection against particles and microorganisms introduced during the setting up of the infusion or while making intravenous additions (Davis *et al.*, 1970a,b; Davis and Turco, 1971; Myers, 1972; Holmes & Allwood, 1979), terminal filters also reduce the risk of an air embolism from air bubbles or when an intravenous infusion runs out (a wetted 0.22-μm membrane filter will not pass air at a pressure below 379 kPa (55p.s.i.)). An early problem associated with in-line filters, namely the formation of airlocks stopping fluid flow, has now been largely overcome, either by increasing the upstream chamber volume of the filter device or, more ingeniously, by incorporating a hydrophobic 0.2-μm membrane filter to permit the continuous venting of accumulated air (Wood & Ward, 1981). The properties of a wetted membrane filter have been further exploited in infusion-burette devices, where they act as an air shut-off 'valve', designed to operate following administration of the required volume.

In-line filter systems have been the subject of several studies, which indicate that their use is not entirely without problems. Turco & Davis (1973b) have shown that, with certain fluids, infusion pumps may be needed to maintain adequate flow rates, especially through a 0.22-μm in-line filter, while Miller & Grogan (1973) have highlighted the increased risk of microbial contamination accompanying the extra manipulations of the giving set associated with the inclusion of an in-line filter. It is likely that their use will be further restricted by the additional burden they impose upon the hospital budget. In-line membrane filters may ultimately be limited to patients receiving long-term intravenous infusion, total parenteral nutrition or dialysis, where the frequency and continuation of administration could compound the problems normally associated with these forms of therapy.

Although conventional wisdom formerly suggested that membrane filtration cannot be employed successfully in the sterilization of emulsions (McKinnon & Avis, 1993), recent reports have shown this not to be so, and both parenteral emulsions (Lidgate *et al.*, 1992) and liposome suspensions (Goldbach *et al.*, 1995) have recently been sterilized by this method.

3.1.2 Sterilization of solid products

The *British Pharmacopoeia* (1998) lists four methods that may be used to sterilize powders: ionizing radiation, dry heat, ethylene oxide and filtration. The principle of the filtration process is that the substance to be sterilized is dissolved in an appropriate solvent, the solution filtered through a membrane filter and the sterile filtrate collected. The solvent is removed aseptically by an appropriate method (evaporation, vacuum evaporation, freeze-drying) and the sterile solid transferred into sterile containers, which are then sealed. Such a method was originally used in the manufacture of sterile penicillin powder.

It appears likely that the probability of contamination occurring during the postfiltration (solid-recovery) stage is higher than that described above for sterilizing solutions.

3.1.3 Sterilization of air and other gases

Air is, of course, the most common gas which is required in a sterile condition, although there is a less frequent, but nevertheless significant, requirement for other sterile gases, e.g. nitrogen for sparging the head-space above oxidation-prone liquids and oxygen administered to patients with breathing difficulties. Filters intended to sterilize air are employed in a variety of industrial applications, often as part of a venting system on fermenters, centrifuges, autoclaves and lyophilizers, or in hospitals to supply sterile air in operating theatres or through respirators to patients vulnerable to infection. In both the industrial and hospital settings, sterile air is also required for 'clean rooms' used for aseptic manufacturing or testing.

Many aspects of liquid filtration have direct parallels in the filtration of gases, although there are certain features specific to the latter. Prominent among these is the fact that particles suspended in a gas are exposed to Brownian motion, as a result of bombardment by the gas molecules. This phenomenon, which operates to an insignificant degree in liquids, means that particles suspended in the gas occupy an effective volume greater than that which would be expected from their real size, and so a filter with a given pore structure will remove much smaller particles from a dry, unwetted gas than it will from a liquid (provided that it is not wetted during use). Filters of up to 1.2-μm pore size have been found suitable for the provision of sterile air. Nevertheless, at these larger pore sizes occasional problems with moisture condensation and subsequent grow-through of bacteria can occur, and GMP regulations generally require a 0.2–0.22-μm filter for air sterilization.

Several methods can be used for reducing the viable microbial count in air (Sykes, 1965; Fifield, 1977). These include ultraviolet radiation (Chapter 19B), chemical aerosols (Chapter 2) and filtration. Air filtration has the greatest practical potential (Decker *et al.*, 1963; Leahy & Gabler, 1984), and air filters may be made of cellulose, glass wool or glass–fibre mixtures, or of PTFE with resin or acrylic binders (Underwood, 1998).

Depths filters, such as those made from fibreglass, are believed to achieve air sterilization because of the tortuous passage through which the air passes, ensuring that any microorganisms present are trapped not only on the filter surface, but also within the interior. The removal of microorganisms from air occurs as a result of interception, sedimentation, impaction, diffusion and electrostatic attraction (White, 1990).

The quality of moving air is described by the maximum level of contamination permitted. In the USA Federal Standard 209D recognizes six classes, namely Class 1, Class 10, Class 100, Class 1000, Class 10 000 and Class 100 000, where the maximum numbers of particles 0.5 μm or larger are, respectively, 1/ft^3 (0.035/l), 10/ft^3, 100/ft^3, 1000/ft^3, 10 000/ft^3 and 100 000/ft^3. Only Class 100 air or better is acceptable for aseptic (sterile-area) purposes and the viable particle count is 0.1/ft^3 (0.0035/l (Avis, 1997; Neiger, 1997). In the UK, environmental cleanliness is stated in terms of size and maximum permitted number of airborne particles, and 4 grades designated A–D now exist (Rules, 1997). Grade A is the equivalent of Class 100 of the Federal Standard, with a particle count not exceeding 3500/m^3 for 0.5 μm size or greater. High-efficiency particulate air (HEPA) filters are available that remove particles of 0.3 μm or larger (Wayne, 1975) and, indeed, for strict aseptic conditions. Phillips & Runkle (1972) state that they will remove particles much smaller than this. Passage of phage particles (0.1 μm diameter) through ultrahigh-efficiency filters is remarkably low and it is considered that these filters provide excellent protecion against virus aerosols (Harstad *et al.*, 1967).

An important type of air filtration incorporates the principle of LAF. This was introduced by Whitfield in 1961 (Whitfield, 1967; Soltis, 1967; Whitfield & Lindell, 1969) and is defined as unidirectional air flow within a confined area moving with uniform velocity and minimum turbulence (Bowman, 1968; Phillips & Brewer, 1968; McDade *et al.*, 1969; Brewer & Phillips, 1971). Close control of airborne contamination may be a difficult problem, partly because of the non-uniform nature of the air-flow patterns in a conventional clean room, partly because they do not carry particulate matter away from critical work areas and partly because airborne contamination is not removed as quickly from the room as it is brought in (Whitfield, 1967; Avis, 1997; Neiger, 1997). Whitfield (1967) concluded that a uniform airflow pattern was needed to carry airborned contamination away from the work area. Laminar air flow was designed originally to remove dust particles from air by filtration, but it will also remove bacteria (Coriell & McGarrity, 1967). It was employed initially in the electronics and aerospace industries for the purpose of producing air with low particulate levels, necessary to prevent instrument and circuitry malfunction, but is now widely used by the pharmaceutical, cosmetic and other industries.

Laminar air flow can be used in the form of:

1 LAF rooms with wall or ceiling units, the air flow originating through one wall or ceiling and exiting at the opposite end, to produce a displacement of air;

2 LAF units (see below) suitable for small-scale operations, such as the LAF bench used for aseptic processing and sterility testing (White, 1990; Avis, 1997).

Thus, airborne contamination is not added to the work space, and any generated by manipulations within that area is swept away by the laminar air currents (Coriell, 1975). Nevertheless, there are limitations to the use of LAF, namely it will not sterilize a contaminated product or area (Wayne, 1975). Laminar air flow controls only airborne particulate contamination and does not remove surface contamination (Phillips & Brewer, 1968; Brewer & Phillips, 1971). Correct techniques must be used, since poor aseptic technique can nullify LAF, and holes in the HEPA filter or air leaks in the system may allow contaminated air to enter the aseptic area (Stockdale, 1987; Neiger, 1997).

Filters that are used in LAF devices are HEPA filters, mentioned above. These have been designed with a bacterial removal efficiency of greater than 99.99% (White, 1990; Avis, 1997; Neiger, 1997) and often possess particle-removal efficiencies in the order of 99.9997% against 0.3 μm particles, a standard sufficient for even the most exacting pharmaceutical purposes. Their life can be prolonged by employing low-efficiency filters upstream to intercept most of the larger particles and some smaller ones before they reach the expensive HEPA filters (Phillips & Runkle, 1972). High-efficiency particulate air filters are most efficient when air passes through them at an average velocity of 100 ft/min (30 m/min; Coriell, 1975).

Laminar-air-flow units providing Class 100

(grade A) clean air are of two types, horizontal and vertical, depending upon the direction of the air flow. In vertical LAF (Fig. 22.14), a supply fan passes air down through an ultrahigh-efficiency filter into the work area, and the air exhausts through a grated work surface, often with the aid of a second fan. A slight negative pressure is maintained by adjusting the fans to exhaust more air than is supplied; this causes ambient air to move from the operator towards the external periphery of the work area, so that a protective curtain of air is created (Favero & Berquist, 1968). A vertical LAF of 100 ft/min maintains a Class 100 condition, whereas 60 ft/min does not (Loughhead & Vellutato, 1969). In horizontal LAF (Fig. 22.15), air passes from back to front through an HEPA filter at an average velocity of 100 ft/min, travels horizontally with minimum turbulence and exits as the front of the unit (Coriell & McGarrity, 1968, 1970).

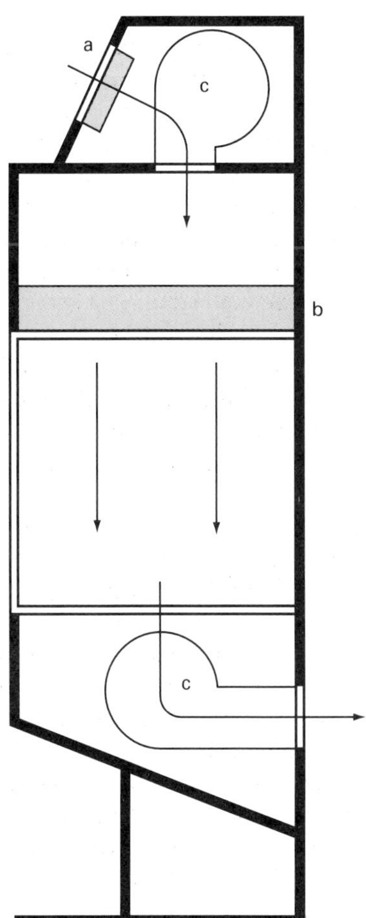

Fig. 22.14 Vertical laminar-air-flow unit. (a) Prefilter; (b) HEPA filter; (c) fan.

Laminar-air-flow units have three general areas of usefulness (Favero & Berquist, 1968; McDade *et al.*, 1968): (i) for product protection, e.g. in sterility testing or aseptic filling; for these purposes, a standard horizontal LAF is suitable; (ii) for personal protection, i.e. protection of personnel processing infectious material, where a horizontal LAF is obviously unsuitable; here, a vertical LAF is essential; and (iii) for product and personnel protection, in which case a vertical LAF must be used.

Additionally, LAF rooms have been used as follows.

1 For conferring protection to patients undergoing bone-marrow transplants. In this procedure, LAF, in conjunction with a strict aseptic technique, produces maximum protection against microbial contamination from the environment (Solberg *et al.*, 1971).

2 For conferring protection from the environment upon leukaemic patients undergoing immunosuppressive (radiomimetic) and anticancer drug

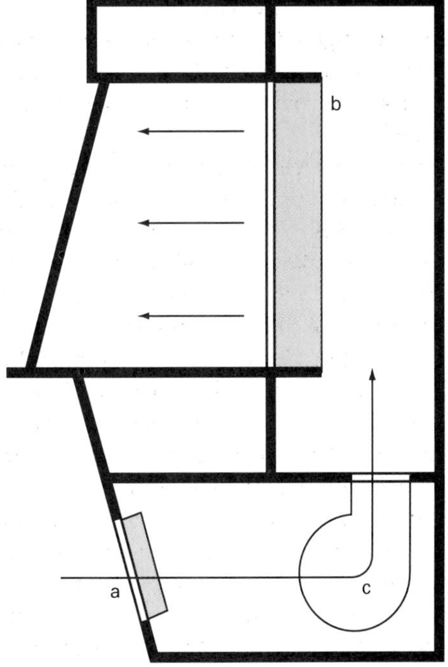

Fig. 22.15 Horizontal laminar-air-flow unit. (a) Prefilter; (b) HEPA filter; (c) fan.

therapy. Results suggest that the incidence of infection of leukaemic patients in LAF rooms is substantially less than for those treated elsewhere (Bodey *et al.*, 1969).

3 For preventing cross-contamination in germ-free mice (van der Waaij & Andres, 1971).

4 For aiding in the treatment of burns (Anon., 1975).

On a smaller scale, the sterile filtration of air (and other gases) for venting, aeration or pressuring purposes can often be accomplished through membrane filters. In line, these filters can also ensure the clarification and sterilization of medical gases. Mechanical patient ventilators may incorporate bacteria-proof filters, which are commonly constructed from hydrophobic glass fibres (Nielsen *et al.*, 1996). Most membranes used are deliberately of the hydrophobic type, so that they will resist wetting by entrained water droplets, which might otherwise cause an airlock. Hydrophobic filters of 0.2 μm have been used to replace the conventional airways needed with rigid infusion and irrigation containers. The hydrophobic material will support the solution but allow filtered sterile air to enter as the fluid is used.

3.1.4 *Microbiological safety cabinets*

Microbiological safety cabinets are of three types: class III, which provides the highest degree of containment for handling category 4 pathogens; class II (laminar-flow recirculating cabinet), which protects both the work and the operator from contamination; and class I (exhaust protective cabinet), which protects the worker against bacterial aerosols possibly generated when handling pathogenic material (Clark, 1980). The cabinets employ HEPA and prefilters, and further information can be obtained by consulting BS 5726 (1979) and Newsom (1979a,b).

3.2 Non-sterilizing uses of membrane filtration

Apart from their use, described above, as a method of sterilization, filters—and especially membrane filters—have wide applications in other microbiological areas.

Membrane filtration in the sterility testing of antibiotics was first described by Holdowsky (1957) and this method is now commonly employed in sterility testing generally (Russell *et al.*, 1979; Akers *et al..*, 1993; Opalchenova & Keuleyan, 1993; *United States Pharmacopoeia*, 1995; *European Pharmacopoeia*, 1997; *British Pharmacopoeia*, 1998).

One method of determining the numbers of colony-forming units (cfu) in bacterial suspensions or in fluids that may be contaminated by microorganisms is by means of membrane filtration. Basically, this procedure consists of filtering a suitable dilution of the suspension through a membrane filter, which retains the organisms and which is then transferred to the surface of an appropriate solid medium. This method has been used for the bacterial examination of water (Windle-Taylor & Burman, 1964) and for the determination of bioburdens in parenteral solutions prior to heat sterilization (Boom *et al.*, 1991) and is routinely employed for evaluating bacterial retention of other sterilizing-grade filters (Carter, 1996). Suitable adaptations have been made to this procedure for determining the numbers of cells surviving treatment with antibiotics (Meers & Churcher, 1974) or disinfectants (Prince *et al.*, 1975). The amounts of disinfectants, for example benzalkonium chloride, phenylmercuric borate or chlorhexidine gluconate, adsorbed on to most types of membrane filters are apparently small (Van Ooteghem & Herbots, 1969; cf. above and Naido *et al.*, 1972, however). Russell (1981) has described a method employing membrane filtration for demonstrating the inactivation of disinfectants by neutralizing agents. The *British Pharmacopoeia* (1998) recommends the use of membrane filtration in preservative-efficacy tests when the preservative cannot be readily inactivated by dilution or specific neutralizing agents. A membrane filter technique has been described for the detection and enumeration of *Escherichia coli* in food (Anderson & Baird-Parker, 1975) and again, in modified form, for the improved detection of damaged cells (Holbrook *et al.*, 1980). Membrane filtration combined with epifluorescent microscopy (known as the direct epifluorescent filtration technique (DEFT)) has been employed for the rapid enumeration of contaminating microorganisms in the water industry (Hobbie *et al.*, 1977), dairy and food products (Pettipher, 1983), ultrapure water

(Mittelman *et al.*, 1983, 1985) and parenteral pharmaceutical products (Denyer & Ward, 1983; Denyer & Lynn, 1987), and as a rapid method in preservative evaluation (Connolly *et al.*, 1993).

A further analytical application for membrane filters is in the bacteriological sampling of moist surfaces, using a simple contact technique (Craythorn *et al.*, 1980). In this method, the sterile membrane (3–5-μm pore size) is placed in direct contact with a contaminated surface for 5 s and then removed, incubated in the conventional manner on the surface of a solid nutrient medium and the resultant colonies counted. A comparison with traditional contact-sampling techniques indicates that the membrane-filter method can be successfully employed for the quantitative bacteriological examination of contaminated clinical surfaces (Craythorn *et al.*, 1980).

Membrane-active antibiotics and disinfectants induce the release of intracellular constituents from bacteria (see Chapter 9). A procedure using membrane filters has been devised for determining the extent of this leakage (Brown *et al.*, 1969). It must be emphasized that, before use, the membrane must be checked for leached impurities which may be present and which could interfere with the assessment of the leakage.

Membrane filtration has been adapted, by means of tangential-flow filter systems, to provide an alternative to centrifugation for the small-scale harvesting of cultures (Tanny *et al.*, 1980; Brock, 1983; Kemken *et al.*, 1996). These filtration devices combine normal fluid flow through the membrane with a washing action, and as a result manage to keep the majority of filtered material in suspension, thereby preventing rapid clogging of the filter (Lukaszewicz *et al.*, 1981b). The technique is reported to have little effect on cell viability and offers a recovery efficiency of up to 75% (Tanny *et al.*, 1980). For the concentration of particularly delicate organisms, a 'reverse-flow' filtration system has been developed (Brock, 1983; Kemken *et al.*, 1996). Other applications of tangential filtration have been described by Genovesi (1983).

Jacobs (1972) describes the use of membrane filters for separating, by zone electrophoresis, individual macromolecular substances from their mixtures, such as the separation of protein fractions in serum or other biological fluids. Jacobs also reports the earlier application of graded collodion (gradocol) membranes (Elford, 1933) to determine the size of virus particles. Nucleic acid hybridization, immunoblotting and protein electrophoresis all exploit membrane technology (Brock, 1983).

Ultrafilter membranes have been used in the purification of water by reverse osmosis (Pohland, 1980). This process may be defined as a reversal of the natural phenomenon of osmosis. If a solution of dissolved salts and pure water is separated by a semipermeable membrane, water will pass through the membrane into the salt solution. This is osmosis itself. Solutes dissolved in the water diffuse less easily and, if their molecular weight is greater than 250, they do not diffuse at all. To reverse the process of osmosis, a pressure in excess of the osmotic pressure of the salt solution is applied and water is thereby forced out of this solution through the membrane in the reverse direction. Since the typical reverse osmosis membrane has pores approaching 2 nm in diameter, this process will remove bacteria, viruses and pyrogens and the purified water produced will be sterile and apyrogenic; it must, however, be added that contamination could occur after production. Ultrafiltration membranes are also exploited in haemodialysis.

4 The testing of filters

Confidence in the integrity and suitability of a filter for its intended task is of paramount importance in filtration sterilization, and this must ultimately rely on stringent testing.

The list of desirable properties which a filter medium should possess (Section 2) gives a guide to the parameters that are controlled during manufacture and the specifications of the finished product. Each manufactured batch of filters should conform to specifications regarding their release of particulate materials, mechanical strength, chemical characteristics, including for example, oxidizable materials and the leaching of materials which may cause a pH shift when flushed with water, and their pyrogenicity. However, filtration performance is of paramount interest, and this, basically, can be tested in two ways. A challenge test is the only true measure of what a filter is capable of removing from suspension, but this is a destructive test and so it cannot be applied to each individual unit in the manufactured batch. What can be, and is, normally applied to each catridge filter is an integrity test, and the data it provides can be correlated with those from a challenge test in order to assess the validity of the non-destructive procedure as a substitute. The tests described below are most frequently applied to membrane filters but the underlying principles will apply equally well in the validation of most other filtration media (Section 2).

4.1 Filters used in liquid sterilization

The challenge test, which is the most severe and direct test to which a bacteria-proof filter can be subjected, involves filtration of a bacterial suspension through a sterile filter assembly, with subsequent collection into a nutrient medium and incubation of the filtrate (Bowman *et al.*, 1967). In the absence of passage of organisms, no growth should be visible.

In the filter industry, such tests are employed for validation purposes (Wallhausser, 1982). They generally use *Serr. marcescens* (minimum dimensions approximately 0.5 μm) and *Saccharomyces cereviseae* to challenge 0.45 μm and 0.8 μm pore-size filters, respectively, while a more rigorous challenge is applied to the 0.2–0.22-μm-rated and 0.1-μm-rated sterilizing filters. Such filters are defined as being capable of removing completely from suspension *Br. diminuta* ATCC 19146 (minimum dimension approximately 0.3 μm) or *A. laidlawii*, respectively. A typical protocol would involve exposure of a sterile filter at a pressure of 276 kPa (40 p.s.i.) to a volume of culture medium containing 10^7/ml *Br. diminuta* cells to result in a total challenge of approximately 10^9 organisms. The filtrate is either passed through a second 0.22-μm membrane disc, which is then placed on an agar plate and incubated for 2 days, or the effluent itself is collected in a sterile flask and incubated for up to 5 days. Any sign of growth would result in failure of the filter. A satisfactory filter would be expected to have a Tr of $\geq 10^7$ (Osumi *et al.*, 1991). Regulatory guidelines for aseptic manufacture of pharmaceuticals recommend validation of sterilizing filters by bacterial challenge under 'worst-case' conditions; a validation protocol applicable to the filter sterilization of high-viscosity fluids at high differential pressures has been described by Aranah & Meeker (1995). While recognizing that such a test should represent the severest challenge possible, Tanny & Meltzer (1979) recommend a realistic approach to selecting a suitable suspension concentration. Details of culture maintenance and handling and factors that govern the final test design have been considered by Reti & Leahy (1979) and Wallhausser (1982).

The bacterial retention tests described above are destructive tests and could not be used by the manufacturers of parenteral products to substantiate the efficacy and integrity of the membrane before and after use, as required by a number of regulatory authorities (Olson, 1980). Similarly, the physical method of mercury intrusion, frequently used to determine pore-size distribution (Marshall & Metzer, 1976), does not offer a satisfactory in-process test. What is required is a simple, rapid, non-destructive test that can be performed under aseptic conditions on sterile membranes to ensure the integrity of the membrane and the use of the correct pore size (Springett, 1981). With this aim in mind a considerable proportion of the industry's research effort has been directed towards validating existing indirect tests and establishing new ones.

The oldest and perhaps most widely used non-destructive test is the bubble-point test (Bechold, 1908), which is the subject of BS 1752 (1983). To understand the principles behind this test, it is necessary to visualize the filter as a series of discrete, uniform capillaries, passing from one side to the other. When wetted, the membrane, will retain liquid in these capillaries by surface tension, and the minimum gas pressure required to force liquid from the largest of these pores is a measure of the maximum pore diameter (d) given by:

$$d = \frac{K\sigma \cos \theta}{P} \tag{22.2}$$

where P = bubble-point pressure, σ = surface tension of the liquid, θ = liquid to capillary-wall contact angle and K = experimental constant.

The pressure (P) will depend in part upon the characteristics of the wetting fluid, which, for hydrophilic filters, would be water but, for hydrophobic filters, may be a variety of solvents (e.g. methanol, isopropanol).

To perform the test, the pressure of gas upstream

from the wetted filter is slowly increased and the pressure at which the largest pore begins to pass gas is the first bubble point (Fig. 22.16). In practice, this value is frequently taken as the lowest pressure required to produce a steady stream of bubbles from an immersed tube on the downstream side. The bubble point for a water-wet 0.22-μm-rated filter is 379 kPa (55 p.s.i.). An automated method for bubble-point testing has been developed (Sechovec, 1989).

The inadequacies of the capillary-pore model for describing the membrane structure have already been discussed (Section 2.4.2). The bubble-point test is unlikely, therefore, to provide an exact indication of pore dimensions (Lukaszewicz *et al.*, 1978; Meltzer & Lukaszewicz, 1979) and it does not, in itself, indicate how efficient the filter is. Instead, its value lies in the knowledge that experimental evidence has allowed the filter manufacturer to correlate bacterial retentivity with a particular bubble point. Thus, any sterilizing-grade filter having a bubble point within the range prescribed by the manufacturer has the support of a rigorous bacterial challenge test regimen to ensure confidence in its suitability. In the words of one manufacturer, 'An observed bubble point which is significantly lower than the bubble point specification for that particular filter indicates a damaged membrane, ineffective seals, or a system leak. A bubble point that meets specifications ensures that the system is integral.'

Small volumes of fluid are often sterilized by passage through a filter unit attached to a hypodermic syringe. The following approximation to the bubble-point test can be applied to such a system to confirm its integrity after use. If the syringe is part-filled with air, then any attempt to force this air through the wet filter should meet appreciable resistance (the bubble-point pressure). Any damage to the membrane would be immediately indicated by the unhindered passsage of air.

The bubble-point test has been criticized because it involves a certain amount of operator judgement and is less precise when applied to filters of large surface area (Trasen, 1979; Johnston *et al.*, 1981; Springett, 1981). Johnston & Meltzer (1980) recognized an additional limitation to the accuracy of this test; commercial membranes often include a wetting agent (see Section 2.4.1, 'Methods of manufacture'), which may well alter the surface-tension characteristics of water held within the filter pores and hence the pressure at which bubbles first appear. This wetting agent is frequently extracted from the membrane during aqueous filtrations, rendering invalid any attempt to make an accurate comparison between before and after bubble-point values (Johnston & Meltzer, 1980). These authors have proposed an additional test based on the flow of air through a filter at pressures above the bubble point. The robust air-flow test examines the applied-pressure/air-flow rate relationship and is amenable to both single-point

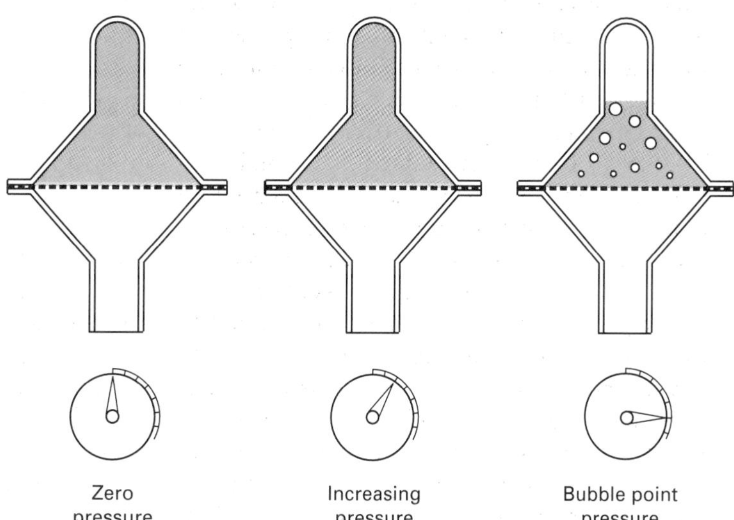

Fig. 22.16 Stages in the bubble-point test.

and multiple-point determinations. This test is described as convenient to use and would, if several readings were taken at different applied air pressures, be more accurate than the single-point bubble-point determination,

The passage of a gas through a wetted filter is not confined solely to bulk flow at applied pressures in excess of the bubble point; it can also occur at lower pressure values by a molecular-diffusion process. With filters of small surface area, this flow is extremely slow, but it increases to significant levels in large-area filters and provides the basis for a sensitive integrity test (Reti, 1977). This test finds its widest application in large-volume systems, where the need to displace a large quantity of downstream water before the detection of bubbles makes the standard bubble-point test impracticable. To perform this diffusion test, gas under pressure is applied at 80% of the bubble-point pressure (Reti, 1977; Olson *et al.*, 1981) for that particular wetted filter and the volumetric gas-flow rate determined by measuring either the rate of flow of displaced water or the volume of gas passed in a specified time (Trasen, 1979). A marked increase in gas flow seen at lower pressures than would normally be expected for that filter type indicates a breakdown in the integrity of the system.

All the major suppliers of cartridge filters have developed and supply to their customers integrity-testing instrumentation, which can evaluate the diffusive flow characteristics of the filters at any time during their working life. The testing procedures tend to be named differently by the various manufacturers, e.g. 'pressure decay test', 'forward flow test' or 'diffusive flow test', but they all operate on similar principles.

The diffusion test can also be combined with bubble-point determination, whereby changes in applied pressure can be measured against gas flow and a break observed at the first bubble point (Olson *et al.*, 1983; Emory, 1989). This approach can be used to assess pore-size distribution; a narrow distribution would be indicated by a significant rise in gas flow at applied pressures only marginally above the bubble-point, while a wide distribution would cause a more gradual increase in gas flow. This approach to integrity testing is amenable to automation and can give diffusion rate, first bubble-point pressure and pore-size distribution (Olson *et al.*, 1983; Hofmann, 1984). The performance of an automated pressure-hold/forward-flow (Cole & Pauli, 1975; Pall, 1975; Price & Pauli, 1976; Schroeder & DeLuca, 1980; Springett, 1981) test system has been evaluated (Lee, 1989).

4.2 Filters used in gas sterilization

The bubble-point and diffusive-flow tests described in the previous section are also applicable, with modifications, to membrane filters used for gas sterilization in venting systems. The major difference is that air filters are hydrophobic, so it is necessary to use a liquid with a lower surface tension than water in order to achieve adequate wetting; isopropyl alcohol mixed with water is most commonly used for this purpose. Water-based testing procedures have been developed for use in situations where alcohol is undesirable, and these are similar in principle to the bubble-point procedure (Dosmar *et al.*, 1992). In these so-called water-intrusion tests, the parameter measured is the pressure required to cause water to be forced through a hydrophobic filter, rather than air to be passed through a wetted filter.

The continuous production of high-quality filtered air by any HEPA filtration system (Section 3.1.3) can be assured by the application of rigorous efficiency tests to the filter, both at the time of installation and at intervals throughout its service life. One of the most exacting test methods available is the diocytylphthalate (DOP) smoke test (Gross, 1976, 1978). In this test, DOP is vaporized upstream of the filter to produce an aerosol of particles which can be detected in the filtered air using a suitable photoelectric device. For efficiency testing by the filter manufacturer, DOP smoke should be thermally generated, to give monosized particles of approximately 0.3 μm diameter, but cold DOP aerosols of larger polydisperse droplet size (Caldwell, 1978) have been recommended for detecting small flaws and leaks that may develop in a filter during use (Gross, 1978). The passage of DOP particles is best examined in a LAF unit by using a small probe to scan the filter-surface closely in an overlapping pattern (Gross, 1976). This will detect any areas of particular weakness, such as pinholes or poor seals (McDade *et al.*, 1969). A HEPA filter is expected to have an overall minimum retention efficiency of 99.97% to hot DOP (Gross, 1978), this value being increased to 99.999% for ultra-HEPA filters (Groves, 1973). Mika (1971) has suggested that filtration efficiency is at a minimum for airborne particles of 0.2–0.3 μm diameter, and the bacterial-retention properties of a HEPA filter (Section 3.1.3) may well be underrated by this test.

Alternatively, filters can be examined using the sodium-flame test (BS 3928, 1969), in which a minimum retention efficiency of 99.995% is expected of all HEPA filters used to prepare air to grade A standard (BS 5295, 1989). An aerosol is produced from a sodium chloride solution, upstream of the filter, and rapid evaporation of these droplets then ensures that the air arriving at the filter contains minute particles of sodium chloride. Retention efficiency is evaluated by downstream sodium-flame photometry. Other testing methods involve discoloration by atmospheric dust or weight gain during filtration, and are generally confined to filters of a coarser grade.

A bacterial aerosol challenge test has been developed to study the filtration efficiency of air and gas filters (Duberstein & Howard, 1978). Other workers (Harstad & Filler, 1969; Mika, 1971; Regamey, 1974) have suggested using phage particles, vegetative organisms and spores as a suitable challenge for HEPA filters.

5 Designing a filtration system for the preparation of medicinal products

Sterilization and clarification by filtration are routinely applied to a variety of liquids, which often differ markedly in their filtration characteristics. The first stage in designing any filtration system, therefore, is to classify the fluid to be processed according to the ease with which it can be filtered. The majority of aqueous solutions for intravenous, ophthalmic and irrigation purposes pass easily through a sterilizing-grade membrane filter, while, at the other end of the spectrum, oils and fluids with a high particulate or protein content (e.g. vaccine, serum, plasma and tissue culture media) will, without exception, require some form of pretreatment before final processing. The early methods of pretreatment, which included centrifugation and settling, have largely been replaced by extensive prefiltration (see Section 2.4.4 and Fig. 22.13) or by sequential filtration through a series of membrane filters of progressively smaller pore size. Often, this series consists of a stack of membrane discs, separated by a support mesh, assembled together in a single filter holder. For ease of handling, it is advisable to arrange the stack of filters in a separate holder from the final sterile, 0.22-μm, sterilizing filter. The serial filters can then be replaced when they become clogged without jeopardizing the sterility of the final filter. The successive filtration of serum through various grades of prefilter, followed by passage through 1.2, 0.8, 0.45 and 0.22-μm membranes, provides a typical example of serial filtration. The pore size of the final filter is dictated by the need to provide a sterile product.

Small-volume parenteral, ophthalmic and other hospital-produced products are routinely passed through single-disc filter systems capable of processing batches in the region of 500 l (Fig. 22.9). Bulk industrial production, however, with its larger volumes and attendant high capital investment, requires a more sophisticated approach to system design. Invariably, this will demand a pilot study, where results obtained from flow-decay tests performed on approximately 0.1% of the batch volume or with small-capacity filters, can be used to provide sufficient information for the scaling-up operation (Meltzer & Lukaszewicz, 1979). Major filter firms may offer an on-site analysis programme, culminating in a computer-assisted appraisal of the filtration process. Any system finally chosen must attempt to optimize total fluid throughput, flow rate and filter and prefilter life.

The ancillary equipment required for an evolving filtration system is determined, at least in part, by the scale of the process. Large industrial systems will make many individual demands for specialized equipment, which may include pumps, holding tanks, cartridge-filter holders and extensive stainless-steel plumbing. This combination of components is rarely found in small-scale hospital units.

Accumulated expertise has now clearly demonstrated that, when selecting equipment for assembly into any filtration system, no matter what its size, the following important points must be taken into consideration.

1 Is filtration to be performed under positive or negative pressure? Vacuum filtration is well suited for small-scale analytical processes, such as sterility testing, but should not be used for production purposes. Positive pressure, provided by syringe, pump or nitrogen gas under pressure, offers the important advantages of high flow rates and easier bubble-point testing, and also protects against the ingress of unsterile air and solvent evaporation. Equipment should be designed, therefore, to withstand the pressures employed during the filtration process.

2 Is filtration to be a batch or continuous process? In a continuously operating large-scale system, provision must be made to allow filter changes without interrupting the process. To do this, a valve must be included to switch flow over to another unit fitted with a fresh filter.

3 The system must be amenable to regular maintenance and cleaning. If not, the filters may well be exposed to challenge levels in excess of their capabilities.

4 The amount of particulate contamination within a system is directly proportional to the number of valves, joints and junctions. It is considered advisable, therefore, to keep any system as simple as possible.

5 All valves shed particles during use and must be placed upstream of the final filter.

6 It is axiomatic that the final membrane filter must be placed at the last possible point in the system.

A system that pays attention to all these points should be capable of providing parenteral products of a standard acceptable to all the regulatory authorities. As a final cautionary word, however, the quality of the finished product does not depend solely upon the design and efficiency of the filtration system; it will also owe a great deal to the standard of the production environment, containers used and personnel employed and must, therefore, depend ultimately upon the continued observance of all pharmaceutical GMP requirements (Anon., 1989; BS 5295, 1989; *Rules*, 1997); see also Chapter 11.

6 Acknowledgements

We are indebted to the Nucleopore Corporation, who originally supplied the photographs for Figs 22.1–22.4 and 22.8–22.11, to Pall Corporation for Fig. 22.12 and to Schleicher & Schull GMBH for Fig. 22.13.

7 References

Akers, M.J., Wright G.E. & Carlson K.A. (1993) Sterility testing of antimicrobial-containing injectable solutions prepared in the pharmacy. *American Journal of Hospital Pharmacy*, **48**, 2414–2418.

Alkan, M.H. & Groves, M.J. (1978) The measurement of membrane filter pore size by a gas permeability technique. *Drug Development and Industrial Pharmacy*, **4**, 225–241.

Anderson, J.M. & Baird-Parker, A.C. (1975) A rapid and direct plate method for enumerating *Escherichia coli* biotype 1 in food. *Journal of Applied Bacteriology*, **39**, 111–117.

Anon. (1975) Clean areas aid treatment of burns. *Laboratory Equipment Digest*, December, 51–52.

Anon. (1989) The rules governing medicinal products in the European Community. In *Guide to Good Manufacturing Practice for Medicinal Products*, Vol. IV. London: HMSO.

Aranah, H. & Meeker, J. (1995) Microbial retention characteristics of 0.2–microns-rated nylon membrane filters during filtration of high viscosity fluids at high differential pressure and varied temperature. *Journal of Pharmaceutical Science and Technology*, **49**, 67–70.

Aranah-Creado, H., Oshima K., Jafari, S., Howard, G. & Brandwein, H. (1996) *Virus Retention by Ultipor VF Grade DV50 Membrane Filters*. Pall Corporation Scientific and Technical Report 1543.

Avis, K.E. (1997) Assuring the quality o. pharmacy-prepared sterile products. *Pharmacopoeial Forum*, **23**, 3567–3576.

Ballew, H.W. & the Staff of Nuclepore Corporation (1978) *Basics of Filtration and Separation*. California: Nuclepore Corporation.

Baumgartner, T.G., Schmidt, G.L., Thakker, K.M. *et al.*, (1986) Bacterial endotoxin retention by in-line intravenous filters. *American Journal of Hospital Pharmacy*, **43**, 681–684.

Bechold, H. (1908) Durchlässigkeit von Ultrafiltern. *Zeitschrift für Physikalische Chemie*, **64**, 328–342.

Bobbit, J.A. & Betts, R.P. (1992) The removal of bacteria from solutions by membrane filtration. *Journal of Microbiological Methods*, **16**, 215–220.

Bodey, G.P., Freireich, E.J. & Frei, E. (1969) Studies of patients in a laminar air flow unit. *Cancer*, **24**, 972–980.

Boom, F.A., Vanbeek, M.A.E.V., Paalman, A.C.A. & Stoutzonneveld, A. (1991) Microbiological aspects of heat sterilization of drugs. 3. Heat resistance of spore-forming bacteria isolated from large-volume parenterals. *Pharmaceutisch Weekblad—Scientific Edition*, **13**, 130–136.

Bower, J.P. & Fox, R. (1985) Definition and testing of a biologically retentive 0.1 micron pore size membrane filter. Presented at the Society of Manufacturing Engineers Conference '*Filtration in Pharmaceutical Manufacturing*', Philadelphia, 26–28 March 1985.

Bowman, F.C. (1968) Laminar air flow for environmental control and sterility testing. *Bulletin of the Parenteral Drug Association*, **22**, 57–63.

Bowman, F.W., Calhoun, M.P. & White, M. (1967) Microbiological methods for quality control of membrane filters. *Journal of Pharmaceutical Sciences*, **56**, 222–225.

Brewer, J.H. & Phillips, G.B. (1971) Environmental control in the pharmaceutical and biological industries. *CRC Critical Reviews in Environmental Control*, **1**, 467–506.

British Pharmacopoeia (1993) London: HMSO.

Brock, T.D. (1983) *Membrane Filtration: A Users' Guide and Reference Manual*. Madison: Science Tech.

Brooks, N. (1979) Filter validation symposium. V. A synopsis of the PDA Panel on Filter Validation. *Journal of the Parenteral Drug Association*, **33**, 280–282.

Brown, M.R.W. & Gilbert, P. (1977) Increasing the probability of sterility of medicinal products. *Journal of Pharmacy and Pharmacology*, **27**, 484–491.

Brown, M.R.W., Farwell, &. & Rosenbluth, S.A. (1969) Use of membrane filters for measurement of 260 µm absorbing substances from bacterial cells. *Analytical Biochemistry*, **27**, 484–491.

BS 1752 (1983) *Laboratory sintered or fritted filters including porosity grading*. London: British Standards Institution.

BS 3928 (1969) *Method for Sodium Flame Test for Air Filters (Other than for Air Supply to I.C. Engines and Compressors)*. London: British Standards Institution.

BS 5726 (1979) *Specification for Microbiological Safety Cabinets and Amendments*. London: British Standards Institution.

BS 5295 (1989) *Environmental Cleanliness in Enclosed Spaces*. London: British Standards Institution.

Caldwell, G.H., Jr (1978) Evaluation of high efficiency filters. *Journal of the Parenteral Drug Association*, **32**, 182–187.

Carazzone, M., Arecco, D., Fava, M. & Saucin, P. (1985) A new type of positively charged filter: preliminary test results. *Journal of Parenteral Science and Technology*, **39**, 69–75.

Carter, J. (1996) Evaluation of recovery filters for use in bacterial retention testing of sterilizing grade filters. *Journal of Pharmaceutical Science and Technology*, **50**, 147–153.

Chamberland, C. (1884) Sur un filtre donnant de l'eau physiologiquement pure. *Compte Rendu Hebdomadaire des Séances de l'Académie des Sciences*, **99**, 247–552.

Chrai, S.S. (1989) Validation of filtration systems: considerations for selecting filter housings. *Pharmaceutical Technology*, **13**, 85–96.

Clark, R.P. (1980) Microbiological safety cabinets. *Medical Laboratory World*, March, 27–33.

Cole, J.C. & Pauli, W.A. (1975) Field experiences in testing membrane filter integrity by the forward flow test method. *Bulletin of the Parenteral Drug Association*, **29**, 296–304.

Cole, J.C., Farris, J.A. & Nickolaus, N. (1979) Cartridge filters. In *Filtration: Principles and Practice*, Part II (ed. Orr, C.), pp. 201–259. New York: Marcel Dekker.

Conacher, J.C. (1976) Membrane filter cartridges for fine particle control in the electronics and pharmaceutical industries. *Filtration and Separation*, May/June, 1–4.

Connolly, P., Bloomfield, S.F. & Denyer, S.P. (1993) A study of the use of rapid methods for preservative efficacy testing of pharmaceuticals and cosmetics. *Journal of Applied Bacteriology*, **75**, 456–462.

Coriell, L.L. (1975) Laboratory applications of laminar air flow. In *Quality Control in Microbiology* (eds Prior, J.E., Bertole, J. & Friedman, H.), pp. 41–46. Baltimore: University Park Press.

Coriell, L.L. & McGarrity, G.J. (1967) Elimination of airborne bacteria in the laboratory and operating room. *Bulletin of the Parenteral Drug Association*, **21**, 46–51.

Coriell, L.L. & McGarrity, G.J. (1968) Biohazard hood to prevent infection during microbiological procedures. *Applied Microbiology*, **16**, 1895–1900.

Corriell, L.L. & McGarrity, G.J. (1970) Evaluation of the Edgegard laminar flow hood. *Applied Microbiology*, **20**, 474–479.

Craythorn, J.M., Barbour, A.G., Matsen, J.M., Britt, M.R. & Garibaldi, R.A. (1980) Membrane filter contract technique for bacteriological sampling of moist surfaces. *Journal of Clinical Microbiology*, **12**, 250–255.

Dahlstrom, D.A. & Silverblatt, C.E. (1986) Continuous vacuum and pressure filtration. In *Solid/Liquid Separation Equipment Scale-up* (eds Purchase, D.B. & Wakeman, R.J.), pp. 510–557. London: Uplands Press, and Filtration Specialists.

Davis, N.M. & Turco, S. (1971) A study of particulate matter in IV infusion fluids – phase 2. *American Journal of Hospital Pharmacy*, **28**, 620–623.

Davis, N.M., Turco, S. & Silvelly, E. (1970a) A study of particulate matter in IV infusion fluids. *American Journal of Hospital Pharmacy*, **27**, 822–826.

Davis, N.M., Turco, S. & Silvelly, E. (1970b) Particulate matter in IV infusion fluids. *Bulletin of the Parenteral Drug Association*, **24**, 257–270.

Decker, H.M., Buchanan, L.M., Hall, L.B. & Goddard, K.R. (1963) Air filtration of microbial particles. *American Journal of Public Health*, **12**, 1982–1988.

De Muynek, C., De Vroe, C., Remon, J.P. & Colardyn, F. (1988) Binding of drugs to end-line filters: a study of four commonly administered drugs in intensive care units. *Journal of Clinical Pharmacy and Therapeutics*, **13**, 335–340.

Denee, P.B. & Stein, R.L. (1971) An evaluation of dust sampling membrane filters for use in the scanning electron microscope. *Powder Technology*, **5**, 201–204.

Denyer, S.P. (1998) Factory and hospital hygiene and good manufacturing practice. In *Pharmaceutical Microbiology* (eds Hugo, W.B. & Russell, A.D.), 6th edn, pp. 426–438. Oxford, Blackwell Scientific Publications.

Denyer, S.P. & Lynn, R. (1987) A sensitive method for the rapid detection of bacterial contaminants in intravenous fluids. *Journal of Parenteral Science and Technology*, **41**, 60–66.

Denyer, S.P. & Ward, K.H. (1983) A rapid method for the detection of bacterial contaminants in intravenous fluids using membrane filtration and epifluorescence microscopy. *Journal of Parenteral Science and Technology*, **37**, 156–158.

Dosmar, M., Wolber, P., Bracht, T., Troger, H. & Waibel, P. (1992) The water pressure integrity test for hydrophobic membrane filters. *Journal of Parenteral Science and Technology*, **46**, 102–106.

Duberstein, R. (1979) Filter Validation Symposium. II. Mechanisms of bacterial removal by filtration. *Journal of the Parenteral Drug Association*, **33**, 251–256.

Duberstein, R. & Howard, G. (1978) Sterile filtration of gases: a bacterial aerosol challenge test. *Journal of the Parenteral Drug Association*, **32**, 192–198.

Ehrlich, R. (1960) Application of membrane filters. *Advances in Applied Microbiology*, **2**, 95–112.

Elford, W.J. (1933) The principles of ultrafiltration as applied in biological studies. *Proceedings of the Royal Society*, **112B**, 384–106.

Elias, W.E. (1975) Panel Discussion. Asbestos and glass fibre regulations. *Bulletin of the Parenteral Drug Association*, **29**, 215.

Emory, S.F. (1989) Principles of integrity-testing hydrophilic microporous membrane filters. Part II. *Pharmaceutical Technology*, **13**, 36–46.

European Pharmacopoeia (1969) p. 54. Sainte-Ruffine: Maisonneuve.

European Pharmacopoeia (1971) Vol. II Test for sterility, Revised text, 1978. Paris: Maisonneuve.

European Pharmacopoeia (1997) Third edition. Maisonneuve.

Fare, G. (1987) Manufacture of Antibiotics. In *Pharmaceutical Microbiology* (eds Hugo, W.B. & Russell, A.D), 4th edn, pp. 151–162. Oxford: Blackwell Scientific Publications.

Favero, M.S. & Berquist, K.R. (1968) Use of laminar airflow equipment in microbiology. *Applied Microbiology*, **16**, 182–183.

FDA (1987) *Guideline on Sterile Drug Products Produced by Aseptic Processing*. United States Food and Drugs Administration.

Fifield, C.W. (1977) Sterilization filtration. In *Disinfection, Sterilization and Filtration* (ed. Block, S.S.), 2nd edn, pp. 562–591. Philadelphia: Lea & Febiger.

Fleischer, R.L., Price, P.B. & Symes, E.M. (1964) Novel filter for biological materials. *Science*, **143**, 249–250.

Gelman, C. (1965) Microporous membrane technology: Part 1. Historical development and applications. *Analytical Chemistry*, **37**, 29A–37A.

Genovesi, C.S. (1983) Several uses for tangential-flow filtration in the pharmaceutical industry. *Journal of Parenteral Science and Technology*, **37**, 81–86.

Gilbert, P. & Allison, D. (1996) Redefining the 'sterility' of sterile products. *European Journal of Parenteral Sciences*, **1**, 19–23.

Goldbach, P., Brochart,, T., Wehrle, P. & Stamm, A. (1995) Sterile filtration of liposomes—retention of encapsulated carboxyfluorescein. *International Journal of Pharmaceutics*, **117**, 225–230.

Gross, R.I. (1976) Laminar flow equipment: performance and testing requirements. *Bulletin of the Parenteral Drug Association*, **30**, 143–151.

Gross, R.I. (1978) Testing of laminar flow equipment. *Journal of the Parenteral Drug Association*, **32**, 174–181.

Groves, M.J. (1973) *Parenteral Products*. London: William Heinemann Medical Books.

Hargreaves, D.P. (1990) Good manufacturing practice in the control of contamination. In *Guide to Microbiological Control in Pharmaceuticals* (eds Denyer, S.P. & Baird, R.), pp. 68 –86. Chichester: Ellis Horwood.

Harstad, J.B. & Filler, M.E. (1969) Evaluation of air filters with submicron viral aerosols and bacterial aerosols. *American Industrial Hygiene Association Journal*, **30**, 280–290.

Harstad, J.B., Decker, H.M., Buchanan, L.S. & Filler, M.E. (1967) Air filtration of submicron virus aerosols. *American Journal of Public Health*, **57**, 2186–2193.

Hawker, R.J. & Hawker, L.M. (1975) Protein losses during sterilization by filtration. *Laboratory Practice*, **24**, 805–807, 818.

Heidam, N.Z. (1981) Review: aerosol fractionation by sequential filtration with Nucleopore filters. *Atmospheric Environment*, **15**, 891–904.

Hobbie, J.E., Daley, R.J. & Jasper, S. (1977) Use of Nucleopore filters for counting bacteria by fluorescence microscopy. *Applied and Environmental Microbiology*, **33**, 1225–1228.

Hofmann, F. (1984) Integrity testing of microfiltration membranes *Journal of Parenteral Science and Technology*, **38**, 148–158.

Holbrook, R., Anderson, J.M. & Baird-Parker, A.C. (1980) Modified direct plate method for counting *Escherichia coli* in foods. *Food Technology in Australia*, **32**, 78–83.

Holdowsky, S. (1957) A new sterility test for antibiotics: an application of the membrane filter technique. *Antibiotics & Chemotherapy*, **7**, 49–54.

Holmes, C.J. & Allwood, M.C. (1979) A review: the microbial contamination of intravenous infusions during clinical use. *Journal of Applied Bacteriology*, **46**, 247–267.

Hou, K., Gerba, C.P., Goyal, S.M. & Zerda, K.S. (1980) Capture of latex beads, bacteria, endotoxin and viruses by charge modified filters. *Applied and Environmental Microbiology*, **40**, 892–896.

Hou, K.L. & Zaniewski, R. (1990) Depyrogenation by endotoxin removal with positively charged depth filter cartridges. *Journal of Parenteral Science and Technology*, **44**, 204–209.

Howard, G., Jr & Duberstein, R. (1980) A case of penetration of 0.2μm rated membrane filters by bacteria. *Journal of the Parenteral Drug Association*, **34**, 95–102.

Jacobs, S. (1972) The distribution of pore diameters in graded ultrafilter membranes. *Filtration and Separation*. September/October, 525–530.

Johnston, P.R. & Meltzer, T.H. (1980) Suggested integrity testing of membranes filters at a robust flow of air. *Pharmaceutical Technology*, **4** (11), 49–59.

Johnston, P.R., Lukaszewicz, R.C. & Meltzer, T.H. (1981) Certain imprecisions in the bubble point measurement. *Journal of Parenteral Science and Technology*, **35**, 36–39.

Jones, H. (1990) Inorganic membrane filter for biological separation applications. *International Labmate*, **15**, 57–58.

Kanke, M., Eubanks, J.L. & Deluca, P.P. (1983) Binding of selected drugs to a 'treated' inline filter. *American Journal of Hospital Pharmacy*, **40**, 1323–1328.

Kempken, R., Rechtsteiner, H., Schäfer, J. *et al.* (1996) *Dynamic Membrane Filtration in Cell Culture Harvest*. Technical report. Portsmouth, UK: Pall Europe

Kesting, R., Murray, A., Jackson, K. & Newman, J. (1981) Highly anisotropic microfiltration membranes. *Pharmaceutical Technology*, **5**, 53–60.

Kesting, R.E., Cunningham, L.K., Morrison, M.C. & Ditter, J.F. (1983) Nylon microfiltration membranes: state of the art. *Journal of Parenteral Science and Technology*, **37**, 97–104.

Kovary, S.J., Agalloco, J.P. & Gordon, B.M. (1983) Validation of the steam-in-place sterilization of disc filter housings and membranes *Journal of Parenteral Science and Technology*, **37**, 55–64.

Kristensen, T., Mortensen, B.T. & Nissen, N.I. (1985) Micropone filters for sterile filtration may leach toxic compounds affecting cell cultures (HL-60). *Experimental Hematology*, **13**, 1188–1191.

Leahy, T.J. & Gabler, R. (1984) Sterile filtration of gases by membrane filters. *Biotechnology and Bioengineering*, **26**, 836–843.

Lee, J.Y, (1989) Validating an automated filter integrity test instrument. *Pharmaceutical Technology*, **13**, 48–56.

Lidgate, D.M., Trattner, T., Schultz, R.M. & Maskiewiez, R. (1992) Sterile filtration of a parenteral emulsion. *Pharmaceutical Research*, **9**, 860–863.

Loughhead, H. & Vellutato, A. (1969) Parenteral production under vertical laminar air flow. *Bulletin of the Parenteral Drug Association*, **23**, 17–22.

Lowe, G.D. (1981) Filtration in IV therapy. Part 1: Clinical aspects of IV fluid filtration. *British Journal of Intravenous Therapy*, **2**, 42–52.

Lukaszewicz, R.C. & Meltzer, T.H. (1979a) Concerning filter validation. *Journal of the Parenteral Drug Association*, **33**, 187–194.

Lukaszewicz, R.C. & Meltzer, T.H. (1979b) Filter Validation Symposium. I. A co-operative address to current filter problems. *Journal of Parenteral Drug Association*, **33** 247–249.

Lukaszewicz, R.C. & Meltzer, T.H. (1980) On the structural compatibilities of membrane filters. *Journal of the Parenteral Drug Association*, **34**, 463–474.

Lukaszewicz, R.C., Tanny, G.B. & Meltzer, T.H. (1978) Membrane filter characterizations and their implications for particulate retention. *Pharmaceutical Technology*, **2** (11), 77–83.

Lukaszewicz, R.C., Johnston, P.R. & Meltzer, T.H. (1981a) Prefilters/final filters: a matter of particle/pore/size distribution. *Journal of Parenteral Science and Technology*, **35**, 40–47.

Lukaszewicz, R.C., Kuvin, A., Hauk, D. & Chrai, S. (1981b) Functionality and economics of tangential flow microfiltration. *Journal of Parenteral Science and Technology*, **35**, 231–236.

McDade, J.J., Sabel, F.L., Akers, R.L. & Walker, R.J. (1968) Microbiological studies on the performance of a laminar airflow biological cabinet. *Applied Microbiology*, **16**, 1086–1092.

McDade, J.J., Phillips, G.B., Sivinski, H.D. & Whitfield, W.J. (1969) Principles and applications of laminar flow devices. In *Methods in Microbiology* (eds Ribbons, D.W. & Norris, J.R.), Vol. 1, pp. 137–168. London and New York: Academic Press.

McKinnon, B.T. & Avis, K.E. (1993) Membrane filtration of pharmaceutical solutions. *American Journal of Hospital Pharmacy*, **50**, 1921–1936.

Maki, D.G. (1976) Preventing infection in intravenous therapy. *Hospital Practice*, **11**, 95–104.

Marshall, J.C. & Meltzer, T.H. (1976) Certain porosity

aspects of membrane filters: their pore-distribution and anisotropy. *Bulletin of the Parenteral Drug Association*, **30**, 214–225.

Meers, P.D. & Churcher, G.M. (1974) Membrane filtration in the study of antimicrobial drugs. *Journal of Clinical Pathology*, **27**, 288–291.

Megaw, W.J. & Wiffen, R.D. (1963) The efficiency of membrane filters. *International Journal of Air and Water Pollution*, **7**, 501–509.

Meltzer, T.H. & Lukaszewicz, R.C. (1979) Filtration sterilization with porous membranes. In *Quality Control in the Pharmaceutical Industry* (ed. Cooper, M.S), Vol. 3, pp. 145–211. London: Academic Press.

Mika, H. (1971) Clean room equipment for pharmaceutical use. *Pharmaceutica Acta Helvetiae*, **46**, 467–482.

Miller, R.C. & Grogan, J.B. (1973) Incidence and source of contamination of intravenous nutritional infusion systems. *Journal of Paediatric Surgery*, **8**, 185–190.

Mittelman, M.W., Geesey, G.G. & Hite, R.R. (1983) Epifluorescence microscopy: a rapid method for enumerating viable and non-viable bacteria in ultrapure water systems. *Microcontamination*, **1**, 32–37, 52.

Mittelman, M.W., Geesey, G.G. & Platt, R.M. (1985) Rapid enumeration of bacteria in purified water systems *Medical Device and Diagnostics Industry*, **7**, 144–149.

Morton, H.E. & Czarnetzky, E.J. (1937) The application of sintered (fritted) glass filters to bacteriological work. *Journal of Bacteriology*, **34**, 461–464.

Myers, J.A. (1972) Millipore infusion filter unit: interim report of a clinical trial. *Pharmaceutical Journal*, **208**, 547–549.

Naido, H.T., Price, C.H. & McCarty, T.J. (1972) Preservative loss from ophthalmic solutions during filtration sterilization. *Australian Journal of Pharmaceutical Sciences*, **NS1**, 16–18.

Neiger, J. (1997) Life with the UK pharmaceutical isolator guidelines: a manufacturer's viewpoint. *European Journal of Parenteral Sciences*, **2**, 13–20.

Newsom, S.W.B. (1979a) The Class II (laminar flow) biological safety cabinet. *Journal of Clinical Pathology*, **32**, 505–513.

Newsom, S.W.B. (1979b) Performance of exhaust-protective (Class I) biological safety cabinets. *Journal of Clinical Pathology*, **32**, 576–583.

Nielsen, H.J., Mecke, P., Tichy, S. & Schmucker, P. (1996) Comparative study of the efficiency of bacterial filters in long-term mechanical ventilation. *Anaesthetist*, **45**, 814–818.

Olson, W. (1980) LVP Filtration conforming with GMP. Communication prepared for Sartorius Symposium 50 Jahre Sartorius Membranfilter held on 7 October 1980 at the Holiday Inn, Frankfurt.

Olson, W.P., Bethel, G. & Parker, C. (1977) Rapid delipidation and particle removal from human serum by membrane filtration in a tangential flow system. *Preparative Biochemistry*, **7**, 333–343.

Olson, W.P., Briggs, R.O., Garanchon, C.M., Ouellet, M.J., Graf, E.A. & Luckhurst, D.G. (1980) Aqueous filter extractables: detection and elution from process filters. *Journal of the Parenteral Drug Association*, **34**, 254–267.

Olson, W.P., Martinez, E.D. & Kern, C.R. (1981) Diffusion and bubble point testing of microporous cartridge filters: preliminary results of production facilities. *Journal of Parenteral Science and Technology*, **35**, 215–222.

Olson, W.P., Gatlin, L.A. & Kern, C.R. (1983) Diffusion and bubble point testing of microporous cartridge filters: electro mechanical methods. *Journal of Parenteral Science and Technology*, **37**, 117–124.

Opalchenova, G. & Keuleyan, E. (1993) Check up for antimicrobial activity of aminoglycoside antibiotics after membrane filtration. *Drug Development and Industrial Pharmacy*, **19**, 1231–1240.

Osumi, M., Yamada, N. & Toya, M. (1991) Bacterial retention mechanisms of membrane filters. *Pharmaceutical Technology (Japan)*, **7**, 11–16.

Pall, D.B. (1975) Quality control of absolute bacteria removal filters. *Bulletin of the Parenteral Drug Association*, **29**, 192–204.

Parks, S.R., Bennett, A.M., Speight, S. & Benbough, J.E. (1996) A system for testing the effectiveness of microbiological air filters. *European Journal of Parenteral Sciences*, **1**, 75–77.

Pettipher, G.L. (1983) *The Direct Epifluorescent Filter Technique for the Rapid Enumeration of Microorganisms*. Letchworth: Research Studies Press.

Phillips, G.B. & Brewer, J.H. (1968) Recent advances in microbiological control. *Development in Industrial Microbiology*, **9**, 105–121.

Phillips, G.B. & Runkle, R.S. (1972) Design of facilities. In *Quality Control in the Pharmaceutical Industry* (ed. Cooper, M.S.), Vol. 1, pp. 73–99. New York and London: Academic Press.

Pitt, A.M. (1987) The non-specific protein binding of polymeric microporous membranes. *Journal of Parenteral Science and Technology*, **41**, 110–113.

Pohland, H.W. (1980) Seawater desalination by reverse osmosis. *Endeavour* (New Series), **4**, 141–147.

Prausnitz, P.H. (1924) Fritted glass filter discs. *Industrial and Engineering Chemistry*, **16**, 370.

Preusser, H.J. (1967) Elektronenmikroskopische Untersuchungen an Oberflachen von Membranfiltern. *Kolloidzeifschrift und Zeitschrift für Polymere*, **218**, 129.

Price, J.M. & Pauli, W.A. (1976) Utilization of new integrity test for membrane filter cartridges. *Bulletin of the Parenteral Drug Association*, **30**, 45–48.

Prince, J., Deverill, C.M.A. & Ayliffe, G.A.J. (1975) A

membrane filter technique for testing disinfectants. *Journal of Clinical Pathology*, **28**, 71–76.

Regamey, R.H. (1974) Application of laminar flow (clean work bench) for purifying the atmosphere. *Developments in Biological Standards*, **23**, 71–78.

Reti, A.R. (1977) An assessment of test criteria for evaluating the performance and integrity of sterilizing filters. *Journal of Parenteral Drug Association*, **31**, 187–194.

Reti, A.R. & Leahy, T.J. (1979) Filter Validation Symposium. III. Validation of bacterially retentive filters by bacterial passage testing. *Journal of the Parenteral Drug Association*, **33**, 257–272.

Rogers, B.G. & Rossmore, H.W. (1970) Determination of membrane filter porosity by microbiological methods. *Developments in Industrial Microbiology*, **11**, 453–458.

Rules and Guidance for Pharmaceutical Manufacturers and Distributors (1997) London: HMSO.

Rusmin, S. & Deluca, P.P. (1976) Effect of in-line intravenous filtration on the potency of potassium penicillin G. *Bulletin of the Parenteral Drug Association*, **30**, 64–71.

Rusmin, S., Althauser, M. & Deluca, P.P. (1975) Consequences of microbial contamination during extended intravenous therapy using in-line filters. *American Journal of Hospital Pharmacy*, **32**, 373–377.

Russell, A.D. (1981) Neutralization procedures in the evaluation of bactericidal activity. In *Disinfectants*, Society for Applied Bacteriology Technical Series. No. 16 (eds Collins, C.H., Allwood, M.C., Fox, A. & Bloomfield, S.F.), pp. 45–59. London and New York: Academic Press.

Russell, A.D., Ahonkhai, I. & Rogers, D.T. (1979) Microbiological applications of the inactivation of antibiotics and other antimicrobial agents. *Journal of Applied Bacteriology*, **46**, 207–245.

Schroeder, H.G. & Deluca, P.P. (1980) Theoretical aspects of sterile filtration and integrity testing. *Pharmaceutical Technology*, **4** (11), 80–85.

Sechovec, K.S. (1989) Validation of an automated filter integrity tester for use in bubble point testing. *Journal of Parenteral Science and Technology*, **43**, 23–26.

Smith, I.P.C. (1944) Sintered glassware: its manufacture and use. *Pharmaceutical Journal*, **152**, 110–111.

Solberg, C.O., Matsen, J.M., Vesley, D., Wheeler, D.J., Good, R.A. & Meuwissen, H.J. (1971) Laminar airflow protection in bone marrow transplantation. *Applied Microbiology*, **21**, 209–216.

Soltis, C. (1967) Construction and use of laminar flow rooms. *Bulletin of the Parenteral Drug Association*, **21**, 55–62.

Springett, D. (1981) The integrity testing of membrane filters. *Manufacturing Chemist and Aerosol News*. February, 41–45.

Stockdale, D. (1987) Clean rooms for aseptic pharmaceutical manufacturing. In *Aseptic Pharmaceutical Manufacturing Technology for the 1990s* (eds Olson, W.P. & Groves, M.J.), pp. 151–160. Prairie View: Interpharm Press.

Sykes, G. (1965) *Disinfection and Sterilization*, 2nd edn. London: E. & F.N. Spon.

Tanny, G.B. & Meltzer, T.H. (1978) The dominance of adsorptive effects in the filtrative purification of a flu vaccine. *Journal of the Parenteral Drug Association*, **32**, 258–267.

Tanny, G.B. & Meltzer, T.H. (1979) A review of sterilization with membrane filters. *Pharmaceutical Technology International*, 44–49.

Tanny, G.B., Strong, D.K., Presswood, W.G. & Meltzer, T.H. (1979) Adsorptive retention of *Pseudomonas diminuta* by membrane filters. *Journal of the Parenteral Drug Association*, **33**, 40–51.

Tanny, G.B., Mirelman, D. & Pistole, T. (1980) Improved filtration technique for concentrating and harvesting bacteria. *Applied and Environmental Microbiology*, **40**, 269–273.

Todd, R.L. & Kerr, T.J. (1972) Scanning electron microscopy of microbial cells on membrane filters. *Applied Microbiology*, **23**, 1160–1162.

Trasen, B. (1979) Filter Validation Symposium, IV. Nondestructive tests for bacterial retentive filters. *Journal of the Parenteral Drug Association*, **33**, 273–279.

Truskey, G.A., Gabler, R. DiLeo, A. & Manter, T. (1987) The effect of membrane filtration upon protein conformation. *Journal of Parenteral Science and Technology*, **41**, 180–193.

Turco, S & Davis, N.M. (1973a) Clinical significance of particulate matter: a review of the literature. *Hospital Pharmacy*, **8**, 137–140.

Turco, S. & Davis, N.M. (1973b) A comparison of commercial final filtration devices. *Hospital Pharmacy*, **8**, 141–160.

Underwood, E. (1998) Ecology of microorganisms as it affects the pharmaceutical industry. In *Pharmaceutical Microbiology* (eds Hugo, W.B. & Russell, A.D., 6th edn, pp. 339–354. Oxford: Blackwell Scientific Publications.

United States Pharmacopoeia (1995) Twenty-second revision. Rockville: United States Pharmacopoeial Convention.

Van der Waaij, D. & Andres, A.H. (1971) Prevention of airborne contamination and cross-contamination in germ-free mice by laminar flow. *Journal of Hygiene, Cambridge*, **69**, 83–89.

Van-Doorne, H. (1993) Sorption of bacterial endotoxin and retention of bacteria by positively charged membrane filters. *Journal of Pharmaceutical Science and Technology*, **47**, 192–198.

Van Ooteghem, M. & Herbots, H. (1969) The adsorption of preservatives on membrane filters. *Pharmaceutica Acta Helvetiae*, **44**, 610–619.

Voorspoels, J., Remon, J.P., Nelis, H. & Vandenbossche, G. (1996) Validation of filter sterilization and autoclaves. *International Journal of Pharmaceutics*, **133**, 9–15.

Wagman, G.H., Bailey, J.V. & Weinstein, M.J. (1975) Binding of aminoglycoside antibiotics to filtration materials. *Antimicrobial Agents and Chemotherapy*, 7, 316–319.

Wallhausser, K.H. (1976) Bacterial filtration in practice. *Drugs Made in Germany*, **19**, 85–98.

Wallhausser, K.H. (1979) Is the removal of microorganisms by filtration really a sterilization method? *Journal of the Parenteral Drug Association*, **33**, 156–170.

Wallhausser, K.H. (1982) Germ removal filtration. In *Advances in Pharmaceutical Sciences* (eds Bean, H.S., Beckett, A.H. & Carless, J.E), pp. 1–116. London: Academic Press.

Wayne, W. (1975) Clean rooms—letting the facts filter through. *Laboratory Equipment Digest*, December, 49.

White, P.J.P. (1990) The design of controlled environments. In *Guide to Microbiological Control in Pharmaceuticals* (eds Denyer, S.P. & Baird, R.), pp. 87–124. Chichester: Ellis Horwood.

Whitfield, W.J. (1967) Microbiological studies of laminar flow rooms. *Bulletin of the Parenteral Drug Association*, **21**, 37–45.

Whitfield, W.J. & Lindell, K.F. (1969) Designing for the laminar flow environment. *Contamination Control*, **8**, 10–21.

Windle-Taylor, F. & Burman, N.P. (1964) The application of membrane filtration techniques to the bacteriological examination of water. *Journal of Applied Bacteriology*, **27**, 294–303.

Wolley, E.L. (1969) Dealing with impurities and pollution. *The Illustrated Carpenter and Builder*, No. 12.

Wood, G.J. & Ward, M.E. (1981) The Pall Ultipor IV filter and air eliminator. *British Journal of Intravenous Therapy*, **2**, 15–16.

Wrasidlo, W. & Mysels, K.J. (1984) The structure and some properties of graded highly asymmetrical porous membranes. *Journal of Parenteral Science and Technology*, **38**, 24–31.

Zsigmondy, R. & Bachmann, W. (1918) Über neue Filter. *Zeitschrift für Anorganische und Allgemeine Chemie*, **103**, 119–128.

CHAPTER 23

New and Emerging Technologies

1 Introduction

While heating remains the technique most extensively employed to inactivate microorganisms in foods, there has been increasing interest recently in the development of alternative approaches. This has occurred mainly in response to the desires of consumers for products that are less organoleptically and nutritionally damaged during processing and less reliant on additives than hitherto. The new approaches, therefore, involve technologies that mostly offer full or partial alternatives to heat for the inactivation of bacteria, yeasts and moulds in foods and non-food materials. The new technologies include high hydrostatic pressure, high-voltage electric discharges, high-intensity laser or non-coherent light pulses, high magnetic-field pulses and manothermosonication (the combination of mild heating with ultrasonication and slightly raised pressure). Of these techniques, high pressure is currently being used commercially to preserve a number of different types of foods, while the other techniques are in various stages of development and commercial evaluation.

2 Ultrahigh pressure

2.1 Effects on microorganisms

Vegetative forms of bacteria were first shown to be inactivated by high pressures above about 100 megapascals (Mpa) by Hite (1899). Bacterial spores were shown to be much more resistant, surviving pressures above 1200 MPa (Larson *et al.*, 1918; Basset and Machebouf, 1932). Pressure was shown to extend the keeping quality of foods, such as milk (Hite, 1899), fruits and vegetables (Hite *et al.*, 1914). However, limitations of the technology prevented commercial use for food preservation until the 1980s (Mertens, 1995). By this time, the technology had advanced to the extent that commercial processes were developed for the non-thermal pressure pasteurization of a number of low-pH foods, in which spores were prevented from outgrowth by the low pH and were therefore not a problem. These foods included jams, fruit juices, jellies, acid sauces and fruit for inclusion in yoghurts (Selman, 1992). More recently, much more attention has been given to the materials science and other food science aspects of pressure (Knorr, 1995), and new pressure-treated foodstuffs have been introduced (chill-stored guacamole, dairy, fish and meat products), including some that have higher pH values than the jams and fruit juices marketed earlier (Palaniappan, 1996).

The effects of high pressure derive from the Le Chatelier principle, in which pressure favours any physical change or chemical reaction associated with a net volume decrease and suppresses any change or reaction involving a volume increase. In biological systems, the volume-decrease reactions that are most important include the denaturation of proteins, gelation, hydrophobic reactions, phase changes in lipids (and therefore in cell membranes) and increases in the ionization of dissociable molecules due to 'electrostriction' (Heremans, 1995). Small molecules are generally less affected than macromolecules, so that low-molecular-weight flavour and odour compounds, etc. in foods tend to survive pressure treatment unchanged, with quality advantages in some types of products (Horie *et al.*, 1991).

A structure as complex as a microorganism will clearly have many potentially pressure-sensitive sites within it, e.g. enzymes, genetic material, macromolecular assemblies, such as membranes, ribosomes, etc. (Isaacs *et al.*, 1995), and pressure has been shown to induce a variety of changes in vegetative bacterial cells that may contribute to their inactivation (Hoover *et al.*, 1989). Kinetic studies have shown some examples of exponential inactivation of cells held at constant pressure (e.g. *Escherichia coli*; Butz & Ludwig, 1986; Ludwig *et al.*, 1992), but the majority of studies have reported 'tails' on survivor curves, i.e. a decreasing death rate with the time of treatment (Fig. 23.1; Metrick *et al.*, 1989; Earnshaw, 1995; Patterson *et al.*, 1995a). It has been proposed that, at higher temperatures (e.g. in the case of 40°C and above for *E. coli* at 250 MPa), inactivation is near first-order, whereas, at lower temperatures (e.g. 30°C for *E. coli*), it is nearer second-order, and that membrane-lipid changes may account for these differences (Eze, 1990).

More generally, over the range -20°C to +20°C pressure is more effective in inactivating vegetative microorganisms at the lower than the higher temperatures, for instance for *Staphylococcus aureus*, *Salmonella bareilly* and *Vibrio parahaemolyticus* in buffers (Takahashi *et al.*, 1991) and for *Citrobacter freundii* in beef (Carlez *et al.* 1992). Reduction in water activity (A_w) resulting from the addition of a range of solutes led to substantial increases in pressure tolerance, as shown in *Rhodotorula rubra* (Oxen & Knorr, 1993). Other factors that are not yet fully understood affect the pressure tolerance of microorganisms in different foods. For instance, *Salmonella typhimurium* was inactivated about 10^6-fold in pork in 10 min at 300 Mpa, but only 10^2-fold in chicken baby food at 350 MPa (Metrick *et al.*, 1989). *Listeria monocytogenes* was more pressure-tolerant in ultraheat-treated (UHT) milk than in phosphate-buffered saline (Styles *et al.*, 1991). Strain-to-strain variability in sensitivity to pressure is greater than the variation with regard to other inactivation techni-

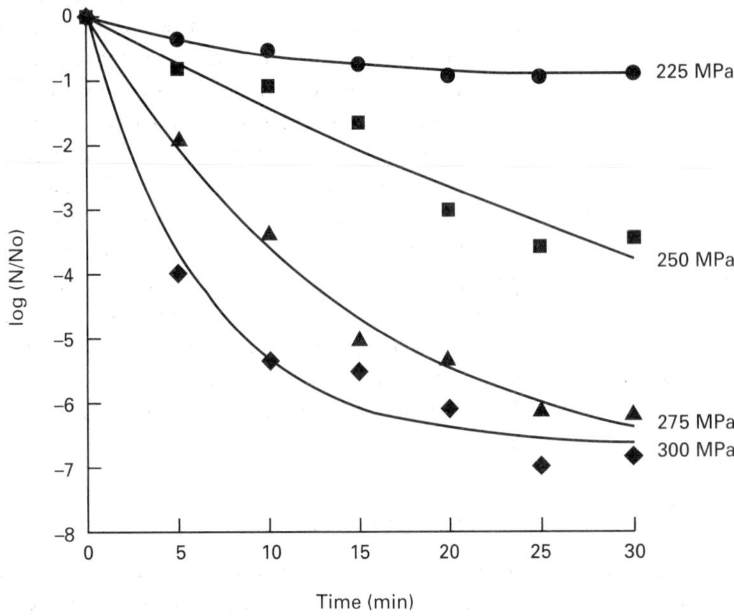

Fig. 23.1 Hydrostatic pressure–survivor curves of *Yersinia enterocolitica* in pH 7 phosphate-buffered saline at 20°C showing the effect of increasing pressure and the non-linearity of survivor curves (from Patterson *et al.*, 1995a).

ques, such as heat. *Listeria monocytogenes* strains NCTC 11994 and Scott A and an isolate from chicken were inactivated by less than 10-fold, just over 10^2-fold and about 10^5-fold, respectively, by a similar 375 MPa pressurization for 10 min in phosphate-buffered saline (Patterson *et al.*, 1995a).

Otherwise, exponential-phase cells are more pressure-sensitive than stationary-phase ones (Dring, 1976) and Gram-positive microorganisms are more pressure-tolerant than Gram-negative ones (Shigahisa *et al.*, 1991). However, there are some important exceptions to this generalization. For example, *E. coli* O157 H7 was found to be extremely pressure-tolerant in some foods; thus, exposure to 800 MPa in UHT milk brought about only a 10^2-fold reduction (Patterson *et al.*, 1995b). Altogether, these various influences of, sometimes poorly understood, environmental factors and strain-to-strain differences make it more difficult to predict accurately the effect of a particular pressure treatment than, for example, a particular heat treatment on microorganisms in foods.

In contrast to vegetative cells, bacterial spores were shown in the earliest studies to be very pressure-tolerant. Pressures up to 1200 MPa failed to inactivate spores of a number of species (Larson *et al.*, 1918; Basset & Machebouf, 1932; Timson & Short, 1965). However, it was shown later that, surprisingly, under certain conditions, inactivation of spores proceeded more rapidly and completely at lower than at higher pressures (Clouston & Wills, 1969; Sale *et al.*, 1970). An explanation for this was found when it was observed that inactivation of spores occurred in two stages (Clouston & Wills, 1969; Gould & Sale, 1970). First, pressure caused spores to germinate and then pressure inactivated the germinated forms. This led to the investigation of the combined use of pressure with raised temperature (Sale *et al.*, 1970) and with low-dose irradiation (Wills, 1974) to achieve a higher level of spore inactivation. The overall pattern of inactivation showed a strong pressure–heat synergism, as illustrated in Fig. 23.2. The effect has been confirmed for a wide range of spore types, although the effectiveness of the combination varies greatly in magnitude for different spores (Murrell & Wills, 1977; Kimugasa *et al.*, 1992; Kowalski *et al.*, 1992; Seyerderholm & Knorr, 1992; Hayakawa *et al.*, 1994). The kinetics of pressure-inactivation was near-exponential for spores of *Bacillus pumilus* (Clouston & Wills, 1970), but for spores of *Bacillus coagulans, Bacillus subtilis* and *Clostridium sporogenes* concave-upward curves or long tails were reported (Sale *et al.*, 1970).

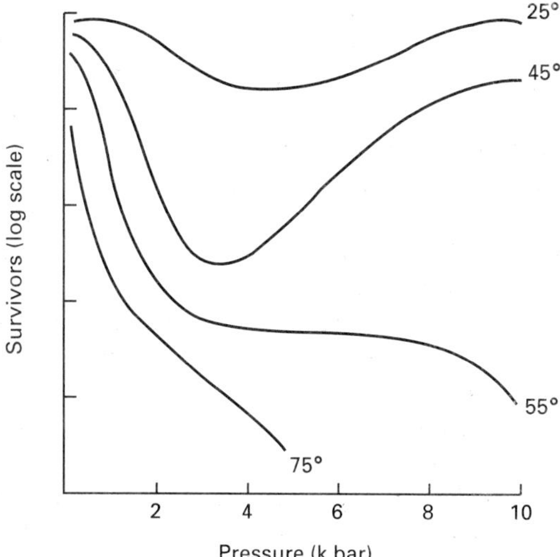

Fig. 23.2 General pattern of inactivation of bacterial spores by combined pressure–temperature treatments. The figure is taken from data for spores of *Bacillus coagulans* pressurized for 30 min in sodium phosphate buffer (100 mnol/l, pH 8). While different types of spores show similar patterns of inactivation, the extent of inactivation varies greatly. (From Sale *et al.*, 1970.)

The fact that, although spores of some species are relatively sensitive to pressure (*Bacillus cereus* is an example), those of others, including some of special importance in foods, such as *Bacillus stearothermophilus* and *Clostridium botulinum*, are very resistant (Knorr, 1995), has so far prevented the use of pressure to sterilize foods (Hoover, 1993). This may change with the development of presses that operate at higher temperature–pressure combinations, or the development of other effective combination techniques. For instance, the presence of bacteriocins, such as nisin, can amplify the effect of pressure against spores, for example those of *B. coagulans* (Roberts & Hoover, 1996).

2.2 High-pressure delivery

The use of high pressure to inactivate microorganisms involves the application of pressure isostatically (that is, the pressure is equal throughout the material being processed; there are no gradients, as commonly occur during other processes, such as the application of heat). Pressure is applied either directly, by forcing liquid into the treatment chamber, or indirectly, by forcing a piston into a liquid-filled vessel containing the material to be treated, usually in prepackaged form. The sealed packages are sufficiently flexible to withstand the compression that occurs during pressurization. The pressure medium and the pack contents are compressed to about 80–90% of their original volumes during pressurization in the 400–800 MPa pressure range, but, of course, return to their original volumes when the pressure is released. There is a transient temperature rise during pressurization of about 11°C at 400 MPa and 23°C at 800 MPa (for water; Farr, 1990), which dissipates at a rate dependent on the volume of the treatment vessel and the conductivity of its materials of construction, etc. The first commercial systems to be used for food processing operate as batch processes, with treatment times commonly between about 0.5 and 5 min. The volumes of treatment vessels are between about 50 and 1000 l (Barbosa–Canovas *et al.*, 1995). Larger vessels are mostly limited to pressures lower than those capable of inactivating microorganisms in foods. Fully continuous processes are not yet used commercially, although cost-effective, semicontinuous systems that can be used with pumpable liquid products have been developed (Barbosa-Canovas *et al.*, 1995, Moreau, 1995).

3 High-voltage electric pulses

3.1 Effects on microorganisms

While the application of electric fields to heat foods has become well established (Palaniappan, 1996)—for instance, through electrical-resistance or 'ohmic' heating (Fryer, 1995) and through microwave heating (Mullin, 1995)—the use of electric pulses to bring about the essentially nonthermal inactivation of microorganisms has only been explored and exploited more recently (Castro *et al.*, 1993). The use of the technique at lower, non-lethal, voltage gradients has become established as the basis for 'electroporation', by which genetic material can be exchanged between protoplasted cells of microorganisms, plants and animals (Neumann *et al.*, 1989). A method was patented by Doevenspeck (1960) for inactivating microorganisms with an electric field. Later studies demonstrated the inactivation of bacteria and yeasts and the lysis of protoplasts and erythrocytes (Sale & Hamilton, 1967, 1968). Still later studies concentrated on varying the electrical parameters (Hulsheger, 1980, 1981, 1983) and the effects of environmental parameters (Mizuno & Hori, 1988; Jayaram *et al.*, 1992).

While the effects of high-voltage fields on microorganisms are not understood at the molecular level, the gross effects and the mechanisms that cause them are well established. They result from the permeabilization of the cell membrane (Hamilton & Sale, 1967), which results when the voltage gradient is high enough to overcome its intrinsic resistance. Breakdown occurs when the potential difference across the membrane exceeds about 1 V (Chernomordik *et al.*, 1987; Glaser *et al.*, 1988). Massive leakage of cell contents occurs and the cell dies (Tsong, 1991).

Pulsed-field inactivation has been reported for *E. coli*, *Sal. typhimurium*, *Salmonella dublin*, *Streptococcus thermophilus*, *Lactobacillus brevis*, *Pseudomonas fragi*, *Klebsiella pneumoniae*, *Staph. aureus*, *L. monocytogenes*, *Saccharomyces cerevisiae* and *Candida albicans* (Barbosa-Canovas *et al.*, 1995). In contrast to vegetative organisms, bacterial spores (Sale & Hamilton, 1967) and yeast ascospores (Mertens & Knorr, 1992) are resistant, even at very high-voltage gradients, i.e. above 30 kV/cm.

A number of intrinsic and extrinsic factors influence the effectiveness of the electrical treatments. Inactivation increased greatly with rise in temperature; examples are provided by *E. coli* (Qin *et al.*, 1996) and *L. brevis* (Jayaram *et al.*, 1992). Low ionic strength favours inactivation. A reduction in the potassium chloride (KCl) concentration in skim milk from 0.17 to 0.03 mol/l resulted in a fall in the surviving fraction of *E. coli* following a 55 kV/cm, 20-pulse treatment, from about 0.3 to about 0.002 (Qin *et al.*, 1996). Reduction in pH increased inactivation, for example a doubling for *E. coli* by reducing the pH of skim milk from 6.8 to 5.7. Log-phase cells were more sensitive than stationary-phase ones (Vega *et al.*, 1996).

Application of electric-pulse treatments to a number of liquid foods has indicated that useful 'cold-pasteurization' inactivation of vegetative bacteria and yeasts can be achieved. For example, treatment of apple juice, at temperatures below 30°C, with fewer than 10 pulses in a continuous-treatment chamber, brought about more than a 10^6-fold reduction in numbers of *Sacch. cerevisiae* at a voltage gradient of 35 kV/cm; 22 kV/cm caused about 10^2-fold inactivation (Qin *et al.*, 1996). Studies of inactivation rates under different conditions have generally indicated kinetics which, on the basis of log survivor versus treatment time or versus number of pulses, show long tails. Near-straight lines are seen when log survivors are plotted against the log of the treatment time or the log of the number of pulses (Zhang *et al.*, 1995). Some potentially useful synergies have been described. For example, electroporated cells of *E. coli, L. monocytogenes* and *Sal. typhimurium* became much more sensitive than untreated cells to nisin and to pediocin (Kalchayanand *et al.*, 1994).

3.2 Electric-pulse delivery

Electric fields may be delivered as oscillating, bipolar, exponentially decaying or square-wave pulses. Bipolar pulses were more lethal than monopolar ones, because, it was presumed, rapid reversal in the direction of movement of charged molecules caused greater damage to cell membranes. Bipolar pulses generate less electrolysis in the material being treated and they are energy-efficient (Qin *et al.*, 1994). It is generally most economic to raise the field strength as high as possible, while reducing the duration of the pulses, without reducing pulse energy (Grahl *et al.*, 1992). On the other hand, the use of very high field strengths demands more complex and expensive engineering (Zhang *et al.*, 1994). As a result of these competing requirements, modern pulse-field devices employ field strengths from about 20 up to about 70 kV/cm, with pulse durations between 1 and about 5 μs. Repetition rates are typically from 1 up to 30 s or so at the higher voltages in order to minimize rises in temperature.

Treatment chambers may operate batchwise or continuously. The earliest versions were not fully enclosed and so were limited to voltage gradients of about 25 kV/cm, because this is the approximate breakdown voltage of air (Sale & Hamilton, 1967; Dunn & Pearlman, 1987). Enclosure and design improvements led to devices that could deliver 30–40 kV/cm (Grahl *et al.*, 1992; Zhang *et al.*, 1994). These were useful for laboratory studies to optimize design parameters for efficient killing of microorganisms. Continuous operation is essential for cost-effective commercial applications able to treat liquids and liquids containing particulates, and a number of such systems, mostly designed around coaxial cylindrical electrodes, have been developed (Boulart, 1983; Hoffman & Evans, 1986; Dunn & Pearlman, 1987; Sato & Kawata, 1991; Bushnell *et al.*, 1993; Qin *et al.*, 1995; Sitzmann, 1995).

4 Other emerging technologies

4.1 High-intensity light pulses

High-intensity laser and non-coherent light has long been known to inactivate microorganisms (Mertens & Knorr, 1992), although it is often unclear to what extent the lethal effects derive from the ultraviolet (UV) component of the radiation and, sometimes, local transient heating. The delivery of light to packaging materials, to food surfaces and to transparent liquid products, in short pulses of high intensity, has been shown to be capable of inactivating vegetative and spore forms of microorganisms in these environments (Dunn *et al.*, 1988) and in the medical area, particularly dentistry (Powell & Wisenant, 1991; Cobb *et al.*, 1992; Rooney *et al.*, 1994).

Commercially practicable machines for treating foods and other materials have been patented (Dunn *et al.*, 1988). These machines use broad-spectrum light with pulse durations from 10^6 to 10^1 s and with energy densities from about 0.1 to about 50 J/cm^2. Different spectral distributions and energies are selected for different applications. For example, UV-rich light, in which about 30% of the energy is at wavelengths shorter than 300 nm, is recommended for treatment of packaging materials, water or other transparent fluids. In contrast, for food surfaces, when high intensities of UV may accelerate lipid oxidation or cause colour loss, etc., the shorter wavelengths are filtered out and the killing effects are largely thermal. The advantage of delivering heat in this manner is that a large amount of thermal energy is transferred to a very thin layer of product surface very quickly, while the temperature rise within the bulk of the product can be very small (Dunn *et al.*, 1988). Overall, therefore, these intense light treatments are effective predominantly because they deliver conventional microorganism-inactivating treatments–UV irradiation or heat–but in an unconventional and sometimes advantageous manner (Mertens & Knorr, 1992).

4.2 High-intensity magnetic-field pulses

Exposure to oscillating magnetic fields has been reported to have a variety of effects on biological systems, ranging from selective inactivation of malignant cells (Costa & Hofmann, 1987) to the inactivation of bacteria on packaging materials and in foods Hofmann, 1985). Treatment times are very short, typically from 25 μs to a few milliseconds and field strengths very high, typically from 2 to about 100 T at frequencies between about 5 and 500 kHz. It has been suggested that the mechanism of action could involve alteration of ion fluxes across cell membranes, but this is not really known (Pothakamury *et al.*, 1993). Efficacies of the treatments did not exceed about 10^2-fold reductions in numbers of vegetative microorganisms inoculated into milk (*Strep. thermophilus*), orange juice (*Saccharomyces*) or bread rolls (mould spores) and no inactivation of bacterial spores has been reported (Hofmann, 1985), so the practical potential for the technique, as it has been developed so far, appears to be limited (Mertens & Knorr, 1992; Barbosa-Canovas *et al.*, 1995).

4.3 Manothermosonication

The use of ultrasound to inactivate microorganisms was first reported nearly 70 years ago (Harvey & Loomis, 1929). The mechanism of action derives from the rapidly alternating compression and decompression zones propagating into the material being treated and the cavitation that these cause. Cavitation involves the formation and collapse of small bubbles, generating shock waves with associated very high temperatures and pressures, which can be sufficiently intense to catalyse chemical reactions and disrupt animal, plant and microbial cells (Scherba, 1991). Generally, large cells are more susceptible than small ones. Rod-shaped bacteria are more sensitive than cocci (Alliger, 1975) and Gram-positive bacteria more sensitive than Gram-negative ones (Ahmed & Russell, 1975), while spores are so resistant as to be essentially non-disruptable (Sanz *et al.*, 1985).

A potentially useful synergy of ultrasound with heat was reported for the inactivation of bacterial spores (*Bacillus cereus* and *B. licheniformis*; Burgos *et al.*, 1972), thermoduric streptococci (Ordonez *et al.*, 1984), *Staph. aureus* and other vegetative microorganisms (Ordonez *et al.*, 1987). However, as the temperature was raised, the potentiating effect of ultrasound became less and less and (for spores) disappeared near to the boiling-point of water (Garcia *et al.*, 1989). The important discovery that led to the development of manothermosonication was that this disappearance of the synergism could be prevented if the pressure was raised slightly (e.g. by only a few tens of MPa; Sala *et al.*, 1995). The combination procedure generally has the effect of reducing the apparent heat resistance of microorganisms by about 5–20°C or so, depending on the temperature, the organism and its *z*-value. While the process has not yet been commercialized, it has been shown to operate in liquid foods for example, milk; Sala *et al.*, 1995), offering the possibility of new sterilization or pasteurization processes for this and other liquid products, with reduced levels of thermal damage.

5 Conclusions

The use of physical techniques to inactivate microorganisms without the the application of heat, or with the use of less heat than would otherwise be necessary, is attractive from the point of view of product quality, and the new and emerging techniques reviewed all aim to do this. Three facts limit their usefulness at the present time. Firstly, bacterial spores remain the organisms most tolerant to all the techniques, so that, with the possible exception of manothermosonication, sterilization, as opposed to pasteurization, is not yet possible. Secondly, the kinetics of inactivation that results from some of the techniques is different from that resulting from heating, so that a careful new approach, for example to product safety, will be needed if application of the techniques continues to be promoted. Thirdly, with the exception of hydrostatic pressure, the efficacy of the other techniques is impaired by product structure, and may therefore be limited to liquid products or products containing small particulates, or (for light pulses) transparent products and surfaces, etc. At the same time, combination techniques, in which the new technologies are only one component of the total preservation system, have already been described, and, if these are further developed and proved to be effective, the opportunities for use of the new techniques are very likely to grow in the future.

6 References

Ahmed, F.I.K. & Russell, C. (1975) Synergism between ultrasonic waves and hydrogen peroxide in the killing of microorganisms. *Journal of Applied Bacteriology*, **39**, 31–40.

Alliger, H. (1975) Ultrasonic disruption. *American Laboratory*, **10**, 75–85.

Barbosa-Canovas, G.V., Pothakamury, U.R. & Swanson, B.G. (1995) State of the art technologies for the sterilization of foods by non-thermal processes: physical methods. In *Food Preservation by Moisture Control: Fundamentals and Applications* (eds Barbosa-Canovas, G.V. & Welti-Chanes, J.), pp. 493–532. Lancaster, Pennsylvania: Technomic Publishing.

Basset, J. & Macheboeuf, M.A. (1932) Étude sur les effets biologiques des ultrapressions: résistance de bactéries, de diastases et de toxines aux pressions très élévées. *Comptes Rendus Hebdomaire Science Acadamie Sciences*, **196**, 1431–1442.

Boulart, J. (1983) *Process for Protecting a Fluid and Installations for Realization of that Process*. French Patent 2,513,087.

Burgos, J., Ordonez, J.A. & Sala, F.J. (1972) Effect of ultrasonic waves on the heat resistance of *Bacillus cereus* and *Bacillus coagulans* spores. *Applied Microbiology*, **24**, 497–498.

Bushnell, A.H., Dunn, J.E., Clark, R.W. & Pearlman, J.S. (1993) *High Pulsed Voltage System for Extending the Shelf Life of Pumpable Food Products*. US Patent 5,235,905.

Butz, P. & Ludwig, H. (1986) Pressure inactivation of microorganisms at moderate temperatures. *Physica*, **139B/140B**, 875–877.

Carlez, A., Cheftel, J.-C., Rosec, J.P., Richard, N., Saldana, J.-L. & Balny, C. (1992) Effects of high pressure and bacteriostatic agents on the destruction of *Citrobacter freundii* in minced beef muscle. In *High Pressure and Biotechnology* (eds Balny, C., Hayashi, R., Heremans, K. & Masson, P., Colloque INSERM/J, pp. 365–368. Libby Eurotech.

Castro, A.I., Barbosa-Canovas, G.V. & Swanson, B.G. (1993) Microbial inactivation in foods by pulsed electric fields. *Journal of Food Processing and Preservation*, **17**, 47–73.

Chernomordik, L.V., Sukharev, S.I., Popov, S.V. *et al.*, (1987) The electrical breakdown of cell and lipid membranes: the similarity of phenomenologies. *Biochimica et Biophysica Acta*, **972**, 360–365.

Clouston, J.G. & Wills, P.A. (1969) Initiation of germination and inactivation of *Bacillus pumilus* spores by hydrostatic pressure. *Journal of Bacteriology*, **97**, 684–690.

Clouston, J.G. & Wills, P.A. (1970) Kinetics of germination and inactivation of *Bacillus pumilus* spores by hydrostatic pressure. *Journal of Bacteriology*, **103**, 140–143.

Cobb, C.M., McCawley, T.K. & Killoy, W.J. (1992) A preliminary study on the effects of the Nd:YAG laser on root surfaces and subgingival microflora *in vivo*. *Journal of Periodontology*, **63**, 701–707.

Costa, J.L. & Hofmann, G.A. (1987) *Malignancy Treatment*. US Patent 4,665,898.

Doevenspeck, H. (1960) German Patent 1,237,541.

Dring, J.G. (1976) Some aspects of the effects of hydrostatic pressure on microorganisms. In *Inhibition and Inactivation of Microorganisms* (eds Skinner, F.A. & Hugo, W.B.), pp. 257–277. London: Academic Press.

Dunn, J.E. & Pearlman, J.S. (1987) *Methods and Apparatus for Extending the Shelf Life of Fluid Food Products*. US Patent 4,695,472.

Dunn, J.E., Clark, R.W., Asmus, J.F., Pearlman, J.S., Boyer, K. & Parrichaud, F. (1988) *Method and Apparatus for Preservation of Foodstuffs*. International Patent WO88/03369.

Earnshaw, R.G. (1995) High pressure microbial inactivation kinetics. In *High Pressure Processing of Foods* (eds Ledward, D.A., Johnston, D.E., Earnshaw, R.G. & Hasting, A.P.M.), pp. 37–46. Nottingham: Nottingham University Press.

Eze, M.O. (1990) Consequences of the lipid bilayer to membrane-associated reactions. *Journal of Chemical Education*, **67**, 17–20.

Farr, D. (1990) High pressure technology in the food industry. *Trends in Food Science and Technology*, **1**, 14–16.

Fryer, P. (1995) Electrical resistanc heating of foods. In *New Methods of Food Preservation* (ed. Gould,

G.W.), pp. 205–235. Glasgow: Blackie Academic & Professional.

Garcia, M.L., Burgos, J., Sanz, B. & Ordonez, J.A. (1989) Effect of heat and ultrasonic waves on the survival of two strains of *Bacillus subtilis*. *Journal of Applied Bacteriology*, **67**, 619–628.

Glaser, R.W., Leikin, S.L., Chernomordik, L.V., Pastushenko, V.F. & Sokirko, A.V. (1988) Reversible electrical breakdown of lipid bilayers: formation and evolution of pores. *Biochimica et Biophysica Acta*, **940**, 275–281.

Gould, G.W. & Sale, A.J.H. (1970) Initiation of germination of bacterial spores by hydrostatic pressure. *Journal of General Microbiology*, **60**, 335–346.

Grahl, T., Sitzmann, W. & Makl, H. (1992) Killing of microorganisms in fluid media by high voltage pulses. *DECHMA Biotechnology Conference Series*, **5B**, 675–678.

Hamilton, W.A. & Sale, A.J.H. (1967) Effects of high electric fields on microorganisms 11. Mechanism of action of the lethal effect. *Biochimica et Biophysica Acta*, **148**, 789–795.

Harvey, E. & Loomis, A. (1929) The destruction of luminous bacteria by high frequency sound waves. *Journal of Bacteriology*, **17**, 373–379.

Hayakawa, I., Kanno, T., Tomita, M. & Figio, Y. (1994) Application of high pressure for spore inactivation and protein denaturation. *Journal of Food Science*, **59**, 159–163.

Heremans, K. (1995) High pressure effects on biomolecules. In *High Pressure Processing of Foods* (eds Ledward, D.A., Johnston, D.E., Earnshaw, R.G. & Hasting, A.P.M.), pp. 81–97. Nottingham: Nottingham University Press.

Hite, B.H. (1899) The effect of pressure in the preservation of milk. *Bulletin of the West Virginia Experiment Station*, **58**, 15–35.

Hite, B.H., Giddings, N.J. & Weakley, C.W. (1914) The effect of pressure on certain microorganisms encountered in the preservation of fruits and vegetables. *Bulletin of the West Virginia Experiment Station*, **146**, 3–67.

Hofmann, G.A. (1985) *Inactivation of Microorganisms by an Oscillating Magnetic Field*. US Patent 4,524,079 and International Patent WO85/02094.

Hofmann, G.A. & Evans, E.G. (1986) Electronic, genetic, physical and biological aspects of electromanipulation. *IEEE Medical Biology Magazine*, **5**, 6–25.

Hoover, D.G. (1993) Pressure effects on biological systems. *Food Technology*, **47(6)**, 150–155.

Hoover, D.G., Metrick, K., Papineau, A.M., Farkas, D.F. & Knorr, D. (1989) Biological effects of high hydrostatic pressure on food microorganisms. *Food Technology*, **43**, 99–107.

Horie, Y., Kimura, K., Ida, M., Yosida, Y. & Ohki, K. (1991) Jam preservation by pressure pasteurization. *Nippon Nogeiki Kaisu*, **65**, 975–980.

Hulsheger, H. &Niemann, E.G. (1980) Lethal effect of high voltage pulses on *E. coli* K12. *Radiation and Environmental Biophysics*, **18**, 281–288.

Hulsheger, H., Potel, J. & Neimann, E.G. (1981) Killing of bacteria with electric pulses of high field strength. *Radiation and Environmental Biophysics*, **20**, 53–61.

Hulsheger, H., Potel, J. & Neimann, E.G. (1983) Electric field effects on bacteria and yeast cells. *Radiation and Environmental Biophysics*, **22**, 149–156.

Isaacs, N.S., Chilton, P. & Mackey, B. (1995) Studies on the inactivation by high pressure of microorganisms. In *High Pressure Processing of Foods* (eds Ledward, D.A., Johnston, D.E., Earnshaw, R.G. & Hasting, A.P.M.), pp. 65–79. Nottingham: Nottingham University Press.

Jayaram, S., Castle, G.S.P. & Margaritis, A. (1992) Kinetics of sterilization of *Lactobacillus brevis* by the application of high voltage pulses. *Biotechnology and Bioengineering*, **40**, 1412–1420.

Kalchayanand, N., Sikes, T., Dunne, C.P. & Ray, B. (1994) Hydrostatic pressure and electroporation have increased bactericidal efficiency in combination with bacteriocins. *Applied and Environmental Microbiology*, **60**, 4174–4177.

Kimugasa, H., Takao, T., Fukumoto, K. & Ishihara, M. (1992) Changes in tea components during processing and preservation of tea extracts by hydrostatic pressure sterilization. *Nippon Nogeiku Kaichi*, **66**, 707–712.

Knorr, D. (1995) Hydrostatic pressure treatment of food: microbiology. In *New Methods of Food Preservation* (ed. Gould, G.W.), pp. 159–175. Glasgow: Blackie Academic and Professional.

Kowalski, E., Ludwig, H. & Tauscher, B. (1992) Hydrostatic pressure to sterilize foods 1. Application to pepper (*Piper nigrum* L). *Deutsche Lebensmittel Rundschau*, **88**, 74–75.

Larson, W.P., Hartzell, T.B. & Diehl, H.S. (1918) The effect of high pressure on bacteria. *Journal of Infectious Diseases*, **22**, 271–279.

Ludwig, H., Bieler, C., Hallbauer, K. & Scigalla, W. (1992) Inactivation of microorganisms by hydrostatic pressure. In *High Pressure Biotechnology* (eds Balny, C., Hayashi, R., Heremans, K. & Masson, P.), pp. 25–32. Colloque INSERM/J, Libby Eurotext: Brussels.

Mertens, B. (1995) Hydrostatic pressure treatment of food: equipment and processing. In *New Methods of Food Preservation* (ed. Gould, G.W.), pp. 135–158. Glasgow: Blackie Academic and Professional.

Mertens, B. & Knorr, D. (1992) Development of nonthermal processes for food preservation. *Food Technology*, **46(5)**, 124–133.

Metrick, C., Hoover, D.G. & Farkas, D.F. (1989) Effects of high hydrostatic pressure on heat-sensitive strains of *Salmonella*. *Journal of Food Science*, **54**, 1547–1564.

Mizuno, A. & Hori, Y. (1988) Destruction of living cells by pulsed high voltage applications. *Transactions IEEE Industrial Applications*, **24**, 387–395.

Moreau, C. (1995) Semicontinuous high pressure cell for liquid processing. In *High Pressure Processing of Foods* (eds Ledward, D.A., Johnston, D.E., Earnshaw, R.G. & Hasting, A.P.M.), pp. 181–197. Nottingham: Nottingham University Press.

Mullin, J. (1995) Microwave processing. In *New Methods of Food Preservation* (ed. Gould, G.W.), pp. 112–134. Glasgow: Blackie Academic and Professional.

Murrell, W.G. & Wills, P.A. (1977) Initiation of *Bacillus* spore germination by hydrostatic pressure: effect of temperature. *Journal of Bacteriology*, **129**, 1272–1280.

Neumann, E., Sowers, A.E. & Jordan, C.A. (eds) (1989) *Electroporation and Electrofusion in Cell Biology*. New York: Plenum Press.

Ordonez, J.A., Sanz, B., Hernandez, P.E. & Lopez-Lorenzo, P. (1984) A note on the effect of combined ultrasonic and heat treatments on the survival of thermoduric streptococci. *Journal of Applied Bacteriology*, **56**, 175–177.

Ordonez, J.A., Aguilera, M.A., Garcia, M.L. & Sanz, B. (1987) Effects of combined ultrasonic and heat treatment (thermosonication) on the survival of a strain of *Staphylococcus aureus*. *Journal of Dairy Research*, **54**, 61–67.

Oxen, P. & Knorr, D. (1993) Baroprotective effects of high solute concentrations against inactivation of *Rhodotorula rubra*. *Lebensmittel Wissenschaft Technologie*, **26**, 220–223.

Palaniappan, S. (1996) High isostatic presure processing of foods. In *New Processing Technologies Yearbook* (ed. Chandarana, P.I.), pp. 51–66. Washington, DC: National Food Processors Association.

Patterson, M.F., Quinn, M., Simpson, R & Gilmour, A. (1995a) Effects of high pressure on vegetative pathogens. In *High Pressure Processing of Foods* (eds Ledward, D.A., Johnston, D.E., Earnshaw, R.G. & Hasting, A.P.M.), pp. 47–63. Nottingham: Nottingham University Press.

Patterson, M.F., Quinn, M., Simpson, R. & Gilmour, A. (1995b) Sensitivity of vegetative pathogens to high hydrostatic pressure treatment in phosphate-buffered saline and foods. *Journal of Food Protection*, **58**, 524–529.

Pothakamury, U.R., Monsalve-Gonzalea, A., Barbosa-Canovas, G.V. & Swanson, B.G. (1993) Magnetic-field inactivation of microorganisms and generation of biological changes. *Food Technology*, **47**(12), 85–92.

Powell, G.L. & Wisenant, B. (1991) Comparison of three lasers for dental instrument sterilization. *Lasers in Surgery and Medicine*, **11**, 69–71.

Qin, B., Pothakamury, U.R., Barbosa-Canovas, G.V. & Swanson, B.G. (1996) Nonthermal pasteurization of liquid foods using high-intensity pulsed electric fields. *Critical Reviews in Food Science and Nutrition*, **36**, 603–607.

Qin, B., Zhang, Q., Barbosa-Canovas, G.V., Swanson, B.G. & Pedrow, P.D. (1994) Inactivation of micro-organisms by pulsed electric fields with different voltage wave forms. *IEEE Transactions Electrical Insulation*, **1**, 1047–1057.

Qin, B., Zhang, Q., Barbosa-Canovas, G.V., Swanson, B.G. & Pedrow, P.D. (1995) Pulsed electric field chamber design using field element method. *Transactions ASAE*, **38**, 557–565.

Roberts, C.M. & Hoover, D.G. (1996) Sensitivity of *Bacillus coagulans* spores to combinations of high hydrostatic pressure, heat, acidity and nisin. *Journal of Applied Bacteriology*, **81**, 363–368.

Rooney, J., Midda, M. & Leeming, J. (1994) A laboratory investigation of the bactericidal effect of a Nd:Yag laser. *British Dental Journal*, **176**, 61–64.

Sala, F.J., Burgos, J., Condon, S., Lopez, P. & Raso (1995) Effect of heat and ultrasound on microorganisms and enzymes. In: *New Methods Of Food Preservation* (ed. Gould, G.W.), pp. 176–204. Glasgow: Blackie Academic and Professional.

Sale, A.J.H. & Hamilton, W.A. (1967) Effects of high electric fields on microorganisms. 1. Killing of bacteria and yeasts. *Biochimica et Biophysica Acta*, **148**, 781–788.

Sale, A.J.H. & Hamilton, W.A. (1968) Effects of high electric fields on microorganisms. II. Lysis of erythrocytes and protoplasts. *Biochimica et Biophysica Acta*, **163**, 37–45.

Sale, A.J.H., Gould, G.W. & Hamilton, W.A. (1970) Inactivation of bacterial spores by hydrostatic pressure. *Journal of General Microbiology*, **60**, 323–334.

Sanz, B., Palacios, P., Lopez, P. & Ordonez, J.A. (1985) Effect of ultrasonic waves on the heat resistance of *Bacillus stearothermophilus* spores. In *Fundamental and Applied Aspects of Bacterial Spores* (eds Dring, G.J., Ellar, D.J. and Gould, G.W.), pp. 215–259. London: Academic Press.

Sato, M. & Kawata, H. (1991) *Pasteurization Method for Liquid Foodstuffs*. Japanese Patent 398, 565.

Scherba, G., Weizel, R.M. & O'Brien, J.R. (1991) Quantitative assessment of the germicidal efficacy of ultrasonic energy. *Applied and Environmental Microbiology*, **57**, 2079–2084.

Selman, J. (1992) New technologies for the food industry. *Food Science and Technology Today*, **6**, 205–209.

Seyerderholm, I. & Knorr, D. (1992) Reduction of *Bacillus stearothermophilus* spores by combined high pressure and temperature treatments. *Journal of Food Industry*, **43**(4), 17–20.

Shigahisa, T., Ohmori, T., Saito, A., Tuji, S. & Hayashi, R. (1991) Effects of high pressure on the characteristics of pork slurries and inactivation of microorganisms associated with meat and meat products. *International Journal of Food Microbiology*, **12**, 207–216.

Sitzmann, W. (1995) High voltage pulse technologies for food preservation. In *New Methods of Food Preservation* (ed. Gould, G.W.), pp. 236–252. Glasgow: Blackie Academic and Professional.

Styles, M.F., Hoover, D.G. & Farkas, D.F. (1991) Response of *Listeria monocytogenes* and *Vibrio parahaemolyticus* to high hydrostatic pressure. *Journal of Food Science*, **56**, 1404–1407.

Takahashi, K., Ishii, H. & Ishikawa, H. (1991) Sterilization of microorganisms by hydrostatic pressure at low temperature. In *High Pressure Science of Food* (ed. Hayashi, R.), pp. 225–232. Kyoto: San-Ei Publishing.

Timson, W.J. & Short, A.J. (1965) Resistance of microorganisms to hydrostatic pressure. *Biotechnology and Bioengineering*, **7**, 139–159.

Tsong, T.Y. (1991) Minireview: electroporation of cell membranes. *Biophysical Journal*, **60**, 297–316.

Wills, P.A. (1974) Effects of hydrostatic pressure and ionizing radiation on bacterial spores. *Atomic Energy Australia*, **17**, 2–10.

Zhang, Q., Barbosa-Canovas, G.V. & Swanson, B.G. (1994) Engineering aspects of pulsed electric field pasteurization. *Journal of Food Engineering*, **25**, 261–268.

Zhang, Q., Qin, B.L., Barbosa-Canovas, G.V. & Swanson, B.G. (1995) Inactivation of *E. coli* for food pasteurization by high strength pulsed electric fields. *Journal of Food Processing and Preservation*, **19**, 103–118.

CHAPTER 24

Reuse of Disposables

1 Introduction

This simple title underlies a simmering controversy that has affected the hospital sectors of most developed countries for a number of years. It has been brought about by a combination of advancing medical technology and the economic constraints placed upon health-care providers by diminishing resources. Before examining in more detail the various reasons why the subject has produced such intense debate, it is appropriate to define what is meant by the different terms involved.

1.1 Reuse

The Medical Devices Agency (MDA) defines 'reuse' as 'repeated episodes of use of a device in circumstances which make some form of reprocessing necessary' (Medical Devices Agency, 1995). The reprocessing might consist of cleaning, disinfection, sterilization, refilling, resharpening or any similar procedure. This is a term which, therefore, embraces a number of different situations. For example, an item which is supplied prepackaged and sterilized by the manufacturers may be opened in the operating theatre, but not used. This is clearly a different scenario from that where such a device is actually used for a diagnostic or therapeutic purpose and different again from that where a device is implanted into a patient and then recovered at a later time. In the first case, the procedures involved would simply be repackaging and resterilizing, while in the other cases additional stages, including cleaning and checking performance, are required.

Kozarek (1995) has defined three categories of disposable items: category I (non-used disposable items; opened or beyond expiration date); category II (disposable items used in non-sterile body areas); and category III (disposable items utilized in sterile body areas). Different criteria are applied to the reprocessing protocols for these three categories of devices. At first, this may not seem to be a particularly controversial practice, since hospitals have been engaged in the business of manufacturing, repairing, cleaning and sterilizing medical equipment for over a century. However, as we shall see, times have changed and we are now faced with an extra dimension of complexity.

1.2 Disposables

In the context of this chapter, the term 'disposables' is used for medical devices which are required to be sterile and are supplied by the manufacturers as being 'for single use only'. Clearly, this definition encompasses a broad range of equipment, for both diagnosis and treatment, and extends from simple syringes to complex electronic components, such as cardiac pacemakers.

Despite the warning by the manufacturers that a piece of equipment is for single use only, there are some instances where, for various reasons, items are safely reused. Such situations can be found where an item of equipment is used on a number of occasions by the same patient; often this occurs in the community and involves minor items, like urethral catheters and plastic insulin syringes.

1.3 Background

It was previously stated that the maintenance and sterilization of medical equipment have been part of the function of hospitals for many years now. Prior to the 1950s, most medical devices were constructed from glass, metals, rubber and fabrics, which readily lent themselves to dismantling, cleaning and heat sterilization (a process which was available in most hospitals). The manufacturing industries confined themselves to the supply of prepackaged and presterilized consumable items, such as dressings and sutures (Greene, 1986).

With the advent of plastics, the manufacturers could make most devices far more cheaply and supply them to the hospitals ready for use. However, because of their heat-labile components, they were now no longer able to be reprocessed using existing techniques. Despite this, hospitals still achieved cost savings by buying disposables and discarding them after single use. The requirement for single-use items was given further impetus when concerns over the transmission of acquired immune deficiency syndrome (AIDS) and hepatitis B grew. However, problems arose as medical technology became more advanced and the devices being supplied by the manufacturers ceased to be cheap alternatives to existing equipment but instead became highly complex and expensive. Hospital departments were also under pressure to maintain a higher throughput of patients, an increasing number of whom required the use of these complex items of equipment for either diagnosis or treatment. Budgets simply did not allow the purchase of the required number of devices and so the temptation arose to reprocess those items which, to all intents and purposes, appeared perfectly serviceable. Ethylene oxide (EO) sterilizers were installed in many hospitals to enable sterilization of these heat-sensitive pieces of equipment, but often the delays imposed by the removal of residuals gave unacceptably long process times and did not solve the problems of backlog. As a consequence, some hospitals went over to less well-validated techniques, such as high-level disinfection (HLD), rather than EO, in order to provide a more rapid means for the removal of contaminant microorganisms and turnover of equipment (Greene, 1986). This departure from normal practice is not necessarily of major significance, in that the final microbiological outcome may still be satisfactory. However, sterilization by steam or EO can be monitored by both physicochemical and biological monitors, while HLD cannot (Greene, 1995; see also Chapter 25).

The ability to validate and monitor all stages of a process is of major significance. Manufacturers are subject to close scrutiny in the production of their medical devices, and the good manufacturing practice (GMP) and quality assurance (QA) procedures (see Chapter 11) required inevitably lead to high cost. As a consequence, they are prepared to accept liability for the product, provided it is used once only and in accordance with instructions. In taking a medical device and subjecting it to cleaning and sterilization processes not recommended by the manufacturer, the hospital is taking a step into the unknown. It has introduced issues not just of sterility but also of toxicity, biocompatibility and potential deterioration in performance.

While the reuse of medical devices is done for the best possible motives, there is now an argument which states that patients are potentially being put at risk and, in addition, that hospitals are exposing themselves to the possibility of expensive litigation, should an adverse event occur.

2 Reprocessing problems

2.1 Operator safety

Technicians who operate any reprocessing procedures potentially put themselves at an increased risk, due both to the handling of contaminated items and to exposure to a variety of toxic cleaning and sterilizing agents. Handling of blood-contacting devices carries a potential risk from both AIDS and hepatitis B, and so, in addition to any device considerations, stringent QA procedures are essential to provide adequate protection for at-risk personnel.

2.2 Cleaning

Examination of many modern medical devices reveals a complex construction, often with different materials and sometimes with tubing of very narrow bore. Such designs, when encrusted with organic matter, such as blood or tissue detritus, can prove extremely difficult to clean. Any residual layers of protein may set up sensitivity reactions when used on another patient, and, if non-pyrogen-free water is used for washing, adsorbed endotoxins may bring about a toxic effect, even if the device has been properly sterilized. The cleaning process must be shown to be compatible with the materials used in the device and, in addition, the agents used to clean the device must not be absorbed or adsorbed; otherwise, these may be released on subsequent use and again set up adverse reactions.

2.3 Sterilization

Of the issues that need to be addressed in this debate the one which appears at first sight to be most obvious is the problem of sterility. The delicate nature of many devices necessitates the use of methods other than heat processes for their sterilization. This was highlighted by Bell & Morgan (1993), who reported a critical incident during a gynaecological operation, concerning a ventilator mask which had been reprocessed and sterilized inappropriately by the use of heat. The distortion which resulted meant that the device could not be connected properly and, after considerable wasted effort, the system had to be abandoned and a new one fitted.

Ethylene oxide would be the most favoured technique for the sterilization of such heat-sensitive devices and this is within the scope of many hospital central sterile-supply departments. However, as has already been said, there are problems of throughput times and residual toxicity to be considered. Hence, although the technology exists to achieve sterility of reuse devices, other less well-documented procedures are often used. If HLD processes are employed, not only must these be validated to ensure they achieve their required effect but, as with the cleaning agents, they must be shown to be compatible and leave no toxic residues.

Proponents of reuse strategy point to the fact that there are few, if any, reported cases in the literature of infection resulting from the use of an improperly sterilized device. An extensive study was carried out by DesCoteaux and co-workers to determine the rate of surgical complications related to the reuse of laparoscopic instruments for procedures carried out in a single hospital department between August 1990 and January 1994 (DesCoteaux *et al.*, 1995). No complications related to disposable-instrument malfunction were recorded and the rate of deep and superficial infections was no greater than for those cases when new equipment was used. Subsequent cost analysis of this study revealed that, even taking into account the cost of reprocessing, the reuse of disposable equipment led to substantial savings (DesCoteaux *et al.*, 1996). The study by DesCoteaux *et al.* (1995) is particularly useful, because it considers a variety of complications and not just infection. In some cases, the lack of infectious episodes has been used as the sole justification for embarking on, or continuing with, a reuse policy, ignoring the other equally valid arguments of functionality, biocompatibility, increased fragility, etc. (Parker *et al.*, 1996). In truth, the chances of a new, sterile device being contaminated by personnel in the operating theatre after opening the package are much higher than a non-sterile reused device being produced.

2.4 Material stability

A manufacturing company produces a limited range of devices, of which it has intimate knowledge. The quality of the raw materials is known, the manufacturing processes fully documented and the sterilization procedures validated for each product. The device has been designed to fulfil a specific function and materials are selected to achieve that purpose. In contrast, a hospital that reuses disposable devices is faced with an extensive range of items, which have had differing histories. They will have little knowledge of the materials from which they are constructed and will probably have no data available concerning the stability of those materials in the face of further chemical processing. This scenario has led to a number of reported incidents of device failure on reuse, some of which have been the subject of major litigation (Jacob *et al.*, 1994). Jayabalan (1995) has reviewed the problems associated with the sterilization of a range of biomedical polymers, highlighting the changes in material properties which can occur during reprocessing. This situation will undoubtedly become more complex with the advent of medical devices which have been surface-modified to achieve enhanced biocompatibility (Hayward & Chapman, 1984).

3 Extent of the practice

The extent of reuse varies from country to country, hospital to hospital and also varies within different hospital departments. In 1994, Collignon *et al.* sent questionnaires to all hospitals in Australia with more than 45 beds where medical or surgical procedures were carried out. The questionnaire requested information about their reuse policies, the types of equipment they reused and details of the cleaning and sterilization protocols. The information requested related only to 'single-use' devices which were used in sterile sites. Forty per cent of hospitals replied and, of those, 38% reused medical devices in sterile sites (58% were carrying out the practice of reuse or had been in the previous 12 months). The figure for reuse increased to 64% in large (> 300-bed) hospitals, but the authors still believe that their study underestimates the extent of reuse in Australia. Over 40% of those reusing devices either had unsatisfactory cleaning/sterilization programmes or did not provide sufficient information (Collignon *et al.*, 1996).

Between 1978 and 1983, the cardiology department at Leiden University Hospital reused 214 pacemakers, or 16–30% of all annually implanted ones (van Hemel, 1993). Of these devices, 80% were functioning normally after a mean follow-up time of 31.5 months, even in those cases where the device had been reused more than once. In Canada, 41% of hospitals regularly reused disposable medical devices (123 surveyed). The rate for hospitals with over 200 beds was 86%, but only 38% had written procedures governing practice (Campbell *et al.*, 1987). In the USA, 82% of hospitals reported that they reused disposables, with 31% reusing cardiac catheters, while 39% of Canadian hospitals-reuse cardiac catheters (Jacob *et al.*, 1994). In 1990, 70% of dialysis units in the USA were reusing dialysers and 75% of patients were in units reusing dialysers. In Japan, the practice of reuse is not permitted, while in 1988 the European Dialysis and Transplant Association reported 10% of patients on haemodialysis being treated with reprocessed dialysers (Held *et al.*, 1994).

4 Specific examples

The subject of reuse is made more complex by the wide range of medical devices available, each of which forms an individual area of discussion, because of its unique structure and application. It is beyond the scope of this chapter to detail all types of devices, and discussion will be limited to two specific examples. Both of these devices are the subject of widespread reuse in different countries, but they highlight different aspects of the problem.

4.1 Balloon catheters for coronary angioplasty

Coronary angioplasty is an important procedure, but one which is expensive to perform. It has been estimated that 800 000 procedures are performed worldwide each year (Plante *et al.*, 1994), and in the USA the average cost per procedure was reported to be $16 000 in 1994, with equipment costs accounting for 15–20% of the total cost (Mak *et al.*, 1996). Not surprisingly, this has been targeted as an area for cost containment by many hospitals, and cardiac catheters, including angioplasty balloon catheters, are the most reused items, after haemodialysis membranes (Bourassa, 1994). Studies in Canada have indicated that, if a reuse policy were implemented, an average of three uses for each angioplasty catheter would result in savings of $100 000 per 100 procedures. However, opinion is divided on the issue of safety of reprocessed catheters. Frank *et al.* (1988) conducted a prospective study, in which 414 patients underwent cardiac catheterization or angiography with either multiple-use or single-use disposable catheters. Using evidence of fever as the sole indicator, the authors concluded that there was no increased risk of infection in patients treated with reused catheters. Plante *et al.* (1994) carried out a prospective study of 693 patients in two centres, one which had a policy of single use only for balloon catheters and the other which reused their catheters many times. The results showed that the success rates were the same at both centres, but the reuse centre had a higher incidence of balloon failure and used more catheters per procedure. This resulted in an increased volume of contrast medium used and longer procedure times.

The risk of equipment breakage is of concern with both new and reprocessed angioplasty equipment and may include catheter breakage, balloon rupture and risk of particulate body contamination (Mak *et al.*, 1996). *In vitro* reports have suggested that repeated use of diagnostic catheters does not itself lead to increased risk of breakage, but their mechanical properties do deteriorate with age. However, balloon rupture occurs at a lower inflation pressure in reused catheters, due to a weakening of the material from which they are constructed (Mak *et al.*, 1996). Such evidence supports the results reported by Plante *et al.* (1994), but is at variance with Rozenman & Gotsman (1995), who reported that angioplasty procedures performed in Israel routinely employ reused catheters and their experience suggests that the number of catheters used per procedure was the same, regardless of whether the catheters were new or used.

The study by Plante *et al.* (1994) also reported a higher rate of adverse clinical events in the reuse centre, particularly in patients with unstable angina. Cost savings resulted from the reuse policy, but these may be offset by the increased costs associated with, among other things, the adverse clinical events. In contrast, the Conseil d'Évaluation des Technologies de la Santé du Québec commissioned a report in 1993 on the reuse of cardiac catheters and concluded that they may be reused without putting patients at increased risk, provided effective cleaning, sterilization and quality-control procedures were adhered to (Jacob & Bentolila, 1994). The report does carry some notes of caution, however, highlighting the fact that EO sterilization may be unsuccessful if the lumen is obstructed with dried blood and also that biological material was found adhering to the inner lumen of the catheters, even when they had been cleaned according to a predetermined protocol. The surface of the lumen of the catheter may also become more irregular with repeated use, due to the passage of guide wires along its length. The consequences of this are not reported but may have an influence on haemocompatibility.

4.2 Haemodialysis membranes

Haemodialysers are not expensive items, like balloon-angioplasty catheters, but they represent a significant medical cost because of the relatively large numbers used. A patient on haemodialysis will need dialysing, on average, three times each week, until the opportunity for transplantation arises. A recent cost analysis carried out in Canada has suggested that adoption of a reuse policy, with each dialyser being used five times, would result in savings of between $5.8 and $8.9 million/year (Baris & McGregor, 1993).

The practice of cleaning and disinfecting dialysers for reuse on the same patient is carried out extensively in the USA where over 70% of patients are being treated with reused equipment. In Western Europe, however, most countries do not reuse dialysers extensively (in Britain, the figure is estimated to be about 16%). In 1989, the figure reported for haemodialysis reuse in Canada was 12%, with the practice mainly concentrated in Quebec (Baris & McGregor, 1993). Discussion on the topic of reuse of haemodialysers is, therefore, particularly heated in the USA with opinions clearly divided. Despite the availability of an extensive literature, the situation is confused, because the earlier data which were published, and are still widely quoted, are now less relevant, due to changes in reuse procedures. The available evidence concerning the efficiency of reprocessed dialysers is ambiguous and many authors suggest that haemodialyses can be reprocessed on a number of occasions and still function correctly. However, Sherman *et al.* (1994) examined the effects of dialyser reuse in a 34-centre study and found that reprocessing did significantly impair dialysis delivery. Nevertheless, with the advent of clearly laid down performance criteria, which are well established, each dialyser should be carefully inspected and tested prior to being used. Automatic reconditioning machines mean that this process should now be even more reliable.

Reprocessing of used dialysers involves cleaning, followed by disinfection with glutaraldehyde, formaldehyde or a peracetic acid–hydrogen peroxide–acetic acid mixture. The process of disinfection would appear to be satisfactory, provided there is strict adherence to accepted protocols, and it is very unusual for patients to become infected when using a reprocessed dialyser (Flaherty *et al.*, 1993). More common are pyrogenic reactions, which, in some cases, have been traced to contaminated water used to prepare the disinfection solutions. During dialysis, patients may experience fever, shivering, nausea, myalgia and hypotension, which are characteristic endotoxin reactions (Baris & McGregor, 1993). It has been suggested that these pyrogenic reactions result from a triggering and release of proinflammatory cytokines by the endotoxin trapped on the dialyser after the reprocessing cycle. This effect has been studied by Pereira *et al.* (1995), using an *in vitro* dialysis system. They found that exposure to reprocessed dialysers did not result in enhanced release of proinflammatory cytokines; indeed, the data suggested that reprocessed dialysers probably induced less cytokine production than new cellulose dialysers. However, Ng *et al.* (1996) used scanning electron microscopy and cytological staining to examine the interaction between blood components and reprocessed synthetic dialyser membranes after formaldehyde treatment. It was shown that various blood components, such as fibrin and blood cells, remained adhering to the membrane after processing and that these could later become detached and gain access to the circulation. The authors argue that this may lead to adverse reactions, such as immunohaemolytic anaemia, due to anti-N-form antibody.

Information comparing death rates of patients on reuse compared with single-use treatment programmes presents a confusing picture, due to the number of variables being investigated. Not only are there three possible types of disinfection programmes, but there are also some treatments which are carried out manually and some which are automated. A recent paper by Held *et al.* (1994) showed that death rates were higher in reuse patients whose dialysers had been disinfected with glutaraldehyde or the peracetic acid–hydrogen peroxide–acetic acid mixture compared with single-use patients. However, death rates in those patients whose dialysers had been reprocessed using formaldehyde were not significantly different from control (single-use). This has led to the regulatory authorities in the USA taking the view that the problem is one of disinfectant type and not reuse itself. Taken overall, however, the data show that the reuse group had a death rate which was significantly higher than in the single-use group. Information such as this has caused one of the pioneers of reuse policy to change his mind and advocate for abandonment of the reprocessing of haemodialysers (Shaldon, 1993a,b).

5 Issues for debate

5.1 Economic/environmental issues

While it is undoubtedly true that the disposal of large amounts of plastic hardware is increasingly becoming an environmental issue and has been cited as an argument for a reuse strategy, the overriding reason for reusing disposable equipment is economy. There is no doubt that, in some countries, if reuse were banned, the additional financial burden on the health systems would create significant problems, and it is probably for this reason that few countries have actually prohibited the practice. In the event of a ban on reuse, either additional resources would need to be provided or funding would have to be diverted from other areas of health care, to allow for the purchase of new devices. This would inevitably lead to a reduction in patient services in some areas.

However, the converse to this argument is that, when calculating the cost of reprocessing equipment compared with buying new, realistic account must be taken of capital expenditure, training costs, materials, labour and record keeping. If hospitals were made to adopt full GMP and QA procedures, with attendant documentation, the additional costs could make reprocessing uneconomic. Daschner (1989) has undertaken a thorough cost–benefit analysis in nosocomial infection control and, in dealing with the issue of reuse, has suggested that much more use be made of reusable devices rather than disposables. Although initially more expensive to purchase, their use is more cost-effective in the long term.

5.2 Ethical issues

In any health-care system where resources are limited and, as a consequence, there is a potential for patients to be denied services, any waste of resources is unjustified. It has, therefore, been argued that it is not unethical to reuse single-use devices, provided it can be established that the performance characteristics of the device are unimpaired and that the patient is at no increased risk compared with the use of a new device.

In most instances, any used devices are recycled for reuse by the same hospital department. However, there is also the necessity to help needy patients in developing countries, who cannot afford many of the more expensive devices commonly found in Western hospitals. For these patients, the use of a reprocessed device is preferable to no device at all (Manders, 1987; Agrawal, 1993).

At the start of this chapter, it was suggested that reuse of single-use items on a same-patient basis may be justified under some circumstances. Indeed, this practice can have some benefits, as some reports have shown haemodialysis filters to have improved properties after recycling. Problems arise when a new device is used on one patient and then reused on a second patient after recycling. A number of questions can then arise.

- Who makes the decision as to which patient receives the new and which the recycled device?
- Is the patient asked his/her opinion or allowed to choose? In Sweden, patient consent is required before a reprocessed medical device is used. This subject has particular relevance in those countries operating private health-care systems, where patients or their insurance companies will be charged for the materials used.
- How do you cost a reused device? Is it the same as a new device or does the cost reduce the more times it is recycled? In the latter case, this would clearly imply that the reused product was inferior.
- How many times will the item be recycled before being discarded and who makes that decision?

Another factor that has emerged recently is one of ownership. If a medical device is implanted in a patient, who, at a later date, dies, can the device be removed and used for another patient? Does the hospital own the implant or does it belong to the patient? In the Netherlands, for example, the law quite clearly states that an implant is the property of the patient and, after death, forms part of the estate of that person, so that it cannot be removed without express permission of the next of kin. A similar situation exists in the USA where the patient or some agency acting on his/her behalf has purchased the device from the hospital, but in other countries, where the state has provided the device, the position is less clear (Silver, 1992).

5.3 Legal/regulatory issues

It has been argued that manufacturers label items 'for single use only' simply to maintain profits. However, if they are to accept liability for the performance of their product, they must be satisfied with all the procedures to which it has been subjected prior to its use. By stating on a label that a product is to be used on a single occasion only, the manufacturer is stating either that the product will not stand repeated processing and still remain fully functional, that not enough information is available to make such a judgement or that they will not take responsibility for any procedures which may be carried out on the product which are outside their control. Hence, if a hospital chooses to ignore this advice and reprocess that device, any manufacturer's warranties on that product are likely to be voided and their liabilities and obligations will cease or be limited. In the event of a reused device causing damage or injury, the hospital concerned will probably become liable. The reprocessor does, of course, have a legal responsibility for reprocessing, irrespective of whether the device is labelled 'for single use only'. However, in the case of single-use items, the manufacturer is specifically recommending that the device not be reprocessed.

The MDA states that, under these circumstances, the reprocessor would be 'exposed to civil liability to pay damages for any injury caused to another person by the device, either on the basis of negligence or under the strict product liability provisions of Part I of the Consumer Protection Act 1987, if the product is found to be defective'. In addition, the hospital could be 'committing a criminal offence under the Health and Safety at Work Act 1974 by contravening the provisions relating to general duties by carrying out activities which expose patients or staff to risk'.

If a label stating that a product was 'for single use only' were not present, it would be incumbent on the manufacturer to state on how many occasions the device might be reprocessed and to lay down clear guidelines on the methods for cleaning, packaging, sterilization and quality control. This would then make them liable in law, should an adverse event occur, even though the reuse procedures were not in their control. It is not surprising, therefore, that the medical-device industry is united in its opposition to the practice of reuse.

From these arguments, it can be seen that regulatory authorities in all countries find themselves in a dilemma. On the one hand, they cannot outwardly support a reuse strategy, because of the legal implications; however, the banning of such a widespread practice could have severe implications for the financing of health care and on the supply of patient services. In Europe, only Italy and Spain have legislation preventing the reuse of single-use devices, while, in the UK and France, this merely takes the form of recommendations. The German authorities have attempted to cope with the problem by publishing standards, with which hospitals would find it difficult to comply (Eucomed, 1995).

The US Food and Drug Administration (FDA) has stated that there is insufficient evidence to support the general reuse of single-use devices, although it does not go so far as to prohibit the practice altogether. It maintains that any institution which reuses a disposable device must be able to demonstrate that it can be adequately cleaned and sterilized, that its physical characteristics or quality will not be adversely affected by these processes and that the device remains safe and effective for use. The FDA also believes that the institution or practitioner must accept full liability for the functioning of the reused device and be responsible for any adverse events which may occur (Jacob & Bentolila, 1994). Various health departments in Australia have made recommendations against reuse but, conscious of the fact that it is practised in hospitals, have put forward guidelines similar to those of the FDA (Collignon *et al.*, 1996).

6 Conclusion

It is evident from the foregoing that there has been much debate in the USA, Canada and Australia on the subject of reuse of disposable equipment, among both health professionals and the general public. However, the situation in Europe is much less clear and, while it would seem that reuse is not as prevalent, there is little quantitative information available in the literature. The MDA in the UK is aware that reuse is occurring in hospitals, but has no real idea of the magnitude of the practice. It is vital that hospital managers are aware of what is going on in their institution and that decisions on reuse are shared within a medical-devices group, which can formulate and monitor the processes used. This group may include clinicians, infection-control staff, reprocessing staff, supplies officer, pharmacists and a risk manager, if available. The problem, even with this scenario, is that individual hospitals are making decisions on reuse policy and deciding for themselves on the protocols necessary for cleaning, testing, repackaging and sterilization, together with decisions on number of recycles, etc.

A prerequisite to solving this problem would therefore be to generate quantitative data on the extent of reuse of single-use devices in hospitals in the UK and Europe, together with qualitative information on the protocols being used for cleaning, performance testing and sterilization. Opponents of reuse strategy advocate the setting of standards requiring absolute proof of safety before use. However, it is pointed out by Woollard (1996) that only a minority of the procedures used in medicine have been fully validated, and he argues that the most appropriate approach might be for all doctors involved in reuse of single-use items to be themselves responsible for ensuring that their activities comply as far as practicable with current guidelines. Given the legal complexities associated with reuse and the potential litigation a hospital will face in the case of an adverse event, this scenario seems somewhat simplistic. The prospect of the regulatory authorities officially sanctioning a reuse strategy is unlikely; however, if the practice is not prohibited, then some hospitals will be prepared to take the risk of litigation in order to cut costs and meet patient demands. Under these circumstances, consultation is necessary between the regulatory authorities, the hospitals and the medical-device industry to ensure that uniform protocols, which have undergone full validation, can be laid down for the reprocessing of specific devices.

The European medical devices industry has put forward a set of guidelines for any organization wishing to reuse single-use devices.

- The procedures used for the reprocessing of the device must be fully validated to ensure a safe and effective product.
- The properties of the materials should remain unchanged and the performance be unaffected by the processing.
- The number of times a device may safely be reused must be determined and records kept to ensure that this number is not exceeded.
- Appropriate records must be made relating to the reprocessing and these must be kept safely.

The records which must be maintained by the institution would include the following.

- Identification of all reprocessed items, including manufacturers, batch numbers and reprocessing batch numbers.
- Information detailing all the steps involved in the reprocessing.
- Identification of all the personnel involved in the reprocessing, including details of their specific training for the task.
- Records of the number of times an item has been reused, together with details of its reuse history.
- Verification that testing has been conducted to ensure that the performance of the device meets the manufacturers, performance criteria (Eucomed, 1995).

Any hospital that wishes to reuse single-use devices could then register as a reprocessing centre and would need to adhere to these overall protocols, together with the specific reprocessing protocols, and to ensure that adequate records are kept. That hospital would also have to accept liability for the performance of the device.

7 References

Agrawal, K. (1993) The reuse of tissue expanders in developing countries. *Plastic and Reconstructive Surgery*, **92**, 372–373.

Baris, E. & McGregor, M. (1993) The reuse of hemodialyzers—an assessment of safety and potential savings. *Canadian Medical Association Journal*, **148**, 175–183.

Bell, M.D.D. & Morgan, P.W. (1993) Critical incident due to inappropriate resterilization. *Anaesthesia*, **49**, 269.

Bourassa, M.G. (1994) Is reuse of coronary angioplasty catheters safe and effective? *Journal of the American College of Cardiology*, **24**, 1482–1483.

Campbell, B.A., Wells, G.A., Palmer, W.N. & Martin, D.L. (1987) Reuse of disposable medical devices in Canadian hospitals. *American Journal of Infection Control*, **15**, 196–200.

Collignon, P.J., Graham, E. & Dreimanis, D.E. (1996) Reuse in sterile sites of single-use medical devices: how common is this in Australia? *Medical Journal of Australia*, **164**, 533–536.

Daschner, F. (1989) Cost-effectiveness in hospital infection control—lessons for the 1990s. *Journal of Hospital Infection*, **13**, 325–336.

DesCoteaux, J.G., Poulin, E.C., Lortie, M., Murray, G. & Gingras, S. (1995) Reuse of disposable laparoscopic instruments: a study of related surgical complications. *Canadian Journal of Surgery*, **38**, 497–500.

DesCoteaux, J.G., Tye, L. & Poulin, E.C. (1996) Reuse of disposable laparoscopic instruments—cost analysis. *Canadian Journal of Surgery*, **39**, 133–139.

Eucomed (1995) The case against the reuse of single use medical devices. Position Document. Brussels: European Commission of Medical Devices Association.

Flaherty, J.P., Garcia-Houchins, S., Chudry, R. & Arnow, P.M. (1993) An outbreak of Gram negative bacteremia traced to contaminated O-rings in reprocessed dialyzers. *Annals of Internal Medicine*, **119**, 1072–1078.

Frank, U., Herz, L. & Daschner, F.D. (1988) Infection risk of cardiac catheterisation and arterial angiography with single and multiple use disposable catheters. *Clinical Cardiology*, **11**, 785–787.

Greene, V.W. (1986) Reuse of disposable medical devices—historical and current aspects. *Infection Control and Hospital Epidemiology*, **7**, 508–513.

Greene, V.W. (1995) Disinfection and sterilization of disposable devices/equipment. In *Chemical Germicides in Health Care* (ed. Rutala, W.A.). Washington,

USA: Association for Professionals in Infection Control and Epidemiology.

Hayward, J.A. and Chapman, D. (1984) Biomembrane surfaces as models for polymer design: the potential for haemocompatibility. *Biomaterials*, **5**, 135–142.

Held, P.J., Wolfe, R.A., Gatlin, D.S., Port, F.K., Levin, N.W. & Turenne, M.N. (1994) Analysis of the association of dialyzer reuse practices and patient outcomes. *American Journal of Kidney Diseases*, **23**, 692–708.

Jacob, R., Bentolila, P., Leroux, T. *et al.* (1994) The reuse of single-use cardiac catheters: safety, economical, ethical and legal issues. *Canadian Journal of Cardiology*, **10**, 413–421.

Jayabalan, M. (1995) Sterilization and reprocessing of materials and medical devices—reusability. *Journal of Biomaterials Applications*, **10**, 97–112.

Kozarek, R.A. (1995) Reuse of disposable equipment—one medical center's approach to the problem. *Gastrointestinal Endoscopy*, **41**, 323.

Mak, K.-H., Eisenberg, M.J., Eccleston, D.S., Cornhill, J.F. & Topol, E.J. 1996 Reuse of coronary angioplasty equipment: technical and clinical issues. *American Heart Journal*, **131**, 624–630.

Manders, E.K. (1987) Used tissue expanders for developing countries: you can help. *Plastic and Reconstructive Surgery*, **80**, 643.

Medical Devices Agency (1995) *The reuse of Medical Devices Supplied for Single-use Only*. Device Bulletin 9501. London: Department of Health.

Ng. Y.Y., Yang, A.H., Wong, K.C. *et al.* (1996) Dialyser reuse—interaction between dialyser membrane, disinfection (formalin), and blood during dialyser reprocessing. *Artificial Organs*, **20**, 53–55.

Parker, A., Kadakia, S.C., Howell, G. & Peserski, J. (1996) Reuse of single-use supplies—the pendulum swings. *Gastrointestinal Endoscopy*, **43**, 319.

Pereira, B.J.G., Snodgrass, B., Barber, G., Perella, C., Chopra, S. & King, A.J. (1995) Cytokine production during *in vitro* hemodialysis with new and formaldehyde-reprocessed or Renalin-reprocessed cellulose dialysers. *Journal of the American Society of Nephrology*, **6**, 1304–1308.

Plante, S., Strauss, B.H., Goulet, G., Watson, R.K. & Chisholm, R.J. (1994) Reuse of balloon catheters for coronary angioplasty—a potential cost-saving strategy. *Journal of the American College of Cardiology*, **24**, 1475–1481.

Rozenman, Y. & Gotsman, M.S. (1995) Reuse of balloon catheters for coronary angioplasty. *Journal of the American College of Cardiology*, **26**, 840.

Shaldon, S. (1993a) Dialyzer reuse—a practice that should be abandoned. *Seminars in Dialysis*, **6**, 11–12.

Shaldon, S. (1993b) Dialyzer reuse—the time has come to stop this practice. *Dialysis and Transplantation*, **22**, 122.

Sherman, R.A., Cody, R.P., Rogers, M.E. & Solanchick, J.C. (1994) The effect of dialyser reuse on dialysis delivery. *American Journal of Kidney Disease*, **24**, 924–926.

Silver, M.D. (1992) Reuse of cardiac pacemakers. *Canadian Journal of Cardiology*, **8**, 1046.

van Hemel, N.M. (1993) The reuse of implantable devices—opinion and practice in the Netherlands. *Canadian Journal of Cardiology*, **9**, 186–187.

Woollard, K. (1996) Reuse of single-use medical devices: who makes the decision? *Medical Journal of Australia*, **164**, 538.

CHAPTER 25

Sterility Assurance: Concepts, Methods and Problems

1 Introduction

Preceding chapters have described in some detail the sterilizing processes and equipment used by industrial manufacturers and hospitals to produce a sterile product. This final chapter considers the effectiveness of those processes and the assurance that may be invested in them.

2 Sterility—a question of semantics

Before discussing the wider issues relating to the concept and practice of sterility assurance, it is necessary to clarify the meaning of some well-known terms. The term sterility is an absolute one, defined in a medical and pharmaceutical sense as the absence of all viable microorganisms. This definition is clear-cut and uncompromising; degrees of sterility do not exist. Sterilization is the process by which sterility is achieved and, in effect, entails the destruction, inactivation or removal of all viable microorganisms, including vegetative and sporing bacteria, fungi (yeasts and moulds), protozoa and viruses. In practice, this is achieved by exposure of the product to a microbicidal agent for a predefined period of time, using physical or chemical methods, individually or in combination. The agents include elevated temperature, ionizing radiation and chemicals in a gaseous state (see Chapters 19A–D, 20A and 21). An alternative method for sterilizing certain liquids and gases utilizes filtration through a microbial-proof filter (Chapter 22). Thus, the purpose of any sterilizing treatment is to render a preparation, material or object completely free of any viable microorganism.

However, while the death of a microorganism can be defined as 'the failure to grow and be detected in culture media previously known to support its growth', demonstration of the 'complete freedom of any viable microorganism' in such a product cannot be proved in practice. Detection of growth involves the production of turbidity in liquid culture media or the presence of colonial surface growth on solid culture media. Such manifestations of microbial life represent many generations of cells which have originated from an individual cell. In practice, we cannot hope to provide the specialized cultural conditions required for the growth of all living cells.

In addition, any cells surviving a potentially lethal treatment may carry so-called sublethal injuries, characterized by a loss of selective permeability of the cell membrane, leakage of intracellular components into the surrounding medium, degradation of ribosomes and ribonucleic acid and decreased enzyme activity. Such damaged cells may require specialized recovery conditions for the repair of these injuries; failure to provide these may result in failure to detect these stressed cells (Busta, 1978). However, should their specialized metabolic requirements be met in the future, these cells may repair the damage and subsequently grow. Thus, on the question of semantics, the term 'freedom from demonstrable forms of life' has been favoured in some quarters as an alternative to the widely accepted definition of sterility as the 'complete freedom from any viable microorganisms'.

3 Mathematical approach to sterility

In recent years, the concept of 'sterility assurance', i.e. assurance that the preparation, material or object which has been subjected to a sterilizing process is indeed sterile, has come to replace our traditional way of viewing sterility. This in turn has originated from the mathematical concept that death of the microbial cell is a probability function, based upon the length of exposure to the lethal agent. The number of organisms decreases exponentially with the time of exposure, to a first approximation. By the same token, however, only by infinite exposure to the lethal agent can absence of all viable organisms be assured with certainty. At the same time, it is acknowledged that indefinite exposure to the lethal agent is likely to have a deleterious effect on end-product quality. In essence, therefore, a compromise must be struck between assuring the sterility of the final product and ensuring that the therapeutic efficacy and acceptability of the product remain unchanged. Thus, the required sterility assurance level (SAL) is derived from what is considered to constitute the maximum acceptable risk, based on the intended use of the product.

This appreciation of the kinetics of microbial inactivation has in turn led to working definitions of the term 'sterile' in the manufacturing industries. In the pharmaceutical and medical-device industries, the definition has been based on a SAL equal to or better than 10^{-6}. In other words, the probability post-sterilization of a non-sterile article is less than or equal to one in one million units processed. The Federation of Industrial Pharmacists (Anon., 1989) has published guidelines on how to achieve the recommended level of sterility assurance. Similarly, current editions of the *British Pharmacopoeia* (BP, 1998), *European Pharmacopoeia* (EP, 1997) and *United States Pharmacopoeia* (USP, 1995) all make reference to this established microbiological definition of sterility assurance. Likewise, the European Standard EN556 (Anon., 1994) specifies that, for terminally sterilized medical devices labelled 'sterile', the SAL should be 10^{-6} or better. This, however, does not infer that one in one million products is allowed to be non-sterile.

A less stringent SAL of 10^{-3} may, however, be acceptable in certain circumstances, owing to the nature of the product or the way in which it is to be used. This is the case for aseptically made preparations, where a heat-sterilization process is inappropriate, owing to the nature of the material. Also, for certain medical devices which only come into contact with intact skin or mucous membranes, this less rigorous standard may be acceptable, as is the case for the regulatory authorities in North America.

4 Factors affecting sterility assurance

A population of organisms exposed to a lethal agent will not die simultaneously. It will exhibit varying sensitivities to the sterilizing agent. As can be seen from Fig. 25.1, some microorganisms are

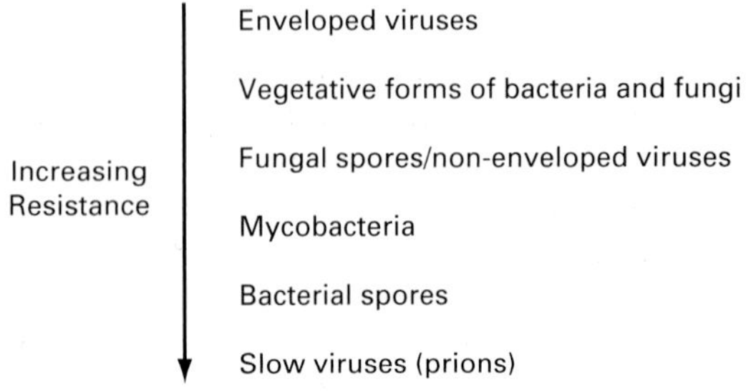

Fig. 25.1 Relative susceptibilities of microorganisms to sterilization processes.

known to be more susceptible to sterilization processes than others, progressing from the more susceptible large viruses, to vegetative forms of bacteria and fungi, to fungal spores and small viruses, to bacterial spores used as reference organisms to determine the efficiency of sterilization processes, and finally to the 'slow' viruses (prions), which have in recent years posed a serious challenge to accepted sterilization processes (see Chapter 7).

The natural bioburden of any pharmaceutical product or medical device undergoing sterilization is likely to be composed of a mixed microbial flora, with varying sensitivities or, conversely, intrinsic resistance to the sterilizing process. On the other hand, laboratory sterilization experiments involving the determination of survivor curves are more likely to use stock cultures with well-characterized resistance patterns.

The initial bioburden of a material prior to sterilization will have a profound effect on the resulting sterility assurance level. Clearly, the higher the bioburden, the greater the challenge to the sterilizing process and, by the same token, the greater the probability of finding microbial survivors. Besides the size of the microbial challenge, there are other factors to be considered: the condition of those cells (age, growth phase and any sublethal injuries); their accessibility to the sterilizing agent, since the presence of any organic matter may act as a buffer and provide physical protection; and the emergence of phenotypically determined resistance mechanisms, resulting from growth under nutrient limitation and, in turn, causing modified cell characteristics.

Sterilization processes differ in their effectiveness in destroying or inactivating microbial challenges. The precise mechanism of action varies with the challenge organism and the target sensitivity, as detailed in Table 25.1.

5 Sterility assurance in practice

The traditional approach to sterility assurance has been based on the time-honoured sterility test, whereby a direct assessment was made of the microbiological status of the article or product in question. A representative sample of the batch purporting to be sterile was selected and either inoculated into a suitable culture medium or passed through a membrane filter and then inoculated into an appropriate culture medium. Following incubation, the culture media were examined for evidence of microbial growth and, based on the

Table 25.1 Mechanisms of inactivation of microorganisms.

Agent*	Destructive event
Elevated temperature	Destruction of essential constituents, including enzymes
Moist heat	Denaturation and hydrolysis reactions
Dry heat	Principally oxidative changes
Ionizing radiation	DNA main target resulting from ionization and free-radical production γ-rays, high-speed electrons
UV radiation	Photoproducts in DNA
Chemicals	Alkylation or other covalent reactions with sulphydryl, amino, hydroxyl and carboxyl group of proteins and imino groups of nucleic acids. Interactions between chemical agent and key structural components may result in loss of structural integrity

*See also Chapters 19A, 19B and 19D (elevated temperatures), 20A (ionizing radiation), 20B (ultraviolet radiation) and 9 (chemical agents).
DNA, deoxyribonucleic acid; UV, ultraviolet.

absence or presence of this visual inspection, the sample passed or failed the test, respectively.

These methods continue to be used today for both terminally sterilized and aseptically made products, there being no alternative test in the case of the latter. However, in terms of status, it must be emphasized that nowadays the sterility test, as applied to the finished product, should only be regarded as the last in a series of control measures by which sterility is assured. Thus, compliance with the test for sterility alone does not constitute absolute assurance of freedom from microbial contamination. Reliable manufacturing procedures provide a greater assurance of sterility.

However, owing to the severe limitations of the sterility test, discussed below, increasing emphasis has been placed in recent years on a different approach to sterility assurance. This has involved not only a detailed monitoring of the sterilization process itself but also using this information to make indirect inferences about the microbiological status of the product, based upon the treatment to which it has been exposed. Both approaches are discussed in detail below.

6 Sterility testing

While the concept of performing a sterility test is simple and straightforward, both in practice and in theory it is fraught with difficulty; furthermore, it presents not only a technical but also a mathematical challenge.

From a technical point of view, the test must be performed under suitable conditions, designed to minimize the risk of accidental microbial contamination. In practice, this involves a suitably qualified, carefully trained and appropriately clad operator (i.e. wearing sterile, clean-room clothing) carrying out the test in a properly maintained laminar-flow cabinet. Dedicated facilities for sterility testing, often of an equivalent environmental standard to that used for preparing the product, have now replaced the traditional method of open-bench testing, previously commonplace in hospital microbiology laboratories. Specialized, approved contract or government laboratories may be used, if suitable facilities are unavailable on site.

Clearly, staff involved in this testing should have a high level of aseptic technique proficiency. This should be regularly monitored and recorded, using sterile broth-filling trials. The USP's Committee of Revision (Anon., 1995) has suggested that a false-positive rate not exceeding 0.5% is desirable. Records of routine failure rates for each operator should also be kept and, if warranted, an individual's requalification in sterility testing may be required.

While samples taken for sterility testing should be representative of the entire batch, it is accepted that the sampling should take particular account of those parts of the batch considered to be most at risk from contamination. Thus, for aseptically filled products, samples should include not only those containers filled at the beginning, middle and end of the batch, but also those filled after any significant interruption in the filling environment. Likewise, for heat-sterilized products in their final container, the sampling scheme should be skewed to account for those samples taken from the coolest part of the load, as determined during commissioning studies.

Detailed sampling instructions and testing procedures are given in the current pharmacopoeias (BP, 1998; USP 1995; EP, 1997). These form the basis of legal referee data in the event of litigation, legal validation or regulatory requirements. The test may be applied not only to parenteral and non-parenteral sterile products, but also to other articles that are required to be sterile.

As alluded to above, the mathematics of sampling pose a number of problems for those involved in sterility testing. As explained in detail below, the results are determined by both the number of samples taken and the incidence of contamination.

In mathematical terms, if n is the number of containers tested, p the proportion of contaminated containers and q the proportion of non-infected containers in a batch, then:

$$p + q = 1$$

From this it can be deduced that:
the probability of rejection $= 1 - (1 - p)^n$

The implications of this are shown in Table 25.2, where it can be seen that, with a constant sample size of 20 containers (the BP-recommended number of samples for a batch of 500 or more paren-

Table 25.2 Sampling in sterility testing.

	Infected items in batch (%)					
	0.1	1	5	10	20	50
p	0.001	0.01	0.05	0.1	0.2	0.5
q	0.999	0.99	0.95	0.9	0.8	0.5
Probability, P, of drawing 20 consecutive sterile items:						
First sterility test*	0.98	0.82	0.36	0.12	0.012	<0.00001
First retest†	0.99	0.99	0.84	0.58	0.11	0.002

*Calculated from $P = 1-p)^{20} = q^{20}$.
†Calculated from $P = (1-p)^{20}[2-(1-p)^{20}]$.
p, proportion of contaminated containers in batch; q, proportion of non-infected containers in batch.

teral preparations) and with varying proportions of the batch contaminated, the probability of drawing 20 consecutive sterile items is given. It can be seen that, with random sampling of the batch, very low levels of contamination cannot be detected with certainty by the test. Hence, if 10 items remained contaminated in a batch of 1000 units (i.e. $p = 0.01$), the probability of accepting the entire batch as sterile, based on a 20 unit sample size, would be $(1-0.01)^{20} = 0.99^{20} = 0.82$. Thus in 82 instances out of 100, all 20 random samples would give negative results and the entire batch would be passed as sterile, although the batch actually contained 10 defective units.

Clearly, the chance of detecting an individual contaminated unit in a batch increases both as the batch contamination rate rises and as the number of samples increases. All pharmacopoeias provide guidance on the number of samples to be tested, depending on the type of product, its intended use and the size of the batch. During its performance, the sterility test is prone to accidental contamination (through faulty aseptic technique or materials), and, again, all current pharmacopoeias make allowance for this by permitting a retest, if the first test is shown to be invalid. In this case, the probability of passing a defective batch on the basis of testing a further 20 samples actually increases, as can be seen from the same table, since a proportion of the contaminated samples have already been removed in the first test.

In mathematical terms, the probability of passing a defective batch at the first retest is:

$$(1-p)^n\,[2-(1-p)^n]$$

The USP (1995) currently requires double the number of samples to be used for the first repeat test, whereas the BP (1998) requires that, if the test is shown to be invalid, it is repeated with the same number of samples as the original test. It should be noted that no retests are permitted where the test has been carried out in an isolator (USP, 1995), although opinions are divided (Anon., 1996a).

A further complication may be introduced where the sample size itself has been reduced, as permitted in all current pharmacopoeias. The BP (1998), for example, states the minimum quantity to be tested per container, varying with the container size. Thus, for parenteral products of less than 1ml volume, the entire contents must be sampled, whereas, if the volume exceeds 1 ml, half the contents of a container but not more than 20 ml it is permitted to be taken as the minimum test volume. Clearly, such testing schemes will have a considerable effect on results where low levels of contamination are expected.

In recent years, there has been considerable progress in terms of harmonizing the individual pharmacopoeia sterility test methods. Current editions of the BP, EP and USP bear a close resemblance to one another in terms of their test requirements. Pharmacopoeial products are nowadays tested for sterility using a membrane-filtration technique (0.45 μm filter-pore size), any contaminating organisms being retained on the surface of the filter. If, however, this proves to be unsuitable, a direct inoculation technique may be used. Similarly, suitable test media are described for the growth of aerobic, anaerobic and fungal organisms. Before use, these must be tested not only for their sterility but also for their ability to support microbial growth, using specified test organisms. In addition, it must be shown that any antimicrobial activity inherent in the preparation under test has been neutralized sufficiently for it to support the growth of a small inoculum of named test organisms (approximately 100 colony-forming units (cfu)).

7 Process monitoring

Owing to the severe limitations of the sterility test, an alternative method of assuring sterility of sterilized products has been sought. The concept has therefore been developed, and has subsequently been widely accepted by the manufacturing industry, that sterility can indeed be assured by adopting an approach based upon process monitoring. In essence, this proposition rests upon the assumptions that if the sterilizing equipment is in proper working order, if the product has been subjected to a validated sterilizing treatment and if good manufacturing practices (GMP) prevail, then the batch will be sterile and can be approved for use.

It follows, therefore, that this approach is based upon three related components.

1 Equipment-function tests, proving proper mechanical operation of the sterilizer.

2 Exposure-verification tests, showing product exposure for the correct sterilizing cycle.

3 Process-validation practices, which indicate bioburden levels, verify the kinetics of microbial inactivation, justify the design of sterilizing treatments and ensure correct pre- and posthandling of the product.

This method of assuring sterility by monitoring only the physical conditions of the sterilization process is termed 'parametric release'. It has been defined as the release of sterile product based on process compliance to physical specification (Hoxey, 1989). It should be noted that, at this point in time, parametric release is acceptable for steam, dry heat and ionizing radiation sterilization processes, where the physical conditions are understood and can be monitored directly.

However, in the case of gaseous or liquid chemical sterilization, parametric release is at present unacceptable, since physical conditions cannot be readily or accurately measured. In these cases, it is a requirement that biological indicators (BIs) are used for each sterilizing cycle. These are removed after processing, incubated and observed for signs of growth, thereby indicating a sterilization failure.

Parametric release is inappropriate for filtration sterilization processes. There is always a probability, albeit remote, that a microorganism can pass through one of the few pores at the larger pore-size extreme of the pore-size distribution of the filter. Additionally, the absorption process in filtration involves a degree of probability of retention. Thus, sterile filtration must be regarded as a probability function and not as absolute. Moreover, filtration is a unit operation, wherein process validation is not practicable, unlike other sterilization methods. Thus, full aseptic precautions must be observed during processing, and a high SAL is dependent upon GMP and an initial low bioburden in the product. Stringent tests for sterility are also required.

7.1 Equipment-function tests

Regardless of the method of sterilization, proper design, construction, installation and operation of the sterilizer is fundamental to sterility assurance. Before being taken into routine use, correct functioning of the equipment must be shown, first by a process of installation qualification and then by a process of operation qualification. The prime responsibility for this task usually rests with the equipment manufacturer. Installation qualification involves the demonstration and certification it must be shown and certified that all parts of the sterilizer have been correctly installed, all measuring instruments have been correctly calibrated and all items of equipment comply with their performance specifications. During operation qualification, it must be demonstrated that, for any given load, the sterilizer performs reliably in at least three consecutive runs, and that sterilizing conditions are attained within every part of the load. Both mechanical operations and automatic cycling must perform as specified. It must also be shown that, within the load, the projected sterilizing conditions are achieved and that these conditions are compatible with the items to be sterilized. Permanent records, in the form of chart recordings or computer printouts, will provide evidence that lethal conditions have been generated in the load;

in the case of a failure, an automatic corrective course of action will be instituted.

Tests carried out during operation-qualification studies will vary according to the method of sterilization used. In the case of heat sterilizers, heat-distribution studies are undertaken, using thermocouples positioned at strategically determined places within the chamber and load. Such tests will need to be repeated if there is any change in routine operations, e.g. product type, shape or size of pack. In the case of irradiation, the penetration of the ionizing radiation within the load is best monitored by the use of an adequate number of dosimeters, again strategically distributed. Where gas sterilizer are used, temperature and relative humidity are measured by physical sensors within the chamber and load. As mentioned above, BIs must also be used to show that sterilizing conditions have been achieved throughout the load.

On the other hand, operation qualification of sterilizing filters is centred upon filter-integrity testing, pressure differentials and flow-rate measurements. Additionally, environmental control and its validation during the filtration process itself must be considered an integral part of the sterile filtration process (Wallhaeusser, 1988). In the USA, the use of a BI, *Pseudomonas diminuta*, is specified for use as a qualifying challenge to certify the proper design and installation of filtration-sterilization equipment (HIMA, 1982; USP, 1995). A minimum challenge of 10^7 cells/cm^2, with no passage into the effluent, is required.

7.2 Exposure-verification tests

Equipment-function tests, discussed above, prove that the sterilizer is performing as expected, thereby generating the required lethal conditions within the chamber. However, it must then be shown that these conditions within the chamber are simultaneously provided within the microenvironment surrounding any microbial contaminant, irrespective of the packaging materials used. Chemical indicators and BIs are widely used to verify this.

7.2.1 *Chemical indicators*

A range of chemical indicators may be used, depending on the method of sterilization employed. They all utilize the principle that, on exposure to heat, ethylene oxide or ionizing radiation, a change in the physical or chemical nature of the indicator is brought about, which can be detected by the naked eye or spectrophotometrically. All chemical indicators are limited in terms of their specificity and sensitivity. Their reliability, stability and safety must also be considered, when choosing which brand is best suited to the particular sterilization method employed. Furthermore, chemical indicators cannot be considered as a substitute for a microbial challenge. They should therefore be viewed as one of several complementary indicators of sterilizing conditions in the load.

Chemical indicators have different functions and these must be considered when making a choice.

1 Temperature-specific indicators show whether a particular temperature has been reached within a pack, but do not indicate the period of time involved. Thus, malfunctions of the sterilizer temperature-control instruments will be detected or perhaps loading or packaging errors will be identified.

2 Multiparameter process indicators are affected by the combined lethal effect of different components, such as heat and time of treatment or gas concentration and exposure time. When placed within a pack, they will provide confirmation that lethal conditions indeed existed within the microenvironment of any contaminants in that pack.

3 Throughput indicators, often in the form of autoclave tape, distinguish between those items which have or have not been subjected to a sterilizing cycle. Since these are applied to the external surface of the pack, they simply reflect existing conditions within the chamber environment and not within the pack itself.

4 Bowie–Dick test indicators are used to monitor the effective removal of air in autoclaves with a prevacuum cycle. The test is based upon an observed colour change in autoclave tape inserted in the centre of a test pack of cotton towels, following sterilization (Bowie *et al.*, 1963; Health Technical Memorandum, 1980; AAMI, 1988). They are required to be used in the first cycle of the day as an equipment-function test.

7.2.2 *Biological indicators*

Biological indicators are used extensively both to validate and to routinely monitor the lethality of a given sterilization process. By integrating all of the sterilization perameters involved, i.e. time, temperature, lethal potential of the sterilizing environment, packaging and loading configuration, these test pieces provide a direct measurement of their combined effect on a population of known bacteria, which has been specially selected for its high resistance to the given sterilization process. Since BIs are placed directly in the container, they will reflect the actual sterilizing conditions in the product itself, rather than just in the sterilizing environment in which the container has been placed. Moreover, since the microbial load on the BI is likely to present considerably more of a challenge, in terms of both numbers and resistance to the sterilization process, than is the expected bioburden of the product, then considerable confidence can be placed in the expected level of sterility assurance associated with the process.

Biological indicators are commercially available preparations containing known numbers of microorganisms deposited on a carrier, often in the form of metal foil, paper strips or discs, or alternatively they may consist of artificially inoculated units of the product. The microbial challenge usually comprises bacterial endospores of *Bacillus* and *Clostridium* spp., selected on the basis of their individual resistance to a given sterilization process. Biological indicators are therefore characterized by the strain of test organism, the number of cfu per test piece, the *D*-value (decimal reduction value), the *z*-value (relating the heat resistance of a microorganisms to changes in temperature in an autoclave or dry-heat sterilizer) and the expiry date. *D*- and *z*-values are presented in Chapters 19B and 19D.

Following exposure to the sterilization process, the BIs are cultured in suitable media and under appropriate recovery conditions, as specified by the manufacturer. If no growth occurs, the sterilization process is deemed to have the required lethality; in the event of growth occurring, this should be identified to establish whether it is derived from the original inoculum or whether it represents accidental contamination during handling or culturing.

A number of factors are known to affect the reliability of BIs. These include the basis of the genotypically determined resistance, environmental influences during growth and sporulation, the environment during storage, the influence of environment during sterilization and finally the influence of recovery conditions. A discussion of these factors is outside the scope of this chapter, but the reader is referred to Quesnel (1984).

Thus, as with all biological systems, because of their inherent variability BIs must be considered as less precise indicators of events than physical perameters. Hence, in the event of failure to comply with a physical specification, a sterilization cycle will be regarded as unsatisfactory, in spite of contrary evidence from the BI none the less supporting the lethality of the sterilizing process.

The test organisms vary with the sterilization process. The following represent the reference organisms listed in the current pharmacopoeias.

1 Steam sterilization: *Bacillus stearothermophilus* NCTC 10007 (ATCC 7953), as in the BP (1998).
2 Dry-heat sterilization: *Bacillus subtilis* var. *niger* NCTC 10073 (ATCC 9372), as in the BP (1998);
3 Ethylene oxide sterilization: *B. subtilis* var. *niger* NCTC 10073 (ATCC 9372), as in the BP (1998).
4 Ionizing-radiation sterilization: *Bacillus pumilus* NCTC 10327 (ATCC 27142), as in the BP (1998).

Further information on the use of BIs in sterilizers employed in the manufacture of sterile medical devices can be obtained from EN 866-1 (general requirements), EN 866-2 and EN 866-8 (ethylene oxide sterilization), EN 866-3 and EN 866-7 (moist heat sterilization), EN 866-4 (irradiation sterilization), EN 866-5 (low-temperature steam and formaldehyde (LTSF)), and EN 866-6 (dry heat sterilization), and also in the following International Organization for Standardization (ISO) publications: ISO 14161 and ISO 11138-1 (general guidance and requirements), ISO 11138-2 (ethylene oxide) and ISO 11138-3 (moist heat sterilization).

Of recent interest, Wright *et al.*, (1995, 1996) have investigated the availability and suitability of BIs for monitoring LTSF sterilization cycles. Currently, this method is used for disinfecting medical equipment and materials and has perceived potential applications for sterilization, particularly in the case of heat-labile items. However, as yet, the method has failed to find acceptance, since there are no acceptable physical or chemical methods of monitoring all the process parameters (temperature, relative humidity, formaldehyde (HCHO) concentration, its distribution and penetration. There is thus a convincing case for reliance on a BI to monitor the efficiency of LTSF sterilization cycles, should a suitable BI be found. Wright *et al.* (1996) reported on the suitability of spores of *B. stearothermophilus* NCIMB 8224 for use as a biological monitor for LTSF sterilization.

Depending on the sterilization process itself, BIs may be used for three purposes: cycle development, validation and monitoring of sterilization processes, as discussed below.

During cycle development, the ability of a given sterilization process to destroy a challenge from resistant contaminants must be assessed. These contaminants can originate from a number of sources, including raw materials, operators or the production environment itself. Once their resistance has been characterized, they can then be used as resistant microbiological reference standards. In effect, such reference organisms in turn become BIs and can be used to evaluate the required cycle to achieve the desired SAL.

The term 'validation' describes tests on a sterilizer and a given product to determine that the sterilization process operates efficiently and performs repeatedly as expected. Any validation exercise must therefore assess not only the physical performance of the sterilizer but also the biological performance of the process on the product. The term 'monitoring', on the other hand, implies the routine control of a process.

With regard to the use of BIs in practice, this depends not only upon the legal requirements of the country in question but also on the efficacy of alternative methods. In some instances, they represent the only practical method of monitoring sterilization cycles, whereas, in others, physical and chemical methods offer a much more reliable and efficient alternative.

Biological indicators are most commonly used in the validation and routine monitoring of ethylene oxide sterilization, owing to the inherent difficulties involved in reliably measuring physical parameters of sterilization, namely gas concentration, temperature and humidity, and because of the wide variety of sterilization cycles involved. The Department of Health (1990) stipulates that a minimum of 10 indicator pieces per cycle should be used for routine control in sterilizers with a capacity of up to 5000 l, with additional indicators being added for larger chambers. Each test piece should have at least 10^6 viable and potentially recoverable spores.

In some circumstances, BIs may be used as part of the validation programme for moist or dry heat sterilization cycles. However, they have little use in routine monitoring cycles, since the required SAL can be defined in terms of easily and reliably measured physical parameters. Occasionally, their use may be justified in performance qualification, when difficulties arise in ensuring adequate contact and penetration of steam in a particular product.

With regard to sterilization by irradiation, BIs are regarded to be of little value in the UK in a monitoring sense, since the process is defined in terms of a minimum absorbed dose of radiation, best and most reliably measured by dosimeters. In other countries, such as France, their use is obligatory for routine monitoring of irradiation sterilization in each batch. During validation work, they may, however, be used for initial characterization of inactivation rates within a given product.

8 Process-validation practices

As discussed previously, sterilization practices nowadays place much greater emphasis upon the concept of sterility assurance, rather than reliance on end-product testing. By understanding the kinetics of microbial inactivation, individual sterilization protocols can be designed to destroy a known and previously determined bioburden with a desired level of confidence in the procedure in question. In other words, by introducing the notion of required margin of safety, the probability of detecting a viable survivor of the sterilizing process can be assessed on a mathematical scale, known as the SAL. As a result, by investing confidence in process-validation practices, a system of parametric release can be used for approval of product.

In theory and in practice, a given microbial population exposed to a given sterilizing cycle has a characteristic response and the death curve follows a logarithmic pattern. This will depend upon the resistance of the organism concerned, the physicochemical environment where the treatment takes place and the lethality of the treatment itself. However, if these do not vary, the number of survivors in a known population can be computed after a given period of exposure to the lethal process. Microbial death can be measured in terms of the *D*-value, which is the time in minutes to reduce the microbial population by 90% or 1 log cycle at a certain temperature (or the dose in kGy when ionizing radiation is used).

As can be seen from Fig. 25.2, if the original population is 10^2 spores/g and if the *D*-value is 1min at 121°C, then after 1 min at 121°C the population will have been reduced to 10^1 spores/g. For each additional minute of exposure to the sterilizing cycle, a further reduction of 1 log cycle in the population will ensue. Thus, after an 8-min cycle at 121°C , the population will have been reduced by a total of 8 log cycles, i.e. from 10^2 to 10^{-6}. In other words, there is a one in a million chance that a viable spore exists in 1g of product. Clearly, this probability of contamination cannot

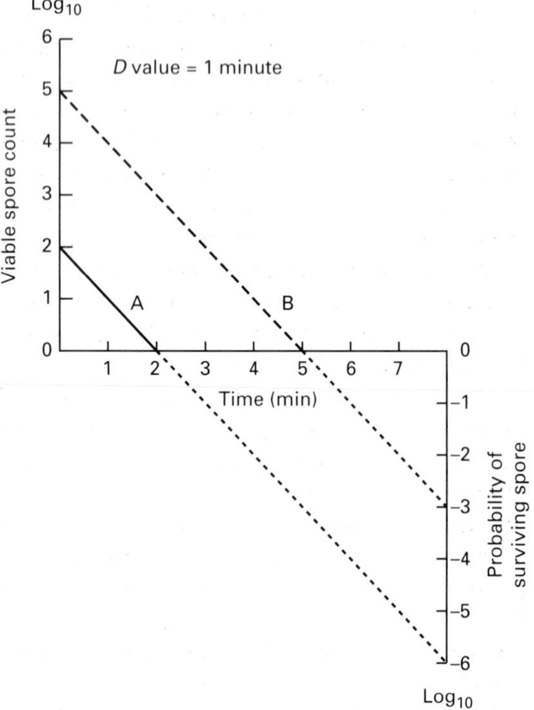

Fig. 25.2 Relationship between *D*-value, initial contamination level and level of sterility assurance.

be demonstrated in practice using end-product testing in the form of a sterility test.

The effect that the bioburden level has on the ensuing SAL of a given process can also be clearly seen from Fig. 25.2. If the original population is 10^5 spores/g, then the same 8-min cycle will result in a SAL of 10^{-3}. The importance of minimizing bioburden levels in any article ready for sterilization is therefore immediately obvious.

In essence, there are three components to process validation: selection and validation of the sterilizing cycle; monitoring of the cycle; and control of the complete process.

8.1 Selection and validation of the sterilizing cycle

In selecting an appropriate sterilizing cycle, account must be taken of the maximum likely bioburden, the *D*-value of the most resistant spore-former in the bioload and the required SAL. With regard to the presterilization bioburden, this requires quantitative evaluation over a period of time. Spore-formers isolated from the bioburden must then be cultured and *D*-values determined for the resulting spore suspensions under the proposed sterilizing conditions. Having decided on the SAL required for the product concerned, the manufacturer must then document fully the sterilizing protocol, including packaging and pre- and post-sterilization handling. Finally, pilot sterilization studies will then be performed, using actual and dummy products, with identical packaging to the process. These packs will previously have been artifically inoculated with either resistant spores from the natural bioburden or BIs, outnumbering the normal spore flora both in terms of inoculum size and *D*-values. Having successfully completed pilot studies, the manufacturer may reasonably assume that the required SAL will be achieved, so long as the process parameters remain unchanged. In this way, the sterilizing cycle is literally designed for the product concerned, balancing the likely bioburden challenge and the required SAL against any deleterious effect of the sterilizing process on the product itself.

In other instances, such an approach may not be practicable and manufacturers may need to adopt an overkill approach. Particularly in hospitals, sterilization cycles are designed in theory to inactivate considerably larger populations, although unlikely to occur in practice. Clearly, in such cases, the additional margin of safety must be balanced against the risk of potentially damaging effects on the product.

8.2 Monitoring the sterilizing cycle

Reproducibility of sterilizing conditions is essential if sterility is to be assured with the required margin of safety. In practice this means that all monitoring equipment, as well as chemical indicators and BIs, must show that the correct sterilizing conditions are being achieved within the microenvironment of the product itself. Additionally, microbiological monitoring of the bioburden challenge and its resistance should be shown not to differ significantly from those of the validation studies. Moreover, the packaging and loading of containers should remain unchanged.

8.3 Control of the complete process

Regardless of the actual treatment involved, no sterilization process can be considered in isolation but must be viewed in the context of GMP (Anon., 1992, 1996b). A discussion of these requirements is outside the scope of this chapter, but essentially it is based on a well-developed system of documentation and record-keeping. Thus, all records associated with the sterilization process itself must be retained for reference purposes, including autoclave planned preventive maintenance (PPM) and breakdown records, temperature, recording charts, chemical and biological indicator readings and experimental data on bioburdens and *D*-values, as well as protocols and their validation. Both medicines inspectors and Food and Drug Administration (FDA) inspectors would expect to scrutinize all such data.

The Health Technical Memorandum on sterilization, known as HTM 2010 (1995), provides advice and guidance not only on management policy for sterilization services in the UK National Health Service (NHS), but also on the design, validation, verification and operational management of sterilizers, as well as a guide to good operational practice.

Besides this, however, the inspectors would expect to see a fully documented support system, which should demonstrate full and complete compliance with GMP requirements. This would include: maintenance, cleaning and microbiological monitoring of any associated controlled-environmental areas; equipment maintenance and calibration; personnel training and qualification; and control over the packaging, labelling, wrapping, handling and storage of sterile items. While not adopting a prescriptive approach, the inspecting authorities place emphasis on the fact that manufacturers themselves must demonstrate that the system is under control at all times and will provide the required SAL.

9 Bioburden estimation

The bioburden of the presterilized product will be determined not only by the microbial flora of incoming raw materials and components and how they are stored, but also by the microbiological control applied to the environment where the product is manufactured, assembled and packed. Reliable, accurate and reproducible bioburden data must be collected; any underestimation of the bioburden population would result in a miscalculation of the sterilization requirements for a given product and possible validation failures; conversely, an overestimation of the bioburden would result in excessive exposure to the sterilizing agent, which in turn could affect the stability or functioning of the product, depending on product type.

As a group, medical devices present a challenge in terms of bioburden testing. They comprise a large, diverse and motley collection of product types and there is no single, universally applicable technique which is appropriaate to all devices. Considerable differences in bioburden levels have been reported (Hoxey, 1993). In one study of a diverse group of medical devices, these ranged from less than 1cfu/device in the case of a syringe to 10^7–10^9 cfu in the raw material of a biological tissue patch of raw material. The microbiologist must therefore use his/her knowledge and judgement to select the most appropriate technique. Ideally, bioburden estimates should be carried out for each product on a regular basis, but this may not always be practicable. In the latter case, selected testing of groups of products with a common raw material or perhaps a common manufacturing process may be acceptable, provided that the rationale behind such decisions is documented and it is shown that the data are representative of all product groups.

Detailed guidance on the estimation of bioburdens in medical devices have recently been published (Anon., 1996c). Five distinct stages are involved: sample selection; removal of microorganisms from device, involving one or a combination of suggested techniques; transfer of microorganisms to recovery conditions; enumeration of microorganisms with specific characteristics; and interpretation of data, involving application of correction factors, determined during validation studies. In addition, where the medical device is shown or known to release inhibitory substances (which may in turn affect bioburden recovery), the method should incorporate a validated neutralization or filtration step.

In contrast to medical devices, the guidance given to pharmaceutical manufacturers for bioburden estimation in presterilization products is nonspecific. A total-viable-count method, such as that described in the BP (1998), the EP (1997) or the USP (1995), would be employed as a reference method, but invariably the method could be adapted to reflect the nature and characteristics of the product itself under test. However, guidelines for the validation of methods for the estimation of bioburden have recently been proposed (Anon., 1996c) and these are currently under discussion.

10 Sterility during storage

The maintenance of sterility during storage is dependent on pack integrity. Provided this is not compromised in any way, sterility will be maintained, irrespective of the time for which it is stored. Klapes *et al.* (1987) showed that the probability of contamination in freshly sterilized packs did not differ statistically from that in packs which had been stored for up to a year.

11 References

AAMI (1988) *Good Hospital Practice: Steam Sterilization and Sterility Assurance.* Arlington, Virginia: Association for the Advancement of Medical Instrumentation.

Anon. (1989) Sterility assurance based on validation of the sterilization process using steam under pressure. *Journal of Parenteral Science and Technology*, **43**, 226–230.

Anon. (1992) *The Rules Governing Medicinal Products in the European Community.* Vol. IV. Office for Official Publications of the EC.

Anon. (1994) *European Standard EN556. Sterilization of Medical Devices. Requirements for a Terminally Sterilized Device to be Labelled 'Sterile'.*

Anon. (1995) *USP Open Conference: Microbiological Compendial Issues.*

Anon. (1996a) PDA comments to USP on proposed changes to (71) sterility tests. *PDA Journal of Pharmaceutical Science and Technology*, **50**, 69–78.

Anon. (1996b) *EC Good Manufacturing Practice for Medicinal Products in the European Community. Annex on the Manufacture of Sterile Medicinal Products.* Office for Official Publications of the EC.

Anon. (1996c) *EN 1174 Medical devices: Estimation of the Population of Micro-organisms on Product.* Part 2: *Guidance.* Office for Official Publications of the EC.

Bowie, J.H., Kelsey, J.C. & Thompson, G.R. (1963) The Bowie and Dick autoclave tape test. *Lancet*, **i**, 586.

British Pharmacopoeia (BP) (1998) London: HMSO.

Busta, F.F. (1978) Introduction to injury and repair of microbial cells. *Advances in Applied Microbiology*, **23**, 195–201.

Department of Health (1990) *Guidance on Ethylene Oxide Sterilization.* London: HMSO.

European Pharmacopoeia. (EP) (1997) 3rd edn. Strasburg: EP Secretariat.

Health Technical Memorandum (HTM) 2010 (1994) *Sterilizers.* Parts 1–5. London: HMSO.

Health Technical Memorandum (HTM) 2010 (1995) *Sterilization*, Parts 2–5. London: HMSO.

HIMA (1982) *Microbiological Evaluation of Filters for Sterilizing Liquids*, No. 3, Vol. 14. Washington, DC. Health Industry Manufacturers Association.

Hoxey, E.V. (1989) The case for parametric release. In *Proceedings of the Eucomed Conference on Ethylene Oxide' Sterilization*, 21–22 April, 1989, Paris. Pp. 25–32. London: Eucomed.

Hoxey, E. (1993) Validation of methods for bioburden estimation In *Sterilization of Medical Products*, Vol. VI (ed. Morrissey, R.F.). pp. 176–180 Morin Heights, Canada: Poly Science.

Klapes, N.A., Greene, V.W., Langholz, A.C. & Hunstiger, C. (1987) Effect of long term storage on sterile status of devices in surgical packs. *Infection Control*, **8**, 289–293.

Quesnel, L.B. (1984) Biological indicators and sterilization processes. In *Revival of Injured Microbes* (eds Andrew, M.H.E. & Russell, A.D.), Society for Applied Bacteriology Symposium Series No. 12, pp. 257–291. London: Academic Press.

United States Pharmacopoeia (USP) XXIII (1995) Rockville, Maryland: USP Convention.

Wallhaeusser, K.-H. (1988) In *Praxis der Sterilisation–Desinfektion–Konservierung*, 4th edn. Stuttgart/New York: Thieme.

Wright, A.M., Hoxey, E.V., Soper, C.J. & Davies, D.J.G. (1995) Biological indicators for low temperature steam and formaldehyde sterilization: the effect of defined media on sporulation, growth index and formaldehyde resistance of spores of *Bacillus stearothemophilus* NCIMB 8224. *Journal of Applied Bacteriology*, **79**, 432–438.

Wright, A.M., Hoxey, E.V., Soper, C.J. & Davies, D.J.G. (1996) Biological indicators for low temperature steam and formaldehyde sterilization: investigation of the effect of change in temperature and formaldehyde concentration on spores of *Bacillus stearothemophilus* NCIMB 8224. *Journal of Applied Bacteriology*, **80**, 259–265.

Index

Note: page numbers in *italics* refer to figures, those in **bold** refer to tables